CURRENT THERAPY IN COLON AND RECTAL SURGERY

SECOND EDITION

CURRENT THERAPY IN COLON AND RECTAL SURGERY

SECOND EDITION

Victor W. Fazio, MB, MS, MD (Hon), FRACS, FRACS (Hon), FACS, FRCS, FRCS (Ed)
Rupert B. Turnbull, Jr., MD, Chair
Chairman, Department of Colorectal Surgery
The Cleveland Clinic Foundation
Cleveland, Ohio

James M. Church, MBChB, M Med Sci, FRACS
Victor W. Fazio Chair in Colorectal Surgery
Staff Colorectal Surgeon
Department of Colorectal Surgery
Head, Sections of Colorectal Endoscopy and Research
Director, David G. Jagelman Inherited Colorectal Cancer Registries
The Cleveland Clinic Foundation
Cleveland, Ohio

Conor P. Delaney, MD, MCh, PhD, FRSCI (Gen), FACS
Staff Surgeon
Department of Colorectal Surgery and
Minimally Invasive Surgical Center
The Cleveland Clinic Foundation
Cleveland, Ohio

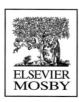

ELSEVIER
MOSBY

ELSEVIER
MOSBY

The Curtis Center
170 S Independence Mall W 300E
Philadelphia, Pennsylvania 19106

CURRENT THERAPY IN COLON AND RECTAL SURGERY   ISBN 1-55664-480-9

Notice

Surgery is an ever-changing field. Standard safety precautions must be followed, but as new research and
clinical experience broaden our knowledge, changes in treatment and drug therapy may become necessary
or appropriate. Readers are advised to check the most current product information provided by the
manufacturer of each drug to be administered to verify the recommended dose, the method and duration
of administration, and contraindications. It is the responsibility of the treating physician, relying on
experience and knowledge of the patient, to determine dosages and the best treatment for each individual
patient. Neither the Publisher nor the author assume any liability for any injury and/or damage to persons
or property arising from this publication.

The Publisher

First Edition 1990.

Library of Congress Cataloging-in-Publication Data
Current therapy in colon and rectal surgery / [edited by] Victor W. Fazio, James M.
   Church, Conor P. Delaney.—2nd ed.
      p.; cm.
   Includes bibliographical references.
   ISBN 1-55664-480-9
      1. Colon (Anatomy)—Surgery. 2. Rectum—Surgery. I. Fazio, Victor W., 1940-II.
Church, James M. III. Delaney, C. P. (Conor Patrick)
      [DNLM: 1. Colonic Diseases—surgery. 2. Rectal Diseases—surgery. 3. Colon—surgery.
   4. Rectum—surgery. WI 650 C976 2004]
   RD34.C87 2004
   617.5¢547—dc22
                                                                                    2003059988

Acquisitions Editor: *Elyse O'Grady*
Developmental Editor: *Janice Gaillard*
Project Manager: *Mary Stermel*

Printed in the United States of America

Last digit is the print number: 9   8   7   6   5   4   3   2

Dedication

To the memory of my mother, Kathleen Eleanor Fazio, whose self-sacrifice resulted in my becoming a surgeon.

—Victor Fazio

To my wife, Lois Church, in appreciation of her selfless love and support.

—James Church

To Clare, for her love and support, and to my parents, without whose direction and support I would not have entered medicine.

—Conor Delaney

Contributors

Hernand Abcarian, MD, FACS
Turi Josefsen Professor and Head, Department
    of Surgery
The University of Chicago
Service Chief, Surgery
University of Illinois Medical Center
Chicago, IL
Rectal Trauma

Neeraj Agrawal, MD
Fellow
Department of Hematology and Medical Oncology
The Cleveland Clinic Foundation
Cleveland, OH
Chemotherapy for Metastatic Colon Cancer

Frederick Alexander, MD, FACS, FAAP
Associate Professor
Case Western Reserve University
MetroHealth Medical Center School of Medicine
Professor
Case Western Reserve University
Cleveland Clinic Lerner School of Medicine
Case Western Reserve University
Chairman, Department of Pediatric Surgery
The Children's Hospital of the Cleveland Clinic
    Foundation
Staff, Department of Pediatric Surgery
Fairview General Hospital; MetroHealth Medical
    Center
Southwest General Hospital
Cleveland, OH
Hillcrest Meridian Hospital
Mayfield Heights, OH
Aultman Hospital
Canton, OH
Hirschsprung's Disease

Jeffrey S. Aronoff, MD
Attending Colorectal Surgeon
Lenox Hill Hospital
New York, NY
Rectal Foreign Bodies

Mirza Khurrum Baig, MBBS, FRCS
Consultant Colorectal Surgeon
Worthing Hospital
Worthing, West Sussex, UK
*Cytomegalovirus Ileocolitis and Kaposi's Sarcoma
    in AIDS*

H. Randolph Bailey, MD
Clinical Professor of Surgery
Program Director, Residency in Colon and Rectal
    Surgery
University of Texas Medical School at Houston
Clinical Professor of Surgery
Baylor College of Medicine
Houston, TX
Endometriosis of the Colon and Rectum

Tricia J. Bardon, BBA, ABA
Assistant Director, Coding and Reimbursement
American Osteopathic Association
Chicago, IL
*Documentation and Use of the CPT Coding System
    for Colorectal Surgery*

Robert W. Beart, Jr., MD
Professor and Chairman
Costello Chair for Colorectal Diseases
Skirball-Kenis Chair for Colorectal Diseases
Keck School of Medicine
University of Southern California
Los Angeles, CA
*Cancer of the Rectum: Operative Management
    and Adjuvant Therapy*

David E. Beck, MD
Clinical Associate Professor of Surgery
F. Edward School of Medicine
Uniformed Services
University of the Health Sciences
Bethesda, MD
Chairman, Department of Colon and Rectal Surgery
Ochsner Clinic Foundation
New Orleans, LA
Perineal Hernia

Paul Belliveau, MD, CM, FRCSC, FACS, FICS
Professor of Surgery (Tenured)
Queens University
Senior Surgeon
Kingston General Hospital
Hotel Dieu Hospital
Kingston, Ontario, Canada
Anal Fistula

Eren Berber, MD
Fellow
Department of General Surgery
The Cleveland Clinic Foundation
Cleveland, OH
Management of Colorectal Liver Metastases

Richard P. Billingham, MD
Clinical Professor
Department of Surgery
University of Washington
Attending Surgeon
Swedish Hospital Medical Center
Attending Surgeon
Northwest Hospital Medical Center
Seattle, WA
Rectocele

David Bimston, MD
Brower Surgical Associates
Fort Lauderdale, FL
Volvulus of the Colon

Mary Sue Brady, MD
Assistant Professor of Surgery
Cornell University Medical College
Assistant Attending Surgeon
Memorial Sloan-Kettering Cancer Center
New York, NY
Melanoma and Basal Cell Carcinoma of the Anus

Marc Brand, MD
Assistant Professor of Surgery
Rush Medical College
Section of Colon and Rectal Surgery
Rush University Medical Center
Chicago, IL
Short Bowel Syndrome

Aaron Brzezinski, MD, FRCP(C)
Staff Gastroenterologist
Department of Gastroenterology
The Cleveland Clinic Foundation
Cleveland, OH
Medical Treatment of Ulcerative Colitis and Other Colitides
Medical Treatment of Crohn's Disease

John L. Cameron, MD
Professor of Surgery
School of Medicine
Johns Hopkins University
Surgeon
The Johns Hopkins Hospital
Baltimore, MD
Small Bowel Neoplasms

Peter A. Cataldo, MD
Associate Professor
University of Vermont
Fletcher Allen Health Care
Burlington, VT
Perianal Crohn's Disease

Javier Cebrian, MD
University of Florida
Orlando, FL
Fecal Impaction

James P. Celebrezze, Jr., MD
Assistant Professor of Surgery
Drexel University School of Medicine
Philadelphia, PA
Senior Attending
Allegheny General Hospital
Pittsburgh, PA
Pseudomembranous Colitis

George K. Chow, MD
Assistant Professor
Mayo Medical School
Consultant
Mayo Medical Clinic
Rochester, MN
Urologic Complications of Colorectal Surgery

James M. Church, MBChB, M Med Sci, FRACS
Victor W. Fazio Chair in Colorectal Surgery
Staff Colorectal Surgeon
Department of Colorectal Surgery
Head, Sections of Colorectal Endoscopy and
  Research
Director, David G. Jagelman Inherited Colorectal
  Cancer Registries
The Cleveland Clinic Foundation
Cleveland, OH
Villous Tumors of the Rectum
Molecular Genetics of Colorectal Cancer
Desmoid Tumors
*Outcomes Analysis and Measurement of Quality of
  Life*

José Cintron, MD, FACS, FASCRS
Associate Professor of Surgery
Director, Surgical Residency Program
University of Illinois College of Medicine at Chicago
Attending Surgeon
University of Illinois Medical Center
Attending Surgeon and Associate Chief of Surgery
VA Chicago Health Care System
Chicago, IL
Anal and Perianal Warts

Jeffrey L. Cohen, MD, FACS, FASCRS
Associate Clinical Professor of Surgery
University of Connecticut
Lead Physical—General and Colorectal Surgery
Connecticut Surgical Group
Hartford, CT
Lower Gastrointestinal Bleeding

Zane Cohen, MD, FRCS(C), FACS
Professor of Surgery
Chairman, Division of General Surgery
University of Toronto
Surgeon in Chief
Mount Sinai Hospital
Toronto, Ontario, Canada
Familial Adenomatous Polyposis

Marvin L. Corman, MD
Professor of Surgery
Albert Einstein College of Medicine
Bronx, NY
The Management of Hemorrhage During Pelvic Surgery

Timothy C. Counihan, MD
Associate Professor of Surgery
University of Massachusetts Medical School
Head of Section of Colon and Rectal Surgery
UMass Memorial Health Care
Worcester, MA
Fecal Incontinence

Jean Couture, MD, FRCSC
Canadian Project Director
Faculty of Medicine
Laval University
Sainte-Foy, Quebec, Canada
Anal Carcinoma

Bernard J. Cummings, MBChB, FRCPC, FRCR, FRANZCR
Professor, Department of Radiation Oncology
University of Toronto
Radiation Oncologist
Princess Margaret Hospital
University Health Network
Toronto, Ontario, Canada
Anal Carcinoma

Conor P. Delaney, MD, MCh, PhD, FRSCI (Gen), FACS
Staff Surgeon
Department of Colorectal Surgery and Minimally
   Invasive Surgical Center
The Cleveland Clinic Foundation
Cleveland, OH
Rectal Prolapse
*Documentation and Use of the CPT Coding System for
   Colorectal Surgery*

David W. Dietz, MD
Assistant Professor of Surgery
Washington University School of Medicine in
   St Louis
Attending Surgeon, Section of Colon and Rectal
   Surgery
Barnes-Jewish Hospital
St. Louis, MO
Small Bowel Obstruction
Radiation Enteritis and Colitis

R. R. Dozois, MD, MS, FACS, FRCS (Glas) (Hon), DSC
Emeritus Professor of Surgery
Mayo Medical School
Emeritus Chair, Division of Colon and Rectal Surgery
Mayo Clinic and Mayo Foundation
Rochester, MN
Chronic Ulcerative Colitis: Surgical Options

John Dvorak, MD
Active Staff Physician
Central Baptist, St. Joseph, and Samaritan Hospitals
Lexington, KY
Radiation Enteritis and Colitis

David M. Einstein, MD
Staff Radiologist, Section of Abnormal Imaging
The Cleveland Clinic Foundation
Cleveland, OH
*Diagnosis and Medical Management of Acute Colonic
   Diverticulitis*

Theodore E. Eisenstat, MD, FACS
Clinical Professor of Surgery
Director of Colon and Rectal Surgery Residency
Robert Wood Johnson Medical School
University of Medicine and Dentistry of New Jersey
Robert Wood Johnson University Hospital
New Brunswick, NJ
Anal Stenosis

Warren E. Enker, MD, FACS
Professor of Surgery
Albert Einstein College of Medicine
Chief, Division of Colorectal Surgery
Vice-Chairman
Department of Surgery
Beth Israel Medical Center
Associate Director
Director of Surgical Oncology
Continuum Cancer Centers of New York
Melanoma and Basal Cell Carcinoma of the Anus

Paula Erwin-Toth, MSN, RN, ET, CWOCN, CNS
Director, Enterostomal Therapy/Wound, Ostomy,
    Continence Nursing and Education
The Cleveland Clinic Foundation
Cleveland, OH
*Stoma and Wound Considerations: Nursing
    Management*

Brent K. Evetts, MD
Legacy Meridian Park Hospital
Tualatin, OR
Rectocele

Linda Farkas, MD
Assistant Professor of Surgery
University of Pittsburgh
Clinical Director of UPMC Hereditary Colorectal
    Tumor Program
Hillman Cancer Institute
Pittsburgh, PA
Rectal Trauma

**Victor W. Fazio, MB, MS, MD (Hon), FRACS,
FRACS (Hon), FACS, FRCS, FRCS (Ed)**
Rupert B. Turnbull, Jr., MD, Chair
Chairman, Department of Colorectal Surgery
The Cleveland Clinic Foundation
Cleveland, OH
Anorectal Abscess
*Diagnosis and Management of Sacral and Retrorectal
    Tumors*

L. Peter Fielding, MB, FRCS, FACS
Professor of Clinical Surgery
The Pennsylvania State University of Medicine
Hershey, PA
University of Pennsylvania Heath Systems
Medical Director, Surgical Service Line
Chairman, Department of Surgery
Director, Surgical Residency Program
York Hospital
York, PA
Large Bowel Obstruction

Josef E. Fischer, MD
Mallinckrodt Professor of Surgery
Harvard Medical School
Chairman, Department of Surgery
Surgeon in Chief
Beth-Israel Deaconess Medical Center
Boston, MA
Enterocutaneous Fistula

James W. Fleshman, MD
Associate Professor of Surgery
Washington University School of Medicine
Department of Surgery
St. Louis, MO
*Prevention and Treatment of Complications of
    Laparoscopic Intestinal Surgery*
Prevention and Management of Stoma Complications

Daniel P. Froese, MBChB, FACS, FASCRS
Attending Surgeon
Swedish Hospital Medical Center
Seattle, WA
Pruritus Ani

Robert Fry, MD
Professor of Surgery
Chief, Division of Colon and Rectal Surgery
Hospital of University of Pennsylvania
Philadelphia, PA
Management of the Malignant Polyp

Susan Galandiuk, MD
Professor and Program Director, Section of Colon
    and Rectal Surgery
University of Louisville
Louisville, KY
*Management and Treatment of Colon and Rectal
    Trauma*
Pneumatosis Cystoides Intestinalis
Acute and Chronic Mesenteric Ischemia

Julio Garcia-Aguilar, MD, PhD
Professor in Residence
University of California, San Francisco
Chief, Department of Colon and Rectal Surgery
Division of General Surgery
UCSF Medical Center
University of California
San Francisco, CA
Rectal Cancer: Local Treatment

Scott W. Gibson, MD
Staff Surgeon
Hackley Hospital
Mercy General Hospital
Muskegon, MI
North Ottawa Community Hospital
Grand Haven, MI
Enterocutaneous Fistula

Robert Gilliland, MD, FRCS (Gen)
Belfast, Ireland
Cytomegalovirus Ileocolitis and Kaposi's Sarcoma in
*   AIDS*

Philip H. Gordon, MD, FRCS(C), FACS
Professor of Surgery and Oncology
McGill University
Director, Colon and Rectal Surgery
Sir Mortimer B. Davis-Jewish General Hospital and
   McGill University
Montreal, Quebec, Canada
Anatomy and Physiology of the Anorectum

Lester Gottesman, MD, FACS, FASCRS
Associate Professor of Clinical Surgery
Columbia University College of Physicians and
   Surgeons
Chief, Colon Rectal Surgery
St. Luke's Roosevelt Hospital
New York, NY
Anorectal Venereal Infections

Suzanne Green, MD
Westfield, NJ ,
Pelvic Pain Syndromes

Sharon Grundfest-Broniatowski, SBEE, MD
Staff Surgeon
Department of General Surgery
The Cleveland Clinic Foundation
Cleveland, OH
Diagnosis and Management of Sacral and Retrorectal
*   Tumors*

José G. Guillem, MD, MPH
Associate Professor of Surgery
Cornell University Medical College
Associate Attending Surgeon
Memorial Sloan-Kettering Cancer Center
New York, NY
Cancer of the Rectum: Follow-up and Management of
*   Local Recurrence*

Dieter Hahnloser, MD
Clinical Assistant Professor, Division of Visceral and
   Transplant Surgery
University Hospital
Zurich, Switzerland
Carcinoid Tumors of the Large and Small Bowel

Thomas E. Hamilton, MD, FACS, FAAP
Assistant Clinical Professor of Surgery and Pediatrics
The University of Vermont School of Medicine
Burlington, VT
Maine Medical Center
Portland, ME
Nutritional Support

Jacqueline Harrison, MD
Attending Surgeon
Provident Hospital of Cook County
Chicago, IL
Pseudo-obstruction (Ogilvie's Syndrome)

Lawrence E. Harrison, MD
Associate Professor, Chief of Division of Surgical
   Oncology
University of Medicine and Dentistry of New Jersey
   Medical School
Newark, NJ
Cancer of the Rectum: Follow-up and Management of
*   Local Recurrence*

Terry C. Hicks, MD, MS
Vice-Chair
Department of Colon and Rectal Surgery
Ochsner Clinic
New Orleans, LA
Preoperative Preparation of the Colon and Rectal
*   Surgical Patient*

Barbara J. Hocevar, BSN, RN, ET, CWOCN
Manager, Enterostomal Therapy/Wound, Ostomy,
   Continence Nursing
The Cleveland Clinic Foundation
Cleveland, OH
Stoma and Wound Considerations: Nursing
*   Management*

Barton Hoexter, MD
St. Francis Hospital
Long Island, NY
Anal Fissure

Philip J. Huber, Jr., MD
Professor of Surgery
University of Texas Southwestern Medical Center
Staff Physician
Zale Lipshy University Hospital
Parkland Memorial Hospital
VA Medical Center
Dallas, TX
Management of Cancer of the Colon (Including Adjuvant Therapy)

Tracy Hull, MD
Staff Colorectal Surgeon
The Cleveland Clinic Foundation
Cleveland, OH
Rectovaginal Fistula

Leif Hultén, MD, PhD, FACS
Professor Emeritus
Sahlgrenska University Hosp/Östra
Department of Surgery—Colorectal Unit
Göteborg, Sweden
The Continent Ileostomy—Management of Complications

Neil H. Hyman, MD
Professor of Surgery
Chief, Division of General Surgery
University of Vermont College of Medicine
Burlington, VT
Unhealed Perineal Wound

Howard S. Kaufman, MD
Associate Professor of Surgery
Keck School of Medicine
University of Southern California
Chief, Division of Colorectal and Pelvic Floor Surgery
USC University Hospital
Los Angeles, CA
Small Bowel Neoplasms

Mark Killingback, AM, MS (Hon), FACS (Hon), FRACS, FRCS, FRCS (Ed)
Visiting Colorectal Surgeon
Sydney Adventist Hospital
Sydney, New South Wales, Australia
Surgical Treatment of Diverticulitis

Ravi P. Kiran, MBBS, MS, FRCS (Eng), FRCS (Glas)
Colorectal Research Fellow
Department of Colorectal Surgery
The Cleveland Clinic Foundation
Cleveland, OH
Anorectal Abscess

Clifford Y. Ko, MD, MS, MSHS
Associate Professor of Surgery
David Geffen School of Medicine at UCLA
Attending Surgeon/Research Scientist (RAND)
UCLA Medical Center
West Los Angeles VA Hospital
Los Angeles, California
RAND
Santa Monica, CA
The Management of Hemorrhage During Pelvic Surgery

Walter A. Koltun, MD
Professor of Surgery
Pennsylvania State University College of Medicine
Chief, Section of Colon and Rectal Surgery
Peter and Marshia Carlino Professor in Inflammatory Bowel Disease
Penn State Milton S. Hershey Medical Center
Hershey, PA
Colorectal Surgery in the High-Risk Patient

Sergio W. Larach, MD, FACS
Associate Professor of Colon and Rectal Surgery
University of Florida
Gainesville, FL
Fecal Impaction

Bret A. Lashner, MD, MPH
Director, Center for Inflammatory Bowel Disease
The Cleveland Clinic Foundation
Cleveland, OH
Medical Treatment of Ulcerative Colitis and Other Colitides
Medical Treatment of Crohn's Disease

Dana P. Launer, MD, FACS
Chief of Staff
Scripps Memorial Hospital
La Jolla, CA
Reoperative Pelvic Surgery

Peter Lee, MD, FRCS (Eng), FRCS (Ed), MBChB
Dean
Penang Medical College
Penang, Malaysia
Rectal Stricture

Kevin M. Lin, MD
Kaiser Permanente Medical Center
Honolulu, HI
Hereditary Nonpolyposis Colorectal Cancer

Walter Longo, MD, MBA, FACS, FASCRS
Professor of Surgery
Chief of Gastrointestinal Surgery
Director of Colon and Rectal Surgery
Yale University School of Medicine
New Haven, CT
Colonic Ischemia

Martin Andrew Luchtefeld, MD
Assistant Clinical Professor
Michigan State University
East Lansing, MI
Michigan Medical PC—Ferguson Clinic
Grand Rapids, MI
Perianal Hidradenitis Suppurativa

John M. MacKeigan, MD, FRCSC, FACS, FASCRS
Associate Clinical Professor
Department of Surgery
Michigan State University School of Human Medicine
Active Staff
Spectrum Health
Grand Rapids, MI
Pilonidal Sinus

Robert D. Madoff, MD
Adjunct Professor of Surgery
University of Minnesota
Minneapolis, MN
Fecal Incontinence

Kenneth Marks, MD
Staff Surgeon
Department of Orthopaedic Surgery
The Cleveland Clinic Foundation
Cleveland, OH
Diagnosis and Management of Sacral and Retrorectal Tumors

P. J. McMurrick, MBBS (Hon), FRACS
Senior Lecturer in Surgery
Cabrini Monash University Academic Surgery Unit
Head of Colorectal Surgical Services
Southern Health Network
Victorian Colorectal Clinic
Victoria, Australia
Chronic Ulcerative Colitis: Surgical Options

David S. Medich, MD
Associate Professor of Surgery
Drexel University School of Medicine
Philadelphia, PA
Director, Colon Rectal Surgery
Allegheny General Hospital
Pittsburgh, PA
Pseudomembranous Colitis

Victor L. Modesto, MD, FACS, FASCRS
Florida Hospital
Winter Park, FL
Anorectal Venereal Infections

Michael A. Moffa, MD
Colon Rectal Associates of CNY, LLP
Liverpool, NY
Bowen's Disease and Paget's Disease

John R. T. Monson, MD, FRCS, FRCSI, FACS, FRCPS (Glas) (Hon)
Professor of Surgery/Head of Department
Academic Surgical Unit
Postgraduate Medical Institute
University of Hull
East Yorkshire, UK
Rectal Stricture

Drogo K. Montague, MD
Professor of Surgery
Cleveland Clinic Lerner College of Medicine of Case Western Reserve University
Head, Section of Prosthetic Surgery and Genitourethral Reconstruction
Glickman Urological Institute
The Cleveland Clinic Foundation
Cleveland, OH
Urologic Complications of Colorectal Surgery

Harvey G. Moore, MD
Clinical Research Fellow
Colorectal Service
Memorial Sloan-Kettering Cancer Center
New York, NY
Cancer of the Rectum: Follow-up and Management of Local Recurrence

H. Moreira, Jr., MD
Professor
Director of Colorectal Residency Program
Colorectal Service
Department of Surgery
Clinical Hospital of the Federal University of Goiás
Colorectal Surgeon
Instituto de Gastroenterologia de Goiânia
Goiás, Brazil
Anatomy and Physiology of the Colon and Rectum

Heidi Nelson, MD, FACS
Professor of Surgery
Mayo Clinic College of Medicine
Chair, Division of Colon and Rectal Surgery
Mayo Clinic
Rochester, MN
Carcinoid Tumors of the Large and Small Bowel

**Graham L. Newstead, MBBS, FRACS, FRCS (Eng),
FACS, FRSCRS, FACP (Hon) (GBI), FRSM (Hon)**
Senior Lecturer
University of New South Wales
Chairman of Medical Staff and Head of Colorectal
    Surgery
Prince of Wales Private Hospital
Sydney, New South Wales, Australia
Complications of Colonoscopy

Santhat Nivatvongs, MD, FACS
Professor of Surgery
Consultant in Colon and Rectal Surgery
Mayo Clinic College of Medicine
Rochester, MN
*Treatment of Colorectal Adenomas: Screening, Follow-
up and Surveillance*

Robert B. Noone, Jr., MD
Assistant Program Director
Department of Surgery
Lankenau Hospital
Wynnewood, PA
Prevention and Management of Sepsis

John R. Oakley, MBBS, FRACS
Clinical Senior Lecturer
School of Medicine
University of Tasmania
Consultant Colorectal Surgeon
Royal Hobart Hospital
Hobart, Tasmania, Australia
Management of Toxic Ulcerative Colitis

Gregory C. Oliver, MD, FACS, FASCRS
Associate Clinical Professor of Surgery
Robert Wood Johnson University School of
    Medicine
University of Medicine and Dentistry of New Jersey
New Brunswick, NJ
Muhlenberg Regional Medical Center
Plainsfield, NJ
John F. Kennedy Hospital
Edison, NJ
Pelvic Pain Syndromes

Guy R. Orangio, MD, FACS, FASCRS
Clinical Associate Professor of Surgery
Medical College of Georgia
Chief of Colon and Rectal Surgery
Dekalb Medical Center
Active Staff Member
Saint Joseph's Hospital
Northside Hospital
Children's Healthcare of Atlanta at Scottish Rite
Atlanta Medical Center
Georgia Colon and Rectal Surgical Associates, PC
Atlanta, GA
Nonepithelial Colorectal Tumors

Robert B. Pelley, MD
Staff Physician
Department of Hematology and Medical Oncology
Taussig Cancer Center
The Cleveland Clinic Foundation
Cleveland, OH
Chemotherapy for Metastatic Colon Cancer

John H. Pemberton, MD
Professor of Surgery
Mayo Clinic College of Medicine
Consultant, Division of Colon and Rectal Surgery
Mayo Clinic
Rochester, MN
Constipation

Alberto Peña, MD
Professor of Surgery and Pediatrics
Albert Einstein College of Medicine
Bronx, NY
Chief, Division of Pediatric Surgery
Schneider Children's Hospital
North Shore-Long Island Jewish Health System
New Hyde Park, NY
Anorectal Congenital Disorders

Jason Penzer, MD
Clinical Instructor in Surgery
New York Medical College
Valhalla, NY
Attending Surgeon
St. Vincent's Hospital and Medical Center
New York, NY
Anal Stenosis

P. Terry Phang, MD
Associate Professor of Surgery
University of British Columbia
Head, Division of General Surgery and Colorectal
    Surgery
St. Paul's Hospital
Vancouver, British Columbia, Canada
*Preoperative Evaluation of the Rectal Cancer Patient:
    Assessment of Operative Risk and Strategy*

Andreas Platz, MD
Lecturer in Trauma Surgery
University of Zurich Medical School
Head of Trauma Division
Department of Surgery
Stadtspital Triemli
Zurich, Switzerland
*Management and Treatment of Colon and Rectal
    Trauma*

Lawrence Prabhakar, MD
Clinical Assistant Professor
University of Illinois
College of Medicine at Rockford
2nd Vice President of Medical Staff
St. Anthony's Medical Center
Active Staff
Swedish American Hospital
Rockford, IL
Courtesy Staff
Rochelle Community Hospital
Rochelle, IL
Formerly of Mayo Clinic
Crohn's Colitis

Elliot Prager, MD
Associate Clinical Professor of Surgery
University of Southern California
Los Angeles, CA
Acute Appendicitis

John A. Procaccino, MD, FACS
Clinical Associate Professor of Surgery
Albert Einstein College of Medicine
Bronx, NY
Chief, Division of Colon and Rectal Surgery
North Shore-Long Island Jewish Health Care System
Great Neck, NY
Bowen's Disease and Paget's Disease

Thomas E. Read, MD, FACS, FASCRS
Associate Professor of Surgery
Temple University School of Medicine
Chief Division of Colon and Rectal Surgery
Western Pennsylvania Hospital
Clinical Campus of Temple University School of
    Medicine
Pittsburgh, PA
*Prevention and Treatment of Complications of
    Laparoscopic Intestinal Surgery*

Feza H. Remzi, MD, FACS, FASCRS
Staff Surgeon, Department of Colorectal Surgery
The Cleveland Clinic Foundation
Cleveland, OH
*Pelvic Pouch Anastomotic Complications and
    Management*

Thomas W. Rice, MD
Head, Section of General Thoracic Surgery
The Cleveland Clinic Foundation
Cleveland, OH
Resection of Colorectal Pulmonary Metastases

John L. Rombeau, MD
Professor of Surgery
University of Pennsylvania School of Medicine
Attending Surgeon
Hospital of the University of Pennsylvania
Philadelphia, PA
Nutritional Support

David Rothenberger, MD
Professor of Surgery and Chief, Divisions of Colon
    and Rectal Surgery and Surgical Oncology
Department of Surgery
University of Minnesota
Associate Director for Clinical Research Programs
University of Minnesota Cancer Center
Minneapolis, MN
Rectal Cancer: Local Treatment

Robert J. Rubin, MD, FACS, FASCRS
Clinical Professor Emeritus of Surgery
Robert Wood Johnson Medical School
New Brunswick, NJ
Attending Surgeon Emeritus
Chief of Surgical Service Emeritus
JFK Medical Center
Edison, NJ
Muhlenberg Hospital
Plainfield, NJ
Robert Wood Johnson Hospital
New Brunswick, NJ
Consultant Surgeon Emeritus
Somerset Hospital
Somerville, NJ
Pelvic Pain Syndromes

Theodore Saclarides, MD
Professor of Surgery
Rush Medical College
Head, Section of Colon and Rectal Surgery
Rush University Medical Center
Chicago, IL
Pseudo-obstruction (Ogilvie's Syndrome)

William J. Sandborn, MD
Professor of Medicine
Mayo College of Medicine
Head, IBD Interest Group and Clinical Research Unit
Mayo Foundation
Rochester, MN
Pouchitis and Functional Complications of the Pelvic Pouch

David J. Schoetz, Jr., MD
Professor of Surgery
Tufts University School of Medicine
Boston, MA
Chairman Emeritus, Department of Colon and Rectal Surgery
Lahey Clinic
Burlington, MA
Crohn's Disease of the Duodenum, Stomach, and Esophagus

Theodore R. Schrock, MD
Professor and Interim Chair
Department of Surgery
University of California, San Francisco
San Francisco, CA
Anastomotic Leak After Colon and Rectal Resections

Douglas Seidner, MD
Associate Professor of Medicine
Ohio State University
Columbus, OH
Staff in Gastroenterology
Department of Gastroenterology and Hepatology
Director, Nutrition Support and Vascular Access Department
Program Director, Fellowship in Clinical Nutrition
Digestive Disease Center
The Cleveland Clinic Foundation
Cleveland, OH
Short Bowel Syndrome

Anthony J. Senagore, MD, MS, MBA, FACS
Staff Physician
Krause-Lieberman Chair in Laparoscopic Colorectal Surgery
Associate Chief of Staff
Medical Director, Office of Medical Operations
The Cleveland Clinic Foundation
Cleveland, OH
Rectal Prolapse
Cecal Ulcer
Documentation and Use of the CPT Coding System for Colorectal Surgery

Clifford L. Simmang, MD, MS
Associate Professor of Surgery
University of Texas Southwestern Medical Center
Staff Physician
Zale Lipshy University Hospital
Parkland Memorial Hospital
VA Medical Center
Dallas, TX
Management of Cancer of the Colon (Including Adjuvant Therapy)

Allan E. Siperstein, MD
Head, Section of Endocrine Surgery
Depatment of General Surgery
The Cleveland Clinic Foundation
Cleveland, OH
Management of Colorectal Liver Metastases

Lee E. Smith, MD, FACS
Clinical Professor of Surgery
Georgetown University
Adjunct Professor of Surgery
Uniformed Services University of the Health Sciences
Director, Section of Colon and Rectal Surgery
Washington Hospital Center
Washington, DC
Hemorrhoids

Norman Sohn, MD, FACS
Clinical Assistant Professor
Department of Surgery
New York University School of Medicine
Attending Surgeon
Lenox Hill Hospital
New York, NY
Rectal Foreign Bodies

Claudio Soravia, MD, MSc
Senior Lecturer in Surgery
Faculty of Medicine
Geneva Medical School
Consultant Colorectal Surgeon
Clinique Générale Beaulieu
Geneva, Switzerland
Familial Adenomatous Polyposis

Ezra Steiger, MD
Associate Professor of Surgery
Case Western Reserve University
Consultant in General Surgery
Co-Director, Nutrition Support and Director,
    Intestinal Rehabilitation Program
The Cleveland Clinic Foundation
Cleveland, OH
Short Bowel Syndrome

Richard J. Strauss, MD, FACS
Associate Professor of Clinical Surgery
Albert Einstein College of Medicine
New York, NY
Attending Surgeon
Long Island Jewish Medical Center
New Hyde Park, NY
Bowen's Disease and Paget's Disease

Scott A. Strong, MD
Staff Surgeon
Department of Colorectal Surgery
The Cleveland Clinic Foundation
Cleveland, OH
Crohn's Disease of the Small Bowel

Steven J. Stryker, MD
Professor of Clinical Surgery
Northwestern University Feinberg School of
    Medicine
Attending Surgeon
Northwestern Memorial Hospital
Chicago, IL
Volvulus of the Colon

Paul H. Sugarbaker, MD, FACS, FRCS, FASAS
Director, Program in Peritoneal Surface Malignancy
Washington Cancer Institute
Washington, DC
*Cancer of the Appendix and Pseudomyxoma Peritonei
    Syndrome*

Alan G. Thorson, MD, FACS
Clinical Associate Professor of Surgery
Program Director
Section of Colon and Rectal Surgery
Creighton University School of Medicine
Clinical Associate Professor of Surgery
University of Nebraska College of Medicine
Omaha, NE
Hereditary Nonpolyposis Colorectal Cancer

Joe J. Tjandra, MBBS, MD, FRACS, FRCS, FRCPS
Associate Professor of Surgery
Royal Melbourne Hospital
Royal Women's Hospital
Epworth Hospital
University of Melbourne
Victoria, Australia
Solitary Rectal Ulcer

Josephine van Helmond, MD
Clinical Staff
Department of Surgery
Marin General Hospital
Greenbrae, CA
Novato Community Hospital
Novato, CA
*Cancer of the Rectum: Operative Management and
    Adjuvant Therapy*

Anthony M. Vernava III, MD, FACS, FASCRS
Clinical Assistant Professor of Surgery
University of South Florida
Tampa, FL
Facility Associate
Florida Gulf Coast University College of Health
    Sciences
Fort Meyers, FL
Chairman, Division of Research and Education
Staff Surgeon, Department of Colon and Rectal
    Surgery
Cleveland Clinic Florida
Naples, FL
Colonic Ischemia

Todd Waltrip, MD
Staff
Department of Surgery
Good Shepherd Medical Center
Longview, TX
Acute and Chronic Mesenteric Ischemia

Steven D. Wexner, MD, FACS, FASCRS
Clinical Professor
Department of Surgery
University of South Florida College of Medicine
Tampa, FL
Professor of Surgery, Ohio State University Health
    Sciences Center at the Cleveland Clinic
    Foundation
Chairman, Department of Colorectal Surgery
Chief of Staff
Cleveland Clinic Florida
Weston, FL
Anatomy and Physiology of the Colon and Rectum
Cytomegalovirus Ileocolitis and Kaposi's Sarcoma in
    AIDS

Bruce G. Wolff, MD
Professor of Surgery
Mayo Medical School
Consultant in Colon and Rectal Surgery
Mayo Clinic and Mayo Foundation
Rochester, MN
Crohn's Colitis

W. Douglas Wong, MD, FACS, FRCS
Professor of Surgery
Cornell University Medical Center
Weill Cornell Medical College
Chief, Colorectal Service
Department of Surgery
Stuart H.Q. Quan Chair in Colorectal Surgery
Memorial Sloan-Kettering Cancer Center
New York, NY
Preoperative Evaluation of the Rectal Cancer Patient:
    Assessment of Operative Risk and Strategy

**Kutt Sing Wong, MD, MBBS, FRCS (Ed), FRCS
(Glas), FAMS**
Clinical Teacher, Faculty of Medicine
National University of Singapore
Consultant Surgeon, Division of Colorectal Surgery
Department of Surgery
National University Hospital
Singapore, Singapore
Clinical Fellow, Department of Colorectal Surgery
The Cleveland Clinic Foundation
Cleveland, OH

Pelvic Pouch Anastomotic Complications and
    Management

Rodney J. Woods, MBBS, FRACS
Staff Surgeon
Department of Colorectal Surgery
Box Hill Hospital
Box Hill, Victoria, Australia
Diverticulitis and Fistula

M. Jonathan Worsey, MA, MBBS, FRCS, FACS
Staff Surgeon
Scripps Memorial Hospital
La Jolla, CA
Reoperative Pelvic Surgery

James S. Wu, MD, PhD
Staff Surgeon
Department of Colorectal Surgery
The Cleveland Clinic Foundation
Cleveland, OH
Diagnosis and Medical Management of Acute Colonic
    Diverticulitis

Douglas Yoder, MD
Blanchard Valley Regional Health Center
Findlay, OH
Perianal Crohn's Disease

Tonia M. Young-Fadok, MD, MS, FACS, FASCRS
Associate Professor of Surgery
Mayo Clinic College of Medicine
Rochester, MN
Consultant Surgeon, Division of Colon and Rectal
    Surgery
Mayo Clinic
Scottsdale, AZ
Constipation

Preface to the Second Edition

In the 14 years since publication of the first edition of this book, there have been significant advances in almost all areas of colorectal surgery. From conditions as minor as an anal fissure to the intricacies of the molecular genetics underlying colorectal cancer, new understanding of pathophysiology has led to new approaches to diagnosis and management; thus almost all chapters underwent major revision and now include the new ideas and methods that have come into the practice of colorectal surgery. We included chapters on CPT coding and outcomes management, topics not often found in colorectal surgical texts, because of the integral part they play in our daily practice as colorectal surgeons. Other chapters were added to cover areas such as laparoscopy and molecular genetics, but the underlying purpose of the book has not changed.

This book is not meant to be an all-inclusive encyclopedia of the literature on colorectal surgery; there are other books that serve this function. We aim to provide for the reader a very practical and helpful aid to the management of patients suffering from the spectrum of colorectal diseases. We chose authors who are experts in their subjects and are experienced in dealing with the various presentations and manifestations of the disease or condition about which they wrote and asked them to focus on the management of colorectal disease, highlighting difficult and controversial issues. They were charged with providing practical advice in the same way that an experienced, worldly-wise surgeon shares his wisdom with a young colleague. We hope that book will not linger on the shelf, but rather will be in constant use in meeting the daily clinical challenges that are our profession.

Victor Fazio
James Church
Conor Delaney

Acknowledgments

We would like to acknowledge, with gratitude, the work of secretaries Jane Sardelle and Linda Libertini, artist Joe Pangrace, and all the contributing authors, whose efforts have made this book a reality.

Contents

SECTION III
THE COLON

SECTION I
ANAL AND PERIANAL REGION

1

ANATOMY AND PHYSIOLOGY OF THE ANORECTUM

Philip H. Gordon, MD, FRCS(C), FACS

Current therapy of diseases of the anorectum relies upon a sound understanding of the anatomy of the region along with an ever-expanding body of knowledge regarding the physiology of the anorectum. This chapter reviews the normal anatomic and physiologic features of the anorectum and describes a variety of techniques for physiologic testing.

■ ANATOMY

Anal Canal

The anal canal (Fig. 1-1) is the terminal portion of the intestinal tract. It begins at the anorectal junction, is 3 to 4 cm long, and terminates at the anal verge. It is surrounded by strong muscles, and as a result of the tonic contraction of these muscles, it is completely collapsed as an anteroposterior slit.

The musculature of the anorectal region consists of two tubes, one surrounding the other. The inner tube, being visceral, is smooth muscle and is innervated by the autonomic nervous system, whereas the outer, funnel-shaped tube is skeletal muscle and has somatic innervation. This short segment of the intestinal tract is of paramount importance because it is essential to the mechanism of continence and is susceptible to many diseases.

Lining

The lining of the anal canal consists of epithelium of different types at different levels. At approximately the midpoint of the anal canal, there is an undulating demarcation referred to as the dentate line. This line is approximately 2 cm from the anal verge. Because the rectum narrows into the anal canal, the tissue above the dentate line takes on a pleated appearance. These longitudinal folds, of which there are 6 to 14, are known as the columns of Morgagni. Between adjacent columns, at the lower end, is a small pocket, or crypt. These crypts are of surgical significance in that foreign material may lodge in them, obstructing the ducts of the anal glands, resulting in sepsis. The mucosa of the upper anal canal is lined with columnar epithelium. Below the dentate line, the anal canal is lined with squamous epithelium. The change, however, is not abrupt. For a distance of 6 to 12 mm above the dentate line, there is a gradual transition where columnar, transitional, or squamous epithelium may be found. This area has been referred to as the cloacogenic zone and is important when neoplasms that arise here are considered.

A color change in the epithelium is also noted. The rectal mucosa is pink, whereas the area just above the dentate line is deep purple or plum in color due to the subjacent internal hemorrhoidal plexus. Subepithelial tissue is loosely attached to and readily distensible by the internal hemorrhoidal plexus. Subepithelial tissue at the anal margin, which contains the external hemorrhoidal plexus, forms a lining that adheres firmly to the underlying tissue. At the level of the valves, the lining is anchored by what Parks called the mucosal suspensory ligament. The perianal space is limited above by this ligament and below by the attachments of the longitudinal muscle to the skin of the anal verge. The area below the dentate line is not true skin, for it is devoid of accessory skin structures (i.e., hair and sebaceous and sweat glands). This pale, delicate, smooth, thin, and shiny stretched tissue is referred to as anoderm, and it runs for approximately 1.5 cm below the dentate line. At the anal verge, the skin becomes thicker and pigmented; it acquires hair follicles and glands and other histologic features of normal skin. In the perianal area there is also a well-marked ring of apocrine glands, which are the site of the anorectal manifestation of a condition called hidradenitis suppurativa. Proximal to the dentate line, the epithelium is supplied by the autonomic nervous system, whereas distally the lining is richly innervated by the somatic nervous system.

Anal Intramuscular Glands

The number of intramuscular glands varies from 4 to 10 in a normal anal canal. Each gland is lined by stratified columnar epithelium and opens directly into an anal crypt. Occasionally, two glands open into the same crypt,

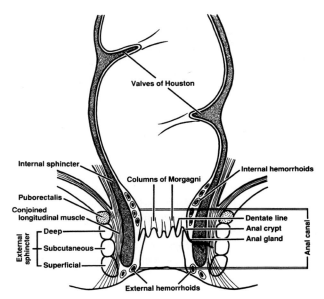

Figure 1-1
Anatomy of the anal canal. (From Gordon PH: The anorectum: Anatomic and physiologic considerations in health and disease. Gastroenterol Clin North Am 1987;16:2.)

whereas half the crypts have no glands. These glands were first described by Chiari in 1878. Their general direction is outward and downward. The importance of their role in the pathogenesis of fistulous abscess was presented by Parks in 1961. Seow-Choen and Ho found that 80% of the anal glands are submucosal, 8% extend to the internal sphincter, 8% extend to the conjoined longitudinal muscle, 2% reach the intersphincteric space, and 1% penetrate the external sphincter. The anal glands are fairly evenly distributed around the circumference of the anal canal, although the greatest numbers are found in the anterior quadrant. The mild to moderate lymphocytic infiltration noted around the anal glands and ducts is sometimes referred to as "anal tonsil." These glands may also be the site of origin of an adenocarcinoma.

■ MUSCLES

Internal Sphincter
The downward continuation of the circular, smooth muscle of the rectum becomes thick and rounded at its lower end where it is referred to as the internal anal sphincter. Its lowest portion is just above the lowest portion of the external sphincter and is 1.0 to 1.5 cm below the dentate line. The lower edge of the internal sphincter is palpable as the intersphincteric groove.

Conjoined Longitudinal Muscle
At the level of the anorectal ring, the longitudinal muscle coat of the rectum is joined by fibers of the levator ani and puborectalis muscles. The conjoined longitudinal muscle so formed descends between the internal and external anal sphincters. Many of these fibers traverse the lower portion

of the external sphincter to gain insertion into the perianal skin and are referred to as the corrugator cutis ani.

External Sphincter
This elliptical cylinder of skeletal muscle that surrounds the anal canal was originally described as consisting of three distinct divisions: the subcutaneous, the superficial, and the deep portions. This account was shown to be invalid by Goligher, who demonstrated that a sheet of muscle runs upward continuous with the puborectalis and levator ani muscles. The lowest portion of the muscle occupies a position below, and slightly lateral to, the internal sphincter. The lowest part (subcutaneous fibers) is traversed by the conjoined longitudinal muscle, with some fibers gaining attachment to the skin. The next portion (superficial) is attached to the coccyx by a posterior extension of muscle fibers, which combine with connective tissue, forming the anococcygeal ligament. Above this level the deep portion of the external sphincter is devoid of a posterior attachment and proximally becomes continuous with the puborectalis muscle. Anteriorly, the higher fibers of the external sphincter are inserted into the perineal body, where some merge and are continuous with a transverse perineal muscles. The external sphincter is supplied by the inferior rectal nerve and a perineal branch of the fourth sacral nerve.

Levator Ani Muscles
The levator ani muscle is a broad, thin muscle that forms the greater part of the floor of the pelvic cavity and is innervated by the fourth sacral nerve. This muscle has been known as pubococcygeus, while puborectalis was considered part of the deep portion of the external sphincter, since the two are fused and have the same nerve supply. However, electrophysiologic studies by Percy and colleagues concluded that stimulation of the sacral nerves resulted in electromyographic activity in the puborectalis but not in the external sphincter. Therefore, these muscles may not have the same nerve supply. Studies by Matzel and coworkers showed the nerve supply of the levator ani to be distinct from that of the external sphincter. The levator is supplied by branches from the sacral nerves proximal to the sacral plexus, whereas the external sphincter is supplied by nerve fibers traveling with the pudendal nerve.

The ileococcygeus muscle arises from the ischial spine and posterior part of the obturator fascia, passes downward, backward, and medially, and becomes inserted on the last two segments of the sacrum and the anococcygeal raphe.

The pubococcygeus muscle arises from the anterior half of the obturator fascia and back of the pubis. Its fibers are directed backward, downward, and medially, where they decussate with fibers from the opposite side.

The puborectalis muscle arises from the back of the symphysis pubis and the superior fascia of the urogenital diaphragm, runs backward alongside the anorectal junction, and joins its fellow muscle of the other side immediately behind the rectum; there they form a U-shaped loop that slings the rectum to the pubes.

The *anorectal ring,* a term coined by Milligan and Morgan, denotes the functionally important ring of muscle that surrounds the junction of the rectum and anal canal. It is composed of the upper borders of the internal and external sphincters and the puborectalis muscle. It is of paramount importance during the treatment of abscesses and fistulas because division of this ring inevitably results in anal incontinence.

Innervation of the Rectum and Anus

The large intestine, including the rectum, is innervated by the sympathetic and parasympathetic nervous systems. The external anal sphincter and the lining of the anal canal, below the dentate line, are supplied by somatic nerves.

Rectum

The sympathetic fibers to the rectum are derived from the first three lumbar segments of the spinal cord, which pass through the ganglionated sympathetic chains. They leave as a lumbar sympathetic nerve that joins the preaortic plexus. From here, a prolongation extends along the inferior mesenteric artery, as the inferior mesenteric plexus, and reaches the upper part of the rectum.

The presacral, or hypogastric, nerve arises from the aortic plexus and the two lateral lumbar splanchnic nerves. The plexus thus formed divides into two branches that separate and pass to each side of the pelvis, where they join branches of the sacral parasympathetic nerves, or nervi erigentes, to form the pelvic plexuses. These nerves supply the lower rectum, anal canal, urinary bladder, and sexual organs. This distribution does not follow the course of the blood vessels.

The parasympathetic nerve supply is from the nervi erigentes, which originate from the second, third, and fourth sacral nerves on either side of the anterior sacral foramina and pass laterally forward and upward to join the pelvic plexuses on the pelvic side walls, from where fibers are distributed to the pelvic organs.

Anal Canal

Motor Innervation. The internal sphincter is supplied by both sympathetic and parasympathetic nerves, which presumably reach the muscle by the same route as that followed to the lower rectum. Contrary to previous belief that the sympathetic nerve supply is motor and the parasympathetic nerve supply is inhibitory to the sphincter, there is some evidence that both systems may be inhibitory. The external sphincter is supplied by the inferior rectal branch of the internal pudendal and the perineal branch of the fourth sacral nerve. As noted earlier, the sacral innervation of the external sphincter has been questioned. The puborectalis muscle is supplied by a branch of the third and fourth sacral nerves. Levator ani muscles are supplied on their pelvic surface by twigs from the fourth sacral nerves and on their perineal aspect by the inferior rectal or perineal branches of the pudendal nerves.

Sensory Innervation. The cutaneous sensation, experienced in the perianal region and wall of the anal canal below the dentate line, is conveyed by the afferent fibers in the inferior rectal nerves; hence, it can be abolished by an inferior rectal nerve block. A poorly defined dull sensation, experienced in the mucosa above the dentate line in response to touching with forceps or injection of hemorrhoids, is possibly mediated via the parasympathetic nerves.

■ PHYSIOLOGY

Physiology of the anorectal region is very complex. Techniques have become available that allow a study of the mechanisms of anal continence. From a review of the works of several investigators, it appears that the maintenance of anal continence depends on a highly integrated series of complicated events about which there is not uniform agreement. The following factors have been considered important in the overall maintenance of continence.

Mechanisms of Continence

Stool Volume and Consistency

Stool weight and volume vary from individual to individual, from one time to another in a given individual, and from one geographic region to another. The frequency of stool may play some role in mechanisms of continence in that colonic transit time is rapid when the bowel content is liquid because the left colon does not store fluid well. However, stool consistency is probably the most important physical characteristic that influences fecal continence. The ability to maintain normal control may depend on whether the rectal contents are solid, liquid, or gas. Some patients may be continent for solid stool, but not for liquid or gas or may be continent for stool but not for gas. This information is important in the management of patients with fecal incontinence, because the maneuver of changing stool consistency from liquid to solid may be enough to allow a patient to recapture fecal control.

Reservoir Function

From a mechanical point of view, the adaptive compliance of the rectum, along with the rectal capacity and distensibility, is important in the maintenance of continence. From a physiologic point of view, motor activity is more frequent and contractile waves are of higher amplitude in the rectum than in the sigmoid colon. This reverse gradient provides a pressure barrier resisting caudad progression of stool. Differences in pressure patterns between the distal and proximal levels of the anal canal result in the development of a force vector in the direction of the rectum. This continuous, differential activity may be of importance in controlling the retention of small amounts of liquid matter and flatus in the rectum.

Sphincteric Factors

The most commonly accepted explanation of anal continence is that the higher pressure zone in the anal canal at rest (average 25 to 120 mm Hg) provides an effective barrier against pressure in the rectum (average 5 to 20 mm Hg). Both the internal and external sphincters contribute to the resting tone, but the resting pressure is largely due to the internal sphincter.

Sensory Components

Duthie and Gairns found an abundance of conventional nerve endings that denote pain, touch, cold, pressure, tension, and friction, together with unnamed conventional receptors in the adult anal canal distal to the dentate line and to a point 0.5 to 1.5 cm cephalad to this level. These receptors are responsible for fine sensory discrimination. No receptors were found in the rectal mucosa. The rectum is insensitive to stimuli other than stretch. Evidence suggests that extrinsic sensory receptors are located in the puborectalis and surrounding pelvic musculature. Because the receptors for this proprioceptive reflex mechanism lie in the parapuborectalis tissues, this reflex remains intact even after amputation of the rectum or low anastomoses.

Duthie suggested that rectal distention results in transient relaxation of the internal sphincter and simultaneous contraction of the external sphincter. This decrease in anal canal pressure would be sufficient to momentarily allow the rectal contents to reach far enough into the anal canal to contact the very sensitive receptors and thus aid in recognition of the physical state of the threatening material, whether solid, liquid, or gas. This recognition of the nature of the content is not only conscious but also subconscious, because flatus can be passed safely during sleep.

The reflex contraction of the external sphincter, which is synchronous with relaxation of the internal sphincter, maintains continence during the time that the simulating material reaches this sensitive sensory area and allows time for impulses to reach conscious awareness (Fig. 1-2); thus, having determined the nature of the material, the individual can decide what to do about it and take appropriate action. Recently, nitric oxide has been identified as the chemical messenger mediating relaxation of the internal sphincter. Voluntary contraction of the external sphincter can extend the period of continence and allow time for compliance mechanisms within the rectum to provide for accommodation to increased intrarectal volumes. As the rectum accommodates to its new volume, stretch receptors are no longer activated, and afferent stimuli and the sensation of urgency disappear. Further rectal distention leads to inhibition of the external sphincter.

Mechanical Factors

In the normal resting state the lumen of the anal canal is occluded by the puborectalis sling and by the resting tone of the internal and external sphincters. Because of the continuous tonic activity of the puborectalis, the angulation of the anorectum is the most important mechanism for the conservation of gross fecal continence. This angle of 80 degrees between the axis of the rectum and the anal canal is present except when the hips are flexed more than 90 degrees or during defecation.

The flap valve theory advanced by Parks suggests that continence is achieved by virtue of the flap of anterior rectal mucosa that comes to lie over the upper end of the anal canal, functioning as an occlusion produced by the pull of the puborectalis muscle at the anorectal angle. Any increased intra-abdominal pressure (e.g., weight lifting, straining, laughing, or coughing) tends to accentuate the angulation and forces the anterior rectal mucosa more firmly over the upper anal canal, producing the flap valve effect. In order for defecation to occur, the flap valve must be broken. This breakage takes place by lengthening of the puborectalis muscle, descending of the pelvic floor, and obliteration of the anorectal angle.

Corpus Cavernosum of the Anus

Stelzner postulated that the vascular architecture in the submucosal and subcutaneous tissues of the anal canal really represents what he called a "corpus cavernosum" of the rectum. This tissue, with its physiologic ability to expand and contract, could contribute to the finest degree of anal continence. This theory might be supported by the fact that after a formal hemorrhoidectomy certain patients have minor alterations in continence, a situation that may arise as a result of the excision of this corpus cavernosum.

Defecation

The stimulus to the initiation of defecation is distention of the rectum. Distention of the left colon initiates peristaltic waves, which propel the fecal mass downward into the rectum. This process normally occurs once or several times a

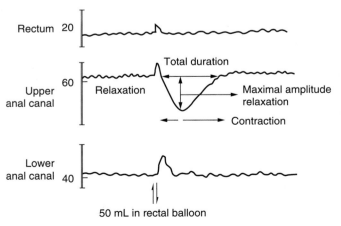

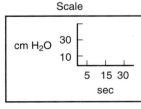

Scale

cm H₂O

Figure 1-2
Anorectal reflex. (From Gordon PH, Nivatvongs S: Principles and Practice of Surgery for the Colon, Rectum, and Anus, 2nd ed. St. Louis, Quality Medical Publishers, 1999.)

day. In many people, a pattern is established so that the urge is felt either upon rising in the morning, or in the evening, or after eating or drinking. This balance can be altered by travel, admission to the hospital, or alterations in diet.

Normally, rectal distention induces relaxation of the internal sphincter. This, in turn, triggers contraction of the external sphincter, and thus sphincter continence is induced. If the decision is made to accede to the urge, the subject assumes the squatting position. In doing so, the angulation between the rectum and the anal canal is straightened out. The second semivoluntary stage is the performance of the Valsalva maneuver, which overcomes the resistance of the external sphincter by voluntarily increasing the intrathoracic and intra-abdominal pressures. The pelvic floor descends, and the resulting pressure on the fecal mass in the rectum increases intrarectal pressure. Inhibition of the external sphincter permits passage of the fecal bolus. Once evacuation has been completed, the pelvic floor and the anal canal muscles regain their resting activity and the anal canal is closed.

The accommodation response consists of receptive relaxation of the rectal ampulla to accommodate the fecal mass. With increasing volume, there is a gradual stepwise increase in rectal pressure, and depending on the age of the patient, an urge to defecate is experienced. The urge, however, abates in a few seconds as the rectum accommodates the stimulus. When volume increases rapidly over a short period, the accommodation response fails and leads to urgent emptying of the rectum. The sampling response consists of transient relaxation of the upper part of the internal sphincter, which permits rectal contents to come into contact with the somatic sensory epithelium of the anal canal in order to assess the nature of the content. Thus, solids can be retained where gas can be passed, thereby relieving the intrarectal pressure. If fluid is present in the rectum, contact with the sensory area of the anal canal excites conscious activity of the external sphincter to maintain control until the rectal accommodation response occurs, and so continence is maintained.

The method of commencement of the act of defecation varies from person to person. If one is exerting anal control during an urge, merely relinquishing this voluntary control allows the reflex to proceed. On the other hand, if the urge abates, voluntary straining with increased intra-abdominal pressure is necessary before defecation can begin. Once it is begun, the act may follow either of two patterns. Expulsion of the rectal contents accompanied by mass peristalsis of the distal colon can occur, clearing the bowel in one continuous movement, or the stool can be passed piecemeal during several bouts of straining. The habit of the individual and the consistency of the feces largely determine which pattern is followed.

If large volumes are rapidly introduced into the rectum, the accommodation response may be overcome, cortical inhibition may be unavailing, and the urgency can be controlled for only 40 to 60 sec by the voluntary external sphincter complex. This time may be long enough to allow some accommodation. If not, leakage temporarily relieves the situation.

Using scintigraphic assessment, Lubowski and colleagues elegantly demonstrated that defecation is not a process of rectal emptying alone but also includes colonic emptying as an integral part of normal defecation. The importance of this finding is twofold: (1) a proctography is an inadequate method of studying patients with defecation disorders because it examines the rectum in isolation; and (2) disorders of defecation may occur in some patients as a result of a disorder of colonic function rather than a disorder of the rectum or pelvic floor muscles.

Physiologic Testing

Certain physiologic techniques have been developed to investigate disorders of function of the anal sphincters, rectum, and pelvic floor. These methods may be used to establish the diagnosis, provide an objective assessment of function, or identify the anatomic site of a lesion. These sophisticated tests are designed to complement but not to substitute for a good clinical examination and sound surgical judgment.

Anal Manometry

Manometry can be used to quantify the function of the internal and external sphincters. Different techniques have been used, including fluid-filled open-tipped catheters, closed multiple balloon systems, and, more recently, microtransducers with readings registered on a recording device. Each method has advantages and disadvantages, and each method has its advocates, but their goals are similar. Anal pressures can be measured at 1-cm intervals, first in the resting state and then during periods of voluntary contraction of the external anal sphincter. In the normal individual, intra-anal pressure is usually doubled during voluntary contraction.

For the assessment of an anal pressure profile, the recording probe must be withdrawn from the rectum, either stepwise or continuously at a constant rate. Although the step-by-step pull-through technique provides reliable measurements of resting anal canal pressure, the continuous pull-through technique allows a more appropriate assessment of the anal pressure profile and functional sphincter length. The length of the high-pressure zone, as determined by the continuous pull-through technique, varies between 2.5 and 5 cm and is shorter in women than in men.

The highest pressure of a pull-through profile is defined as a maximal resting anal pressure. Normal values of the maximal resting anal pressure are poorly defined because a variety of different techniques have been used, because normal values have been reported only for small control populations, and because there is a large range of normal maximal resting anal pressure. Using the microballoon technique, the normal maximal resting pressure ranges from 70 to 120 cm H_2O for men and 60 to 100 cm H_2O for women, with a maximum resting pressure located 1.5 cm from the anal verge. Resting pressure in the anal canal exhibits regular fluctuations varying from day to night by the presence or absence of fecal material in the rectum and by posture. Furthermore, based on the results of a manometric study, using a rigid recording device and a step-by-step pull-through technique, it has been concluded that intra-anal pressure exhibits longitudinal and radial variations. In the proximal part of the anal canal, the pressure recorded in the dorsal segment is higher than the pressure in the anterior segment. This finding has been ascribed to the activity of the puborectalis muscle. In the midanal canal the pressure is equally distributed in all segments, whereas in the lower anal canal the pressure is highest anteriorly. With the aid of a microcomputer and using an eight-channel multilumen probe, Coller calculated the radial cross-sectional pressure in five segments of the sphincter and found a gradient of pressure changing from posterior to lateral to anterior proceeding from the proximal to the distal end.

Voluntary contraction of the external sphincter produces an increase in anal pressure, superimposed on the basal tone. This increase in pressure is maximal in the distal part of the anal canal, where the bulk of the external sphincter is situated. To determine the functional activity of the different parts of the external sphincter, the recording device has to be withdrawn stepwise. After each step, the patient is asked to squeeze at full strength. In this way, it is possible to measure the maximal squeeze anal pressure at every level of the anal canal. It has been shown that maximal squeeze anal pressure is higher in male than in female subjects and that it is reduced as subjects get older. This age-related reduction is more significant in women.

The internal sphincter reflex in response to rectal distention can be mimicked by inflation of a rectal balloon. Transient inflation of a balloon with relatively small volume of air results in an initial rise in pressure, caused by a transient contraction of the external sphincter. Almost immediately after this initial increase in pressure, a transient reduction in anal canal pressure can be observed as a result of relaxation of the internal sphincter. Inflation of a rectal balloon with 30 cc of air results in a pressure reduction of about 50% for a mean duration of 19 sec. However, as the balloon is inflated with larger volumes, the amplitude as well as the duration of the relaxation reflex increases.

Disorders such as Hirschsprung's disease may be diagnosed using this noninvasive test. Other causes of severe chronic constipation can be assessed by manometry. Patients with anal incontinence, rectal procidentia, and the descending perineum syndrome have been investigated with manometry. Biofeedback therapy using anal manometry has been found to be an effective method of correcting or at least improving fecal incontinence in many patients. Patients with anal fissures demonstrate a characteristic overshoot contraction of the internal sphincter, whereas it has been suggested that patients with hemorrhoids have a dysrhythmia of the internal sphincter. Patients undergoing repair of a fistula-in-ano have been found to have lower resting pressures when their external sphincter has been divided, and disturbances in continence are related to these abnormally low resting pressures. The study of the sphincter mechanism preoperatively might be helpful to determine whether a patient will be continent following a pouch-anal anastomosis.

Defecography and Balloon Proctography

In the 1960s, cineradiography was used in the dynamic investigation of the defecation mechanism. A contrast medium with a semisolid consistency is introduced into the rectum and the subject is seated on a radiolucent commode to void the contrast agent. With this technique, the distal rectum and anal canal are outlined. The anorectal angle can be measured by drawing the axes of the anal canal and the floor of the rectum posteriorly. This angle depends on the tone of the puborectalis muscle and is normally 92 degrees (±1.5) at rest and 137 degrees (±1.5) during straining. Another application of defecography is determining the position of the pelvic floor by calculating the distance between the anorectal junction and the pubococcygeal line. In this way perineal descent at rest and during straining can be measured. The pubococcygeal line is drawn from the tip of the coccyx to the posteroinferior margin of the pubic ramus. Normally, the pelvic floor lies on a plane approximately 1 cm below that of the pubococcygeal line. A modification of this technique using a simple barium and air mixture has recently been described.

In an attempt to simplify the procedure and make it more acceptable for the patient, the balloon proctogram has been developed. It provides a visual assessment of the pelvic floor both in the resting state and during defecation. The examination is conducted by inserting a special shaped balloon filled with a barium suspension into the rectum. Lateral view radiographs are taken with the patient on a commode; thus, the rectum and anal canal can be outlined at rest and during straining. Evacuation of the balloon rather than of feces is more esthetically acceptable for patient and staff. The examination is well tolerated, quick, and clean and involves a relatively low radiation dose.

For the evaluation of defecation disorders that are associated with abnormalities such as anterior rectal wall prolapse, incomplete or complete rectal procidentia, rectocele, and solitary rectal ulcer syndrome, defecography is more sensitive than balloon proctography. Another determination that can be made is the patient's ability to expel rectal contents. A scintigraphic method using a balloon filled with a ^{99m}Tc-labeled suspension has been developed that allows the anorectal angle to be measured with minimal radiation exposure. Other conditions that can be studied are the detailed investigation of the physiologic aspects of normal continence, defecation, perineal descent, and enterocele. Defecography has also been used to study postoperative function after pouch-anal anastomoses. Poor functional results are caused by rapid pouch filling and impaired pouch evacuation, which lead to increased stool frequency. Patients with inflammatory bowel diseases, especially in the active phase, suffer from a decreased distensibility of the rectum, which could be the result of either decreased muscle compliance or increased sensitivity. Knowledge of this decreased rectal capacity may be of practical value in predicting which patients with Crohn's disease would benefit from an ileorectal anastomosis.

In summary, defecography is a useful imaging modality for assessing anorectal function, detecting anatomic abnormalities, and for performing anatomically guided anorectal surgery. The main contribution of defecography is its specific ability to reveal rectal intussusception and enterocele as well as sigmoidocele. However, the wide range of morphologic variations among healthy individuals and a large interobserver variation in measurements prevent defecography from being an ideal examination of anorectal defecation disturbance.

Simultaneous Dynamic Proctography and Peritoneography

Simultaneous dynamic proctography and peritoneography identifies both rectal and pelvic floor pathology and provides a qualitative assessment of its severity, allowing for better treatment planning in selected patients with obstructed defecation, pelvic fullness/prolapse, or chronic intermittent pelvic floor pain. The method consists of injection of 50 mL of nonionic contrast material intraperitoneally. The patients are immediately given 100 to 120 mL of barium rectal contrast and 20 to 25 mL of liquid barium intravaginally. On a radiolucent commode, lateral radiographs are taken at rest and at maximal anal squeeze. Patients are asked to evacuate rectal contrast material, which is observed on videotape using fluoroscopy. The evacuation videotape is used to identify rectocele, enteroceles, and rectal prolapse. An enterocele is present if peritoneal contrast material separates the rectum from the vagina, either at rest or during straining.

Balloon Expulsion Test

The balloon expulsion test was designed to demonstrate impaired rectal evacuation. However, many patients with electromyographic evidence of anismus are able to pass an inflated balloon. Inability to expel a balloon may represent insufficient colonic and rectal contractility or the failure to adequately raise intrarectal pressure by weak contraction of the diaphragm and abdominal muscles.

Saline Continence Test

This test was developed to obtain a more dynamic assessment of the continence mechanism. To gain insight into sphincter function, patients who were incontinent to liquids only were compared with patients who were incontinent to both solids and liquids. A method was devised by Bartolo and colleagues for assessing the function of the continence mechanism under stress by measuring the leakage that occurs when 1.5 L of saline is infused into the rectum. By recording anorectal pressures and obtaining external sphincter electromyogram during saline infusion, it was found that patients with incontinence to liquids only had peak anal pressures that did not differ from those of control subjects; this finding suggests a functional weakness of the internal sphincter only. The addition of external sphincter weakness rendered patients incontinent to solid stools. The technique has been used to study patients with hemorrhoids and the descending perineum syndrome.

Colonic Transit Studies

Although they are not directly related to anorectal function in all cases, colonic transit studies are helpful in understanding patients suffering from constipation. The technique may establish an abnormality but may also demonstrate a normal transit time in a patient with a bowel neurosis or in the occasional patient who denies having bowel actions. Methods for the study of intestinal transit times have been well described. Patients swallow 20 radiopaque markers, and abdominal x-ray films are obtained in a serial manner to determine the progression or lack of progression of these markers through the intestinal tract. The patient is instructed to consume a daily intake of 30 g of dietary fiber and to refrain from laxatives, enemas, and all nonessential medications for at least 48 hours prior to and during investigation. The progression of the markers is followed by daily films of the abdomen until complete expulsion of the markers occurs, or for a maximum of 7 days after ingestion. The markers are counted in three segments of the large bowel—right, left, and rectosigmoid. For this purpose, the spinal processes and two lines from the fifth lumbar vertebra to the pelvic outlet serve as landmarks. The transit times of the whole gut and of each segment of the colon are compared with normal transit time values. In this way, one may distinguish the patients with colonic inertia in whom a prolonged whole-gut transit time is found by means of markers distributed throughout the large bowel from the cecum to the rectum from those suffering from anorectal outlet obstruction, in whom the markers proceed quickly along the colon but accumulate in the rectum. Another group of patients exhibit a pattern in which the markers proceed to and then accumulate along the left colon. In this way a better understanding of the cause of the constipation or the segment of bowel most severely affected in a given patient may be determined.

Anorectal Sensitivity

Interest in the physiologic significance of anorectal sensation has spawned a technique that involves placing a bipolar ring electrode into the rectum or the anal canal and incrementally increasing the current until a threshold of sensation is reported by the patient. Conflicting information is available regarding gender and age variations. Rectal sensitivity seems to be reduced in constipated patients, especially those with objective evidence of prolonged colonic transit. Abnormal rectal sensation assessed by filling a rectal balloon reflects impaired viscoelastic properties of the rectal wall rather than disturbed sensation.

Rectal Compliance

Rectal compliance reflects the distensibility of the rectal wall, meaning the volumetric response of the rectum to stretch when subjected to an increased intraluminal pressure. After introduction into the rectum, a balloon is continuously inflated to selected pressure plateaus, and the volume changes at the various levels of distending pressures are recorded. A volume-pressure curve is plotted, and the slope of this curve represents the compliance. A deficit of rectal sensory function together with an increased compliance has been observed in women with intractable constipation following hysterectomy. Other investigators have found a decreased rectal compliance in patients with obstructed defecation. Significant inter- and intraindividual variations in pressure-volume profile in normal subjects indicates that rectal compliance measurements should be interpreted with caution.

Electrophysiologic Techniques

Electromyography records action potentials derived from motor units within contracting muscles. The external sphincter and probably the puborectalis muscle are unique skeletal muscles, as they show continuous tonic contractions at rest, with activity present even during sleep. During defecation, sphincter activity ceases.

Conventional Concentric Electromyography

By inserting a needle into the external sphincter or puborectalis without a local anesthetic, the normal resting continuous or basal action potentials can be obtained. This phenomenon is usually not displayed by skeletal muscle, which is characteristically electrically silent at rest. During voluntary contraction there is a burst of activity that is the consequence of increase frequency of motor unit firing and recruitment of new motor units. Contraction reflexly induced by balloon distention of the rectum or by perianal pin prick can also be recorded electromyographically.

Single-Fiber Electromyography

An even more sophisticated technique identifies the muscle action potential from a single muscle fiber. The technique provides a means of assessing innervation and reinnervation of the skeletal muscle under investigation. An assessment can be made quantitatively using the fiber density that represents the mean of a number of muscle fibers in one motor unit within the uptake area of the electrode averaged from 20 different electrode positions. A raised fiber density may be used as an index of collateral sprouting and reinnervation of muscle fibers within the muscle and is evidence of denervation.

In the past the most useful clinical application of electromyography was sphincter mapping of incontinent patients. Now other techniques such as endoanal sonography and endoanal magnetic resonance imaging seem to be more accurate for the detection of sphincter defects. Furthermore, the latter techniques obviate the need for the painful insertion of a needle at several locations around the anal canal. Jost and colleagues reported on the use of surface versus needle electrodes in the determination of motor conduction time to the external anal sphincter. They compared surface electrodes with needle electrodes and believe the surface electrodes are preferable.

Nerve Stimulation Techniques

Even more sophisticated techniques have been described to develop a better understanding of perineal functional abnormalities that may be of neurogenic origin.

Spinal Nerve Latency

A stimulus is applied to the spine initially at the level of L1 and is repeated at the L4 level. The induced response within the pelvic floor can be detected either by a surface anal plug electrode or by an intramuscular needle electrode. The mean latency to the external sphincter and to the puborectalis muscle can be determined.

The difference in the latencies from L1 to L4 has been called the spinal latency ratio. In patients with anal incontinence caused by a proximal lesion in the innervation, this spinal latency ratio is increased. Such a proximal lesion may be the result of damage to the motor nerve roots of S3 and S4 often due to disk disease. Stenosis of the spinal canal from osteoarthritis may also disturb proximal motor conduction.

Pudendal Nerve Terminal Motor Latency

By means of a rectal examination using a specially designed glove, a fingertip containing a stimulating electrode is brought into contact with the ischial spine on each side. A square wave stimulus is delivered, and a tracing is examined for evidence of contraction as detected in the external anal sphincter by the surface electrodes, thereby indicating accurate localization of the pudendal nerve. A supramaximal stimulus is delivered, and the motor latency of the terminal portion of the nerve is measured on each side.

The pudendal nerve terminal motor latency is increased in patients with pelvic floor disorders such as anal incontinence due to pudendal neuropathy with or without rectal prolapse, solitary rectal ulcer syndrome, and traumatic division of the external sphincter. The same phenomenon has been found in patients with intractable constipation. However, this increase in pudendal nerve latency is most impressive in patients with fecal incontinence.

Perineal Nerve Terminal Motor Latency

A similar technique can be employed for determining the distal motor latency in the perineal branch of the pudendal nerve by measuring the latency from pudendal nerve stimulation to the periurethral striated muscles.

The techniques of nerve stimulation provide objective assessment of neuromuscular function as well as a more precise identification of the anatomic site of the nerve or muscle lesion. The methods used allow evaluation of both the distal and proximal motor innervations of the perianal striated sphincter muscle.

Nerve stimulation techniques have been employed to study patients with pelvic floor disorders, especially anal incontinence. They have proved useful in the determination of the site of conduction delay and in the investigation of differential innervation of the puborectalis muscle and the external sphincter.

Suggested Readings

Carty NJ, Moran B, Johnson CD: Anorectal physiology measurements are of no value in clinical practice. True or false? Ann R Coll Surg Engl 1994;76:276–280.

Gordon PH, Nivatvongs S: Principles and Practice of Surgery for the Colon, Rectum, and Anus. St Louis, Quality Medical Publishing, 1999, chapters 1–2.

Lubowski DZ, Meagher AP, Smart RC, Butler SP: Scintigraphic assessment of colonic function during defecation. Int J Colorectal Dis 1995;10:91–93.

Matzel KE, Schmidt RA, Tanagho EA: Neuroanatomy of the striated muscular and anal continence mechanism. Implications for the use of neurostimulation. Dis Colon Rectum 1990;33:666–673.

Sentovich SM, Rivela, LJ, Thorson AG, et al: Simultaneous dynamic proctography and peritoneography for pelvic floor disorders. Dis Colon Rectum 1995;38:912–915.

Sultan AH, Kamm MA, Bartram CI, Hudson CN: Third-degree obstructive anal sphincter tears: Risk factors and outcome of primary repair. BMJ 1994;308:887–891.

Toma TP, Zighelboim J, Phillips SF, Talley NJ: Methods for studying intestinal sensitivity and compliance: In vivo studies of balloons and a barostat. Neurogastroenterol Mot 1996;8:19–28.

2

HEMORRHOIDS

Lee E. Smith, MD, FACS

Symptomatic hemorrhoids are one of the most common conditions that bring a patient to see a physician. Prior to seeing the physician, the patient often has self-diagnosed the problem and attempted treatment using some of the many over-the-counter products available. Unfortunately, diseases and disorders such as abscesses, fistulas, fissures, condylomata acuminata, and carcinomas may be mistaken by the patient for hemorrhoids. Ordinarily, the symptoms are pain, bleeding, or prolapse when internal hemorrhoids are enlarged, or pain when external hemorrhoids are thrombosed. Itching is usually of idiopathic origin and is unrelated to hemorrhoids, and pain can be the result of a fissure or a fistulous abscess.

Hemorrhoids enlarge as a result of pressures exerted from the hemorrhoidal arteries, portal veins, and systemic veins through an arteriovenous shunt system at the level of the hemorrhoids. This shunt system accounts for the finding of the bright red, freshly oxygenated blood of the internal hemorrhoids. However, bright red blood may result from other, more dangerous, pathologic conditions. The workup of outlet-type rectal bleeding should, therefore, include sigmoidoscopy to rule out neoplasm, even though large internal hemorrhoids are an obvious source of bleeding. This chapter addresses the author's approach to assessment and management of hemorrhoids. Patients first must be classified properly, then therapy appropriate for the severity of the hemorrhoids can be employed (Fig. 2-1).

■ EXTERNAL HEMORRHOIDS

Patients who have a thrombosed external hemorrhoid present with a painful lump at the anal verge. They are often fearful that this is a carcinoma; therefore, reassurance that hemorrhoids are unrelated to cancer alleviates much anxiety. Thrombosed hemorrhoids are often associated with pregnancy or physical exertion by young active males. Increased abdominal pressures transmitted to the hemorrhoidal veins may be a precipitating factor. The patient who is the best candidate for surgical excision of the thrombosed, external hemorrhoid has had recent development of symptoms, preferably within 72 hours, and no lessening of pain during that time. Once 72 hours have elapsed, the clots begin to soften spontaneously, shrink, and become less painful. Patients who have reached this stage can be allowed to continue to resolve their problem spontaneously without a surgical procedure. The nonsurgical treatment consists of pain medication, a stool softener, and sitz baths.

■ INTERNAL HEMORRHOIDS

Patients who have symptomatic internal hemorrhoids are classified on the basis of the degree of prolapse that is present (Table 2-1). This classification is ranked in four degrees. First-degree hemorrhoids are maintained in their normal position but may occasionally bleed a little. Second-degree hemorrhoids have begun to prolapse during defecation but reduce spontaneously at the end of the effort. The patient may note blood on the toilet paper or in the toilet water but may not recognize that there is prolapse. The physician can verify prolapse by having the patient sit on the toilet and strain to produce maximal exertion; the physician can then look at the hemorrhoidal area by having the patient lean forward for direct inspection or by observing via a mirror system. Third-degree hemorrhoids have begun to stay entrapped by the sphincter outside the anal canal. They are easily palpable and the patient is usually aware of them. Symptoms may be reduced by manually pushing the internal hemorrhoids back into the anus. These hemorrhoids often squirt and drip blood into the toilet water. Neglected hemorrhage from such hemorrhoids can result in marked anemia. Fourth-degree hemorrhoids are trapped outside the anal canal and cannot be reduced by manual pressure. They are often clotted, are exquisitely tender, and may eventually become gangrenous. Fortunately, they are not common.

Asymptomatic hemorrhoids do not merit treatment. The cosmetic appearance, as judged by the physician, is not an indication for treatment. However, fastidious individuals may demand that even minimal symptoms be addressed by some form of therapy.

■ TIMING OF SURGERY

Thrombosed external hemorrhoids that are seen early (within 72 hours) and are accompanied by persistent, severe pain should be operated on immediately. Medical management, which consists of hot sitz baths and bulk stool softeners, can be instituted at once as part of the treatment regimen for external or internal hemorrhoids. If an outpatient ambulatory procedure is recommended by the physician, it can be performed under local anesthesia immediately if the patient agrees with the potential risks and benefits and accepts the complications and inconvenience that may ensue. Fourth-degree hemorrhoids that are clotted, swollen, and markedly painful are a relative emergency. The best approach is to admit the patient to the hospital and perform an emergency operation.

■ PREOPERATIVE PREPARATION

Disorders that have been discovered during the patient history and physical and laboratory examinations should

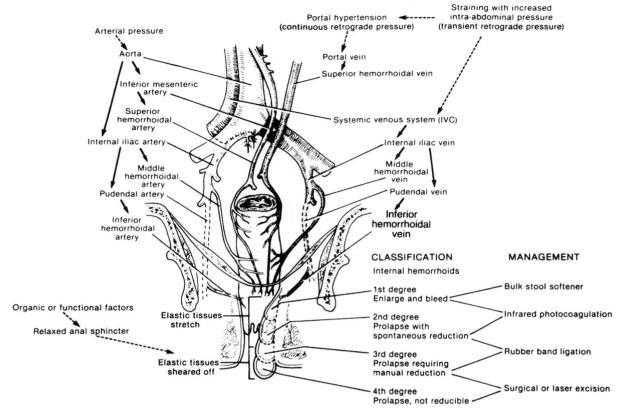

Figure 2-1
Pathogenesis, classification, and management of prolapsing hemorrhoids. The systemic and portal venous pressures as well as the arterial pressures are exerted on the hemorrhoids. When the sphincter is relaxed, the hemorrhoids dilate under these pressures.

be completely evaluated prior to beginning elective surgery. Special attention should be paid to investigating cardiorespiratory problems, medications that might interfere with anesthesia or promote surgical complications, and bleeding disorders. Abnormal laboratory values should at least be repeated and verified so that the source of the abnormality can be addressed. In this age of shortened hospital stays and ambulatory surgical procedures, much of the preoperative preparation is left to the patient. Ordinarily, the history, physical examination, and laboratory studies are done on an outpatient basis. The patient is asked not to eat or drink anything after midnight on the

night prior to surgery. Prior to the patient's surgery, the rectum can be cleaned by two small enemas. A responsible adult must accompany the patient at the time of discharge, especially after an outpatient surgical procedure.

■ CHOICE OF PROCEDURE

Internal hemorrhoids are managed based on the classification of prolapse (Fig. 2-2). In general, three basic factors will improve the hemorrhoidal condition. First, reducing straining at stool relieves the pressure on the hemor-

Table 2-1 Classification and Symptoms of Internal Hemorrhoids		
STAGE	PROLAPSE	SYMPTOMS
1	None	Bleeding
2	Occurs with bowel movements but reduces spontaneously	Prolapse, bleeding, mild discomfort
3	Occurs readily with bowel movements, sometimes with exertion; requires manual reduction	Prolapse, bleeding, discomfort, soiling, occasional pruritus and discharge
4	Persistent; reduction is not possible	Prolapse, bleeding, pain, thrombosis, soiling and discharge

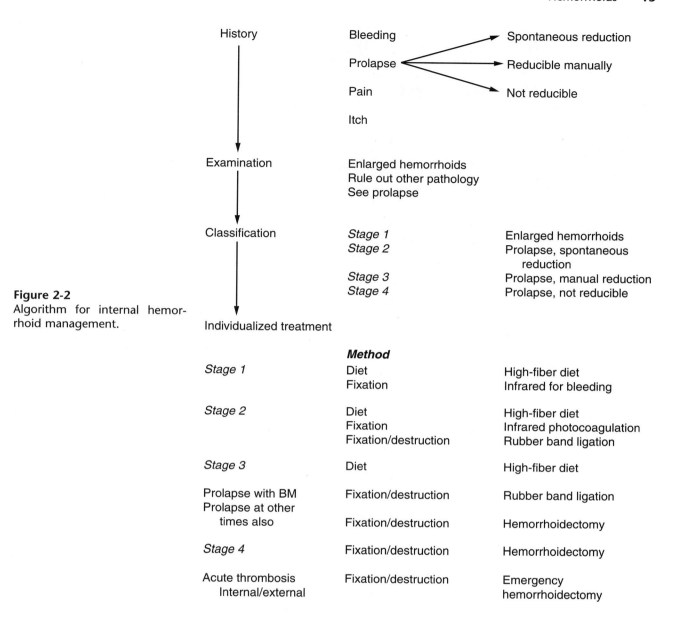

Figure 2-2
Algorithm for internal hemorrhoid management.

rhoids. The second factor is the removal or destruction of the redundant mucosa and hemorroidal tissues. Third, if scars are created to fixate the adjacent tissues, prolapse can be limited or prevented.

In general, bulk stool softeners may be utilized in the treatment of any type of hemorrhoids. However, this choice may be the primary treatment modality for first-degree hemorrhoids and minor second-degree hemorrhoids. Diet modification is the only treatment employed in approximately 50% of the author's patients. High-fiber diets promote a bulky, soft stool that decreases the amount of straining required to achieve a bowel movement.

Second-degree hemorrhoids and minor third-degree hemorrhoids can be treated by fixation procedures that destroy minor amounts of tissue and create scarring to fixate the tissues. These same procedures may also be applied to greater degrees of prolapse in elderly and high-risk

patients. The fixation procedures include sclerotherapy, rubber band ligation, infrared photocoagulation, cryodestruction, laser vaporization, monopolar electrocautery, and bipolar electrocautery.

Preferred fixation procedures include rubber band ligation and infrared photocoagulation because of the ease and convenience of achieving the fixation by these procedures (Figs. 2-3 to 2-6). Rubber band ligation employs a special gun on which a rubber band is fitted and from which it can be released by a trigger mechanism. This gun, which has a barrel at the tip on which the rubber band is placed, allows the hemorrhoidal tissues to be drawn by a forceps into the barrel. The released band encompasses the tissue, which then sloughs, creating necrosis at its base and subsequently a scar.

The procedure may be accomplished easily in the clinic setting. An anoscope is inserted and withdrawn to allow

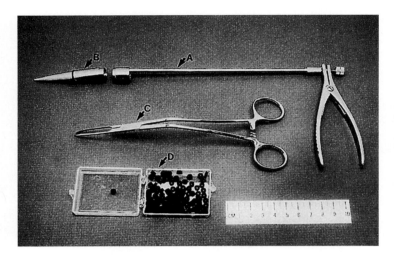

Figure 2-3
The rubber band ligator system contains the following parts: ligating gun (*A*); loading cone (*B*); tenaculum (*C*); rubber (elastic) bands (*D*).

inspection of the hemorrhoidal columns. The largest hemorrhoidal column is selected. The dentate line is observed, and a point is selected 2 to 3 cm proximal to that point. A forceps is passed through the barrel of the gun, and the hemorrhoid is teased into the barrel. The rubber band application can be followed with an injection of 0.25% bupivacaine with 1:200,000 epinephrine solution

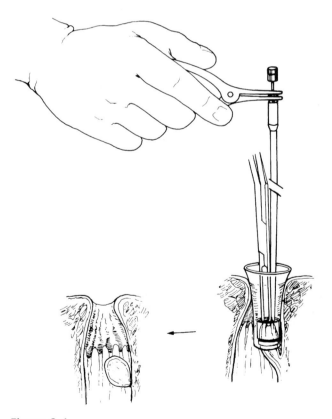

Figure 2-4
The internal hemorrhoid is teased into the barrel of the ligating gun. The point chosen is well above the dentate line in order to minimize pain.

into the ligated tissue. A small volume of local anesthesia may decrease the discomfort that accompanies the rubber band ligation; in addition, the swollen tissue keeps the rubber band from sliding off. One rubber band is applied and the patient is observed for the effect. If there is negligible discomfort, another band is applied. Before the procedure, the patient is told that four to six rubber bands may be required before symptoms are relieved. Appointments are scheduled approximately 1 month apart, which allows healing and time for the patient to decide whether the symptoms have been alleviated.

Infrared photocoagulation is a procedure that is rapid, causes little pain, and is inexpensive. The infrared photocoagulation applications should be applied well above the dentate line in the area where sensory fibers are minimal (Fig. 2-5). However, it should not be touted as a painless procedure, because virtually every patient feels some initial heat when the infrared photocoagulator is turned on, usually for 1 second. Ordinarily, the coagulator is applied to four sites on each column chosen: one at the apex, one at the midportion of the hemorrhoidal column, and one each on the right and left lateral sides between the two previously mentioned points.

The infrared photocoagulator is most effective for hemorrhoids that have fine serpiginous venules on the surface of the columns. These tiny bleeders may be obliterated by this form of teatment with minimal outlay of time and money.

In general, third- and fourth-degree hemorrhoids require an operative procedure involving excision of tissue that results in a well-formed linear scar to fixate larger bundles of tissue (Fig. 2-7). The formal hemorrhoidectomy, performed with laser or with standard cutting surgical instruments, provides the best linear fixation. In addition, these procedures permit removal of the columns of hemorrhoids and tailoring of the anal skin, resulting in a smooth surface.

Operative treatment is reserved for patients with major degrees of prolapse. At Washington Hospital Center this procedure normally is performed on an outpatient basis in the ambulatory surgical unit. Traditionally, the patient

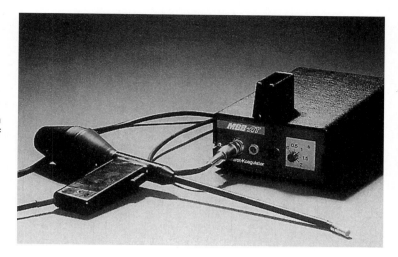

Figure 2-5
The infrared photocoagulator. Note the timer (in seconds), which is set to determine the time of tissue exposure.

was hospitalized for about 4 days and kept until he or she produced the first bowel movement. In this period of cost consciousness, it is hard to justify keeping a patient in the hospital even one day for this type of an anorectal procedure. In order to accomplish hemorrhoidectomy successfully in the outpatient setting, informed patient consent preceded by careful explanation of the preoperative, operative, and postoperative courses must be obtained. In addition, during the postoperative period, the physician must be readily available to answer questions and deal with complications.

The patient may be operated on in the prone jack-knife or lithotomy position. It is not necessary to shave or clip the hair unless it is very dense. Intravenous fluids are begun, and the patient's vital signs are monitored. The buttocks are taped apart so that the anal area is effaced and

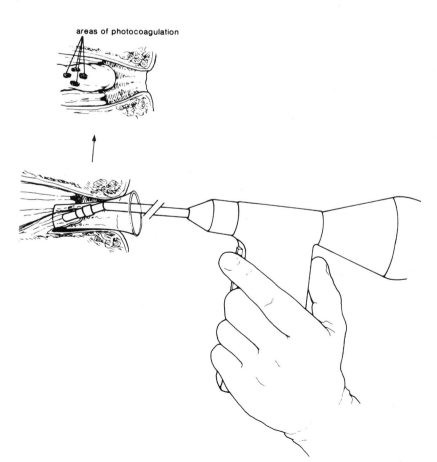

Figure 2-6
The infrared photocoagulator creates a small, thermal injury. Thus, several applications are required for each hemorrhoidal column.

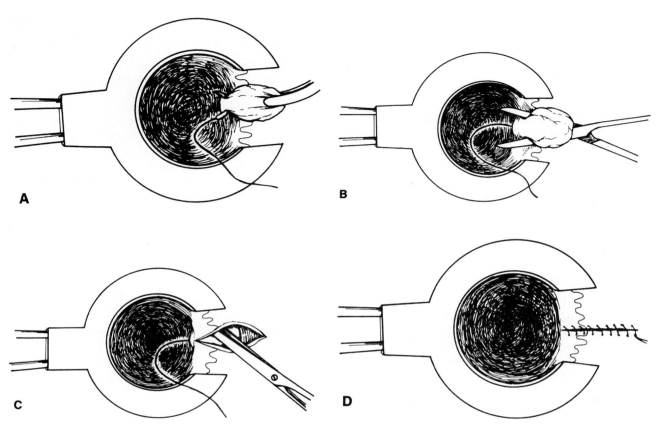

Figure 2-7
Operative hemorrhoidectomy. *A*, After injection of local anesthesia and epinephrine, the largest column of hemorrhoids is selected for excision. The operating anoscope isolates the hemorrhoid. At the apex of the hemorrhoidal column, a chromic suture is placed to mark the extent of proposed excision and to occlude arterial circulation. *B*, The hemorrhoidal column, including the skin tag, anoderm, and mucosa with underlying hemorrhoids, is excised down to the sphincter muscle. *C*, The internal and subcutaneous external sphincters are partially exposed during dissection. Additional hemorrhoids may be excised from beneath the margins of the excision site. *D*, The previously applied suture is used to close the entire wound.

readily observable. This places the external hemorrhoids and external tags, if they are present, in relief. Local anesthesia is used; a combination of hydrochloride solution (Xylocaine) and bupivacaine works well. Hydrochloride 1% mixed with epinephrine to a strength of 1:200,000 is used to inject the skin circumferentially, with a 30-gauge needle. A spinal needle is used to inject the local anesthetic up to the level of the levator muscles at eight points around the anus. Hydrochloride is selected because its action is almost instantaneous in onset, and there is no pain secondary to the chemical contact with tissues. The bupivacaine with ephinephrine is slow-acting and is irritating to the tissues, but its redeeming feature is its long duration of action. This combination of local anesthetics offers excellent analgesia, muscle relaxation, and hemostasis for venous bleeding. Preceding injection, the author gives the patient a combination of narcotic (meperidine) and tranquilizer (midazolam), in a dosage appropriate to the patient's age and health status.

Good exposure is imperative, and the author's choice of retractors is the slotted Fansler operating anoscope. The hemorrhoids are treated in order of size: The largest column is excised first and then the next largest in serial fashion. Ordinarily, the right anterior column is the largest. Usually, both internal and external enlarged hemorrhoidal tissues are found. A suture is placed at the apex of the internal column using a number 3-0 chromic. This apical suture is used for two reasons. First, the arteries that attend the column are usually located in the submucosal planes; thus, they are ligated early in the procedure. Second, the extent of the hemorrhoidal columns is most evident prior to beginning the actual dissection. Therefore, the resection of tissue is defined before the anatomy is distorted. The apical suture of 3-0 chromic is not cut but retracted aside for subsequent closure of the excision. Metzenbaum scissors are excellent for excision. Tissues that are to be cut are grasped and pulled between the blades of the scissors. Simultaneously, the blades of the scissors must be pressed down flat against the muscle to make the loose tissues bulge between the scissors' blades. The intact circular sphincter muscle tissue is automatically held away and below the cutting edges. As the ellipse of skin, anoderm, and mucosa is excised, the internal sphincter and margin of the subcutaneous portions of the external sphincter are seen in the base of the wound. Additional hemorrhoidal tissues may be excised by elevating flaps off the muscle on both sides of the primary excision. Then those tissues between the muscle and the mucosa or skin may be excised. Wide bridges of normal skin, anoderm, and mucosa are left intact. Arterial bleeders may be electrocoagulated or suture ligated. The previously applied 3-0 chromic suture is used as a running, locked stitch for closure of the elliptical wound to the level of the dentate line. The remainder of the anoderm and skin is closed with a simple running suture. Avoid pulling on the sutures and prolapsing the mucosa out as it is closed to prevent an ectropion. Each of the columns of hemorrhoids, whether there are two, three, or four, is treated in the same fashion, but the removed strips must be narrower as the number of excisions increases.

After closure, additional 0.25% bupivacaine with epinephrine is injected along the margins of the incisions for long-term pain relief. A simple external dressing is applied to collect any spillage of mucus or blood. Specifically, no intra-anal packing is inserted. Anorectal packing may be responsible for marked spasm, pain, and hence urinary retention. Refer to Figure 2-2 for an overview of the management of internal hemorrhoids.

In recent years, a new technology has been introduced: A circular stapler has been designed for application at the level just above the internal hemorrhoids. This stapler excises a circular segment of mucosa and submucosa, resulting in a circular scar. The safety and efficacy of this technique require the test of time; however, the cost of the stapler markedly increases the cost of the procedure. There were early reports of bleeding and sepsis, but with experience, these complications rates are reduced. The positive effect of the procedure is a significant decrease in pain.

■ POSTOPERATIVE COURSE

The patient must be accompanied home by a responsible adult. He or she is instructed to begin sitz baths at the first hint of localized pain. The bathtub should be filled to the level of the umbilicus with hot water. Sitz baths are done for 10 minutes four times per day. A bulk stool softener can be begun that evening. Pain relief by oral medication is necessary, especially during the first night. On the following morning, the patient usually feels much better.

Pain is the most common problem: The patient is encouraged to take pain medication for the first 2 days. Thereafter, he or she is asked to taper such medications rapidly. Urinary retention is a major problem in young males; women and older men seldom have this problem. Formerly, it was believed that older men had difficulty resuming urination because of their enlarged prostates, but interestingly, it is more commonly the young male with a hypertonic sphincter who fails to urinate. Patients are kept relatively dehydrated during surgery so that the bladder will not be overdistended. In addition, the patient is instructed to begin trying to urinate early, while the anal area is still anesthetized. It is of great importance to assure the patient that he or she will not injure the operative sites by straining to urinate or defecate. In fact, the patient is expected to make a great effort to strain and push down to evacuate, even if pain is produced by such efforts. During preoperative counseling, the patient is informed that there may be a small amount of bleeding postoperatively. He or she is instructed to call the surgeon if there is persistent bleeding or fever, which may indicate infection. The patient is followed up in the office in 1 week to ensure that healing is proceeding properly. To avoid causing pain, do not place a finger or anoscope into the anal canal prior to 3 weeks after the procedure.

The open-tip yttrium-aluminum-garnet (YAG) laser, the contact-tip YAG laser, or the carbon dioxide (CO_2) laser may be used as the instrument for dissection. It has been alleged that laser treatment is less painful, but the author has not been able to prove this. If the CO_2 laser is used to excise tissue that has been clamped, sometimes a welding phenomenon occurs.

■ COMPLICATIONS

Diet modification has few, if any, complications. Infrared photocoagulation causes local pain, and occasionally bleeding can ensue. Rubber band ligation has the disadvantage of causing a dull, aching tenesmus, which often requires pain medication for 1 or 2 days. Approximately 1% of these patients have major secondary bleeding that requires some form of anesthesia and suture ligation. Rare reports have noted infection following rubber band ligation. These patients have the common finding of increasing rather than decreasing pain after the second postoperative day. These patients also develop urinary retention after having been able to urinate initially. This complex of symptoms, which is associated with fever, points to an infection, which must be diagnosed early for possible debridement and administration of broad-spectrum parenteral antibiotics. The physician who does not acknowledge these symptoms and decides that the patient is simply pain-intolerant may fail to recognize this serious sequela. Therefore, the patient may not be seen and treated early enough to interrupt the septic spiral that can result in death.

Operative hemorrhoidectomy has the serious drawback of causing extreme pain postoperatively. By using the stool softeners, analgesics, and sitz baths, this discomfort can be minimized. A survey of the author's patients showed that one third had less pain than expected, one third had the pain that was expected, and one third had more pain than was expected. Unfortunately, no common identifying factor suggests which of these groups a patient will fall into. In general, a positive attitude that pain can be managed is important, and avoidance of packing minimizes the pain. For ambulatory patients, the use of long-term local anesthetics allows the patient to get home and to prepare for any ensuing pain.

On occasion, minor degrees of incontinence, especially for gas and liquid, are reported. Infections are extremely rare because suture lines disrupt enough to allow self-drainage. Frequently, if large skin tags are present prior to the procedure, minor residual ones may persist. As with rubber band ligation, 1% of patients who are operated on have a significant primary or secondary hemorrhage that requires additional suture ligations. If the apical suture is placed and either it is cut out accidentally or the knot is broken, bleeding will occur and a significant hematoma can be created in the submucosal tissues at the apex of the excision. Deep excisions could conceivably enter the rectovaginal septum and result in a rectovaginal fistula. Stenosis is relatively rare, especially if a large operating anoscope is utilized for the operative closures. If the operating scope fits into the anal canal, the final canal size is at least of that diameter. Even though bridges of normal tissue are left between the columns, some stenosis has been reported. In general, this stenosis can be treated by minor dilations. Rarely, stenosis requires an anoplasty to gain circumference by advancing skin into the anal canal. Because several linear scars are created in operative hemorrhoidectomy, recurrence is unusual, and deaths are rare for this procedure.

Suggested Readings

Ambrose NS, Hares MM, Alexander-Williams J, et al. Prospective randomized comparison of photocoagulation and rubber band ligation in treatment of hemorrhoids. BMJ 1983;286:1389–1391.

Barron J. Office ligation of internal hemorrhoids. Am J Surg 1963;105:563–569.

Buls JG, Goldberg SM. Modern management of hemorrhoids. Surg Clin North Am 1978;58:469.

Leicester RJ, Nicholls RJ, Mann CV. Infrared coagulation. Dis Colon Rectum 1981;24:602.

Moesgaard F, Nielsen ML, Hansen JB, et al. High-fiber diet reduces bleeding and pain in patients with hemorrhoids. Dis Colon Rectum 1982;25:454–456.

Queredo-Bonilla G, Farkas AM, Abcarian H, et al. Septic complications of hemorrhoidal banding. Arch Surg 1988;123:650–651.

3

ANAL FISSURE

Barton Hoexter, MD

An anal fissure is a small linear tear in the anal mucosa. Surprisingly, such a small lesion can produce symptoms severe enough to incapacitate the human body. The majority of fissures occur in the posterior midline. In women, 10% are found in the anterior midline (less than 1% in males). Other locations are usually associated with systemic disease such as Crohn's disease, tuberculosis, and previous surgery. Recent investigations have proposed explanations for this preponderance of posterior tears, including the following:

1. Defecating through the posterior epicenter with the use of our commode toilets, rather than the squatting of primitive societies
2. Anatomic configuration of the sphincter mechanism with the elliptical anterior-posterior direction of the muscles (Lockhart-Mummery's lack of posterior muscle support)
3. Decrease in mucosal blood supply to the posterior commissure (Shouten's Doppler laser flow studies)

In the past decade, the etiology of fissures itself has been attributed to higher resting sphincter pressures and a decrease in anodermal blood flow, rather than local sepsis and caustic irritation (Coller and Karulf). With these newer etiologic concepts, new medical treatments have evolved, such as topical nitroglycerin, diltiazem, botulinum A toxin, and local injections. Further refinements have occurred in surgery also, in open or closed lateral sphincterotomies, controlled posterior sphincterotomy, or sliding flap anoplasties and controlled anal dilation.

Arguments exist in today's managed care environment as to whether cure rates of 80% after medical treatment are real, or whether they reflect procrastination or convenience delays for elective surgery.

■ DIAGNOSIS

The designation of acute and chronic fissure varies, according to duration of symptoms and response to therapy. History alone usually renders the diagnosis, with symptoms of tearing, knife-like pain, with or without bleeding, usually associated with forceful hard stool or diarrhea. Pain starting with defecation lasts minutes to hours. Fear of subsequent symptoms causes the patient to withhold stooling, causing an exacerbation of constipation, impaction, and pain.

Examination requires gentle retraction of the buttocks without any sudden pulling. Pain is noted as the fissure is exposed. An edematous sentinel tag may be present. White fibers of the internal sphincter may be seen in the base of the fissure or they may be covered by a thin epithelium. This rolling epithelium may hide the fissure. Digital examination may be attempted with a very well lubricated finger pressing away from the fissure, either anteriorly or laterally for a posterior fissure. Lidocaine (Xylocaine) 2% jelly or local anesthetic injection may make the examination more comfortable. If anoscopic examination is possible, the rectal mucosa may be examined for infections or proctitis, and the presence of the fissure confirmed. Overhanging edges suggest chronicity. Gentle sigmoidoscopies with a narrow scope (11 mm) may be used to further evaluate the rectal mucosa.

■ ETIOLOGY

The anal canal consists of epithelium overlying sphincter muscles and, when closed, is a few millimeters in diameter. However, it opens to accommodate large fecal masses and is capable of being dilated to eight fingers (Lord Procedure). Occasionally a linear tear along the longitudinal axis occurs, exposing the underlying internal sphincter (not external sphincter as shown by Eisenhammer in 1953).

Normal maximal resting anal pressure (MRAP) in females is 60 to 100 cm H_2O and in males is 75 to 125 cm H_2O, although pressures decreases with age. Higher resting internal sphincter pressures are found in people with fissures. A sawtooth pattern may be seen on these high-pressure manometry tracings. Sphincterotomy and nitric oxide donors have been shown to decrease these pressures.

More recently, Shouten and associates have also suggested a decrease in blood flow as the cause of fissures, accounting for the pain, which appears to be out of proportion to the small fissure present. Klosferhalfen has injected the inferior rectal artery and has noted the terminal capillaries are in the posterior commissure, making ischemia a possibility. Because increased MRAP is associated with decreased mucosal blood flow, the two may be related. Therapy decreases MRAP and increases blood flow. Local therapy with antibiotics is futile, and hygiene alone is adequate. In chronic cases, there is a lack of inflammatory response, again showing infection to be a secondary problem (not true of HIV, etc.). Sentinel tags are the result of lymphatic obstruction and edema, not infection. Studies by Eisenhammer show that the external sphincter plays a part in hypertonicity as in fissures themselves.

On anal manometry an "overshoot" phenomenon can be seen in the anorectal inhibitory reflex. This overshoot phenomenon, unlike the anorectal reflex, returns to normal in 20 seconds. It has not been shown to be a cause of pain. Preoperative manometry has little use in the investigation or treatment of fissures. Most prefer now to use it in patients who have failed initial treatment.

NONOPERATIVE TREATMENT

In typical acute anal fissures, many patients respond to medical therapy. The mainstays of therapy are avoidance of straining at stool and use of warm sitz baths multiple times a day. Hydrocortisone creams may help, but suppositories are of no value, because they act well above the affected area (Coller and Karulf), and they cause pain on insertion.

Jensen and coworkers found local anesthetic ointments such as 2% lidocaine, which should be given before defecation in a squatting position and allowed to reside for 2 minutes (they can cause allergic reactions if continuously used), were associated with healing in 60%; 82% healed with hydrocortisone, but 87% healed with bran alone.

Clostridium botulinum toxin, when injected (0.1 mL diluted toxin 2.5 u) in two doses into the external anal sphincter on both sides of the fissure (Jost and Schimrigk, 1993) provided complete healing in 21 of 26 patients after 3 months. Two patients had mild incontinence, which subsided, and 5 patients developed perianal thrombosis. As with other uses of this toxin, paralysis helped heal resistant fissures.

By far, the most popular topical treatment today is the application of topical nitroglycerin ointment ranging from 0.15 to 0.8% three to four times per day. Watson and coworkers demonstrated that a concentration greater than 0.2% was required to decrease MRAP by 25%, but the headaches increased accordingly. Nitric oxide donors (glyceryl trinitrate and isosorbide dinitrate) have the same physiologic effects on the internal sphincter as sphincterotomy. Championed by Gorfine, topical nitroglycerin has been suggested for thrombosed hemorrhoids and levator spasms as well. Pain from fissure resolves, but many of the fissures do not heal.

Diltiazem has also been used in recent years as a means of "chemical sphincterotomy." Success rates in the order of 65 to 70% have been described, and the drug is best used as a 2% topical preparation. Oral preparations have been tried, but to less effect. Side effects are generally less frequent with this medication than with nitroglycerin, particularly that of headache (Knight and coworkers).

Anal dilation varies from gentle dilation to 3 or 4 fingers to 8 or 9 fingers of the traditional Lord procedure. Recent controlled dilation using the rectosigmoid balloon, 40 mm in diameter and 6 cm in length at 20 psi for 6 minutes under anorectal local anesthesia, has been championed by Sohn and Weinstein. A smaller balloon is used for patients over 60 years of age.

OPERATIVE TECHNIQUES

The division of the pectin band was essential for fissure healing (credited to Brodie in 1835). Eisenhammer described posterior internal sphincterotomy in 1951 with excision of the fissure, but 40% of his patients in this series developed some degree of flatus, fluid, or stool incontinence. A keyhole deformity resulted from a posterior incision and caused this soiling. Eisenhammer next developed

the lateral sphincterotomy. Mazier popularized multiple superficial sphincterotomies as causing less incontinence. Notaras developed the subcutaneous distal internal sphincterotomy most popular today. In our hands and many others, permanent incontinence of feces, fluid, or flatus is rare, with only occasional temporary loss of flatus control. Rarely, a repeat sphincterotomy is necessary.

TECHNIQUE

Most sphincterotomies are done as outpatient procedures with sedation and intravenous anesthesia (Versed, ketamine, droperidol, propofol, etc.). The author prefers the prone jack-knife position because of the lack of engorgement of the anal tissues, although the lithotomy and lateral positions are also acceptable. Local perianal injection of lidocaine 1% with 1:100,000 epinephrine combined with equal parts bupivacaine 0.5% with 1:200,000 epinephrine start posteriorly, then either in four quadrants or behind the three primary hemorrhoids.

The intersphincteric groove is palpated laterally (many prefer right lateral to avoid the hemorrhoid plexus, but if done on the left, the hemorrhoid can be taken if desired). A radial incision no more than 5 mm is made. Subcutaneous tissues are gently mobilized away from the sphincter, and the transverse fibers of the internal sphincter are picked up with an Allis clamp. The lower third of the internal sphincter is divided superficially by knife, cautery, or scissors. The ability to insert an extra large Hill-Ferguson retractor signifies completeness. Hemostasis and complete division are accomplished with gentle pressure. The incision can be closed with absorbable chromic sutures or left open.

The closed subcutaneous internal sphincterotomy can be performed similarly. Local anesthetic is placed in both lateral positions. The intersphincteric groove is palpated and a cataract knife (No. 15 or 11 can also be used) is inserted into it. A finger is placed in the canal and the blade is advanced up to the lower third of internal sphincter. Then the knife is turned toward the finger, gently dividing the fibers. The remaining fibers are broken with the finger after the knife is removed. Adequacy is again checked with the retractors. This method requires special care and it is better to make several shallow passes with the knife, cutting only on withdrawal.

Relief from the fissure pain is often felt immediately or at least within a few days. Recurrence or prolongation of pain may be associated with a hematoma or abscess. Gordon's text is pessimistic concerning postoperative soiling and incontinence, but more recent articles described nearly no problems. Caveats include the following:

1. Do not cross the dentate line.
2. Hemostasis must be excellent.
3. Avoid taking too much internal sphincter, especially in women and patients over 60 years old.
4. Avoid the external sphincter.

In patients with mucosal stenosis or a fissure and low MRAP (even clinically), the use of sutured anoplasty or sliding island flap anoplasty as done for stenosis is advised by Farouk, Bartolo, and others.

If a fissure recurs, biopsies should be taken to rule out Crohn's disease, human immunodeficiency virus (HIV), neoplasia, or other diseases. Cultures should be taken for HIV, herpes simplex virus (HSV), cytomegalovirus (CMV), syphilis, and *Hemophilus ducreyi*. Postoperative manometry is indicated to look for persistent sphincter hypertonia, and anal ultrasonography will validate the remaining internal sphincter. Contralateral sphincterotomy may be indicated.

Although other chapters will cover Crohn's disease, anal stenosis, and AIDS-related anal disease, their relationship to fissures should be noted. In Crohn's disease, most fissures are posterior, but the findings of multiplicity (14 to 37%), aberrant position (up to 20%), and painful fissures (20 to 40%) mandate investigation with endoscopy and radiographic studies. Many Crohn's-related fissures will progress to fistulas. Primary therapy is conservative use of bulking agents, sitz baths, and anesthetic creams. Gottesman advocates

Depo-Medrol intralesional injection (80 mg) every 2 weeks. Anti-inflammatory agents (NSAIDs), metronidazole, 6-mercaptopurine, and steroids give a 50% healing rate. Many advocate proximal control of abdominal processes in resistant cases, including surgical extirpation. Recent studies show no major advantages for this, however.

Today, local control is most accepted with sphincterotomy and fissure debridement giving excellent results, especially when combined with postoperative use of metronidazole. The success of anal dilatation (up to 4 fingers) in England is not shared in the United States because of the associated incontinence and high recurrence rate, a particular concern in patients with inflammatory bowel disease.

Anorectal disease is found in up to 60% of HIV patients, usually condyloma and fissures (both benign fissures and HIV-infected fissures). Repeated anoreceptive intercourse causes hypotonic sphincters, so the hypertonic etiology of ulcer does not apply. Trauma and diarrhea (infection) have been implicated. Benignity is usually

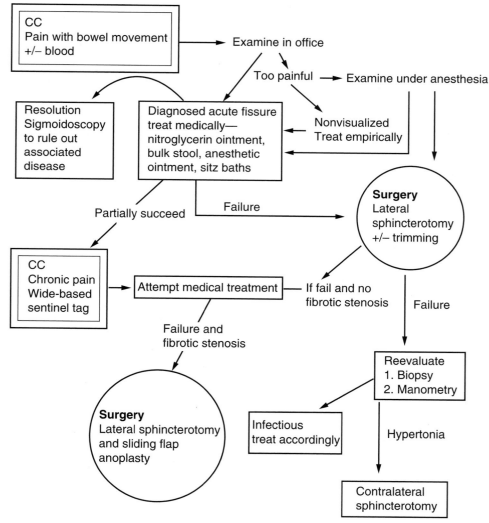

Figure 3-1
Algorithm summarizing treatment of anal fissures.

associated with shallow ulcers with or without sentinel tags, both posterior and anterior midline, never going cephalad to the dentate line.

Idiopathic AIDS/HIV-related ulcers, are usually cephalad to the dentate line, broad-based, deeply erosive, transgressing normal sphincter planes with mucosal bridging, occasionally burrowing into the external sphincter with a patulous anus, usually in patients with advanced AIDS (CD4 counts of less than 200 cells/mm^3). Occasionally, they cause severe bleeding, eroding the inferior rectal artery. Treatment generally involves bulking agents, sitz baths, and local ointments. Suppositories are of minimal use. Steroid injections may be used.

■ SUMMARY

Figure 3-1 shows a treatment algorithm for anal fissures.

1. Medical history is important, especially if there is pain with and after defecating.
2. Examination to rule out HIV infection or neoplasm should be done very gently.
3. Conservative medical treatment consists of bulking agents, sitz baths, local anesthetic, and buffered hydrocortisone creams.
4. Surgical treatment of fissures with hypertonic sphincter involves sphincterotomy with or without debridement of ulcer or biopsy and culture of ulcer.
5. If fissures are HIV-related, provide appropriate medical therapy, with possible sliding flap anoplasty.
6. If sphincter tone is low, perform a sliding flap anoplasty.

Suggested Readings

Abcarian H: Lateral internal sphincterotomy: A new technique for treatment of chronic fissure-in-ano. Surg Clin North Am 1975;55:143–50.

Brisinda G, Maria G, Bentivoglio AR, et al: A comparison of injections of botulinum toxin and topical nitroglycerin ointment for the treatment of chronic anal fissure. N Engl J Med 1999;341:65–69.

Coller JA, Karulf RE: Anal fissure. In Fazio VW (Ed.). Current Therapy of Colon and Rectal Surgery. Philadelphia, BC Decker, 1989, pp 15–19.

Eisenhammer S: The evaluation of the internal anal sphincterotomy operation with special reference to anal fissure. Surg Gynecol Obstet 1959;109:583–590.

Fleshner P: Anal fissure in Crohn's disease. Semin Colon Rectal Surg 1997;8(1):36–39.

Gordon PH. Fissure in ano. In Gordon PH, Nivatvongs S (Eds.). Principles and Practice of Surgery of the Colon, Rectum and Anus. St. Louis, Quality Medical Publishers, 1992, pp 199–219.

Gorfine S: Treatment of benign anal disease with topical nitroglycerin. Dis Colon Rectum 1995;48:453–456.

Jensen SI, Lund R, Nielson OV, Tange G: Lateral subcutaneous sphincterotomy vs. dilatation. BMJ 1984;289:528–530.

Jost WH, Schimrigk K: Use of botulinum toxin in anal fissure. Dis Colon Rectum 1993;36:974.

Knight JS, Birks M, Farouk R: Topical diltiazem ointment in the treatment of chronic anal fissure. Br J Surg 2001;88:553–556.

Lewis TH, Corman ML, Prager ED, Robertson WG: Long-term results of open and closed sphincterotomy for anal fissure. Dis Colon Rectum 1988;31:368–371.

Lund JN, Scholefield JH: A randomised, prospective, double-blind, placebo controlled trial of glyceryl trinitrate ointment in treatment of anal fissure. Lancet 1997;349:11–14.

Nelson R: Meta-analysis of operative techniques for fissure in ano. Dis Colon Rectum 1999;42:1424–1428.

Nyam PC, Wilson RG, Stewart KJ, et al: Island advancement flaps in the management of anal fissures. Br J Surg 1995;82:326–328.

Rosen L, Abel M, et al: Practice parameters for management of anal fissure. Standard Task Force of American Society CRS. Dis Colon Rectum 1992;15:206–208.

Sharp FR: Patient selection and treatment modalities for chronic anal fissure. Am J Surg 1996;171:512–515.

Shouten WR, Briel JW, Auwerda SS, Boerma MO: Anal fissure: New concepts in pathogenesis and treatment. Scand J Gastroenterol Suppl 1996;218(Suppl):78–81.

Viamonte M, Dailey T, Gottesman L: Anorectal surgery in HIV positive patient. Dis Colon Rectum 1991;34:299–304.

Watson SJ, Kamm MA, Nicholls RJ, Phillips RK: Topical glyceryl trinitrate in treatment of chronic anal fissure. Br J Surg 1996;83:771–775.

Wexner SD, Smithy WB, Milton J, et al: The surgical management of anal rectal disease in AIDS. Dis Colon Rectum 1986;29:19–23.

4

ANORECTAL ABSCESS

Ravi P. Kiran, MBBS, MS, FRCS (Eng), FRCS (Glas)

Victor W. Fazio, MB, MS, MD (Hon), FRACS, FRACS (Hon), FACS, FRCS, FRCS (Ed)

Abscesses in the anorectal region occur in all age groups and are a common distressing problem. Predisposing factors include diabetes, Crohn's disease, previous perianal surgery, and impairment of immunity, as occurs in human immunodeficiency virus (HIV) infection. The majority of abscesses, however, occur spontaneously in healthy individuals. Diagnosis is usually established by clinical examination, and as with abscesses elsewhere in the body, adequate drainage is the treatment of choice. Drainage results in healing in more than half of cases, and persistence or recurrence is due to inadequate drainage or the presence of predisposing factors such as systemic disorders or the development of fistula in ano.

Based on a study of patients treated for anorectal abscesses at the Cook County Hospital and followed for a 35-month period, Read and Abcarian reported in 1979 that the peak incidence was in the third decade, with males being affected 1.76 times more frequently than females. The most common anatomic location of the abscess in this series was perianal, which occurred in 42% of patients, followed by ischiorectal in 20% and supralevator in 7%. An anal fistula could be demonstrated in 34% of patients. A subsequent report from the hospital in 1984 confirmed a similar relative frequency of anorectal abscesses (42.7% perianal, 22.7% ischiorectal, 21.4% intersphincteric, and 7.3% supralevator). Intersphincteric and supralevator abscesses had a higher incidence of fistulas identified at the time of abscess drainage. Other studies also found the perianal variety to be the most common type of anorectal abscess and the intersphincteric the most commonly associated with a fistula in ano.

A brief knowledge of the anatomy of the spaces surrounding the anorectum helps in the understanding of the etiology, pathways of spread of infection, and clinical presentation, all of which have a bearing on the management of anorectal abscesses.

■ SURGICAL ANATOMY

The perianal space surrounds the anus and becomes continuous with the fat of the buttocks. The intersphincteric space separates the external and internal sphincter muscles, is continuous with the perianal space, and extends superiorly into the rectal wall. Anal glands are found in the intersphincteric plane, traverse the internal sphincter, and empty into the anal crypts in the anal canal at the level of the dentate line (Fig. 4-1). Lateral to the anus is the ischiorectal space, which is bounded superiorly by the levators, medially by the external sphincter, laterally by the ischial tuberosity, and inferiorly by the transverse perineal septum. The two ischiorectal fossae are connected posteriorly by the deep postanal space between the levators and the anococcygeal ligament. The supralevator space lies superior to the levator ani on either side of the rectum.

■ ETIOLOGY

The most widely accepted theory of etiology of perineal abcess is the cryptoglandular theory, which postulates that sepsis originates in the anal crypts located at the dentate line. The crypts extend into the surrounding sphincter muscles, and hence, when there is infection, sepsis may extend to a variable extent into these muscles and track along lines of least resistance. The findings of one study in the United Kingdom suggest that patients with fistula in ano, in addition to an abscess, are more likely to have gut aerobes (predominantly *Escherichia coli* or gut-specific anaerobes like *Bacteroides fragili*) isolated from the pus than those without fistulas.

■ NATURAL HISTORY OF THE DISEASE AND PATHWAYS OF SPREAD

As infection of anal glands is the primary event for most anorectal abscesses, the intersphincteric plane is involved first, leading to an intersphincteric abscess. Spread of infection in a downward direction in this plane leads to presentation as a perianal abscess. When pus penetrates the external sphincter below the puborectalis and expands into the ischiorectal fossa, it may point further laterally as an ischiorectal abscess. From here, pus may track into the postanal space and into the opposite ischiorectal space, leading to the formation of a horseshoe abscess. Upward extension of an intersphincteric abscess results in a supralevator abscess. Abscesses may enlarge and burst spontaneously in the perianal or ischiorectal area or into the rectum. Once drained, healing occurs most of the time but occasionally a persistent fistula may develop. This may in turn lead to recurrence of the abscess.

■ CLINICAL FEATURES

The four cardinal clinical signs of inflammation, described by Celsus as rubor (redness), calor (warmth), dolor (pain), and tumor (swelling), and the additional sign of functio laesa (difficulty in sitting down and painful defecation) are usually seen. Patients sometimes present with a partially burst abscess and persistent residual sepsis, and examination may reveal induration. The findings

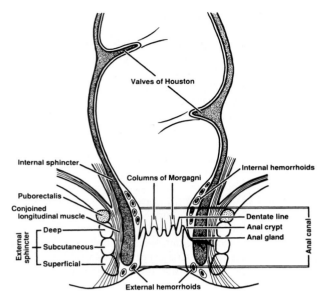

Figure 4-1
Anatomy of the anal canal. (From Gordon PH: The anorectum: Anatomic and physiologic considerations in health and disease. Gastroenterol Clin North Am 1987;16:2.)

on physical examination depend on the location of the abscess and associated disease.

Perianal Abscess

Perianal abscess accounts for the majority of abscesses in the anorectal region and is seen in 40 to 45% of these patients. Patients present with perianal pain, swelling, and fever. Examination reveals an erythematous, tender swelling adjacent to the external opening, and varying amounts of induration, cellulitis, and fluctuation. Rectal examination usually does not demonstrate any fluctuation or tenderness above the dentate line. In some patients only tenderness may be demonstrated, and fluctuation or swelling may be absent.

Ischiorectal Abscess

Ischiorectal abscess presents further laterally than a perianal abscess in the region of the ischiorectal fossa, which is bounded laterally by the ischial tuberosity. As there is greater room for the abscess to expand in the area occupied by the ischiorectal pad of fat and surrounding fibroareolar tissue, it may present as a diffuse swelling in the gluteal region. The abscess may extend posteriorly to communicate with the opposite ischiorectal fossa, thus forming a horseshoe abscess. The deep anterior anal space may also be involved.

Intersphincteric Abscess

The relative incidence of this variety of anorectal abscess is 2 to 5%. Intersphincteric abscesses were first described by Eisenhammer and subsequently divided into high and low types. Symptoms and signs are similar to those for other anorectal abscesses, but findings are not as prominent. Patients complain of dull anal or rectal pain and may occasionally present with a high temperature. A sense of

fullness in the rectum and painful defecation may be present. Mucous discharge from the anus may also occur. There are usually no external findings but on rectal examination exquisite tenderness and swelling may be present in the region of the abscess. Adequate examination may be precluded by patient discomfort. Intersphincteric abscesses are most commonly associated with fistulas and are also most likely to recur.

Supralevator Abscess

This variety of anorectal abscess is uncommon, with incidence ranging from 2.5 to 9.1% in different studies. A supralevator abscess results from the upward spread of infection from a low intermuscular abscess above the level of the puborectalis muscle secondary to an infected anal crypt gland or from the downward spread of infection from diverticulitis or pelvic inflammatory disease. Presentation is similar to an intersphincteric abscess, and diagnosis is difficult because of the absence of significant local findings. Symptoms may be in the form of a dull aching rectal pain accompanied by fever with chills. Urinary symptoms may be present due to local pressure effects. Digital rectal examination may suggest the presence of an abscess or diffuse anorectal fullness. Imaging usually plays an important role in the diagnosis of this variety of abscess.

Postanal Abscess

Postanal abscess involves the postanal space, which is bounded by the levators superiorly and the external sphincter inferiorly. The postanal space communicates with the ischiorectal fossa bilaterally; thus, spread of infection usually results in a horseshoe abscess.

Submucous Abscess

These high intermuscular abscesses may present after rupture into the rectum. A symptom may be a dull ache with sense of fullness in the rectum. The only finding may be a tender, smooth submucosal swelling.

■ DIAGNOSIS

Diagnosis of anorectal abscesses is based on clinical findings in the majority of instances. Patients usually present with a combination of symptoms, including perianal pain, swelling, discharge, fever, and painful defecation. There may be a previous history of anorectal abscess or history of absence of response to antibiotics. Clinical examination may reveal a fluctuant swelling, induration, or exquisite tenderness in the region of the abscess. Aspiration with a wide-bore needle may be needed to confirm the diagnosis. Sigmoidoscopy helps to rule out Crohn's disease and to identify the internal opening of a fistula. It is also useful in ruling out other conditions that predispose to anorectal abscess such as HIV infection and carcinoma. Imaging modalities including intrarectal ultrasound, computed tomography (CT), and magnetic resonance imaging (MRI) have been reported to be useful adjuncts in diagnosis, especially for deep or complex anorectal abscesses.

Differential diagnosis of anorectal abscesses includes hidradenitis suppurativa, pilonidal abscess, tuberculosis, and actinomycosis.

■ TREATMENT

Anorectal abscesses should be drained before the development of fluctuance. The traditional method of treatment involves adequate drainage by deroofing, using a cruciate incision followed by loose packing of the abscess cavity. Because the acidic medium of pus reduces the effectiveness of local anesthetic agents, general anesthesia may be required for adequate drainage in some cases. An alternate procedure that is particularly useful in the office setting is the placement of a catheter into the abscess after a small incision at the site of maximal pointing. This approach obviates the need for an extensive skin incision and hence can be done under local anesthesia. Satisfactory results following drainage of anorectal abscesses by a de Pezzer catheter were reported by Isbister in 1987 and by means of a mushroom catheter by Beck and associates in 1988. Catheter drainage is safe, convenient, and well tolerated by patients and compares favorably with the more traditional method of treating anorectal abscesses.

Perianal abscesses are managed by incision and drainage combined with a primary fistulotomy if a fistula is identified. A cruciate incision is made over the site of pointing and the skin edges trimmed in order to prevent premature closure of the skin, which results in recurrence. The resulting cavity is either loosely packed with iodoform gauze or alternatively drained with a 10F to 16F mushroom or de Pezzer catheter. Patients are advised to take frequent sitz baths and change dressings regularly, and are followed up in the office. If a drain is placed, it is removed when the cavity shows signs of healing.

Ischiorectal abscesses are managed in the same way as perianal abscesses. Concomitant involvement of the deep anterior or posterior anal spaces and horseshoe abscesses is managed by additional incisions. Deep anterior or posterior anal space abscesses are managed by midline fistulotomy in men, but in women a staged fistulotomy is effected by the placement of a seton in order to minimize separation of sphincter muscles. Horseshoe abscesses are managed by drainage of the postanal space with bilateral counterincisions in the ischiorectal fossae.

Intersphincteric abscesses are treated by an internal sphincterotomy, which unroofs the abscess, permitting drainage. The mucosa at the site may need to be sutured to establish hemostasis.

The cause of a supralevator abscess must be identified because optimal management depends upon knowing the source of infection. Supralevator abscesses originating from cephalad spread of infection from perianal and ischiorectal abscesses are drained by means of an initial internal sphincterotomy exposing the abscess cavity, which may in turn be drained into the rectum. Extensive abscesses and those originating from a pelvic source, such as diverticulitis or inflammatory bowel disease, may need to be drained through the rectum or ischiorectal fossa or by CT-guided transabdominal drainage. Persistent and complex supralevator abscesses may sometimes respond only to proximal diversion of the fecal stream by means of a colostomy or ileostomy, especially in patients with inflammatory bowel disease.

Submucosal abscess is managed by drainage into the rectum.

Role of Antibiotics and Biopsy

Antibiotic cover is not routinely indicated during drainage of anorectal abscesses in healthy individuals. Immunocompromised individuals and diabetics who are at high risk for spread of infection and sepsis and those with cardiac prostheses require perioperative broad-spectrum antibiotics. The need for extensive débridement at the time of drainage and the presence of residual surrounding cellulitis are also indications for antibiotic cover. Culture of pus and biopsy of the cavity wall are performed for persistent sepsis or recurrence of abscess despite adequate initial treatment. Biopsy may also be indicated at the time of initial drainage of abscess if Crohn's disease or neoplasia must be ruled out.

Postoperative Care

Following drainage of pus, patients are managed by regular dressings and sitz baths. Laxatives help prevent constipation and reduce the effort and pain of defecation. If recurrence or fistula develops, examination under anesthesia and treatment of the abscess or fistulotomy is indicated.

Complications

Urinary retention is a common complication after operations for benign anorectal conditions including abscesses. Severe disease, older age group, and use of perioperative fluids were identified as risk factors in a study at the Mayo Clinic.

■ RECURRENCE AND THE DEVELOPMENT OF FISTULA IN ANO

Hamalainen and Sainio followed patients who underwent drainage of anorectal abscesses over a period of 99 months and found that 37% developed a fistula and 10% developed a recurrent abscess. The study in Cook County Hospital referred to earlier in this chapter found that patients who underwent only abscess drainage had a recurrence rate of 3.7%, but those who had a simultaneous fistulotomy with drainage had a lower recurrence rate of 1.8% during a mean follow-up period of 36 months. Chrabot and colleagues studied anorectal abscesses prospectively and noted that causes for recurrence included insufficient prior treatment (68%), wrong diagnosis (hidradenitis suppurativa), and missed components. Vasilevsky and Gordon reported that 11% of patients with perianal or ischiorectal abscesses developed recurrent abscess and 37% developed persistent fistula in ano after isolated drainage of anorectal abscesses. They advocated the policy of selective secondary fistulotomy based on these results because more than half of all patients with anorectal abscesses are cured by simple drainage of the abscess. Schouten and van Vroonhoven compared primary fistulotomy with drainage alone for perianal abscesses in a randomized controlled trial and reported a similar combined persistence or recurrence rate (40.6%) after isolated abscess drainage over a median follow-up period of 42.5 months. Recurrence was lower but disturbances of anal function were higher in the fistulectomy group than in the isolated drainage group. The authors also advocate reserving fistulectomy as a second procedure in order to obviate the risk of anal functional disturbances in the remaining 60% of patients. In contrast, other studies recommend primary fistulotomy at the time of drainage of perianal abscesses as the preferable treatment to reduce persistent fistulas, because there was no added risk to fecal incontinence in their series.

Suggested Readings

Abcarian H: Acute suppurations of the anorectum. Surg Annu 1976;8:305–333.

Beck DE, Fazio VW, Lavery IC, et al: Catheter drainage of ischiorectal abscesses. South Med J 1988;81:444–446.

Cataldo PA, Senagore A, Luchtefeld MA: Intrarectal ultrasound in the evaluation of perirectal abscesses. Dis Colon Rectum 1993; 36:554–558.

Chrabot CM, Prasad ML, Abcarian H: Recurrent anorectal abscesses. Dis Colon Rectum 1983;26:105–108.

Corman ML: Colon and Rectal Surgery, 2nd ed. Philadelphia, JB Lippincott, 1989, pp 128–131.

Eykyn SJ, Grace RH: The relevance of microbiology in the management of anorectal sepsis. Ann R Coll Surg Engl 1986;68:237–239.

Goligher JC: Surgery of the Anus, Rectum and Colon, 5th ed. London, Balliere Tindall, 1984, p 171.

Hamalainen KP, Sainio AP: Incidence of fistulas after drainage of acute anorectal abscesses. Dis Colon Rectum 1998;41:1357–1361.

Hanley PH: Anorectal supralevator abscess: Fistula in ano. Surg Gynecol Obstet 1979;148:899–904.

Ho YH, Tan M, Chui CH, et al: Randomized controlled trial of primary fistulotomy with drainage alone for perianal abscesses. Dis Colon Rectum 1997;40:1435–1438.

Isbister WH: A simple method for the management of anorectal abscess. Aust NZ J Surg 1987;57:771–774.

Maruyama R, Noguchi T, Takano M, et al: Usefulness of magnetic resonance imaging for diagnosing deep anorectal abscesses. Dis Colon Rectum 2000;43(10 suppl):S2–S5.

McElwain JW, Maclean MD, Alexander RM, et al: Experience with primary fistulectomy for anorectal abscess: A report of 1000 cases. Dis Colon Rectum 1975;18:646–649.

Ramanujam PS, Prasad ML, Abcarian H, Tan AB: Perianal abscesses and fistulas: A study of 1023 patients. Dis Colon Rectum 1984; 27:593–597.

Read DR, Abcarian H: A prospective study of 474 patients with anorectal abscess. Dis Colon Rectum 1979;22:566–568.

Schouten WR, van Vroonhoven TJ: Treatment of anorectal abscess with or without primary fistulectomy. Results of a prospective randomized trial. Dis Colon Rectum 1991;34:60–63.

Vasilevsky CA, Gordon PH: The incidence of recurrent abscesses or fistula-in-ano following anorectal suppuration. Dis Colon Rectum 1984;27:126–130.

Zaheer S, Reilly WT, Pemberton JH, Ilstrup D: Urinary retention after operations for benign anorectal diseases. Dis Colon Rectum 1998;41:696–704.

5

ANAL FISTULA

Paul Belliveau, MD, CM, FRCSC, FACS, FICS

Fistula in ano is a common disease that in most circumstances lends itself to surgical treatment with gratifying results. It is widely held that anal gland infection is the principal cause of anal fistulas, whereas other causes, such as inflammatory bowel disease, trauma, fungal or mycobacterial infections, and neoplasm, account for unusual presentations. Symptoms should always guide the need for intervention in that patients without pain, discharge, bleeding, or recurrent abscesses should be observed rather than subjected to surgery. When it is indicated, the surgical management of anal fistulas is centered around an understanding of the anatomy of the anorectal sphincter mechanism and a complete exploration of the avenues of spread of sepsis according to the classification proposed by Parks (Table 5-1).

■ THERAPEUTIC ALTERNATIVES

Medical Therapy
In general, antibiotics have little to offer in the early management of anal fistulas. However, they may be of benefit in occasional cases such as prolonged healing of a well-drained abscess, or following a satisfactory surgical approach. Metronidazole may be used in a dose of 250 mg three times a day for 10 days. Immunosuppressed or diabetic patients should be given adjuvant antibiotics at the time of intervention and for several days thereafter.

Surgical Therapy
There are several surgical options for the treatment of anal fistulas, and the best choice is determined by the anatomy of the fistula. Fistulotomy with opening and unroofing of

the fibrous portion of the tract and fistulectomy with excision of the tract are two options for relatively low transsphincteric tracks. Excision should be used when an obliterated tract is encountered or when a definite cord, lying superficially, is palpated. This procedure should always be combined with excision of the internal opening and division of the distal fibers of the internal sphincter in order to adequately drain the intersphincteric plane. In most cases a form of unroofing with or without marsupialization of the fistula is applicable, with gentle curettage of the base of the wound. A seton may be used either as a drain to allow the track to mature or epithelialize, or as a way of slowly cutting through muscle while preventing separation of the ends. Cutting setons are silk, to promote localized fibrosis in the muscle fiber. Drainage setons are silicone, to allow satisfactory drainage while limiting the degree of reaction and fibrosis. When the silicone thread (small vessel loop or thin silicone tubing) is removed, the muscle enclosed within may not have to be divided to obtain a good result.

Another alternative is to excise the fibrous lining of the internal opening and the external tract, without division of external sphincter muscle, to reapproximate the internal sphincter muscle fibers and to cover the repair with a mucosal advancement flap or an island flap anoplasty. This technique must be accompanied by adequate external drainage with wide saucerization.

Drainage of acute abscesses with primary anal fistulotomy should be reserved for cases in which an internal opening is easily identified and in which there is not a complex high fistula. In these latter cases, drainage alone is preferable, with close observation for the delineation of the fistula tract.

■ PREFERRED APPROACH

Patient Selection
Careful surgical intervention offers patients with anal fistulas relief of discomfort and an end to soiling from perianal discharge. Asymptomatic fistulas are best left alone unless the fear of a recurrent abscess by the patient dictates a more radical approach. Patients should be made aware of the possibility of a temporary reduction in the control of flatus that can result from division of part of the internal sphincter and some of the external sphincter. In more complex fistulas cases an open discussion with the patient often brings out his or her fears regarding incontinence. The option of a conservative surgical approach with muscle preservation is reassuring. The problem of recurrent fistulas can be dealt with surgically; recurrences usually indicate failure to recognize or adequately deal with the internal opening. Occasionally a second, separate fistula develops. Suspect such patients of having Crohn's disease. Patients with a history of inflammatory bowel disease are approached with caution. Although most low anal fistulas in these patients will heal with standard treatment, complex fistulas or extrasphincteric fistulas may best be treated with antibiotics or by a technique that allows the tract to be brought closer to the anal orifice, thus making

Table 5-1 Types of Anal Fistula in 249 Cases*		
FISTULA	NO. OF CASES	PERCENTAGE
Intersphincteric	149	60
Trans-sphincteric	70	28
Low	46	
High	24	
Suprasphincteric	25	10
Extrasphincteric	5	2

*Personal series.

the care of the fistula by the patient much easier than if it were situated several centimeters onto the buttock.

Patients with immunodeficient states such as neutropenia, myeloproliferative diseases, transplants, leukemia, and acquired immune deficiency syndrome (AIDS) deserve special comment. In these circumstances perianal sepsis may indicate a worsening of their general disease state, and drainage procedures are indicated even though very little true pus can be found. Poor healing of tissue is the rule, and antibiotic coverage for both aerobes and anaerobes is warranted for several days. Depending on the healing rate of the patient, fistulotomy may be performed if symptoms are incapacitating. However, in most cases it is preferable to accept minor symptoms and adopt a conservative approach, with sitz baths and possibly long-term antibiotics, because poor healing and ulceration of the wound may lead to local and systemic sepsis.

Timing of Surgery

Once the diagnosis of an anal fistula is made, the patient can be offered surgery. If the patient presents with an abscess, it is adequately drained. Then a period of at least 6 weeks should be allowed to pass to determine if a fistula will become evident by persistent or recurrent symptoms. If symptoms suggest this is the case, and examination in the office reveals an external opening, an examination under anesthesia is scheduled to confirm the diagnosis and drain the fistula by laying it open (if it is superficial) or by seton (if it is deep). Adequate drainage allows the surrounding edema, cellulitis, and discomfort to disappear. The majority of cases can be treated electively, with many low fistulas treated in an outpatient setting.

Preoperative Preparation

The routine use of preoperative fistulography to determine the course of the tract is not warranted, because careful probing under anesthesia will usually show the track and its internal opening. Fistulography is used in rare cases when there may be an extrasphincteric fistula from an intra-abdominal source such as inflammatory bowel disease (Crohn's disease affecting the small bowel or colon, diverticulitis with perforation and abscess, or postoperative anastomotic leaks) or when attempts to localize the internal opening by probing or injecting are unsuccessful. Magnetic resonance imaging (MRI) or endorectal ultrasound has also been used in this situation. MRI uses a specially designed endoanal coil applicable to patients with anorectal sepsis. In one study, this method was reported to correctly identify the site of the internal opening of the fistula in 80% of cases. It also demonstrated disease that had been unsuspected at surgery.

Most fistula surgery can be performed as day surgery in a standard operating room. Routine hematologic, biochemical, and radiologic investigations are no longer indicated for general or regional anesthesia, except for an electrocardiogram in patients over 40 years of age. The patient fasts overnight and a small enema may be prescribed on the morning of the planned operation. Because most wounds are left open, the enema is not mandatory. More complex cases may require a short

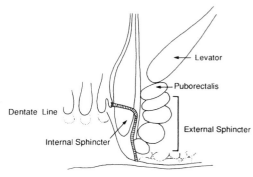

Figure 5-1
Intersphincteric fistula.

hospitalization. The area is disinfected topically with povidone-iodine or chlorhexidine solution, and shaving is rarely necessary. The patient is best positioned prone on gel rolls to support the chest and pelvis, with generous padding of pressure points, or in the lithotomy position, with avoidance of pressure in the popliteal fossa or on the feet. Bladder catheters are unnecessary.

Choice of Procedure

Once muscle relaxation has been achieved by regional or general anesthesia, the external opening is probed with a gently curved stylet. A finger in the anus allows control of the probe and gives an appreciation of its position relative to the anus. False passages must be avoided. A Pratt's bivalve speculum is inserted and the area of the dentate line is inspected for purulent discharge or for a dimple indicating the internal opening. Defining the trajectory of the fistula in relation to the external sphincter establishes the type according to the following classification:

1. Intersphincteric fistula (Fig. 5-1)
2. Trans-sphincteric (low or high) fistula (Fig. 5-2)
3. Suprasphincteric fistula (with or without supralevator abscess) (Fig. 5-3)
4. Extrasphincteric fistula (with an internal opening above the level of the levators) (Fig. 5-4)

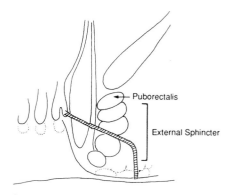

Figure 5-2
Trans-sphincteric fistula.

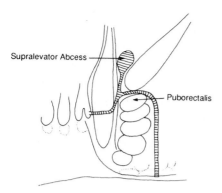

Figure 5-3
Suprasphincteric fistula.

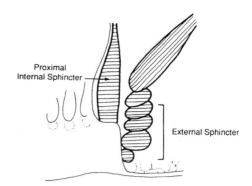

Figure 5-5
Intersphincteric fistulotomy.

Intersphincteric Fistula

Typically the external opening is close to the anal verge. The probe will pass in a direction parallel to the longitudinal axis of the anal canal upward to enter the intersphincteric plane and exit at the dentate line in the base of a crypt (see Fig. 5-1). Occasionally the tract will curve before it reaches the internal opening, or indeed it may cross the midline to the contralateral side (horseshoe). The area is then infiltrated with bupivacaine 0.25% with 1:200,000 epinephrine for postoperative analgesia and reduction of bleeding. The anoderm and segment of internal sphincter overlying the probe are sharply incised (Fig. 5-5). It is usually not necessary to excise the edges, as they will be marsupialized to the edge of the fibrous tract using 3-0 chromic catgut suture. The base of the tract is curetted of granulation tissue and any residual anal gland in that area. Suspicious firm tissue should be biopsied; occasional carcinomas have been diagnosed at the time of fistulotomy in very long-standing fistulas. If the tract does not admit the probe, it is wise to excise this tract using a circular local dissection, to then apply traction on the fibrosed cord, and to identify the internal opening, which can then be opened by incising the distal portion of the

internal sphincter. Upward proximal intermuscular extensions should be unroofed at the same sitting and the edges marsupialized. In these cases, the distal portion of the internal sphincter should also be divided to provide adequate drainage.

Trans-sphincteric Fistula

Low trans-sphincteric fistulas can be recognized initially by an external opening usually situated more than 2 cm from the anal verge and with a trajectory of the probe that is at an angle to the long axis of the anal canal (see Fig. 5-2). The tissues are infiltrated with the local anesthetic supplement (bupivacaine), and the Pratt bivalve retractor is positioned to expose the area of the dentate line near the tract of the fistula. Anterior fistulas commonly enter in a radial fashion, whereas more posterior fistulas enter in a curved tract leading to the posterior midline. If the probe does not pass readily into the internal opening, injection of the track with hydrogen peroxide solution with one drop of methylene blue may identify the internal opening. Once the tract has been identified, the anoderm and internal sphincter are divided just distal to the internal opening, and the skin overlying the external sphincter is divided to expose the external sphincter. The subcutaneous portion can be divided, and the small amount of superficial external sphincter overlying the probe can be divided to expose the tract, which is laid open (Fig. 5-6).

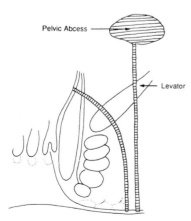

Figure 5-4
Extrasphincteric fistula.

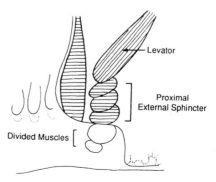

Figure 5-6
Trans-sphincteric fistulotomy.

Granulation tissue is curetted, and the skin is marsupialized to the edges of the open fibrous tract with running absorbable sutures. A moist gauze is placed over the wound, but no packing is introduced into the anal canal.

When the tract appears to cross a more significant portion of the external sphincter, a high trans-sphincteric fistula must be suspected. Manometric studies have shown that division of the external sphincter in these cases reduces anal pressures and may be associated with partial incontinence. Hence, it is better to incise the anoderm and internal sphincter just distal to the internal opening and to incise the skin leading to the external opening. The external tract is then opened to the point at which it crosses the external sphincter and curetted as much as possible. The remaining mass of external sphincter is not divided but instead is loosely surrounded with a silicone band (single or double, 2-mm loop [Surg-i-Loop]) passed with the probe through the residual deep tract (Fig. 5-7). This allows identification of the tract and encourages ongoing drainage of the deep portion of the fistula. The superficial and external parts of the open wound are marsupialized to the edges of the deep tract, and the seton is left free. The seton in these cases is not used as a cutting seton, as the muscle enclosed is not divided when the seton is removed 6 to 8 weeks later. A success rate of 75% can be expected. This procedure is applicable in most cases of trans-sphincteric fistula in female patients, in whom muscle preservation to maintain adequate continence is important. When infralevator abscesses are found, drainage and curettage through the external wound are adequate. In recurrent or improperly resolving tracts, it is possible to use a technique of excision of part of the internal tract and closure with a flap of muscle and musosa in two layers, advanced locally to allow coverage. Adequate external drainage and curettage of the tract are essential.

Suprasphincteric Fistula

The diagnosis and recognition of these fistulas are often difficult. Induration felt above the levators and probing of a deep tract often leading to the deep postanal space should alert the surgeon to this complex fistula. The search for the internal opening should concentrate in the posterior midline, where it will most often be found leading to the deep cavity in the region of the coccyx (see Fig. 5-3). Horseshoe patterns of external tracts are often present, and bilateral external openings are not unusual. If the internal opening cannot be found, methylene blue peroxide solution may prove helpful. Occasionally all efforts to locate the intemal opening fail, and probing the external tract leads deeply above the dentate line; in these circumstances, it is wiser to obtain adequate drainage of the cavity and not to create an artificial intra-anal opening, which may be obliterated at the time of surgery. Recurrent symptoms may indicate reappearance of the internal communication. Often, the internal opening in the posterior midline is found. The anoderm and internal sphincter are then divided, and the cutaneous incision is carried over the area of the anococcygeal raphe. Using a blunt hemostat, the fibers of the raphe are split and the deep postanal space abscess or cavity, if present, is entered. The tract is seen communicating deep to the sphincter mechanism with the external opening, which has been opened until it is seen to cross the muscle and lead to the posterior cavity. The tract is curetted, and scrapings are sent to the pathology laboratory. A Silastic seton is then loosely tied around the external sphincter by passing through the exposed internal opening, and the anococcygeal raphe is split to expose the deep postanal abscess (Fig. 5-8). The seton drains the area and marks the depth of the tract, which can be better assesed when the anesthesia has worn off. The edges of the external tract are marsupialized to make a smaller wound and for hemostasis.

In dealing with recurrent fistulas of this type, anorectal manometry may help in determining the anal pressures at various levels and in documenting areas of deficiency that should be left intact for fear of worsening the state of continence. Using a technique of perfused catheters attached to a set of transducers, one can measure basal pressure at rest and voluntary contraction pressure. Since most of the voluntary contraction or squeeze pressure is expressed as the amplitude of the wave over baseline pressure levels measured at rest, this becomes a measure of the external sphincter function and contribution to the rise in pressure observed during a squeeze effort. The resulting reduction in pressure demonstrated in cases in which external sphincter muscle has been severed may account for anal soiling and certain degrees of incontinence.

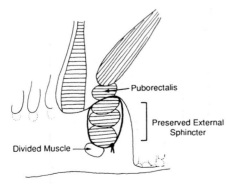

Figure 5-7
High trans-sphincteric fistulotomy with seton.

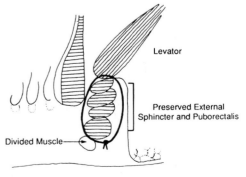

Figure 5-8
Suprasphincteric fistulotomy with seton.

Very complex fistulas and some recurrent fistulas may require a temporary loop sigmoid colostomy for fecal diversion when delicate intrarectal repairs with flaps or wide debridement are employed. These circumstances are rare, but may be more frequent in diabetic patients. Obtaining expert advice on these difficult cases would be prudent.

Extrasphincteric Fistula

These fistulas are caused by pelvic disease (appendiceal abscess, diverticulitis, Crohn's disease), by foreign body impalement in the lower rectum, or by external penetrating trauma to the perirectal tissues (see Fig. 5-4). In some cases, they may be iatrogenic. Typically, the external opening communicates with an opening in the rectum well above the dentate line, indeed at the level of the levator muscles. When there is no rectal communication, correction of the pelvic disease solves the pararectal problem. In patients in whom there is no pelvic disease and yet there is a high opening, the creation of a colostomy usually is indicated to control ongoing sepsis, as some of these fistulas will heal with diversion. Endorectal partial excision of the edges of the internal opening with primary closure using fine wire sutures and adequate curettage of the external tract has been successful without a sigmoid diverting colostomy. If this approach fails, however, a colostomy may be a helpful adjunct in management with another attempt at closing the internal opening. Occasionally, a retained foreign body, such as a piece of clothing pushed in by impalement on sharp objects, may explain continued purulent discharge despite otherwise adequate drainage. Removal of this material helps to accelerate healing.

■ POSTOPERATIVE COURSE

The flat dressing applied to all cases of fistulotomy should be removed the following day and hot sitz baths initiated three to four times a day for 15 to 20 minutes. Analgesia in the form of moderate-strength narcotics or nonsteroidal anti-inflammatory drugs may be used for the first 2 to 3 days combined with bulk laxatives twice daily. In hospitalized patients, intravenous fluids should be discontinued soon after surgery to reduce the incidence of urinary retention. This approach would apply for patients with complex, high fistulas in whom much dissection in the postanal space has taken place. Following discharge from the hospital, the patient is examined every 2 to 3 weeks to ensure proper healing by granulation tissue in a flat wound. Packing is not used, because it may delay healing and possibly lead to persistence of the fistula.

In cases in which a seton has been employed, the elastic properties of silicone allow the patient to be comfortable and reduce the local irritant effect, thus stimulating less granulation tissue within the tract itself. Ordinarily, discharge will continue but in decreasing amounts, as long as the seton is in place. The principle in the use of silicone is to convert the anal gland infection into a foreign body reaction, which in most cases will subside spontaneously once the seton is removed. In fact, after a period of 8 to 12

weeks, this type of seton is simply removed in the office without dividing any external sphincter muscle. The area is reassessed at one month, and in the majority of cases (75%) there is satisfactory healing without further need for intervention. In cases with ongoing drainage, a persistent internal opening can be suspected, and these patients are then examined under anesthesia. If an internal opening is found, excision of the fibrosed lining within the anal canal with primary suture transversely, with or without a mucosal-muscular flap, leads to further healing. Occasionally, when this technique fails, division of the distal fibrosed portion of the external sphincter may succeed in healing these difficult fistulas.

Postoperative surveillance in all cases is necessary to detect persistence of sepsis. In complex fistulas with deep abscesses, the addition of metronidazole in the initial 2 to 3 weeks may reduce the amount of discharge and possibly shorten the period of morbidity, although no controlled studies have been carried out on this treatment. Topical creams probably have no effect on healing and are not indicated in the care of these wounds. Proper hygiene with warm water baths definitely reduces pain and discomfort and soiling of the incisions. In general, complete healing of intersphincteric or low trans-sphincteric fistulas is observed at 6 weeks, whereas high trans-sphincteric and suprasphincteric fistulas require 12 to 14 weeks.

■ COMPLICATIONS AND SEQUELAE

Postoperative complications include bleeding, pyrexia, urinary retention, cellulitis, fecal impaction, partial fecal incontinence, and persistent discharge. Immediate problems that may be encountered following surgery are bleeding, fever, urinary retention, cellulitis, and fecal impaction. The incidence of bleeding from the operative site is reduced by marsupialization of the wound or by meticulous electrocautery at the time of surgery. Occasionally, brisk bleeding may occur the night of the surgery; it usually subsides with topical pressure. If this is not adequate, direct suture of the bleeding point, at the bedside, with the help of parenteral analgesia, controls the problem. Rarely, the patient may have to be returned to the operating suite to correct the problem using better lighting and muscle relaxants.

Fever is rarely seen following the opening of low anal fistulas. It may, however, be encountered for the first 2 to 3 days following drainage and curettage of high extensions into the infralevator, supralevator, or postrectal spaces. For temperatures higher than 38.5° C, blood cultures are indicated, and the other usual causes such as atelectasis and pneumonitis should be excluded. Antibiotics should be considered if the fever persists, if blood culture results are positive, or if progressive cellulitis is seen.

Urinary retention is infrequently seen in ambulatory patients, although in-hospital patients undergoing more extensive dissections may have a problem in approximately 5% of cases. These patients require brief catheterization of the bladder and analgesia. It has been proposed that stopping intravenous fluids and withholding oral intake until the patient has voided may reduce the incidence of this problem.

It is not unusual to see edema of the anorectal tissues following surgery as well as purulent exudate from the wound. Discoloration of the skin, progressive edema, and increasing pain are signs of cellulitis, which should be treated with broad-spectrum antibiotics. Clostridial cellulitis is extremely rare but devastating when it occurs and should be recognized quickly and treated aggressively with operative débridement and high-dose penicillin.

Fecal impaction is more common in elderly patients but may be troublesome in younger individuals as well. It is fortunately infrequent compared with its rate of incidence following hemorrhoidectomy. Use of bulk-forming agents and mild laxatives usually avoids the problem. Once impaction occurs, however, a gentle tap-water enema relieves the pressure caused by the fecal mass.

Partial fecal incontinence is reported to occur in 5 to 30% of patients. Incontinence develops as a consequence of sphincter division, performed to provide adequate drainage of the fistula tract. It has been shown manometrically that quadrants of decreased pressure correspond to zones of muscle division. When the external sphincter muscle was cut, lower resting pressure and lower voluntary contraction pressure were associated with a higher incidence of patients with impaired continence to flatus and liquid stool. Conversely, when efforts were made to preserve the external sphincter, with drainage of secondary tracts, both resting and voluntary contraction pressures were higher, and fewer patients had impaired control. The use of a seton to drain the area and mark the tract for proper identification of the level of the muscle affected is encouraged in high fistulas and in anterior trans-sphincteric fistulas in women. Drainage of the intersphincteric plane must always be accomplished, however, in order to obtain proper healing without necessarily dividing the enclosed external sphincter several weeks later. This technique also reduces the formation of a deep groove or keyhole deformity, which has been associated with minor degrees of mucous seepage through the anal canal.

Persistent drainage from the wound or scar usually indicates failure of the internal opening to close following otherwise adequate fistulotomy. The most common cause is to have missed the true primary opening while possibly creating one during probing of the external tract. Palpation in the posterior midline often identifies the fibrosis and pitting that is suggestive of the primary opening. With the patient under anesthesia the external tract should again be opened and curetted, and the internal opening may be freshened, closed, and covered with a mucosal-muscular flap. If the tract is posterior and is now surrounded by dense fibrosis, a complete laying open with curettage of the base of the tract (as long as this does not involve division of the puborectalis muscle) offers the best chance for cure. The muscles generally do not retract significantly, but a groove may often persist, and without the hemorrhoidal cushion, the patient should be warned of the possibility of partial incontinence, at least on a temporary basis.

■ OTHER OPTIONS

Advancement Flap Repair

This repair seeks to heal the fistula by healing the internal opening, thus preventing the egress of bacteria from the rectum. If the internal opening can be healed, the track will heal. The principles of the advancement flap repair are to operate when the fistula is well established and has no active extensions and no uncontrolled sepsis, and to repair in two layers.

Preoperative preparation includes an antegrade gut lavage, intravenous antibiotics and predrainage of the fistula for at least 6 weeks. The operation is performed with the patient in lithotomy for posterior internal openings and in the Kraske position for anterior openings. The internal opening is circumcised and the incision is extended for 1 cm on each side along the dentate line. The track is de-epithelialized and curetted, and muscular-mucosal flaps are raised 1 cm top and bottom. The defect in the muscle is closed with interrupted absorbable sutures and tested by saline injection through the external opening. The muscular-mucosal flaps are then closed over the muscle repair. If the external track is long, it is drained with a mushroom-tipped catheter.

Postoperatively, patients are maintained on antibiotics for 1 week and ice only by mouth for 2 days to limit bowel movements.

Fibrin glue may be used for fistulas with a straight tract without extensions or sepsis. Trans-, supra-, or extra-sphincteric fistulas are suitable, but a short track is better. After the track has been curetted, glue is injected through the track so that a bead is seen at the internal opening. A dressing is applied. This procedure can often be done in an outpatient setting.

■ PROS AND CONS OF TREATMENT

It should be remembered that the surgical approaches to the treatment of anal fistulas are based on alleviation of symptoms of pain, discharge, recurrent swelling, bleeding, and irritation. If a fistula is discovered incidentally, it should be pointed out to the patient but is best left alone if there are no referable symptoms. The majority of symptomatic fistulas respond satisfactorily to the previously outlined treatment principles that afford comfortable, dry anal skin with good fecal continence (Fig. 5-9).

■ OUTCOMES

Table 5-2 shows results of some recent series in which anal fistulas are being treated. Cutting setons clearly can cause a problem with impaired continence, and flap repairs have patchy results. Fibrin glue procedures have the highest recurrence rates.

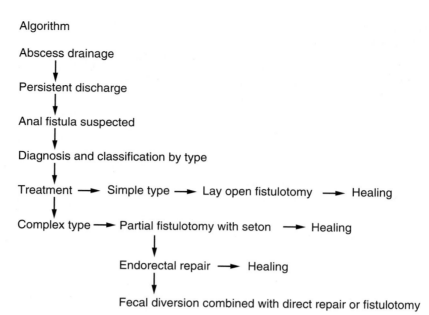

Figure 5-9
Algorithm for treatment of anal fistula.

Table 5-2 Outcome of Recent Series for Treatment of Anal Fistula

AUTHOR	METHOD	NO. OF PATIENTS	RECURRENCE	INCONTINENCE SOLID	INCONTINENCE LIQUID	FLATUS	SOILING
Hamalainen and Sainio (1997)	Cutting seton	35	6%	0		51%	51%
Garcia Olmo, Vazquez Aragon, and Lopez Fando (1994)	Cutting seton	12	0	0	0	33%	NS
Dziki and Bartos (1998)	Cutting seton	32	0	5%	9%	14%	24%
Aguilar, Plasencia, and Hardy Jr. (1985)	Advancement flap	151	2%	0	6	7	8
Hyman (1999)	Advancement flap	33	19%	0	0	0	0
Schouten, Zimmerman, and Briel (1999)	Advancement flap	44	25%	12%	ns	38%	38%
Jun and Choi (1999)	Anocutaneous flap	40	0	0	0	0	0
Robertson and Mangione (1998)	Anocutaneous flap	20	20%	0	0	5%	0
Park, Cintron, and Orsay (2000)	Fibrin glue	29	32%				
Cintron, Park, Orsay, et al. (1999)	Fibrin glue	26	19%				
Venkatesh and Ramanujam (1999)	Fibrin glue		40%				

Suggested Readings

Aguilar PS, Plasencia G, Hardy Jr TG, et al: Mucosal advancement flap in the treatment of anal fistula. Dis Colon Rectum 1985;28:496–498.

Belliveau P, Thomson IPS, Parks AG: Fistula-in ano: A manometric study. Dis Colon Rectum 1983;26:152–154.

Cintron JR, Park JJ, Orsay CP, et al: Repair of fistulas-in-ano using autologous fibrin tissue adhesive. Dis Colon Rectum 1999;42:607–613.

Del Pino A, Nelson RL, Abcarian H: Island flap anoplasty for treatment of transsphincteric fistula-in-ano. Dis Colon Rectum 1996;39:224–226.

deSouza NM, Hall AS, Puni R, et al: High resolution magnetic resonance imaging of the anal sphincter using a dedicated endoanal coil. Comparison of magnetic resonance imaging with surgical findings. Dis Colon Rectum 1996;39:926–934.

Dziki A, Bartos M: Seton treatment of anal fistula: Experience with a new modification. Eur J Surg 1998;164:543–548.

Fazio VW: Complex anal fistulae. Gastroenterol Clin North Am 1987;16:93–114.

Felt-Bersma RJ, van Baren R, Koorevaar M, et al: Unsuspected sphincter defects shown by anal endosonography after anorectal surgery. A prospective study. Dis Colon Rectum 1995;38:249–253.

Garcia Olmo D, Vazquez Aragon P, Lopez Fando J: Multiple setons in the treatment of high perianal fistula. Br J Surg 1994;81:136–137.

Hamalainen KP, Sainio AP: Cutting seton for anal fistulas: High risk of minor control defects. Dis Colon Rectum 1997;40:1443–1446.

Hyman N: Endoanal advancement flap repair for complex anorectal fistulas. Am J Surg 1999;178:337–340.

Jun SH, Choi GS: Anocutaneous advancement flap closure of high anal fistulas. Br J Surg 1999;86:490–492.

Lewis WG, Finan PJ, Holdsworth PJ, et al: Clinical results and manometric studies after rectal flap advancement for infra-levator transsphincteric fistula-in-ano. Int J Colorect Dis 1995;10:189–192.

Lunniss PJ, Barker PG, Sultan AH, et al: Magnetic resonance imaging of fistula-in-ano. Dis Colon Rectum 1994;37:708–718.

Park JJ, Cintron JR, Orsay CP, et al: Repair of chronic fistulae using commercial fibrin sealant. Arch Surg 2000;135:166–169.

Parks AG, Gordon PH, Hardcastle JD: A classification of fistula-in-ano. Br I Surg 1976;63:1–12.

Robertson WG, Mangione JS: Cutaneous advancement flap closure: Alternative method for treatment of complicated anal fistulas. Dis Colon Rectum 1998;41:884–886.

Schouten WR, Zimmerman DD, Briel JW: Transanal advancement flap repair of transsphincteric fistulas. Dis Colon Rectum 1999;42:1419–1422.

Venkatesh KS, Ramanujam P: Fibrin glue application in the treatment of recurrent anorectal fistulas. Dis Colon Rectum 1999;42:1136–1139.

Weisman RI, Orsay CP, Pearl RK, et al: The role of fistulography in fistula-in-ano. Dis Colon Rectum 1991;34:181–184.

6

RECTOVAGINAL FISTULA

Tracy Hull, MD

Fistulas from the anorectal region to the posterior vagina are traditionally termed *rectovaginal*. True rectovaginal fistulas are rare and typically result from inflammatory bowel disease, iatrogenic injury, or trauma. This chapter will deal with anovaginal or very low rectovaginal fistulas; however, the term *rectovaginal fistula* will be used.

■ PRESENTATION AND DIAGNOSIS

The initial problem in women with rectovaginal fistulas may be to verify the diagnosis. Women can present with classic symptoms such as the passage of air or stool per vagina and examination of the area may show nothing abnormal. Other symptoms include purulent drainage from the perineal area, recurring vaginitis, or a foul odor. When symptoms raise suspicion of a fistula with a "normal" anorectal examination, carefully instilling methylene blue into the rectum with a tampon in the vagina and leaving the patient for 15 minutes may demonstrate blue staining on the tampon when removed. Alternatively, an examination in the operating room may be needed to fully evaluate the patient. A narrow probe is used to explore any vaginal fold that cannot be smoothed out. Sometimes a faintly darker pink coloration or a slight pucker in the mucosa may be the only clues to the location of the fistula opening. It is usually easier to locate the fistula via the vaginal surface, but if this approach is unsuccessful, a careful examination of the anal surface may demonstrate an opening. If the fistula still cannot be found while in the operating room, the patient (in the lithotomy position) is placed in the Trendelenburg position and the vagina is filled with water. Then air is insufflated into the anorectum via a proctoscope or a bulb syringe while the surgeon looks for bubbles in the vagina.

Before treatment, there should be a thorough history and physical examination. The physical examination should include a thorough inspection of the anus, rectum, and vagina. The cause of the fistula can be important, as associated conditions sometimes influence treatment options. Table 6-1 lists causes of rectovaginal fistula. Important related issues include the pliability of the surrounding tissue, associated proctitis, exclusion of cancer, and state of the anal sphincters.

■ TREATMENT

Prior to repair all sepsis must be drained and local inflammation associated with the initial injury resolved. This may take up to 3 to 6 months after an injury (such as obstetric trauma). Fistulas associated with radiation may require initial fecal diversion for up to 12 months while the inflammation decreases.

Simple Fistulotomy

In a few select superficial fistulas, simple fistulotomy can be performed. Virtually no sphincter muscle must be involved for fistulotomy to be considered. However, this circumstance is rare and the possibility of dividing sphincter muscle or creating a groove in the anterior anal margin would discourage this form of treatment.

Transanal Approaches

Advancement Rectal Flap

When the sphincter muscle has not been otherwise injured (e.g., during a vaginal delivery) and the rectum is pliable, a common form of treatment involves a sliding advancement flap. Traditionally, the flap is raised primarily from the rectal lining. Patients are prepared with an antegrade bowel lavage and preoperative intravenous antibiotics. Anesthesia can be general, epidural, or spinal. After a Foley catheter is placed the patient is placed in prone jack-knife position and adequately padded. The anus, perineum, and vagina are prepared for surgery. To keep the perineum displayed, perianal traction sutures are circumferentially placed. (Some surgeons prefer the Lone Star retractor. A lighted retractor such as a Hill-Ferguson gives intra-anal exposure. A probe is passed through the fistula. A solution of 1:200,000 epinephrine is injected into the submucosal plane to assist in hemostasis and help raise the flap. Limited amounts are infiltrated to minimize ischemia. A curvilinear or "smiley face" flap is outlined, starting just distal to the fistula opening. The curved configuration decreases the occurrence of ischemia laterally. A flap consisting of mucosa, submucosa, and a few fibers of internal sphincter muscle is raised cephalad using cutting electrocautery. As the flap is raised, the probe is removed. Saline injection can be used to aid in the dissection. During the flap construction the wound is irrigated with a tetracycline-based fluid, and point electrocautery is used to maintain strict hemostasis. The flap is usually mobilized 4 to 5 cm cephalad. If there is a lot of scarring, starting the dissection laterally and working medially may help achieve the correct plane. When the flap is sufficiently mobilized, the fistula is cored out and the edges of the defect in the sphincter muscle are approximated with

---

Table 6-1 Causes of Rectovaginal Fistula

Obstetric injury
Inflammatory bowel disease (Crohn's disease)
Radiation injury
Infection (cryptoglandular, Bartholin's gland, tuberculosis, lymphogranuloma venereum)
Neoplasm—anal, rectal, vaginal, hematologic (leukemia)
Trauma—foreign body injury, surgical injury (vaginal and anorectal)
Congenital

absorbable suture such as 2-0 polyglycolic suture. Usually this is accomplished in layers (Fig. 6-1). The vaginal side is left open. Next, the apex of the flap containing the fistula opening is trimmed, and the flap is advanced down and sutured to the distal cut surface of the anoderm without tension using 3-0 polyglycolic suture (Fig. 6-2). At times sutures placed from the undersurface of the flap to the sphincters will relieve tension on the sutured edges and obliterate the dead space. A complete closure is essential to avoid the potential for recurrence. Postoperatively, the patient receives 2 to 5 days of intravenous antibiotics and nothing by mouth for several days or until stooling resumes. It is important to maintain soft stool after discharge because impaction or straining during defecation could disrupt the repair. A range of success rates has been reported from 78% to 92%.

Sleeve Advancement Flap

A sleeve (circumferential) advancement flap may be needed if the fistula is large (greater than 2.5 cm), if there is significant anterior scarring, or if there have been previous flap repairs. Patient preparation is identical to the advancement flap just described. After the anal everting sutures have been placed, the anal canal and lower rectal submucosa are injected with 1:200,000 epinephrine. Using electrocautery (and scissors if needed) a 90 to 100% sleeve of mucosa and submucosa is dissected (similar to a mucosectomy). The dissection is continued proximally, reaching into the supralevator space (Fig. 6-3) until the sleeve of tissue will easily advance to the neodentate line after trimming the terminal portion (Fig. 6-4). Closure of the fistula tract is the same as described previously. The ends are then anastomosed at the neodentate line with a circumferential

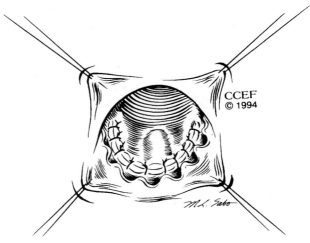

Figure 6-2
Advancement rectal flap: The diseased portion of the flap is trimmed before the flap is sutured to the mucosal edge of the anus. (From Hull TL, Fazio VW: Surgical approaches to low anovaginal fistula in Crohn's disease. Am J Surg 1997;173:95–98.)

3-0 polyglycolic suture. Consideration is given for a temporary diverting stoma.

Transperineal Approaches

Episioproctotomy

When fecal incontinence coexists with the fistula or the anterior anal sphincter complex is extremely thin, an episioproctotomy (dividing the tissue above the fistula and creating a defect similar to a fourth degree perineal laceration during childbirth) may be the best treatment option. Preparation is similar to that previously described. For this repair the author still prefers the prone position. A probe is placed through the fistula, and all tissue anteriorly is divided with electrocautery. The tract is débrided of chronic granulation tissue from the fistula. Then dissection is carried laterally and the sphincter muscles are identified and mobilized. An overlapping sphincter repair is then performed. It is sometimes is necessary to partially close the rectal mucosa with a mattress suture of 3-0 polyglycolic acid suture before completing the sphincter wrap; otherwise, it can be difficult to visualize the upper anal canal to reapproximate its edges without stretching the repair.

Transverse Transperineal Repair

Particularly in the gynecologic literature, an incision transversely through the perineal body is advocated to repair rectovaginal fistula. Saline injection facilitates dissection, which is carried past scar into fresh, healthy tissue above the fistula. The fistula tract is completely transected by sharp dissection, and the posterior vaginal wall and anterior rectal wall are widely mobilized. Scar tissue from the tract and os is excised. The vagina is closed longitudinally and the rectal wall closed transversely with 3-0 delayed

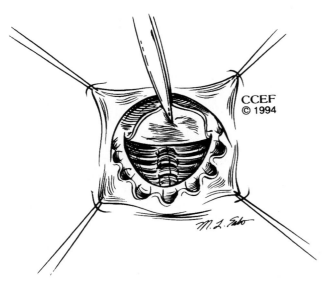

Figure 6-1
Advancement rectal flap: Everting sutures are placed. A semicircular flap has been raised. The fistula has been cored out and closed in layers. (From Hull TL, Fazio VW: Surgical approaches to low anovaginal fistula in Crohn's disease. Am J Surg 1997;173:95–98.)

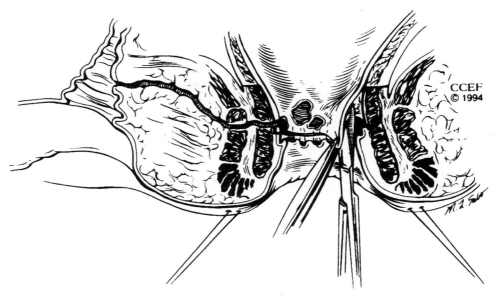

Figure 6-3
Sleeve advancement flap: A 90 to 100% sleeve of mucosa and submucosa is dissected, breaching into the supralevator space. (From Hull TL, Fazio VW: Surgical approaches to low anovaginal fistula in Crohn's disease. Am J Surg 1997;173:95–98.)

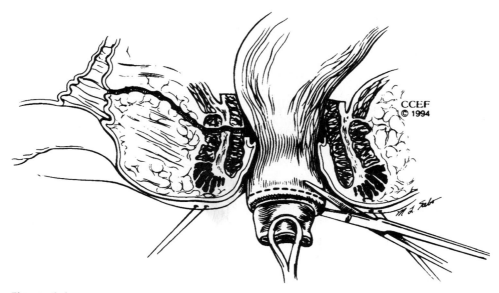

Figure 6-4
Sleeve advancement flap: The distal cuff of diseased tissue is trimmed, the fistula tract is cored out and closed, and the cylinder of rectal tissue is sutured to the remaining ridge of anoderm. (From Hull TL, Fazio VW: Surgical approaches to low anovaginal fistula in Crohn's disease. Am J Surg 1997;173:95–98.)

absorbable sutures. A second layer is placed to imbricate the mucosal layers. The puborectalis muscles are approximated in the midline with 2-0 delayed absorbable sutures. If needed, a bulbocavernosus flap or gracilis muscle can be mobilized and transposed beneath the posterior vaginal wall. If there is a defect in the external sphincter, it can also be reapproximated at this point.

Transvaginal Repair

Inversion of Fistula

If the fistula is small and low, inversion may be an option. A circular incision is made around the vaginal os, and the surrounding flap of vaginal mucosa is mobilized. Several concentric purse-string sutures are placed to invert the fistula into the rectum. The vaginal mucosa is then reapproximated. All surrounding tissue must be soft and pliable for this approach to be successful.

Advancement Vaginal Flap

Some surgeons advocate an advancement flap of vaginal mucosa. They feel that it eliminates operating in the confines of the anal canal and in patients with Crohn's disease prevents disturbing the anorectal area. However, others oppose this approach, noting that it does not address the high-pressure side of the fistula (the anorectal side). Usually this repair is done with the patient in the lithotomy position. Epinephrine solution (1:200,000) is injected into the vaginal submucosa. A curvilinear flap is mapped out and dissection is extended laterally to the ischial tuberosities and cephalad. If it is impossible to raise a flap that is long enough without shortening the vagina, a caudad flap is also raised. The vaginal defect is approximated with absorbable suture and the levator ani muscle is approximated. Excessive flap and the fistula site are excised and the flap and cut edges are reapproximated using absorbable suture.

Miscellaneous Repairs

Coloanal Anastomosis

Rarely, it is impossible to mobilize a sleeve of rectum from the transanal approach. In these patients transabdominal mobilization of the rectum and mucosectomy with a coloanal anastomosis may be a treatment option. Circumstances that require this type of repair are rare, but this approach may be useful in a few individuals.

Fibrin Glue

Fibrin glue has been used to treat rectovaginal fistula. Patients are given a mechanical bowel preparation and

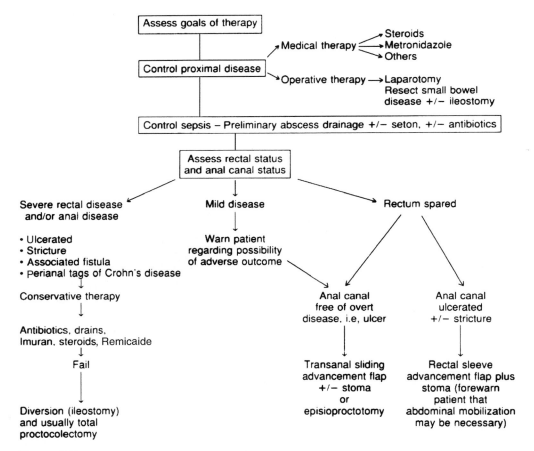

Figure 6-5
An algorithm for treatment of rectovaginal fistula in patients with Crohn's disease. (From Hull TL, Fazio VW: Rectovaginal fistula in Crohn's disease. In Phillips RKS, Lunniss PJ (Eds.). Anal Fistula. London, Chapman and Hall, 1996.)

perioperative antibiotics. While the glue is being prepared the patient is examined in the prone position and granulation tissue is debrided from the tract. Thrombin (Thrombinar) is reconstituted at 1000 U/mL. Equal volumes of each solution (the thrombin and fibrinogen) are connected to a Y-connector. A plastic catheter (14 gauge) is attached to the end and equal amounts of each solution are tested by injecting each down the Y-catheter and assessing the coagulum. A coagulum is immediately formed, but the concentration of fibrinogen is variable, so the amount injected into each limb of the Y-catheter may need to be adjusted to create a coagulum with the consistency of warm melted candle wax. When the concentrations to be mixed are adjusted, a new catheter is attached to the end of the Y-connector and the mixture is injected into the fistula tract. Postoperative oral intake is restricted for about 2 days.

■ FECAL DIVERSION

The use of a stoma as part of repairing a rectovaginal fistula remains controversial. Fecal diversion does not guar-antee success and is not probably required for every repair. Consideration for a stoma should be given if there have been other previous failed repairs, when an abdominal repair is to be performed, or with a complicated type of repair such as a sleeve advancement or muscle interposition. Additionally, a stoma should be considered with any repair where the procedure was technically unsatisfying.

■ DIFFICULT FISTULA

Fistula from Radiation
Pelvic irradiation, especially for cervical malignancy, can produce a fistula that is usually located high in the rectum. These fistulas must be carefully examined in the operating room to rule out residual or recurrent neoplasm as the etiology. Rectal or vaginal advancement flaps are usually not a good treatment option because the tissue used for the flaps has been irradiated. Sometimes the entire area is indurated and a stoma is required for up to a year to allow a decrease in the tissue thickness before any type of repair can be considered. When a repair is undertaken, nonradi-

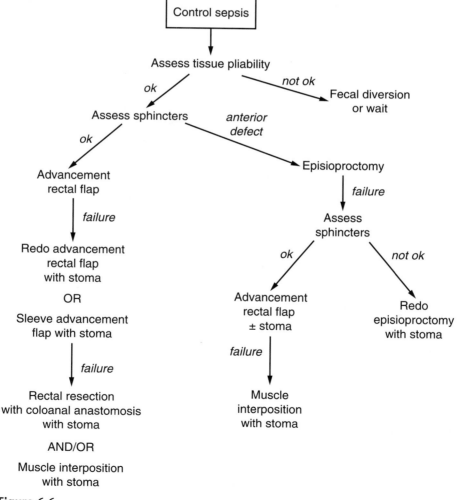

Figure 6-6
An algorithmic approach to treatment options in rectovaginal fistula.

ated tissue is used. Several approaches have been used successfully, including rectal resection with a coloanal anastomosis; a layered closure utilizing muscle interposition with gracilis or other nonradiated muscle; and a vascular pedicle graft of bowel. Usually a stoma is employed after one of these repairs while healing occurs.

Crohn's Disease and Rectovaginal Fistula

In the past patients with fistula from Crohn's disease were not offered any type of repair. Indeed, if the fistula is associated with severe rectal disease, a proctocolectomy is probably the best treatment option.

In some women with minimal symptoms from their fistula, a chronic loosely tied indwelling seton prevents sepsis and delays a permanent stoma. However, in selected patients repair can be offered. If there is minimal anal and rectal disease, advancement rectal flap can be done. If the anal canal is ulcerated or strictured but the rectum is spared, a sleeve advancement flap is an option. Some prefer to do a transvaginal repair in patients with Crohn's disease—associated fistula because it prevents tissue manipulation on the diseased anal side. In patients without severe anorectal disease, but with a sphincter deformity, an episioproctotomy allows simultaneous sphincter and fistula repair. Success rates for most repairs in these patients are about 70%. Multiple repairs are sometimes necessary for success.

The issue of active Crohn's disease elsewhere in the bowel is unresolved. Aggressive treatment, usually with steroids, should be done in an attempt to induce remission. Immunosuppressive agents can be considered if steroids are poorly tolerated, but sustained healing of the fistula usually does not occur. Sometimes resection of small bowel disease is done before fistula surgery is planned or if an initial attempt at fistula repair has failed.

For colonic disease, 5-ASA compounds and metronidazole may help induce remission. Patients with moderate to severe colonic disease that does not respond to treatment seem to have less successful fistula repairs. Figure 6-5 provides an algorithm for treatment of patients with Crohn's disease and rectovaginal fistula.

■ CONCLUSION

Rectovaginal and anovaginal fistulas remain a challenge for the surgeon who needs to be familiar with multiple treatment options to give these patients the best chance of a successful repair. Figure 6-6 shows an algorithmic approach when considering treatment options.

Suggested Readings

Able ME, Chiu YSY, Russell TR, Volpe PA: Autologous fibrin flue in the treatment of rectovaginal and complex fistulas. Dis Colon Rectum 1993;36:447–449.

Halverson AL, Hull TL, Fazio VW, et al: Repair of recurrent rectovaginal fistulas. Surgery 2001;130:753–757.

Hull TL, Fazio VW: Rectovaginal Fistula in Crohn's Disease. In Phillips RKS, Lunniss PJ (Eds.). Anal Fistula: London, Chapman and Hall, 1996.

Hull TL, Fazio VW: Surgical approaches to low anovaginal fistula in Crohn's disease. Am J Surg 1997;173:95–98.

Khanduja KS, Padmanabhan A, Kerner BA, et al: Reconstruction of rectovaginal fistula with sphincter disruption by combining rectal mucosal advancement flap with anal sphincteroplasty. Dis Colon Rectum 1999;42:1432–1437.

Senatore PJ: Anovaginal fistulae. Surg Clin North Am 1994;74:1361–1375.

Tsang CB, Madoff RD, Wong WD, et al: Anal sphincter integrity and function influences outcome in rectovaginal fistula repair. Dis Colon Rectum 1998;41:1141–1146.

Wiskind AK, Thompson JD: Transverse transperineal repair of rectovaginal fistulas in the lower vagina. Am J Obstet Gynecol 1992;167:694–699.

7

PILONIDAL SINUS

John M. MacKeigan, MD, FRCSC, FACS, FASCRS

■ ETIOLOGY

Pilonidal sinus is an acquired subcutaneous chronic infection secondary to hair implantation. Congenital theories of etiology include medullary canal remnants, dermal inclusions, or vestigial sex glands. The distribution in the sacral region and the disease's occurrence more frequently in hirsute white males support the acquired theories, however. A sex hormone influence may be a factor predominantly in males under 40 years of age. It is unknown whether the pilonidal sinus is related to a foreign body reaction to implanted hairs or to hair follicle infection with rupture into the subcutaneous fat. The occasional occurrence of a pilonidal sinus in other locations such as the perineum, finger, and amputation stumps, along with recurrence in the natal cleft following wide excision, also support the acquired theories.

■ PRESENTATION AND DIAGNOSIS

Pilonidal sepsis presents either acutely, as an abscess or an infected sinus with intermittent episodes of swelling and spontaneous drainage, or chronically, as poorly draining abscesses or chronic sinuses. Diagnosis is suggested by the site and appearance of the infection. Almost always, there are primary pits in the midline of the natal cleft, one of which appears to be the site of origin. The primary openings are almost always in the midline with squamous epithelium lining the superficial portion of the sinus tract. These pits are an important clue to the diagnosis. There may be surrounding induration with or without abscess formation.

Chronic pilonidal sinuses present with recurring swelling, abscess, or drainage. The primary openings are in the midline and commonly lead to a cavity full of infected hairs and granulations. More complex fistulization of the primary tract with multiple secondary openings may occur. Secondary openings have an elevated and slightly erythematous coloration. Unusual presentations include multiple tracts and openings simulating severe hidradenitis suppurativa. The process may extend into the perineum from the sacral region, and isolated anterior perineal sinuses have been seen and described. Surgical intervention can be performed in either the left lateral position or the jack-knife position with good access to most pilonidal sinuses.

■ DIFFERENTIAL DIAGNOSIS

Any acute abscess presenting in the sacral or coccygeal region with a midline sinus opening is likely to be a pilonidal infection. A small abscess may have minimal erythema and no fluctuance. Other causes of infection in the natal cleft include hidradenitis suppurativa, or cryptoglandular sepsis. It is essential that the latter be excluded because of the different approaches to surgical treatment. Sinuses extending caudad, toward the anal canal, raise the suspicion of a communication with the anus.

A gentle digital examination with care to palpate the retrorectal and posterior perineal region for tenderness or mass should be performed as part of the process of differential diagnosis. If palpation of the perianal tissue posteriorly and inspection for an internal fistula tract opening show no abnormality, cryptoglandular infection is unlikely. It is uncomfortable for the patient to have the tract probed in the office; this procedure is better done in the operating room before definitive surgery. Proctoscopy helps rule out inflammatory bowel disease, especially in patients with low caudal abscesses or patients with chronic complex sinuses. Actinomycosis, tuberculosis, syphilis, and sacral osteomyelitis should be considered when there are unusual, complex, recurrent sinuses, but such infections are extremely rare.

■ CHOICE OF PROCEDURE

The choice of procedure is based on a consideration of the complexity of the sinus, cost, healing time, and recurrence rate (Table 7-1). Comfort and limiting time lost from work are also major factors. Most simple sinuses can be laid open, and complex and recurrent sinuses may be excised with reconstruction.

As pilonidal sinus is either an acute or chronic abscess, incision and drainage offer the simplest procedure that allows early comfort and mobility. The author's preference in most simple sinuses is a lateral incision with drainage of the tract. The midline sinus openings are elliptically excised as a part of that incision and drainage, leaving the base of the wound in place. Incision and marsupialization may have a slightly shorter healing time and lower recurrence but is associated with more pain in the early postoperative phase. Excision of the tracts is rarely done and is reserved for the most complex

---

Table 7-1 Treatments of Pilonidal Sinus

Incision and drainage
Superficial excision and drainage
Marsupialization with or without excision
Sinus excision and lateral drainage (Bascom)
Excision with primary closure
Sclerosing injection
Excision with skin grafting
Excision with lateral advancement flap
Excision with Z-plasty
Excision with buttock apposition
Rotation flaps with or without gluteus muscle

and recurrent sinuses. Excision with primary closure for the simple, common pilonidal sinus is significantly more painful than laying the sinus open and usually requires the patient to be admitted to hospital. The author has reserved primary closure for the rare circumstance of a sinus that persists or recurs after multiple incisions and drainage. Complex and recurrent sinuses may be better treated with excision and creation of a flap, closure of the cleft, or a Z-plasty, all of which are described later in this chapter. If the sinus is extensive, a myocutaneous flap may be the only significant choice. Whatever the procedure, close follow-up of the healing wound is as important in ensuring a satisfactory outcome as the choice and conduct of the primary procedure.

■ TREATMENT

Abscess

Superficial abscesses may be drained in the office with a field block of 1 to 2% lidocaine. Adequate drainage of deeper abscesses or large and extensive abscesses requires an anesthetic. If an abscess can be widely drained, recurrence is reduced and a more definitive initial procedure is performed (Fig. 7-1).

Twenty to 30 mL of 1 to 2% lidocaine with 1:200,000 epinephrine is infiltrated slowly in a field block using a No. 30 gauge needle. A linear incision is made parallel to and just lateral to the midline. An elliptical excision of a narrow portion of skin overlying the track, including the central midline pits, is performed. The excision is superficial and is made only to facilitate drainage, leaving the base of the sinus. The ends of the narrow excision or drainage are kept to one side of the midline to facilitate healing. The distal or caudal end of any incision in the midline is a common site of persistence or recurrence. Chances of healing are better if the incision is lateral to the midline. The base of the wound is curetted, and the wound is packed lightly with gauze. The gauze is removed the next day by soaking in the bath or shower.

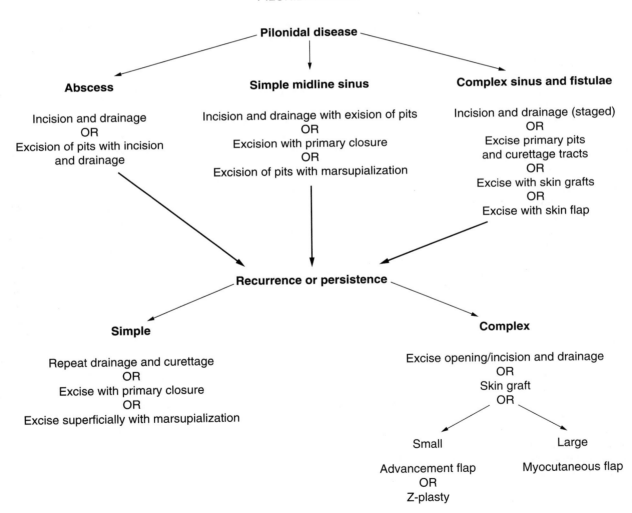

PILONIDAL SINUS

Figure 7-1
Algorithm for the management of pilonidal disease.

Postoperative care includes light gauze packing of the wound several times per day to keep the wound clean of debris. Showers, a Water Pik, or sitz baths are used two or three times daily to clean the wound. A cotton-tipped applicator may be useful to clean the depths of some wounds. Use of a hair dryer improves comfort after showering or bathing. Follow-up every 1 or 2 weeks makes sure that the skin edges do not come together prematurely.

Uncomplicated Midline Chronic Sinus

The simple common pilonidal sinus with one or two midline openings and one to two secondary sinus tracts or openings is usually treated like the acute abscess. The anesthetic, preparation, and suturing principles are the same. A narrow elliptical excision of the primary openings, leaving the base, is performed. The ends of the ellipse are kept away from the midline. All extensions must be probed and opened, or the disease will recur. Generally, with epinephrine included in the local anesthetic, good hemostasis and visualization of the granulating sinus is possible. Debris and hair are removed, and the base of the sinus is curettaged to remove excess granulation tissue. Hemostasis is achieved with cautery, and light gauze packing is applied. The postoperative care is the same as that for abscesses.

Marsupialization of the wound using an absorbable suture such as 3-0 chromic catgut or 4-0 polyglycolic acid (Vicryl, Dexon) is used for the uncommon deep wound. A continuous suture from skin to the margin of the fibrotic sinus base is performed. Gauze packing and postoperative care are as described previously.

Complex or Lateral Sinus

Very extensive pilonidal sinuses with large areas of multiple tracts are often suspicious for Crohn's disease, tuberculosis, or hidradenitis. Rarely, a bone scan, magnetic resonance imaging, or sacral x-rays are necessary to rule out osteomyelitis.

Large areas with multiple tracts may need staged surgeries for incision and drainage of sinuses to control the sepsis. Multiple tracts within 5 to 6 cm of the midline may be simply opened, curettaged, and incorporated into the main central wound, excising the primary opening. Again, excision of tracts or sinuses is rarely necessary. Wide excision of skin is to be avoided.

Lateral tracts more than a few centimeters from the midline may be treated similarly to horseshoe anal fistulas. The principle is to open and drain or excise the primary pits as for the uncomplicated sinus. The lateral extensions are treated with small elliptical excision of the external openings or opening the lateral aspect of the sinus. The intervening sinus leading to the midline area is curettaged and then left open. The lateral extension generally heals when the primary midline site is adequately drained. If it does persist or fail to heal, it may be opened later in stages to minimize the extent of the wound.

Recurrent Pilonidal Sinus

Recurrence of pilonidal disease after good primary healing is rare. Persistence or early recurrence within 6 to 12 months is related to unsuccessful initial control of the condition and is more common. It occurs because the conditions that contributed to the first pilonidal sinus are still present. Pilonidal disease, if not curable, can usually be managed successfully.

Recurrence rates for simple incision and drainage range from 15 to 60%. When sinuses and abscesses are treated definitively early, avoiding small drainage incisions, recurrence is reduced.

Recurrent pilonidal sinuses should be treated in the same way as the initial sinus. If there is a third or fourth recurrence, a different approach might be suggested, such as excision and closure. If primary excision and closure are performed, the skin incision should be kept off the midline as much as possible. Keeping it off the midline avoids fixation of the healing scar to the coccyx. Primary closure is often performed in layers with large sutures acting much in the fashion as retention sutures. These sutures are tied over a roll of gauze to help tamponade enclosed dead space. The closure is associated with a significant degree of pain and generally requires hospitalization. Extensive recurrence is discussed later.

Persistent or Slow-Healing Wounds

Occasionally, persistent or slow-healing wounds are related to inadequate drainage or failure of recognition of the true nature of the condition. Many slow-healing wounds occur in the midline, especially distally over the coccygeal region. Deep wounds between large buttocks also have problems with delayed healing. The motion of the buttocks may contribute to this.

Some patients cannot seem to clean or open their wound well enough to allow gauze or other direct treatment to the wound. Taping the buttocks to prevent persistence does not seem useful, although hairs in the skin around the wound need to be periodically clipped or shaved. The best way to prevent recurrence is to tailor the wound off the midline. Frequent follow-up with periodic light curettage of the wounds reduces granulation tissue buildup. Occasionally, overlying skin margins may have to be opened and the shape of the wound revised to prevent the formation of deep isolated segments.

Persistence of a sinus for longer than 6 to 9 months may be an indication for further surgery. Usually, the wound is cleaned and laid open as described for the primary surgery. If the sinus still persists, then excision and primary closure are attempted (Keighley and Williams, 1993).

When patients have deep buttocks, there may be an indication to obliterate the upper portion of the intergluteal fold. The buttocks are closely apposed and then a line is drawn on either buttock medially. The site is then excised with a portion of the intergluteal fold. The buttocks are approximated and closed primarily. Absorbable sutures are used, such as 3-0 to 4-0 Dexon or Vicryl.

Many of the same results may be obtained by developing a lateral-based skin flap using one side of the medial aspect of the buttock. This flap is advanced a short distance across the midline and the wound is closed vertically and laterally. It has been called a Karydakis flap and was first described by Karydakis. A Z-plasty accomplishes some of the same effects but is more extensive and complicated, and requires more mobilization. Mansory and Dixon described 120 cases with one recurrence.

Any primary closure or flap-type procedure is preceded by good skin preparation and is not done if there is significant cellulitis or surrounding infection. Preoperative antibiotics are given intravenously prophylactically and may include cefotetan or quinolones and metronidazole.

Extensive and Recurrent Disease

The management of recurrent pilonidal sinus is intended to reduce intergluteal cleft depth and reduce friction or gluteal motion in the process. The goal is to achieve healing in the simplest and least complicated way possible.

If the area of recurrence is relatively small with a shallow intergluteal cleft, open the tracts. Excision of the areas is performed if there is a large amount of firm, fibrinous induration in the surrounding tissue. The wound is monitored closely and lightly packed with fine gauze to allow granulation tissue to form and allow contraction of the wound. In time, many wounds will ultimately heal. If healing stops, then areas that are shallow can be skin grafted. Recurrence rate less than 2% and graft failure rates below 5% have been reported.

If the original excised area is smaller than 10 to 12 cm in circumference and if there is a moderate amount of buttock adipose tissue and laxity, a simple rotation cutaneous flap or lateral advancement flap is sufficient. If areas are larger than 10 to 12 cm and deep, a myocutaneous flap is needed to maintain blood supply and to fill the deep intergluteal cleft.

The myocutaneous flap is based inferiorly and laterally. The area of the pilonidal sinus is excised to fresh tissue in an elliptical fashion. The large flap is created with a curvilinear incision along the superior aspect of the buttock. The upper aspect of the gluteus maximus is detached from its fascial insertion superiorly and included in the rotational flap. A surgeon comfortable with similar flap surgery for pressure ulcerations is of assistance to design the flap. The procedure was first described for pressure ulcerations by Minami and coworkers, and Perez-Gurriand coworkers described its use for pilonidal sinuses in 1984.

The flaps require good preoperative planning and design. A clean wound without surrounding cellulitis is an obvious prerequisite. Intravenous antibiotics with aerobic and anaerobic coverage are utilized. The flap is designed to be as broad as it is long. A closed drain is inserted under the myocutaneous flap. Close observation for infections and to assess the vascular supply is important.

Other Methods of Therapy

Bascom has described a technique of excising the primary midline pits in a diamond-shape fashion and draining the main cavity with a vertical lateral incision. Meticulous and specific care of the wound is advocated. This method is well described in the prior edition of this textbook and by Bascom in a 1980 article in *Diseases of the Colon and Rectum*. The author's personal experiences were not as successful as Bascom's, and the author has abandoned this method as a primary therapy.

Cryosurgical destruction has been described but should be abandoned. Cryosurgery generally destroys tissue in an uncontrolled fashion. It often leaves a large open wound with excessive reactive drainage. The technique was advocated by J. J. O'Connor in the late 1970s and described in a 1979 article in *Diseases of the Colon and Rectum*.

Sclerosing injection using 80% phenol into the tract after drainage has been described with good results. A low recurrence rate has been reported by Hegge and associates, although the technique has not been widely adopted.

■ CONCLUSION

Management of most pilonidal abscesses and sinuses is relatively straightforward. A complex and large persistent or recurrent pilonidal sinus requires good wound control and careful design of corrective skin flaps. However, patience and repeated simple opening of recurrent areas with close postoperative wound management controls and cures most situations.

Suggested Readings

Aydede H, Erhan Y, Sakarya A, Kumkumoglu Y: Comparison of three methods in surgical treatment of pilonidal disease. Aust NZ J Surg 2001;71(6):362–364.

Bascom J: Pilonidal disease: Long-term results of follicle removal. Dis Colon Rectum 1983;26:800–807.

Bascom JU: Pilonidal disease: Origins from follicles of hairs and results of follicle removal as treatment. Surgery 1980;87:567–572.

da Silva JH: Pilonidal cyst: Cause and treatment. Dis Colon Rectum 2000;43(8):1146–1156.

de Bree E, Zoetmulder FA, Christodoulakis M, et al: Treatment of malignancy arising in pilonidal disease. Ann Surg Oncol 2001;8(1):60–64.

Hegge HG, Vos GA, Patka P, Hoitsma HF: Treatment of complicated or infected pilonidal sinus by local application of phenol. Surgery 1987;102:52–54.

Karulf RE: Hidradenitis suppurativa and pilonidal disease. In Beck DE, Wexner SD (Eds.). Fundamentals of Anorectal Surgery. New York, McGraw-Hill, 1992, Chap. 13, pp 183–191.

Karydakis GE: New approach to the problem of pilonidal sinus. Lancet 1973;2:1414–1415.

Keighley M, Williams D: Pilonidal disease. In Surgery of Anus, Rectum and Colon. London, WB Saunders, 1993, Chap. 11, pp 467–489.

Khoury DA: Surgery for pilonidal disease and hidradenitis suppurativa. In Hicks T, Beck D, Opelka F, Timmcke A (Eds.). Complications of Colon and Rectal Surgery. Baltimore, Williams & Wilkins, 1996, pp 203–221.

Minami RT, Mills R, Pardoe R: Gluteus maximus myocutaneous flaps for repair of pressure sores. Plast Reconstr Surg 1977;60:242–249.

Nivatvongs S: Pilonidal disease. In Gordon P, Nivatvongs S (Eds.). Principles and Practice of Surgery for the Colon, Rectum and Anus. St. Louis, Quality Medical Publishers, 1992, pp 267–279.

O'Connor JJ: Surgery plus freezing as a technique for treating pilonidal disease. Dis Colon Rectum 1979;22:306–307.

Perez-Gurri JA, Temple WS, Ketcham AS: Gluteus maximus myocutaneous flap for treatment of recalcitrant pilonidal disease. Dis Colon Rectum 27:262–264.

Senapati A, Cripps NP, Thompson MR: Bascom's operation in the day-surgical management of symptomatic pilonidal sinus. Br J Surg 2000;87(8):1067–1070.

8

PERIANAL HIDRADENITIS SUPPURATIVA

Martin Andrew Luchtefeld, MD

Hidradenitis suppurativa is a chronic recurring inflammatory condition of the apocrine glands and adjacent skin and connective tissue. Because apocrine glands are found primarily in the axillary, groin, and perianal regions, this condition is most often found in these areas. In the perianal and perineal area, hidradenitis suppurativa is a relatively uncommon condition and can be easily mistaken for a number of other infectious/inflammatory conditions.

■ PATHOGENESIS

It has been postulated that this condition starts with the obstruction of an apocrine gland duct that then allows the gland to become infected. The infected gland ruptures within the dermis, resulting in sinus and abscess formation. Eventually dermal scarring and chronic sinuses can form as a result of the acute infection. Infection does seem to be a secondary event in that in at least one large series bacteria could be identified in less than half of the active hidradenitis lesions. When bacteria are present, numerous types of organisms have been cultured from the wounds of hidradenitis suppurativa. Skin organisms such as staphylococci are commonly involved. In the perianal region there are coliforms as well as anaerobic organisms. It is clear that no one organism is responsible for the majority of these cases.

The inciting factor that starts this inflammatory process is not known. Deodorant has been suggested to be the cause of an inflammation of the axillary region but obviously not in the groin or perineum. Clearly this condition requires a postpubertal hormonal milieu, as hidradenitis occurs only after hormones have stimulated apocrine gland secretion. Also, hidradenitis suppurativa has been associated with severe acne, obesity, and a hot environment. It appears to be more common in blacks than in whites. The incidence in men and women is relatively equal, although the male-female ratio has varied widely in different series.

■ PRESENTATION

The presentation of perianal hidradenitis suppurativa depends on the stage at which patients present to the treating physician. The picture is always that of perianal inflammation/sepsis, but this condition can be acute or chronic. The severity can range from very minimal to widely extensive disease.

In the very early stages of disease, patients can present with a firm, subcutaneous nodule that is tender and may at some point develop fluctuance. This nodule can drain spontaneously or may seem to wax and wane somewhat without any specific treatment. The area involved in this process can initially be very small but can expand to involve widely varying amounts of the perianal region. In the more chronic phase, the disease is usually marked by multiple draining sinuses a well as a wide area of scarred and indurated skin and subcutaneous tissue. A clinical staging system has been described for hidradenitis suppurativa, which can be helpful when deciding on therapy (Table 8-1).

Hidradenitis suppurativa is commonly misdiagnosed on its initial presentation. It can be very difficult to distinguish this disorder from a straightforward anal fistula, pilonidal disease, or perianal Crohn's disease. It can, in fact, coexist with Crohn's disease. It is important to note that invasive squamous cell carcinoma has been seen in patients with chronic hidradenitis suppurativa. The duration of the disease in these cases was 16 years or more. In patients who present with an extremely long history of this disorder, squamous cell carcinoma should be considered as a possibility.

Differentiating hidradenitis suppurativa from other disorders can be difficult; however, a careful examination under anesthesia is often helpful. Because apocrine glands are related to the hair-bearing portion of the perianal area, the location of the suppuration can help differentiate hidradenitis suppurativa from other disorders. In addition, because of their anatomic origin, the superficial fistulas and sinuses associated with hidradenitis suppurativa can extend up into the anal canal but typically do not track all the way up to the dentate line.

■ MANAGEMENT: GENERAL PRINCIPLES

Many different forms of medical management have been used for the treatment of perianal hidradenitis suppurativa. Although they may be useful as adjuncts, generally these treatments are either unsuccessful or have very high recurrence rates for anything other than stage I disease (see Table 8-1 for staging system). The treatments include topical antibacterial soaps, antiacne medications such as cis-retinoic acid, cyclosporine, immunotherapy (staphage lysate), and hormonal therapy. Antibiotics can play an important role in the treatment of hidradenitis suppurativa, but long-term use does not prevent ongoing abscess and sinus tract formation. These treatment modalities sometimes can be useful in clearing acute infection or moderating the disease in preparation for surgery. Rather than divide the therapy into medical and surgical treatments, it is more useful to consider the therapy in its acute and chronic phases and review the surgical options in the context of the clinical staging.

Table 8-1 Clinical Staging of Hidradenitis Suppurativa

STAGE	DESCRIPTION
I	Isolated abscess formation, single or multiple, without scarring or sinus tracts
II	Recurrent abscesses with tract formation and cicatrization; single or multiple, widely separated lesions
III	Diffuse or near-diffuse involvement, or multiple interconnected tracts and abscesses across an entire area

Source: Hurley HJ: Diseases of the apocrine sweat glands. In Moschella SL, Hurley HJ (Eds.). Dermatology, Vol. 2. Philadelphia, WB Saunders, 1992, p 1509.

■ INITIAL THERAPY AND EVALUATION

When a patient first presents with perineal hidradenitis, the emphasis should be on establishing a diagnosis and controlling any acute infection. In addition to taking a thorough history, the physician must perform a careful examination that includes anoscopy and sigmoidoscopy. The extent of involvement of the anal canal should be documented. Examination under anesthesia may be necessary to determine the anatomic relationships of sinuses and potential fistulas. If any other diagnoses are being entertained (i.e., Crohn's disease or squamous cell cancer), appropriate evaluation should be initiated.

Once the diagnosis of hidradenitis suppurativa is made, any acute infection should be dealt with by a combination of antibiotics as well as incision and drainage of any abscesses. Antibiotics are one of the most useful of the nonsurgical therapies. Both short- and long-term dosing schedules have been used and seem to be associated with improvement. Ideally, the agent of choice would be determined by cultures and sensitivities. In the absence of such information, a broad-spectrum antibiotic such as erythromycin, tetracycline, or ciprofloxacin can be effective.

In addition to treatment with one of the foregoing antibiotics, incision and drainage of any obvious fluctuant abscesses can bring significant relief. Use of the antibiotics as well as draining any large collections of purulence can be effective in limiting the immediate propagation of the inflammation and scarring in the surrounding areas.

For stage I disease, the preceding interventions sometimes can be curative. In stage II and III disease, the benefit of this regimen is that it allows the tissues to be in an optimal, minimally infected state prior to starting definitive surgical treatment.

■ DEFINITIVE TREATMENT

Although antibiotics and incision and drainage of abscesses associated with hidradenitis suppurativa can be helpful in management of the acute phase, eradication of stage II and III disease always requires surgical intervention. Definitive surgery is usually planned after the judicious use of antibiotics and incision and drainage have controlled any acute infection.

Most authors would agree that the best chance for cure is a wide excision of the involved area down to soft, pliable, and obviously noninvolved tissues. The actual depth of the excision will vary, depending on the depth of the inflammation. If necessary, the excision can be brought all the way down to the underlying fascia. Any controversy or decision making revolves around the handling of the resulting wound once the wide local excision has been done.

Stage II disease with a relatively limited amount of surface area involved is one circumstance in which primary closure can be considered. Heavy contamination of the wound would mandate leaving the wound open. Primary closure has the obvious advantage of quick wound healing but tends to have a higher recurrence rate than when the wound is left open.

For stage III disease with a larger area involved or if one chooses not to do primary closure for stage II lesions, several options are available. The simplest and most straightforward of these options is to allow the wound to heal by secondary intention. The primary drawback of this approach is the long healing times that are required. However, in patients with hidradenitis suppurativa healing is often surprisingly fast, and it is this author's experience that very large areas can be excised with much lower morbidity rates than expected and ultimate successful healing of large areas.

■ SUMMARY

Diagnosis of perianal hidradenitis suppurativa depends on a high index of suspicion and exclusion of other causes of sepsis. Superficial sinuses and fistulas, and evidence of chronic scarring in the area, are suggestive. The most effective treatment is surgical, with drainage and laying open small abscesses and fistulas. Larger areas of infected skin can be excised, with the defect left to heal by second intention.

Suggested Readings

Brown TJ, Rosen T, Orengo IF: Hidradenitis suppurativa. Southern Med J 1998;91(12):1107–1114.

Bohn J, Svensson H: Surgical treatment of hidradenitis suppurativa. Scand J Plast Reconstruct Surg Hand Surg 2001;35(3):305–309.

Endo Y, Tamura A, Ishikawa O, Miyachi Y: Perianal hidradenitis suppurativa: Early surgical treatment gives good results in chronic or recurrent cases. Br J Derm 1998;139(5):906–910.

Jemec GB, Wendelboe P: Topical clindamycin versus systemic tetracycline in the treatment of hidradenitis suppurativa. J Am Acad Derm 1998;39(6):971–974.

Lapins J, Ye W, Nyren O, Emtestam L: Incidence of cancer among patients with hidradenitis suppurativa. Arch Derm 2001;137(6):730–734.

Martinez F, Nos P, Benlloch S, Ponce J: Hidradenitis suppurativa and Crohn's disease: Response to treatment with infliximab. Inflam Bowel Dis 2001;7(4):323–326.

Mortimer PS, Lunniss PJ: Hidradenitis suppurativa. J R Soc Med 2000; 93(8):420–422.

Nadgir R, Rubesin SE, Levine MS: Perirectal sinus tracks and fistulas caused by hidradenitis suppurativa. AJR 2001;177(2):476–477.

Parks RW, Parks TG: Pathogenesis, clinical features and management of hidradenitis suppurativa. Ann R Coll Surg Eng 1997;79(2):83–89.

Ritz JP, Runkel N, Haier J, Buhr HJ: Extent of surgery and recurrence rate of hidradenitis suppurativa. Int J Colorect Dis 1998;13(4): 164–168.

von der Werth JM, Jemec GB: Morbidity in patients with hidradenitis suppurativa. Br J Derm 2001;144(4):809–813.

9

PRURITUS ANI

Daniel P. Froese, MBChB, FACS, FASCRS

Patients with pruritus ani experience symptoms of perianal itching, burning, or soreness. These symptoms may occur during the day or night, with higher intensity after bowel movements; at night they may even interfere with sleep. The prevalence may increase during the warm summer months with increased sweating and moisture. Pruritus ani afflicts 1 to 5% of the population, with men experiencing symptoms more often than women. It predominantly affects those 20 to 40 years in age and is rarely seen in the elderly despite their more frequent perianal soilage. Classically the patient starts to itch and naturally scratches the region, which eases the symptoms. However, this relief is short lived. Continued scratching damages the protective skin surface, causing seepage from damaged skin and possibly allowing infection. This result accentuates the problem, thus setting up a vicious circle of escalating symptoms.

■ ETIOLOGY

The etiology of pruritus ani is readily divided into primary (idiopathic) and secondary categories (Table 9-1). Conditions causing secondary pruritus ani are as follows:

1. Anorectal conditions causing pruritus ani include rectal prolapse, hemorrhoids, fistula in ano, fissure, skin tags, mucosal ectropion, villous adenoma, and hidradenitis suppurativa. Some conditions create the problem by preventing the anus from closing effectively, leading to seepage or inadequate cleanliness and then to pruritus. In addition, rectal prolapse, villous adenoma, and mucosal ectropion may result in mucus seepage, aggravating the problem.
2. Numerous infections, including viral conditions such as herpes simplex and condyloma acuminatum, may cause pruritus ani. Symptoms relate to underlying irritation or the inability to maintain perianal hygiene. Bacterial infections include gonorrhea (*Neisseria gonorrhoeae*), syphilis (*Treponema pallidum*), tuberculosis (*Mycobacterium tuberculosis*), and rarely erythrasma caused by *Corynebacterium minutissimum*. The normal microflora of the perianal skin has not itself been described as a factor. Fungal infectious agents include *Candida albicans*, which can cause infection primarily or secondary to other systemic disorders, and other fungi, including any of the dermatophytes such as *Epidermophyton floccosum*, *Trichophyton mentagro-*

phytes, and *Trichophyton rubrum*. These infections cause a characteristic unilateral ringworm appearance with clear-cut margins. Parasites such as pinworms (*Enterobius vermicularis*), pubic louse (*Pediculosis pubis*), and scabies (*Sarcoptes scabiei*) are more unusual and require exact identification and specific treatment.

3. Pruritus ani may also result from surgical procedures that involve weakening the anus and removal of the rectum, causing seepage and frequent stools. Restorative proctocolectomy with hand-sewn ileo-anal anastomosis and proctosigmoidectomy with coloanal anastomosis are examples of procedures that may cause pruritus.
4. Primary skin disorders include contact dermatitis secondary to such allergens as washing soaps, clothing detergents, bleaches, perfumes, and even fiberglass. Ironically, many over-the-counter preparations meant to treat these symptoms contain agents that can act as allergens and exacerbate symptoms. More rarely, primary dermatologic conditions including psoriasis, eczema, lichen planus, lichen sclerosis et atrophicus, lichen simplex, and leukoplakia may be identified. These conditions give classical dermatologic appearances that are usually associated with similar skin complaints and changes elsewhere.
5. Primary neoplastic disorders of the skin may be intensely pruritic and include extramammary Paget's disease and Bowen's disease. They may have a characteristic appearance yet persistent symptoms; even in the absence of the typical appearance, biopsy is warranted to rule out these conditions.
6. Ingested drugs that may induce pruritus include mineral oil, colchicine, quinidine, anabolic hormones, and antibiotics such as tetracycline and erythromycin. The antibiotics are implicated because of the diarrhea they cause. Itching from constant perianal contamination may be due to this or some other diarrheal condition or simply inadequate hygiene by the patient following a bowel movement. This poor hygiene results in itching with secondary scratching and subsequent infection. Of note, pruritus ani is not seen in constipated patients.
7. Systemic disorders such as obstructive jaundice and uremia usually result in generalized pruritus but may present with a more localized problem. Diabetes mellitus, which if untreated results in excess hyperglycemia, may cause pruritus as a result of either internal sphincter weakening or fungal overgrowth. Stress is not felt to be a cause of symptoms.

Once this large group of etiologic agents is ruled out, the remaining subgroup is idiopathic disease. Most primary pruritus ani is diet-induced. By far the most common agent is coffee, including freshly brewed, freeze-dried, decaffeinated, espresso, and even coffee ice cream. Other dietary agents include tea, colas, chocolate, beer, milk, tomatoes, citrus fruits, and vitamin C. Each of these foods has an intake threshold above which susceptible patients will have pruritus ani and below which they will not. This amount varies among individuals.

Some patients are frequently compulsive anal cleaners. Continuous and excess cleaning and wiping sets up an irritation and a secondary bacterial infection that

---

Table 9-1 Etiology of Pruritus Ani

Primary (idiopathic)
  1. Diet: coffee, tea, colas, chocolate, beer, milk, tomatoes, citrus fruits, vitamin C
Secondary
  1. Anal pathology: rectal prolapse, hemorrhoids, fistula in ano, fissure, skin tags, ectropion, villous adenoma, hidradenitis suppurativa
  2. Infection
    a. Viral: herpes simplex, human papilloma
    b. Bacterial: gonorrhea, syphilis, tuberculosis, erythrasma
    c. Fungal: *Candida albicans* infection, dermatophytes
    d. Parasitic: pinworms, pubic louse, scabies
  3. Surgery: restorative proctocolectomy, hand-sewn coloanal or ileoanal anastomoses, transanal procedures such as rectal polypectomy, pouch advancement
  4. Contact dermatitis: soaps, detergents, bleaches, perfumes, fiberglass, topical anesthetics
  5. Dermatologic skin conditions: psoriasis, eczema, lichen sclerosis et atrophicus, lichen simplex, lichen planus, leukoplakia, Bowen's disease, extramammary Paget's disease
  6. Drugs: mineral oil, colchicine, quinidine, anabolic hormones, tetracycline, erythromycin
  7. Systemic diseases: diabetes mellitus, obstructive jaundice, uremia

---

perpetuates and intensifies the problem. These patients are often the most difficult to treat as no underlying etiology is identified, but symptoms have persisted and sadly are often resistant to therapy. Recent work on pathophysiology has helped in understanding the underlying disorder. Eyres and Thompson noted that symptomatic patients had an exaggerated rectal anal inhibitory reflex with rectal distention, leading to subsequent soiling. Allan and coworkers, in comparing symptomatic patients with control subjects, identified earlier leakage from the anal canal in pruritic patients when the rectum was filled with saline. In keeping with our experience with coffee, Smith and coworkers used anal manometry to demonstrate diminished sphincter tone after coffee ingestion. However, the most notable study was the ambulatory monitoring carried out by Farouk and coworkers, who noted three important observations: first, an internal sphincter pressure decrease, which was greater in pruritus ani patients compared with control subjects; second, a prolonged duration of internal sphincter relaxation after rectal distention; and third, symptoms of seepage which correlated with abnormal sphincter relaxation. All these observations describe an abnormality in internal sphincter function either as a primary defect or following coffee ingestion.

HISTORY

The investigation of pruritus ani is centered on possible etiologies. A complete history is important in narrowing down the investigative window. It is important to note the duration and timing of the symptoms and any obvious precipitating factors, such as exposure to other people with intense itching, pets, strange environments, or chemicals, along with the use of soaps, tissue papers, and even the types of underclothes worn. Contact allergens are ruled out by addressing the agents mentioned earlier, and in addition, the use of any cream or ointment that may contain anesthetic agents which act as allergens is asked for. Hygiene habits are noted, as is the presence of chronic

diarrhea, which may be primary or secondary. A complete drug history is taken to determine any possible pharmaceutical cause, especially relating to the use of antibiotics. Dermatologic conditions must be discussed, as any previously diagnosed systemic condition may aid in identifying a rash in the perineum. Diabetes mellitus, biliary disease, or uremia would be important to note, but these conditions tend to cause more generalized itching. Finally, and most important, is a history of dietary habits, including the intake of any type of coffees, tea, colas, chocolate, beer, milk, tomatoes, citrus fruits, and vitamin C, even in amounts that may not be expected to cause symptoms.

EXAMINATION

Examination involves careful inspection of the perianal skin for the presence of any seepage or soiling. The appearance of the skin changes may be classified as stage 0 (skin normal), stage 1 (skin red and inflamed), stage 2 (white, lichenified skin), and stage 3 (coarse ridging of the skin with ulceration superimposed on lichenification). The distribution of the rash is important in that diet-induced pruritus ani is centered symmetrically around the anus, yet infection surrounds the anal orifice asymmetrically. The diagnosis of specific infections including scabies and the dermatophytoses is possible with a discerning eye. Further inspection should note the presence of anal pathologic changes, including prolapsing hemorrhoids, anal fissure or fistula, skin tags, rectal prolapse, or mucosal ectropion. Suspicion of any dermatologic condition mandates examination of the entire body to aid in the diagnosis.

A thorough examination includes a digital rectal examination, anoscopy, and rigid sigmoidoscopy. In the difficult cases blood testing including a complete blood cell count, liver and renal tests, glucose testing, and thyroid function tests may be considered. A glucose tolerance test is usually not necessary, as symptoms in the diabetic occur with excessive hyperglycemia. If no obvious cause is found on inspection and endoscopy, referral to a dermatologist is reasonable. Skin scrapings for mycologic examination may be helpful, and in suspicious cases skin biopsy will rule out neoplastic changes. In most situations histologic examination reveals chronic inflammation with skin hypertrophy. If erythrasma is suggested, Wood's lamp testing will reveal the classic pink fluorescence due to porphyrin production by *C. minutissimum.* If pinworm infestation is suspected by nocturnal itching, then morning testing by applying cellulose tape to the perianal skin may reveal egg deposition. This testing may need to be repeated up to five times to obtain a high degree of accuracy. In the truly difficult case, anorectal manometry may be useful to assess internal sphincter function, and it has been suggested that total colonoscopy to rule out proximal neoplasia can be helpful if the pruritus is refractory to extended treatment.

■ TREATMENT

Secondary Pruritus Ani

Once a cause is established or excluded, then treatment may begin (Fig. 9-1). Certain therapies can be initiated that will help in all cases. Adding a bulking agent (e.g., Metamucil wafers) to the patient's diet absorbs liquid from the stool and helps to diminish any seepage associated with minor internal sphincter weakness. The patient is advised to stop taking any oral antibiotics or other drugs that are felt to be causative and to stop applying any types of soaps, topical antipruritic agents, or other therapies to the perianal skin. It is important to stress the necessity to stop scratching the skin, even when intense itching is present. It is useful to remind them that the scratching, although it temporarily relieves the itch, is actually perpetuating the problem. After a bowel movement patients are advised to either bathe or wash the area using water without any soap. The skin is then gently patted dry with a cotton towel, not rubbed vigorously with toilet paper. Scented toilet paper is discouraged. Loose underclothes allow the skin to remain dry afterward.

Specific treatment of any cause is undertaken. Symptoms secondary to bacterial infections, such as gonorrhea, are treated by either ceftriaxone (250 mg IM) or ciprofloxacin (500 mg PO) followed by a 7-day course of doxycycline (100 mg PO bid). Syphilis is treated using benzathine penicillin (2.4 million IU IM weekly for three doses) in addition to a 21-day course of doxycycline (200 mg PO bid). Erythrasma responds to a 10-day course of erythromycin (250 mg PO tid). The rare case of tuberculosis will require a full 6-month treatment schedule of isoniazid, rifampin, and pyrazinamide, in addition to either streptomycin or ethambutol. This treatment is best undertaken by an infectious disease consultant. Secondary bacterial infection from excess scratching is usually staphylococcal and is best treated by a course of oral dicloxacillin.

Herpes simplex is treated by a 10-day course of acyclovir (400 mg PO bid), which will diminish the symptoms of the primary attack but will have little effect in preventing recurrence. Condyloma acuminatum is treated by destructive techniques using podophyllin, bichloroacetic acid, or topical 5-fluorouracil painted directly on the lesions, or by excision or fulguration (see Chapter 12).

Parasitic infections, mostly commonly due to pinworms, are easily treated by mebendazole (Vermox) 100 mg orally in a single dose with a repeat in 2 weeks. This results in at least a 90% cure but must include follow-up and treatment of the family members as the infestation commonly involves others in the household. Both pediculosis pubis and scabies infestations are treated using lindane 1% (Kwell) cream or lotion, which is applied to the infected area and left in place for 8 to 12 hours, then washed off to prevent side effects from systemic absorption. This application is repeated 1 week later. Other options include pyrethrin and permethrin creams.

Finally, fungal infections are predominantly caused by *Candida,* so it is important to treat any underlying systemic conditions allowing this overgrowth. Specific treatment is best accomplished with topical nystatin, clotrimazole, miconazole, or similar antifungal agents.

Dermatophytic infections require a more specific therapy using Whitfield's ointment (a salicylic and benzoic acid compound) if it does not respond to any of the azole agents mentioned earlier. All these therapies are topical.

Should a dermatologic disorder be diagnosed, the perianal irritation is often only part of a larger condition involving other parts of the body. In this situation the aid of a dermatologist is invaluable. A brief discussion will be given in case this is not available. If the clinical appearance and biopsy report are consistent with eczema (atopic dermatitis), then the careful skin care outlined earlier is used in addition to application of topical steroids and coal tars followed by a covering of petroleum gel. Similar methodology is also used for psoriasis, lichen planus, lichen simplex, and lichen sclerosis et atrophicus. Leukoplakia in itself does not require any treatment other than ruling out neoplasia, but it responds well to removing the irritating etiology.

It is extremely important to remember Paget's and Bowen's diseases. These diseases are covered in detail in Chapter 13. A high index of suspicion is necessary to biopsy any unusual area of skin that may be itchy. Once diagnosed, complete excision is mandatory to prevent the possibility of malignant degeneration. Anal intraepithelial neoplasia (AIN) may present with significant pruritus ani. Only AIN 3 with severe dysplasia requires surgical excision; lesser grades may be followed clinically.

Contact dermatitis requires removal of the allergen and the use of topical steroids. Topical anesthetics are contraindicated as they only hide the symptoms. The same applies for the use of topical antihistamines that may actually result in sensitization. Any local infection is treated with systemic antibiotics. Diabetes mellitus, jaundice, and uremia require therapy of those disorders to bring blood levels closer to a normal range. The addition of cholestyramine (4 g PO tid) may be useful to ease symptoms in biliary disease and uremia.

ALGORITHM

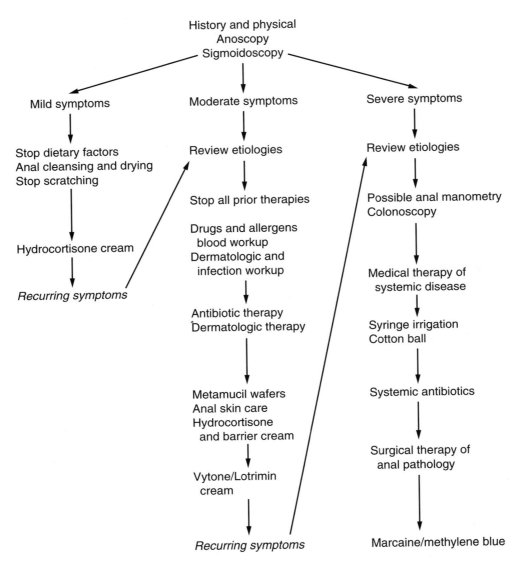

Figure 9-1
Treatment algorithm for pruritus ani.

Primary Pruritus Ani

Dietary factors are the main cause of idiopathic pruritus ani. They can be identified only by obtaining a thorough and systematic dietary history. The patient is then instructed to completely eliminate from the diet the substance that is being taken in the largest quantity. In most circumstances, it will take 2 to 3 weeks before the itching ceases, so perseverance is encouraged. If the itching is not relieved, then the next most likely item is eliminated from the diet while the patient continues to refrain from ingesting the first item. This process continues until either a dietary cause is established or dietary factors are ruled out as a cause. Once the causative dietary factor is identified, that item may be reintroduced gradually until the threshold level is noted. That level must not be exceeded in the future or the symptoms will recur. If compliance is a problem, only the severity of symptoms will drive the patient to comply.

If symptoms remain severe despite this approach, the patient will need to follow further steps to obtain relief. After a bowel movement a bulb tip syringe is used to irrigate the rectum to flush out any fecal residue. Following this, a small cotton ball may be placed on the anal canal to absorb any further seepage and perianal skin contamination.

A steroidal anti-inflammatory cream (preferably acid-based) is then applied, over which a second layer of barrier cream (calamine, calmoseptine, zinc oxide) is placed. Generally, the steroid use should not exceed 3 weeks in order to prevent skin atrophy. Talcum powder is then applied to the area to keep the skin dry. It is important to emphasize to the patient that excessive cleaning is not helpful but rather may damage the skin barrier and set up an underlying infection. Patients are encouraged to persevere with the treatment regimen because it may take several days to a few weeks to see results. If there is failure at this point, a secondary bacterial or yeast infection may be the cause or the patient may be surreptitiously relapsing in his or her dietary intake. If infection is suspected, then a combination of Vytone and Lotrimin may be used to combat a bacterial and fungal infection. If the infection is more severe, then an oral agent such as dicloxacillin (250 mg PO tid) is recommended. Should a patient continue to suffer despite this exhaustive approach, then a dermatology consultation would be helpful to rule out any other possible etiology.

Surgical treatment falls into two categories. First, correction of any anorectal abnormalities thought to be a source of either fecal contamination or inadequate cleanliness is undertaken. This procedure includes repair of rectal prolapse or excision of hemorrhoids, tags, rectal villous adenoma, hidradenitis suppurativa, or ectropion. Fistulotomy or sphincterotomy is indicated for the treatment of fistulas or anal fissures, respectively. Second, surgical treatment involves the subcutaneous injection of an anesthetic agent and methylene blue into the perianal skin. This procedure has typically had poor results causing sepsis and skin necrosis in up to 25% of patients. However, the topic has recently been revisited in an article in which six patients with intractable pruritus ani were given general anesthesia and intravenous antibiotics, and then a combination of 10 mL of methylene blue (1%) mixed with 7.5 mL of marcaine with epinephrine was infiltrated intradermally around the perianal skin. All the patients reported numbness of the skin, and five of the six had substantial reduction of symptoms. No skin necrosis was noted, and the authors felt this was due to the use of smaller volumes of the agents than previously described. This author includes this for interest only, as he has no experience with this technique and has not come across any cases of such severity that it would be indicated.

In summary, pruritus ani is common. In almost all cases the cause may be identified by a careful history and examination of the perianal area. Treatment in most cases consists of three measures: (1) careful but not excessive perianal hygiene, (2) specific treatment of the primary cause, and (3) careful and gentle care of the perianal area in addition to antibiotic therapy if infection has set in. Surgery can allow the anus to close better and helps the patient to maintain cleanliness. Dermatology consultation should be considered when the usual remedies are unsuccessful.

Suggested Readings

Allan A, Ambrose NS, Silverman S, Keighley MRB: Physiological study of pruritus ani. Br J Surg 1987;74:576–579.

Daniel GL, Longo WE, Vemava AM: Pruritus ani: Causes and concerns. Dis Colon Rectum 1994;37:670.

Dasan S, Neill SM, Donaldson DR, Scott HJ: Treatment of persistent pruritus ani in a combined colorectal and dermatological clinic. Br J Surg 1999;86:1337–1340.

Eyres AA, Thompson JPS: Pruritus ani: Is anal sphincter dysfunction important in etiology? BMJ 1979;2:1549–1551.

Farouk R, Lee PWR: Intradermal methylene blue injection for the treatment of intractable idiopathic pruritus ani. Br J Surg 1997;84:670.

Farouk R, Duthie GS, Pryde A, Bartolo DCC: Abnormal transient internal sphincter relaxation in idiopathic pruritus ani: Physiological evidence from ambulatory monitoring. Br J Surg 1994;81:603–606.

Friend WG: The causes and treatment of idiopathic pruritus ani. Dis Colon Rectum 1977;20:40–42.

Pirone E, Infantino A, Masin A, et al: Can proctologic procedures resolve perianal pruritus and mycosis? Int J Colorect Dis 1992;7:18–20.

Smith LE, Henrichs D, McCullah RD: Prospective studies in the etiology and treatment of pruritus ani. Dis Colon Rectum 1982;25:358–363.

10

ANAL STENOSIS

Theodore E. Eisenstat, MD, FACS
Jason Penzer, MD

Anal stenosis (anal stricture) is a common problem in colon and rectal surgery. The diagnosis of anal stenosis is suggested by a history of constipation, occasional bleeding, and difficulty with passage of stool. Pain is frequently associated with anal spasm secondary to fissure, but this condition is not a true stenosis. The diagnosis is confirmed by physical examination. The anal canal may be defined as that part of the alimentary tract from the anal verge to the level of the levator muscle, or anorectal ring. Scarring and contracture may occur in a narrow band-like fashion at the anal verge or occasionally may involve the entire anal canal with a thick unyielding contracture. Severe stenosis may be defined by the inability to pass an 11-mm scope or the index finger into the anal canal. Stenosis of this degree is usually symptomatic and frequently requires operative treatment.

Anal stenosis may be broadly classified with regard to its etiology. An apparent stenosis of the anal canal may be due to anatomic contracture or spasm. Pain may mean that examination under anesthesia is necessary to determine the etiology. Narrowing associated with spasm will be apparent as anesthesia relaxes the sphincters; stricture due to contracture will persist. Stenosis caused by the relative narrowing of the anal canal associated with hypertrophy of the internal sphincter secondary to painful anal fissure is generally treated by lateral internal sphincterotomy, which is discussed in Chapter 3.

Excision of excessive amounts of anoderm during anorectal operations or overambitious electrocoagulation of anal warts resulting in scarring and contracture are the next most frequent causes of anal stenosis. Less common causes of stenosis are listed in Table 10-1.

Postoperative anal stenosis is preventable. Good surgical technique dictates that adequate anoderm be preserved during operative procedures, such as hemorrhoidectomy, in order to prevent postoperative stenosis. In performing the classic closed Ferguson hemorrhoidectomy, three (at most four) hemorrhoids may be removed. During the procedure, adequate bridges of anoderm between excisions must be preserved. If at the completion of the procedure the largest Hill-Ferguson (3.5 cm) anoscope can be introduced into the anal canal, postoperative stricturing will be unlikely. Severe postoperative stenoses, historically, have occurred following the "Whitehead" hemorrhoidectomy. When performed correctly, the "Whitehead" operation should not result in anal

stenosis or ectropion. However, lack of attention to details and poorly performed procedures can result in severe deformities. Do not try to remove all hemorrhoidal disease; later banding of residual internal hemorrhoids and excision of skin tags is preferable to stenosis from over aggressive excision. Be especially conservative when operating on acute hemorrhoidal disease. Postoperatively, fiber or bulking agent should be prescribed in order to assure daily bowel movements. The best way to prevent postoperative stenosis is to pass a formed stool daily.

Inflammatory bowel disease (Crohn's colitis and ulcerative colitis) as well as any condition that predisposes patients to chronic diarrhea, may result in stenosis of the anal canal. The presence of active inflammatory bowel disease, especially with rectal involvement or suppuration, may preclude surgical correction of a stricture. Occasionally, fecal diversion will be required in this group of patients. Gentle dilation under anesthesia with a lubricated dilator has been reported to have good effect in these patients. This success is thought to be related to the absence of new wounds in these inflammatory bowel disease patients, and carries the caveat of using minimal dilation, just adequate to allow the passage of semiliquid stool without disrupting the sphincters.

The elderly and senile, or patients with Alzheimer's disease who chronically abuse laxatives, may develop anal stenosis. Care must be taken to avoid operative intervention in these patients whose continence may, in part, depend upon the presence of anal stenosis. Both the anal stenosis and the atrophy of the sphincters are due to passage of only liquid stools and the lack of natural dilatation by formed movements. Mineral oil has been implicated frequently in these patients. Caution is advised in the management of these patients because correction of the anal stenosis may result in severe incontinence. Education with regard to bowel habits and diet may alleviate symptoms. Anal manometry and biofeedback may also be of value.

■ TREATMENT

Nonoperative Management
Treatment of anal stenosis depends upon its severity and symptoms. Minimal anal stenosis without symptoms requires no treatment at all. Mild to moderate symptoms may require only dietary adjustment and counseling. In patients with these degrees of stenosis, nonoperative management should be initially employed. Dietary manipulation and the use of bulk agents and stool softeners will frequently provide gentle dilatation and symptomatic relief. Severe stenosis and symptoms usually require surgical correction.

Surgical Management
Surgery is indicated for symptomatic patients who do not obtain appropriate benefits from conservative treatment. A lateral sphincterotomy may be all that is required for a stenosis associated with chronic anal fissure.

For moderate stenosis, simple release of the stricture only (anotomy) may suffice (Fig. 10-1), often with a lateral

Table 10-1 Common Causes of Anal Stenosis

Anal fissure
Operative trauma and scarring
Inflammatory bowel disease
Chronic suppuration
Chronic diarrhea
Radiation
Venereal disease
Congenital malformation (imperforate anus, stenosis, or
  membrane)
Neoplasm (benign or malignant anal, perianal, or rectal
  lesions)
Trauma (lacerations, crush, thermal injury, chemical injury)
Infection (tuberculosis, lymphogranuloma venereum,
  schistosomiasis, syphilis, actinomycosis)
Ischemia

sphincterotomy. The lateral sphincterotomy is generally performed in an open fashion, with the wound left open to heal by secondary intention. Granulation of this wound may result in a more adequate orifice in contrast to primary closure. Occasionally, restricture will occur with healing, and multiple anotomies are sometimes necessary (Fig. 10-2).

Stenosis and stricturing that occur following anorectal surgery should initially be managed conservatively. A waiting period of 3 to 6 months is appropriate; frequently, symptoms will resolve with conservative management and gentle office dilatation on a regular basis. Rectal dilators may be employed, but the index finger used on a frequent basis is preferable.

As previously mentioned, active inflammatory bowel disease within the rectum may preclude operative correction. Radiation strictures present a unique problem and are difficult to approach surgically. Fortunately, they are rare.

When stenosis secondary to contracture and scarring requires excision and anoplasty, viable healthy tissues must be moved into the anal canal in order to prevent recurrent scarring and stricture. Mucosal ectropion and scar tissue should be excised prior to advancement of flaps into the anal canal. For severe anal strictures, simple release of the stricture or scar tissue, by anotomy, is usually inadequate. As healing occurs, the contracture reforms. Therefore, transposition of healthy viable tissue into the defect that results after release of the stricture is required. This transposition can be accomplished either by advancing the mucosa or by moving skin into the

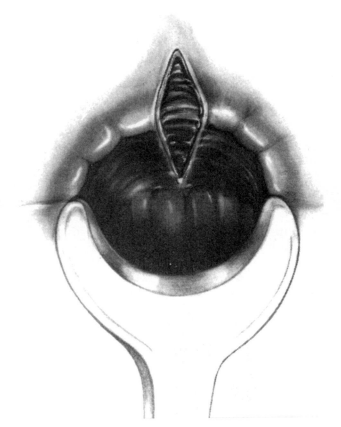

Figure 10-1
Simple anotomy. (From Oliver GC, Rubin RJ: Anoplasty. In Fielding LP, Goldberg, SM (Eds.). Rob & Smith's Operative Surgery. Surgery of the Colon, Rectum and Anus, 5th ed. London, Butterworth-Heinemann, 1993.)

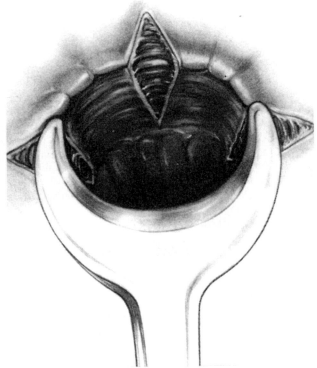

Figure 10-2
Multiple anotomies. (From Oliver GC, Rubin RJ: Anoplasty. In Fielding LP, Goldberg, SM (Eds.). Rob & Smith's Operative Surgery. Surgery of the Colon, Rectum and Anus, 5th ed. London, Butterworth-Heinemann, 1993.)

defect. Because advancement of the mucosa beyond the dentate line will create an ectropion, it is usually preferable to bring skin into the anal canal.

When loss of anoderm is significant and stricture is severe, anoplasty is required. Depending on the severity of the stricture and the resultant deformity following excision of the scar tissue, one of several flap-type procedures may be used. In order of magnitude, these procedures may be described as a "Y-V" advancement flap, "island" advancement flaps, or "S" plasties. The advancement flaps provide viable tissue to fill the defect left after stricture excision and prevent recurrent contracture. Local anesthesia, with the patient in the knee-chest position, can be used for all but the most extensive procedures.

Historically, a "Y-V"–type advancement flap has been used to replace anoderm. An anotomy is performed and continued into a Y-shaped incision to create a flap, which may be advanced into the anal canal. This procedure can be performed in any of the four anal quadrants. Although we most frequently use a single lateral site, the procedure may be performed bilaterally. Limitations relate to the distance this flap can be moved and the resultant tension on the flap. Occasionally, necrosis of the tip may occur, but will not result in restenosis, as long as the width of the interposed flap remains viable

"Island" flaps are recommended for larger defects that require further advancement of viable tissue. "Island" flaps should be constructed such that they include the attached subcutaneous tissue and adaquate blood supply. Closure of the skin defect behind these flaps aids in securing the flap within the anal canal and relieving tension; this maneuver also tends to push the flap into the anal canal. Grafts may be configured as a triangle (Fig. 10-3A and B) or a "house" flap (Fig. 10-4A and B). Care must be taken to ensure that the length of the flap is no longer than its width. Beveling the lateral aspects of the flap is helpful to maintain adequate blood supply. Extensive dissection into the perirectal fat is occasionally required. The graft is mobilized into the anal canal and secured with sutures of 3-0 polyglycolic acid. Multiple flaps can be constructed for severe stenosis, although they probably should be limited to two.

For more severe strictures associated with even greater loss of anoderm, a rotational-type "S" plasty (Fig. 10-5A

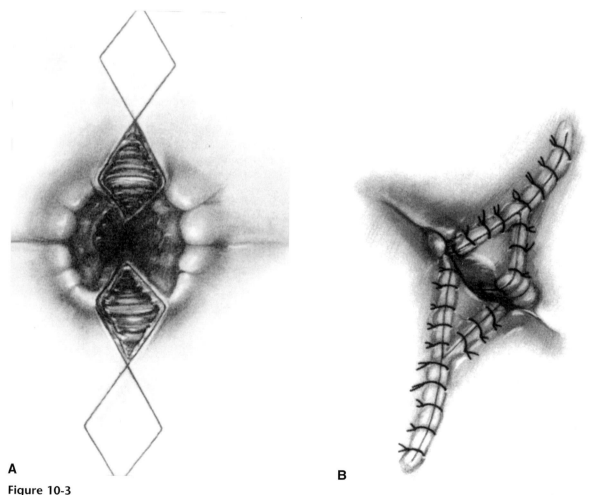

A

B

Figure 10-3
"Triangle" island flap. *A*, Diamond-shaped defects are created by excision of scar. *B*, Triangular flaps are moved into the defects and sutured in place.

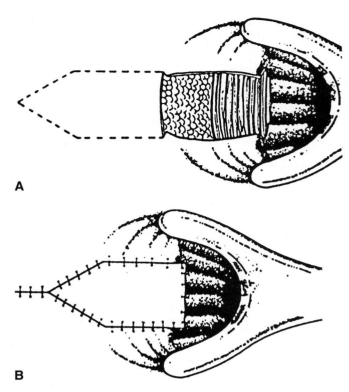

A

B

Figure 10-4
"House" island flap. *A,* Excision of scar leaves a rectangular defect. A "house-shaped" flap is outlined. *B,* The flap is advanced into the anus to cover the defect. Its site of origin is closed directly.

and *B*) may be required. This operation is the procedure of choice for the mucosal ectropion which occurs as the Whitehead deformity after injudicious hemorrhoidectomy.

The two most common postoperative complications that will lead to failure of anoplasty are infection and hematoma. Meticulous surgical technique, therefore, as well as appropriate bowel preparation, is required. For procedures such as simple anotomy and lateral sphincterotomy, bowel preparation is limited to phosphate ene-

mas preoperatively. For the more extensive procedures, oral cathartics as well as oral and intravenous antibiotics should be considered. A short period of a "bowel lock" postoperatively is not required because the preoperative bowel preparation usually precludes bowel activity for 24 to 72 hours. Postoperatively, anoplasty patients should be maintained on a high-fiber diet and bulking agents. Dietary management of this type may be required on a prolonged basis.

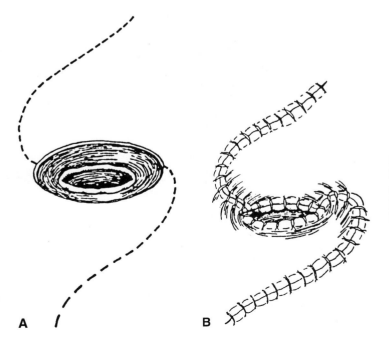

A   **B**

Figure 10-5
Rotational flap (S-plasty). *A,* Circumferential scar is excised, leaving a ring-shaped defect. S-shaped incisions are marked. *B,* The flaps created by the incisions are rotated to cover the defect.

Postoperative follow-up of anorectal surgery patients should include the following:

1. Frequent office visits to assess wound healing and bowel function.
2. Examinations to be sure patients are not impacted and are not having diarrhea from inappropriate use of laxatives.
3. Occasional frequent gentle dilatation by use of the index finger or small sigmoidoscope. (The best dilators are normal postoperative bowel movements.)
4. Follow-up visits until wound healing is complete.

A final issue is the occasional patient with a high anal stenosis, extending from the dentate line to the anorectal ring. Sphincterotomy, either single or multiple, may be quite useful for this cohort. The involvement of mucosa and not anoderm appears to confer an improved prognosis on these patients.

Suggested Readings

Christensen MA, Pitsch RM, Cali RI, et al: House advancement pedicle flap for anal stenosis. Dis Colon Rectum 1992;35:201–203.

Corman ML: Colon and Rectal Surgery, 3rd ed. Philadelphia, Lippincott, 2001.

Oliver GC, Rubin RJ: Anoplasty. In Fielding LP, Goldberg SM (Eds.). Rob & Smith's Operative Surgery. Surgery of the Colon, Rectum and Anus, 5th ed. London, Butterworth-Heinemann, 1993.

Pidala MJ, Slezak FA, Porter JA: Island flap anoplasty for anal canal stenosis and mucosal ectropion. Am Surg 1994;3:194–196.

11

ANAL AND PERIANAL WARTS

José Cintron, MD, FACS, FASCRS

Anal and perianal warts (condylomata acuminata) constitute a significant health problem in the United States, being the most common viral sexually transmitted disease (STD) with an incidence that continues to increase rapidly. In addition, condylomata acuminata probably represent the most common venereal disease seen in a surgical practice. These warts occur with greatest frequency in male homosexual patients but can also be seen in bisexual individuals and in heterosexual men, women, and even children. With respect to children, perianal warts encountered in infants not yet 1 year old may represent vertical transmission from the mother. However, when perianal warts are found in children who are older than 1 year of age, sexual abuse must be considered. It is estimated that approximately half a million individuals each year acquire symptomatic genital warts.

Human papillomavirus (HPV) is the cause of anal and perianal condylomata acuminata. This virus contains a double-stranded circular DNA genome. The virus produces epithelial tumors of the skin and mucous membranes, and is closely associated with genital tract malignancies. More than 70 subtypes of human papillomavirus have been identified, and although the same virus is implicated in warts in other locations, certain subtypes are usually associated with specific sites. HPV subtypes 6, 11, 16, and 18 are most commonly associated with perianal condylomata. Subtypes 6 and 11 are typically encountered with benign condylomata, whereas types 18 and in particular 16 are more commonly seen with severe dysplasia or invasive squamous cell carcinoma. Typing alone, however, is not sufficient for distinguishing benign from malignant disease. The significance of the HPV type is unclear because HPV infection can be multicentric, and two or more types can coexist.

Close personal contact is assumed to be an important factor for the transmission of most cutaneous warts. Furthermore, evidence suggests that anogenital warts are sexually transmitted because the age of onset is similar to that for other STDs, and two thirds of sexual contacts of patients with anogenital warts subsequently develop the disease. Minor trauma at the site of inoculation also seems to be important in the transmission of this disease. Once inoculation occurs, the incubation period usually ranges from 1 to 6 months. All types of squamous epithelium may be infected by HPV, but other tissues seem to be relatively resistant. Infection is thought to begin with the entrance of viral particles into the nuclei of basal cells located in the stratum germinativum, at which time viral replication commences. As the basal cells differentiate and migrate to the surface of the epithelium, HPV DNA replicates and transcribes, and virus particles are assembled in the nucleus.

Condylomata acuminata are usually located in the perianal region, anal canal, perineum, vulva, vagina, cervix, penis, and urethra. Other less common sites include the scrotum, groin, and pubic area. Approximately 50 to 90% of patients with perianal warts also harbor intra-anal warts. Associated genital warts are also commonly seen in 80% of women and 16% of men as reported by Abcarian and Sharon.

Patients with anal warts often present with minor complaints. In fact, when questioned closely, almost all patients note visible or palpable lesions and complain of bleeding, pruritus, irritation, discharge, pain, and difficulty with anal hygiene. Anal and perianal warts have a characteristic appearance that usually allows diagnosis on visual inspection alone. Macroscopically, condylomata acuminata have a papilliform, almost cauliflower-like surface and are usually pink to grayish white. The warts can vary in size and extent from less than a millimeter and hardly visible with the naked eye to extensive circumferential and confluent growths that can occlude the anal aperture (Fig.11-1). The warts may reach considerable size, particularly during pregnancy or immunosuppression. Lesions can be described as flat, sessile, pedunculated, or exophytic.

Microscopically, acanthosis, parakeratosis, and hyperkeratosis can be seen and are due to excessive proliferation of the epidermal layers caused by viral replication. Additionally, some infected cells characteristically transform into koilocytes, which are large, polygonal shaped squamous cells with shrunken nuclei within a large cytoplasmic vacuole (Fig. 11-2).

Perianal and anal warts rarely undergo malignant degeneration, with isolated reports putting the incidence at less than 2%. The spectrum of neoplasia associated with

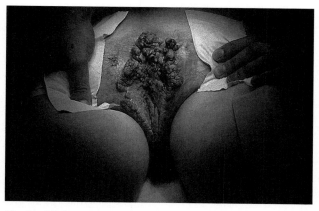

Figure 11-1
Photograph of female patient in prone jack-knife position with extensive circumferential perianal and vulvar warts. The anal opening is nearly occluded. (Courtesy of Richard Nelson, MD.)

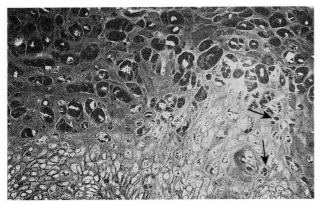

Figure 11-2
Koilocytes (*arrows*) are characteristically seen in condylomata acuminata and represent large, polygonal shaped squamous cells with a hyperchromatic, pleomorphic nucleus and perinuclear halo representing a large cytoplasmic vacuole. (H&E, X235)

HPV ranges from subclinical infection through condylomata to anal intraepithelial neoplasia (AIN) and ultimately invasive squamous cell carcinoma (SCC). Large condylomas that show histologic features of local destructive invasion or malignant behavior without metastases are called Buschke-Loewenstein tumors, giant condylomas, or verrucous carcinomas (Fig.11-3). This rare tumor appears as a large, rapidly enlarging growth that behaves in a malignant fashion. Microscopically, it is difficult to prove the existence of a malignancy despite a malignant transformation rate of greater than 50% and a recurrence rate after excision of approximately 66%. Early wide local excision is the most effective form of treatment despite the high recurrence rate.

In recent years, the use of the colposcope and prior soaking of examined tissues with 3 to 5% acetic acid has expanded the clinical spectrum of anogenital warts. It is well known that HPV infection is associated with carcinoma of the female genital tract, and a parallel relationship has been suggested in the anal canal in the form of AIN. It is possible that AIN lesions could further evolve into invasive SCC, and in fact, HPV has been identified in approximately 60% of anal cancers. Unfortunately, AIN is a relatively recently recognized clinical problem. As yet its prevalence is largely unknown and its malignant potential is uncertain. Because the natural history of AIN is not known, treatment is a clinical dilemma. Levels I and II are usually observed, and Level III may be treated topically. Wide excision of Level III AIN is an option, but recurrence is almost universal.

Condyloma acuminatum of the external anogenital tract is rarely confused with other STDs, such as condyloma latum of syphilis, nodular scabies, genital herpes, lymphogranuloma venereum, chancroid, or granuloma inguinale. However, molluscum contagiosum, particularly in its more atypical presentations, may be difficult to distinguish from anogenital warts. Other conditions considered in the differential diagnosis of condylomata acuminata include keratoses, nevocellular nevi, penile and vestibular papules, the condyloma lata of syphilis, and neoplasia.

■ TREATMENT

Many methods of treating condylomata acuminata have been employed. The treatment can be exceptionally frustrating to both patient and physician owing to the high recurrence rate. Treatment essentially can be categorized into cytotoxic, physically ablative methods and immunotherapy (Table 11-1). The algorithm in Figure 11-4 represents the author's approach in the management and treatment of perianal and anal condylomata acuminata.

Medical Treatment

Cytotoxic podophyllin is the most common topical agent used to treat warts. It is a resin extract from the root of the May apple plant. The active agent, podophyllotoxin, is antimitotic, although its mode of action in warts is unknown. It is usually applied as a 25% suspension in a vehicle, such as tincture of benzoin, which provides better adherence to the warts. Podophyllin is applied directly to the warts, avoiding adjacent normal skin, and then washed off by the patient in 6 to 8 hours to minimize local reactions. It should not be used in the anal canal.

The treatment is repeated at weekly intervals as required, and, therefore, its best use is in the treatment of a very small number of warts. Disadvantages to its use include skin irritation, teratogenic effects in animals contraindicating its use in pregnancy, and the need for repeated applications. Additionally, podophyllin is poorly absorbed by highly keratinized lesions and hence may be ineffective in treating long-standing warts. Lack of regression after four applications suggests the need for different therapy. The application of large amounts of podophyllin may result in severe systemic toxic effects involving the hematologic, hepatic, renal, gastrointestinal, respiratory,

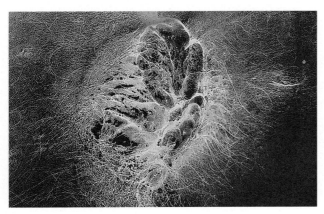

Figure 11-3
Photograph of perianal Buschke-Loewenstein tumor, biopsies of which were always read as condyloma yet clinically behaved in a malignant fashion.

| Table 11-1 | Treatment Methods for Condylomata Acuminata | |
CYTOTOXIC	PHYSICAL	IMMUNOTHERAPY
Podophyllin solution, 25%	Scissors excision	Autologous vaccine
Trichloracetic acid	Electrocoagulation	Alpha-interferon
Bichloracetic acid	Cryotherapy	Imiquimod
5-Fluorouracil cream 5%	Laser fulguration	Cimetidine

and central nervous systems. Other reported complications include severe necrosis, scarring, and fistula in ano. Prolonged treatment with podophyllin is undesirable because it produces dysplasia and may induce temporary cell changes that are difficult to differentiate histologically from carcinoma. These histologic abnormalities will reverse completely within a few weeks of discontinuation of the drug. Unfortunately, results have been disappointing, with recurrence rates reported as high as 30 to 65%. A relatively recent advance is the availability of purified podophyllotoxin (Podofilox) in emulsions of 0.25 and 0.50%, which has the advantage of being the only treatment that is approved for use by patients at home. It is chemically uniform and of standardized potency and is more efficacious and less toxic than podophyllin.

Caustic acids, such as trichloracetic acid and bichloracetic acid, are also used to treat condylomata acuminata.

These acids function by causing tissue sloughing and are applied on a weekly basis until satisfactory results are obtained. Lesions change from pink to frosty white (Figs. 11-5 and 11-6). This agent can be applied to warts within the anal canal but should be dabbed gently with a cotton ball before the walls of the anal canal are allowed to fall back together to limit contralateral burns. If too much acid is applied, the area should be washed with water, and bicarbonate may be applied as a local antidote. Acid is best used when small to moderate numbers of warts are present. Side effects are local in nature, primarily due to skin irritation. Skin ulceration can occur if excess solution is not removed. Reported recurrence rates have been around 25%.

Topical 5-fluorouracil (5-FU) is an antimetabolite and immunostimulative agent that inhibits DNA synthesis. It has been used effectively in the treatment of anogenital

ANAL AND PERIANAL WARTS

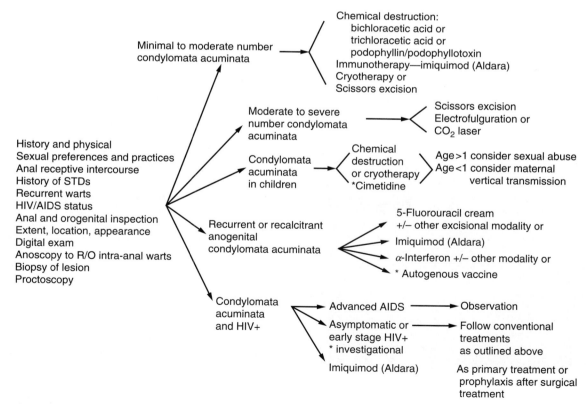

Figure 11-4
Algorithm for the management of perianal warts.

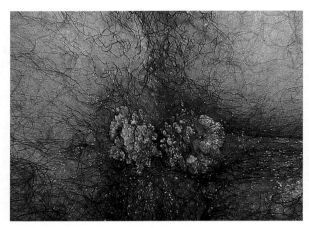

Figure 11-5
Perianal warts prior to application of bichloracetic acid. (Courtesy of The American Society of Colon and Rectal Surgeons.)

warts. Most commonly used in a 5% cream, it is administered daily or periodically over approximately 10 weeks. The Food and Drug Administration, however, has not approved 5-FU for treating genital warts. Mild local discomfort, responsive to cortisone cream, is the usual side effect. Prolonged use can result in erosive dermatitis or mucositis. Like other antimetabolites, 5-FU is contraindicated during pregnancy. It has been used most often in the management of genital warts in women and urethral warts in men, with 40 to 70% response rates and recurrence rates less than 20%. Experience in recurrent perianal warts refractory to other treatments has been favorable. Additionally, it has been used with success in the prevention of recurrence after condylomata ablation, especially in immunocompromised patients, in whom biweekly applications resulted in a 66% decrease in recurrence rate compared to control subjects.

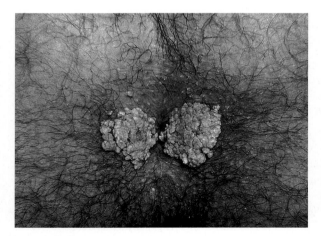

Figure 11-6
Perianal warts after the application of bichloracetic acid. Warts take on a frosty white appearance. (Courtesy of The American Society of Colon and Rectal Surgeons.)

Immunotherapy has been directed predominantly at the treatment of recalcitrant warts. Autogenous vaccination with an extract of the patient's own warts appeared promising in initial studies but was not effective in a subsequent controlled trial. Further randomized controlled studies are needed prior to recommending general application of this promising technique. Imiquimod is an immune response modifier that induces interferon, interleukin, and tumor necrosis factor-alpha (TNF-α). A placebo-controlled trial of a 5% imiquimod cream showed a significant benefit for the cream, although there was a 19% recurrence rate at 12 weeks.

Cimetidine is a histamine receptor antagonist that has immunomodulatory effects at high doses. It has been used to treat common warts with variable success but has also been shown to be useful for treating condylomata acuminata. The daily dose is 30 to 40 mg/kg (up to 3.5 g per day) in three divided doses, for 3 months. Franco reported success in all four children treated.

Interferons are naturally produced proteins with antiviral, immunomodulatory, and antiproliferative properties. Interferon has been evaluated for systemic, topical, and intralesional use. Encouraging results have been supported by four randomized double-blind trials of intralesionally administered interferon. Interferon-α is approved by the Food and Drug Administration for injection in refractory condylomata acuminatum. Current recommendations are to inject 1×10^6 IU under each of a maximum of five lesions three times per week for 3 to 8 weeks. For larger lesions, the total dose should be distributed equally. Side effects of interferon are usually mild and may include viral syndrome symptoms, gastrointestinal complaints, leukopenia, thrombocytopenia, and abnormal liver function. Viral symptoms can be treated effectively with acetaminophen or nonsteroidal anti-inflammatory drugs. Human immunodeficiency virus (HIV)-infected patients do not respond to this treatment. Recurrence rates range from 20 to 40%. Disadvantages include high cost and need for repeated office visits.

Surgical Treatment

Electrocoagulation is an effective method of destroying perianal, anal, and genital warts. It requires anesthesia, the method of which depends on the extent of involvement and the patient's comorbid medical problems. The operator must control the depth and width of the wound to avoid third-degree burns; therefore, the benefits and complications vary according to the surgeon's skill. The area involved with warts can be infiltrated with an epinephrine-containing local anesthetic to control blood loss and splay out lesions so that normal epithelium is preserved. Scissors excision of one or more representative warts should be sent for pathologic evaluation. The warts should be individually fulgurated and curetted, and the base refulgurated with the aim of obtaining a white coagulum. Circumferential burns, especially in the anoderm, should be avoided to prevent anal stenosis and underlying sphincter damage. Complications include pain and discharge, but bleeding, scarring, and anal stenosis occur infrequently. Recurrence rates are approximately 30%.

Postoperatively, patients are instructed to take sitz baths in warm water two to three times daily for 1 week following the procedure. They are prescribed analgesics and told to expect some discomfort. Patients are seen in the office 10 to 14 days postoperatively.

Laser therapy works by physically destroying the warts. Initial enthusiasm was based on reports of less postoperative pain and fewer recurrences, especially in the obstetric and gynecologic literature. Billingham and Lewis, however, studied 38 patients with anal warts, comparing CO_2 laser and electrocoagulation in the same patients, and noted similar pain with both modalities and higher recurrences for the warts treated with laser. Although the laser is rapid and relatively easy to use, it is very expensive and requires special knowledge and experience in its use. Furthermore, consideration should be given regarding vapor transmission of virus particles, and, hence, proper precautions should be taken with the use of goggles, laser mask, and laser smoke evacuator. Postoperative care is similar to that for electrocoagulation.

Cryotherapy has been effectively utilized for anal and perianal warts provided they are small to moderate in size. No anesthetic is necessary and the cold is administered utilizing a cotton-tipped applicator and either liquid nitrogen or CO_2 snow. Alternatively, a cryoprobe may be used. Lesions should be treated on a weekly basis. It is safe to use in the anal canal and can also be used safely during pregnancy. Recurrence rates range from 24 to 37%. Side effects such as burning and ulceration are tolerable. There is little or no scarring, but patients are informed that there can be considerable discharge from the wound postoperatively. Patients are prescribed analgesics and are seen in the office 7 to 10 days after the procedure.

Surgical excision can be performed precisely with the use of fine-tipped scissors and fine-toothed forceps. It is especially useful when there is massive involvement, when excision can be performed quickly and accurately under general or regional anesthesia. This method usually avoids the use of cautery except for control of bleeding. The type of anesthesia required usually depends on the extent of the warts. The patient can be prepared for surgery simply with an enema given that morning. The involved region should be infiltrated with an epinephrine-containing local anesthetic (i.e., 0.25% bupivacaine with 1:200,000 solution of epinephrine) to control bleeding and splay out the lesions to preserve normal epithelium during excision. In the majority of patients it is possible to remove all the warts in one procedure, but if there are too many warts, removal may be done in two stages at an interval of approximately 1 month. Side effects are primarily pain and discharge from the wounds. Postoperative complications include bleeding, prolonged convalescence, scarring, and, rarely, anal stenosis. Recurrence rates have been reported to range between 9 and 42%. Postoperative care is as outlined for electrocoagulation.

Immunocompromised patients have a higher incidence of condylomata acuminata and anogenital neoplasia than the general population. The increase in survival of both transplant recipients and HIV-positive individuals has increased the prevalence of genital warts in these groups. In a prospective study of HIV-positive patients, the most frequent anorectal disease was condylomata, seen in 30%. Anogenital warts in these patients tend to be more aggressive, recur earlier, and are more often dysplastic. Although podophyllin, laser, and fulguration have been used with success, disadvantages include podophyllin-induced pseudoneoplastic changes in an already high-risk group, possible transmission of viral particles in fumes, and high recurrence rates. Despite these disadvantages, studies have shown that patients do well with appropriate treatment. Repeated treatments and close follow-up are needed in immunodeficient patients owing to an increased risk of recurrence and cancer. Topical 5-FU has emerged as one of the best treatment options for decreasing recurrence in this population. Interferon currently is not recommended in this group of patients, and for most patients with advanced AIDS (acquired immune deficiency syndrome), dysplastic lesions should be observed because of potential problems with poor perineal healing.

In summary, patience on the part of the physician and patient is encouraged in the treatment of anal and perianal warts. Patients are counseled as to the high recurrence rate, the need for frequent follow-up in the immediate post-treatment period, and ways to minimize reinfection such as use of condoms, abstinence from anal-receptive or sexual intercourse during treatment, and treatment of recent sexual contacts.

Suggested Readings

Abcarian H, Sharon N: Long-term effectiveness of the immunotherapy of anal condyloma acuminatum. Dis Colon Rectum 1982; 25:648–651.

Beutner KR, Spruance SL, Hougham AJ, et al: Treatment of gential warts with an immune-response modifier (imiquimod). J Am Acad Dermatol 1998;38:230–239.

Billingham RP, Lewis FG: Laser versus electrical cautery in the treatment of condylomata acuminata of the anus. Surg Gynecol Obstet 1982;155:865–867.

Cintron JR: Buschke-Loewenstein tumor of the perianal and anorectal region. Semin Colon Rectal Surg 1995;6:135–139.

Congilosi SM, Madoff RD: Current therapy for recurrent and extensive anal warts. Dis Colon Rectum 1995;38:1101–1107.

Fleshner PR, Freilich MI: Adjuvant interferon for anal condyloma: A prospective randomized trial. Dis Colon Rectum 1994;37:1255–1259.

Franco I: Oral cimetidine for the management of genital and perigenital warts in children. J Urol 2000;164:1074–1075.

Gilson R, Mindel A: Sexually transmitted infections. Recent advances. BMJ 2001;322:1160–1164.

Gordon PH: Condyloma acuminata. In Gordon PH, Nivatvongs S (Eds.). Principles and Practice of Surgery for the Colon, Rectum, and Anus. St. Louis, Quality Medical Publishing, 1992, pp 301–316.

Luchtefeld MA: Perianal condylomata acuminata. Surg Clin North Am 1994;74:1327–1338.

McMillan A: The management of difficult anogential warts. Sex Transmit Infect 1999;75:192–194.

12

ANORECTAL VENEREAL INFECTIONS

Victor L. Modesto, MD, FACS, FASCRS
Lester Gottesman, MD, FACS, FASCRS

"I am the love that dare not speak its name."
—*Lord Alfred Douglas, 1894*

The anorectum has been used with increasing frequency for sexual fulfillment. In both sexes this has resulted in a subsequent growth in the incidence and variety of sexually transmitted diseases (STDs). The promiscuity that is often associated with the homosexual lifestyle is a definite risk factor for STD. Monogamous homosexuals have no higher risk than do monogamous heterosexuals.

Anorectal venereal infections also afflict women who practice anal receptive intercourse (ARI). Heterosexual anal intercourse is far more common than generally realized; more than 10% of American women and their male consorts engage in the act with some regularity.

The diagnosis and treatment of STD is often hampered by the harboring of multiple organisms, only some of which are pathogenic.

■ BACTERIAL INFECTIONS

Gonorrhea
Gonorrhea is caused by *Neisseria gonorrhoeae*, a gram-negative intracellular diplococcus. Anoreceptive transmission, after a 5- to 7-day incubation period, causes proctitis and cryptitis. In women, gonorrhea can result from ARI or by autoinoculation of vaginal gonorrhea into the lower rectum.

When symptoms occur, patients present with severe tenesmus, pruritus, and bloody or mucoid rectal discharge. Initial infection, if untreated, can progress on rare occasions to more advanced disease, such as perihepatitis, meningitis, endocarditis, pericarditis, and probably the most common disseminated form, gonococcal arthritis.

A thick yellow mucopurulent discharge with or without proctitis is highly suggestive of gonorrhea. One classic finding is the ability to express the mucopus from the anal crypts by applying gentle external pressure while the anoscope is in place. Swabbing the mucopus under direct visualization causes a positive yield on Gram's stain in 34 to 79% of cases. The diagnosis is made by culture that has been placed on Thayer-Martin medium.

Preferred Clinical Approach
Empiric treatment is started on clinical suspicion while awaiting definitive culture results because nondiagnostic, or false-negative, Gram's stains do occur. Screening at 3 months post-treatment is an important part of the management, as 35% of patients will suffer recurrent disease. Treatment of all sexual contacts decreases the recurrence rate.

Because of the tremendous rise in the prevalence of penicillinase-producing strains of *Neisseria gonorrhoeae*, penicillin-based therapies are no longer suggested. Uncomplicated gonococcal disease can be treated with 400 mg po of cefixime, 125 mg IM of ceftriaxone, 500 mg po ciprofloxacin, 400 mg po ofloxacin, or 250 mg po levofloxacin. All are given in a single dose and are the currently recommended regimens. Alternative regimens include 2 g IM cefoxitin with 1 g of oral probenecid, 400 mg po single-dose gatifloxacin, 800 mg po single-dose norfloxacin, 400 mg po single-dose lomefloxacin, or 2 g IM single-dose spectinomycin. Since concomitant chlamydial infections are common, a single-dose of azithromycin 1 g is added. With close follow-up and treatment of all sexual partners, a 95% cure rate is a reasonable expectation. Evaluation for other sexually transmitted pathogens, such as syphilis and HIV (human immuno-deficiency virus), is also required, because multiple organisms are often present. Guidance by regional public health services should dictate prevalence of emerging resistant strains of gonorrhea and dictate therapeutic choices.

Chlamydia trachomatis and Lymphogranuloma Venereum
Chlamydia infection is the *most* common STD in the United States. Approximately 4 million chlamydial infections occur yearly in the United States. The incidence is on the rise in both men and women who practice ARI.

Chlamydia proctitis typically occurs within 10 days of penetrating anal sexual contact and may coexist with other STDs, especially gonorrhea. Up to 15% of asymptomatic homosexuals harbor chlamydial organisms. Fifteen immunotypes are known—serovars D through K are responsible for proctitis, and serovars L_1, L_2, and L_3 are responsible for lymphogranuloma venereum (LGV).

Following either ARI or oral-anal intercourse, non-LGV proctitis presents with pain, tenesmus, fever, and an erythematous rectal mucosa, but rarely with mucosal ulcerations. Inguinal nodes may be enlarged and matted. LGV patients also experience pain and tenesmus, but with associated mucosal ulcerations and a more pronounced friability resembling Crohn's proctitis. The inguinal lymphadenopathy plays an important role in differentiating LGV from Crohn's proctitis. Untreated disease can progress to ulceration, causing rectovaginal or rectovesical fistulas, abscesses, and, as a late finding, rectal strictures.

The organism is hard to grow in the laboratory. Antichlamydial antibody titers, as determined by complement fixation test, should be 1:80 or greater to establish the diagnosis. Unfortunately, the titer elevation generally occurs 1 month or more after an infection. The most sensitive serotyping test, the microimmunofluorescent antibody titer, is not universally available. The enzyme immunoassay is the most readily available test, but the diagnosis is best made by nucleic acid amplification tests—either ligase chain reaction (LCR) or polymerase chain reaction (PCR).

Biopsy reveals infectious proctitis with crypt abscesses, infectious granuloma, and giant cells. The presence of granulomas can lead to an erroneous diagnosis of Crohn's proctitis.

Preferred Clinical Approach

Chlamydia trachomatis infections generally respond to oral doxycycline, 100 mg twice a day for 7 days, but a single dose of azithromycin, 1 g po, yields similar success rates and may be more convenient because of better adherence. Alternative regimens include erythromycin base, 500 mg po qid times 7 days; erythromycin ethysuccinate, 800 mg po qid times 7 days; ofloxacin, 300 mg bid times 7 days; or levofloxacin, 500 mg po qid times 7 days. With LGV, treatment course should be extended to 21 days.

Treatment of the strictures is often complicated, because they can be multiple and of varying segments. Many extend to the splenic flexure and must be differentiated from inflammatory bowel disease, ischemia, and cancer.

The treatment of symptomatic strictures should initially include a 3-week course of the appropriate antibiotics. A proximal diversion or sphincter-saving excisional surgery may be the only alternative for treatment failures. Asymptomatic strictures require no treatment.

Chancroid

Chancroid is caused by *Haemophilus ducreyi*, a small gram-negative, nonmotile, non–spore-forming aerobic bacillus. It is characterized by painful adenopathy, multiple perianal abscesses, and tender genital or anorectal ulcers. The soft nature of the ulcers can make it difficult to distinguish from herpes. Lymphadenopathy is present in approximately 50% of cases and sometimes the lymph nodes become suppurative. Chancroid is common in developing countries and facilitates HIV transmission. Effective and early treatment is therefore an important part of any strategy to control spread of HIV infection. Diagnosis is determined by culture. Several different media have been used, but GC agar (GIBCO Laboratories, Grand Island, NY) has the highest sensitivity for the isolation of *H. ducreyi*. Isolation of *H. ducreyi* on selective media is relatively insensitive; however, recent advances in nonculture diagnostic tests have enhanced our ability to diagnose chancroid.

Preferred Clinical Approach

The recommended treatment regimens include azithromycin, 1 g orally (single dose), ceftriaxone, 250 mg IM (single dose), ciprofloxacin, 500 mg po bid times 3 days, or erythromycin base, 500 mg po tid times 7 days. Resolution of the adenopathy lags behind resolution of the ulcers.

Granuloma Inguinale

Granuloma inguinale is a chronic granulomatous infection caused by a gram-negative bacillus, *Calymmatobacterium granulomatis* (*Donovania granulomatis*). The disease is insidious, taking several months before red, shiny, hard masses develop on the genitals or around the anorectum. Scarring can lead to stenosis of the anorectum. Biopsy confirms the diagnosis. The differential diagnosis includes carcinoma, secondary syphilis, and amebiasis. This disease is fairly rare in the United States.

Preferred Clinical Approach

Recommended regimens include doxycycline, 100 mg twice daily for at least 3 weeks, or trimethoprim-sulfamethoxazole, one double-strength tablet (800 mg/160 mg) orally twice daily for at least 3 weeks. Alternative regimens include ciprofloxacin, 750 mg po bid; erythromycin base, 500 mg po qid; or azithromycin, 1 g po q week, all for at least 3 weeks.

Syphilis

The organism (*Treponema pallidum*) enters the anus during ARI, and anal ulcers usually appear within 2 to 6 weeks, but may occur up to 3 months later. In 10 to 20% of cases, the primary lesion, referred to as a chancre, may be hidden within the anal canal. The chancre is usually at the anal verge and is classically painless. In some instances, especially if the lesion becomes secondarily infected, it may cause exquisite pain and be mistaken for an anal fissure. Unlike classic fissures, the lesion may be situated off the midline, peripherally on the anal skin, or proximally above the dentate line. Chancres may be multiple and appear opposite each other, as in a "mirror image" or "kissing" configuration.

With untreated chancres, the ulcer heals spontaneously in 3 to 4 weeks. This stage is followed "classically" 2 to 10 weeks later by secondary lesions in the guise of a diffuse red maculopapular rash on the palms of the hands and soles of the feet.

Secondary syphilis may also present as a pale brown or pink flat verrucous lesion called condyloma latum, a large perianal mass composed of many raised smooth warts, which tend to secrete mucus, and are associated with pruritus and a foul odor. This lesion can coexist with a primary chancre. The differential diagnosis includes condyloma acuminatum, which is often more desiccated and keratinized. Spirochetes are usually demonstrated in condyloma latum on darkfield examination. Both primary and secondary lesions are infectious.

Proctitis in the absence of anogenital lesions has also been reported. Rectal syphilis with inguinal adenopathy has been mistaken for lymphoma, because both diseases present with rubbery inguinal lymphadenopathy and submucosal rectal irregularities. Syphilitic rectal gummas are exceedingly rare and can be confused with malignant growths. Like lymphoma, rectal syphilis is generally accompanied by tenesmus, mucoid discharge, and rectal pain.

In one third of patients, anal syphilis proceeds to spontaneous cure with an additional third remaining latent. About a third of the cases will progress to late or tertiary syphilis (occurring more than 1 year after infection). Asymptomatic central nervous system involvement is demonstrated in up to 25% of patients with late or latent syphilis.

Because of the variable manifestations of syphilitic ulcers, any ulcer in a homosexual or bisexual man must be viewed with suspicion. Women with anal ulcers should be questioned regarding ARI. Anoscopy with darkfield examination of scrapings from the base of the chancre reveals early syphilis.

Serologic tests are defined as either treponemal or nontreponemal. Nontreponemal tests include VDRL (Venereal Disease Research Laboratory) and the RPR (rapid plasma reagin) tests, which vary according to disease activity; hence, titers can reflect persistent disease or responsiveness to treatment. The VDRL is used predominantly for screening, and false positive results have been reported with rheumatologic disorders, Epstein-Barr virus (EBV) infections, and cancer.

T. pallidum–specific assays usually use the fluorescent treponemal antibody absorption test (FTA-ABS). The FTA-ABS becomes positive earlier than the nontreponemal tests and is confirmatory for syphilis.

Preferred Clinical Approach

The treatment of primary syphilis is a single dose of long-acting benzathine penicillin (Bicillin), 2.4 million units intramuscularly. For patients with latent syphilis of less than a one-year duration (early latent syphilis), a single dose of benzathine penicillin is still recommended. However, if the latent period is greater than one year or of unknown duration, then the patient is classified as having late latent syphilis and the 2.4 million unit injection of Bicillin is repeated every week for 3 consecutive weeks for a total of 7.2 million units. In nonpregnant patients allergic to penicillin, doxycycline, 100 mg po bid, or tetracycline, 500 mg po qid, has been used for many years with good results. Ceftriaxone and azithromycin have also been used, but data on efficacy is limited. Follow-up is recommended for all patients, but is especially important in those patients receiving regimens other than penicillin. In patients reporting penicillin allergy, whose adherence and follow-up are deemed unreliable, skin testing and possible desensitization to penicillin is suggested. Pregnant patients reporting penicillin allergy should undergo skin testing and possible desensitization to penicillin as no other therapy is considered reliable. Follow-up testing with the VDRL or RPR should be undertaken at 3-month intervals for 1 year.

■ VIRAL INFECTIONS

Molluscum Contagiosum

Molluscum contagiosum is caused by a poxvirus and transmitted by direct body contact. A painless 3-mm flattened, round, umbilicated lesion develops after an incubation period of 3 to 6 weeks. The disease is benign and self-limiting, but treatment (including local destruction with phenol, surgical treatment, or preferably cryotherapy) is used to prevent spread or for cosmesis.

Preferred Clinical Approach

In the acquired immune deficiency syndrome (AIDS) patient, extensive lesions involving mainly the face and neck are seen. Cutaneous cryptococcal infections in AIDS patients may mimic molluscum contagiosum. Because of similar appearance, the diagnosis is often delayed, as is the institution of systemic antifungal therapy. Therefore, confirmatory biopsy and staining for molluscum bodies appear prudent, especially in HIV-positive patients.

Herpes Simplex Virus

Recently, herpes simples virus (HSV) infections of the anorectal region have become more frequent. Once local inoculation occurs, the virus is transported along the peripheral nerves to the neuronal nucleus. This viral invasion of neurons leads to a latency state that is not well understood.

The risk of recurrence with genital herpes is greater than 80%. In many immunocompetent hosts, recurrence may be subclinical and infrequent or may not occur at all, whereas others may recur monthly. Cell-mediated responses appear to be important in controlling the severity of mucocutaneous outbreaks of the virus, which explains the severe infections observed in HIV-positive patients.

HSV infection begins 4 to 21 days after ARI. The infection usually presents with severe, constant pain in the anorectal region and proctitis, which can be severe, manifesting as constipation, tenesmus, and a mucopurulent discharge. The pain is so intense that it leads to inhibition of the desire to defecate (psychogenic constipation), with subsequent fecal impaction. Systemic manifestations include fever, chills, and malaise. Occasionally, bilateral tender inguinal lymphadenopathy may occur. Neurologic symptoms due to sacral nerve root involvement, such as paresthesia, neuralgia, and pain radiating down the posterior thighs, may be observed. Dyspareunia, urinary retention, and impotence may also occur. The clinical course generally lasts 7 to 21 days, with recurrent infections being mild and rarely associated with systemic symptoms. The disease is highly contagious from the first appearance of the vesicles until perianal re-epithelialization is complete.

During the acute phase, the anorectum is often exquisitely tender, and thus, accurate examination requires topical or regional anesthesia. Inspection may reveal acute lesions ranging from small vesicles with red areolae to larger ruptured vesicles of aphthous coalesced ulcers on the perianal skin or in the anal canal. Shallow perianal ulcers may coalesce and extend to the sacrococcygeal area in a butterfly distribution.

Anoscopy reveals friable epithelium, ulceration, and mucopurulent discharge. Proctoscopy reveals friable mucosa, diffuse ulcerations, and occasional vesicles and pustules limited to the distal 10 cm of the rectum (the extent to which the ejaculum can reach).

Viral cultures of a suspicious vesicle are positive in up to 90% of clinical HSV-2 infections. Scrapings of the ulcerations stained with Giemsa's stain reveal the multinucleated giant cells typical of herpetic infection (Tzanck preparation). A direct biopsy may also reveal the typical giant cells or intranuclear inclusion bodies. Trauma and Behçet's syndrome may mimic the painful anorectal lesions seen in anorectal herpes.

Preferred Clinical Approach

Treatment includes both the acute infection and suppressive therapy to diminish recurrence. Management of the acute infection includes palliative measures, such as sitz bath, stool softeners, and analgesics.

No effective cure for HSV-2 infection is known. Antiviral agents, particularly acyclovir, shorten the clinical course, decrease the severity, and suppress HSV-2 infection in most patients. Newer agents such as valacyclovir and famciclovir (Famvir) have superior bioavailability in oral formulations. Acyclovir is available in topical (5%), oral, and intravenous formulations.

The recommended regimens for an initial episode of HSV include acyclovir, 400 mg po tid times 7–10 days; acyclovir, 200 mg po five times daily for 7–10 days; famciclovir, 250 po tid times 7–10 days; or valacyclovir, 1 g po tid times 7–10 days.

Effective episodic treatment of recurrent disease is most effective when administered within 1 day of lesion outbreaks and may require that the patient include acyclovir, 400 mg po tid or 800 mg po bid both for 5 days; famciclovir, 125 mg po bid times 5 days; valacyclovir, 500 mg po mg po bid times 3–5 days; or valacyclovir, 1 g po qd for 5 days.

For patients with recurrent outbreaks, consider suppressive therapy with acyclovir, 400 mg po bid; famciclovir, 250 mg po bid; valacyclovir, either 500 mg or 1 g po qd indefinitely.

Condylomata Acuminata

Condylomata acuminata (anal and perianal warts) is the most common sexually transmitted disease seen by the colon and rectal surgeon. The issue is discussed in detail in Chapter 11.

The disease is caused by human papillomavirus (HPV), of which more than 70 different types have been identified, each exhibiting some tissue and disease specificity. HPV types 6 and 11 are most commonly associated with benign, exophytic condylomata acuminata of the anogenital region, as well as low-grade dysplasia. Types 16 and 18 have been associated with anogenital condylomata and the more severe forms of dysplasia, including invasive squamous cell carcinoma. This emphasizes the need for HPV typing to assess the malignant potential of the HPV lesion and to identify those patients requiring closer surveillance. Homosexual men (in whom HPV is prevalent) are at increased risk for the development of invasive anal carcinoma.

The typical patient is a sexually active homosexual or bisexual man, although lesions in the perianal region may be seen in heterosexual men, women, and even children. The primary mode of transmission of anogenital HPV infection is sexual intercourse, although spread may occur through close nonsexual contact.

Clinical Manifestations

After a 1- to 3-month period of incubation, condylomata acuminata are easily recognizable as either pinhead-sized lesions or projecting cauliflower-like masses. Individual warts may be sessile or pedunculated, having a tendency to grow in radial rows that may become confluent and form almost an entire sheet around the anal orifice, sometimes obscuring the anal aperture. Symptoms may include pruritus ani, bleeding, discharge, persistent perianal wetness, and pain. Some patients complain of a lump or mass. In symptomatic homosexual men condylomata are confined to the perianal area in only 6%, whereas both perianal and intra-anal lesions are noted in 84%. Furthermore, 10% of symptomatic patients have only intra-anal condylomata, emphasizing the importance of anoscopy. The condylomata are usually confined below the dentate line except in immunocompromised patients. Acetic acid enhances visualization. Isolated treatment of perianal condylomata acuminata without coincidental treatment of the concomitant anal canal condylomata acuminata is doomed to failure.

A variant of anal condylomata is the giant condyloma acuminatum (Buschke-Loewenstein tumor, verrucous carcinoma). Clinically, it appears as a rapidly growing, fungating squamous cell carcinoma that histologically shows no evidence of invasion. The aggressive nature of the lesion may cause multiple sinuses or fistulous tracts that can invade fascia, muscle, or rectum and cause inflammation, infection, and hemorrhage. Microscopically, the lesions bear a strong resemblance to condyloma acuminatum, and there is no evidence of invasion of lymphatics or blood vessels or other histopathologic criteria of malignancy. The treatment for verrucous carcinoma is surgical, and the extent of the operation should be individualized. Wide local excision with clear margins is recommended. If the anal sphincter is involved, then abdominoperineal resection should be performed, as it offers the only hope of permanent cure.

Treatment

Anal and perianal warts are notorious for their recurrence. All patients should undergo anoscopy, proctosigmoidoscopy, and either vaginal or penile examination. Treatment includes excisional therapy, immunotherapy, and destructive therapy. Reported recurrence rates range from 10 to 75%. Accuracy in determining recurrence rates is not easily achieved because it is often difficult to distinguish cases of true recurrence from reinfection. The prevalence of anal squamous intraepithelial lesions is high among HIV-positive homosexual males and to a lesser extent among HIV-negative homosexual males. The natural history of anal intraepithelial neoplasm (AIN) has not been fully established, and this prevents clinicians form defining clear management protocols. Treatment options are often limited by morbidity and high recurrence rates. Early detection may permit better tolerance of therapy. Therefore, individuals who engage in anal receptive intercourse should have high-resolution anoscopy and aggressive biopsy of abnormal areas because of a high prevalence of AIN.

Preferred Clinical Approach

Electrocautery. Most patients are treated in the office setting, with more extensive lesions reserved for the operating room. In the office, patients are placed in the prone jack-knife position; pulse oximetry is used, and the buttocks are held apart by adhesive tape. Intravenous sedation can be used depending on the need; however, all patients receive local anesthesia with a lidocaine-marcaine preparation mixed with sodium bicarbonate to eliminate the burning sensation associated with administration. A headlight is used for good direct lighting and a 3 to 5% solution of acetic acid is applied to the warts for better visualization. The HPV-infected lesions are prone to aceto-whitening and stand out from the surrounding mucosa or skin.

Either a circumferential field block is administered or each wart is individually injected, depending on the extensiveness of the disease. Excision of several condylomata is performed for histopathologic evaluation if the lesion appears suspicious for neoplasm.

Electrocautery is then used for the remainder of the warts. The aim is to produce a white coagulum, which is the equivalent of a superficial second-degree burn. After adequate anesthesia, the cautery tip is placed near, but not into, the wart and a "spark gap" is created, producing a white coagulum. One must be careful not to allow too deep a burn or fibrous scarring may result. A wheal can be created with local anesthesia to elevate the warty tissue and spare normal skin. Intense pain and sphincter spasm may occur both during and after the procedure, requiring oral analgesics. Patients are usually seen 4 to 6 weeks later. They are followed until they remain recurrence-free for 1 year. Anal stenosis is a potential complication.

Electrocautery is a rapid method for treating multiple small warts, that is, less than 5 mm. This method is often combined with scissor excision of larger warts. Recurrence rates range from 10 to 25%.

For patients with extensive recurrent disease, a single injection of 10 million IU of interferon-α2b is used in combination with electrocautery. The injection is given into the operative bed. Five percent aldara (Imiquimod) ointment can be used as an adjunct to surgical treatment in patients with recurrent disease. Treatment is three times a week for 12 weeks.

Sexually Transmitted Diseases in AIDS Patients

HIV infection influences the acquisition rates, severity, transmission, and host response for a variety of STDs. In many situations, rates of acquisition are increased, severity is worsened, persistence is prolonged, and treatment response is impaired in the HIV-positive persons. STDs, as mentioned previously, are managed accordingly in HIV-positive and AIDS patients, with the exception of chancroid, syphilis, HSV, condylomata acuminata, and those STDs specific for AIDS patients (e.g., cytomegalovirus, *Mycobacterium avium-intracellulare* infection).

HIV infection results in increased ease of acquisition of chancroid; larger, more persistent ulcers; and increased resistance to single-dose treatment. As a result, the preva-lence of chancroid is increased among HIV-seropositive patients. Treatment failures are six times more common in the HIV-positive patient. Evidence suggests that genital ulcers (principally chancroid) play a role in the sexual transmission of HIV, not only by providing a mechanical portal for shedding and entry of HIV, but also by biologically enhancing transmission.

Syphilis may also have an atypical presentation, and serologic tests may be falsely positive or negative. Early progression to central nervous system (CNS) disease can occur. Treatment failures are also more common when standard therapy is used; therefore, many experts advocate more intensive therapy for HIV-positive persons with syphilis. Routine examination of cerebrospinal fluid (CSF) is also advocated by some experts for patients with concomitant HIV infection who have any form of syphilis. Others simply treat all HIV-positive patients using the neurosyphilis protocol (intramuscular benzathine penicillin G weekly for 3 weeks). However, the clear consensus is that all patients with syphilis should be tested for HIV infections to assist in clinical management and that serologic tests for syphilis are indicated in all HIV-positive patients.

The development of acyclovir-resistant strains of HSV-2 (thymidine kinase–deficient HSV-2) should be considered if lesions fail to improve and if they remain culture positive after 1 full week of treatment on adequate doses of acyclovir. Successful treatment of acyclovir-resistant HSV-2 infections in AIDS patients has been reported using the drug foscarnet and to a lesser extent monophosphate (ARA-A). Resistance to foscarnet has been reported. Once treatment is discontinued, however, the relapse rate is high.

HPV infection in immunocompromised patients shows a propensity for dysplastic and neoplastic changes. Anal condylomata are more aggressive in the immunosuppressed patient, and recurrence rates are higher. Intralesional interferon has not been shown to benefit HIV-seropositive patients with anogenital warts, and warts treated with topical agents also appear to require a longer course of therapy in HIV-positive than in HIV-negative patients.

Anal condylomata in HIV-positive patients are managed in the following manner: Observation alone is appropriate for those with late-stage disease. Symptomatic patients with warts limited to the anal margin are treated with one or two applications of podophyllin (5% in benzoin), BCAA, or fulguration. Those with anal canal lesions are offered excision and/or fulguration, with either general or regional anesthesia.

Patients with HIV are predisposed to develop dysplasia or even invasive cancer in tissue involved by condylomata. Thus, patients are followed carefully and regularly. Whether the optimal treatment for those with high-grade dysplasia should include wide excision, or whether simple local excision and close postoperative monitoring is adequate is unclear at present.

Although many of the preceding conditions may present as ulcers in the HIV-positive patient, simple anal fissures remain the most common acutely ulcerative process seen in these patients. However, patients with HIV may also develop AIDS-specific ulcers of the anal canal. These tend to be wider and longer than benign fissures. They are frequently deeply erosive, and may be more proximal in the anal canal than traditional fissures. Retained pus and stool within the fissures and the cavities underlying them cause acute pain, which is best treated by débridement and unroofing of any cavity, with additional intralesional injection of depot steroids.

■ INFECTIOUS DIARRHEAL DISORDERS

Many infections are seen with impressive regularity in the homosexual and bisexual male population. These diseases include amebiasis, giardiasis, and infections with *Enterobius vermicularis* and other helminths. The mode of transmission is fecal-oral.

Amebiasis

Entamoeba histolytica is a protozoan that commonly infects humans. Transmission is related to sanitation measures or sexual activity. The prevalence rate for infection with *E. histolytica* among homosexual and bisexual men ranges between 20 and 30%. Twenty to 70% of the homosexual population with diarrhea is found to harbor one or more protozoan organisms in the stool. Amebic cysts may be ingested in contaminated food or drink, but in the homosexual population, transmission is usually via oral-anal intercourse with an infected partner.

Preferred Clinical Approach

Diagnosis is made by examining the stool for amebas. A number of serologic tests can be used to diagnose amebic infection, including the indirect hemagglutination test, the indirect immunoelectrophoresis test, and an enzyme-linked immunosorbent assay (ELISA). Endoscopic evaluation of the colon can be performed. Sigmoidoscopy is adequate for the majority of patients because distal disease is seen in up to 85%. The "classic" finding is round ulcerations, 2 mm to 2 cm in diameter, covered with exudate and with normal mucosa between the ulcers. Examination of endoscopically obtained stool and mucus samples reveal trophozoites in about 85% of cases. Metronidazole is the treatment of choice. It is the only orally administered drug that provides amebicidal concentrations both systemically and in the bowel lumen. The dose is 500–750 mg orally three times a day for 10 days. Intravenous metronidazole does not provide amebicidal levels in the intestinal lumen.

Giardiasis

Giardia lamblia organisms are intestinal flagellates that inhabit the upper small intestine and biliary tract of infected individuals and are transmitted via oral-anal intercourse with an infected partner. Anoscopic and sigmoidoscopic findings are usually normal, but could reveal diffuse ulcerations. Identification of trophozoites in a fresh stool specimen, in the scrapings from an ulcer base,

or in jejunal biopsies will make the diagnosis. Treatment consists of 250 mg metronidazole by mouth three times a day for 5 days.

Shigellosis

The true incidence of *Shigella* infection in the homosexual population is unknown, but 30 to 50% of shigellosis occurring in New York City, San Francisco, and Seattle is found in homosexuals. Transmitted by direct or indirect fecal-oral route, patients can present with lower abdominal pain, the onset of bloody mucoid diarrhea, urgency, and tenesmus. A significant percentage will mimic acute appendicitis. Shigellosis should be suspected whenever an acute diarrheal illness productive of bloody mucoid stools lasts longer than 2 days. Sigmoidoscopy often reveals inflamed, ecchymotic, friable, or ulcerated mucosa. The diagnosis is made by stool culture. Most laboratories routinely culture fecal specimens for *Shigella* organisms.

Preferred Clinical Approach

The illness is self-limiting, lasting on the average 1 week. However, untreated patients shed viable organisms for up to 1 month after resolution of symptoms. Antibiotic treatment shortens the clinical illness and limits the time of active shedding of the organisms. We recommend antibiotic treatment with 500 mg of ciprofloxacin given by mouth twice a day for 3 to 5 days. Alternately, double-strength trimethoprin-sulfamethoxazole, twice a day for 3 days is an acceptable regimen. All patients should have follow-up cultures to document eradication of the organism.

Campylobacter Infection

Campylobacter jejuni is recognized as a common cause of enterocolitis or infectious diarrhea. Although no proof of sexual transmission exists, *Campylobacter jejuni*, *Campylobacter fetus*, and *Campylobacter intestinalis* infections are seen in homosexual men more frequently than in matched heterosexual control subjects.

The most common symptoms are diarrhea, abdominal pain, and fever. Diarrhea may or may not be bloody and varies in severity. Abdominal pain tends to be colicky and can be localized to any part of the abdomen. It can be confused with appendicitis. Sigmoidoscopy reveals nonspecific colitis characterized by erythema and edema; aphthous ulcerations may also be seen. Histologically, a nonspecific acute inflammatory infiltrate in the lamina propria with crypt abscesses, ulceration, and atrophy may be observed. Microscopic examination of fecal smears reveals polymorphonuclear leukocytes and red blood cells. A presumptive diagnosis can be made if phase-contrast or darkfield microscopy of fresh fecal specimens demonstrates rapidly moving, curved, rod-shaped organisms. Similarly, Gram's stains demonstrate *Vibrio* forms suggestive of *Campylobacter* infections. Stool culture is the only means of definitively establishing the diagnosis. Many laboratories do not routinely culture for *Campylobacter*; therefore, specific requests are necessary.

Preferred Clinical Approach

The illness is usually self-limited; antimotility agents should be avoided, because toxic megacolon has been reported. Although antibiotic therapy is not necessary for all cases, patients who are very sick or at high risk (immunocompromised) should be treated. The preferred regimen is azithromycin, 500 mg orally a day for 3 days, or ciprofloxin, 500 mg orally twice a day. Alternatively, 500 g erythromycin may be given orally four times a day for 5 days. Relapses occur in 5 to 10% of cases.

Cryptosporidiosis

Cryptosporidial colitis is usually a self-limited infection in nonimmunocompromised patients; however, in patients with AIDS, it produces a life-threatening colitis. Patients present with a profuse (5 to 10 L per day), often bloody mucoid diarrhea. Electrolyte imbalance, dehydration, and prostration ensues. The diagnosis is established from histopathologic examination of rectal biopsy specimens, which demonstrate the characteristic oocysts. Alternatively the organisms may be seen on either routine or modified acid-fast (Kenyoun) stain. Very thin tissue sections and proper fixation are necessary to identify these minuscule protozoans.

Preferred Clinical Approach

Treatment is largely supportive with rehydration and nutritional support. Since cryptosporidiosis is not commonly seen in non-HIV-infected homosexuals, its presence should alert the physician to the need for HIV testing.

Isosporiasis

Isospora belli, an opportunistic protozoan, has much lower prevalence than does *Cryptosporidium* in patients with AIDS. *Isospora belli* causes symptoms similar to those caused by *Cryptosporidium*: diarrhea, vomiting, fever, and abdominal pain. However, the quantity of diarrhea tends to be less with *Isospora belli*.

Preferred Clinical Approach

The diagnosis is made by using a modified acid-fast stain on a fresh stool specimen. Endoscopic biopsy followed by histopathologic tissue examination may also reveal the organism. In contrast to cryptosporidiosis, isosporiasis responds promptly to antiprotozoal therapy. Treatment is initiated with double-strength trimethoprim-sulfamethoxazole twice a day for 10 days. Because relapse rates are high, prophylaxis with a nightly dose of double-strength trimethoprim-sulfamethoxazole twice a day for an additional 3 weeks in patients with AIDS is suggested.

Mycobacterium avium-intracellulare

Mycobacterium avium-intracellulare (MAI) is an opportunistic microbial pathogen causing a disseminated infection, noted in virtually 100% of AIDS patients at autopsy. Some patients remain asymptomatic carriers, and others develop profuse watery diarrhea with its associated dehydration, malabsorption, and severe abdominal pain. The diagnosis can be made by examining the stool with acid-fast stains; if it is negative, ileocolonic biopsies should be obtained by colonoscopy with the tissue stained for acid-fast bacilli. Granuloma formation is rare because of the lack of T cells; however, macrophages filled with acid-fast mycobacteria can be seen.

Computed tomographic (CT) scan findings include diffuse bowel wall thickening, enlarged soft-tissue densities (lymph nodes), and marked hepatic and splenic enlargement.

The complications of abdominal MAI infections include obstruction (30%), fistulas (2% to 20%), perforation (5%), and bleeding (20%).

Medical treatment is discouraging. Resistance to standard antituberculosis drugs is common. Newer agents are being tried, such as quinolines, amikacin sulfate, and macrolide antibiotics.

Acknowledgment. Special acknowledgment to Jason C. Sniffen, DO, infectious disease consultant, for his assistance with this chapter.

Suggested Readings

Centers for Disease Control: 2002 Sexually Transmitted Diseases Treatment Guidelines. MMWR May 10, 2002;51:RR-6.

Gottesman L: Ulcerative disease of the anorectum in AIDS. Int J STD AIDS 1995;6:4–6.

Modesto VL, Gottesman L: Sexually transmitted diseases and anal manifestations of AIDS. Surg Clin North Am 1994;74(6):1433–1464.

Modesto VL, Gottesman L: Sexually transmitted diseases. In Wexner SD, Vernava AM III (Eds.): Clinical Decision Making in Colorectal Surgery. New York, IGAKU-SHOIN, 1995, pp 195–198.

Sobhani I, Vuagnat A, Walker F, et al: Prevalence of high-grade dysplasia and cancer in the anal canal in human papillomavirus–infected individuals. Gastroenterology 2001;120:857–866.

Wexner SD, Beck DE: Sexually transmitted and infectious diseases. In Beck DE, Wexner SD (Eds.): Fundamentals of Anorectal Surgery. New York, McGraw-Hill, 1992, pp 402–422.

13

BOWEN'S DISEASE AND PAGET'S DISEASE

Richard J. Strauss, MD, FACS
John A. Procaccino, MD, FACS
Michael A. Moffa, MD

Malignant neoplasms of the anal margin and perianal skin include basal cell cancer, extramammary Paget's disease (intraepithelial adenocarcinoma), Bowen's disease (intraepithelial squamous cell carcinoma), malignant melanoma, and epidermoid cancer. As a group they account for 3 to 4% of all anorectal cancers. This chapter deals with Bowen's and Paget's diseases.

A correct diagnosis is based on a high index of suspicion on the part of the surgeon. A biopsy of all nonhealing lesions and all perianal growths must be performed with microscopic tissue analysis.

Symptoms produced by an anal neoplasm, regardless of histologic type, are similar to those seen with more common inflammatory and benign conditions and are usually nonspecific. A patient with either condition may describe pruritus, burning, pain, bleeding, drainage, or sensation of a mass. Lack of attention to these common complaints may delay diagnosis of a malignant tumor of the anal region.

■ BOWEN'S DISEASE

Although the clinical appearance of perianal Bowen's disease may be dismissed as a vague skin irritation, recognition and treatment of the condition are important because of its potential for becoming an invasive, keratinizing squamous cell cancer.

Bowen's disease of the perianal skin is a rare, slow-growing, intraepidermal squamous cell cancer (carcinoma in situ) occurring most often in patients who are 50 to 60 years of age. It often masquerades as a chronic dermatosis and may be so small or nondescript that it is found only incidentally during histologic examination of perianal tissue removed during another anorectal procedure. Alternatively, the lesion may be a large, irregular, erythematous or pigmented zone of scaly, fissured plaques that slowly extend over a wide area (Fig. 13-1).

When Bowen first described this entity in 1913, he designated it a precancerous dermatosis. Now, however, Bowen's disease is considered to be a slowly maturing intraepidermal squamous cell carcinoma from its very beginning, with a tendency to invade and metastasize in less than 5% of cases.

Histologically, the perianal epidermal lesion may show hyperkeratosis, parakeratosis, and marked acanthosis. The malpighian cells have a disorderly type of hyperplasia, with atypism and malignant dyskeratotic cells. Characteristic of this disease is the Bowen cell, a large, atypical cell with a haloed, giant, or "clumped" hyperchromatic nucleus produced by amitotic cell division. Both mitotic and amitotic figures are often numerous. Intracellular edema produces a haloed effect on the large hyperchromatic nuclei of the atypical cells. The cells vary in size and shape. A chronic round cell and plasma cell inflammatory infiltrate is always present in the dermis. The gross appearance is often that of a raised, irregular, scaly, brownish red plaque with eczematoid characteristics. However, the lesion is usually not characteristic or diagnostic in itself, and biopsy is necessary for diagnosis.

The differential diagnosis of these lesions includes leukoplakia, perianal Paget's disease, squamous cell cancer, condyloma acuminatum, dermatitis, eczema, and downward spread of rectal carcinoma. There also exists an entity known as bowenoid papulosis that appears much the same histologically. These lesions are multiple and discrete and are associated with human papillomavirus (HPV) types 16 and 18. Treatment consists of eradication in a fashion similar to that used for condyloma.

Any suspicious anal lesion, or one that fails to respond to conventional therapy within a month, should be biopsied. An adequate biopsy is essential both to confirm the diagnosis and to exclude an invasive carcinoma. A proper biopsy entails several full-thickness samples from the central portion and the edges of the lesion. Biopsy techniques are discussed later in this chapter.

In a study of 33 patients with perianal Bowen's disease reported by Beck and colleagues from the Cleveland Clinic, 13 patients (39%) were diagnosed after histologic examination of hemorrhoidectomy specimens, whereas the remaining 20 patients (61%) had symptomatic perianal lesions for from 1 month to 10 years.

A curiosity of Bowen's disease has been its supposed relationship to other systemic and cutaneous cancers. In

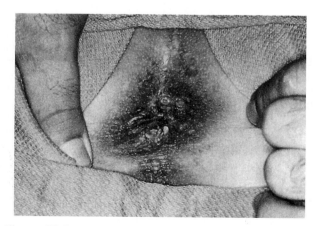

Figure 13-1
Bowen's disease, a chronic intraepithelial squamous cell carcinoma.

1961 Graham and Helwig found that systemic malignant neoplasms developed in one third of the patients with Bowen' s disease within 10 years of the original diagnosis. This was also the case in Beck's study in which 10 of 33 patients had histories of prior cancer. This paraneoplastic nature of Bowen's disease is supported by the recent independent work of Hughes and Takata, who concluded that accumulation of the p53 tumor suppressor protein might be an important mechanism of oncogenesis in these neoplasms.

■ MANAGEMENT

We have described a systematic approach to the diagnosis and treatment of perianal Bowen's disease. This type of approach is important when the surgeon encounters a patient who has recently undergone hemorrhoidectomy with the pathology report having revealed Bowen's disease. The surgeon needs to apply a systematic approach to biopsy the distorted anal area. Biopsies are performed to map affected areas so that during subsequent wide local excision, as much of the anal mucosa and skin can be preserved as possible. According to Goligher, the sensitive anal and lower rectal mucosa are as important in the mechanism of continence as the sphincter musculature itself, and he considers retention of the anal skin important for continence. When this method of treatment was used, no patients demonstrated local recurrence, invasive anal cancer, or metastasis.

The techniques include the administration of laxatives and enemas preoperatively so that if skin grafting is necessary, the patient will not have an early bowel movement that may soil the graft.

At operation the patient is placed in the Kraske position, and the buttocks are taped apart. After antiseptic skin preparation of the thighs and buttocks, the perianal skin and anal canal are carefully examined to evaluate any gross lesions.

A systematic four-quadrant biopsy of the anal canal, anal verge, and perianal skin is performed in addition to biopsy of any abnormal-appearing skin; therefore, at least 12 biopsies are performed (Fig. 13-2). This procedure is done under local anesthesia with intravenous sedation.

The biopsy specimens are about 4 mm by 4 mm in size. They are carefully labeled as to their origin and sent for immediate frozen section evaluation. If any of the specimens show intraepidermal cancer, additional biopsies are taken to define the limits of the disease. Many of the samples appear to be normal skin, but it is impossible to determine the limits of the lesion by gross inspection. After mapping the limits of the disease, all the involved skin is removed, with wide local excision of any gross lesions. This area often includes the skin of the entire circumference of the perianal and anal regions.

The wound can be handled in several ways. Small defects can be closed primarily or left open to heal by secondary intention. Defects greater than 50% of the circumference of the anus are covered by split-thickness skin graft to avoid anal stenosis. If grafting is required, these

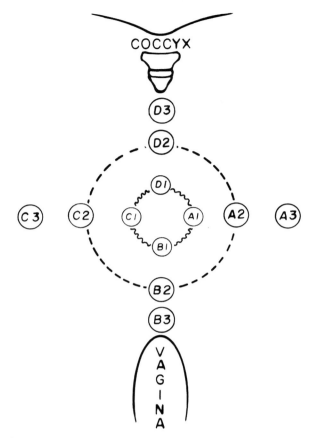

Figure 13-2
Technique of four-quadrant biopsy of the perineum: 1, dentate line; 2, anal verge; 3, perineum.

patients are put on a postoperative regimen of bed rest for 1 week and a clear liquid diet for 5 to 7 days. Additionally, they are given tincture of opium (0.6 mL every 4 hours) and diphenoxylate atropine (Lomotil) elixir (5 mg every 6 hours) to help prevent a bowel movement causing soilage of the graft.

Follow-up visits at intervals of 6 months are recommended. If recurrent Bowen's disease is found at follow-up examination and is confined to the skin, local excision is again the treatment of choice. This procedure may be repeated as often as necessary.

If there is no gross evidence of recurrent Bowen's disease after 1 year, we recommend that the patient have random biopsies taken (as described). Long-term follow-up is then necessary to identify other potential malignancies or recurrences in the patient with perianal Bowen' s disease.

■ PAGET'S DISEASE

Darier and Coulillaud first described perianal Paget's disease or extramammary Paget's disease of the perianal region in 1893. It is an extremely rare tumor arising from the dermal apocrine sweat glands and is an intraepithelial adenocarcinoma. Unlike Paget's disease of the nipple, which virtually always overlies a mammary duct cancer, in many cases extramammary Paget's disease is not associated with invasive tumor.

Since the report by Darier and Coulillaud, approximately 150 cases of perianal Paget's disease have been reported, although the true incidence is probably higher. Extramammary Paget's disease may be found in the axillary or anogenital region. It is a malignant neoplasm of the intraepidermal portion of the apocrine glands with or without associated dermal involvement. Morson believes that Paget's disease of the perianal skin has a long preinvasive stage, ultimately leading to an adenocarcinoma of the apocrine gland type.

Like perianal Bowen's disease, perianal Paget's disease is more common in women than in men. The average age of affected people is in their 60s and a significant number have an associated malignancy. Grodsky reported a 50% incidence of underlying carcinoma in such patients. Fazio and Tjandra reported a 69% incidence. Associated cancers included apocrine or eccrine carcinoma (36%), rectal adenocarcinoma (22%), and anal carcinoma (11%). The remaining 31% of patients without malignancy are evidence of a biologic difference between perianal Paget's disease and its mammary counterpart, which is almost universally associated with underlying invasive carcinoma.

The most prominent clinical feature of the condition is an intractable itch that has often been present for months. There may also be discharge, ulceration, and occasionally bleeding and pain. The lesions are usually erythematous, raised, crusted, scaly, or eczematoid and plaque-like and are similar to other cutaneous lesions, making clinical diagnosis difficult (Fig. 13-3). These lesions may sometimes have a gross appearance similar to that of leukoplakia, squamous cell cancer, condyloma acuminatum, dermatitis, eczema, and downward spread of rectal cancer. In addition, perianal Paget's disease is sometimes diagnosed only after histologic examination of hemorrhoids or perianal tissue excised for other reasons.

The diagnosis of perianal Paget's disease is made by biopsy, which should be performed within 1 month in any patient with chronic perianal dermatosis that is resistant to treatment. The histologic examination shows the characteristic Paget's cells: large, pale, vacuolated cells with hyperchromatic eccentric nuclei. There is also hyperkeratosis, parakeratosis, and acanthosis of the epidermal cells. Sialomucin may be identified by periodic acid–Schiff (PAS) stain, whereas Bowen's disease does not show this positive staining.

An accurate diagnosis is important for prognosis and therapy. In distinction to Bowen's disease, in which the progression to invasive cancer occurs in about 5% of cases, invasive carcinoma has been reported in up to 40% of those with untreated Paget's disease.

Diagnosis is obtained by full-thickness biopsies into the subcutaneous tissue, including the edge and central portion of the lesion. We also take 3 mm to 4 mm biopsy specimens at the dentate line, anal verge, and perineum approximately 3 cm from the anal verge in all four quadrants to map the exact extent of the lesion. This technique is also used to map the lesion in Bowen's disease and has

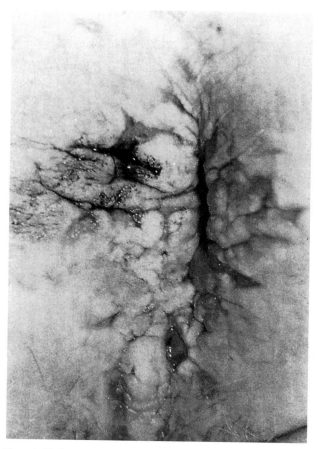

Figure 13-3
Perianal Paget's disease with raised, crusted scaly lesions.

been described earlier (see Fig. 13-2). Biopsies are performed several days before definitive treatment because traditional frozen section without histochemical staining may show false negative results.

■ MANAGEMENT

In a case of noninvasive disease, a wide local excision is performed and the edges of the resection are checked by frozen section to confirm total excision. The defect is closed primarily if it is small, but if it is large, a split-thickness skin graft may be required. In more extensive lesions, Murakami and Tanimura report four wide local excisions subsequently reconstructed with bilateral gluteus maximus rotation flaps with good result. When a skin graft is used, the patient is pharmacologically constipated as previously described to prevent graft loss.

If evaluation demonstrates Paget's disease with an invasive cancer without metastasis, an aggressive approach is employed. An abdominoperineal resection is indicated, followed by postoperative radiotherapy and chemotherapy. Groin lymph node dissection should be considered if these nodes are involved. Because of the commonly delayed diagnosis, 25% of patients with perianal Paget's disease have metastases at the time of diagnosis.

There are scattered reports in the medical literature of the use of radiation to treat extramammary Paget's disease. However, these are case reports only and this should not be considered the standard of care.

As recommended by Beck and Fazio, long-term follow-up is mandatory in order to exclude recurrence of the Paget's disease and development of an associated cancer. This follow-up includes a complete physical examination, proctosigmoidoscopy, a biopsy of any new lesions, and a random biopsy at the edges of the split-thickness skin graft at yearly intervals. Colonoscopy is performed at 2- to 3-year intervals.

Suggested Readings

Amin R: Perianal Paget's disease. Br J Radiol 1999;72(858):610–612.

Beck DE, Fazio VW: Perianal Paget's disease. Dis Colon Rectum 1987;30:263.

Beck DE, Fazio VW, Jagelman DG, Lavery IC: Perianal Bowen's disease. Dis Colon Rectum 1988;31:419.

Bowen JT: Precancerous dermatosis: A study of two cases of chronic atypical epithelial proliferation. J Cutan Dis 1912;30:241.

Brown RS, Lankester KJ, Spittle MF: Radiotherapy or surgery in perianal Paget's disease? Br J Radiol 2000;73(867):340.

Butler JD, Hersham MJ, Wilson CA, Bryson JR: Perianal Paget's disease. J R Soc Med 1997;90(12):688–689, 1997.

Cleary RK, Schaldenbrand JD, Fowler JJ, et al: Treatment options for perianal Bowen's disease: Survey of American Society of Colon and Rectal Surgeons members. Am Surg 2000;66(7):686–688.

Cleary RK, Schaldenbrand JD, Fowler JJ, et al: Perianal Bowen's disease and anal intraepithelial neoplasia: Review of the literature. Dis Colon Rectum 1999;42(7):945–951.

Darier J, Coulillaud P: Sur un cas de maladie de Paget de la region penneo-anale et scrotale. Societe-Francaise de Permatologie et de Syphiligraphie, 1893, p 425.

Goligher JC: Surgery of the Anus, Rectum and Colon, 4th ed. London, Bailliere Tindall, 1980, p 675.

Graham JH, Helwig EB: Bowen's disease and its relationship to systemic cancer. Arch Dermatol 1961;83:738.

Grodsky L: Bowen's disease of the anal region (squamous cell carcinoma in situ). Am J Surg 1954;88:710.

Grodsky L: Intraepidermal cancer of the anus: Evolution to invasive growth. Calif Med J 1957;87:412.

Grodsky L: Extramammary Paget's disease of the perianal region. Dis Colon Rectum 1960;3:502.

Grodsky L: Uncommon non-keratinizing cancers of the anal canal and perianal region. NY State J Med 1965;65:894.

Helwig EB, Graham JH: Anogenital (extramammary) Paget's disease. Cancer 1963;16:387.

Hughes JH, Robinson RA: p53 expression in Bowen's disease and in microinvasive squamous cell carcinoma of the skin. Mod Pathol 1995;8(5):526.

Jabbar AS: Perianal extramammary Paget's disease. Eur J Surg Oncol 2000;26(6):612–614.

Jones RE, Austin C, Ackerman AB: Extramammary Paget's disease: A critical reexamination. Am J Dermatopathol 1979;1:101.

Kwan WH; Teo PM: Perianal Paget's disease: Effective treatment with fractionated high dose rate brachytherapy. Clin Oncol (R Coll Radiol) 1995;7(6):400–401.

Lam DT, Batista O, Weiss EG, et al: Staged excision and split-thickness skin graft for circumferential perianal Paget's disease. Dis Colon Rectum 2001;44(6):868–870.

Marchesa P, Fazio VW, Oliart S, et al: Perianal Bowen's disease: A clinicopathologic study of 47 patients. Dis Colon Rectum 1997;40(11):1286–1293.

Marfing TE, Abel ME, Gallagher DM: Perianal Bowen's disease and associated malignancies: Results of a survey. Dis Colon Rectum 1987;30:782.

Morson BC, Dawson MP: Gastrointestinal Pathology. Oxford, Blackwell Scientific Publications, 1972, p 625.

Morson BC, Pang LSC: Pathology of anal cancer. Proc R Soc Med 1968;61:623.

Murakami K, Tanimura H: Reconstruction with bilateral gluteus maximus myocutaneous rotation flaps after wide local excision for perianal extramammary Paget's disease. Dis Colon Rectum 1996;39:227.

Sarmiento JM, Wolff BG, Burgart LJ, et al: Perianal Bowen's disease: Associated tumors, human papillomavirus, surgery, and other controversies. Dis Colon Rectum 1997;40(8):912–918.

Stearns MW, Grodsky L, Harrison EG, et al: Malignant anal lesions. Panel discussion. Dis Colon Rectum 1966;9:315.

Strauss RJ, Fazio VW: Bowen's disease of the anal and perianal area: A report and analysis of twelve cases. Am J Surg 1979;137:231.

Takata M, Matsui Y: Proliferating cell nuclear antigen and p53 protein expression in Bowen's disease. J Dermatol 1994;21(12):947.

Tjandra JJ, Fazio VW: Perianal disease. In Cohen AM, Winawer SJ (Eds.): Cancer of the Colon, Rectum and Anus. New York, McGraw-Hill (in press).

14

MELANOMA AND BASAL CELL CARCINOMA OF THE ANUS

Warren E. Enker, MD, FACS
Mary Sue Brady, MD

■ ANORECTAL MELANOMA

The anorectal region is an uncommon area for the development of melanoma, but when it occurs it is usually fatal. Significant controversy exists regarding the surgical management of patients with anorectal melanoma. On the one hand, many surgeons feel that the disease is largely incurable and that only local procedures are indicated. At the other extreme, abdominoperineal resection (APR) with pelvic or even inguinal lymphadenectomy may be justified in an attempt to cure a small subset of patients with relatively early disease. There are data to support both views, and operative management must be individualized. Preoperative staging is under investigation.

Demographics and Epidemiology

Patients with anorectal melanoma account for approximately 0.5 to 4% of all patients with anal tumors, and only 0.04 to 0.4% of all patients with melanoma. Demographic features of patients reported in the largest clinical series are listed in Table 14-1 and are characterized by a slight female preponderance and an older median age than that of patients with cutaneous melanoma (60 to 70 years versus 54 years of age, respectively). Most patients in reported series are Caucasian. A review of the SEER database (Surveillance, Epidemiology and End Results) suggests that there is now a bimodal age distribution, in younger men and older women. The incidence in younger men, especially in the San Francisco area, tripled when compared to other locations. This raises the possibility of an association with HIV (human immunodeficiency virus) infection.

Pathology

Anorectal melanoma is a mucosal melanoma that arises in the anal canal or rectum near the dentate line. It is distinct from cutaneous melanoma arising in the perianal region. The tumor has a propensity for proximal growth via submucosal extension into the rectum and frequently presents as a polypoid tumor at the anorectal ring (Fig. 14-1). True rectal melanoma is much less common than anal melanoma. These lesions arise at a significant distance from the anorectal junction without evidence of submucosal extension. Anorectal melanoma is characterized pathologically by deep infiltration with a propensity for lymphatic and vascular invasion. A dense, lymphocytic infiltrate around the tumor is common. Most tumors (approximately 66%) are either grossly or histologically pigmented.

Clinical Presentation

A delay in diagnosis is common because initial symptoms, such as bleeding, are often attributed to hemorrhoidal disease. Persistent bleeding as well as the growth of an anal mass, pain, and obstruction lead to diagnostic biopsy. Seven of our 85 patients had anorectal melanoma incidentally discovered upon the pathologic review of hemorrhoidectomy specimens. Three of these patients were long-term (>5 years) survivors following APR. Between 30 and 40% of patients with anorectal melanoma present with localized disease (no evidence of regional or distant metastases). More than half of these patients have evidence of regional or distant metastasis at presentation.

Prognostic Variables

Most clinical series of patients with anorectal melanoma report 5-year survival rates of 6 to 21% with median survival periods of 4 to 19 months (Table 14-2). Unlike cutaneous melanoma, the depth of invasion is often difficult to determine in patients with anorectal melanoma, and the prognosis is determined by the presence or absence of positive mesenteric or pelvic lymph nodes or of distant metastasis. Large primary tumors are more commonly associated with advanced stages of disease. As in cutaneous melanoma, evidence suggests that females fare better than males. Reports from Memorial Sloan-Kettering Cancer Center, the largest single institution experience with anorectal melanoma, indicate a 5-year survival rate of 17%, with a median survival time of 19 months in 85 patients.

Surgical Management

Significant controversy exists regarding the surgical approach to patients with localized anorectal melanoma. Many surgeons advocate local excision with sphincter preservation as the treatment of choice, as most reports describe a similar survival experience in patients managed with wide local excision (WLE) compared to those managed with APR (see Table 14-2). At some centers, patients are treated by WLE followed by adjuvant radiation therapy to the pelvis and/or inguinal lymph nodes. In our experience, APR is more commonly associated with long-term survival in patients with localized anorectal melanoma ($p < .05$). Indeed, 9 of our 10 long-term survivors ($n = 85$) had undergone APR with pelvic-mesenteric lymphadenectomy. All long-term survivors were women, and 8 of 9 survivors who had undergone APR had negative mesenteric lymph nodes (Ward et al).

Patients with anorectal melanoma who present with distant metastases should undergo local excision of their tumors, when this is technically feasible. Local control is important for effective palliation. APR is indicated when local procedures will not allow sphincter preservation, or for symptomatic local recurrence in patients who have failed initial local treatment with WLE.

Table 14-1 Demographic Characteristics of Patients with Anorectal Melanoma

AUTHORS	YEAR	FEMALES	MALES	RACE	AGE	MEDIAN SIZE	INITIAL SYMPTOM
Ooi et al	2001	2	4		31–81	2.5cm	Rectal bleeding
Ward et al	1986	9	12	NA	NA	5 cm*	Bleeding, pain, mass
Konstadoulakis et al	1995	11	4	NA	63	NA	Mass, bleeding
Goldman et al	1990	31	18	NA	71	2–3.9 cm	Bleeding
Slingluff et al	1990	17	7	22 white 2 black	64*	NA	Bleeding
Brady et al (1995)	1995	46	39	81 white 3 black 1 Asian	60	3.3 cm	Bleeding
Roumen	1996	36	27	NA	66	3.8 cm	Bleeding
Ben-Izhak et al	1997	12	6	white	60	NA	Bleeding

NA = not available
*mean

Patients who present with clinically apparent pelvic or inguinal metastases should undergo transanal, sphincter-preserving excision of their tumors, when technically feasible, as these patients are unlikely to survive long term, and major resections are likely to leave residual pelvic disease. Some surgeons advocate at least a 2-cm margin of normal-appearing mucosa surrounding the lesion to minimize the chance of a local recurrence. In most patients this much margin is impractical and runs the risk of functional impairment. In addition, therapeutic inguinal lymphadenectomy may be appropriate for palliative control of bulky nodal metastases that will enlarge and cause lymphedema and ulceration. Some patients with large primary tumors may be best served by an APR for palliation from obstruction, pain, and bleeding.

APR with pelvic lymphadenectomy should be considered in patients with no clinical evidence of nodal metas-tases, especially in the setting of a relatively small primary lesion (2 to 3 cm in size). This subset of patients may be curable with aggressive operative management of the anorectal primary tumor as well as the draining lymph nodes. Because anorectal melanoma grows proximally, it is more likely to involve the pelvic and mesenteric lymph nodes than the inguinal nodes. In our experience, 42% of patients undergoing APR had positive mesenteric nodes. Of these, one survived long term. In contrast, 25 patients found to have negative mesenteric lymph nodes following APR had a relatively favorable prognosis; 40% survived disease free at 5 years. In a series of 15 patients from Roswell Park Cancer Institute, 6 of 9 patients treated with APR had positive pericolic lymph nodes. In patients with distal lesions, where inguinal lymph node drainage is more likely, lymphatic mapping to identify drainage to the inguinal lymph nodes may be considered (Brady and

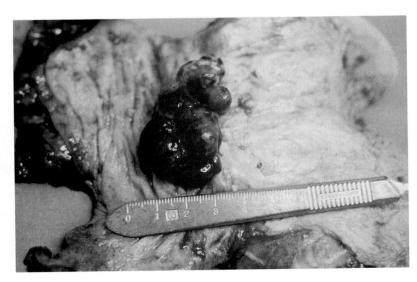

Figure 14-1
Gross appearance of a typical pigmented anal melanoma after abdominoperineal resection. The polypoid tumor arising within the anal canal extends proximally into the rectum.

Table 14-2 Clinical Series of Anorectal Melanoma

AUTHOR	YEAR	NO. OF PATIENTS	MEDIAN SURVIVAL	COMMENTS
Ooi et al	2001	6	50% alive	All APR
Chiu et al	1986	34	13 mo; 21% 5-yr survival	All APR
Ward et al	1986	21	4 mo	No difference APR vs. WLE
Goldman et al	1990	49	12 mo	No difference APR vs. WLE
Ross et al	1990	32	19 mo	No difference APR vs. WLE
Slingluff et al	1990	24	1.5 yr	No difference APR vs. WLE
Brady et al	1995	85	19 mo; females, 29% 5-yr survival; males, no 5-yr survivors	
				9 of 10 long-term survivors had APR
Roumen	1996	63	28 mo (Stage I), 6% 5-yr survival; 16 mo (Stage II), 4 mo (Stage III)	
Konstadoulakis et al	1995	15	16 mo; 9% 5-yr survival	9% 5-yr survival
Ben-Izhak et al	1997	12	16 mo	

NA = not available, NA APR = abdominoperineal resection, WLE = wide local excision.

Coit). An inguinofemoral lymphadenectomy for a positive sentinel lymph node in the groin of a patient undergoing APR should be considered.

Patterns of Failure

No data suggest any difference in the rates of local recurrence in patients treated with WLE compared to those treated with APR. Local failure is almost invariably associated with simultaneous regional or distant relapse and is rarely an isolated event. In our experience after APR, distant or multiple sites of recurrence occurred in 65% (n = 17) of patients who developed recurrence. Isolated inguinal recurrence was the second most common pattern (occurring in approximately 25% of patients, n = 7), followed by isolated local recurrence (8% of patients, n = 2). In patients who underwent WLE of their primary lesion, the most common pattern of failure was multiple sites of recurrence (including local recurrence) and isolated inguinal recurrence. In our experience and that of others, WLE is not associated with a significantly higher rate of local recurrence than APR. In contrast, local recurrence as the initial site of failure is common in patients (4 of 7 patients, 57%) who undergo an incomplete excision, either a biopsy or fulguration only.

Summary

The surgical management of patients with anorectal melanoma must be individualized. A thorough discussion of the alternatives and controversies is essential. Patients with potentially curable lesions (small primary tumors without evidence of metastasis) should be offered APR with pelvic lymphadenectomy. In our experience, and that of Konstadoulakis and colleagues, this approach is more commonly associated with long-term survival. Patients with bulky primary lesions or evidence of regional or distant disease should undergo transanal excision with clear margins when technically feasible. Under such circumstances, abdominoperineal resection may be of benefit, even if only to achieve local control.

■ BASAL CELL CARCINOMA OF THE ANUS

Basal cell carcinomas of the anus are rarer than melanomas, accounting for approximately 0.02% of anal and rectal neoplasms. The gender distribution is equal, and the majority of patients are over 50 years of age. Most patients present with a mass at the anal margin or the anal verge, and the lesion is often mistaken for a hemorrhoid. The lesion often has the same characteristics as basal cell carcinomas elsewhere in the body—a curled or rolled edge, chronic induration, and ulceration. Early biopsy is warranted for any mass lesion in this region. Most lesions can be locally excised and only rarely metastasize. Excisional biopsy is warranted and involved margins may be re-excised if the specimen is properly marked. In larger or neglected lesions, abdominoperineal excision of the rectum may be required, even if only to accomplish local control. In some cases, excision may be supplemented by external radiation, but damage to sphincter function may be a long-term consequence.

Of 200 anal cancers reported in 1976, only six cases involved basal cell cancer at the anal margin. As with most anal margin lesions, treatment is usually local excision, except in rare cases of locally advanced, large tumors. Treatment contrasts sharply with anal canal cancers, which primarily require combined radiation and chemotherapy, and in some cases, abdominoperineal excision of the rectum. Inguinal lymph node dissection is rarely needed. With an early diagnosis most lesions can be treated by excision alone, with good outlook.

Basal cell carcinoma may arise in longstanding perianal fistulas, and should be distinguished from small cell carcinomas, which usually carry an ominous prognosis. Nielsen and Jensen report on 34 patients with basal cell cancers treated between 1943 and 1974. Tumors were usually between 1 and 2 cm in diameter and were localized to the anal margin. Twenty-seven of the 34 patients were treated by local excision. Local recurrences were mostly treated by re-excision, and no further recurrences were seen after 5 years of observation. The 5-year crude survival rate was 73%.

Suggested Readings

Beahrs OH, Wilson SM: Carcinoma of the anus. Ann Surg 1976;184:422–428.

Ben-Izhak O, Levy R, Weill S, et al: Anorectal malignant melanoma. Cancer 1997;79:18–25.

Brady MS, Coit DG: Lymphatic mapping in the management of the patient with cutaneous melanoma. Cancer J 1997;2:87–93.

Brady MS, Kavolius JP, Quan SHQ: Anorectal melanoma: A 64-year experience at Memorial Sloan-Kettering Cancer Center. Dis Colon Rectum 1995;38:146–151.

Cagir B, Whiteford MH, Topham A, et al: Changing epidemiology of anorectal melanoma. Dis Colon Rectum 1999;42:1203–1208.

Chiu, YS, Unni, KK, Heart, RW: Malignant melanoma of the anorectum. Dis Colon Rectum 1986;23:122–124.

Cooper PH, Mills SE, Allen S: Malignant melanoma of the anus: Report of 12 patients and analysis of 255 additional cases. Dis Colon Rectum 1982;25:693–703.

Goldman S, Glimelius B, Pahlman L: Anorectal malignant melanoma in Sweden: Report of 49 patients. Dis Colon Rectum 1990;33:874–877.

Klas JV, Rothenberger DA, Wong WD, Madoff RD: Malignant melanomas of the anal canal: Spectrum of disease, treatment and outcomes. Cancer 1999;85:1686–1693.

Konstadoulakis MM, Ricaniadis N, Walsh D, Karakousis CP: Malignant melanoma of the anorectal region. J Surg Oncol 1995;58:118–120.

Kosary CL, Ries LAG, Miller BA, et al (Eds.): SEER Cancer Statistics Review, 1973–1992: Tables and Graphs, National Cancer Institute. NIH Pub. No.96-2789. Bethesda, MD, 1995.

McNamara, MJ: Melanoma and basal cell carcinoma. In Fazio VW (Ed.). Current Therapy in Colon and Rectal Surgery. Toronto, BC Decker, 1990, pp 62–64.

Nielsen OV, Jensen, SL: Basal cell carcinoma of the anus—A clinical study of 34 patients. Br J Surg 1981;68:856–857.

Ooi BS, Eu KW, Seow-Choen F: Primary anorectal malignant melanoma: Clinical features and results of surgical therapy in Singapore—A case series. Ann Acad Med Sing 2001;30:203–205.

Quan SH, Deddish MR: Noncutaneous melanoma: Malignant melanoma of the anorectum. Cancer 1966;16:111–114.

Ross M, Pezzi C, Pezzi T, et al: Patterns of failure in anorectal melanoma. Arch Surg 1990;125:313–316.

Roumen RMH: Anorectal melanomas in the Netherlands: A report of 63 patients. Eur J Surg Oncol 1996;22:598–601.

Slingluff CL Jr, Vollmer RT, Seigler HF: Anorectal melanoma: Clinical characteristics and results of surgical management in twenty-four patients. Surgery 1990;107:1–9.

Ward MWN, Romano G, Nicholls RJ: The surgical treatment of anorectal malignant melanoma. Br J Surg 1986;73:68–69.

15

ANAL CARCINOMA

Bernard J. Cummings, MBChB, FRCPC,
FRCR, FRANZCR
Jean Couture, MD, FRCSC

Anal carcinomas are classified according to whether they arise in the anal canal or the perianal skin. The canal extends from the upper border of the anal sphincter and puborectalis muscle to the junction with the hair-bearing perianal skin. The perianal skin covers a radius of 5 cm around the anal verge. Cancers that arise in the canal are more likely to spread to regional lymph nodes or metastasize beyond the pelvis. The regional node groups for the anal canal are the perirectal, internal iliac, and inguinal nodes. For the perianal skin, the ipsilateral inguinal nodes are designated as the regional nodes by the major Cancer Staging Committees. Although there are some differences in the approach to treatment for anal and perianal cancers, the intent for both should be cure with preservation of anorectal function whenever possible.

■ ANAL CANAL

Four out of five cancers that arise in the anal canal are epidermoid, the remainder being adenocarcinomas, undifferentiated cancers, and small cell cancers. Epidermoid cancers collectively include all variants of squamous cell cancer (cloacogenic cancer)—keratinizing, nonkeratinizing, and basaloid. For the most part, no distinction need be made between the subtypes of epidermoid cancer when considering treatment.

The key to successful management is the initial assessment. The extent of the cancer, and the possibility of conserving anorectal function, should be considered. The common symptoms of anal bleeding, discharge, a palpable lump, or discomfort on defecation are nonspecific and frequently attributed wrongly to benign conditions such as hemorrhoids. Diagnosis is often delayed, so that epidermoid cancers are found to have infiltrated the sphincter muscles or beyond in up to 90% of patients, and lymph node metastases are present in one third. We offer conservative therapy to all patients except the few who have gross incontinence or a malignant fistula.

Patients with anal discharge or occasional soiling are not considered incontinent. Similarly, fixation of the cancer to the pelvic sidewalls or prostate, infiltration of the vaginal mucosa without fistulization, or the presence of nodal or extrapelvic metastases are not contraindications to conservative therapy.

Nigro, Vaitkevicius, and Considine first described treatment with radiation and concurrent 5-fluorouracil (5-FU) and mitomycin C (MTC) in 1974. The ability of this combination to eradicate epidermoid anal cancer without the need to sacrifice anorectal function is now well established. Two randomized trials, one conducted in the United Kingdom and the other in Europe, have confirmed the superiority of combined modality treatment over radiation alone, in the radiation schedules used, with respect to local tumor control and cause-specific survival rates. In these trials, anorectal excision was reserved for the management of residual or recurrent cancer. A North American randomized trial found that superior levels of tumor control and colostomy-free survival were achieved by combining both 5-FU and MTC with radiation, rather than 5-FU only. The only other cytotoxic drug known to produce significant response in anal cancer is cisplatin and its analogues. Clinical trials in which 5-FU and MTC with radiation are compared to 5-FU and cisplatin with radiation are in progress.

We have studied the effectiveness and toxicity of radiation with concurrent 5-FU and MTC in a series of nonrandomized protocols. Although it has been suggested that interruptions in radiation therapy may allow a cancer to repopulate, we have found that breaks in treatment because of acute tenesmus and perineal radiodermatitis are often needed. We therefore prefer planned split-course schedules.

A well-tolerated schedule was 24 Gy in 12 fractions in 16 days, with a concurrent 96-hour continuous intravenous infusion of 5-FU, 1000 mg/m^2/24 hours (maximum 1500 mg/24 hours), starting on the first day of pelvic radiation, together with a single bolus injection of MTC, 10 mg/m^2 (no maximum), on day 1. Following a 3.5-week break, treatment resumed with a radiation dose of 28 Gy in 14 fractions in 18 days, the chemotherapy being repeated as before. The radiation fields for the first phase covered the inguinal, external and internal iliac, and pararectal lymph nodes, up to the lower border of the sacroiliac joints. In patients with no clinical evidence of lymph node metastases, the second phase of radiation was directed to the anal canal region only. Various techniques were used to irradiate regions of known node involvement to the same dose as the primary tumor. Between 1991 and 1993, 48 of 58 (83%) patients treated by this schedule achieved local-tumor control for 2 years or longer. Anorectal function was preserved in 75% overall and in 94% of those whose primary tumor was controlled by chemoradiation. The actuarial 5-year cause-specific survival rate was 75%. Our subsequent protocols have examined different total doses of radiation graded according to the size of the primary cancer, daily fractions of 1.8 Gy rather than the 2.5 Gy or 2.0 Gy used previously, a shorter interval between the courses of radiation and chemotherapy, and changes in radiation technique in efforts to reduce late morbidity. We do not yet have long-term results for these protocols.

The schedules of concurrent 5-FU, MTC, and radiation therapy used in different centers vary in their details, but the results are consistent. The primary cancer has been controlled in 75 to 95% of patients. Differences appear due more to variations in tumor size and stage than to any major advantage of one schedule over another. The U.K. randomized trial resulted in a relative improvement of 18% in the 3-year cause-specific survival rate for those treated by radiation and chemotherapy, compared with radiation alone (72% versus 61%, $p = 0.02$). There has not been, nor is there now likely to be, a direct randomized comparison of chemoradiation with radical surgery. Overall survival rates in series treated by chemoradiation are in the same general range as those reported in the past following treatment by radical surgery or radiation alone.

Current investigational protocols seek principally to improve local-regional control rates and, secondarily, to reduce extrapelvic metastases. Local-regional recurrences, either alone or accompanied by distant metastases, are the most common failure pattern and have been reported in up to about 30% of cases in many series after chemoradiation. Extrapelvic metastases alone are reported in no more than 10% of patients. Although some investigational protocols aim to deliver higher doses of radiation therapy, of the order of 60 to 65 Gy in 6 weeks or equivalent, there is some evidence that increasing the number of courses of chemotherapy rather than the dose of radiation may be associated with a lower risk of late morbidity.

The primary cancer has generally regressed completely by about 6 to 12 weeks after the completion of treatment but may take longer. A pale, irregular scar is usually visible at the site of the primary tumor. The base and edges of this fibrotic scar have a rubbery texture, but any hard, tender, or ulcerated area should be regarded as suspicious for residual cancer. We do not routinely biopsy or excise all scars, because the fibrosed areas following treatment are often fairly extensive, and random biopsies may not only fail to include residual cancer but may also be slow to heal. The false negative biopsy rates in patients with complete clinical regression of the primary tumor range up to 15%. There is no convincing evidence that identifying residual cancer histologically by early elective biopsy, when it is not detectable clinically, results in better long-term local control or cure rates than delaying biopsy and salvage treatment until recurrence is clinically apparent.

When residual or recurrent cancer is identified, anorectal excision, usually in the form of abdominoperineal resection and colostomy (APR), is most often necessary. Some authors have found that, provided the initial radiation dose had not been to the limit of normal tissue tolerance, further radiation and chemotherapy may occasionally be effective, and successful local excision of small areas of recurrence has also been reported. Since we began combining 5-FU and MTC with radiation, lasting local control has been achieved by radical salvage surgery in only 4 of 22 residual cancers treated between 1978 and 1989. Several groups have reported similar poor salvage rates, perhaps because those cancers not eradicated by chemoradiation are more aggressive biologically. A treatment algorithm for anal canal cancer is outlined in Figure 15-1.

The technique of anal excision by the combined abdominoperineal route includes a wider perianal excision than that used for low-lying adenocarcinomas of the rectum. We take this approach, as many cancers exhibit extensive subcutaneous lymphatic involvement and are often accompanied by an in situ component. A preliminary diverting stoma is usually not necessary unless there is significant anorectal sepsis. Care is taken to stay away from fistulas or sinuses during dissection in the ischiorectal space. Posteriorly, the coccyx can easily be removed if necessary. Anteriorly, the dissection is carried immediately posterior to the urethra in males. When cancerous infiltration of the prostatic capsule is suspected, an exenterative procedure is considered. In females, a posterior vaginectomy is performed if the lesion is in the anterior half of the anal circumference. The levator muscles are taken down as far laterally as possible. We prefer to do all dissection sharply, with cautery, under direct vision. The abdominal portion of the procedure is similar in technique and extent to an excision for rectal cancer, including a total mesorectal excision down to the pelvic floor. We do not dissect the internal iliac nodes unless they appear to be involved with cancer. The perineum is closed primarily and generally heals despite prior radiation and chemotherapy as long as there is no tension. The extent of in situ disease, the tumor size, presence or absence of a fistula, and the need for a vaginectomy influence the choice of primary closure or use of a flap. Myocutaneous flaps have the double advantage of bringing in fresh nonradiated tissue and filling the pelvic cavity.

Preoperative imaging studies such as computerized tomography or magnetic resonance imaging are helpful in determining the extent of disease, but radiation-induced changes may affect the interpretation of these studies and also make assessment difficult during surgery. Intraoperative frozen-section histologic examination is obtained freely. Even with this aid, scattered islands of apparently viable cancer may be identified in the final pathologic specimen, and assurance of tumor-free margins is difficult.

Late treatment-related damage of such severity that surgical intervention is necessary is uncommon. A few patients with near or fully circumferential cancers develop anal strictures, although these strictures do not occur in all patients and, even if present, are often well tolerated, so that we do not regard a circumferential cancer as a contraindication to attempting anorectal conservation. Anal strictures may sometimes be managed by dilation under anesthesia followed by regular dilation by the patient. Rectal or rectosigmoid strictures are uncommon, but are more difficult to manage. Endoscopic balloon dilation should be attempted first. In unusually severe rectal strictures or high fistulas, a variety of abdominal procedures may be feasible. Areas of perforation or stricture can sometimes be resected without a colostomy. Care should be taken to select unirradiated colon for the proximal arm of the anastomosis. Consideration should be given to a diverting stoma if the anastomosis is very low in the pelvis. The amount of small bowel irradiated by our technique is quite limited, and serious small bowel damage is rare. Of the 120 patients in our series to 1993 whose primary cancer was controlled by radiation and chemotherapy, 7 (6%) have had surgery for treatment-associated morbidity.

Mild or moderate degrees of late morbidity which do not require surgical management are relatively common, particularly urgency of defecation and frequent bowel

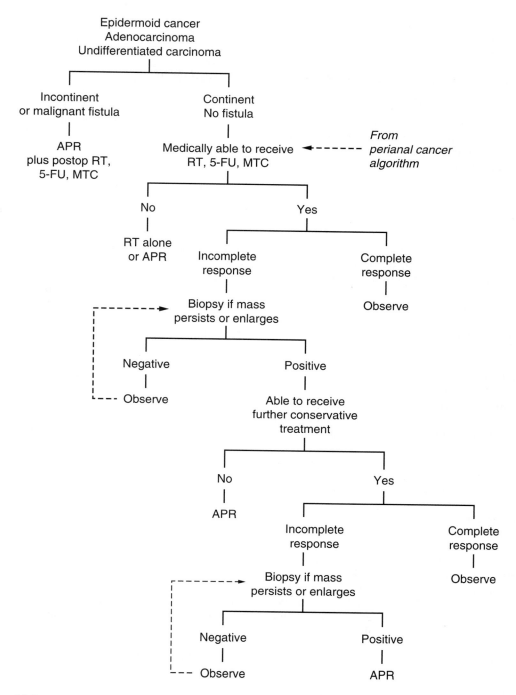

APR = abdominoperineal resection
        and colostomy
RT   = radiation therapy
5-FU = 5-fluorouracil
MTC = mitomycin C

Figure 15-1
Treatment algorithm for anal canal cancer.

motions. These symptoms can generally be improved by antidiarrheal medication and by exclusion of foods that are found to exacerbate them. Dyspareunia is common and the response to systemic or vaginal hormone therapy is only fair. Sitz baths and skin emollients relieve perianal dermatitis and pruritus ani, but long-term use of topical steroids should be avoided. Slight bleeding with defecation from radiation-induced telangiectasia in the distal rectum and anal canal is common but usually requires no treatment; it is important to exclude a more proximal cause if there is any doubt about the source of bleeding.

In most series, no more than 5% of patients are incontinent or have a draining malignant fistula at first presentation. When incontinence is clearly due to irreversible destruction of the anal sphincter mechanism or anovaginal fistula, we prefer elective APR. Because the risk of pelvic recurrence after primary surgery was about one in three in large series, we recommend postoperative adjuvant radiation with concurrent 5-FU and MTC. An alternative approach for these patients is to perform a diverting colostomy prior to radiation and chemotherapy, but we have found that it is usually not possible to close the colostomy subsequently because of persistent incontinence or fistula, even when the cancer is eradicated.

Local Excision

We rarely consider local excision for carcinomas of the anal canal. Limited excision is appropriate only when the risk of regional nodal metastasis is low and local excision will not compromise sphincter function. The likelihood of nodal metastasis is related to the histologic subtype, size, and depth of infiltration of the primary cancer. In series treated by primary APR, the risk of metastases to the pararectal and superior hemorrhoidal chain was less than 5% only in superficial squamous cell carcinomas less than 2 cm in size, but ranged from 30 to 50% for larger cancers. The risk of nodal involvement was about 10% when the cancer was confined to the mucosa and submucosa, but increased to 30% when the sphincters were invaded. Local excision is recommended by some authors for superficial or moderate well-differentiated squamous cell cancers of the distal canal, less than 2 cm in diameter. We do not use this treatment in patients who are medically able to receive radiation and chemotherapy.

Local excision is said to be adequate treatment for those occasional patients found to have histologically superficial cancer as an incidental finding at the time of treatment of a benign anal condition. However, in our experience it is often not possible to identify the site from which the malignant tissue was removed, and to assess the surgical margins properly. Usually, the entire surgical field is at risk of implantation if the cancer was transected; therefore, wide local re-excision is rarely practical. We treat these patients with combined radiation and chemotherapy as described previously, but limit the total radiation dose.

Regional Node Metastases

Regional pelvic or inguinal node metastases are present when the cancer is first diagnosed in up to 35% of patients, although they are often not detectable by cur-

rently available imaging techniques. These nodes are managed by principles similar to those for the primary cancer. The likelihood of conserving anorectal function is not reduced in most series by the presence of nodal metastases. However, the prognosis for cure is worse when the cancer has spread to regional nodes.

Histologic confirmation of cancer as the cause of enlargement of inguinal nodes should be obtained whenever possible, because the nodes may be affected by reactive hyperplasia only. We prefer an excisional biopsy of inguinal nodes larger than about 2 to 3 cm prior to chemoradiation because it appears to improve local control. More extended groin dissections are avoided because of the risks of infection and leg edema. The local control rate in the inguinal region in patients with confirmed nodal metastases treated with selective excision biopsy, radiation, 5-FU and MTC in the various schedules we have used was 89% (17 of 19). We irradiate the inguinal node regions electively for the first half of the treatment program in patients who do not have clinical evidence of nodal enlargement. Node metastases have occurred later in the irradiated groin in fewer than 5%, whereas most centers that do not electively treat the inguinal nodes report subsequent groin metastases in 10 to 25% of patients.

Histopathologic studies from surgical series suggest that spread to the superior hemorrhoidal and internal iliac node chains is somewhat more common than inguinal node metastases. Imaging techniques demonstrate these node metastases imperfectly, and histologic confirmation of metastasis in enlarged pelvic nodes by fine needle aspiration biopsy, while technically feasible, is rarely undertaken. The very low rate of tumor recurrence in pelvic nodes following chemoradiation provides indirect evidence that metastases in these nodes are eradicated as readily as inguinal metastases and the primary tumor.

Extrapelvic Metastases

The risk of extrapelvic metastases is low and in the range of 10 to 20%. The metastases are often accompanied by local-regional failure. There have so far been no formal studies of long-term systemic adjuvant therapy. The most effective palliative chemotherapy is cisplatin, sometimes given in combination with 5-FU, but responses are rarely complete and are short-lived. Focal symptoms may often be palliated by radiation alone or by radiation combined with cytotoxic drugs. Isolated extrapelvic spread is very uncommon, and there are only a small number of anecdotal reports of potentially curative resection of hepatic or pulmonary metastases.

Adenocarcinoma of the Anal Canal

Adenocarcinomas of the anal canal are uncommon. Those in the proximal canal probably arise from the columnar epithelium of the rectum, and we generally treat them as cancers of the rectum. Adenocarcinomas of the middle and lower canal arise mainly from anal ducts or fistulas. Although most authors recommend anorectal excision, we have chosen to treat these cancers, particularly when they are relatively small, by the same programs of combined radiation and chemotherapy used for epidermoid cancers.

Five of 11 patients have had local tumor control for 5 years or longer with preservation of anorectal function.

CARCINOMA OF THE PERIANAL SKIN

The perianal region is defined as the skin within a 5-cm radius of the anal verge, and lymphatic drainage is principally to the inguinal nodes. The most common cancers in this region are squamous cell carcinomas, usually well or moderately well differentiated. Provided that a squamous cell cancer can be removed without risk of loss of continence, we recommend local excision. For more extensive lesions, we use combined modality treatment programs similar to those used for anal canal cancers.

The randomized trial conducted in the United Kingdom included patients with cancers of both the anal canal and perianal regions. The results of that trial favor treatment by radiation, 5-FU, and MTC rather than radiation alone. We have achieved local control with preservation of anorectal function by chemoradiation in 80% of perianal cancers 3 cm or more in diameter. We also recommend elective treatment of the inguinal node regions when the primary cancer is 5 cm or larger, or when it is deeply infiltrating or poorly differentiated. We apply similar principles in the management of the rare perianal basal cell cancers and adenocarcinomas. A decision pathway for perianal cancer is summarized in Figure 15-2.

ANAL CANCER AND HIV INFECTION

Sexually transmitted substances or infections, particularly some types of human papillomavirus (HPV), have been implicated as a risk factor for anal cancer. Although not an AIDS-defining illness, the incidence of anal cancer is

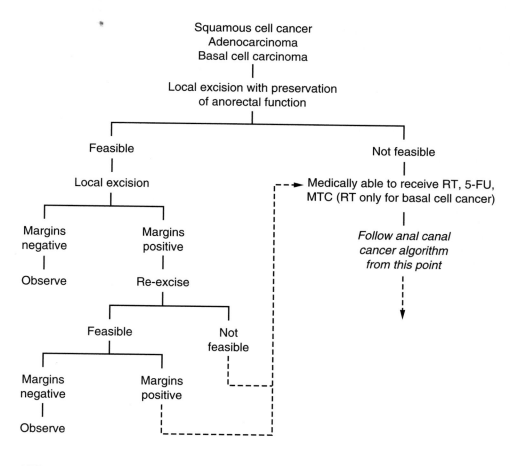

APR = abdominoperineal resection
        and colostomy
RT   = radiation therapy
5-FU = 5-fluorouracil
MTC = mitomycin C

Figure 15-2
Treatment algorithm for perianal cancer.

increased in those who have HIV (human immunodeficiency virus) infection. Patients infected with HIV who have not progressed to AIDS (acquired immune deficiency syndrome) usually tolerate radiation and cytotoxic chemotherapy normally. Those with AIDS may develop severe reactions in normal tissues at unexpectedly low radiation doses. We pursue a conservative protocol for the management of epidermoid cancers of the canal or perianal area in patients with HIV infection or AIDS. If local excision preserving anorectal function is feasible, this procedure is our treatment of choice. If conservative surgery is not feasible but the cancer is causing minimal symptoms and not growing rapidly, we examine the patient regularly but do not start specific anticancer treatment. When a small cancer is symptomatic or clearly enlarging, we treat the primary tumor with radiation alone and do not electively treat clinically uninvolved regional lymph nodes. Cytotoxic chemotherapy in the form of 5-FU and MTC, and more extensive radiation fields, are recommended to patients who have large or deeply invasive cancers, or nodal metastases. Standard doses and treatment schedules are used, modified according to pretreatment blood counts and liver and renal function, and the severity of the reactions seen. Radical surgery is recommended for the same indications as in patients not infected by HIV.

Suggested Readings

Bartelink H, Roelofsen F, Eschwege F, et al: Concomitant radiotherapy and chemotherapy is superior to radiotherapy alone in the treatment of locally advanced anal cancer: results of a Phase III randomized trial of the European Organisation for Research and Treatment of Cancer Radiotherapy and Gastrointestinal Cooperative Groups. J Clin Oncol 1997;15:2040–2049.

Cummings BJ: Anal canal. In Perez CA, Brady LW (Eds.). Principles and Practice of Radiation Oncology, 3rd ed. Philadelphia, Lippincott-Raven, 1997, pp 1511–1524.

Cummings BJ: Anal cancer: Treatment with and without chemotherapy. In Cohen AM, Winawer SJ (Eds.). Cancer of the Colon, Rectum and Anus. New York, McGraw-Hill, 1995, pp 1025–1042.

Flam M, John M, Pajak TF, et al: The role of mitomycin C in combination with 5-fluorouracil and radiotherapy, and of salvage chemoradiation in the definitive nonsurgical treatment of epidermoid carcinoma of the anal canal: Results of a phase III randomized Intergroup study. J Clin Oncol 1996;14:2527–2539.

Gerard JP, Chapet O, Samiei F, et al: Management of inguinal lymph node metastases in patients with carcinoma of the anal canal: Experience in a series of 270 patients treated in Lyon and review of the literature. Cancer 2001;92:77–84.

Giovannini M, Bardou VJ, Barclay R, et al: Anal carcinoma: prognostic value of endorectal ultrasound (ERUS). Results of a prospective multicentre study. Endoscopy 2001;33:231–236.

Goldie SJ, Kuntz KM, Weinstein MC, et al: Cost-effectiveness of screening for anal squamous intraepithelial lesions and anal cancer in human immunodeficiency virus-negative homosexual and bisexual men. Am J Med 2000;108:634–641.

Herrera L, Luna P, Garcia C: Surgical therapy of recurrent epidermoid carcinoma of the anal canal. In Cohen AM, Winawer SJ (Eds.). Cancer of the Colon, Rectum and Anus. New York, McGraw-Hill, 1995, pp 1043–1050.

Kim JH, Sarani B, Orkin BA, et al: HIV-positive patients with anal carcinoma have poorer treatment tolerance and outcome than HIV-negative patients. Dis Colon Rectum 2001;44:1496–1502.

Nilsson PJ, Svensson C, Goldman S, et al. Salvage abdominoperineal resection in anal epidermoid cancer. Br J Surg 2002;89:1425–1429.

Peiffert D, Giovannini M, Ducreux M, et al: High-dose radiation therapy and neoadjuvant plus concomitant chemotherapy with 5-fluorouracil and cisplatin in patients with locally advanced squamous-cell anal canal cancer: Final results of a phase II study. Ann Oncol 2001;12:397–404.

Place RJ, Gregorcyk SG, Huker PJ, et al: Outcome analysis of HIV-positive patients with anal squamous cell carcinoma. Dis Colon Rectum 2001;44:506–512.

Ryan DP, Compton CC, Mayer RJ: Carcinoma of the anal canal. N Engl J Med 2000;342:792–800.

Smith AJ, Whelan P, Cummings BJ, et al: Management of persistent or locally recurrent epidermoid cancer of the anal canal with abdominoperineal resection. Acta Oncol 2001;40:34–36.

Tarantino D, Bernstein MA: Endoanal ultrasound in the staging and management of squamous-cell carcinoma of the anal canal: Potential implications of a new ultrasound staging system. Dis Colon Rectum 2002;45:16–22.

UKCCCR Anal Canal Cancer Trial Working Party: Epidermoid anal cancer: Results from the UKCCCR randomized trial of radiotherapy alone versus radiotherapy, 5-fluorouracil and mitomycin. Lancet 1996;348:1049–1054.

Winburn GB: Anal carcinoma or "just hemorrhoids"? Am Surg 2001;67:1048–1058.

16

PELVIC PAIN SYNDROMES

Robert J. Rubin, MD, FACS, FASCRS
Gregory C. Oliver, MD, FACS, FASCRS
Suzanne Green, MD

Pelvic pain syndromes have often been considered enigmatic. This group of disorders falls into a generalized area of misunderstanding, and their cause and management have remained obscure. Despite multiple innovative anatomic, radiologic, and physiologic studies that have become almost routine in the evaluation of anorectal function and pelvic floor disorders, pelvic pain syndromes are largely considered to be functional. Pelvic pain without a uniform demonstrable organic origin has yet to be defined.

■ INCIDENCE

Specific types of anorectal and pelvic pain can be identified, treated, and cured. The number of patients who have rectal pain without any distinguishing anatomic or pathologic problems other than spasm or tenderness of the puborectalis portion of the levator muscle is surprisingly high. It is estimated that between 8% and 19% of the population experiences intermittent functional rectal pain. There is a great deal of overlap in patients who experience functional gastrointestinal symptoms as well as functional rectal pain. It is reported that only about 20% of patients with this pain syndrome have sought medical care.

■ PRESENTATION

In order to understand this group of patients, it is necessary to identify and remove those who have organic pain syndromes and then to deal with the larger group of patients who have pain without specific organic cause.

■ LEVATOR SYNDROME

Often, significant confusion has been caused by authors who misidentify or blur the pain syndromes with which we deal. We group all the patients with spastic levator muscles as having levator syndrome. These patients are a clinically distinct group with recognizable common denominators, both historically and on physical examination.

Tenderness of the levator sling on transanal palpation is found in all these patients. If pressure on one or both levator muscles does not reproduce the pain or if this tenderness is absent, levator syndrome is not the diagnosis. Historically, patients with levator syndrome are more often women (2:1 vs. men). They are usually middle-aged or older, and sometimes have associated symptoms of depression and functional gastrointestinal distress. These patients complain of a dull, inconstant rectal discomfort, which frequently radiates to the coccyx. It is most often associated with a feeling of pressure within the rectum and has been likened to "sitting on a ball." The discomfort is deep-seated and may radiate not only to the coccyx but also into the buttock and sometimes down the leg in a sciatic distribution. In men the pain may radiate to the base of the scrotum and can be associated with ejaculation. In women there can be dyspareunia when the muscle is in spasm. The pain that these people experience is deep-rooted, inconsistent, and accentuated by sitting. It is often relieved by ambulation or recumbency. The combination of all or part of this symptom complex, with the finding of a tender levator sling, is a requisite in making the diagnosis. Actual muscle spasm may be absent on examination if the patient is symptom-free at this time. However, symptoms must be duplicated by palpation of the affected side or sides. For reasons unclear to us, the left levator is affected about 70% of the time.

■ PROCTALGIA FUGAX

Another functional entity is proctalgia fugax, a variant of levator syndrome that can best be described as lancinating, short-lived anorectal pain. The pain most often awakens the patient from sleep and yet occurs infrequently, no more than once every 1 or 2 months. The pain abates spontaneously before an analgesic can be taken, flatus can be passed, or a hot tub initiated.

■ COCCYGODYNIA

Coccygodynia is the third syndrome of anorectal pain, but is separate from levator syndrome because its origin is organic and not functional. This pain follows coccygeal trauma. It exists in and about the coccyx and can be triggered by transanal digital manipulation of the coccyx. It may follow a previous fracture, trauma, or arthritis in the area. This extremely rare finding is the only pelvic pain syndrome that is improved by coccygectomy. Functional pain secondary to muscle spasm that radiates to the coccyx has often incorrectly been labeled coccygodynia.

■ INVESTIGATIONS

In attempting to make an objective diagnosis, studies of the pelvic floor have often been carried out. Anal manometry has a low diagnostic yield in patients with levator syndrome. Electromyography and nerve conduction studies of patients with rectal pain have shown some mild, variable abnormalities with prolongation of pudendal nerve latency being the most common finding. A more common finding has been the demonstration of paradoxic puborectalis contraction. Paradoxic contraction of the puborectalis is also found in a large group of patients who have absolutely no pain symptoms, and its presence in 45% of patients with rectal pain syndromes may not be causally linked. It is difficult to determine why most patients with paradoxic puborectalis contraction do not have rectal pain if it is truly related to the levator muscle syndrome. Clinical significance of the above-mentioned laboratory findings is uncertain, and they are neither a basis for the diagnosis of the disorder nor for therapeutic intervention. Undoubtedly, the most important underlying finding in levator syndrome is a tender, spastic pelvic floor. The precise cause of the spasm is unknown and, at the present time, most therapies are directed at relieving the spasm rather than at blocking the cause of the spasm (Table 16-1). In making an accurate diagnosis of functional anorectal pain, a detailed history is important. Determination of the nature of the pain, its location, type, and radiation are all important in suggesting the diagnosis. All patients should undergo complete anorectal examination. Digital examination with movement of the coccyx by the examining index finger and a sweeping of the puborectalis margin of the levator sling bilaterally should be carried out to determine if spasm or tenderness is present. In men, prostatic examination is essential because levator spasm may be secondary to prostatitis. Following digital and anoscopic examination, sigmoidoscopy (preferably flexible fiberoptic sigmoidoscopy) should be carried out so that the area in which the painful symptoms arise can be readily visualized and determined to be organically normal. In women, a pelvic examination should also be performed. If the only positive findings are spasm or tenderness of the levator sling, then the diagnosis of levator muscle syndrome can be made. It is not necessary to perform computed tomographic (CT) scans, magnetic resonance imaging (MRI), rectal ultrasound, and complete anorectal physiologic tresting unless other signs or symptoms pointing to anatomic or organic disorders of these areas are indicated (Fig. 16-1).

■ SECONDARY ANORECTAL PAIN SYNDROME

There are three groups of surgical patients who often exhibit signs and symptoms of levator muscle syndrome. We have found that patients who have undergone a low pelvic anastomosis after a low anterior resection of the rectum and sigmoid may exhibit rectal pressure, tailbone pain, and rectal urgency for a period of up to 6 months. This spasticity of the pelvic floor seems to dissipate with time. These patients can be reassured by their physicians. Their discomfort can be duplicated by digital pelvic pressure, and their symptoms are often alleviated by the use of local heat, nonsteroidal anti-inflammatory drugs, and analgesics. Women who have undergone pelvic surgery, particularly hysterectomy, are also prone to have a postoperative levator muscle syndrome variant that may last from 6 months to a year after their pelvic surgery. We're uncertain why this occurs but believe it may be due to the loss of lateral pelvic support, which usually affords stability to the levator floor.

The last group of patients who develop secondary levator muscle and pelvic floor spasm are those who have just had anorectal surgery or who have painful conditions of the anus. Patients with an acute anal fissure or perianal abscess sometimes have more pain from their levator muscles than they do from the fissure itself. Patients who are in the early postoperative period following hemorrhoidectomy often have severe levator muscle spasm that is relieved only by the use of local heat and diazepam. Abscesses and other painful conditions of the anus seem to initiate anismus and spasm of the levator muscle complex. However, primary idiopathic levator syndrome in which there is no recognizable anatomic or pathologic abnormality encompasses the vast majority of patients of the symptomatic group.

Secondary levator syndromes may be associated with inflammation and sepsis of pelvic organs in women and the prostate in men. Mechanical factors such as excessive physical activity, vigorous athletic workouts, and disorders of the pelvic floor comprise another group of mechanical causes. Patients who have had previous neoplasms of the rectum, prostate, or ovary and who have recurrence of their disease constitute a very small group of individuals with a pelvic pain syndrome in which there is tumor infiltration of the levator muscles or metastases to the pelvic bones or nerves by tumor. A levator syndrome–like condition may occur. Musculoskeletal disorders such as arthritis and fractures of the coccyx, neurologic disease involving the chorda equina, and psychiatric disorders, particularly severe depression, can be associated with pelvic pain syndromes. To this group must be added the group of postoperative patients who have transient postoperative levator syndrome following

---

Table 16-1 Classification of Levator Syndromes

Primary idiopathic
    No recognizable anatomic or pathologic abnormality
    Secondary levator syndromes
Inflammatory
    Septic
    Others
Mechanical
    Disorders of pelvic floor
    Excessive physical activity
Neoplastic
    Rectal
    Prostatic
    Ovarian
Neuroskeletal
    Osseous
    Neurologic
    Psychiatric
Postoperative

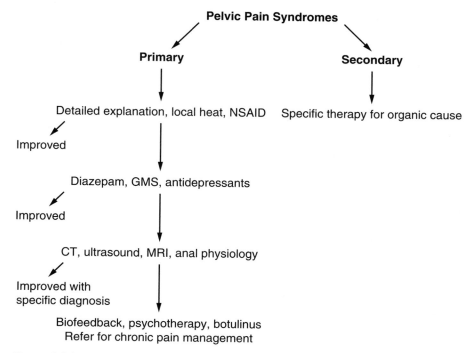

Figure 16-1
Algorithm for treatment of pelvic pain syndromes.

low anterior resection of the rectum, abdominal hysterectomy, and anorectal surgery. In the neoplastic group, one must consider chordomas and retrorectal presacral tumors. Presacral cysts may also be a cause of pelvic pain complaints.

■ THERAPY

A large group of the patients with levator syndrome seek medical help because they are concerned that this poorly localized deep visceral discomfort is a result of some underlying cause. When they have been adequately examined digitally, anoscopically, and with a flexible sigmoidoscope and reassured that no cause is present, their fears are often allayed. A significant amount of time must be spent explaining this syndrome to patients who suffer with it and giving them insight into how it may be improved and relieved. The realization that there is not an occult incurable disease is extremely important to a large number of our patients and seems to benefit the vast majority of patients whom we see.

Patients who require treatment are directed to use warm tub baths, sit on a heating pad, and take oral nonsteroidal anti-inflammatory pain relievers (NSAIDs) (ibuprofen in doses of 600 mg to 800 mg every 6 to 8 hours or diflunisal every 8 hours as necessary) as a first line of therapy.

If the patient's discomfort still persists and there is a spastic element recognized digitally, we then recommend diazepam and galvanic muscle stimulation as a second line of therapy. More than two thirds of our patients respond to the first-line regimen outlined here. Those who do not improve and who have spasm of the levator muscles are offered an opportunity to be treated by electrogalvanic muscle stimulation (EGS) using a rectal probe. The physiatric principle is that a slow-frequency oscillating current will induce muscle fasciculation and produce fatigue in a spastic muscle group. The treatment may be uncomfortable but is not painful. We use the EGS model 100 (Electro-Med Health Industries, Inc., Miami, FL) at a frequency of 80 cps starting at zero voltage. This level is increased until discomfort is produced and then it is reduced to a comfortable range. Best results are obtained if the patient can tolerate 250 to 300 V at this cycle. We utilize a self-retaining rectal probe and follow Sohn's recommendation of three treatments lasting 1 hour within a 10-day period. Others have recommended 15- to 30-minute treatments every other day until there is symptom resolution. We have had good success in relieving four of every five patients who had previously failed to improve after the simpler treatments already outlined and subsequently had been treated with EGS. Patients who show improvement but then experience recurrence of their symptoms may be re-treated and often improve again with EGS. Diazepam used sparingly is also effective during this time.

Reports on the use of galvanic stimulation have varied from less than 50% improvement to over 90% of patients being improved. Several factors may explain this. In series in which lower improvement levels are reported, the series have uniformly been small. Patients were not specifically selected out with spastic levator muscles. Simple treatment measures have not been outlined to the patients to try to improve their lot before they were placed on galvanic muscle stimulation. In all the series in which the response was poor, a percentage (usually at least 10%) of those who did poorly had subsequent diagnoses that were organic in nature. These patients would not be expected to improve with galvanic muscle stimulation. Overall, it is fair to say that about two thirds of properly selected patients will show a response to galvanic muscle stimulation. This treatment may have to be repeated over the long term. EGS remains an excellent treatment modality when conservative first-line measures have failed.

Patients who remain symptomatic following attempts at treatment with NSAIDs, analgesic, local heat, galvanic muscle stimulation, and diazepam deserve further study and workup. Considerations include pelvis or rectal ultrasonography, CT scanning of the abdomen and pelvis and MRI evaluation of the pelvis to seek out overlooked causes of the pain. Occasionally, pudendal nerve latency studies and defecography are beneficial because some patients with severe internal prolapse or perineal descent may exhibit the levator muscle syndrome.

Not all patients with pelvic pain need extensive workups beyond local examination and evaluation if they fall into the category of recognizable levator muscle syndrome both by history and by physical examination. If the history is at variance with this disorder or the physical examination demonstrates retrorectal, perirectal, or intrarectal abnormalities, then certainly these findings must be studied, evaluated, and treated. If the treatments outlined here are not effective, we have utilized outpatient levator muscle stretching and levator massage as well as rectal divulsion with puborectalis stretching under general anesthesia. This approach has occasionally been beneficial, but if it remains fruitless, biofeedback has been described as being helpful in some patients. Patients who are not willing to work with biofeedback or who appear to be profoundly depressed should be evaluated psychiatrically to determine whether they are in need of skilled supportive therapy.

We have recently started to use botulinum toxin in very refractory levator muscle syndromes but have generally avoided it because of the potential of transient anal incontinence which may follow botulinum-induced paralysis of the levator muscles. Our greatest success has been with the instillation of 100 units of botulinum toxin into the spastic levator muscle via a CT-directed needle. It has been used on patients who have undergone proctectomy when incontinence will not be a problem but levator muscle syndrome has been extreme and has received a very good response. Although we are concerned about the potential of producing temporary anal incontinence, we have not noted this development in over 20 cases so treated. We have been dissatisfied with attempts to deliver it transanally or perianally utilizing direct injection techniques. The CT scan with its excellent demonstration of the levator muscles that are in spasm has been our most effective means of guiding delivery of the toxin. Whether this will remain a valid form of therapy and whether it is a reasonable therapy to project into the future is uncertain at this time.

■ CONCLUSIONS

1. Not all patients with a pelvic pain syndrome that does not have a demonstrable cause require extensive workup of the pelvic pain syndrome.
2. Patients with the typical history and physical findings of levator muscle spasm may be treated empirically with NSAIDs and local heat, with galvanic muscle stimulation and diazepam reserved for failures. If symptoms remain refractory, further workup for organic sources of pain and then ultimately psychiatric evaluation or biofeedback is indicated. We have all but abandoned use of Botox in idiopathic levator syndrome due to consistently poor outcomes.

Suggested Readings

Eckardt VF, Dodt O, Kanzler G, Bernhard G: Anorectal function and morphology in patients with sporadic proctalgia fugax. Dis Colon Rectum 1996:755–762.

Ger GC, Wexner SG, Jorge JMN, et al: Evaluation and treatment of chronic intractable rectal pain—A frustrating endeavor. Dis Colon Rectum 1993;36:139–145.

Grant SR, Salvati EP, Rubin RJ: Levator syndrome: An analysis of 316 cases. Dis Colon Rectum 1975;18:161–163.

Hull T, Milsom JW, Church J, et al: Electrogalvanic stimulation for levator syndrome: How effective is it in the long term? Dis Colon Rectum 1993;36:731–733.

Joo IS, Agachan F, Wolff B, et al: Initial North American experience with botulinum toxin type A for treatment of anismus. Dis Colon Rectum 1996;39:1107–1111.

Oliver GC, Rubin RJ, Salvati EP, Eisenstat TE: Electrogalvanic stimulation in the treatment of levator syndrome. Dis Colon Rectum 1985;28:662–663.

Sohn N, Weinstein MA, Robbins RD: The levator syndrome and its treatment with high-voltage electrogalvanic stimulation. Am J Surg 1982;144:580–582.

17

ANORECTAL CONGENITAL DISORDERS

Alberto Peña, MD

Anorectal congenital malformations include a wide spectrum of defects; each one requires a specific treatment and has a different functional prognosis. The main and most feared sequel is fecal incontinence, which is a devastating problem, although anal stenosis may complicate some repairs.

In the author's experience, roughly 70% of all patients, properly treated, will enjoy voluntary bowel movements by the age of 3 years, although a significant portion of them will still suffer from some degree of occasional soiling. About 40% of all patients are considered totally continent, meaning that they enjoy voluntary bowel movements and never soil their underwear. Our goal in the treatment of patients born with potential for bowel control is to repair their malformation by preserving the anatomic elements that the patient was born with in order to achieve fecal continence. For those patients who are born without potential for bowel control, our goal is the anatomic repair of the defect followed by the implementation of a bowel management program aimed to keep the patients constantly clean, giving them the best possible socially acceptable quality of life. This chapter is designed to help clinicians and surgeons find quick answers to practical therapeutic questions.

Because we are dealing with a spectrum of defects, any attempt to classify these malformations risks false generalizations. Figure 17-1 shows a list of the most conspicuous and common defects seen in everyday practice. This list may serve as a practical classification based on therapeutic and prognostic implications and includes benign defects (traditionally known as low defects), which are treated without a colostomy and with a small operation (anoplasty), achieving 100% bowel control and associated with a very low frequency of urinary malformations. On the other extreme of the spectrum are complex anorectal defects that are treated with a preliminary protective colostomy, followed by a major repair, with a high incidence of fecal incontinence. These patients also suffer from a high incidence of associated urinary malformations. The term *high imperforate anus* is not used here because it includes malformations that require different treatments and have completely different prognoses (see Table 17-1).

A significant portion of patients born with anorectal malformations suffer also from other associated defects including mainly genitourinary, sacrospinal, gastrointestinal, and cardiovascular defects. Early suspicion and expedited diagnosis and treatment of these defects will help to avoid significant numbers of deaths as well as increased morbidity. Genitourinary defects represent the main source of death and morbidity, and therefore their presence should always be kept in mind. The frequency of associated defects varies depending on the specific type of anorectal defect (see Table 17-1).

Establishing the final functional prognosis in patients with anorectal malformations is an important step in their management; it avoids false expectations from the parents and allows the early implementation of a bowel management program in those patients with poor functional prognosis. This approach also avoids the traditional saga of fecally incontinent patients in search of a remedy that never comes, guided by a hope that has no factual basis. The prognosis can be established fairly accurately based on the type of defect. In addition, the accuracy of this prognosis can be enhanced by evaluating the integrity of the sacrum.

■ DESCRIPTION OF DEFECTS

Perineal Fistula

Perineal fistula is the simplest of all defects and is seen with similar characteristics in male and female patients. The rectum opens into the perineum, always anterior to the location of the sphincter, into an abnormal orifice, which is usually stenotic and therefore is called a fistula. Most of the rectum is surrounded by a good sphincter mechanism, except in its most distal part, where the rectum deviates anteriorly. The sacrum is almost always normal, the incidence of associated defects is low, and the functional prognosis is excellent (see Table 17-1).

Males

Perineal (cutaneous) fistula

Rectourethral fistula
Bulbar
Prostatic
Recto–bladder–neck fistula
Imperforate anus without fistula
Rectal atresia

Females

Perineal (cutaneous) fistula

Vestibular fistula
Persistent cloaca
Imperforate anus without fistula
Rectal atresia

Figure 17-1
Classification of congenital anorectal disorders in males and females.

Table 17-1 Common Congenital Anorectal Defects, Their Treatment, and Prognosis

TYPE OF DEFECT	COLOSTOMY	MAIN REPAIR	PROGNOSIS OF VOLUNTARY BOWEL MOVEMENTS	FREQUENCY OF URINARY ASSOCIATED DEFECTS
Perineal fistula (male & female)	No	Anoplasty	100%	< 10%
Rectal atresia (male & female)	Yes	PSARP	100%	0 %
Vestibular fistula (female)	Yes	Limited PSARP	93%	30%
Imperforate anus with no fistula (male & female)	Yes	PSARP	76.5%	26.4%
Rectourethral bulbar fistula (males)	Yes	PSARP	81%	25%
Rectourethral prostatic fistula (male)	Yes	PSARP	67%	66%
Cloaca (Common channel < 3 cm)	Yes	PSARVUP	70%	60%
Cloaca (Common channel > 3 cm)	Yes	PSARVUP plus laparotomy	50%	90%
Recto-bladder-neck fistula (male)	Yes	PSARP plus laparotomy	15%	92%

PSARP = posterior sagittal anorectoplasty; PSARVUP = posterior sagittal anorectovaginourethroplasty

Rectal Atresia

This defect occurs in only 1% of all male or female patients. Externally the anus looks normal, but an atresia or stenosis is located about 1 to 2 cm above the anal verge, at the junction of the anal canal with the rectum. The sphincter mechanism is normal, as is the sacrum. The incidence of associated defects is very low and the prognosis is excellent (see Table 17-1).

Vestibular Fistula

This fistula is the most frequently seen defect in female patients. The rectum opens into the vestibule of the female genitalia immediately external to the hymen. It is frequently erroneously called vaginal fistula. Most of the rectum is surrounded by a good sphincter mechanism, except for the lower part, which is frequently stenotic and is called a fistula. A very thin wall separates the rectum from the vagina. The sacrum is usually normal, the frequency of association with urologic defects is low, and the prognosis is very good (see Table 17-1).

Imperforate Anus Without Fistula

This defect occurs in only 5% of all male and female patients. It is very frequently associated with Down syndrome. The rectum ends blindly about 1 to 2 cm above the perineal skin. The sphincter mechanism is fairly well developed, the sacrum is usually normal, and the prognosis is good (see Table 17-1).

Rectourethral Bulbar Fistula

This fistula is perhaps the most frequently seen defect in male patients. The rectum opens into the lower part (bulbar) of the posterior urethra. The sphincter mechanism, quality of the sacrum, and functional prognosis are similar to those of imperforate anus without fistula (see Table 17-1).

Rectourethral Prostatic Fistula

This defect is fairly common in male patients. The rectum opens into the upper part (prostatic) of the posterior urethra. The sphincter mechanism is frequently underdeveloped, the sacrum is frequently abnormal, the perineum tends to be flat, and the scrotum is frequently bifid. The prognosis is not as good as in cases of bulbar fistula (see Table 17-1).

Cloaca

Cloaca is a complex malformation seen in female patients. Rectum, vagina, and urethra are fused, forming a single common channel that opens into a single orifice located where the female urethra normally is. The frequency of association with urologic defects is extremely high. The length of the common channel varies from 1 to 10 cm, and it has important prognostic implications. The author's series indicate that when the common channel is shorter than 3 cm the prognosis is remarkably better than in cases with longer channels (see Table 17-1).

Recto-bladder-neck Fistula

Recto-bladder-neck fistula is the highest defect seen in male patients. It occurs in 10% of all male cases. The rectum opens into the bladder neck. Most of these patients suffer from other associated defects, and the functional prognosis is poor (see Table 17-1).

◼ NEONATAL MANAGEMENT

When confronted with a newborn baby with an anorectal malformation, the surgeon must consider two important questions:

1. Does the baby need a diverting colostomy as a temporary management or a small primary operation (anoplasty)?
2. Does the baby suffer from an associated defect (mainly genitourinary) that threatens his (her) life and requires immediate treatment?

These two questions can be answered by following relatively easy decision-making algorithms (Figs. 17-2 and 17-3).

A golden rule that must always be observed concerning the opening of a colostomy is to wait 20 to 24 hours after

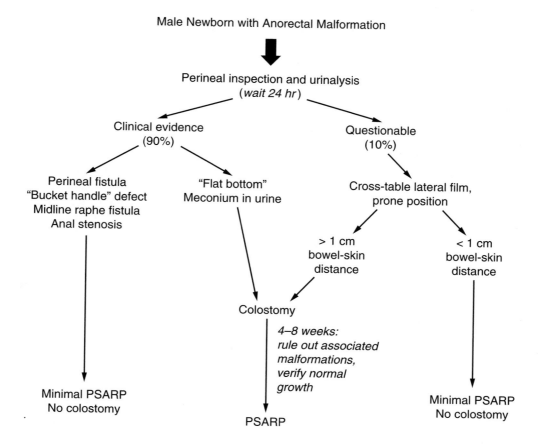

Male Newborn with Anorectal Malformation

Figure 17-2
Algorithm for congenital anorectal malformations in males. (PSARP = posterior sagittal anorectoplasty.)

birth before making a decision. The reason for this is that it takes a significant increase in the intrarectal pressure to force the passing of the meconium through a usually narrow fistula. Knowing the origin of the meconium, one learns about the location of the fistula (perineum, vestibule, or urinary tract) or the absence of fistula, and those facts help one to decide the best treatment for the patient.

A protective colostomy is still the best initial treatment for most patients with anorectal malformations because it decompresses the gastrointestinal tract, avoids the contamination of the urinary tract, and has minimal morbidity when properly done. Patients with perineal fistulas (traditionally known as low defects) are treated with a primary anoplasty without a protective colostomy. The diagnosis of a perineal fistula is a clinical one and is established by a careful examination of the baby's perineum. These babies have a good-looking perineum, meaning that both buttocks are well formed with a conspicuous midline groove and a prominent anal dimple that represents the center of the sphincter and, therefore, the place where the anus should be located. Anterior to that site, one can almost always identify a narrow orifice through which meconium comes out, usually between 12 and 24 hours after birth. The fistula is located somewhere between the genitalia and the center of the sphincter. Male patients may have peculiar perineal

findings that include a prominent skin tag below which an instrument can be passed and is, therefore, called bucket handle malformation. The perineal fistula is to be found below the "handle." Sometimes the fistula runs subepithelially in the midline raphe, opening at the base of the scrotum or even at the base of the penis; the layer of epithelial cells that covers the fistula is so thin that one can see the meconium and, therefore, the baby seems to have a midline black ribbon. The perineal fistula sometimes is very small and can be undetected for the first 24 hours. Therefore, before accepting that there is no perineal fistula, one must wait 24 hours because sometimes, after that time, meconium comes out through a pinhole orifice.

The absence of a perineal fistula, as well as the presence of meconium in the urine, or a vestibular fistula, or a single perineal orifice (cloaca), is an indication for a colostomy. Other perineal findings are greatly suggestive of a very high defect and are also indications for a colostomy. These include a flat bottom, meaning an absence of the midline groove and an absence of an anal dimple.

About 85 to 90% of the time one can find enough clinical evidence by the examination of the perineum to be able to make an decision concerning the opening of a colostomy or the performance of an anoplasty. In the remaining 10 to 15% of the cases a radiologic evaluation

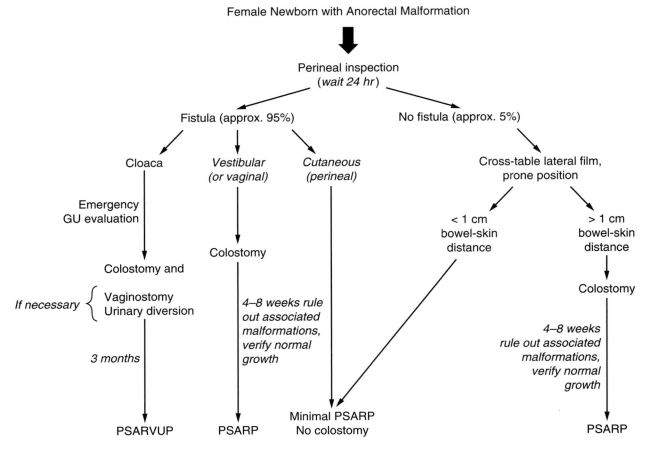

Figure 17-3
Algorithm for congenital anorectal malformations in females. (PSARP = posterior sagittal anorectoplasty; PSARVUP = posterior sagittal anorectovaginourethroplasty.)

is indicated. The traditional invertogram (upside-down film) is no longer done because of the risks of vomiting and bronchial aspiration. The same image can be obtained by taking a cross table lateral film of the pelvis with the patient in prone position with the pelvis elevated and with a lead marker in the anal dimple. The distal end of the rectum can be seen full of air, and the distance from the rectum to the anal dimple can be measured. If this distance is longer than 1 cm it is an indication for a colostomy because the patient likely has an imperforate anus without a fistula. The very unusual instance of a distance shorter than 1 cm usually means that the patient has a perineal fistula that was missed during the examination of the perineum, and, therefore, the patient can be treated with a primary anoplasty without a colostomy. Figures 17-2 and 17-3 show the decision-making algorithms used in the management of newborn babies with anorectal malformations.

During the waiting period of 24 hours the presence of associated defects, particularly urinary malformations, must be ruled out. An ultrasound study of the abdomen and pelvis is mandatory and is the best initial screen test to rule out the presence of hydronephrosis, megaureter,

and hydrocolpos in female patients. If this study produces normal findings, no further examinations are indicated to evaluate the urinary tract. On the other hand, an abnormality found in the ultrasound represents an indication for further urologic evaluation. A plain x-ray film of the sacrum is also very useful; an absent sacrum or a very hypotrophic one usually means that the patient has a high and rather complex malformation and, therefore, needs a diverting colostomy. Cardiac or gastrointestinal evaluation are done if the patient shows related symptoms.

A colostomy in patients with anorectal malformations is an important source of complications when not done properly. The surgeon must keep in mind that the colostomy should be totally diverting (separated stomas) to avoid fecal contamination of the urinary tract. Also, when deciding the portion of colon to be exteriorized, one must be sure to leave enough length of colon distal to the colostomy to allow the pull-through of the rectum to be done at a later time. In the author's experience the best type of colostomy is a descending one with separated stomas. The mucous fistula (distal stoma) is created intentionally narrow to avoid prolapse, because it is used only for irrigations and diagnostic tests.

■ MAIN REPAIR

Anoplasty

This operation is used to repair minor anal defects (perineal fistula) in both male and female patients. In both, the goal of the procedure is to move the anal orifice back and place it within the bounds of the external sphincter, which is the lowest part of the funnel-like sphincter mechanism.

The operation is usually done during the newborn period; at that stage of life it does not require any kind of bowel preparation. When done later in life, patients require a strict bowel preparation, which is not easy to achieve owing to the fact that these patients suffer from constipation.

With the patient in the prone position and the pelvis elevated, multiple fine sutures are placed at the mucocutaneous junction of the fistula, in order to exert a uniform traction to facilitate the dissection of the rectum. The external sphincter is divided in the midline and the rectum is positioned within its limits. In male patients, it is imperative to place a Foley catheter in the urethra to avoid urethral injury because the anterior wall of the rectum is intimately attached to the urethra.

A cut-back procedure is another alternative for patients with perineal fistulas and can be done when one is dealing with very small (premature) or very sick babies. It consists of making a deep cut in the posterior wall and the sphincter and suturing rectal wall to the skin. The functional results seem to be as good as an anoplasty although cosmetically the results are less than optimal. If the surgeon is not familiar with the delicate, meticulous technique required for an anoplasty, it is preferable to perform a cut-back procedure.

Limited Posterior Sagittal Anorectoplasty

This operation is used to repair vestibular fistulas. These patients require only irrigations of the colon distal to the colostomy preoperatively. The patient is placed in prone position with the pelvis elevated. A midline, posterior sagittal incision is used, extending from the vestibule to a point located halfway along the distance to the coccyx. The sphincter mechanism is divided, including only the muscle complex and the external sphincter. Uniform traction is applied to the fistula, and the lower rectum is meticulously mobilized posteriorly to be placed within the limits of the sphincter mechanism. Special attention is paid to the separation of rectum from the vagina, because both structures share a common wall. One must create two walls out of one; this is a very delicate maneuver and may be the main source of complications when it is not done properly.

Posterior Sagittal Anorectoplasty with or Without Laparotomy

This technique is used to repair all other defects except for cloacas. A Foley catheter is placed in the bladder. The patient is also placed in the prone position with the pelvis elevated. The midsagittal incision extends from the middle portion of the sacrum down through the anal dimple. The entire sphincter mechanism is divided, and the rectum is then meticulously separated from the urinary tract, preserving the urethra intact, as well as the vas deferens, seminal vesicles, and prostate. The most delicate part of the operation is the separation of the rectum from the urinary tract because both structures share a common wall, without a plane of separation, for about 5 to 20 mm above the fistula site. This common wall also exists between the rectum and the posterior urethra, even in patients without a fistula.

Once the rectum has been separated it is mobilized down to the perineum, placed within the funnel-like sphincter, and an anoplasty is performed. Sometimes, it is necessary to tailor the rectum in order to be placed within the limits of the sphincter mechanism.

In cases with a recto-bladder-neck fistula (which represents 10% of all male patients), it is necessary to find and mobilize the rectum by using a laparotomy. The patient is first approached posteriorly and sagittally to create the path through which the rectum will be pulled down, within the limits of the sphincter mechanism. This path is marked with a rubber tube, which subsequently is identified during laparotomy. Next, the rectum is separated from the bladderneck, is tapered when necessary, attached to the rubber tube, and pulled down into the perineum using the rubber tube that traverses the sphincter mechanism. An anoplasty represents the last part of the operation.

Posterior Sagittal Anorectovaginourethroplasty with or Without Laparotomy

This operation is used to repair a cloaca. These operations are usually long, technically demanding procedures that must be done by surgeons with special dedication and experience. Via a posterior sagittal approach, the rectum is separated from the genitourinary tract; the urethra and vagina frequently are separated from one another and mobilized down, or both may be mobilized together to create a separate urethra, vagina, and rectum.

About 40% of the time, it is necessary to open the abdomen to reach a very high rectum, a very high vagina, or both. Patients with very small or absent vaginas may require a form of vaginal replacement, which is usually done with colon or small bowel. A significant number of patients require a ureteral reimplantation. Others need a bladder augmentation and some form of continent diversion, which means the creation of a tube (appendix, ureter, fallopian tube, or tubularized bowel) implanted in the bladder with an antireflux mechanism to avoid leakage of urine and allow the emptying of the bladder by use of intermittent catheterization.

Management of Functional Sequelae

The most devastating functional sequela seen in patients with anorectal malformations is fecal incontinence, which occurs in at least 30% of these patients. This complication occurs either because the patients are born without potential for bowel control, as previously mentioned, or because some form of damage occurs during the repair of a defect with a good prognosis. A special form of bowel management program has been designed to keep these patients clean and improve their quality of life. Most patients suffer from fecal incontinence and a tendency toward constipation. The bowel management implemented in that kind of patient includes the use of large enemas given every day, aimed to clean the colon. The fact that these patients tend to suffer from constipation happens to be serendipitously good, because it keeps the patient completely clean in between enemas.

In some patients the rectosigmoid or some other portion of their colon was resected at the time of the main repair. This procedure was used in patients who underwent endorectal techniques, or else a portion of the colon was sometimes resected for various other reasons. The final consequence is a tendency to suffer diarrhea. In these types of cases, the bowel management implemented includes not only the use of enemas every day to clean the colon, but also the administration of a constipating diet or medications to slow down the colon motility in order to keep the patient clean. This last group of patients is, in general, more difficult to manage. Overall, in the author's experience, 90% of the patients can be kept clean by using a form of bowel management.

Recently, an operation called continent appendicostomy allows the patient to receive the enemas through the cecal appendix, which is implanted at the patient's umbilicus. The cecum is usually plicated around the appendix to create a one-way valve mechanism. This operation provides a great deal of independence to adolescent patients, because this way they do not need assistance to receive the enemas. For those patients who lost their appendix in the past, a continent neoappendicostomy is created by making a neoappendix with a tubularized flap of cecum plus a plication of the cecum around it, to provide continence.

Constipation is the most common sequela suffered by patients who were born with imperforate anus and underwent a repair in which the original rectum and colon of the patient were preserved. Paradoxically, the lower the defect, the worse the constipation experienced by the patient. This symptom must be treated energetically because untreated constipation creates more constipation. The degree of constipation also correlates with the degree of megarectum that the patient suffered from originally. The megarectum is more severe in patients subjected to a transverse colostomy and is the worst in patients with loop colostomies that allow the spillage of stool from proximal to distal stoma. Severe constipation and chronic fecal impaction may subsequently provoke overflow pseudoincontinence, and that is another reason to treat the constipation to be sure that the rectum empties every day.

Urinary incontinence in male patients with imperforate anus occurs only in those born with absent sacrum or in those who suffered nerve damage during the repair of their otherwise benign anorectal malformation. In female patients, on the other hand, it occurs in 20% of those girls with a cloaca with a common channel shorter than 3 cm and in 70% of those girls with a cloaca and a common channel longer than 3 cm. Most of these patients can be kept dry by the use of intermittent catheterization.

Suggested Readings

Hendren, WH: Repair of cloacal anomalies. Current techniques. J Pediatr Surg 1996; 21:115–176.

Peña A: Posterior sagittal anorectoplasty: Results in the management of 322 cases of anorectal malformations. Pediatr Surg Int 1988; 3:94–104.

Peña A: Surgical management of persistent cloaca: Results in 54 patients treated with a posterior sagittal approach. J Pediatr Surg 1989; 24(6):590–598.

Peña A: Anorectal Malformations. Semin Pediatr Surg 1995; 4(1):35–47.

Peña A, deVries PA: Posterior sagittal anorectoplasty. Important technical considerations and new applications. J Pediatr Surg 1982; 17:796–811.

Rich M, Brock W, Peña P: Spectrum of genitourinary malformations in patients with imperforate anus. Pediatr Surg Int 1988; 3:110–113.

18

HIRSCHSPRUNG'S DISEASE

Frederick Alexander, MD, FACS, FAAP

Hirschsprung's disease (HD) or congenital aganglionosis of the colon is a common cause of intestinal obstruction in infants and children, occurring in 1 of every 5000 live births. It is characterized by absent ganglion cells and hypertrophy of adrenergic and cholinergic nerves in the submucosal and myenteric plexus of the bowel, extending proximally from the internal anal sphincter a variable distance into the rectum or colon.

■ PATHOPHYSIOLOGY

Although the pathophysiology of HD is not fully understood, the aganglionic bowel exhibits tonic contraction resulting in functional obstruction of the colon with proximal dilatation and an abrupt or gradual transition to the relatively narrow distal bowel. Normally, neuroblasts from the vagal neural crest migrate from the primitive esophagus to the distal anal canal by the 12th week of gestation. HD occurs when the normal migration or differentiation of enteric neuroblasts is interrupted by a possible alteration of enteric extracellular matrices or underlying immunologic mechanism.

Several clinical observations suggest that HD has a genetic etiology. For example, approximately 10 to 15% of all cases occur in infants with Down syndrome (trisomy 21), and 5% occur in infants with other serious neurologic abnormalities. Thirty percent of cases have a family history of HD. Recent genetic research has demonstrated a link between HD and mutations in the RET gene (10q 11.2) and in the endothelin-B receptor (EDNRB) gene (13q 22). Further, it has been demonstrated that deletion of RET causes total aganglionosis in mouse mutants. Aganglionic bowel taken from patients with HD expresses a significantly less intense signal for RET mRNA compared to normal ganglionic bowel. Thus, it appears that controlled and regulated expression of the RET gene among others is essential for normal migration and differentiation of vagal neural crest–derived cells. Future genetic research may explain the variety of clinical states and unusual inheritance patterns in HD.

■ CLINICAL FEATURES AND DIAGNOSIS

The clinical presentation of HD varies widely from complete obstruction or enterocolitis in newborns to chronic constipation in older children and adults. This wide clinical spectrum is not explained by the variable length of aganglionic bowel, because there is no definite correlation between the length of aganglionosis and the severity of symptoms. Other factors may affect smooth muscle function in the aganglionic segment and thus contribute to the degree of bowel obstruction. For example, recent studies have shown that intestinal relaxation may be mediated by several neurotransmitters normally released from nonadrenergic and noncholinergic (NANC) inhibitory nerves. Nitric oxide (NO), a potent smooth muscle relaxant synthesized from L-arginine in NANC nerves, may be the most important of these neurotransmitters and is variably diminished or absent in aganglionic bowel.

The mean age at diagnosis of HD has steadily decreased to approximately 6 months, with 40 to 60% of cases diagnosed at less than 1 month of age. The principal symptoms in the newborn period are abdominal distention, vomiting, and failure to pass meconium within 24 hours of birth. Plain films virtually always demonstrate dilated loops of bowel, and the rectum is frequently devoid of gas. Gaseous intestinal distention with abrupt cutoff at the level of the pelvic brim (intestinal cutoff sign) on plain film is highly indicative of Hirschsprung's associated enterocolitis. Barium enema is diagnostic of HD in nearly 90% of cases. The hallmark of HD on barium enema is a transition or change in caliber from proximal dilated bowel to distal contracted bowel, usually in the upper rectum or lower sigmoid. In some neonates with HD a transition may not be evident, but delayed plain films invariably show abnormal retention of barium at 24 to 48 hours.

Barium enema is a valuable screening tool for other problems with a similar clinical presentation such as ileal atresia, meconium ileus, meconium plug syndrome, and small left colon syndrome. Ileal atresia results from an intrauterine mesenteric vascular occlusion indicated on barium enema by an unused or microcolon. Meconium ileus is an early manifestation of cystic fibrosis wherein abnormally thickened meconium plugs the ileum and colon producing a dense filling defect on barium enema. Meconium ileus frequently requires laparotomy for evacuation and decompression of the bowel. Meconium plug syndrome is unrelated to cystic fibrosis and rarely requires surgical therapy. This condition is characterized by inspissated lumps of meconium in the colon which usually evacuate following the enema. In some cases, HD initially may be mistaken for meconium plug syndrome, and is suggested by persistent obstructive symptoms. Small left colon syndrome is a transient dysmotility disorder that occurs most often in infants of diabetic mothers. Barium enema demonstrates a small rectum and left colon with proximal dilatation. Most patients evacuate spontaneously, but diverting colostomy is occasionally required for persistent functional obstruction.

Histologic confirmation of HD is obtained either by submucosal or by full-thickness punch biopsy of the anal canal. Ganglion cells in the submucosal or myenteric plexus 1.5 to 2 cm above the dentate line exclude the diagnosis of HD. Conversely, absence of ganglion cells in the same zone examined by an experienced pathologist confirms the diagnosis of HD. The suction rectal biopsy tool devised by Noblett provides an excellent sample of (submucosal) tissue at bedside in patients less than 2 years of age. In older patients, sampling errors with this tool lead to a false negative response rate approaching 10%. Acetylcholinesterase stain for hypertrophied cholinergic nerves has been shown to enhance the accuracy of suction biopsies from 84 to 99%. Nevertheless, full-thickness punch biopsies obtained by direct visualization in the operating room consistently provide the most reliable specimens in patients older than 2 years. Another tool used to diagnose HD is anorectal manometry. This device is less accurate than full-thickness rectal biopsy but is also less invasive, and is particularly useful in older patients with suspected ultrashort segment disease. HD is confirmed by anorectal manometry when rectal distention fails to produce relaxation of the internal anal sphincter. In a patient with a megarectum, however, lack of a rectoanal inhibitory reflex is not conclusive evidence of HD, as the dilated rectum may be too insensitive for the reflex to be stimulated. A normal reflex does rule out HD.

Several variations of HD deserve special mention here. "Ultrashort segment" HD is an uncommon condition, occurring in 5% of patients with HD. In this condition, the transition zone is located within the anal canal, causing constipation without obstructive episodes. For this reason, the diagnosis is usually made in older children. Barium enema is usually nondiagnostic, and rectal biopsies may be misleading because of the close proximity of ganglion cells to the internal anal sphincter. A suspicion of ultrashort segment HD is best confirmed by anorectal manometry. Another relatively rare condition, occurring in 1 to 5% of patients with HD is total colonic aganglionosis (TCA). Patients with TCA present in the newborn period with severe small bowel obstruction. Barium enema usually demonstrates a normal-appearing colon, but plain films taken 24 hours later invariably show abnormal retention of barium. The diagnosis is confirmed at laparotomy by frozen section analysis of multiple biopsies. TCA differs from the typical form of HD in that it may encompass "skip areas" of zonal ganglionic innervation, usually in the terminal ileum and transverse colon, surrounded by aganglionic bowel. Also, histochemical studies of TCA usually demonstrate little or no evidence of neural hypertrophy usually associated with typical HD.

Fifteen percent of patients with HD present with enterocolitis, a syndrome comprising explosive diarrhea, abdominal distention, and fever. More than two thirds of these patients are infants less than 3 months of age, and up to one third have trisomy 21. Enterocolitis is the major cause of death in children with HD, associated with a mortality rate of 5 to 30%. Many studies have shown that enterocolitis and its complications may be avoided completely if HD is diagnosed and treated in the first week of life. Thus, the diagnosis of HD should be seriously entertained in any newborn who fails to pass meconium within the first 24 hours of life.

■ SURGICAL TREATMENT

The surgical treatment of HD has evolved since the first definitive repair was reported by Swenson and Bill in 1948. The Swenson rectosigmoidectomy utilizes circumferential dissection on the muscular coat of the aganglionic rectum in order to avoid injury to the splanchnic nerves. This extramuscular dissection is carried down to the internal anal sphincter, which is preserved. The rectum is divided and then everted through the anus. The anal canal is transected on a diagonal plane 1.5 cm from the dentate line on the anterior border and 1.0 cm on the posterior border. As the anal canal is transected, an anastomosis is performed between the pulled-through ganglionic bowel and the cut edge of the anal canal.

An alternative reconstructive procedure devised by Duhamel and modified by Martin preserves the anterior aganglionic wall of the rectum. In this procedure, the aganglionic bowel is resected down to the peritoneal reflection where the rectal stump is closed. The retrorectal space is bluntly opened to within 1 cm of the dentate line where full-thickness incision is made 180 degrees along the posterior margin of the anal canal. The ganglionic bowel is pulled through and its posterior rim anastomosed to the cut edge of the anal canal. A side-to-side anastomosis of the anterior aganglionic rectal wall and the posterior ganglionic rectal wall is performed using the GIA stapler. The proximal end of the aganglionic rectum is opened in order to complete the side-to-side anastomosis from above and to confirm that the division of the anterior and posterior rectum is complete. The proximal aganglionic rectum is then trimmed and tapered as it is closed in order to eliminate formation of a blind rectal pouch. The Martin-Duhamel procedure is ideally suited to the treatment of TCA. In patients with TCA, the procedure is modified to preserve the aganglionic left colon. Using the GIA stapler, a long side-to-side anastomosis is constructed between the ganglion-containing ileum and aganglionic left colon, extending all the way down to the anal canal.

A third reconstructive approach utilizes an endorectal dissection first described by Ravitch and Sabiston, then applied to the treatment of HD by Soave, and finally modified by Boley. The Soave-Boley procedure is performed by resection of the aganglionic bowel to the peritoneal reflection, whereupon a circumferential seromuscular incision is made and a submucosal plane is dissected down to the anal canal. A circumferential mucosal incision is made in the anal canal 1 cm from the dentate line on the anterior margin and 0.5 cm on the posterior margin. The submucosal dissection is continued in a proximal direction through the anus and the entire mucosal sleeve is everted and removed from below. The muscular cuff is then incised vertically along its posterior midline axis. Finally, the cut end of the ganglionic bowel is pulled through and anastomosed to the cut edge of the mucosa within the anal canal.

In the past, most newly diagnosed patients with HD underwent preliminary colostomy before reconstruction for the following reasons: (1) early diversion prevents or treats enterocolitis in newborns, (2) diversion averts the complications of reconstructive surgery, such as leak or stricture, and (3) diversion permits complete pathologic evaluation of the bowel prior to definitive repair. Initially, most patients underwent three-stage repair including right transverse colostomy followed (at 1 year of age in the newborn) by definitive repair and subsequent colostomy closure. As surgical techniques improved, two-stage repairs could be performed safely and were adopted as standard practice. In a two-stage repair, a divided colostomy is performed just above the transition zone guided by frozen section analysis of partial-thickness biopsies. Biopsy results are confirmed by permanent section analysis of the full-thickness stomal edge, and stomal function is carefully assessed. At a second procedure, the colostomy is taken down and a pull-through procedure is performed without a covering colostomy. The time interval between the first and second stages is variable, depending upon the patient's age at diagnosis and the surgeon's preference. In the newborn, the time interval between the two stages has gradually diminished from 1 year to 3 to 6 months, as it appears that younger children tolerate reconstructive surgery with less perianal excoriation, fewer septic complications, and shorter recovery time than older children.

More recently, major reconstruction has been successfully performed in newborns in one step without preliminary colostomy. Once the diagnosis of HD is made, colonic irrigations are performed once or twice a day using 60 mL warm saline via a 16 Fr Foley catheter until the infant is 3 to 4 weeks old. A primary one-stage pull-through is then performed, the level of transection being determined by frozen section analysis of partial-thickness biopsies. The principal advantage of this procedure is avoidance of a colostomy and restoration of anorectal function as early as possible. The principal risk of this procedure is mistaken analysis of frozen sections leading to retention of the transition zone in the pulled-through bowel. Contraindications to this technique include unavailability of pediatric pathologic expertise, previous enterocolitis, and inability of the parents to perform irrigations at home.

The latest development in the treatment of HD is the primary laparoscopic assisted pull-through. This procedure combines a single-stage approach with advanced laparoscopic techniques that permit mobilization of the colon. As described by Georgeson, the patient is placed in a modified lithotomy position and the abdomen is insufflated with a Varess needle. Three 5-mm trocars are inserted in the upper abdomen, two on the right side and one on the left. A 5-mm laparoscopic camera is used to visualize the transition zone and the mesentery of the sigmoid colon is mobilized, preserving the marginal vessels. Laparoscopic dissection is carried out on the rectal wall to the level of the prostate or cervix. Transanal circumferential submucosal dissection is performed from a level 5 to 10 mm proximal to the dentate line to the distal margin of the intra-abdominal dissection. The mucosal cuff is pulled downward, and the intussuscepted muscular cuff is incised circumferentially, allowing the colon to be pulled down and through the anus. A full-thickness biopsy is obtained to check for ganglion cells, and the colon is transected at the appropriate level. The procedure is completed with a single-layer coloanal anastomosis. Although ideally suited to the Soave-Boley endorectal pull-through, laparoscopic techniques have also been applied to the Duhamel procedure.

In some cases, HD may be successfully managed by transanal myomectomy rather than the pull-through procedure. For example, "ultrashort segment" HD is an excellent indication for myomectomy. Another indication is recurrent constipation following the pull-through procedure. This development may occur as a result of retained transition zone or ischemic "dropout" of ganglion cells in the distal margin of the pulled-through bowel. In this instance, it is important to distinguish between anastomotic stricture and abnormal or absent ganglion cells, because the former responds to anal dilatation and the latter does not. Thus, it is important to obtain full-thickness punch biopsies before attempting myomectomy. Transanal myomectomy is performed through a transverse incision 0.5 cm above the dentate line on the posterior aspect of the anal canal. A mucosal flap is raised allowing visualization of the muscle complex of the posterior anal canal. A vertical strip of muscle 1 cm wide and 1 cm deep is excised along the length of the anal canal. The excised muscle is labeled, and a frozen section of the proximal cut edge is analyzed for ganglion cells. If no ganglion cells are identified, the myomectomy may be extended, taking care not to create a buttonhole of the mucosal flap. After the myomectomy is complete and hemostasis achieved, the flap is closed transversely with interrupted dissolvable sutures. No drains are used with this procedure, but placement of a rectal pack is useful to prevent submucosal hemorrhage and flap dehiscence.

Anal achalasia can cause significant difficulty with defecation after definitive surgery for HD. Some patients have responded well to topical nitric oxide in isosorbide dinitrate paste, applied topically (1 mg/kg/day in two separate doses for a minimum of 3 weeks).

■ OUTCOME

Outcome comparisons of the major reconstructive procedures are difficult to make because of variable surgical technique, irregular levels of transection with respect to the transition zone, and inconsistent follow-up and documentation of bowel function. The best comparative figures are provided by a survey of the members of the Surgical Section of the American Academy of Pediatrics. In this report of 1196 patients, the Swenson procedure had the highest rate of postoperative enterocolitis (15.6%), anal stenosis (9.5%), and fecal soiling (3.2%). By comparison, the Soave-Boley procedure had the lowest rate of enterocolitis (2.1%) and fecal soiling (1.1%). However, the Soave-Boley procedure had a higher rate of anal stenosis (9.4%) and postoperative perianal excoriation. The Duhamel procedure had a relatively low rate of anal stenosis (5.5%) and fecal soiling (1.1%) and a moderately low rate of enterocolitis (6%). Recurrent constipation was not surveyed in this study, but more recent studies indicate that it occurs in 7 to 8% of cases following the Duhamel procedure and less often following the other procedures. Behavioral therapy may help to minimize residual defecation problems after surgery. Instruments are being developed to measure quality of life in these patients.

Because the preceding differences in outcome are actually quite minor, the choice of operation depends largely upon surgeon's preference. Properly performed, all procedures should yield a 90 to 95% success rate with minimal morbidity and mortality rates, and virtually no need for permanent enterostomy. The exception is TCA, which entails a higher morbidity and mortality rate than does typical HD. For example, in the preceding survey, the overall mortality rate of patients with TCA was 47%, with a high percentage of deaths occurring following enterostomy. Postoperative mortality rate was 21% following definitive repair. It is hoped that advances in surgical technique and nutrition will lead to improvement in the outcome of patients with TCA in the future.

The long-term results of primary pull-through are not yet available. However, short-term complications occur in 6 to 30% of cases following primary pull-through. These complications include anastomotic leak and stricture, bowel obstruction, and retained transition zone (i.e., transection of the bowel through the transition zone). Approximately 3 to 10% of patients require a stoma or redo pull-through, and 6 to 30% develop postoperative enterocolitis. Several comparative studies indicate no significant difference in morbidity rate between one-stage and two-stage procedures; however, the overall complication rate of staged procedures cited in these studies (18 to 32%) appears to be higher than in other reports. For example, at the Cleveland Clinic Foundation, the overall length of stay and complication rate following two-stage Soave-Boley pull-through is 4 days and 6%, respectively, and only 6% of patients have developed postoperative enterocolitis (unpublished data). Similarly, short-term results of primary laparoscopic pull-through appear to be excellent, with low morbidity rate and average postoperative stay of 4 days; however, long-term results are not available. The question remains whether short- and long-term results—open or laparoscopic—will match or improve upon those staged procedures.

Postoperative enterocolitis is a major cause of morbidity and death, occurring in 15 to 20% of patients. It was once assumed that preoperative enterocolitis predisposed to further episodes, but this has been disproved recently. In most cases, it occurs in association with an anastomotic stricture or anorectal dysfunction related to retained transition zone in the distal margin of the pulled-through bowel. Initial management consists of prompt rectal tube decompression, intravenous hydration, and broad-spectrum antibiotic therapy. Subsequently, secondary procedures are commonly required to relieve stricture or dysfunction. Within the past decade, the mortality rate of postoperative enterocolitis has fallen to less than 5%, while the mortality rate of enterocolitis at diagnosis has remained nearly 30%. Further improvement in the outcome of HD must now depend upon early diagnosis and treatment in order to avert the life-threatening complications of enterocolitis.

Suggested Readings

Boley SJ: New modification of the surgical treatment of Hirschsprung's disease. Surgery 1964;56:1015–1017.

Burleigh, DE: N^G-Nitro-L-arginine reduces nonadrenergic noncholinergic relaxations of human gut. Gastroenterology 1992;102:679–683.

Duhamel B: A new operation for the treatment of Hirschsprung's disease. Arch Dis Child 1960;35:38–39.

Ederyl P, Lyonnet S, Mulligan L, et al: Mutations of the RET proto-oncogene in Hirschsprung's disease. Nature 1994;367:378–380.

Fujimoto T, Hata J, Yokoyama, Mitomi T: A study of the extracellular matrix protein as the migration pathway of neural crest cells in the gut: analysis of human embryos with special reference to the pathogenesis of Hirschsprung's disease. J Pediatr Surg 1989;24:550.

Gabriel SB, Salomon R, Pelet A, et al: Segregation at three loci explains familial and population risk in Hirschsprung's disease. Nat Genet 2002;31:89–93.

Garrett JR, Howard ER, Nixon HH: Autonomic nerves in rectum and colon in Hirschsprung's disease. Arch Dis Child 1969;44:406–417.

Georgeson KE, Fuenfer MM, Hardin DH: Primary laparoscopic pull-through for Hirschsprung's disease in infants and children. J Pediatr Surg 1995;30:1017–1022.

Hackam DJ, Superina RA, Pearl RH: Single-stage repair of Hirschsprung's disease: A comparison of 109 patients over 5 years. J Pediatr Surg 1997;7:1028–1032.

Hannman MJ, Sprangers MA, De Mik EL, et al: Quality of life in patients with anorectal malformation or Hirschsprung's disease: Development of a disease-specific questionnaire. Dis Colon Rectum 2001;44:1650–1660.

Kapur RP: Hirschsprung's disease: Pathology and molecular pathogenesis. Adv Pathol Lab Med 1995;8:201–221.

Klein MD, Coran AG, Wesley JR, Drongowski RA: Hirschsprung's disease in the newborn. J Pediatr Surg 1984;19:370–374.

Kleinhaus S, Boley SJ, Sheron M, Sieber WK: Hirschsprung's disease: A survey of the members of the Surgical Section of the American Academy of Pediatrics. J Pediatr Surg 1979;14:588–597.

Kobayashi H, Hirakawa H, Surana R, et al: Intestinal neuronal dysplasia is a possible cause of persistent bowel symptoms after pull-through operation for Hirschsprung's disease. J Pediatr Surg 1995;30:253–259.

Kuroda T, Doody DP, Donahoe PK: Aberrant colonic expression of MHC class II antigens in Hirschsprung's disease. Aust NZ J Surg 1991;61:373.

Kusafuka T, Puri P: Altered RET Gene in RNA expression in Hirschsprung's disease. J Pediatr Surg 1997;32:600–604.

Martin LW, Altemeier WA: Clinical experience with a new operation (modified Duhamel procedure) for Hirschsprung's disease. Ann Surg 1962;156:678–681.

Marty TL, Seo T, Mallak ME, et al: Gastrointestinal function after surgical correction of Hirschsprung's disease: Long-term follow-up in 135 patients. J Pediatr Surg 1995;30:655–658.

Meier-Ruge W: Hirschsprung's disease: Its aetiology, pathogenesis and differential diagnosis. Curr Topics Pathol 1974;59:131.

Millar AJ, Steinberg RM, Raad J, Rode H: Anal achalasia after pull-through operations for Hirschsprung's disease—Preliminary experience with topical nitric oxide. Eur J Pediatr Surg 2002;12:207–211.

Nixon HH: Hirschsprung's disease: Progress in management and diagnostics. World J Surg 1985;9:189–202.

Noblett HR: A rectal suction biopsy tube for use in the diagnosis of Hirschsprung's disease. J Pediatr Surg 1969;4:406–409.

Okamoto E, Veda T: Embryogenesis of intramural ganglia of the gut and its relation to Hirschsprung's disease. J Pediatr Surg 1967;2:437.

Passarge E: The genetics of Hirschsprung's disease. N Engl J Med 1967;276:138.

Pierro A, Fasoli L, Kiely EM, Spitz L: Staged pull-through for rectosigmoid Hirschsprung's disease is not safer than primary pull-through. J Pediatr Surg 1997;32:505–509.

Puffenberger AG, Hosoda K, Washington SS, et al: A missense mutation of the endothelin-B receptor gene in multigenic Hirschsprung's disease. Cell 1994;79:1257–1266.

Puri P: Hirschsprung's disease: Clinical and experimental observations. World J Surg 1993;7:374.

Qualman SJ, Pysher T, Schauer G: Hirschsprung disease: Differential diagnosis and sequelae. In Dahms BB, Qualman SJ (Eds.). Gastrointestinal diseases. Perspect Pediatr Pathol 1997;20:110–126.

Ravitch MM, Sabiston DC: Anal ileostomy with preservation of the sphincter. Surg Gynecol Obstet 1947;84:1095–1099.

Rescorla FJ, Morrison AM, Engles D, et al: Hirschsprung's disease: Evaluation of mortality and long-term function in 260 cases. Arch Surg 1992;27:934–942.

Romeo GF, Ronchetto P, Luo Y, et al: Point mutations affecting the tyrosine-kinase domain of the RET proto-oncogene in Hirschsprung's disease. Nature 1994;367:378–380.

Rothenberg SS, Chong JHT: Laparoscopic pull-through procedures using the harmonic scalpel in infants and children with Hirschsprung's disease. J Pediatr Surg 1997;32:894–896.

Schuchardt A, D'Agati V, Larsson-Blomberg L, et al: Defects in the kidney and enteric nervous system of mice lacking the tyrosine-receptor RET. Nature 1994;367:380–383.

Smith BM, Steiner RB, Lobe TE: Laparoscopic Duhamel pull-through procedure for Hirschsprung's disease in childhood. J Laparosc Surg 1994;4:273–276.

So HB, Schwartz DL, Becker JM, et al: Endorectal "pull-through" without preliminary colostomy in neonates with Hirschsprung's disease. J Pediatr Surg 1980;15:470–471.

Soave F: A new surgical technique for the treatment of Hirschsprung's disease. Surgery 1964;56:1007–1044.

Swenson O: Hirschsprung's disease: A review. Pediatrics 2002;109:914–918.

Swenson O, Bill AH Jr: Resection of rectum and rectosigmoid with preservation of anal sphincter for benign spastic lesions producing megacolon: An experimental study. Surgery 1948;24:212–220.

Teitlebaum DH, Qualman SJ, Caniano DA: Hirschsprung's disease: Identification of risk factors for enterocolitis. Ann Surg 1988;207:240–244.

Tiffin ME, Chandler LR, Faber HK: Localized absence of ganglion cells of the myenteric plexus in congenital megacolon. Am J Dis Childhood 1940;59:1071–1082.

Van Kuyk EM, Brugman-Boezeman AT, Wissink-Essink M, et al: Defecation problems in children with Hirschsprung's disease: A prospective controlled study of a multidisciplinary behavioural treatment. Acta Paediatr 2001;90:1154–1159.

Vanderwinden JM, Delaet MH, et al: Nitric oxide synthase in the enteric nervous system of Hirschsprung's disease. Gastroenterology 1993;105:969–973.

Wakely PE, McAdams AJ: Acetylcholinesterase activity and the diagnosis of Hirschsprung's disease: A 3½ year experience. Pediatr Pathol 1984;2:35–46.

Welch KJ, Randolph JG, Ravitch MM, et al (Eds.): Pediatric Surgery, 4th ed. Year Book Medical Publishers, 1986, pp 995–1020.

19

FECAL INCONTINENCE

Timothy C. Counihan, MD
Robert D. Madoff, MD

Fecal incontinence, the inability to control the release of flatus or stool, is a clinical problem that is commonly encountered by the colorectal surgeon. The prevalence of fecal incontinence in the United States was recently reported as 2.3%, based upon a community survey. This figure soars to 30 to 40% in certain institutionalized populations such as nursing home residents.

Although fecal incontinence is a benign condition, its social consequences are frequently devastating. Because of the embarrassing nature of the problem, many patients are reluctant to admit its presence or seek medical attention. The overall cost of fecal incontinence to society is unknown, but the magnitude of the problem can be appreciated by the fact that Americans spend $400 million per year on adult diapers alone. Fecal incontinence is the second leading reason for admission of elderly patients to nursing homes, and is more common than dementia.

Fecal incontinence depends upon a wide variety of anatomic and physiologic factors. Colonic transit and stool consistency, rectal reservoir function, anorectal sensation, muscle innervation, and function of the internal and external anal sphincter all contribute to maintenance of normal continence. The causes of fecal incontinence are described in Table 19-1. In general, the three main etiologic categories are (1) abnormal stool consistency and volume; (2) neurologic disorders leading to sphincter weakness; and (3) anatomic defects in the sphincter. These problems often overlap, but accurate diagnosis and effective treatment depend upon addressing each area.

■ ASSESSMENT

Many scoring systems have been proposed to categorize the severity of fecal incontinence. The use of such systems is important for accurate patient assessment, medical/legal documentation, and objective evaluation of treatment outcomes. Although each scoring system has strengths and weaknesses, the ideal system would accurately and

Table 19-1 Causes of Fecal Incontinence
NORMAL PELVIC FLOOR
Diarrheal states
Infectious diarrhea
Inflammatory bowel disease
Short-gut syndrome
Laxative abuse
Radiation enteritis
Overflow
Impaction
Encopresis
Rectal neoplasms
Neurologic conditions
Congenital anomalies (e.g., myelomeningocele)
Multiple sclerosis
Dementia, strokes, tabes dorsalis
Neuropathy (e.g., diabetes)
Neoplasms of brain, spinal cord, cauda equina
ABNORMAL PELVIC FLOOR
Congenital anorectal malformation
Trauma
Accidental injury (e.g., impalement, pelvic fracture)
Anorectal surgery
Obstetrical injury
Aging
Pelvic-floor denervation (idiopathic neurogenic incontinence)
Vaginal delivery
Chronic straining at stool
Rectal prolapse
Descending-perineum syndrome

From Madoff RD, Williams JG, Caushaj PF: Fecal incontinence. N Engl J Med 1992;326:1002–1007.

reproducibly describe the frequency of incontinent episodes; the degree to which patients are incontinent of gas, liquid, and solid stool; and the effect of incontinence on the patient's lifestyle. At present, severity and quality-of-life scores should be determined independently. Use of the recently validated FIQL symptom-specific quality-of-life score is encouraged.

Evaluation of fecal incontinence begins with the detailed interview that includes a careful medical, surgical, and obstetric history. The timing and type of incontinence should be noted, as well as the use of pads, diapers, or medicine. Physical examination should include flexible sigmoidoscopy to rule out neoplastic and inflammatory disorders, with further evaluation of the small and large bowel as is clinically indicated. The perineum is inspected for scars, fistulas, and adequacy of the perineal body. The presence of rectal prolapse or perineal descent is appreciated by asking the patient to bear down. Digital examination at rest and with squeeze effort permits qualitative assessment of internal and external sphincter function.

Patients whose incontinence is severe enough to be considered for surgical therapy should undergo anorectal physiologic assessment. Anal manometry documents resting and squeeze pressures, indicating internal and external sphincter function, respectively. Rectal sensation is assessed using balloon distention. Pudendal nerve function is evaluated noninvasively by determining the terminal motor latency with a glove-mounted electrode. Defecography provides a dynamic view of rectal function and permits identification of pelvic floor disorders such rectocele or internal intussusception.

Endoanal ultrasonography is the best technique currently available to evaluate patients for possible anatomic anal sphincter defects. Use of a rotating probe with an anal cap easily demonstrates the internal and external sphincters, as well as location and severity of specific sphincter defects. Occult fistulas and other less common pathologic conditions may also be identified with this examination.

■ TREATMENT

Treatment should be individualized based on the severity of the symptoms, the patient's overall condition, and the degree to which the incontinence is affecting the patient's quality of life. Figure 19-1 shows an algorithm for the evaluation and treatment of fecal incontinence.

Medical Management

True incontinence must be differentiated from pseudoincontinence, soiling of mucus or pus caused by prolapsing hemorrhoids, full-thickness rectal prolapse, or occult fistulas. In these instances, therapy is directed at the primary cause itself. Conservative management is appropriate for mild true incontinence and is focused on optimizing stool consistency and frequency. Fiber supplements are prescribed to be taken once or twice daily in order to provide a soft, bulky stool. Patients with loose stools should be instructed to take only enough water to dissolve the bulking agent, thus permitting maximal absorption for excess stool water. Judicial use of antidiarrheals such as loperamide or diphenoxylate with atropine is appropriate to decrease stool frequency. Frequently, these drugs are most helpful at bedtime or prior to planned social engagements. Some patients, particularly those with chronic seepage, may also benefit from regular emptying of the rectum with a small tap-water enema.

Management of specific factors that may be contributory to fecal incontinence should be optimized before addressing the anal sphincter. Such therapy may be medical (e.g., infectious diarrhea, inflammatory bowel disease) or surgical (e.g., small bowel resection for Crohn's disease, rectopexy or perineal rectosigmoidectomy with levatoroplasty for full-thickness rectal prolapse).

Biofeedback

Biofeedback is a dynamic technique that allows an individual to learn of and respond to physiologic changes in the body. In the case of fecal incontinence, patients are trained to improve voluntary sphincter contraction, improve rectal sensation, and coordinate squeeze efforts with rectal distention. Biofeedback represents a qualitative improvement over simple pelvic floor exercises, such as those popularized by Kegel, because the biofeedback patient learns to focus efforts upon the appropriate target, the external anal sphincter, rather than the gluteus maximus. Biofeedback also has a number of appealing features in contrast to surgery: it is painless, noninvasive, relatively inexpensive, and risk-free.

Although anorectal biofeedback was originally devised using the Schuster triple balloon system, most centers now employ systems based on electromyography (EMG). An anal sensor is used to detect sphincter activity, which is displayed to the patient on a computer monitor. Gluteal surface electrodes may also be used to help focus contraction efforts exclusively upon the sphincter. Rectal sensory training is accomplished by instillation of progressively smaller quantities of air into a rectal balloon.

Requirements for biofeedback therapy include motivation, the ability to process instructions, and the ability to contract the sphincter muscle to a detectable degree. Specific indications for biofeedback include neurogenic fecal incontinence, inability to undergo surgery, and failure of operative sphincteroplasty. Patients with keyhole anal deformities tend to do poorly. Most centers now perform biofeedback on an outpatient basis; in our practice patients typically require three or four weekly sessions that last approximately 1 hour each. Patients are required to maintain a continence diary and are asked to exercise twice daily at home with the assistance of an audiotape.

The results of biofeedback for incontinence are impressive. In our series of 291 patients, 112 (38%) became completely continent, and an additional 123 patients (42%) achieved at least a 90% decrease in incontinent episodes. Abnormal pudendal nerve function did not appear to compromise results. Long-term follow-up demonstrated less than 10% deterioration after initial success after 1 to 5 years. A recent systematic review showed that 49% of incontinent patients were cured following biofeedback; 72% were cured or improved. However, studies varied

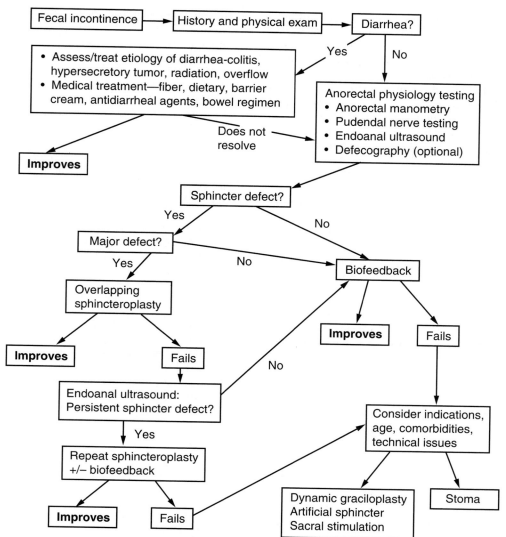

Figure 19-1
Algorithm for treating fecal incontinence.

with respect to biofeedback method, outcome measure, and criteria for success, and few series included control groups.

Surgery

Sphincter Repair

For fit patients, direct repair of sphincter defects is generally indicated. Sphincter injury is most commonly due to obstetric trauma in which the site of injury is in the anterior midline. In other patients, such as those who have had previous anorectal surgery, perineal injury, or pelvic fractures, the site and extent of a suspected sphincter injury may be less obvious on clinical examination; these patients should undergo endorectal ultrasonography to accurately define their sphincter anatomy. Several centers have reported inferior results of sphincter repair in the face of pudendal neuropathy, but others, including ours, have not observed this association. Although it is probably appropriate to discuss

the potential adverse impact of neuropathy on results with patients, most surgeons still advocate repair of obvious clinical defects, even in the face of neuropathy.

Acute sphincter injuries, particularly those that occur during childbirth, are best repaired primarily at the time of injury. When a significant injury has occurred, this repair is best performed under optimal conditions in the operating room, rather than attempting to do the best one can with imperfect lighting, inadequate assistance, and incomplete supplies in a birthing room. After the immediate postinjury phase, sphincter repair should be delayed a minimum of 6 months to permit complete resolution of the local inflammation and edema.

Sphincteroplasty patients should undergo full mechanical bowel preparation and receive preoperative broad-spectrum parenteral antibiotics. The operation is easiest to perform with the patient in the prone jack-knife position and the buttocks taped apart. A curvilinear incision is created between the anus and vagina and the anal and vaginal mucosa are elevated from the sphincter complex and associated scar. The sphincter mechanism is dissected laterally to the midcoronal line; posterolateral dissection is to be avoided because this area is where the branches of the pudendal nerve travel to innervate the sphincter. Cephalad dissection continues until the levators are identified as parallel muscle bands running anteriorly toward the pubis. It is often easiest to identify normal sphincter in the ischiorectal fossa, away from the area of maximal scarring in the anterior midline, and dissect medially. In most instances, an overlapping sphincteroplasty is preferred. The attenuated muscle and scar are divided (preserving the scar to help prevent the suture from tearing through the muscle) and wrapped to recreate a snug anal canal (Fig. 19-2). The repair is then effected with a series of absorbable horizontal mattress sutures. Many surgeons also perform an anterior levatoroplasty in an effort to lengthen the anal canal. Other authorities, however, advise against levatoroplasty because it is a potential cause of dyspareunia.

Occasionally, the area of sphincter injury may show only thinning rather than a complete disruption. Under these circumstances some surgeons prefer to simply plicate the muscle rather than divide it and overlap the ends. Data supporting this approach are limited. Colostomy or other fecal diversion is not necessary for the great majority of sphincter repairs, but may be considered under special circumstances such as the failure of previous repair efforts.

One important aspect of sphincter repair following obstetric injury is re-creation of an adequate perineal body. For routine repairs, vertical closure of the anterior portion of the incision is generally adequate. When more severe injuries are present, for example, when a complete cloacal defect is present, additional skin can be brought into the area by use of a cruciate incision followed by a Z-plasty closure (Fig. 19-3).

Postoperative management following sphincter repair varies considerably among surgeons. Narcotic analgesics are needed, and are best delivered in the postoperative period either by epidural catheter or by patient-controlled analgesia (PCA) pump. Although some advocate a clear liquid diet and bowel confinement, little convincing evidence exists to suggest that such a regimen is in fact necessary or of benefit. More important, both for patient comfort and for avoiding disruption of the repair, is the avoidance of constipation with a consequent fecal impaction. Patients should be maintained on a high-fiber diet with stool-bulking supplements and must be encouraged to drink adequate quantities of fluid. Mild laxatives such as milk of magnesia are often beneficial to counteract the constipating effects of oral narcotic analgesics. Patients should be taught how to self-administer tap-water enemas with a soft rubber catheter. Many surgeons instruct their patients to perform a daily tap-water enema for the first month postoperatively; at a minimum, patients should be instructed to perform an enema in the absence of a spontaneous daily bowel movement.

Approximately 60 to 80% of patients can expect a good or excellent result following sphincter repair, although minor defects in control, such as leakage of gas or mild

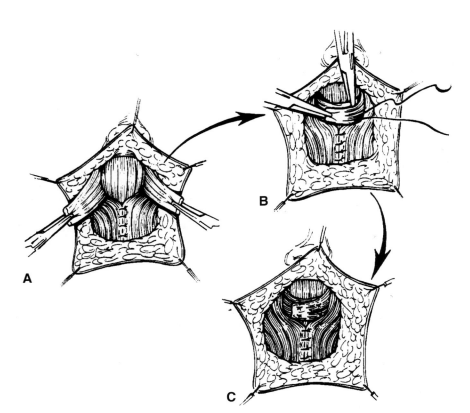

Figure 19-2
Overlapping sphincteroplasty.

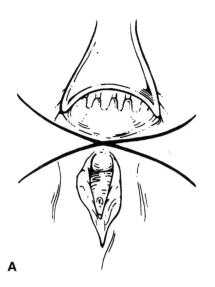

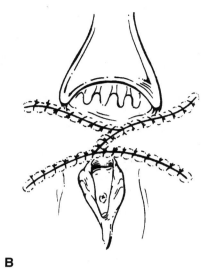

A

B

Figure 19-3
Reconstruction of the perineal body.

seepage, are not uncommon (Table 19-2). However, recently presented long-term studies have shown that results may deteriorate over time to 50% good or excellent results. Adverse prognostic factors include multiple previous failed repairs, severe preoperative incontinence (to solid versus liquid stool), and possibly pudendal neuropathy.

Postanal Repair

Parks devised the postanal repair for patients with anatomically intact but poorly functioning anal sphincters. The goals of the operation are to lengthen and narrow the anal canal and to provide a more acute anorectal angle. The procedure is accomplished via a posterior intersphincteric dissection and is carried above the rectosacral fascia, which provides access to plicate the puborectalis

and external anal sphincter. Results following this procedure have been highly variable, and evidence suggests that function continues to deteriorate after surgery. The operation is now rarely performed.

Anal Encirclement

Thiersch described the first anal encirclement procedure for rectal prolapse in 1891, and the technique has been adopted by subsequent surgeons for treating incontinence in high-risk surgical patients. The principle of the technique is to tighten the anal orifice by use of a simple subcutaneous suture. Thiersch advocated the use of silver wire, but high rates of disruption, erosion, fecal impaction, and reoperation have led to a search for softer and more pliable encircling materials. Over the past 50

Table 19-2 Results of Sphincteroplasty for Fecal Incontinence

STUDY	NUMBER OF PATIENTS	EXCELLENT/GOOD RESULTS (%)	FAIR RESULTS (%)	POOR RESULTS (%)
Fang, 1984	76	58	38	4
Hawley, 1985	100	52	32	18
Morgan, 1987	45	82	9	9
Ctercteko, 1988	44	54	32	18
Yoshioka, 1989	27	26	48	26
Jacobs, 1990	30	83	17	—
Fleshman, 1991	55	72	22	6
Wexner, 1991	16	76	19	5
Gibbs, 1993	33	73	15	12
Londono-Schimmer, 1994	60*	60	18	22
Engel, 1994	55	79	17	4
Sangalli, 1994	36	78	19	3
Sitzler, 1996	31	74	—	—
Oliveira, 1996	55	71	9	20
Nikiteas, 1996	42	67	14	19
Gilliland, 1998	100	60	19	21
Rasmussen, 1999	38	68	13	18
Buie, 2001	158	62	26	12

*Anterior repairs

years a large number of these alternatives have been described, ranging from synthetic suture to various forms of silicone rubber. Although these materials are undoubtedly superior to wire, they all remain prone to the same variety of local complications. Despite the attraction of a simple operation that can be performed under local anesthesia in infirm patients, the persistently high complication rate precludes routine use of this procedure.

Muscle Transposition

The most popular muscle transposition for fecal incontinence was described by Pickrell in 1952. Although the transposed muscle was meant to serve as a replacement sphincter, functional results following the operation proved to be poor. At present, most authorities consider the transposed gracilis to be a "living Thiersch," providing supple vascularized tissue that is less prone to complication than foreign material but acting poorly as a functional sphincter mechanism. Meanwhile, a number of centers over the past century have gained experience with transposition of the gluteus maximus. Several technical modifications of this operation have been proposed, using one or two muscles (unilateral or bilateral), partially detached either from the sacrum or the femur. Results of gluteus muscle transposition appear to be superior to those seen after gracilis transposition, probably due to the greater bulk of muscle available to surround the anus.

Two principal problems are responsible for the poor functional results of the Pickrell operation. First, continuous contraction of the transposed gracilis requires continuous volition on the part of the patient, who must concentrate on "adducting" his donor leg to contract the muscle. Even if such attention were possible, the gracilis muscle is physiologically poorly suited to tonic contraction because it comprises predominantly type 2 "fast-twitch" muscle fibers, which are rapidly fatigable.

The observation that fast-twitch muscle can be converted to slow-twitch, fatigue-resistant, type 1 fibers by continuous electrical stimulation, and the development of implantable electrical pulse generators capable of providing such stimulation, has led to the development of the electrically stimulated skeletal muscle neosphincter or dynamic graciloplasty.

While success rates of approximately 50 to 70% have been reported for patients with refractory fecal incontinence, dynamic graciloplasty has been associated with prohibitively high complication and failure rates except in the most experienced hands. Dynamic graciloplasty continues to be practiced in a small number of centers, but the device has not been approved for use for this indication in the United States by the Food and Drug Administration (FDA).

Artificial anal sphincter (AAS) represents an alternate approach to dynamic anal encirclement. The device is an adaptation of the artificial urinary sphincter that has already seen wide clinical use. It consists of three components: an inflatable cuff, a pressure-regulating balloon reservoir, and a patient-activated control pump. An appropriate size of cuff is selected and positioned extrasphincterically by means of bilateral circumanal incisions. The balloon is implanted in the space of Retzius by means of a short Pfannenstihl incision. The pump is positioned in the labia majora in women and in the scrotum in men. The system is filled with radiopaque fluid and its components are attached to one another by connecting tubing (Fig. 19-4). The cuff is left in a deflated position postoperatively by use of a deactivating button on the control pump. Provided healing is complete, the cuff is activated after 6 weeks, and under normal circumstances the cuff is inflated. When the patient wishes to defecate, he or she pumps the fluid from the cuff. The cuff spontaneously refills from the pressure-regulating balloon over 7 to 10 minutes.

Experience with the artificial anal sphincter continues to grow, and the device has recently been approved for use in the United States by the FDA. As in the case of dynamic graciloplasty, local complications, especially infection and erosion, remain problematic. Thus, while approximately 80% of patients who retain their implanted AAS have a successful result, the total intention to treat success rate is only about 50% because of a significant complication and explantation rate.

Sacral Nerve Stimulation

Sacral nerve stimulation (SNS) is a novel approach to the treatment of fecal incontinence. This technique is identical to that used in urology practice, where considerable success has been reported for voiding dysfunction. Patients undergo acute percutaneous nerve testing to confirm pelvic floor contraction and identify the optimal site of stimulation. The optimal site of stimulation causes maximal pelvic floor contraction with minimal associated contraction of the leg and foot. Once this site is identified (most commonly S3), a temporary lead is secured in position and the patient undergoes test stimulation with an external pulse generator. If the incontinence improves significantly, permanent lead implantation with subcutaneous attachment to an implantable pulse generator is performed.

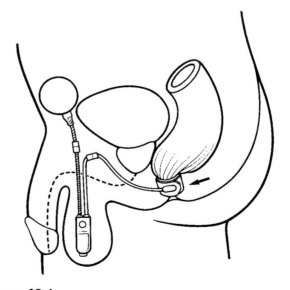

Figure 19-4
Artificial anal sphincter implanted in a male patient. (Acticon® Neosphincter, Courtesy of American Medical Systems, Inc., Minnetonka, Minnesota, www.American MedicalSystems.com)

Current indications for SNS include refractory fecal incontinence with an intact anal sphincter. The procedure is available in Europe and is currently under FDA protocol in the United States. Although the total number of patients reported upon following SNS for fecal incontinence remains relatively low, excellent functional outcomes with minimal morbidity have been reported. Several studies have shown improved quality of life associated with SNS therapy.

The mechanism of action of sacral nerve stimulation for improving fecal incontinence is unknown. Physiology studies demonstrate increases in both resting and squeeze anal pressures, as well as improved rectal sensation. Ambulatory manometry shows decreased rectal motor complexes and a decreased number of spontaneous episodes of anal relaxation. However, which, if any, of these alterations is responsible for the improvement is uncertain.

Fecal Diversion

Patients with severe fecal incontinence who have no further therapeutic options should be strongly encouraged to consider fecal diversion. Many patients, sometimes including those with debilitating symptoms, are reluctant to even consider this option. However, the decision should be considered in the context of converting an unmanageable perineal stoma into a manageable abdominal one. Patients have unlimited time to make this decision, and referral to an enterostomal therapist, ostomy patient, or both is invaluable. Patients can predictably expect to regain control of their bowel function and return to normal function in society without the fear of embarrassing accidents.

For most patients, the appropriate choice of stoma is an end-sigmoid colostomy. The stoma site should be marked preoperatively by the enterostomal therapist, taking into consideration patient habitus, scars, and other abdominal wall deformities. Patients with severe associated bowel dysfunction such as slow transit constipation may be better served by an end-ileostomy. The procedure itself can be expeditiously performed using minilaparotomy, trocar procedure, or laparoscopic techniques.

■ CONCLUSIONS

Fecal incontinence is a distressing condition that is underreported and undertreated. The cause of the incontinence dictates its therapy. Although the diagnosis is usually evident from the history and physical examination, laboratory tests provide useful confirmation and may uncover additional occult pathology. Endoanal ultrasonography plays a particularly important role in defining the anatomy of both normal and disrupted anal sphincters.

The treatment of incontinence depends both on its cause and its severity. Mild incontinence is best treated by conservative management and sometimes biofeedback. Direct sphincter repair is indicated for more severe incontinence when an anatomic sphincter defect is present. When the sphincter is anatomically intact, biofeedback is the initial treatment of choice. When standard therapy is not appropriate or has failed, salvage therapy using either the artificial anal sphincter or sacral nerve stimulation can be considered. Fecal diversion remains an excellent solution for the incontinent patient who has failed or is not a candidate for standard or salvage therapy.

Suggested Readings

Baeten CGMI, Geerdes BP, Adang EMM, et al: Anal dynamic graciloplasty in the treatment of intractable fecal incontinence. New Engl J Med 1999;332:1600–1605.

Blatchford GJ: The evaluation of incontinence. Semin Colon Rectal Surg 1997;8:61–72.

Buie WD, Lowry AC, Rothenberger DA, et al: Clinical rather than laboratory assessment predicts continence after anterior sphincteroplasty. Dis Colon Rectum 2001;44(9):1255–1260.

Ctercteko GC, Fazio VW, Jagelman DG, et al: Anal sphincter repair: a report of 60 cases and review of the literature. Aust N Z J Surg 1988;58:703–710.

Engel AF, Kamm MA, Sultan AH, et al: Anterior anal sphincter repair in patients with obstetric trauma. Br J Surg 1994;81:1231–1234.

Fang DT, Nivatvongs S, Vermeulen FD, et al: Overlapping sphincteroplasty for acquired anal incontinence. Dis Colon Rectum 1984;27:720–722.

Fleshman JW, Dreznick Z, Fry RD, Kodner IJ. Anal sphincter repair for obstetric injury: Manometric evaluation of functional results. Dis Colon Rectum 1991;34:1061–1067.

Fleshman JW, Peters WR, Shemesh EI, et al: Anal sphincter reconstruction: Anterior overlapping muscle repair. Dis Colon Rectum 1991;34:739–743.

Ganio E, Masin A, Ratto C, et al: Short-term sacral nerve stimulation for functional anorectal and urinary disturbances: results in 40 patients: Evaluation of a new option for anorectal functional disorders. Dis Colon Rectum 2001;44(9):1261–1267.

Gibbs DH, Hooks VH: Overlapping sphincteroplasty for acquired anal incontinence. South Med J 1993;86:1376–1380.

Gilliland R, Altomare DF, Moreira H, Jr, et al: Pudendal neuropathy is predictive of failure following anterior overlapping sphincteroplasty. Dis Colon Rectum 1998;41:1516–1522.

Halverson AL, Hull TL: Long-term outcome of overlapping anal sphincter repair. Dis Colon Rectum 2002;45:345–348.

Hawley PR: Anal sphincter reconstruction. Langenbecks Arch Chir 1985;366:269–272.

Jacobs PP, Scheuer M, Kuijpers JH, Vingerhoets MH: Obstetric fecal incontinence. Role of pelvic floor denervation and results of delayed sphincter repair. Dis Colon Rectum 1990;33:494–497.

Jensen LL, Lowry AC: Biofeedback improves functional outcome after sphincteroplasty. Dis Colon Rectum 1997;40(2):197–200.

Kenefick NJ, Nicholls RJ, Cohen RG, Kamm MA: Permanent sacral nerve stimulation for treatment of idiopathic constipation. Br J Surg 2002;89:882–888.

Lehur PA, Roig JV, Duinslaeger M: Artificial anal sphincter: prospective clinical and manometric evaluation. Dis Colon Rectum 2000;43(8):1100–1106.

Londono-Schimmer EE, Garcia-Duperly R, Nicholls RJ, et al: Overlapping anal sphincter repair for faecal incontinence due to sphincter trauma: Five year follow-up functional results. Int J Colorectal Dis 1994;9:110–113.

Madoff RD, Rosen HR, Baeten CG, et al: Safety and efficacy of dynamic muscle plasty for anal incontinence: Lessons from a prospective, multicenter trial. Gastroenterology 1999;116(3):549–556.

Madoff RD, Williams JG, Caushaj PF: Current concepts: Fecal incontinence. New Engl J Med 1992;326:1002–1007.

Malouf AJ, Norton CS, Engel AF, et al: Long-term results of overlapping anterior anal-sphincter repair for obstetric trauma. Lancet 2000;355:260–265.

Marcello PW, Coller JA: Neuromuscular re-education and the management of fecal incontinence. Semin Colon Rectal Surg 1997;8:84–92.

Matzel KE, Stadelmaier U, Hohenfellner M, Hohenberger W: Chronic sacral spinal nerve stimulation for fecal incontinence: Long-term results with foramen and cuff electrodes. Dis Colon Rectum 2001;44:59–66.

Morgan S, Bernard D, Tasse D, et al: Results of Parks' sphincteroplasty for post traumatic anal incontinence (abstract). Can J Surg 1987;30:299.

Nikiteas N, Korsgen S, Kumar D, Keighley MR: Audit of sphincter repair. Factors associated with poor outcome. Dis Colon Rectum 1996;39:1164–1170.

Norton C, Kamm MA: Anal sphincter biofeedback and pelvic floor exercises for faecal incontinence in adults—a systematic review. Aliment Pharmacol Ther 2001;15:1147–1154.

Oliveira L, Pfeifer J, Wexner SD: Physiological and clinical outcome of anterior sphincteroplasty. Br J Surg 1996;83:502–505.

Rasmussen OO, Puggaard L, Christiansen J: Anal sphincter repair in patients with obstetric trauma: Age affects outcome. Dis Colon Rectum 1999;42:193–195.

Rockwood TH, Church JM, Fleshman JW, et al: Fecal Incontinence Quality of Life Scale: Quality of life instrument for patients with fecal incontinence. Dis Colon Rectum 2000;43(1):9–16; discussion 7.

Sangalli MR, Marti MC: Results of sphincter repair in postobstetric fecal incontinence. J Am Coll Surg 1994;179:583–586.

Shelton AA, Madoff RD: Defining anal incontinence: Establishing a uniform continence scale. Semin Colon Rectal Surg 1997;8:54–60.

Sitzler PJ, Thomson JP: Overlap repair of damaged anal sphincter. A single surgeon's series. Dis Colon Rectum 1996;39:1356–1360.

Wexner SD, Marchetti F, Jagelman DG: The role of sphincteroplasty for fecal incontinence reevaluated: A prospective physiologic and functional review. Dis Colon Rectum 1991;34:22–30.

Wong WD, Jensen LL, Bartolo DCC, Rothenberger DA: Artificial anal sphincter. Dis Colon Rectum 1996;39:1345–1351.

Wong WD, Congliosi SM, Spencer MP, et al: The safety and efficacy of the artificial bowel sphincter for fecal incontinence: Results from a multicenter cohort study. Dis Colon Rectum 2002;45:1139–1153.

Yoshioka K, Keighley MR: Sphincter repair for fecal incontinence. Dis Colon Rectum 1989;32:39–42.

20

ANATOMY AND PHYSIOLOGY OF THE COLON AND RECTUM

H. Moreira, Jr., MD
Steven D. Wexner, MD, FACS, FASCRS

A complete knowledge of colonic and rectal anatomy is essential to successful surgical treatment of colorectal disease. However, the precise anatomy of the pelvic floor is still a subject of discussion. Dynamic study of the pelvic floor is limited because *postmortem* muscle tone may not reflect *in vivo* status. Conventional dissection with histologic and histochemical studies and dynamic studies of the mechanism of evacuation using cinedefecography have helped to clarify deficiencies. This chapter will provide a succinct description of the anatomy and physiology of the colon and rectum.

■ RELATIONSHIPS OF THE COLON AND RECTUM IN THE ABDOMINAL CAVITY AND PELVIS

The colon represents the terminal segment of the digestive tract, and is approximately 1.50 m (5 to 6 ft) in length. The proximal colon is larger in diameter than the distal colon (7.5 cm in the cecum to 2.5 cm in the sigmoid) (Fig. 20-1).

The cecum represents the beginning of the large bowel. The ileocecal valve is located in the posteromedial surface of the cecum, and is sustained in place by the superior and inferior ileocecal ligaments, which help maintain the angulation between the ileum and cecum, preventing cecal reflux. The appendix arises also from the posteromedial surface of the cecum approximately 3 cm below the ileocecal valve. It ranges from 2 to 20 cm in length and, due to its mobility, can be in different positions: retrocecal (65%), pelvic (31%), subcecal (2.3%), preileal (1.0%), and postileal (0.4%). The blood supply of the appendix is provided by vessels located at the mesoappendix originating from 16 ileocolic vessels (see Fig. 20-1). The cecum lays down on the lumbar musculature and usually has a short mesocecum that gives little mobility to this portion of the colon. However, an abnormally mobile cecum and ascending colon can be found in 10 to 22% of the cases and predisposes to volvulus.

The ascending colon extends from the ileocecal valve proximally to the hepatic flexure distally. It is usually covered by peritoneum on its anterior and lateral surfaces and has little or no mobility. Mobilization of the right colon should occur through Toldt's fascia, an avascular areolar tissue derived from coalescence of the posterior parietal peritoneum and the serosa that reflects off the posterior wall of the ascending and descending colon posteriorly and laterally. The right ureter lays over the psoas muscle, and is anteriorly crossed by the spermatic vessels and genitofemoral nerve. It is also lateral to the inferior vena cava and anteriorly crossed by the right colic and ileocolic arteries, the mesenteric root, and the terminal ileum. At the pelvis, anterior and slightly lateral to the common iliac artery bifurcation, the ureter descends abruptly between the peritoneum and the internal iliac artery. In females, it traverses the posterior layer of the broad ligament and parametrium, then runs alongside the neck of the uterus and upper third of the vagina. Here, the uterine artery crosses the ureter above and lateromedially.

As the colon ascends, it reaches the undersurface of the right lobe of the liver, lateral to the gallbladder, where it angulates acutely medially, downward, and anteriorly to the hepatic flexure. This angle is supported by the nephrocolic ligament anterior to the right kidney, and covering the second part of the duodenum. The second portion of duodenum and right kidney are exposed during mobilization of this flexure.

The transverse colon is the longest segment of the colon, very mobile, and enveloped by both layers of the transverse mesocolon attaching the posterosuperior border of the colon to the lower border of the pancreas. Moreover, the posterior and inferior layers of the greater omentum are fused on the anterosuperior aspect of the transverse colon. A dissection between the omentum and the mesentery is required to mobilize the transverse colon. This dissection is easy on the left, where the structures are naturally separated by the lesser sac of the peritoneum. It is harder on the right, where the omentum and the transverse mesocolon are fused. These peculiarities make laparoscopic dissection of the transverse colon difficult, increasing the risk of injury to important nearby structures.

The splenic flexure, the highest and deepest segment of the colon, is attached to the undersurface of the diaphragm at the level of the 10th and 11th ribs by the phrenocolic ligament and represents the distal limit of the transverse colon. Some attachments of mesentery of appendices epiploicae to the splenic capsule make traction on the splenic flexure potentially dangerous. At the time of mobilization, the surgeon should take care to avoid inadvertent splenic injury.

The descending colon passes over the lateral border of the left kidney, then descends medially between the psoas and the quadratus lumborum muscles to the junction with the sigmoid, which usually begins at the pelvic brim and the transversus abdominal muscle. Similar to the ascending colon, the descending colon is covered by peritoneum in the anterior, lateral, and medial surface.

The length of the sigmoid colon varies from 15 to 50 cm. It is mobile, with a generous inverted V-shaped mesosigmoid, creating a recessed intersigmoid fossa. The left ureter lies immediately beneath this fossa and is

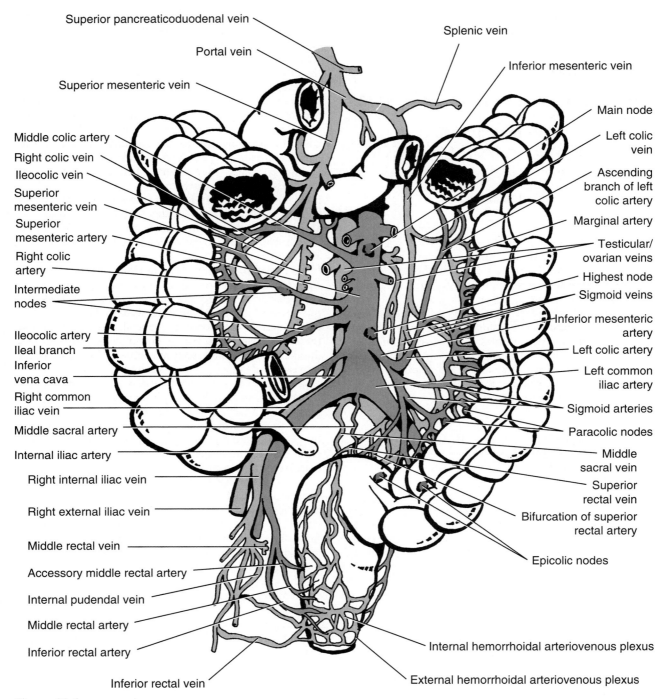

Superior pancreaticoduodenal vein

Portal vein

Superior mesenteric vein

Splenic vein

Inferior mesenteric vein

Main node

Left colic vein

Ascending branch of left colic artery

Marginal artery

Testicular/ovarian veins

Highest node

Sigmoid veins

Inferior mesenteric artery

Left colic artery

Left common iliac artery

Sigmoid arteries

Paracolic nodes

Middle sacral vein

Superior rectal vein

Bifurcation of superior rectal artery

Epicolic nodes

Internal hemorrhoidal arteriovenous plexus

External hemorrhoidal arteriovenous plexus

Middle colic artery

Right colic vein

Ileocolic vein

Superior mesenteric vein

Superior mesenteric artery

Right colic artery

Intermediate nodes

Ileocolic artery

Ileal branch

Inferior vena cava

Right common iliac vein

Middle sacral artery

Internal iliac artery

Right internal iliac vein

Right external iliac vein

Middle rectal vein

Accessory middle rectal artery

Internal pudendal vein

Middle rectal artery

Inferior rectal artery

Inferior rectal vein

Figure 20-1
Vascular and lymphatic anatomy of the colon and rectum.

crossed anteriorly by the spermatic vessels and left colic and sigmoid vessels. The mesosigmoid recess on its lateral surface gives guidance to the left ureter, which is situated posteriorly. The ureter should be seen before any ligation of colonic vessels is attempted. If distorted anatomy is suspected preoperatively, the placement of ureteric stents can help to localize the ureters.

The rectum is 12 to 15 cm in length and is divided into an upper third, middle third, and lower third. The anterolateral surface of the upper third is covered by peritoneum, while the middle third is covered only anteriorly; the lower third is completely extraperitoneal. The rectum descends, following the curvature of the sacrum and coccyx, and ending as it passes through the levator muscle

(Fig. 20-2). In males, the proximal two thirds are related to the small bowel loops and sigmoid colon while the lower third is related anteriorly to the prostate and seminal vesicles, vasa deferens, ureters, and urinary bladder. In females, the distal third is related anteriorly to the posterior vaginal wall. The upper and middle thirds are related to the upper part of the vagina, uterus, fallopian tubes, ovaries, small bowel, and sigmoid colon. Below the peritoneal reflection, lateral relations of the rectum are the ureters and iliac vessels. The rectal lumen shows three folds known as the valves of Houston; the upper and lower with the convexity to the right and the middle to the left, this being a landmark of the anterior reflection of the peritoneum. After complete mobilization, the rectum straightens and its length increases by 4 cm.

The rectum is surrounded by a fatty mesentery, which is most prominent posterolaterally. Superiorly, it is continuous with the sigmoid mesentery. In the pelvis, it is encapsulated by a fascial layer, the fascia propria. A lateral condensation of this fascia, known as lateral stalks or lateral ligaments, which attaches the rectum to the endopelvic fascia, has been described by Goligher. However, this is controversial. Although the middle rectal artery does not traverse the lateral stalks, it can send minor branches along one or both sides in approximately 25% of cases. Therefore, there is a 1:4 chance of minor bleeding when the lateral ligaments are cut. A strong presacral fascia covers the sacrum and coccyx, with the middle sacral artery, nerves, and the presacral veins underneath. Intraoperative rupture of the presacral fascia may cause a hemorrhage from these veins that is difficult to control. Waldeyer's fascia runs from the presacral fascia over the fourth sacral segment forward and down to the fascia propria of the rectum. During rectal mobilization, this avascular tissue should be deliberately divided. Anteriorly, the extraperitoneal portion of the rectum is covered by Denonvilliers' fascia, a layer of connective tissue which extends from the anterior peritoneal reflection to the urogenital diaphragm, separating the rectum from the vagina in females and the seminal vesicles in males.

The proximal margin of the anatomic anal canal is the dentate line at 2 cm from the anal verge. The surgical anal canal extends 2 cm above the dentate line to the level of the anorectal sling (Fig. 20-3). The anal canal is surrounded by two distinct muscle tubes, which completely collapse the lumen. The inner layer, which has autonomic innervation, is the internal sphincter, a continuation of the circular muscle of the rectum that becomes thickened and rounded at its lower end. The outer layer is composed of skeletal muscle: the puborectalis and the external sphincter. Between these two muscles is the conjoined longitudinal muscle, which is a continuation of the longitudinal muscle layer of the rectum. As it passes downward, some of its terminal

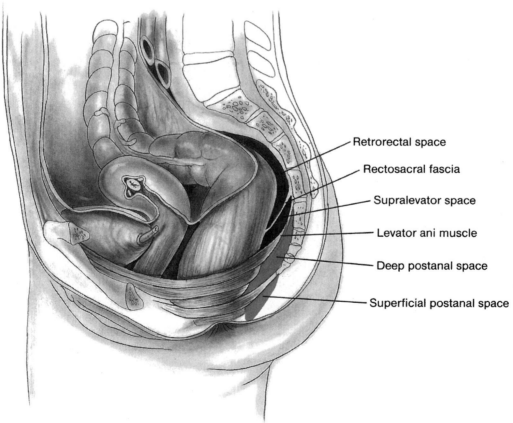

Figure 20-2
Sagittal view of the rectum and illustration of perianal and perirectal spaces.

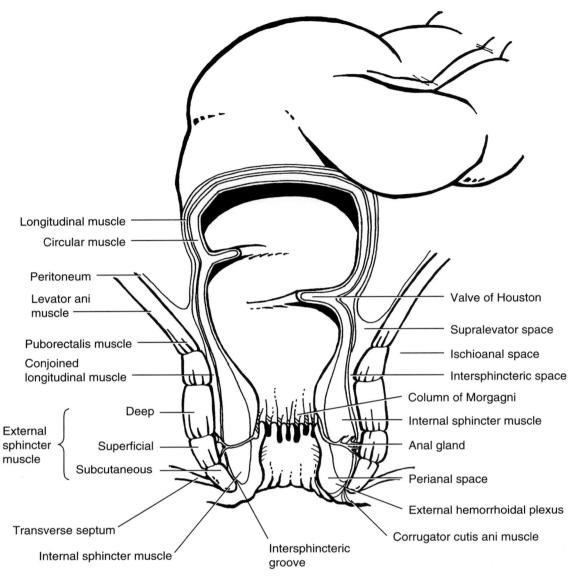

Figure 20-3
Anal canal and perianal and perirectal spaces.

fibers will cross the external sphincter and gain insertion on the perianal skin; this muscle is referred to as the corrugator cutis ani (see Fig. 20-3). The intersphincteric space is the preferable plane of dissection during an abdominal perineal resection for a patient with Crohn's disease, as it will facilitate wound healing. Moreover, it is the same plane that should be entered while a closed sphincterotomy is performed in the treatment of anal fissure. The lining of the anal canal corresponds to the different anatomic structures. A monostratified columnar epithelium in the rectum is followed by 0.5 to 1 cm of transitional epithelium. This includes columnar, transitional, and squamous epithelium, with a predominance of stratified columnar epithelium. Above the dentate line are 6 to 14 columns of Morgagni. Between the dentate

line and the distal portion of these columns, there are crypts that can be obstructed by foreign material causing sepsis. The anoderm is a squamous epithelium below the dentate line that in its proximal half is devoid of hair, sebaceous glands, and sweat glands (see Fig. 20-3).

■ ANORECTAL SPACES

The perianal space is limited laterally by the conjoined longitudinal muscle and extends medially around the anal canal. The superior limit is the mucosal suspensory ligament, which are transverse fibers of the conjoined longitudinal muscle that traverse the internal sphincter just below the anal valves. The external hemorrhoidal plexus, lymphatics, and terminal branches of the inferior rectal artery are located in this space (see Fig. 20-3).

The ischiorectal space is a pyramid-shaped space that contains the internal pudendal vessels and the pudendal nerve, which are lateral to the obturator fascia, inside the Alcock's canal. Medially, it is limited by the levator ani and external sphincter muscles and posteriorly by the sacrotuberous ligament and the lower border of the gluteus maximus muscle. The anterior boundary is composed of the superficial and deep transverse perineal muscles (see Fig. 20-3).

The intersphincteric space is between the internal and external sphincters, extending superiorly along the rectal wall and limited inferiorly by the mucosal suspensory ligament. It is a common site of cryptoglandular abscesses because two thirds of the anal glands end at this site without crossing the external sphincter (see Fig. 20-3).

The supralevator space is situated above the levator ani, limited superiorly by the peritoneum, laterally by the pelvic wall, and medially by the rectum. Abscesses in this area can be caused by extension of cryptoglandular abscess or pelvic sepsis (see Fig. 20-2).

The submucosal space is located between the mucosa and the internal sphincter.

The superficial postanal space is the posterior communication between the two ischiorectal spaces, below the anococcygeal ligament (see Fig. 20-2).

The deep postanal space is also a posterior communication of the right and left ischiorectal space, but it is above the anococcygeal ligament and below the levator muscle. Sepsis here may result in a horseshoe abscess (see Fig. 20-2).

The retrorectal space is limited, anteriorly by the fascia propria of the rectum, posteriorly by the presacral fascia, superiorly by the retroperitoneum, and inferiorly by Waldeyer's fascia. Below this area is the supralevator space. This is an area of embryologic fusion; therefore, unusual neoplasms derived from embryologic remnants may arise (see Fig. 20-2).

■ BLOOD SUPPLY

The blood supply of the right colon to the middle of the transverse colon is provided by the superior mesenteric artery, while the distal transverse colon, left colon, and superior third of the rectum are supplied by the inferior mesenteric artery (see Fig. 20-1).

The pattern of vascular distribution is variable. The superior mesenteric artery arises from the aorta, below the celiac trunk. Its first branch is the middle colic artery, which subdivides into two or three arcades in the mesentery of the transverse colon. The next branch is the right colic artery, which divides into an ascending branch joining the right branch of the middle colic and a descending branch that will anastomose with the arcades of the ileocolic artery. The ileocolic artery is the last colonic branch of the superior mesenteric artery, although sometimes it can arise from the right colic artery. It divides into four terminal branches: anterior and posterior cecal branch, the appendicular artery, and an ileal branch that forms arcades with the ileal branches from the superior mesen-

teric artery. This particular arcade pattern allows the construction of an ileal J-pouch after division of the ileocolic artery, because there are patent ileal branches.

The inferior mesenteric artery arises from the aorta below the third part of the duodenum. The first branch is the left colic artery, which divides into a descending and an ascending branch directed toward the splenic flexure. This ascending branch of the left colic artery joins with the left branch of the middle colic, while the descending branch of the left colic anastomoses with the sigmoid arteries. Three to four sigmoid branches of the inferior mesenteric artery give continuity to a marginal artery known as the marginal artery of Drummond. This marginal artery can provide blood supply to the entire left colon in case of occlusion of the inferior mesenteric artery. In about 7% of the population, another artery connects the middle colic artery with the left colic. This is the arc of Riolan (meandering mesenteric artery), and, on occasion, it may be the main blood supply to the left colon. The inferior mesenteric artery becomes the superior rectal artery as it crosses the pelvic brim, running downward in the mesorectum and dividing into the right and left branches. These branches subdivide into anterior and posterior arteries supplying the upper third of rectum. The lower two thirds of the rectum are supplied by the middle rectal artery and inferior rectal artery; the first is a direct branch of the internal iliac and the second derives from the pudendal artery, a subsidiary of the anterior division of the internal iliac artery. The inferior rectal artery passes downward surrounded by the endopelvic fascia as it exits the pelvis through the greater sciatic foramen. After a short distance, it reenters the pelvis through Alcock's canal in the lateral wall of the ischiorectal fossa. As it crosses this space, it can cause bleeding during abdominal perineal resection.

Venous drainage generally follows the arterial pattern, with three exceptions: (1) the contribution of the middle rectal vein to the drainage of the rectum is minimal; (2) there is an intense communication between the superior and inferior rectal vein through the rectal venous plexus; and (3) the inferior rectal vein drains to the systemic circulation through the internal iliac vein while the inferior mesenteric vein unites with the splenic vein at the lower border of the pancreas to join the portal vein.

■ LYMPHATIC DRAINAGE

The lymphatic drainage of the colon and rectum starts at the level of the lamina propria, becomes more significant at the level of submucosa and muscle wall, and finally reaches the extramural lymphatics. This network explains why tumors confined to the mucosa will not spread. Lymphatic vessels and nodes pair with the regional arteries. The lymph nodes can be classified into four types: epicolic, paracolic, intermediate, and main nodes (see Fig. 20-1). The first group represents the extramural nodes under the peritoneum, usually at the appendices epiploicae. Paracolic nodes are at the mesenteric border of the colon. Intermediate nodes lie around the main colic arteries, before their point of division. Main lymph nodes are located at the origin of the superior and inferior mesenteric arteries, in front of the aorta.

The pararectal lymph nodes are contained in the mesorectal tissue mainly at the posterior and lateral surfaces of the rectum. The proximal two thirds of the rectum drain to the inferior mesenteric lymph nodes, following the course of the superior rectal artery. The lower third of the rectum drains in two directions: cephalad, through the same lymphatics as the upper and middle thirds, and laterally, through the middle rectal lymphatic to the internal iliac nodes (Fig. 20-4A).

Total mesorectal excision can be safely performed, even through the lateral stalks, where occasionally some small vessels can cause minor bleeding. Posterior dissection of the rectum should be between the presacral fascia and fascia propria of the rectum through Waldeyer's fascia, to the level of the levator ani muscle.

The anal canal lymphatics drain in all directions: upward to the superior rectal lymphatic and inferior mesenteric nodes, laterally to the middle rectal nodes, and inferiorly to the internal iliac nodes. Below the dentate line, they usually drain to the inguinal nodes (Fig. 20-4B).

■ INNERVATION

Colon

The colon is innervated by inhibitory sympathetic nerves and excitatory parasympathetic nerves, which stimulate motor activity and gland secretion. The distribution of these fibers follows the regional arteries.

Sympathetic Innervation

The sympathetic trunk lies on the medial margin of the psoas muscle, in the retroperitoneal space, as it goes down and posteriorly to the common iliac artery. Here it presents four enlarged nodes denoting the sympathetic ganglia. Below this point, the sympathetic trunk continues downward as the sacral sympathetic trunk that may present up to four ganglia. It ends at the coccyx joining the opposite trunk, as a single ganglia.

The preaortic ganglia receive splanchnic nerves as preganglionic fibers, named from the adjacent arterial trunks. The fibers emerging at this point are postganglionic. The superior hypogastric plexus or presacral nerve, at the bifurcation of the aorta, arises from the aortic plexus and two lateral lumbar splanchnic nerves. The inferior hypogastric plexus is located together with the internal iliac arteries (Fig. 20-5A and B).

Parasympathetic Innervation

There are two distinct levels of innervation: vagal nerve and sacral outflow. The posterior vagal nerves descend to the preaortic plexus and are distributed to the regional vessels of the superior mesenteric artery, supplying the right colon to the middle of the transverse colon. The sacral outflow from the second, third, and fourth sacral nerves passes laterally, upward, and forward to join the superior hypogastric

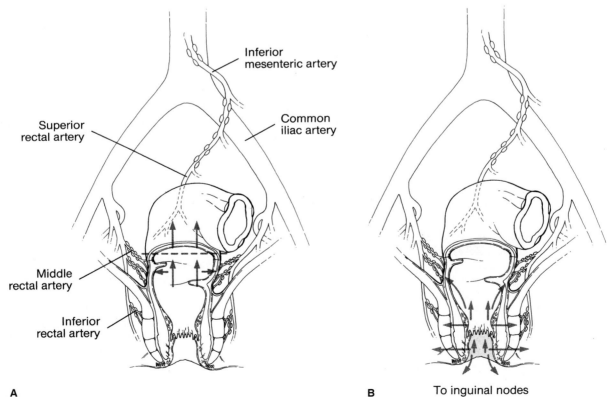

A

B   To inguinal nodes

Figure 20-4
Lymphatic drainage of the rectum (*A*) and anal canal (*B*).

plexuses (see Fig. 20-5*A* and *B*). These preganglionic fibers will form synapses in the myenteric plexus of Auerbach and Meissner located in the colon wall.

Rectum

The sympathetic innervation of the rectum originates from the first three lumbar segments of the spinal cord, which reach the upper third of the rectum, and by the presacral nerves, which divide into two branches that run on each side of the pelvis, innervating the lower third of the rectum, the anal canal, urinary bladder, and the sexual organs.

The presacral nerve or superior hypogastric plexus lies behind the inferior mesenteric vessels, between the

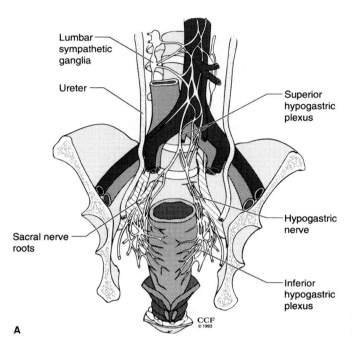

Lumbar sympathetic ganglia

Ureter

Superior hypogastric plexus

Sacral nerve roots

Hypogastric nerve

Inferior hypogastric plexus

CCF © 1993

A

Figure 20-5
Pelvic innervation.

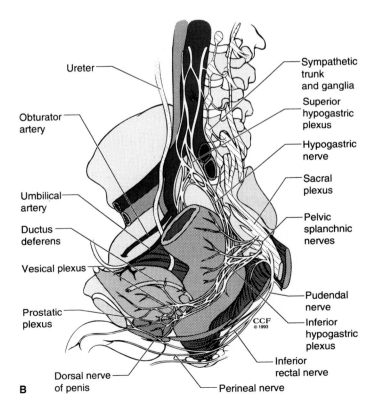

Ureter

Obturator artery

Umbilical artery

Ductus deferens

Vesical plexus

Prostatic plexus

Dorsal nerve of penis

Perineal nerve

Sympathetic trunk and ganglia

Superior hypogastric plexus

Hypogastric nerve

Sacral plexus

Pelvic splanchnic nerves

Pudendal nerve

Inferior hypogastric plexus

Inferior rectal nerve

CCF © 1993

B

ureters, and gets closely applied to the iliac artery and lumbar artery. Once the lateral branches reach the lateral pelvic wall, the sacral parasympathetic nerve or nervi erigentes joins these fibers, forming the pelvic plexus. The risk of nerve damage at this level is low, unless the endopelvic fascia is breached, or dissection of the internal iliac lymph nodes is performed. Both sympathetic and parasympathetic innervation are involved in erection. Depending on which nerve has been damaged, different deficiencies can become apparent, including incomplete erection, lack of ejaculation, retrograde ejaculation, or even impotence. These fibers are located anterior to Denonvilliers' fascia, between the rectum and prostate. The pelvic plexus also provides visceral branches to the bladder, ureters, seminal vesicles, prostate, rectum, membranous urethra, and corpora cavernosa and somatic innervation to the levator ani, coccygeus, and striated urethral musculature.

Pudendal Nerve

The pudendal nerve originates in the sacral plexus, from S2 to S4, leaves the pelvis through the greater sciatic foramen, takes a short descending route through the buttocks, and re-enters the pelvic floor through Alcock's canal. It has three major branches: inferior rectal, perineal, and dorsal nerves of the penis or clitoris (see Fig. 20-5B). The external sphincter is supplied by the inferior rectal and perineal branches. The inferior rectal branch crosses the ischiorectal fossa together with the inferior rectal vessels to reach the external sphincter. It also carries fibers responsible for the sensitivity of the anal canal, particularly in the vicinity of the dentate line. The puborectalis is also innervated by the pudendal nerve and by a direct branch from the third and fourth sacral nerves, just above the pelvic floor. The remaining levator muscles receive fibers from the fourth sacral nerves and inferior rectal or perineal branches.

■ PHYSIOLOGY OF THE COLON, RECTUM, AND ANAL CANAL

The colon, the terminal segment of the digestive tract, functions by absorbing water and electrolytes from fecal material; it can absorb up to 5 L of water in 24 hours. The motility of the colon is more complex than observed in either the stomach or the small bowel. Two functional units can be identified in colonic motility: rhythmic peristalsis and tonic contractions. In the proximal colon, from the hepatic flexure to the cecum, the rhythmic antiperistalsis predominates and helps retain the material entering the cecum for a longer period. These contractions exert a churning or mixing effect on the colonic contents, extracting most of the water and electrolytes. Radiopaque markers in patients undergoing colonic transit studies are retained in the right colon for 12 hours or more, thereby suggesting the mixing process occurs at this point in digestion. In the distal left colon, this pattern is changed to a rhythmic peristalsis, or antegrade movement. These two patterns of colonic motility, although found in different segments of the colon, are similar in maximal frequency, velocity, and magnitude. Segmental contractions are similar throughout the proximal and distal colon, in the form of narrowing rings, known as haustrae. The effect of these contractions remains unclear but they probably retard the axial flow of the fecal material induced by rhythmic peristalsis and knead the semisolid fecal mass to expel water from it. A purely propulsive contraction (mass movement) occurs only two or three times a day. By the time the stool reaches the transverse colon it is usually solid. Solid stool then passes around the left colon to reach the high pressure zone at the rectosigmoid junction. Here, stool accumulates until a mass movement expels the entire contents of the left colon into the rectum. The high pressures and strong muscle of the sigmoid make it prone to disease.

The rectum exhibits a different mode of motor activity as rhythmic peristalsis is absent most of the time. The mechanism of evacuation is complex and involves voluntary and involuntary muscle activity, mediated by mucosal and pelvic receptors. When the rectum is distended, a sensation of fullness occurs, followed by the rectoanal inhibitory reflex (RAIR). This important reflex consists of relaxation of the internal sphincter due to the distention of the rectal wall. This mechanism is mediated by the myenteric plexuses of Meissner and Auerbach, at the level of the submucosa and circumferential musculature of the distal rectum, respectively. If evacuation is desired, a squatting position is adopted, the intra-abdominal pressure increases, the pelvic floor relaxes, the rectal muscular wall contracts, and the rectum is emptied. If a bowel movement is inappropriate at that time, the external sphincter contracts for up to 50 seconds, in order to achieve continence. After this period, rectal accommodation will occur, directing part of the contents back to the upper third of the rectum, and restoring the resting tone of the internal sphincter.

■ PHYSIOLOGIC TESTING

Physiologic studies such as colonic transit, small bowel transit, manometry, cinedefecography, anal ultrasound, electromyography (EMG) of the external anal sphincters and puborectalis muscle, and pudendal nerve terminal motor latency (PNTML) assessment are available to assist in the diagnosis and treatment of functional disorders of the large bowel.

In constipated patients, dietary management (intake of at least 30 g of fiber and 3 L of liquids per day) along with routine physical activity, should be offered before submitting the patient to any physiologic testing. All other systemic, infectious, and neurologic causes of constipation should be considered before any further investigation is undertaken. However, for patients who continue to have problems, colonic transit time, small bowel transit time, manometry, cinedefecography, and EMG are important tools to determine the cause and treatment.

Colonic transit studies consist of ingestion of a capsule containing 20 to 24 radiopaque markers and abdominal x-rays taken on the third and fifth days after ingestion. In an individual with normal colon transit, all the markers should be expelled by the fifth day. Conversely, retention of 80% of the rings may be an indication of colonic inertia (Fig. 20-6). Although total colectomy with ileoproctostomy is the standard treatment for colonic inertia, biofeedback should be offered prior to colectomy if paradoxical puborectalis contraction is demonstrated by cinedefecography.

Small bowel transit time should be undertaken to exclude panenteric hypomotility. There are different ways to measure the small bowel transit time. Most prefer the hydrogen breath test, which consists of ingestion of 10 g of lactulose (lactulose syrup); by the time the lactulose reaches the terminal ileum, it will be fermented by bacteria, producing molecules of hydrogen, which is quickly diffused through the blood to the lungs and exhaled. Breath samples are taken every 10 minutes after lactulose ingestion and the parts per million of hydrogen (ppm) are counted by a gas chromatography analyzer. The rise of hydrogen in the breath sample is the end point of measuring the small bowel transit time. Normal transit time varies from 60 to 100 minutes. Dietary factors that can interfere with the results of this test are cabbage, beans, peanuts, milk, yogurt, spices, and cheese. Therefore, the patient should abstain from these foods along with any

tobacco products on the day of the test. Moreover, 5 to 20% of the general population do not produce hydrogen. Despite these disadvantages, it is a noninvasive, easy, inexpensive, and reproducible test that does not expose the patient to radiation.

Manometry can be useful in patients who have been chronically constipated since childhood, in order to elicit the RAIR and thus exclude Hirschsprung's disease. A positive RAIR excludes Hirschsprung's disease, but an absent RAIR does not confirm the diagnosis. Other causes of constipation such as scleroderma and megarectum can also cause an absent RAIR. Manometry provides information regarding the resting and squeeze pressures, rectal capacity, compliance, and sensation. Different techniques may be used when performing manometry: stationary technique, continuous pull-through technique, and stationary pull-through technique. Our preference is for the latter, which consists of placing a four-radial-channel catheter inside the anal canal, which is continuously perfused with water using a microperfusion device and manually withdrawn at constant 1-cm intervals. The pressure of water necessary to overcome the sphincter pressure is measured by a transducer that converts it into electrical signals sent to a microcomputer that reads the signals as the resting and squeeze pressure. Measure of the rectal capacity and compliance follows, and finally, the RAIR is elicited.

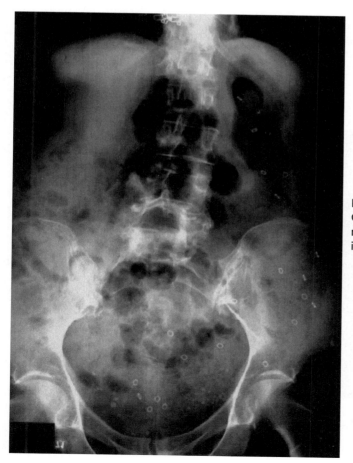

Figure 20-6
Colonic transit time showing retention of the radiopaque markers at the fifth day, suggesting colonic inertia.

Cinedefecography is a useful test to identify different causes of outlet obstruction, including paradoxical puborectalis contraction, rectocele (Fig. 20-7), sigmoidocele, rectoanal intussusception, megarectum, and perineal descent. However, findings that suggest intussusception, rectocele, or sigmoidocele should be analyzed with caution because they may be present in a population with no symptoms. Cinedefecography is a dynamic study in which the mechanism of evacuation is recorded by a fluoroscopic unit. After rectal injection of barium paste, the patient is seated on a radiolucent commode and x-rays are obtained during resting, squeezing, pushing, and, in the post-evacuatory phase, allowing the measure of the anorectal angle, puborectalis length, perineal descent, and the variation of such parameters between the resting and pushing phases. The mechanism of evacuation is then recorded for further analysis.

Anal ultrasound is a very useful test in the evaluation of incontinent patients as it provides a 360-degree image of the anal canal and surrounding structures. For didactic purposes, the anal canal is divided into upper, middle, and distal thirds. The upper third begins when the puborectalis is identified as a "V"-shaped structure of mixed echogenicity surrounding the posterior wall of the anal canal. As the probe is withdrawn caudally, the internal sphincter is seen as a hyperechoic structure surrounding the anal canal. Lateral to this muscle, the external sphincter is identified as a structure with similar echogenicity to the puborectalis muscle (Fig. 20-8A). The distal anal canal begins when the internal anal sphincter ends. The lower two thirds of the anal canal are the most common sites of sphincter defects and are the easiest to interpret (Fig. 20-8B).

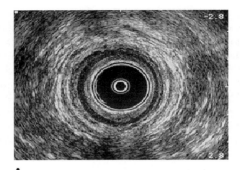

A

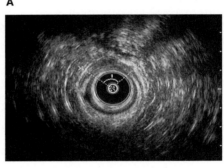

B

Figure 20-8
Normal anatomy of the midanal canal (*A*) and anterior defect of external sphincter in the midanal canal (*B*).

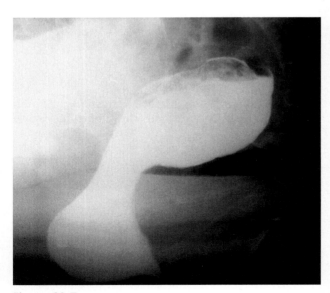

Figure 20-7
Paradoxical puborectalis contraction with secondary anterior rectocele causing outlet obstruction.

Electromyography (EMG) of the anal sphincters consists of inserting an electromyographic needle at different sites around the anal canal to detect the motor unit potential, which is increased in injured muscles. Detecting areas with neuromuscular damage (despite normal anatomy) can be crucial in identifying the cause of fecal incontinence. Although the study offers excellent information, it is complementary to the data yielded by anal ultrasound. Whereas ultrasound shows gross anatomic structure, EMG yields functional information. Owing to the discomfort of the needle, EMG studies in constipated patients should be used only to confirm the diagnosis of paradoxical puborectalis contraction (PPC). In this setting, an intra-anal plug or sponge EMG device or cutaneous patch electrodes are good options in the evaluation of constipated patients.

Pudendal nerve terminal motor latency (PNTML) identifies pudendal neuropathy that may be associated with a sphincter defect. Many reports in the literature have cited that PNTML is the only physiologic test predictive of the outcome of patients who undergo sphincteroplasty. Specifically, while bilaterally normal pudendal nerves correlate with success, unilateral or bilateral neuropathy predict failure. Thus, in incontinent patients, anal ultrasound and PNTML form the cornerstones of diagnosis; conversely, in constipated patients colonic and small bowel transit combined with cinedefecography, manometry, and surface EMG are the important diagnostic tools.

Suggested Readings

Beck DE, Wexner SD: Fundamentals of Anorectal Surgery. New York, McGraw Hill, 1992.

Christensen J: The motor function of the colon. In Yamada T, Alpers DH, Owyang C, et al (Eds.). Gastroenterology. Philadelphia, J.B. Lippincott, 1991, pp 180–194.

Jorge JMN, Wexner SD: Surgical anatomy of the colon, rectum and anus—Part I. Contemp Surg 1996;48(2):71–79.

Jorge JMN, Wexner SD: Surgical anatomy of the colon, rectum and anus—Part II. Contemp Surg 1996;48(3):141–148.

Jorge JMN, Yang YK, Wexner SD: Incidence and clinical significance of sigmoidoceles as determined by a new classification system. Dis Colon Rectum 1994;37:1112–1117.

Keighley MRB: Anatomy and physiology. In Keighley MRB, Williams NS (Eds.). Surgery of the Anus, Rectum and Colon. London, WB Saunders LTD, 1993, pp 1–18.

Nivatvongs S, Gordon PH: Surgical anatomy. In Nivatvongs S, Gordon PH (Eds.). Principles and Practice of Surgery for the Colon, Rectum and Anus. St. Louis, Quality Medical Publishing, 1992, pp 3–38.

Nogueras JJ, Wexner SD: Biofeedback for nonrelaxing puborectalis syndrome. Semin Colon Rectal Surg 1992;3(2):120–124.

Pfeifer F, Agachan F, Weiss EG, Wexner SD: Surgery for constipation: A review. Dis Colon Rectum 1996;39:444–460.

Wexner SD, Bartolo DDC: Constipation. Etiology, Evaluation and Management. London, Butterworth Heinemann, 1995.

Wexner SD, Jorge JML: Colorectal physiological tests: Use or abuse of technology? Eur J Surg 1994;160:167–174.

21

RECTAL STRICTURE

Peter Lee, MD, FRCS (Eng), FRCS (Ed), MBChB

John R. T. Monson, MD, FRCS, FRCSI, FACS

■ DEFINITION AND CLASSIFICATION

The *Oxford English Dictionary* defines a stricture as a morbid narrowing of a canal, duct, or passage. Some would define a rectal stricture as the inability to allow passage of a standard 15-mm rigid sigmoidoscope or a standard flexible sigmoidoscope. In terms of diagnosis and treatment it is probably better to define the narrowing as being significant only if producing symptoms, rather than in terms of diameter. The stricture can be classified as benign or malignant, short or long, annular, tubular, intrinsic or extrinsic, all of which will have direct relevance to treatment.

■ INCIDENCE AND DIAGNOSIS

If the newly presenting annular or stenosing adenocarcinoma of the rectum is excluded, rectal stricture is a relatively uncommon condition. The majority are due to anastomotic stenosis, radiotherapy, or inflammatory bowel disease. Other etiologic factors are given in Table 21-1. Diagnosis of the stricture and its etiology can usually be made by history and examination. Obstructive or local symptoms may be predominant with colicky abdominal pain, increasing constipation, intermittent diarrhea, bleeding, leakage, and rectal pain present to a varying degree. The stricture is either digitally palpable or visible with the rigid sigmoidoscope but should always be defined by contrast enema and, if indicated, magnetic resonance image (MRI) scanning. Histologic diagnosis is essential and may involve repeated biopsy, needle aspiration, and brush cytology. The diagnosis and definition of type and extent of the stricture may be aided by examination under anesthesia. In our practice this approach is almost always used.

■ BENIGN ANASTOMOTIC STRICTURE

The incidence of symptomatic anastomotic stricture after anterior resection of the rectum is about 8%; this figure is higher in anastomoses that leak, those with a covering stoma, and possibly when the double-staple technique is

used. A high percentage of stapled rectal anastomoses appear narrow at 4 to 6 weeks. This appearance is caused by a narrow fibrous band (or web) along the line of the staples, which, when subjected to digital pressure or the sigmoidoscope with introducer in place, gives way. Any residual early narrowing is rarely a clinical problem, and passage of stool usually provides the necessary dilatation. When a covering stoma is in place a routine water-soluble contrast enema done before operative closure will identify the occasional significant anastomotic stricture. At operation for stoma closure the anastomosis should always be examined. This examination will identify the occasional early recurrence and allow simple dilatation of a benign stricture. A degree of benign narrowing does not preclude stoma closure.

Practical points to remember in evaluating anastomotic strictures are as follows:

1. Exclude malignancy.
2. Do not treat unless symptomatic.
3. Define the length and configuration of stricture.
4. Always check anastomosis before closure of stoma.

Therapy

The time-honored outpatient dilation of a benign low rectal stricture, digitally or with dilators (Hagar, Eder-Peustow) usually helps and rarely will cause harm. For higher strictures, skilled interventional radiologic or endoscopic help is now readily available and should be sought. Balloon dilatation has the advantage of producing controlled incremental radial pressure rather than the actual tearing of metal bougie dilatation. Individual techniques vary: The following highlight the advantages of radiologic balloon dilatation in definition of the stricture, safety, and effectiveness of the procedure when compared to rigid dilatation.

Dilatation Technique

The patient is placed in the left lateral position and may be sedated. The rectum is initially opacified with water-soluble contrast medium and air is introduced to achieve double-contrast visualization of the entire length of the stricture. At this point a straight 6 Fr catheter is introduced per rectum across the stricture with the aid of an 0.035-inch angiographic J-tipped guidewire. If the anatomy is more complex, C-arm fluoroscopy can help to clarify the situation. In addition, tight and more complex strictures can be crossed using hydrophilic angled guidewires. The initial guidewire is exchanged for a stiffer guidewire, such as an Amplatz wire. A 2- to 3-cm balloon is placed across the stricture under fluoroscopic guidance. Subsequent gentle dilatation is then undertaken and abolition of the balloon "waiting" is clearly seen as the stricture opens up.

It is preferable for the patient to have received full bowel preparation and covering antibiotics before the procedure in case perforation occurs; under these circumstances perforation may be initially treated conservatively. The patient should be observed for 12 hours after the procedure, even if there is no suspected complication.

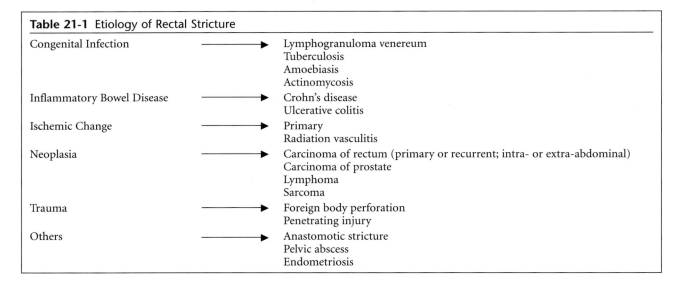

Table 21-1 Etiology of Rectal Stricture

Congenital Infection ⟶	Lymphogranuloma venereum
	Tuberculosis
	Amoebiasis
	Actinomycosis
Inflammatory Bowel Disease ⟶	Crohn's disease
	Ulcerative colitis
Ischemic Change ⟶	Primary
	Radiation vasculitis
Neoplasia ⟶	Carcinoma of rectum (primary or recurrent; intra- or extra-abdominal)
	Carcinoma of prostate
	Lymphoma
	Sarcoma
Trauma ⟶	Foreign body perforation
	Penetrating injury
Others ⟶	Anastomotic stricture
	Pelvic abscess
	Endometriosis

Repeated dilatations may be necessary. However, these should be based on symptomatic recurrence rather than either endoscopic findings or time.

Failed Balloon Dilatation

A wide spectrum of interventional surgical techniques are available when balloon dilatation has failed, including laser stricturoplasty, urethrotome or ERCP papillotomy knife, the urologic resectoscope, and the circular stapling instrument, used to debulk or divide the fibrous part of the stricture. Failure of these widening techniques in the short stricture or, more commonly, the nonresponding or restenosing longer stricture will necessitate resection and anastomosis. It should be remembered that the patient's general medical condition or preference may dictate the use of a simple loop stoma which will prove effective without significant risk.

Practical points to remember in treating benign anastomotic strictures are as follows:

1. Do not treat stricture unless symptomatic.
2. Use radiologic balloon dilatation under controlled circumstances.
3. Other stricturoplasty techniques are suitable only for short strictures.
4. Repeat surgery may be difficult and complicated.
5. Do not forget simple stoma.

A suggested therapy plan for benign anastomotic strictures is outlined in Figure 21-1.

■ MALIGNANT RECTAL STRICTURES

Narrowing of the rectum by adenocarcinoma or its recurrence at an anastomosis is common, in the form of either a stenosing lesion or a bulky exfoliative tumor. Primary treatment by resection and anastomosis is covered elsewhere. Palliation of a primary cancer in the unfit or elderly patient or in the rarer younger patient with con-

comitant disease that dictates against excisional surgery (e.g., extensive metastatic disease) is achievable by a number of techniques, either in isolation or combined with intracavity or external beam irradiation.

The particular modality used is dictated by available expertise, instrumentation, and the configuration of the stenosis. Thus, a truly stenotic primary or anastomotic recurrence can be widened by laser, urethroscope resection, or heater probe. The laser can be used via the flexible sigmoidoscope, a proctoscope, or the ports of the

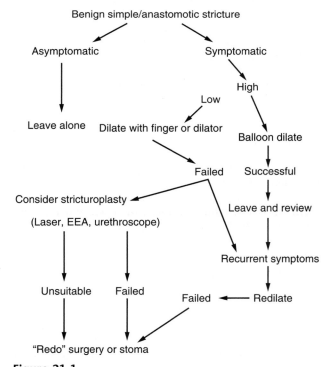

Figure 21-1
Algorithm representing a therapy plan for benign anastomotic strictures.

transanal endoscopic microsurgery apparatus and can be performed under either local or general anesthesia. We have favored the Nd:YAG (neodymium:yttrium-aluminum-garnet) laser via an open approach for lower cancers (under general anesthesia) or via the flexible sigmoidoscope if higher (under local anesthesia). The patient should have bowel preparation and be given antibiotics. The focused beam at 20 to 30 watts of power is applied to the tumor circumferentially until sloughing (black/white appearance) occurs. The treatment is repeated every 4 to 6 weeks using a "little and often" technique to avoid the complications of perforation and bleeding.

■ RECTOSIGMOID STENTING FOR OBSTRUCTING RECTOSIGMOID NEOPLASM AND PALLIATION OF RECTAL TUMORS

Self-expanding metal stents have been used successfully for rectal/rectosigmoid neoplastic strictures in the following circumstances:

1. As palliation in advanced rectal cancer
2. For temporary relief of obstructive symptoms prior to planned resection

A variety of stents have been used:

- 40-mm Giantorco Z stent
- 0-mm, 25-mm covered Wallstent
- 20-mm uncovered Wallstent
- 18-mm Nitinol stent

The stent is placed under fluoroscopic control. Complications consist of external migration, perforation, and tumor overgrowth. It would appear that adequate short-term palliation is achievable, although no direct comparison with other modalities (e.g., laser) is available. Successful laser therapy for stent overgrowth has been reported.

A 25-mm covered Wall stent, 25-mm uncovered Wall stent, or 18-mm Giantorco stent has been used for temporary relief of obstructing rectosigmoid neoplasm. Elective, one-stage resection has then been performed without problems from the stent. A new, self-expanding, stainless steel uncovered rectal stent with flared ends is available in diameters of 18 to 22 mm and lengths of 6 to 9 cm, specifically for treatment of rectal and rectosigmoid stricture. Numbers of reported patients are low, however.

■ POSTRADIATION RECTAL STRICTURE

Radiation damage to the large bowel is likely to occur in approximately 15% of irradiated patients. Most radiation-induced rectal strictures are after radiotherapy for nonrectal cancers, such as prostate or cervical cancer. Malignant recurrence must be ruled out before a stricture is labeled postradiation.

Therapy

Medical

Therapy with the use of low-residue diet, antispasmodics, anticholinergic drugs, and stool softeners should be instituted. Sulfasalazine, systemic steroids, antibiotics, and local steroid enemas and suppositories can all be helpful.

Surgery

Commonly, metal bougie dilatation has been used, and few data are available on balloon dilatation. Formal resection should be avoided when possible because of the high complication rate. Failure of conservative management and impending obstruction is the main indication for surgery, which should consist of a defunctioning stoma made in healthy large or small bowel. Only if the patient refuses to accept a long-term stoma and has a good long-term prognosis should resection and anastomosis be considered. The choice of operation for rectal stricture lies between rectal excision with coloanal anastomosis and colonic J-pouch or the Bricker-type operation with an onlay graft of healthy sigmoid colon onto the split rectum. If an operative approach becomes necessary, the following general principles should be adhered to:

1. Provide optimal preoperative nutritional status.
2. Preoperative mechanical bowel preparation with antibiotic prophylaxis is necessary.
3. Avoid incisions through irradiated skin, if possible (including stoma).
4. Insert ureteric stents to aid pelvic dissection.
5. Limit adhesiolysis to avoid unnecessary fistulas.
6. Practice meticulous anastomotic technique using non-irradiated healthy bowel (always mobilize the splenic flexure and use mid-descending colon).
7. Always cover using loop stoma in nonirradiated bowel.
8. Delay postoperative oral feeding, using total parenteral nutrition for 10 to 14 days.
9. Initial long tube decompression may help.

■ RECTAL STENOSIS IN INFLAMMATORY BOWEL DISEASE

Crohn's Disease

Two types of rectal stricture occur in Crohn's disease. Stricture of the lower 1 to 2 cm of the rectum as a direct extension of perianal Crohn's disease may cause either a low membranous-type stricture at the anorectal junction, a broad extrarectal stricture due to perirectal extension of sepsis, or a broad extrarectal band caused by perirectal extension of anal sepsis. The typical "colonic" Crohn's disease type of stricture occurs higher in the rectum due to severe rectal Crohn's disease.

In long-standing cases malignancy should always be excluded. The low membranous type of stricture has a much better prognosis and is best treated by digital dilatation, on a repeated basis if necessary. Self-dilatation can also be effective. Balloon dilatation may be necessary for the denser band stricture. The higher Crohn's disease bowel-related rectal strictures do not respond well to either medical treatment or dilatation (which may be dangerous) and will often require proctectomy.

Ulcerative Colitis

Strictures that occur in the rectum are more frequently benign than those occurring more proximal to the splenic flexure (10% versus 86%). If the rectal stricture occurs late in the disease or with symptoms of intestinal obstruction, it is more likely to be malignant (60% probability after 20 years).

Unless malignancy can be confidently excluded, the rectal stricture is better treated by excisional surgery. The presence of the stricture need not alter the traditional approach to choice of operation.

Suggested Readings

Chia YW, Ngoi SS, Tung KH: Use of the optical urethrotome knife in treatment of benign low rectal anastomotic stricture. Dis Colon Rectum 1991;34:717–719.

Gumaste V, Sachar DB, Greenstein AJ: Benign and malignant colorectal strictures in ulcerative colitis. Gut 1992;22:938–941.

Keighley MRB, Williams NS: Surgical treatment of colorectal Crohn's disease. In Keighley MRB, Williams NS (Eds.). Surgery of the Anus, Rectum, and Colon. Philadelphia, WB Saunders, 1993, p 1757.

Kelly MJ: Use of the urological resectoscope in benign and malignant rectal lesions. R Soc Med 1989;82:588–590.

Lee PWR: Endoscopic palliation of rectal malignancy. In Tytgat GNJ, Classen M (Eds.). Practice of Therapeutic Endoscopy. Edinburgh, Churchill Livingstone, 1994, pp 236–239.

Maclennan AC, Moss JG: Palliative treatment of a rectal tumour with self-expanding metallic stent. Clin Radiol 1997;52:633–635.

McKeown BJ, Blake H, Swift I: Use of metal stents to relieve malignant obstruction of the colon. J Vasc Int Radiol 1996;7(suppl):200.

McLean RAH: Rectal stricture resection using EEA autostapler. Br J Surg 1980;67:281–282.

Meloni GB, Proali S, Bifulco V: Dilatation of benign colo-colonic and colorectal anastomotic stenosis with radiology-guided balloon catheter. Radiol Med 1995;89:554–557.

Smith LE: Anastomosis with EEA stapler after anterior colonic resection. Dis Colon Rectum 1981;24:236–242.

Venkatesh KS, Ramanujam PS, McGee S: Hydrostatic balloon dilatation of benign colonic anastomotic strictures. Dis Colon Rectum 1992;35:789–791.

22

FECAL IMPACTION

Sergio W. Larach, MD, FACS
Javier Cebrian, MD

Fecal impaction may be defined as a large compacted mass of feces in the rectum, which cannot be evacuated by the patient. Fecal impaction may be the result of incomplete bowel movements over a period of time. It can occur in any age group, but elderly institutionalized patients and children are most commonly afflicted.

Ninety-eight percent of all fecal impactions occur in the rectum. Etiologies include drugs (see Table 22-1), chronic and systemic diseases (cystic fibrosis, chronic renal failure, Chagas' infection), neurologic diseases (Hirschsprung's disease, Parkinson's disease, multiple sclerosis, spinal cord injuries), painful anorectal problems, and postoperative anorectal surgery. Proper assessment includes identifying risks factors (advanced age, prolonged inactivity, mental illness and cancer patients).

The most common disease underlying fecal impaction is constipation. The most common symptom is fecal incontinence (also known as overflow incontinence) due to a ball-valve effect of the impacted fecal bolus. Other symptoms include rectal discomfort, lower abdominal pain, rectal fullness, and tenesmus. Presenting symptoms are not specific, masking the diagnosis. Rectal examination is the most important diagnostic tool in these patients. Although most impactions are in the rectal vault, the absence of palpable stool on rectal examination does not rule out a fecal impaction, because fecal impactions can occur anywhere in the colon. When fecal impaction is suspected, and digital rectal examination is negative, then a plain abdominal radiograph, to look for masses of stool or signs of obstruction, is indicated. If underlying disease is suspected, particularly malignancy, a barium enema and proctosigmoidoscopy or colonoscopy should be performed after treatment.

Fecal impaction can have multiple complications. Debilitated patients with fecal incontinence due to an impaction can develop decubitus ulceration and urinary infections. Large bowel obstruction is also common, especially in patients with spinal cord injuries. The long-term presence of a fecal mass leads to an ischemic necrosis on the wall of the colon, causing stercoral ulceration. Many of these problems are clinically silent unless a further complication occurs. Bleeding or perforation is associated with significant risk of death; this complication can be life-threatening for patients who are older or in poor general condition. Clinical presentation of a perforated stercoral ulcer is usually that of an acute abdomen.

■ TREATMENT

The aggressiveness of treatment can vary, depending on the extent of the impaction, how long the condition has existed, general condition of the patient, and presence or absence of acute abdominal signs. Basically, six therapeutic modalities can be used in the treatment of patients with fecal impaction: manual fragmentation, mineral oil, oral lavage, colonic irrigation, pulsed irrigation enhanced evacuation, and surgery. These modalities can be used alone or in combination. Figure 22-1 shows an algorithm for the treatment of fecal impaction.

Although enemas and suppositories alone may eliminate the impaction, manual fragmentation and extraction of the fecal mass are almost always indicated first. The procedure can usually be performed without anesthesia; however, occasionally local, spinal, or even general anesthesia is required. The procedure initiates with progressive anal dilatation, first with one finger and then with two fingers; but care must be taken in order to avoid damage to the sphincters during the manual disimpaction. A scissoring action is used to fragment the impaction. In women transvaginal pressure may be useful in disimpaction and expulsion of the fecal mass. Once fragmentation and partial expulsion have occurred, bisacodyl suppositories, water enemas, or rectal lavage may be used. An enema with mineral oil is also recommended. Soap, hydrogen peroxide, and hot-water enemas are not advised because they may irritate the mucosa and cause bleeding.

When manual disimpaction is attempted but the mass is beyond the reach of the fingers, a colonic irrigation directed by sigmoidoscopy visualization can be useful. The most helpful solution used is water-soluble contrast medium (meglumine diatrizoate, or Gastrografin) because this agent stimulates peristalsis, draws water into the colon, and lubricates the fecal mass. Large volumes of normal saline solution via enema can also be used to lubricate, hydrate, and facilitate the expulsion of the fecal mass.

Table 22-1 Drugs That Can Cause Fecal Impaction
Narcotics
Drugs used to treat psychiatric disorders
Tricyclic antidepressants
Phenothiazines
Antihypertensive drugs
Beta-adrenergic blockers
Calcium-channel blockers
Diuretics
Drugs used in the treatment of gastrointestinal disorders
Antacids containing aluminum
Sucralfate
Long-term use of laxatives ("cathartic syndrome")
Psyllium seed (with insufficient hydration)
Miscellaneous Agents
Iron
Drugs used in chemotherapy

FECAL IMPACTION

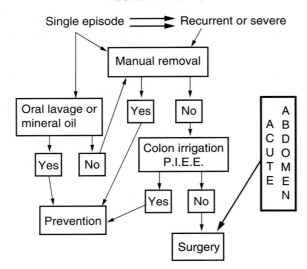

Figure 22-1
Algorithm for the treatment of fecal impaction.

Mineral oil and oral lavage solutions have been shown to be extremely useful in the treatment of fecal impaction, and are safe for both children over 2 years of age and elderly patients. Patients with prior medical history of recurrent vomiting or aspiration, central nervous system problems, liver or kidney disease, and conscience disorders should not be treated with these modalities. The dose of mineral oil is 30 mL/10 kg of body weight given orally in two divided doses for 2 days. Its major disadvantage is the bad taste; therefore, administration in 100 to 150 mL of fruit juice is recommended. Oral lavage comes as a fruit-flavored balanced oral lavage solution, or polyethylene glycol solution (Colyte), and is given at a dose of 20 mL/kg body weight on 2 consecutive days. The maximum amount of lavage solution in children must not exceed 1 L of oral solution per hour. Oral solutions have been shown to be more effective and quicker in achieving fecal disimpaction than mineral oil therapy. Moreover, the oral lavage solutions can be used in the treatment of patients with chronic constipation who are prone to have repeated fecal impactions.

The pulse irrigation enhanced evacuation (PIEE) (Medic Mark, Inc., Buffalo Grove, IL) system utilizes the mechanical action of pulsed water to disrupt dehydrated stool and to stimulate colonic peristalsis. The irrigant used is water at a temperature between 93° and 104° F, for both patient comfort and success of treatment. The patient is placed in the left lateral decubitus position, and the rectal speculum in placed within the anorectum. The balloon of the speculum is then inflated to secure a watertight seal at the level of the puborectalis. A pulsatile irrigation of water is started with an initial instillation time of 2 seconds with a volume of 40 mL/sec. This step is followed with a passive drainage time of 4 seconds. The duration of one entire session is generally 1 hour. If complete emptying of the colon was not achieved with the initial treatment, it can be repeated. This procedure is a safe and inexpensive treatment, and is useful in both distal and proximal impactions.

When all these procedures have failed, surgery may be necessary, usually in an unprepared colon. Surgical options include the following:

1. Milking forward the fecal mass trying to expulse it out the anus.
2. A colotomy for extraction of the hard mass.
3. A segmental resection with a diversion, or with a colonic anastomosis, based on the general and local condition of the patient and surgeon's preference.
4. Acute perforation of the colon as a result of stercoral ulceration must be treated with segmental resection of the involved area, or with a subtotal colectomy and diversion.
5. In patients with chronic severe constipation and colonic inertia, with repetitive episodes of fecal impaction, when colon preparation is permitted, a subtotal colectomy with ileorectal anastomosis has been successful.
6. A sigmoid colon resection is indicated when an isolated distended sigmoid colon is the cause of fecal impaction.
7. Segmental colon resection with low colorectal anastomosis or a modified Duhamel procedure is indicated in patients with Hirschsprung's disease and Chagas' disease.

The best treatment is prevention. Aggressive treatment of constipation should be undertaken, modifying fiber intake, water intake, and physical activities of patients. A bulk laxative (such as hydrophilic mucilloid) and stool softeners (such as dioctyl sodium: 50 mg three times daily) must be taken by the patient. Changes in patient environment, medication, and treatment of underlying disorders must be made in order to avoid additional episodes of fecal impaction.

Suggested Readings

Cefalu CA, McKnight GT, Pike JI: Treating impaction: A practical approach to an unpleasant problem. Geriatrics 1981;36:143–146.

Kokoszka J, Nelson R, Falconio M, Abcarian H: Treatment of fecal impaction with pulsed irrigation enhanced evacuation. Dis Colon Rectum 1994;37:161–164.

Pfeifer J, Agachan F, Wexner SD: Surgery for constipation. A review. Dis Colon Rectum 1996;39:444–460.

Wrenn K: Fecal impaction. N Engl J Med 1989;321:658–662.

23

RECTAL PROLAPSE

Conor P. Delaney, MD, MCh, PhD,
FRCSI (Gen), FACS
Anthony J. Senagore, MD, MBA, MS, FACS

Rectal prolapse occurs when the full thickness of the rectal wall protrudes through the anal canal. The condition is most commonly seen in older females, but may occur in both sexes and at any age. Although rectal prolapse has fascinated surgeons for many years, the optimal surgical approach has not been determined. Over 100 surgical operations have been reported, and these procedures can be grouped into perineal and abdominal approaches. Choosing the optimal repair for an individual patient involves consideration of many factors, including the patient's general health and whether there is a history of constipation (present in 25 to 50%) or fecal incontinence (present in approximately 75%).

■ PATHOPHYSIOLOGY

The mechanisms by which prolapse occur remain poorly understood. Broden and Snellman suggested that prolapse is initiated by a midrectal intussusception, which commences 8 to 10 cm inside the rectum. One initiating factor may be chronic straining, which might explain the association with colitis cystica profunda and solitary rectal ulcer. Prolapse is also thought to be related to abnormal intestinal motility, such as is seen in slow-transit constipation.

Low anal resting pressures are frequently observed in patients with prolapse and may be caused by continuous rectoanal inhibition, or by the dilating effect of the prolapse itself, with or without pudendal neuropathy. However, others feel that an initial increase in external sphincter tone may cause a cycle of outlet obstruction, constipation, and straining. An impaired tolerance to distention, with reduced compliance and tone, may contribute to incontinence. Obviously it is difficult to determine which physiologic alterations are direct etiologic factors and which are secondary to the progressive prolapse of the rectum, especially a reduced internal sphincter pressure.

Internal intussusception, also called internal or hidden prolapse, occurs when the prolapse does not protrude through the anal orifice. Mucosal prolapse is diagnosed when the mucosa slides on the submucosa and protrudes through the anal canal. It is generally treated along the lines of hemorrhoidal disease.

■ CLINICAL FEATURES

Except when occurring in infants or the senile elderly patient, the patient is immediately aware of the prolapse. Prolapse initially occurs only with defecation and straining. Later as the tissues become more lax, the rectum may prolapse with the mildest straining, or even when the patient stands up. Tenesmus, bleeding, and mucus discharge are associated symptoms. Incontinence may range from mucus leakage to complete fecal incontinence. A history of bladder and gynecologic dysfunction and prolapse should be sought in appropriate cases.

On examination, the anus may be patulous. Visualization of everted bowel with concentric folds allows definitive diagnosis. If prolapse is not evident, the patient should be examined while straining on the commode. The left lateral and jack-knife positions are frequently inadequate to reproduce the prolapse, and more important, they are inadequate to rule out a diagnosis of prolapse. Occasionally the prolapse is incarcerated and requires the application of hypertonic sugar or honey to allow shrinkage and reduction. If a small prolapse is difficult to distinguish from hemorrhoids, the index finger should be introduced to display the sulcus between the layers of prolapsed bowel.

As well as confirming the diagnosis of prolapse, examination is performed to check for an anterior enterocele or rectocele. The sphincters are carefully examined. Proctosigmoidoscopy is the minimum requirement to look at the mucosa and evaluate for a lead point or other pathologic change. The majority of patients have already been examined by colonoscopy because of their age and the presence of rectal bleeding that is associated with their presentation.

The diagnosis of rectal prolapse is usually straightforward, but hemorrhoids, prolapsing polyps, and anorectal neoplasia must be excluded. Conditions such as solitary rectal ulcer and colitis cystica profunda may present with similar symptoms, but may also coexist in the patient with prolapse.

Some authors advocate evaluating transit time in those with constipation. We do not do this routinely, but only in those with a history of severe constipation and associated sphincter weakness, in order to get evidence to avoid colectomy in patients without definite slow transit. Those with chronic straining at stool should have evaluation for paradoxic contraction of the anal sphincters, or anismus, so that biofeedback therapy may be instituted prior to repair of the prolapse. The clinical and cost benefit of routine preoperative studies, including anal manometry, pudendal nerve terminal motor latency, colonic transit studies, and defecography is unclear.

■ PREOPERATIVE CONSIDERATIONS

The general health of the patient is of great importance in preoperative decision making. The elderly with extremely poor health may be more suitable for a perineal approach. However, increasing experience with the laparoscopic approach suggests that the benefits of abdominal prolapse repair may be conferred with greatly reduced morbidity rate.

Continence may be impaired in patients with rectal prolapse, but both resting and squeeze pressures frequently improve after prolapse repair. This improvement is likely related to prevention of the dilating effect of the prolapse, and also cessation of the constant rectoanal inhibitory reflex. The improvement is generally reported to be better after abdominal repair (0 to 90% chance) than perineal repair (45 to 60%). Only rarely do we perform concomitant sphincter repair at the time of prolapse surgery, the option being reserved for those with complete or near-complete incontinence.

Constipation is also a concern because of frequent reports of exacerbated constipation after prolapse repair. This development is likely to be related to a redundant sigmoid loop flopping forward over the mesh or sutures holding the rectum to the sacral promontory, causing partial obstruction at the rectosigmoid junction. Because of this we favor sigmoid colectomy with a sutured rectopexy in constipated patients. In this manner, we have found improvement of preoperative constipation in 95% of those having laparoscopic rectal prolapse surgery. Conversely, a laparoscopic Wells procedure for those with diarrhea or incontinence can improve continence in more than 80% of these patients. Constipation may also may be precipitated by lateral ligament division during rectal mobilization, which we do not advocate.

■ SURGICAL OPTIONS

The goals of surgery are to prevent recurrent prolapse and improve continence and bowel function. Prolapse repair may be achieved using either a perineal or an abdominal approach, and the primary techniques and alternatives are discussed here. Colonic resection is reserved for those with significant constipation because of the potential increase in morbidity by the addition of an anastomosis and the risk of exacerbating this symptom when rectopexy is performed.

1. *Perineal repairs.* One benefit of perineal repairs is that they can be performed using local anesthesia and intravenous sedation. The main alternatives are devices encircling the anal canal, perineal rectosigmoidectomy, and the mucosal stripping procedure described by Delorme.
   a. Anal encircling procedures have generally fallen out of practice owing to high failure and complication rates. They are usually reserved for those with the most comorbidities in whom one would not wish to perform perineal resection. Examples of candidates for these precedures are patients with ascites and hepatic failure who are not suitable for the TIPS (transjugular intrahepatic portosystemic shunt) procedure, followed by abdominal repair. Encirclement procedures, like the Thiersch wire, are associated with 20 to 60% prolapse recurrence rates and the additional complications of breakage, infection, and

erosion. Thus, some surgeons favor the use of a soft encircling drain when this operation is performed.
   b. Altmeier popularized the procedure of perineal rectosigmoidectomy in the 1960s. Recurrence rates between 0 and 50% have been reported. Altmeier initially combined the operation with a levatorplasty, which may further improve continence. The technique attempts to remove the prolapsing segment and use the subsequent fibrosis to fix the rectum in position in the pelvis. This operation remains the ideal option for patients presenting with an incarcerated, gangrenous prolapse.
   c. A less invasive alternative was suggested by Delorme. In this version of perineal rectosigmoidectomy, the mucosa is stripped starting 1 cm above the dentate line and continuing right up above the prolapsing segment. The rectal muscle is then plicated with concertina-type stitches, and the proximal mucosa is anastomosed to the distal margin of mucosal resection. Submucosal infiltration with diluted epinephrine during mucosal mobilization may reduce perioperative bleeding. Variable recurrence rates have been reported, but they are generally in the order of 5 to 20%.
2. *Abdominal procedures.* In contrast, abdominal procedures for rectal prolapse are generally associated with a recurrence rate in the order of 5%, although recurrence rates between 0 and 20% have been reported. Abdominal repairs involve mobilization of the rectum and its fixation to the sacral promontory with suture or a prosthetic material or mesh. In an anterior repair, such as the Ripstein procedure, the mesh is wrapped around the anterior aspect of the rectum, and fixed on both sides to the sacral promontory. Posterior repairs involve the mesh being placed behind the rectum and superior rectal artery and fixed to the sacrum, before being wrapped around both sides and fixed to the lateral mesorectum. Although recurrence rates are generally less than 10%, anterior wraps may be complicated by stenosis and obstruction. Posterior fixation, as per Wells, avoids stenosis and may reduce constipation. Although a variety of materials have been used, such as the Ivalon sponge, we favor polypropylene mesh to reduce the risk of septic complications, which are reported in 3 to 4% of cases using the Ivalon sponge.

The rectum is usually mobilized by dissecting posteriorly in the presacral space down to the pelvic floor; however, the extent of lateral dissection is controversial. Division of the lateral ligaments has been evaluated in two prospective randomized trials (with 26 and 18 patients, respectively). One study suggested no change in postoperative functional outcome, but the other revealed significantly less constipation with lateral ligament preservation, at the cost of an increased recurrence rate.

Abdominal repairs may be performed with or without a concomitant bowel resection. Thus, resection rectopexy incorporates resection of the sigmoid and upper rectum. Fixation of the rectum is achieved by the perianastomotic fibrosis, with sutures providing additional fixation of the lateral tails of the mesorectum to the sacral promontory. Recurrence rates are generally in the order of 2 to 8%, but there is the added potential morbidity of a colorectal anastomosis. Some authors have advocated a formal anterior resection, but this operation provides an increased potential for morbidity without reducing recurrence rates.

It is increasingly obvious that laparoscopic colorectal procedures accelerate recovery after major abdominal surgery. Laparoscopy reduces postoperative pain, allows earlier introduction and tolerance of diet, and shortens the length of hospital stay. When laparoscopy is used, the surgeon can perform exactly the same operation as when using the open approach. The primary difference is that the largest wound is the 10-mm incision for the camera port. When a laparoscopic resection rectopexy is performed, then a 4-cm left lower quadrant muscle-splitting incision is also used.

The rectum is fixed to the sacral promontory using a suture or stapled technique. A mesh can be used as in open surgery. Many series describe no cases of recurrence. An excellent outcome can be achieved when rectopexy is associated with sigmoid resection, giving the reduced constipation, incontinence, and outlet obstruction rates seen after open surgery. Several authors have experience with the laparoscopic Wells procedure, and have found this to be associated with reduced constipation and no recurrences, with a reduction in length of stay and costs compared to open repair. When laparoscopic suture rectopexy is performed without mesh or resection, it has been associated with a 7% recurrence rate.

The laparoscopic approach is the same as that for open surgery. The presacral space is entered and a posterior rectal mobilization is performed to the level of the pelvic floor. We do not divide the lateral ligaments. For Wells rectopexy, a precut mesh is passed down a port and tacked or sutured to the sacral promontory in the midline. The edges are then sutured to the lateral mesorectal tissue to maintain rectal support. In patients having a resection, the upper rectum is transected with an endoscopic stapler and passed out through a 4-cm left lower quadrant muscle splitting incision. The proctosigmoidectomy is completed and the anvil of a circular stapler is inserted in the proximal bowel before it is returned to the abdomen. The anastomosis to the rectal stump is completed before suturing the lateral mesorectal tissue to the sacral promontory for additional support. We have recently described a series of 24 laparoscopic rectopexy repairs, using the Wells or resection rectopexy, depending on symptoms (Madbouly et al). Median hospital stay was 2.3 days for Wells and 3.6 days for resection rectopexy patients, and there have been no recurrences to date.

■ RECOMMENDATIONS

Clearly, many options are possible for repair of rectal prolapse. A major review by Kim and coworkers over a 19-year period studied 188 perineal rectosigmoidectomies and 160 abdominal resection rectopexy patients. Although the morbidity rate was lower for perineal repairs, recur-rence rates ranged from 5 to 16%. In our opinion, laparoscopy helps reduce postoperative morbidity rates, allowing for a safe abdominal repair in more patients. This approach reduces recurrence rates of abdominal surgery in the older patient, who traditionally would be offered a perineal repair.

Thus, patients who present to us are managed by laparoscopic Wells rectopexy if they have no constipation, or in the presence of diarrhea or incontinence. Those with constipation are managed by laparoscopic resection rectopexy. Perineal approaches are reserved for those who are medically very unfit, and Delorme and Altmeier approaches are used, with a preference for the Delorme approach, in patients with poor continence.

■ COMPLICATIONS

If mucosal prolapse persists or occurs after repair, as may happen in 5 to 10% of patients, it is not considered to be a true recurrence. This prolapse is treated with elastic banding, or excision under local anesthesia. Patients with persisting difficulties with continence should be observed for improvement for 6 to 12 months, unless symptoms are extremely severe and warrant earlier operative sphincter repair.

Solitary rectal ulcer, present in approximately 12% of prolapse patients, is often considered as a complicating issue. Solitary ulcer should be treated as a separate issue. If the ulcer is associated with prolapse, then repair the prolapse. If not, then initial treatment of the ulcer involves correction of straining and defecation habit, and may include biofeedback.

Internal intussusception, diagnosed by barium studies or defecating proctography, is a diagnosis to be wary of as an indication for surgical repair. In fact, many asymptomatic patients may have an internal intussusception on defecating proctography. Thus, surgical repair may not relieve their symptoms. These patients should be fully evaluated for other possible causes of their symptoms, including an evaluation for anismus. Surgical repair is generally avoided.

When rectal prolapse occurs in conjunction with urogenital prolapse or other pelvic floor disorders, a combined approach by colorectal, gynecologic, and urologic surgeons may be indicated. For this patient cohort, Sullivan and coworkers have reported total pelvic mesh repair in 236 patients, involving the placement of mesh from the sacrum to the perineal body and around the vagina. In this report there were no recurrences, and patients had a 70% satisfaction rate, but 10% required reoperation for problems with mesh. A perineal approach to the rectal prolapse can also be used, combined with a perineal colporrhapy.

■ MANAGEMENT OF RECURRENT PROLAPSE

Recurrent prolapse generally occurs a mean of 18 to 24 months postoperatively. A repeat repair usually provides an excellent outcome for treatment of the prolapse, but there is often little improvement in other functional problems, such as constipation and incontinence. These patients should be extensively investigated prior to repeat repair to elucidate factors that might predispose to recurrence, such as slow-transit constipation and anismus.

Additional operative considerations must be observed. If a resection is performed, any prior anastomoses must be resected in order to avoid leaving an ischemic segment. Some authors would suggest a perineal repair after a failed abdominal repair, and vice versa. In fact, both types of repair are feasible, and there is inadequate evidence in the literature to determine strategy. Our preference is to perform repeat abdominal repair except in the most unfit patient, reserving laparoscopy for those with a failed perineal approach.

Suggested Readings

Baker R, Senagore AJ, Luchtefeld MA: Laparoscopic-assisted vs. open resection. Rectopexy offers excellent results. Dis Colon Rectum 1995;38:199–201.

Boccasanta P, Venturi M, Reitano MC, et al: Laparotomic vs laparoscopic rectopexy in complete rectal prolapse. Dis Surg 1999;16:415–419.

Bruch HP, Herold A, Schiedeck T, Schwandner O: Laparoscopic surgery for rectal prolapse and outlet obstruction. Dis Colon Rectum 1999;42:1189–1194.

Eu KW, Seow-Choen F: Functional problems in adult rectal prolapse and controversies in surgical treatment. Br J Surg 1997;84:904–911.

Himpens J, Cadiere GB, Bruyns J, Vertruyen M: Laparoscopic rectopexy according to Wells. Surg Endosc 1999;13:139–1341.

Hool GR, Hull TR, Fazio VW: Surgical treatment of recurrent complete rectal prolapse: A thirty-year experience. Dis Colon Rectum 1997;40:270–272.

Kim DS, Tsang CB, Wong WD, et al: Complete rectal prolapse: Evolution of management and results. Dis Colon Rectum 1999;42:460–466.

Madbouly KM, Senagore AJ, Delaney CP, et al: Clinically-based management of rectal prolapse: A comparison of laparoscopic Wells procedure versus resection/rectopexy. Surg Endosc 2003;17:99–103.

Mollen RM, Kuijpers JH, van Hoek F: Effects of rectal mobilization and lateral ligaments division on colonic and anorectal function. Dis Colon Rectum 2000;43:1283–1287.

Sullivan ES, Longaker CJ, Lee PY: Total pelvic mesh repair: A ten-year experience. Dis Colon Rectum 2001;44:857–863.

24

SOLITARY RECTAL ULCER

Joe J. Tjandra, MBBS, MD,
FRACS, FRCS, FRCPS

Solitary rectal ulcer (SRU) is a severe variant of mucosal prolapse syndrome, in which the mucosa of the large bowel becomes loose and redundant, and is driven caudally by peristalsis. The diagnosis of SRU can be suspected clinically, but there is a specific histologic diagnosis, defined by fibromuscular obliteration of the lamina propria of the rectum with thickening of the muscularis mucosa. The clinical features of SRU can be variable.

■ HISTOLOGY

In SRU, there is intense submucosal fibrosis with a predominance of sialomucins. The epithelium is hyperplastic and mucus glands may be displaced deep to the muscularis mucosa. These submucosal cysts account for the appearances of colitis cystica profunda and may be confused with mucinous adenocarcinoma. Sometimes, the cyst epithelium disappears completely, leaving lakes of mucus within the submucosa. Description of SRU is further confused because of a large number of other terms used for the condition. These terms include colitis cystica profunda, solitary ulcer, benign solitary rectal ulcer, solitary rectal ulcer syndrome, mucosal prolapse syndrome, enterogenous cyst of the rectum, and hamartomatous inverted polyp of the rectum. Colitis cystica profunda is not specific to SRU but is associated with changes in the submucosa secondary to some traumatic process and has been described in association with radiation therapy, stomas, adenomas, malignancies, and inflammatory bowel disease.

■ CLINICAL SPECTRUM

The term *solitary rectal ulcer* does not adequately describe the clinical spectrum of the disease. The rectal lesions may include an ulcer, an area of hyperemia, a polypoid mass, or a combination of these. Thus, SRU may be neither "solitary" nor "ulcerated." A typical "ulcer" is shallow (without the rolled edges of a malignant ulcer), with a white fibrous base, surrounded by a thickened rectal wall.

Most SRUs are on the anterior wall about 7 cm from the anal verge. However, they may be multiple or circumferential and may be located anywhere within the rectum. The macroscopic appearances of the SRU seem to be associated with its clinical course. The polypoid variety is different from the nonpolypoid variety in that it is usually associated with mild symptoms and tends to respond more favorably to therapy. In contrast, the ulcerating variety tends to be associated with intractable and severe symptoms.

Symptomatic SRU is most common in the second and third decades of life and affects females more than males. The most common symptoms are chronic constipation, rectal pain, and a feeling of incomplete evacuation. This feeling is associated with straining at defecation, tenesmus, and rectal bleeding. About 10% of patients admit to digital evacuation of stool. Both complete (20%) and mucosal (20%) rectal prolapse may be present. Diagnosis of occult mucosal prolapse can be made if the patient is asked to strain during proctoscopy or with defecography.

■ PATHOGENESIS

The etiology of SRU is probably multifactorial. In many patients, it is due to a combination of direct trauma and ischemia of the rectal mucosa. These injuries may be caused by repeated episodes of occult or complete rectal prolapse or by self-digitation or use of enemas. Many patients with SRU have pelvic floor disfunction, strain excessively at defecation, and have incomplete defecation. Intense and prolonged straining exposes the rectal wall to intraluminal pressures of up to 300 mm Hg and is often associated with an inappropriate reflex contraction of the external anal sphincter and pelvic floor, rendering the tip of the prolapsing mucosa ischemic. Evidence of pathophysiologic disturbances associated with SRU is, however, conflicting. Although rectal prolapse is causally related to a proportion of SRUs, it is not the predominant cause. Inappropriate puborectalis contraction on attempted defecation is noted in about 25% of patients only. Elaborate anorectal physiology testing does not yield consistent results and should be used selectively in patients with severe symptoms of obstructed defecation.

In a large series of 80 patients with histologically proven SRU from the Cleveland Clinic, 26% had none or trivial symptoms and the rectal biopsy was obtained "incidentally." A polypoid rectal lesion was the predominant finding in this asymptomatic group. The natural history of this asymptomatic group is unclear, although it may represent a presymptomatic phase of SRU.

■ CLINICAL EVALUATION

The diagnosis of SRU is often delayed, sometimes for several years. The differential diagnosis includes rectal neoplasm, Crohn's disease, suppository-induced rectal ulcer, and HIV-associated rectal ulcer. An unusual rectal lesion with atypical presentation should raise the possibility of SRU. The presence of rectal prolapse should further suggest a diagnosis of SRU. To achieve a correct diagnosis of SRU, both the clinician and the pathologist should maintain a high index of suspicion for the condition.

Initial diagnostic efforts should include a thorough history and anorectal examination, including proctoscopy and sigmoidoscopy with biopsy. A large biopsy specimen from the edge of the rectal ulcer or from the center of the hyperemic and polypoid lesion is essential to show the characteristic fibromuscular obliteration of the lamina propria. Straining on a commode may elicit an overt rectal prolapse and perineal descent. It is essential to establish the diagnosis histologically and exclude malignancy and other causes of a rectal ulcer. If the endoscopic biopsy is inadequate, a specimen should be obtained during examination under anesthetic.

Defecography may reveal incomplete rectal evacuation and the presence of rectocele or occult mucosal prolapse. Physiologic assessment may be performed in patients with chronic constipation using anorectal manometry, electromyography, balloon expulsion, and colonic transit study. If indicated, colonoscopy or barium enema is performed to exclude a proximal colonic lesion.

■ THERAPEUTIC OPTIONS

Once the diagnosis is established and malignancy is excluded, patients can be reassured. Therapeutic alternatives are selected based on the severity and chronicity of symptoms and any associated disorders (Fig. 24-1). Spontaneous resolution of SRU is not common but may

occur. A few heal for a while, then recur. In patients with mild or moderate symptoms, without significant rectal prolapse, nonoperative treatment should be first attempted. If the SRU is associated with a rectal prolapse, as demonstrated clinically or by defecography, good results can be expected from repair of the prolapse.

■ NONOPERATIVE TREATMENT

Dietary and Bowel Habit Modifications

The mainstay of conservative therapy involves dietary and bowel habit modifications. A high-fiber diet (30 to 35 g fiber per day) or stool-bulking agents containing psyllium products (2 tsp in a glass of water or juice twice daily) are initially prescribed. Fluid intake is increased, and caffeinated and alcoholic beverages are avoided to prevent dehydration of the stool. Patients are counseled as to the nature of the problem and to avoid prolonged straining at stool. In a large series (Tjandra and coworkers), about half the patients improved with these conservative measures, although these improvements were maintained over the long term in only 20%. Patients with the polypoid variety of SRU tend to have a better response than do patients with an ulcerated or hyperemic rectal lesion. In addition, bowel symptoms may persist despite healing of the rectal lesion. Other treatments with variable success rates include topical steroids, sucralfate enema, and oral sulfasalazine.

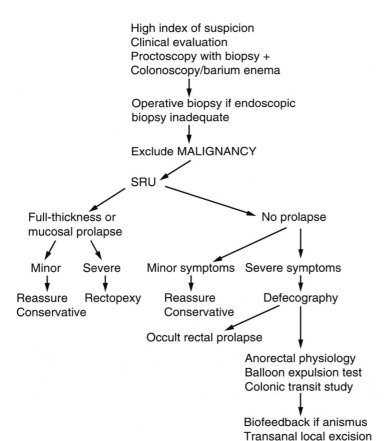

Figure 24-1
Management of solitary rectal ulcer (SRU).

Biofeedback Therapy

Management is particularly difficult in patients with refractory symptoms who do not have rectal prolapse. Pelvic floor retraining, using biofeedback techniques, has a small role in patients with nonrelaxing puborectalis proved on electromyography. Biofeedback is performed by monitoring the manometric and electromyographic activity of the external anal sphincter and pelvic floor during straining and squeeze, using an audiovisual signal display system. A relearning program is initiated using the anorectal manometry and electromyography equipment. Psychologic counseling and behavior modification techniques may be a useful adjunct to biofeedback therapy.

■ SURGICAL TREATMENT

Although the success rate of nonoperative management is low, less than half of symptomatic SRUs ultimately require surgery because of intractable symptoms or significant rectal prolapse. Overall, symptomatic improvement occurred in two thirds of patients after surgery, and the best results are obtained in patients with rectal prolapse or the polypoid variety of SRU. Few centers have extensive experience with the surgical management of SRU.

Repair of Occult and Full-Thickness Rectal Prolapse

Surgical results are most satisfactory if full-thickness rectal prolapse is present. Symptoms improve in more than 85% of patients. With longer follow-up, some patients develop recurrent symptoms, even if there is no prolapse. Rectopexy is done only if there is rectal prolapse associated with significant symptoms. We do not support rectopexy as the universal treatment for SRU as proposed by Nicholls and colleagues. We favor a suture rectopexy because of its simplicity and a lower incidence of constipation compared to a Ripstein rectopexy with a mesh. A full posterior mobilization of the rectum to the level of the coccyx is essential. The lateral ligaments are mobilized but not divided. Others recommend anterior mobilization of the rectum as well, which should be performed with care if there is a large anterior rectal ulcer and intense surrounding fibrosis and scarring. Some investigators routinely perform an anterior resection with rectopexy. Because of a slightly higher morbidity rate associated with a colorectal anastomosis, we tend to reserve anterior resection for those patients with preoperative constipation. In selected patients, rectopexy/resection may be performed by laparoscopic-assisted techniques. If the patient is very old or frail, a Delorme repair or perineal resection of the rectal prolapse may be a better option. The results of surgery in patients with occult mucosal prolapse are less predictable.

Preoperatively, a full medical and colonic evaluation should be performed. A full mechanical bowel preparation is done, and antibiotic prophylaxis is administered. After induction of anesthesia, a urinary catheter is inserted. Postoperatively, a closed suction drain is kept in the pelvis for 24 to 48 hours to evacuate any serous fluid and blood. After rectopexy, patients are maintained on bowel rest and intravenous fluids until bowel function returns, usually around days 4 to 6. The urinary catheter is left in place until the patient is mobile. Intraoperative complications include massive pelvic hemorrhage from trauma to the presacral veins. This trauma usually occurs because of mobilization in the wrong plane, breaching the presacral fascia. In most circumstances, bleeding will cease with packing, patience, cautery, and at times, suture ligation. With persistent hemorrhage, a sterilized thumbtack or endoscopic hernia tacker directed to the bleeding site in the sacrum is helpful. With uncontrolled hemorrhage, pressure packing with a large gauze roll is almost always effective in controlling the bleeding and allowing closure of the wound. The gauze roll may be removed 48 hours later under general anesthesia. Surgical complications are otherwise uncommon after a suture rectopexy.

Despite healing of the SRU after rectopexy, bowel symptoms often persist or recur because of chronic straining at stool. Fecal incontinence often improves after surgery for rectal prolapse. Full-thickness rectal prolapse recurs in 10% of cases after rectopexy; one third of these occurred 3 to 14 years after surgery in one series.

Transanal Local Excision

Symptomatic localized SRUs without a rectal prolapse often benefit from a transanal local excision, at least in the short term, in 75% of patients. This procedure is most suitable for patients complaining of rectal bleeding or excessive mucus discharge. Local excision is not appropriate if the rectal lesion is circumferential because of technical difficulties. Simple transanal excision of the prolapsing anterior mucosal prolapse will not alter the underlying defection disorder and the prolapse almost always recurs.

A full mechanical bowel preparation and antibiotic prophylaxis are given, as the local excision plane may sometimes be extended deeper beyond the submucosa because of intense fibrosis. The patient is placed in the prone position if the rectal lesion is primarily anterior in location and in the lithotomy position if the involvement is mainly posterior. With a small defect, a longitudinal closure is satisfactory. With a larger defect, a horizontal closure may be preferred to minimize rectal narrowing.

Postoperatively, patients are placed on a fluid diet for 48 hours. Prior to discharge, patients are counseled on a new bowel habit and avoidance of straining at stool. Complications include bleeding, infection, rectal stricture, and recurrence.

Low Anterior Resection

This resection is considered in complicated situations with a large rectal ulcer or when local excision or rectopexy has failed. In extreme cases, a complete proctectomy and a coloanal anastomosis are performed. It has been reported that low anterior resection benefits half the patients with or without a rectal prolapse, although surgical morbidity is substantial, including fecal incontinence, bladder dysfunction, and dyspareunia. This surgical option should be reserved for extreme situations with severe intractable symptoms.

Fecal Diversion

Fecal diversion with either a diverting colostomy or loop ileostomy provides some relief for severe incapacitating symptoms, although rectal bleeding and mucus discharge often persist. This option is often the last resort for patients with intractable symptoms despite various other surgical procedures.

Abdominoperineal Excision of the Rectum

This procedure is the ultimate last resort when all else has failed. Few patients will accept a permanent stoma for a benign condition. However, the author has two patients who remain symptom-free after abdominoperineal excision when all other procedures had failed.

Suggested Readings

Bogomeltz WV: Solitary rectal ulcer syndrome: Mucosal prolapse syndrome. Pathol Ann 1992;27(Pt1):75–86.

Felt-Bersma RJ, Cuesta MA: Rectal prolapse, rectal intussusception, rectocele, and solitary rectal ulcer syndrome. Gastroenterol Clin North Am 2001;30(1):199–222.

Gopal DV, Young C, Katon RM: Solitary rectal ulcer syndrome presenting with rectal prolapse, severe mucorrhea and eroded polypoid hyperplasia: Case report and review of the literature. Can J Gastroenterol 2001;15(7):479–483.

Haray PN, Morris-Stiff GJ, Foster ME: Solitary rectal ulcer syndrome—An underdiagnosed condition. Int J Colorect Dis 1997;12(5):313–315.

Li SC, Hamilton SR: Malignant tumors in the rectum simulating solitary rectal ulcer syndrome in endoscopic biopsy specimens. Am J Surg Pathol 1998;22(1):106–112.

Madigan MR, Morson BC: Solitary ulcer of the rectum. Gut 1969;10:871–881.

Reilly WT, Pemberton JH: Solitary rectal ulcer. In Wexner SD, Vernava AM III (Eds.). Clinical Decision Making in Colorectal Surgery. New York, Igaku-Shoin, 1995, pp 177–182.

Sitzler PJ, Kamm MA, Nicholls RJ, McKee RF: Long-term clinical outcome of surgery for solitary rectal ulcer syndrome. Br J Surg 1998;85(9):1246–1250.

Tjandra JJ, Fazio VW, Church JM, et al: Clinical conundrum of solitary rectal ulcer. Dis Colon Rectum 1992;35:227–234.

Tjandra JJ, Fazio VW, Petras RE: Clinical and pathologic factors associated with delayed diagnosis in solitary rectal ulcer syndrome. Dis Colon Rectum 1993;36:146–153.

Vaizey CJ, Roy AJ, Kamm MA: Prospective evaluation of the treatment of solitary rectal ulcer syndrome with biofeedback. Gut 1997;41(6):817–820.

Vaizey CJ, van den Bogaerde JB, Emmanuel AV, et al: Solitary rectal ulcer syndrome. Br J Surg 1998;85(12):1617–1623.

25

RECTOCELE

Brent K. Evetts, MD
Richard P. Billingham, MD

■ DEFINITION

A rectocele is a herniation of the rectovaginal septum anteriorly into the lumen of the vagina. It involves the anterior rectal wall as well as the posterior aspect of the vaginal wall. This herniation begins as a gradual thinning of this structure, which is first noticeable just above the anal sphincter anteriorly, and may extend as far superiorly as the cul-de-sac. The specific etiology is unknown, though the condition is clearly acquired, as opposed to congenital. The stresses of vaginal delivery, or of chronically straining to defecate in the setting of paradoxic contraction (nonrelaxation) of the levator muscle or the anal sphincter, result in increased pressure anteriorly in the rectum and the formation of what is in essence a pulsion diverticulum (Fig. 25-1).

■ SYMPTOMS

A patient with a rectocele will often complain of difficulty or inability to empty the rectum during defecation, a feeling of perineal or vaginal fullness, or a protrusion of tissue through the introitus on straining or even while walking. The hallmark of the patient with a symptomatic rectocele will often be the patient's need to push upward on the perineal body, or to apply backward pressure on the posterior wall of the vagina, to aid in rectal emptying. The straining associated with defecation may also be associated with internal or external rectal prolapse. Associated symptoms may be bleeding (from associated hemorrhoids or rectal prolapse), fecal incontinence (either from incomplete emptying or from any associated sphincter dysfunction), or pruritus.

■ DIAGNOSIS

On digital rectal examination, one can easily feel the anterior wall defect present with a rectocele. In order to rule out other possible causes of difficulty with defecation, such as occult intussusception or nonrelaxing puborectalis syndrome, videodefecography is usually the most helpful diagnostic study. Defecography will show the size of a rectocele, as well as the degree to which emptying will occur with defecation. Further, defecography helps to determine the presence of any associated rectal prolapse, sigmoido-

cele, nonrelaxing puborectalis muscle, or, when done with oral contrast medium to opacify the small bowel, enterocele. Anal manometry, endorectal ultrasound, and pudendal nerve conduction studies may help to delineate the cause of any associated sphincter dysfunction. Computed tomographic (CT) scan is rarely useful in the diagnosis and management of these conditions. A dynamic magnetic resonance imaging (MRI) scan with vaginal and rectal contrast medium is becoming useful in the diagnosis of pelvic floor dysfunction and may be helpful in the workings of suspected rectocele.

■ TREATMENT

Because the usual complaint is difficulty with defecation, the first priority in treating patients with rectocele is conservative treatment for this and associated conditions. If stool consistency and frequency are believed to be contributory, treatment usually begins with bulk laxatives. Patients with paradoxic contraction of the puborectalis muscle may benefit from biofeedback, though success with this technique is highly variable and depends on the skill and attitude of the therapist as well as the cooperation of the patient. Rubber band ligation of associated hemorrhoids may also be helpful, if they are felt to be contributory to symptoms. If conservative measures fail to provide relief, operative treatment of rectocele can be beneficial in up to 90% of symptomatic patients.

Operative Approaches

Transvaginal Approach

The transvaginal approach, which has traditionally been the procedure of choice by the gynecologist, involves utilizing the lithotomy position, making an incision just inside the fourchette, and extending the incision as far as the apex of the vagina. The vaginal mucosa is separated by blunt dissection from the underlying tissues of the rectovaginal septum. When this is combined with perineorrhaphy to build up the perineal body, the incision may be extended through the fourchette into the perineum. This technique historically has provided improvement of preoperative constipation symptoms by 44 to 69%, with very low morbidity.

Rectoceles with accompanying vaginal defects requiring operative repair, such as cystoceles, enteroceles, or uterine descensus, are usually best suited for repair via the transvaginal approach. When the high form of a rectocele includes an enterocele, one must consider the transabdominal approach.

Transrectal Repair

The low- and mid-form of a rectocele, which is an isolated defect in the suprasphincteric portion of the rectovaginal wall and contains only the rectovaginal septal defect, begins just above the anal sphincter anteriorly and can extend the length of the anal canal. This is best treated with the transrectal approach.

The majority of patients can undergo repair as an outpatient. We routinely have our patients undergo a complete

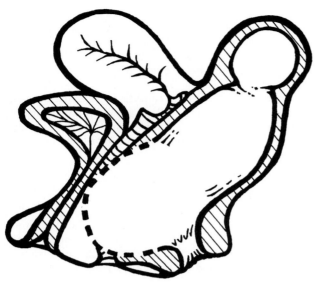

Figure 25-1
Sagittal view showing relationship of rectocele (*dashed line*) to posterior vaginal wall.

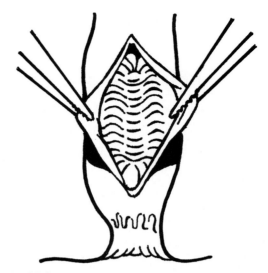

Figure 25-3
Dissection of mucosa and submucosa laterally to expose septal defect.

mechanical bowel preparation as well as antibiotic prophylaxis with a second-generation cephalosporin. Unless the patient has other preferences, spinal anesthesia with mild sedation has been quite satisfactory. With the patient in the prone jack-knife position, and utilizing a large Sawyer retractor in the anus, we begin by making a vertical incision from the dentate line to the apex of the palpable septal defect, which can be as high as 7 to 8 cm from the anal verge (Fig. 25-2). Dissection of mucosa and submucosa is carried out bilaterally, for a radial extent of about 90 degrees, with particular attention paid to hemo-

stasis (Fig. 25-3). The needlepoint cautery is often helpful here for both dissection and hemostasis. Some feel that submucosal infiltration of a solution containing epinephrine, 1:200,000, is helpful in facilitating both dissection and hemostasis.

Once an adequate amount of dissection has been carried out to expose the rectovaginal septum with enough solid tissue surrounding the defect to hold sutures, we use interrupted figure-of-eight, 0 polyglycolic acid sutures placed every 1 to 2 cm to imbricate the musculofascial defect vertically (Fig. 25-4). Smaller bites are taken superiorly with the first one or two sutures to taper the upper levels of the repair in order to avoid the creation of a shelf

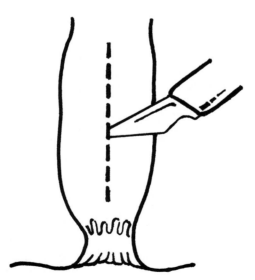

Figure 25-2
Initial incision from dentate line vertically to apex of rectovaginal septal defect.

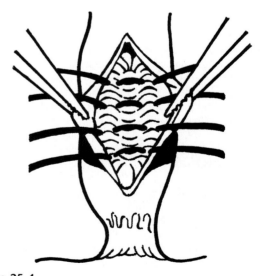

Figure 25-4
Initial layer of suture used to reapproximate musculofascial defect.

in the anterior midrectum. A second row of imbricating sutures may be used if needed (Fig. 25-5). Alternatively, the defect can be imbricated transversely, or a combination of these techniques can be used, as dictated by the size and shape of the defect.

Levatoroplasty is not usually performed because it is not feasible from this approach to identify the muscles. Excess mucosa is then excised and the mucosal defect closed with a running 3-0 polyglycolic acid suture (Fig. 25-6). A large (size 100) piece of Gelfoam is then rolled up and placed in the rectum at the end of the procedure, which may aid in obliterating the dead space in the early postoperative period, and is passed spontaneously with the first bowel movement.

Another variation in technique is to make a 180-degree transverse incision just above the dentate line, then two vertical incisions proximately to the apex of the defect, and then to repair the defect as described earlier, excising the excess mucosa.

Postoperatively, the patients are given bulk laxatives and an oral narcotic for pain and sent home. We make no effort to confine the bowels or limit dietary intake; in fact, we encourage normal diet and bowel activity. We usually see patients in the office at approximately 3 weeks and 2 months after the procedure.

Overall, the results of transrectal repair of rectocele are excellent in 79 to 98% of individuals. Associated morbidity is essentially zero. In those patients in whom repair does not relieve preoperative symptoms, continued symptoms are usually due to unrecognized associated pathology such as prolonged colonic transit time, nonrelaxing puborectalis syndrome, or possible pudendal nerve damage. Thus, we emphasize the importance of a careful and thoughtful preoperative evaluation prior to undertaking operative treatment. Patients who have had a vaginal hysterectomy tend not to have as high a success rate.

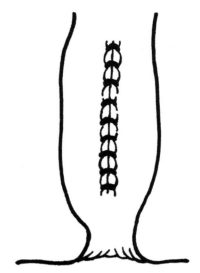

Figure 25-6
Completed repair.

Repair of Combined Problems

Generally other common anorectal problems, if present and symptomatic, can and should be repaired at the same time as rectocele repair. Internal hemorrhoids can be treated by closed or open hemorrhoidectomy in combination with rectocele repair. When it is necessary to remove the right anterior hemorrhoid, we will often begin our mucosal dissection in this location. There is usually enough redundancy of the mucosa after the rectocele repair to allow easy closure. Complete rectal prolapse and rectocele can be repaired with the Altemeier-type perineal proctectomy, which is our usual preference, or by a Delorme procedure, repairing the rectocele in the course of doing either procedure. Alternatively, an intra-abdominal procedure for rectal prolapse, if indicated, can be employed without compromising the rectocele repair. When faced with internal rectal prolapse and rectocele, it is important to keep in mind that internal rectal prolapse may be an early precursor to complete procidentia, and some form of transanal repair of this problem should be considered. The combination of rectocele and sigmoidocele is only corrected via the abdominal approach to repair the sigmoidocele.

The combination of cystocele and rectocele are probably best served by the transvaginal approach, as mentioned earlier. If an enterocele repair is needed, and an associated rectocele is present, both can often be repaired transvaginally, so as to be able to reach the apex of the musculofascial defect, although one may need to consider a transabdominal approach. If sphincteric disruption is an associated problem, sphincteroplasty may be combined with a transanal approach to rectocele repair.

Transperineal Approach

Although this approach has been described, with or without the insertion of a buttressing material, such as autogenous fascia lata or even polypropylene mesh, it is more

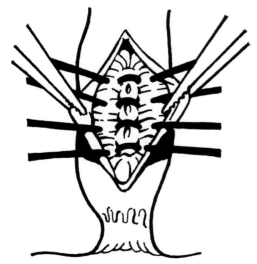

Figure 25-5
Completed initial layer as well as second row of sutures.

technically difficult than the approaches described previously, and we are unable to see any advantage to performing the procedure in this way.

Suggested Readings

Ayabaca SM, Zbar AP, Pescatori M: Anal continence after rectocele repair. Dis Colon Rectum 2002;45:63–69.

Ho YH, Ang M, Nyam D, et al: Transanal approach to rectocele repair may compromise anal sphincter pressures. Dis Colon Rectum 1998;41:354–358.

Janssen LWM, van Dijke CF: Selection criteria for anterior rectal wall repair in symptomatic rectocele and anterior rectal wall prolapse. Dis Colon Rectum 1994;37:1100–1107.

Kahn MA, Stanton SL: Techniques of rectocele repair and their effects on bowel function. Int Urogynecol J Pelvic Floor Dysfunct 1998;9: 37–47.

Khubchandani IT, Clancy JP, Rosen L, et al: Endorectal repair of rectocele revisited. Br J Surg 1997;84:89–91.

Mellgren A, Lopez A, Schultz I, Anzen B: Rectocele is associated with paradoxical anal sphincter reaction. Dis Colon Rectum 1998;41:354–358.

Murthy VK, Orkin BA, Smith LE, et al: Excellent outcome using selective criteria for rectocele repair. Dis Colon Rectum 1996;39:374–378.

Sehapayak S: Transrectal repair of rectocele: An extended armamentarium of colorectal surgeons. A report of 355 cases. Dis Colon Rectum 1985;28:422–433.

Van Dam JH, Hop WC, Schouten WR: Analysis of patients with poor outcome of rectocele repair. Dis Colon Rectum 2000;43:1556–1560.

Van Dam JH, Huisman, WM, Hop WC, Schouten WR: Fecal continence after rectocele repair: A prospective study. Int J Colorectal Dis 2000;15:54–57.

Van Laarhoven CJ, Kamm MA, Bartram CI, et al: Relationship between anatomic and symptomatic long-term results after rectocele repair for impaired defecation. Dis Colon Rectum 1999;42:204–210.

26

RECTAL TRAUMA

Linda M. Farkas, MD
Herand Abcarian, MD, FACS

Rectal trauma is rare in comparison to the solid organ injury in blunt trauma and other hollow viscus injuries in penetrating trauma. These injuries are unique in that they cannot be easily visualized during the usual trauma secondary surveys. Surgeons may also overlook rectal injuries during celiotomy if they occur below the peritoneal reflection. Therefore, to prevent the significant morbidity and potential for fatality, a high index of suspicion is necessary.

■ ETIOLOGY

Penetrating trauma is the most common cause of rectal trauma, accounting for at least 95% of rectal injuries (Table 26-1). In inner-city hospitals, gunshot wounds account for 70% of colon and rectal perforations. Shotgun pellets are less likely to injure the rectum as the velocity decreases during penetration of the buttocks or the abdominal wall. Stab wounds of the pelvis and buttock due to ice picks or stilettos can produce small rectal perforations which may be easily overlooked.

Rectal perforation secondary to blunt trauma is much less common in urban areas, accounting for only 4% of colorectal injuries. These injuries may also be more difficult to diagnose. An example is a motor vehicle accident patient suffering from crushed pelvis with bone spicules penetrating the rectum. These injuries may go unnoticed in light of massive pelvic bleeding and bladder injuries. On the other hand, motorcycle accident victims may be dragged on the pavement which can cause obvious severe perineal or sphincter injuries with significant tissue destruction. Impalement by straddle injuries can cause severe anorectal lacerations, but such trauma is relatively rare (1%). Impalement injuries due to criminal sexual assault are uncommon. Rectal foreign bodies are listed for the sake of completeness but will be discussed in more detail in another chapter.

Iatrogenic injuries sometimes occur during diagnostic procedures, such as endoscopy or barium enema. Iatrogenic perforations during pelvic operations such as radical prostatectomy, prostatic biopsy, or gynecologic procedures are uncommon, and their true incidence is unknown. Perforation of the rectum during internal fixation of a hip fracture has been reported.

■ DIAGNOSIS: TRAUMA PATIENTS

Except for the obvious anorectal lacerations, most rectal injuries are not readily noticeable. A high index of suspicion is necessary when a penetrating injury crosses the pelvic midline. The presence of a pelvic fracture, hematuria, passage of blood per rectum or vagina, or blood on the examining glove are indications for proctosigmoidoscopy (Table 26-2).

The value of hemoccult testing to detect occult rectal injuries due to penetrating trauma has been addressed by Levine and coworkers. Of their 19 patients with suspected rectal injuries, guaiac testing was only 69% sensitive and 33% specific. On the other hand, sigmoidoscopy was 100% sensitive and 67% specific. In fact, no rectal injuries were found solely where the guaiac was positive and the proctoscopy negative. Each time, either proctoscopy or other obvious findings led the examiners to the correct conclusions. The guaiac test alone did not lead to the diagnosis. In fact, 5 of 17 patients had a negative test despite rectal injuries, so a negative test does not mean no further workup is needed.

Rigid proctosigmoidoscopy is the preferred diagnostic test. Because the bowel is unprepared, the large caliber of the rigid scope allows better visualization and evacuation of stool. Rectal injuries may be seen as an obvious tear, but more frequently there is only a bluish discoloration, submucosal hematoma, or active bleeding. At times, lack of patient cooperation or presence of the stool does not permit a thorough examination. If the patient needs to go to the operating room for other injuries, endoscopy should

---

Table 26-1 Etiology of Rectal Injuries

Rectal Traumas

Penetrating (gunshot, shotgun, stab wounds, watercraft accidents)
Nonpenetrating (blunt)
Impalement (straddle injuries)

Iatrogenic Traumas

Endoscopic and electrosurgery
Barium enema
Pelvic surgery
Other operations

Rectal Foreign Bodies

Self-induced (autoeroticism)
Impalement (criminal assault)

Table 26-2 Injuries and Symptoms Frequently Associated with Rectal Trauma

Penetrating injury crossing the pelvic midline
Pelvic fracture
Hematuria
Blood per rectum
Blood per vagina
Blood on examining glove after digital examination

be performed under anesthesia. The patient should be positioned in a low lithotomy position for proctoscopy in preparation for possible rectal repair, anastomosis, external drainage, or washout.

Most patients with rectal injuries have other associated injuries, commonly of the small bowel and the genitourinary system. Therefore, each trauma patient needs to undergo the initial "ABCs" (Airway, Breathing, Circulation) of resuscitation. Once stabilized, the secondary survey may alert the trauma team to the possibility of rectal injury, which in itself is an indication for proctoscopy.

■ ENDOSCOPIC INJURIES

Iatrogenic injuries during diagnostic endoscopy most often occur at the rectosigmoid junction. This area tends to be most tethered by previous pelvic operations and, therefore, undergoes the most tension during the endoscopy. Suspicion should be aroused when the patient has sharp abdominal pain followed by increasing pain and tenderness after diagnostic endoscopy, biopsy, or electrosurgery. An upright chest x-ray may reveal free air under the diaphragm. A water-soluble contrast enema may be helpful in localizing the area of perforation to the extra or intraperitoneal rectum. Reviewing colorectal perforations due to diagnostic procedures, Nelson and coworkers reported 13 cases in an 8-year period. The incidence of perforation from proctosigmoidoscopy was 0.18%, those secondary to colonoscopy 0.24%, and from barium enema 0.16%. Barium enema perforations were uniformly fatal.

■ TREATMENT OF TRAUMATIC INJURIES: PRINCIPLES

In a traumatized patient, an injury with a trajectory that crosses the pelvic midline mandates proctoscopy. If the patient is uncooperative, too unstable in the emergency room, or stool obscures visualization, proctoscopy can be performed intraoperatively. Hemodynamic instability secondary to blood loss, neurogenic shock, or tension pneumothorax must be addressed first. Whether this is accomplished in the emergency room or operating room is a matter of logistics and preference. Broad-spectrum antibiotics should be given preoperatively, and once anesthetized, the patient is placed in a low lithotomy position. Intra-abdominal or intrathoracic bleeding should be managed first. Then rectal injuries can be found or ruled out with rigid proctoscopy.

■ MANAGEMENT OF RECTAL WOUNDS

If the rectal wound is greater than 1 cm in width it should be repaired. It is best to leave smaller injuries alone rather than risk enlarging or injuring an alternate site with extensive manipulation and mobilization. Tuggle and Huber treated 47 major rectal injuries with proximal diversion

but repaired only 19 wounds. Unrepaired rectal injuries were not associated with higher morbidity or longer hospitalization. An exception to this may be the presence of a genitourinary injury. Franko and coworkers found in their study of simultaneous rectal and genitourinary injuries, only those (7 out of 16) that did not have a rectal repair later were complicated by rectovesical and rectourethral fistulas. Furthermore, although Tuggle and Huber showed no overall increase in morbidity associated with leaving rectal wounds unrepaired, the one rectoprostatic and the two rectovesical fistulas in their study occurred in patients who did not have a rectal repair. Therefore, in such circumstances it seems wise to repair both rectal and urinary injuries and interpose healthy tissue (e.g., omentum) between the repairs.

Regardless of whether the rectal injury is repaired or not, a proximal diverting colostomy is placed as close to the injury as possible. Many studies have shown no difference in morbidity whether an end or loop colostomy is made. Fontes and Morris both showed by barium studies that loop colostomies divert completely as long as the ends are not retracted. Winset, using radioisotope and dye techniques, showed that loop ileostomies are completely diverting. We prefer the end-loop colostomy described by Prasad and associates. This procedure accomplishes complete diversion and prevents distal limb prolapse. Because the stoma is similar in size and shape to an end-colostomy, it is easier to care for than a loop stoma. Also, unlike an end-colostomy, an end-loop stoma can be closed through a peristomal incision, and a formal laparotomy is unnecessary. This procedure decreases associated morbidity and length of stay. Some authors have suggested that upper third (intraperitoneal) rectal injuries may be managed using guidelines for colonic injuries and that diversion may not be mandatory.

■ PRESACRAL DRAINAGE

With the patient in the low lithotomy position, a transverse incision is made over the anococcygeal raphe through skin and subcutaneous (Fig. 26-1). There is no advantage in disconnecting the external sphincter at the coccyx. Instead, dissection on either side of the anococcygeal raphe allows placement of drains without division of the coccygeal attachments. Three to four Penrose drains or a closed drainage system can be brought out through this incision and secured to the skin and left in place for 5 to 7 days. Coccygectomy is unnecessary and may result in septic complications or incontinence postoperatively. A recent randomized controlled trial by Gonzalez and colleagues has suggested that routine presacral drainage may be unnecessary, although they do recommend drainage for those with extensive soft tissue or military-type injuries such as bullet wounds.

■ DISTAL RECTAL WASHOUT

Evacuation of stool from the injured rectum has resulted in fewer septic complications. In the technique is described by

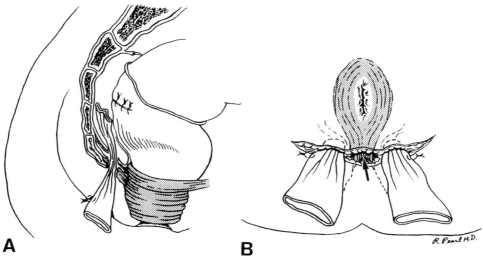

Figure 26-1
A, Lateral view; *B,* view from above of presacral drains.

Franko and coworkers, a Foley catheter is inserted in a small opening made in the stapled distal rectal stump and the rectum is then irrigated with 4 to 5 L of saline. To prevent backflow into the abdomen, the anus must be kept open. Although some authors advocate manual dilation of the anus, Franko describes using anesthesia tubing, which is large enough to keep the anus open during irrigation. No advantage to using antimicrobial solutions instead of saline has been reported.

Tuggle and Huber recommend washout only for high-velocity missile wounds. On the other hand, Mangiante and coworkers reported no intra-abdominal infectious complications using rectal washout, and they had three cases of infection in those who had not had rectal washout. They concluded overall that civilian and military wounds are unique in terms of their postoperative complications, mortality rate, and management techniques. In the study by Shannon, the patients with rectal washout had a significantly lower incidence of pelvic abscesses (46% versus 8%), rectal fistulas (23% versus 7%), and sepsis (15% versus 8%). The only death in the series occurred in the nonwashed-out group. In the last decade, a dramatic rise in the use of automatic handguns makes it likely that rectal washout will be used more frequently as more civilians are injured with these high-velocity weapons.

■ PERITONEAL LAVAGE

At the completion of laparotomy, the pelvic and abdominal cavities should be thoroughly washed out with saline to remove all particulate matter, especially clotted blood. The presence of hemoglobin in the peritoneal cavity lowers intraperitoneal leukocyte counts, inhibits in vivo chemotaxis, and results in increasing bacterial colony counts. If the rectum is perforated during barium enema, the perirectal and pelvic soft tissue must be carefully debrided to remove as much of the barium as possible.

■ ANTIBIOTICS

All patients with suspected or proved rectal injuries should receive preoperative broad-spectrum antibiotics. Many centers use cefoxitin or ampicillin/sulbactam. There is good evidence that second- or third-generation cephalosporins may be just as effective and produce fewer antibiotic-related complication than an aminogycoside-clindamycin combination. There is no evidence to support more than 72 hours of perioperative antibiotic therapy in penetrating abdominal trauma. If postoperative fever persists, it is best to discontinue the antibiotic after 3 days, reculture the patient, and begin a second course of therapy with the appropriate antibiotics.

■ MANAGEMENT OF SURGICAL WOUNDS

After the fascia is closed with monofilament suture, the skin and subcutaneous tissues may be left open and treated with wet to dry dressings. One or two sutures can be placed in the skin around the umbilicus to facilitate application of the stoma appliance and for cosmetic purposes. After 4 to 5 days, if there is no evidence of infection, the edges can be approximated with skin tapes. If small, perineal lacerations can be left open and treated like a fistulotomy wound. Dirty wounds, especially large perineal lacerations compounded by the contaminated tattooing of asphalt into the skin, must be extensively debrided. Long lacerations may be closed over suction irrigation catheters. Diverting colostomy and distal rectal washout must be added to reduce infectious complications.

■ RESULTS

Lowe and associates reported 212 patients with colorectal injuries, with 6.12% overall mortality rate and 3.3% mor-tality rate from septic complications. Twenty-one patients with rectal injuries were treated with closure, drainage, proximal colostomy, and rectal washout. In these patients there were no deaths and no septic complications. Our results, as well as those of other institutions, confirm that there is a direct correlation between death from rectal wounds and trauma severity index or mean number of associated injuries. In one series of patients with blunt col-orectal trauma, the survivors and nonsurvivors had an average of 1.9 and 3.8 injuries per patient, respectively.

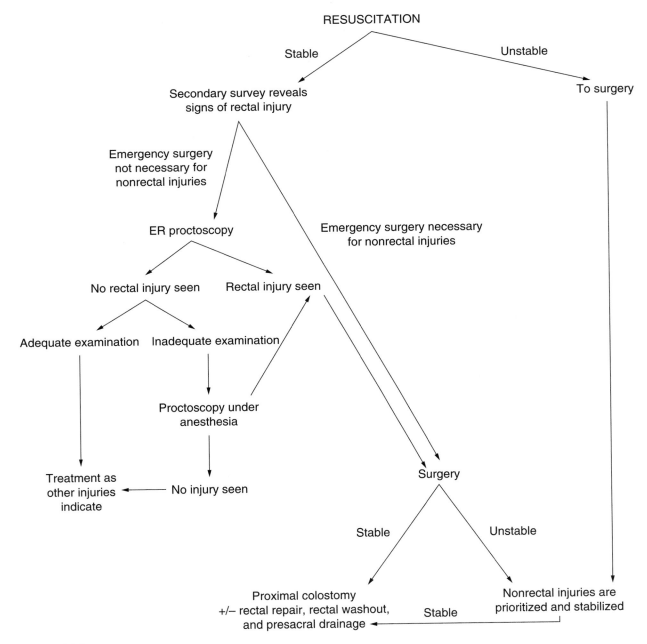

Figure 26-2
Proposed algorithm for treatment of rectal injuries.

■ TREATMENT OF IATROGENIC INJURIES

Iatrogenic perforations are treated in the same manner as other colorectal perforations. An exception is a small perforation created during colonoscopic biopsy or polypectomy. In these instances, if bowel preparation is excellent and there are no signs of peritonitis, the patient may be placed NPO (given nothing by mouth), receive intravenous antibiotics, and undergo serial examinations. If diffuse peritonitis occurs, then the patient needs surgical intervention. If a perforation occurs during a diagnostic colonoscopy, the hole is usually larger and the patients tend to fail nonsurgical therapy. When the perforation is diagnosed early with minimal contamination, a primary repair can be performed without a diverting colostomy. These patients should be continued on intravenous antibiotics for 3 days.

In contrast, barium enema perforations, even though diagnosed early and operated on urgently, continue to have a high mortality rate. Clearly the single element in this catastrophic event that distinguishes it from the other forms of rectal trauma is the presence of barium sulfate. Barium rapidly and tenaciously adheres to the peritoneal and retroperitoneal tissues and is impossible to remove by lavage. Therefore, extensive débridement should be part of the surgical treatment of barium extravasation if postoperative complications are to be kept to a minimum.

■ CONCLUSION

Surgical treatment of rectal trauma must follow specific plans for the management of rectal wounds, external drainage, distal rectal washout, pelvic/peritoneal irrigation, broad-spectrum antibiotics, and care of surgical wounds (Fig. 26-2). Adherence to the aforementioned principles should result in satisfactory functional outcome with low complication rate and no deaths.

Suggested Readings

Franko ER, Ivantury RR, Schwalb DM: Combined penetrating rectal and genitourinary injuries: A challenge in management. J Trauma 1993;34:347–353.

Gonzalez RP, Falimirski ME, Holevar MR: The role of presacral drainage in the management of penetrating rectal injuries. J Trauma 1998;54:656–661.

Levine H, Simon RJ, Smith TR, et al: Guaiac testing in the diagnosis of rectal trauma: What is its value? J Trauma 1992;32:210–212.

McGrath V, Fabian TC, Croce MA, et al: Rectal trauma: Management based on anatomic distinction. Am Surg 1998;64:1136–1141.

Morken JJ, Kraatz JJ, Balcos EG, et al : Civilian rectal trauma: A changing perspective. Surgery 1999;126:693–698.

Prasad ML, Abcarian H, Pearl PK: End-loop colostomy. Surg Gynecol Obstet 1984;158:380–382.

Rowlands BJ, Ericcson CD, Fischer RP: Penetrating abdominal trauma: The use of operative finding to determine the length of antibiotic therapy. J Trauma 1987;27:250–254.

Shannon FL, Moore EE, Moore FA, et al: Value of distal colon washout in civilian rectal trauma-reducing gut bacterial translocation. J Trauma 1988;28:989–994.

Tuggle D, Huber PJ: Management of rectal trauma. Am J Surg 1984;148:806–808.

Velmahos GC, Gomez H, Falabella A, Demetriades D: Operative management of civilian rectal gunshot wounds: Simpler is better. World J Surg 2000;24:114–118.

27

RECTAL FOREIGN BODIES

Norman Sohn, MD, FACS
Jeffrey S. Aronoff, MD

A retained rectal foreign body is an infrequent and potentially difficult clinical problem that can test maximally the imagination, ingenuity, and resourcefulness of the surgeon who seeks to achieve a solution. Additionally, most retained rectal foreign bodies are the result of anal erotic behavior, and therefore, they can be a source of embarrassment and emotional discomfort to the patient. In this chapter, the common retained rectal foreign bodies and a standardized technique for their removal will be discussed first. Then, more unusual foreign bodies and the innovative and imaginative techniques for their extraction will be discussed.

■ ETIOLOGY

Retained rectal foreign bodies can be divided into two broad categories—sexual and nonsexual. The sexual category can be divided into voluntary and involuntary. The latter involves rape, assault, and homicide. Many cases of the involuntary sexual variety have been reported in the pediatric population. The voluntary sexual act as a cause of retained rectal foreign bodies is the most common. In many cases it is autoerotic. Although retained foreign bodies are found in males and females, both heterosexual and homosexual, in our experience, they are most common in homosexual males. However, heterosexual males and females as well as homosexual females are also represented. The most common foreign bodies seen in this group of patients are vibrators and dildos. The latter are usually latex, phallus-shaped objects. Fruits and vegetables including carrots, cucumbers, and bananas are also common.

Nonsexual rectal foreign bodies include ingested foreign objects such as chicken bones, toothpicks, and fish bones, as well as disposable enema tip protectors and thermometers. In addition, the entire gastrointestinal tract and particularly the rectum are used to conceal contraband. More recently, this mode of transport has been utilized in the international transportation of illicit drugs. The patient, referred to as a "mule," ingests latex condoms that have been packed with cocaine or heroin. These large ingested objects can cause a small bowel obstruction or become impacted in the rectum. Breakage of the latex container can result in a substantial drug overdose and can cause death.

■ SYMPTOMS

The symptoms of a retained foreign body include its presence and the inability to evacuate it. However, a retained rectal foreign body can also cause rectal pain, bleeding, or discharge or may result in perforation of the rectum or sigmoid colon. The presence of abdominal pain alerts the physician to the possibility of an intraperitonal perforation. In assessing patients with retained rectal foreign bodies, the associated symptoms, the type of foreign body, and the duration of the history are important. In one case, a foreign body was reported to be present for 6 months before an effort was made to remove it. Occasionally, rectal abscesses and vulvar abscesses have been associated with intrarectal foreign bodies. This development has occurred particularly with chicken bone and fish bone perforations. Rectal pain without any abscess can be due to a fish bone or chicken bone or toothpick that has been ingested innocently. Complications of rectal foreign bodies have been reported in which there has been migration intraspinally or to the vulva or urinary tract. Ooi and coworkers reported a series of 30 cases in which 10 admitted to inserting the foreign object. Clues to the presence of a rectal foreign body in the other 20 included atypical gender behavior, lax anal sphincters, and a bloody or mucoid discharge.

■ PHYSICAL EXAMINATION

Physical examination should include examination of the abdomen to search for tenderness and a palpable mass. Rectal examination is more important. In general, most foreign bodies can be palpated in the midrectum. A long object cannot negotiate the anterior curve of the rectum and becomes lodged at that location. If the foreign body is not palpable, its presence should be ascertained either with appropriate endoscopy or x-ray examination. If the foreign body is not palpable but is certain to be present, we prefer to wait several hours for the foreign body to descend into the rectum. If appropriate, the patient can be hospitalized for this period of time. In most cases the foreign object is at the point just described or will migrate to that point.

Obviously, it is advantageous to remove the foreign body in an outpatient setting. This approach avoids the need for hospitalization and exposure of the patient to many different observers of this embarrassing and emotionally compromising situation. Equipment not normally stocked in an ambulatory facility is helpful for retained rectal foreign body removal. Facilities likely to care for such patients should have this equipment, including Parks' and narrow Deaver retractors, large Kocher clamps, and uterine tenacula, available.

■ STANDARD TECHNIQUE OF REMOVAL

After the retained rectal foreign body is palpated in the midrectum, local anesthesia is administered in a manner analogous to that administered for anal surgery in general. The patient is placed in the prone jack-knife position on the operating or examining table. Any other position can be used according to the surgeon's preference. Unlike most other cases of anorectal surgery performed under local anesthesia, it is usually unnecessary to provide supplemental conscious sedation. However, this can easily be administered if necessary. Two and a half mL of 0.5% bupivacaine (0.5% lidocaine can be substituted) is injected in the right and left midlateral positions and in the anterior and posterior midline positions by inserting a 1½-inch needle up to its hub and depositing 2.5 mL at each site. Thereafter, a subcutaneous wheal of local anesthetic is raised around the anus utilizing the same solution with a 30-gauge needle. Complete anesthesia and sphincter relaxation are thereby achieved. After the local anesthetic is administered, a Parks' retractor is inserted, with its third blade positioned anteriorly. Occasionally, a narrow Deaver retractor is placed posteriorly to facilitate exposure. A large Kocher clamp or uterine tenaculum is then used to grasp the foreign body, with care being taken to avoid clamping the adjacent rectal mucosa. Other clamps may be used, but we have found those mentioned here to be most satisfactory. The foreign body is then deflected posteriorly and removed from the rectum. Proctosigmoidoscopy is performed to make sure that there has been no rectal or sigmoid colon perforation and that there is no active bleeding.

Less Common Retained Rectal Foreign Bodies

Besides vibrators, dildos, carrots, cucumbers, and bananas, many other objects whose shape permits placement within the rectum have been inserted and occasionally require a physician's assistance for removal. A partial list has been collated from the authors' experience and a search of the medical literature as well as an analysis of several Internet sites that deal with that subject matter. The list includes apples, ax handles, baby powder boxes, ball bearings, balloons, baseballs, beer glasses, billiard balls, bottle caps, bottles, broomsticks, candle boxes, candles, cattle horns, cold cream jars, cups, flashlights, frozen fish, frozen pig's tail, glasses, ice picks, iron rods, jars, knife sharpeners, knives, light bulbs, microwave egg boilers, onions, parsnips, pears, pens, pepper mills, plantains, potatoes, rubber tubes, salamis, screwdrivers, snuff boxes, soap bars, spoons, stones, tennis balls, test tubes, toothbrush holders, toothbrushes, turnips, umbrella handles, wire springs, yams, and zucchini. Perhaps the most daring foreign body that has been inserted into a rectum is an artillery shell, reportedly live.

Despite rumors of gerbils or other rodents being placed in the rectum of male homosexuals for sexual stimulation, this practice has not been documented. A Medline search as well as an Internet search regarding rectal insertion of rodents also failed to document the existence of this type of perverted activity.

Other Techniques of Removal

The authors have not found rigid anoscopy or proctosigmoidoscopy or flexible colonoscopy useful in removing the retained rectal foreign body with the exception of very thin or small objects such as thermometers or disposable enema nozzle protectors. Although visualization of the foreign body is desirable, the examiner must recognize that in most situations, attempts to remove the retained rectal foreign body with rigid or flexible sigmoidoscopes may displace it more proximally and confound attempts to remove it.

Many ingenious techniques have been devised to remove retained rectal foreign bodies. Yet, one of the most useful tools is simply the hand. A surgeon or an assistant with a small hand may be able to insert that hand into the rectum and grasp the retained rectal foreign body and remove it. Often, a female surgeon or other health care worker may have the right size of hand needed to accomplish this maneuver. With the increased number and availability of female surgeons and residents, this technique is assuming an important place in the management of difficult retained rectal foreign bodies.

The removal of glass objects without breakage presents another challenge to the surgeon. Obstetric forceps and suction vacuum extractors have been helpful in some cases. One author reported filling a retained hollow glass container with plaster of Paris into which a gauze wick had been placed. After the plaster had set it was a simple matter to remove this glass foreign body by withdrawing it with the gauze wick. In another case, the esophageal balloon portion of a Blakemore-Sengstaken tube was placed in a retained test tube. Inflating the balloon caused sufficient traction to enable the test tube to be extracted.

In some cases the foreign object fits snugly in the rectum or rectosigmoid and attempts at its removal cause a proximal negative pressure and suction effect. This pressure can be of sufficient magnitude to prevent extraction of the retained rectal foreign body. One author reports being able to pass a colonoscope alongside the retained rectal foreign body, enabling air to be inserted and eliminating the suction effect and thereby facilitating removal of the retained rectal foreign body. Others have been able to pass a Foley catheter alongside the retained rectal foreign body, permitting the insufflation of air and thereby overcoming the suction effect.

A modification of Yorke-Mason's operation also has been successfully employed to remove a large, retained rectal foreign body. In this technique the entire sphincter mechanism is divided. Prior to division of the sphincter, all its components are identified and marked with sutures to enable subsequent reconstruction after the retained rectal foreign body is removed.

Corkscrews and gimlets have been successfully employed in the removal of retained rectal foreign bodies. In one case managed by one of the authors (NS) a huge yam had been in place for over 24 hours. The yam was readily palpated as a mass in the lower abdomen. The technique that enabled its removal consisted of having the assistant apply abdominal pressure to the yam and manually push it into the pelvis. Simultaneously, the surgeon passed a 1½-inch-diameter operating proctoscope and was able to visualize the yam. Through the proctoscope he whittled the yam down, by shaving off slices with a uterine curette, until it was small enough to be passed rectally.

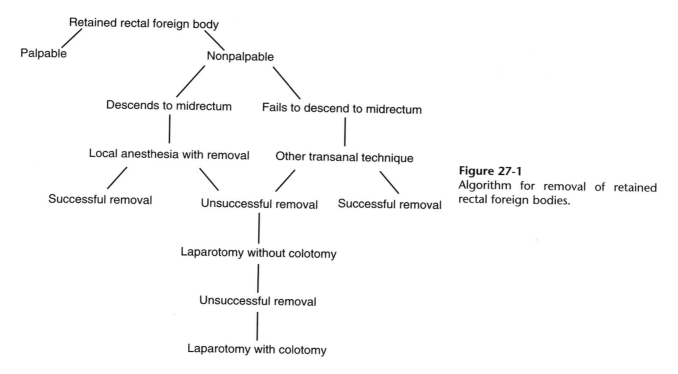

Figure 27-1
Algorithm for removal of retained rectal foreign bodies.

The surgeon has many options for removing retained rectal foreign bodies and may be limited only by imagination. The overwhelming majority of retained rectal foreign bodies can be removed transanally without resorting to a laparotomy. Every effort should be made to remove a retained rectal foreign body transanally. Nevertheless, infrequently the surgeon will have no other option and will have to perform a laparotomy. Ideally, at laparotomy, the retained rectal foreign body will be able to be milked toward the rectum where it could be removed transanally. In a rare circumstance, a colotomy with removal of the retained rectal foreign body will be necessary. This approach obviously has a greater potential for postoperative complications.

In the 30 cases reported by Ooi and coworkers, transanal recovery was possible in 25 (12 under sedation, 13 with general anesthesia). Laparotomy was needed in 3 cases and in 2 cases the foreign object was passed with an enema. The authors reported that at a median follow-up of 63 (8 to 96) months there was no instance of reimpaction.

■ CONCLUSION

Retained rectal foreign bodies can be managed according to the algorithm in Figure 27-1. Efforts are made to remove the retained rectal foreign body transanally, reserving laparotomy for failures and even then attempting to avoid a colotomy. The ingenuity of people in finding new, unique, and interesting articles to insert into the rectum will present a continuing challenge to the further ingenuity and resourcefulness of physicians who extract them.

Suggested Readings

Cohen JS, Sackier JM: Management of colorectal foreign bodies. J R Coll Surg Edinburgh 1996;41(5):312–315.
Fry RD: Anorectal trauma and foreign bodies. Surg Clin North Am 1994;74(6):1491–1505.
Ooi BS, Ho YH, Eu KW, et al: Management of anorectal foreign bodies: A cause of obscure anal pain. Aust NZ J Surg 1998;68:852–855.

28

DIAGNOSIS AND MANAGEMENT OF SACRAL AND RETRORECTAL TUMORS

Sharon Grundfest-Broniatowski, SBEE, MD
Kenneth Marks, MD
Victor W. Fazio, MB, MS, MD (Hon), FRACS, FRACS (Hon), FACS, FRCS, FRCS (Ed)

Tumors of the sacrum and retrorectal space are rare. Only 50 such tumors were encountered at the Cleveland Clinic between 1929 and 1985 (Table 28-1). The incidence of retrorectal tumors at the Mayo Clinic has been reported to be approximately 1 in 40,000 general hospital admissions. The annual incidence of congenital retrorectal tumors is estimated to be 0.0023 to 0.015%.

It is useful to consider the sacrum and the retrorectal space as a functional anatomic unit. The retrorectal space is bounded by the rectum anteriorly, the sacrum and coccyx posteriorly, the peritoneal reflection superiorly, and the levator ani and coccygeal muscles inferiorly. Laterally, the boundaries are the iliac muscles and the ureters (Fig. 28-1). Tumors may arise from the hindgut and proctodeum, neural elements, or bone. Masses found in this area may be either congenital or acquired, and can be classified as (1) developmental anomalies, (2) inflammatory lesions, (3) neoplastic lesions, or (4) metastatic lesions. Tumors such as chordomas, which have commonly been classified as originating in the retrorectal space, probably arise within the sacrum. Symptoms from these lesions are variable and depend on the size and location of the tumor. Common complaints are lower back or rectal pain, a feeling of heaviness or pressure in the pelvis or rectum, and a change in bowel habits. Small, benign developmental cysts may remain asymptomatic. Larger cysts may cause symptoms of incomplete defecation or obstructed labor. Infection is common, leading to local pain, drainage, fever, and chills. Thus, patients suspected of having perianal abscess, pilonidal abscess, or pelvic abscess should undergo digital rectal examination to exclude a presacral mass. Neurologic symptoms such as perianal or lower extremity paresthesias, urinary retention, or incontinence should lead the examiner to suspect malignancy.

■ DEVELOPMENTAL LESIONS

Developmental lesions may arise from embryonic mishaps involving primitive gut or neural structures. Sacrococcygeal teratoma (SCT) is the most common presacral tumor of the newborn, with an incidence of about 1 in 40,000 live births. Although it is possible that these tumors may arise from germ cells or may represent a form of fetus in fetu, current thinking is that SCT orignates from totipotent somatic cells in the primitive knot (Hensen's node) or caudal cell mass.

Difficulty may be encountered in distinguishing the cystic lesions of the retrorectal space, which include germ cell tumors, tailgut cysts, and duplication cysts. Endoluminal ultrasound, computed tomographic (CT) scanning, and magnetic resonance imaging (MRI) are useful in diagnosing the extent of these lesions. MRI is particularly helpful in assessing bone invasion and metastases. Advances in obstetric ultrasound have made it possible to diagnose sacrococcygeal teratomas in early gestation. The imaging appearance of a tumor cannot reliably predict its histology; however, benign tumors are more commonly cystic, and malignant lesions are more likely to be solid.

Germ Cell Tumors

Germ cell tumors in the retrorectal space may be pure or mixed. The pure tumors include teratoma (mature or immature) (Fig. 28-2), yolk sac tumor (endodermal sinus tumor), germinoma (histologically identical to seminoma), embryonal carcinoma, and choriocarcinoma. Only the first two are commonly seen in the sacrococcygeal region. Mixed germ cell tumors are composed of combinations of the preceding types. Teratomas, which include all three germ layers, may undergo malignant transformation, for example, squamous cell carcinoma originating in squamous epithelium, or rhabdomyosarcoma developing in mesenchymal tissue.

Sacrococcygeal teratomas have been classified according to their location by the American Academy of Pediatrics Surgical Section as follows: type I, completely external with no presacral component; type II, manifest

Table 28-1 Cleveland Clinic: Sacral and Retrorectal Tumors, 1929–1985	
TUMOR	**NUMBER**
Chordoma	17
Germ cell tumors	16
Squamous cell carcinoma developing in a teratoma (teratoma with malignant transformation) (1)	
Endodermal sinus tumor (yolk sac tumor) (2)	
Mature teratoma (13)	
Tailgut cysts	6
Duplication cyst	1
Fibrosarcoma	1
Giant cell tumor of the sacrum	3
Aneurysmal bone cyst of the sacrum	1
Ewing's sarcoma	1
Hemangiopericytoma	1
Neurogenic tumors	3
Myxopapillary ependymoma (1)	
Lipomeningocele (2)	
Total	50

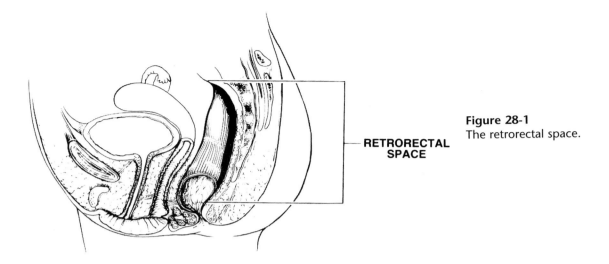

Figure 28-1
The retrorectal space.

RETRORECTAL
SPACE

externally with a minimal pelvic extension; type III, apparent externally but predominantly pelvic or abdominal; type IV, no external manifestation. Tumors with an external component are more commonly diagnosed early in life and are more commonly mature. The terms "mature" and "immature" reflect histologic differentiation of teratomas. They are preferred to the words "benign" and "malignant" which imply behavior and are not invariably correct. For example, mature teratomas may recur and occasionally, may metastasize. Malignant degeneration from remnants of histologically mature teratomas has been reported as long as 40 years after resection.

The natural history of SCT diagnosed in utero is unclear. The prognosis of fetal SCT is worse than neonatal SCT and is dependent on the physiologic consequences of the tumor. SCT may produce uterine enlargement, polyhydramnios, placentomegaly, and fetal hydrops. The latter two findings are associated with

poor survival. Large tumor-associated arteriovenous fistulae can shunt blood away from the placenta and result in high output failure. Successful in utero devascularization followed by staged resection has been reported, but fetal surgery does not always reverse the placental changes.

Teratomas are more common in females than males (5:1), and are often associated with anomalies of the vertebrae, urinary tract, or anorectum. Immature teratomas are more commonly diagnosed after the age of 2 months and have an increased risk of local recurrence compared to those diagnosed before that age. The 5-year survival rate is around 80% after complete resection of a localized tumor, but if residual disease is present, the chance of survival decreases markedly. Germinomas are very sensitive to radiotherapy and respond well to treatment. Mixed malignant teratomas and endodermal sinus tumors usually metastasize to lung, liver, regional nodes, and the central nervous system. Less frequently, they may involve bone or other distant sites. Before the 1980s the long-term survival rate was only 20%. Since the introduction of more aggressive multidrug chemotherapy with etoposide, bleomycin, carboplatin, and other CIS-platinum based chemotherapies, the survival rate has improved to about 90%.

Tailgut Cysts

Tailgut cysts, also called retrorectal cystic hamartomas, are multilocular cysts having histologic features similar to and consistent with derivation from embryonic tailgut. Early in fetal development, the primitive gut extends caudal to the point where the anus develops and then subsequently regresses. Remnants of this structure may then give rise to congenital cysts. The neurenteric canal, which connects the amnion to the yolk sac around the 16th day of development, may also be a source of some lesions. Tailgut cysts may be lined by squamous, transitional, or columnar epithelium. The columnar epithelium may be ciliated or mucin-containing. Often there is an abrupt change from one type of epithelium to another. Muscle bundles in the

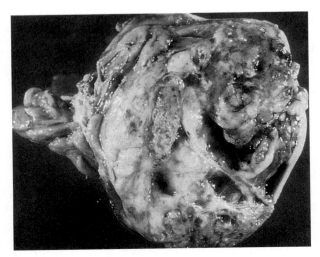

Figure 28-2
Sacrococcygeal teratoma resected from a 3-day-old girl.

cyst wall are disorganized. Tailgut cysts lack dermal appendages, mesenchymal derivatives other than smooth muscle, fibrous tissue, and blood vessels, and do not contain immature elements. Most so-called "dermoid cysts" fall into this category, as dermal appendages are rarely seen. When hair or sweat glands are found, tissues derived from other cell layers are usually identified, leading to a diagnosis of teratoma. Tailgut cysts may become quite large and occasionally develop adenocarcinomas or carcinoid tumors (Fig. 28-3). There is a strong female predominance (3:1), and the average age at presentation is 36 years. Tailgut cysts are frequently misdiagnosed as perirectal abscess, leading to misguided attempts at incision and drainage. A history of recurrent abscesses or perianal fistulas without an internal opening should alert the surgeon to the possibility of a retrorectal cystic lesion. Recurrence occurs frequently and is a result of incomplete excision.

Duplication Cysts

The hindgut is an uncommon site for duplication anomalies. Presenting symptoms and signs include distention, vomiting, failure to thrive, constipation, diarrhea, and hematochezia. Two forms are recognized: (1) a limited tubular duplication on the mesenteric aspect of the gastrointestinal tract with squamous, columnar, or mixed epithelium, and (2) an abortive caudal twinning with duplication of the rectum, anus, genitalia. Complete duplication of the colon, rectum, urinary tract, and external genitalia is extremely rare. There may be associated cleft vertebrae, intraspinal cysts, or a dorsal sinus tract. Unlike retrorectal cystic hamartomas, duplication cysts are generally surrounded by a well-formed smooth muscle coat. The tubular duplication may communicate with the intestine with stagnation of intestinal contents within the blind pouch. Gastric mucosa with fistula formation and malignant tumors have been reported in duplication cysts. Therefore, it is suggested that the mucosa be excised if the cyst cannot be removed.

Management of the caudal twinning anomaly is quite complex. Smith has classified these lesions as three types. Type 1 consists of duplications with two separate perineal ani; type 2 includes duplications with one or both rectums terminating in a fistula to the urogenital tract (and frequently duplication of the external genitalia); and type 3 includes duplications with one external anus and one anal atresia in the pelvis. Asymptomatic type 1 lesions may not require treatment. Type 2 lesions usually present as neonatal intestinal obstruction. If there is one normal anus, the fistula can be closed and the duplication anastomosed to the other colon. If both colons end in a fistula, a diverting colostomy should be performed. External urinary diversion may also be required for incontinence. If a functional puborectalis sling exists, the bowel may be brought down to the perineum at a later date. Patients with type 3 anomalies are difficult to diagnosis and, for that reason, often do poorly. Treatment consists of dividing the common septum between the two lumens or excising the blind colon.

Anterior Sacral Meningocele

Approximately 150 cases of anterior sacral meningocele have been reported. The meningocele sac is located in the presacral space and contains cerebrospinal fluid and sometimes neural elements. It may be associated with spina bifida, a tethered spinal cord, uterine and vaginal duplication, urinary tract malformation, anal malformations, germ cell tumors and presacral lipomas. Patients may complain of headache associated with straining. The finding of a "scimitar" sacrum, characterized by a rounded, concave border without bone destruction is pathognomonic. In patients with Marfan's syndrome or neurofibromatosis, the sacral foramen may simply be widened and the scimitar sign may be absent. If communication with the dura is in doubt after CT or MRI scanning, myelography with metrizamide is recommended. Aspiration is avoided because of the risk of meningitis. Treatment consists of opening the dura mater and obliterating the neck of the meningocele. This procedure usually does not require the participation of an abdominal surgeon unless the sac is too large to be closed securely from the posterior approach or unless there is an associated tumor.

■ INFLAMMATORY LESIONS

Inflammatory lesions usually can be diagnosed by history and physical examination. Lipid granulomas can result from sclerosing hemorrhoids with injections of oil-based phenol solutions. These lesions have been treated by application of heat and by curettage. Perforation of the posterior rectal wall during a barium enema can also lead to a chronic inflammatory mass. The usual treatment is a diverting colostomy, lavage of the presacral space, and insertion of drains. Postpartum hematomas in the retrorectal space may calcify and be confused with tumor. The most common inflammatory lesion is, of course, the perianal abscess, which is usually apparent from the history of fever and pain. As mentioned earlier, any recurrent abscess without an internal opening must be suspected to be a retrorectal tumor. Endoluminal rectal ultrasound should be helpful in making the diagnosis in such cases.

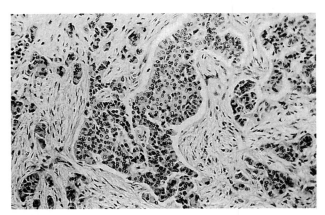

Figure 28-3
Carcinoid tumor arising in a tailgut cyst (H & E stain, ×41).

■ NEOPLASTIC LESIONS

Chordomas

The most common malignant tumor is the chordoma. This lesion derives from remnants of the fetal notochord. Normally, the notochord is manifest in the adult as the nucleus pulposus of the intervertebral disks, but rests of notochordal tissue may remain in ectopic positions. Chordomas represent approximately 1 to 5% of primary bone tumors and less than 1% of all central nervous system tumors. From 50 to 60% of chordomas occur within the sacrococcygeal area. Other common sites are the base of the skull and the vertebrae. Most series have noted a male predominance for the sacrococcygeal lesions with a ratio of approximately 2:1. Although they may occur at any age, the greatest incidence is between the ages of 40 and 70 years.

Chordomas may be gelatinous or firm, depending upon the amount of mucinous material present. Hemorrhage and necrosis may lead to cyst formation or secondary calcification. A pseudocapsule is often present, and bone invasion is common. Microscopically, one sees a lobular framework with fibrous septa containing variable amounts of vacuolated physaliferous cells and extracellular mucin.

Common presenting complaints include buttock or back pain; numbness in the perianal region, buttock, or leg; muscle weakness; difficulty voiding; and constipation. A mass is usually palpable, but it is difficult to assess tumor size on digital rectal examination. Radiographs of the pelvis will show abnormalities such as sacral bone erosion or calcification in approximately 50% of patients. CT scanning and MRI give an accurate assessment of size and bone invasion (Fig. 28-4).

Chordomas are slow-growing and locally invasive. Median survival times of 5 years or more are commonly reported (Fig. 28-5). Metastases have been reported to have an incidence of 10 to 50% and usually involve bone or lung.

The recommended treatment is complete surgical excision. Tumors that are incompletely removed will recur. The role of radiotherapy remains controversial. Although

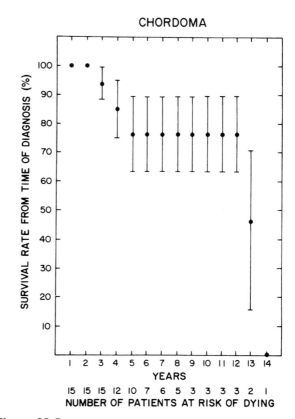

Figure 28-5
Actuarial survival rates of 15 patients treated for chordoma at the Cleveland Clinic between 1927 and 1983. Five-year survival rate is 76%.

palliation is commonly reported after radiotherapy, cures are not. High-dose radiation (48 to 80 Gy) improves the disease-free interval compared to doses less than 40 Gy but is associated with an increased risk of radiation proctitis, neuritis, and bone necrosis. Preoperative radiotherapy has been recommended by some, but there is no documentation of improved survival. Chemotherapy has not been proved to be useful, although there are isolated reports of palliation.

Osseous Tumors

Tumors which involve bone may arise from cartilage, bone, fibrous tissue, or marrow. A list of the more frequently found sacral tumors is given in Table 28-2. The behavior of bony tumors of the sacrum is similar to that of bony tumors elsewhere in the body, and only a brief discussion can be given here.

Giant cell tumors usually arise in the third and fourth decades of life. They have a predilection for the epiphyses of long bones, but are not rare in the sacrum. Approximately 10% of these lesions behave in a malignant manner. On x-ray, they are radiolucent, and one may see thinning and expansion of the overlying cortex. Grossly, they are reddish gray with areas of necrosis. Microscopically, one finds numerous multinucleated giant cells within a fibrous stroma. Reactive bone formation may lead to a mis-

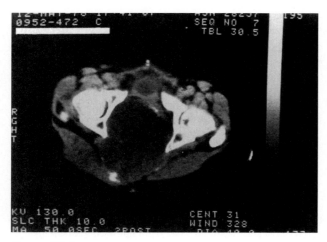

Figure 28-4
Chordoma. The tumor is eroding through the sacrum and filling the pelvis.

Table 28-2 Common Sacral Tumors
BENIGN
Osteochondroma
Giant cell tumor
Osteoid osteoma
Eosinophilic granuloma
Chondroblastoma
Osteoblastoma
MALIGNANT
Chondrosarcoma
Fibrosarcoma
Osteosarcoma
Ewing's tumor
Fibrous histiocytoma
Lymphoma
Myeloma

taken diagnosis of osteosarcoma. Extensive sampling is necessary to determine whether a given lesion is malignant because the histologic appearance is variable within these tumors. The usual treatment is wide resection. Radiation is not beneficial and may induce malignant change, but sarcomas have also been noted after surgical resection alone. Metastases are characterized by a "benign" histologic appearance and most commonly appear in the lungs.

Aneurysmal bone cysts are benign lesions that may recur if incompletely removed. They are more common in patients under 20 years of age. These tumors may also contain foci of benign giant cells, but they are characterized by prominent blood-filled spaces. This lesion may be treated by local curettage and does not metastasize.

Malignant bone tumors are treated by wide resection, if feasible, often combined with adjunctive chemotherapy or radiotherapy. The most common lesion is the osteosarcoma. Characteristically, lytic areas are seen on x-ray accompanied by subperiosteal new bone formation. Histologically, osteosarcomas may demonstrate not only malignant bone cells (osteoblasts) but also areas of malignant cartilage and fibrous tissue. Pulmonary metastases are common.

Neurogenic Tumors

Neurogenic tumors account for approximately 5 to 15% of tumors in the retrorectal space. The most frequent of these is the ependymoma. Ependymomas are classified into the myxopapillary, papillary, subependymoma, and anaplastic variants. The myxopapillary tumors usually arise near the cauda equina, but may be found in the presacral space or in the skin of the sacrococcygeal area without any apparent connection to the spinal cord or filum terminale. They show a predilection for males and may occur at any age. Back pain is frequently is a presenting symptom. Metastases occur in about 17% of patients and may involve the subarachnoid space or lungs. If the lesion is well encapsulated and can be totally excised, a long survival is to be anticipated. Tumors that cannot be completely removed have a higher rate of recurrence and a shorter survival period. Radiotherapy may be palliative.

The neurilemmoma is a rare benign lesion which usually causes symptoms by reason of its bulk. Occasionally, it can cause sacral bone destruction by pressure erosion. Complete excision is curative.

Malignant neurogenic tumors occurring in this area include neuroblastomas, malignant schwannomas, and ganglioneuroblastomas.

Nonosseous Mesenchymal Tumors

Other soft tissue tumors that may involve the retrorectal space include chondromyxosarcoma, lipoma, liposarcoma, leiomyoma, and leiomyosarcoma.

Vascular lesions reported in the retrorectal space include hemangioendotheliomas and hemangiopericytomas. Hemangiopericytomas can occur at any age and have no sex predilection. Symptoms are related to the site and size of the tumor. Rarely, hypoglycemia has been reported in association with these lesions. The biologic behavior is difficult to predict. Tumors having more than four mitoses per high-power field, tumors greater than 6.1 cm in greatest dimension, and tumors with necrosis or hemorrhage have an increased rate of metastasis. Radiotherapy or chemotherapy do not affect survival.

■ METASTATIC LESIONS

Lymphomas, myeloma, and adenocarcinoma can all involve the retrorectal space. Generally such lesions are part of a diffuse disease process and the diagnosis is obvious. Occasionally, a myeloma may be present only in the retrorectal space.

Lesions in this area require a multidisciplinary approach to staging and therapy. As mentioned earlier, the history and physical examination give important clues in distinguishing benign from malignant lesions. The preoperative workup includes a thorough physical examination including digital rectal examination, neurologic examination, and proctosigmoidoscopy. Staging is aided by endoluminal ultrasound, CT scan, or MRI of the pelvis and abdomen and a chest x-ray. MRI gives a very detailed picture of anatomic relationships in the pelvis and is probably superior to CT scanning for establishing the extent of spinal disease. A technetium-99m bone scan and a CT scan of the lungs may be useful for the detection of metastases in patients with suspected malignancy.

When there are signs of neurologic injury or bone invasion, the surgeon should suspect malignant disease and an orthopedic surgeon or a neurosurgeon should be consulted. Digital subtraction angiography or MRI with gadolinium is performed if a malignant bone tumor is suspected. In the event that the angiogram shows a highly vascular lesion, preoperative arterial embolization is recommended to minimize blood loss.

Biopsy may cause seeding of tumor through previously unaffected tissue planes and should be approached with caution. Smaller tumors are probably best removed intact without a preliminary biopsy. For tumors that would require a large and complicated resection or when metastatic disease is suspected, fine needle aspiration can be performed through a posterior route, which can subsequently be excised. If an open biopsy is to be done, perineal tumors may be approached via a longitudinal midline posterior incision. Transrectal needle biopsy is condemned because seeding of a noninvolved rectum might occur. For bony tumors, a limited amount of posterior cortex of the sacrum can be removed and a biopsy obtained. The ultimate treatment depends on the type of tumor, its histologic grade, and the presence or absence of regional or distant metastases. Benign tumors (e.g., aneurysmal bone cysts) may be adequately treated by intralesional excision; however, aggressive benign and malignant tumors require a wide margin of resection.

■ POSTERIOR APPROACH FOR SMALL TUMORS

If a false tract has been established between a benign teratoma or tailgut cyst and the colon because of previous diagnostic error of a supralevator abscess, it may be necessary to administer antibiotics for several weeks prior to definitive resection in order to allow the inflammation to subside. Occasionally, a diverting colostomy may be required.

Small tumors less than 4 to 5 cm may be excised through a posterior approach. After preoperative mechanical and antibiotic colonic preparation, the patient is given spinal or general anesthesia and placed in the prone jackknife position. The buttocks are spread apart and the operative site is prepared. A transverse or a vertical presacral incision is then made over the coccyx. In most cases, coccygectomy is performed to facilitate access, although a parasacrococcygeal approach has been described by Abel and associates. The anococcygeal ligament is divided transversely. If necessary, further exposure is achieved by detachment of the gluteus maximus muscle from its sacral attachments. Mobilization of the tumor can then be carried out with relative ease. Using head-down tilt of the table and lighted retractors, the cephalad portion of the tumor can be delivered. It is always preferable to remove benign cystic lesions intact, but if the lesion is difficult to remove, aspiration may collapse the cyst enough to allow easier dissection, especially of the anterior attachment. The wound is then closed in layers over a closed suction drain.

■ APPROACH FOR LARGE RETRORECTAL TUMORS

Larger tumors, those exhibiting bone erosion, and those producing symptoms of nerve compression should be approached both anteriorly and posteriorly. Wide excisions may be very hazardous if performed solely through the posterior approach. Tumors involving the lower sacrum may be removed using a combined abdominosacral approach with the patient in a lateral position, as described by Localio. The abdomen is entered through an oblique left lower quadrant incision. The rectum is mobilized from the sacral hollow and any intra-abdominal tumor is mobilized while a second team works through a posterior midline or paracoccygeal incision to widely excise the tumor one segment above any suspected bony involvement.

For very large tumors or for those exhibiting involvement of the upper sacrum, we prefer the following approach. The anterior dissection is performed first with the patient supine (Fig. 28-6). For tumors having no significant posterior component, the anterior approach can be combined with the biopsy. Packs should be placed around the lesion to avoid intraperitoneal seeding, and the biopsy surface should be cauterized. If the frozen section demonstrates a benign tumor such as an aneurysmal bone cyst, an intralesional excision can then be performed, negating the necessity for a posterior dissection. During the anterior dissection, the full extent of the tumor can be visualized. The rectum is mobilized out of the sacral hollow, and the middle sacral artery and vein are ligated. Control of the internal iliac artery and vein can be achieved with vessel loops to decrease blood loss. For tumors involving the rectal wall or for those patients who have previously undergone a transrectal biopsy, a rectal resection is done at this time. Colostomy is recommended for patients with extensive infection, contamination, or blood loss or when extensive rectal involvement makes anastomosis hazardous or impractical. Depending on the extent of the tumor, the resection can then be completed either in one stage, or rarely, in two stages. If the resection is to be done in two stages, the patient is then closed and rescheduled for completion in 3 to 7 days. If, as is usual, the anterior approach is not overly time-consuming and the patient is in good physical condition, the posterior phase of the surgery is performed during the same anesthetic.

It is important that the posterior approach be extensive enough to provide good visualization of the sacrum, blood vessels, and the major neurologic structures. Preservation of S1–S5 nerve roots on one side preserves continence, but with hemisensory loss and some leg weakness. If both S3 nerve roots can be preserved, continence and sensation will be near normal. Even sacrifice of one S3 root is generally well tolerated. Resection of both S2 nerve roots often requires the patient to practice intermittent catheterization and bowel training, and male patients will suffer impotence. Some authors have actually resected S1 nerve roots with success, but incontinence and some weakness of the leg is noted. Preservation of the upper half of the S1 vertebra is generally considered necessary for stability of the spine and pelvis, although modern orthopedic techniques may soon allow vertebral replacement.

The patient is then turned prone for the posterior approach. If a biopsy has been performed previously, the scar is totally ellipsed, and the skin surrounding the scar is included in the resected specimen (Fig. 28-7). The incision is begun at approximately the level of L4 and extended distally to the junction of the coccyx and sacrum. Lateral extensions of the incision are made in line with the fibers of the gluteus maximus muscle toward the greater trochanters. The dissection is then carried through the

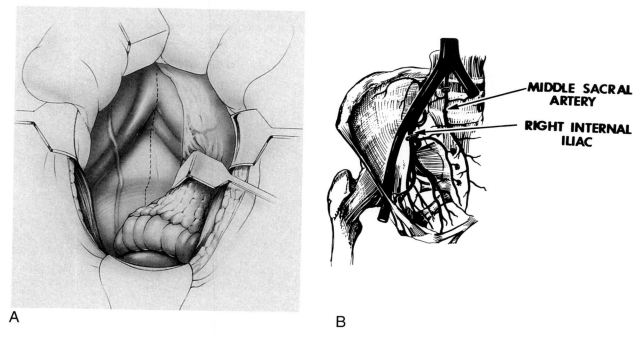

A   B

Figure 28-6
For large retrorectal and sacral tumors, the anterior dissection is performed first. *A,* The rectosigmoid is mobilized, and the retroperitoneum incised in order to ligate the middle sacral artery and vein. *B,* The internal iliac artery and vein are surrounded by vessel loops. If the tumor is exceedingly vascular, ligation of the posterior branches of the internal iliac artery and vein may be performed at this time.

gluteal fascia, and the fibers of the gluteus maximus are split, identifying the piriformis muscle (Fig. 28-8). The piriformis tendon is transected, and the muscle is retracted medially. If muscle invasion is suspected, then a portion of the gluteus maximus must also be taken. At

least 2 cm should be taken with the specimen on all sides to achieve a wide margin of dissection. The sciatic nerve and the nerve supply to the gluteus maximus can be visualized after mobilization of the piriformis muscle, allowing transverse sectioning of the gluteus maximus without sacrifice of its nerve supply. The sacrospinous and

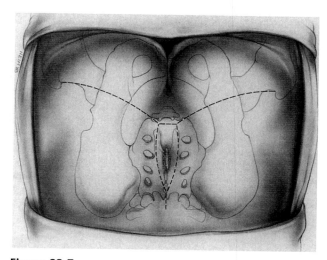

Figure 28-7
Posterior approach to sacral and retrorectal tumors. The biopsy scar is ellipsed and carried up to approximately the level of L4. Distally the incision is carried to the junction of the sacrum and coccyx. Lateral extensions are then made toward the greater trochanters of the femurs.

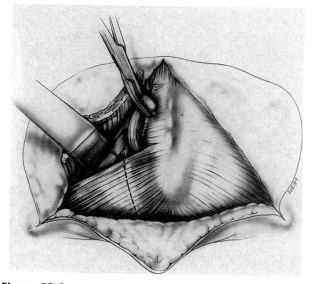

Figure 28-8
The gluteal fascia is divided, and the fibers of the gluteus maximus are split. The piriformis tendon is transected.

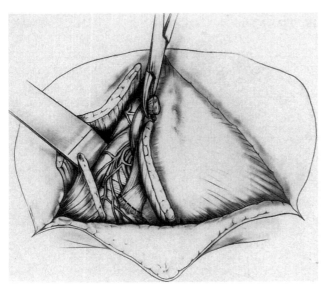

Figure 28-9
The sacrospinous and sacrotuberous ligaments are divided under direct vision.

sacrotuberous ligaments are divided under direct vision as far laterally as possible (Fig. 28-9). The level of the sacral resection will have been previously determined by scanning techniques and observations obtained during the anterior approach. The neurosurgeon or orthopedist may then enter the spinal canal one segment above the anticipated superior extent of the tumor, and inspect the canal for tumor extension and to identify the nerve roots to be saved (Fig. 28-10). An osteotome is placed distal to the nerve root, and a V-shaped osteotomy is performed. During this maneuver the anterior structures are protected by a large pack. The anterior longitudinal ligament is usually divided and mobilized during the anterior dissection, and the blood vessels, having previously been con-

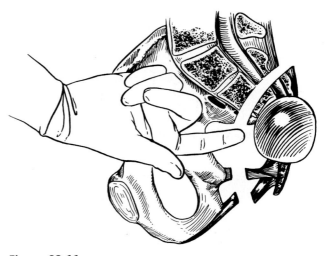

Figure 28-11
The tumor is removed by making an osteotomy through the sacral segment above the tumor. Severed nerve roots are clipped.

trolled by preoperative embolization, or tied and clipped during anterior phase of the surgery, should present no problems. The remaining fascial and muscular structures are then divided through the posterior approach, and the specimen is removed (Fig. 28-11). Severed nerve roots are surgically clipped to prevent spinal fluid leaks. The anterior pack is then removed through the posterior incision, and hemostasis is achieved. If postoperative radiation therapy is planned in women of childbearing age or younger, then the ovaries are mobilized during the anterior phase of the operation and moved out of the projected radiation field. Multiple suction drains are inserted, and the gluteal muscles are reapproximated. The skin is then closed in a routine fashion over the drains, which are kept in place until the daily output is less then 60 mL per day. The drains should not be removed too early to prevent formation of a seroma, which may become infected.

The day after surgery the patient is allowed to sit at the bedside, and is then progressively ambulated during the next 3 to 7 days. The bladder is drained with a Foley catheter, which in large resections is removed on the fifth to seventh day. A low-residue diet is prescribed.

Suggested Readings

Cummings BJ, Esses S, Harwood AR: The treatment of chordomas. Cancer Treat Rev 1982;9:299–311.

Hjermstad BM, Elwig EB: Tailgut cysts. Report of 53 cases. Am J Clin Pathol 1988;89:139–147.

Jao SW, Beart RW, Spencer RJ, et al: Retrorectal tumors: Mayo Clinic experience, 1960–1979. Dis Colon Rectum 1985;28:644–652.

Keslar PJ, Buck JL, Suarez ES: Germ cell tumors of the sacrococcygeal region: radiologic-pathologic correlation. Radiographics 1994;14:607–620.

Robertson FM, Crombleholme TM, Frantz ID, et al: Devascularization and staged resection of giant sacrococcygeal teratoma in the premature infant. J Pediatr Surg 1995;30:309–311.

Romero J, Cardenes H, la Torre A, et al: Chordoma: Results of radiation therapy in eighteen patients. Radiat Oncol 1993;29:27–32.

Smith ED: Duplication of the anus and genitourinary tract. Surgery 1969;66:909–921.

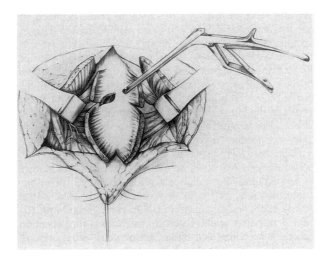

Figure 28-10
A laminectomy is begun at L5 and is continued distally to S1 if necessary.

29

VILLOUS TUMORS OF THE RECTUM

James M. Church, MBChB, M Med Sci, FRACS

The rectum and the cecum, at opposite ends of the large bowel, have notable similarities. They are both capacious organs, without regular throughput of stool, and are both liable to produce large flat adenomatous polyps with villous histology. Such soft flat polyps rarely cause significant symptoms because of their low profile and resistance to abrasion by feces. They can therefore grow to considerable size before being diagnosed. Rectal villous adenomas are easier to treat than those in the cecum because the rectum is a thicker-walled organ, because the rectum is substantially extraperitoneal, and because the accessibility of rectal polyps allows a wider range of therapeutic options. Treatment of rectal villous adenomas consists of a thorough assessment to exclude carcinoma, documentation of dimensions and position in the rectum, and a consideration of the various options for treatment.

■ PRESENTATION AND DIAGNOSIS

The presentation of rectal villous adenomas depends on their size and position in the rectum. Ultra low-lying polyps may prolapse through the anus, while bulky lesions in the rectal ampulla may present with a false urge to defecate or unsatisfactory defecation. Rectal bleeding is the most common symptom, and some polyps produce large amounts of mucus. Clinically significant electrolyte imbalances can occur from losses in the mucus. Diagnosis is usually made with endoscopy, although a careful digital rectal examination may pick up a soft lesion in the low rectum.

■ ASSESSMENT

Rigid proctoscopy is the best way of determining the position, size, and softness of the polyp. Its distance from the dentate line and its cephalad extent are important in deciding the best method of treatment. Any areas of firmness or fragility in the polyp raise the suspicion of malignancy. Several biopsies are taken, with the understanding that a negative result of biopsy doesn't necessarily exclude cancer. Full colonoscopy is needed to exclude synchronous lesions. Endorectal ultrasound is the best way of detecting invasion of the neoplasm out of the mucosa. If there is any suspicion of invasion, the polyp is treated as a cancer.

■ TREATMENT OPTIONS

There are six treatment options:

1. Endoscopic polypectomy
   a. By fiberoptic endoscope
   b. By operating proctoscope
2. Formal transanal excision
   a. Simple
   b. Delorme-type
3. Transanal endoscopic microsurgery
4. Transabdominal proctectomy

Endoscopic Polypectomy

Fiberoptic Endoscopy

Endoscopic polypectomy is a good choice for smaller upper rectal lesions that are clearly benign. Resection is by piecemeal snare excision. Injection of 1:100,000 epinephrine solution under the polyp minimizes the chance of immediate bleeding but is not always necessary.

Operating Proctoscope

Snare polypectomy through an operating proctoscope is a useful technique for handling large midrectal adenomas—those that are too high for transanal resection and too large for easy colonoscopic snare. The patient is put in the Kraske position with a degree of Trendelenburg that helps drain the blood away from the lesion. A large operating proctoscope is inserted and positioned to give maximum exposure to the polyp. The polyp is then snared piecemeal using a Frankenfeld snare. Small areas of residual adenoma can be tidied up with a suction diathermy probe. This probe is also useful for obtaining hemostasis.

Formal Transanal Excision

Simple Procedure

Simple transanal excision is suitable for polyps up to 7 cm in diameter situated in the lower rectum. Patients are positioned according to the location of the polyp (anterior = Kraske, posterior = lithotomy), and it is helpful to use either a "Lone Star"-type retractor or a series of anal everting sutures. These devices bring the dentate line close to the anal verge. A lighted retractor is placed and a small gauze sponge is inserted above the polyp to expose its cephalad extent. Diathermy with coagulation current is used to incise the rectal mucosa, leaving a clear margin circumferentially around the polyp. If the polyp is clearly benign, a mucosal resection is done. If there is suspicion of cancer, a full-thickness excision of the rectal wall is done. After excision, the wound in the rectum is irrigated with betadine and then saline. The wound can be left open, as long as it is extraperitoneal (in the lower rectum, or posterior midrectum). Alternatively, the wound can be closed for hemostasis and quicker healing, as long as the closure is secure (a poorly and partially closed wound is a setup for an abscess and worse than a wound that is not closed at all). Suturing the defect from top to bottom rather than from side to side avoids a narrowing of the lower rectal lumen by leaving a transverse suture line in the rectum. The polyp is pinned out on a piece of cardboard and oriented for the pathologist.

Delorme-type Transanal Excision

A Delorme-type transanal excision is best suited for large circumferential adenomas that extend distally close to the dentate line and that do not extend higher than about 10 cm from the anal verge. This procedure is best done with the patient in the Kraske position. Coagulating diathermy current is used to make a circumferential incision in the mucosa just below the adenoma. The mucosa is then dissected from the underlying muscle from the incision to a level just above the most cephalad extent of the polyp. As dissection proceeds circumferentially a stage is usually reached where the rectum can be prolapsed through the anus and further dissection is done on the outside, rather than through a retractor. Pulling down on the midrectal valve with noncrushing forceps can assist in this eversion. Injecting dilute (1:200,000) epinephrine solution to open the plane of dissection can minimize blood loss. Once the mucosa and polyp have been resected, the mucosa is approximated to the anoderm. A plication of the rectal muscle can be done if the denuded area is more than an inch or so wide. This folding helps to narrow the gap between mucosa and anoderm.

Transanal Endoscopic Microsurgery

Transanal endoscopic microsurgery is a relatively new technique using a closed operating proctoscope with CO_2 insufflation to keep the rectum open and laparoscopic-type instruments. Special techniques, instruments, and sutures have been devised to allow sharp excision of the polyp (mucosal or full thickness) with primary suture closure of the defect. The technique has been used to treat not only rectal adenomas but also rectal cancers. Its downside is the cost of the instrumentation and the learning curve inherent in use. In addition, most rectal polyps can be dealt with by other, less expensive options.

Transabdominal Proctectomy. The main reason for a transabdominal proctectomy is a suspicion of cancer. The second common reason is the sheer size of the polyp. The approach is similar to that for an obvious cancer, using wide margins, high ligation of the inferior mesenteric artery, and intraluminal irrigation with a cytocidal agent. Reconstruction with a colorectal or coloanal anastomosis is performed as indicated by the extent of the lesion.

■ PREPARATION FOR SURGERY

A full antegrade mechanical bowel preparation is routine for all options. Intravenous antibiotic prophylaxis and anti–deep vein thrombosis prophylaxis are used for options 2 through 4.

■ COMPLICATIONS

Three serious complications that may occur are bleeding, perforation, and inadequate treatment of a cancer. Because of the rectum's rich vasculature, bleeding can be severe and persistent. This bleeding must be controlled intraoperatively so an accurate operation can be done. Postoperative bleeding is usually an indication for a return to the operating room, evacuation of clot, and suture of the bleeder. A secure, hemostatic closure of the rectal wound will help prevent a postoperative bleed.

An intraperitoneal perforation is possible when the polypectomy is in an intraperitoneal part of the rectum. Anterior lesions are more at risk than posterior, and those above the lower rectal valve anteriorly are at the highest risk of all. Perforation can occur immediately if there is direct full-thickness damage to the rectal wall, or may occur later when rectal wall necrosis results from excessive diathermy use. Postoperative pain, fever, and free intraperitoneal gas suggest a perforation. Laparotomy with repair +/– diversion is indicated.

Inadequate treatment of a cancer is, in practice, equivalent to perforation of the cancer. Cancer cells then have the opportunity to escape the rectum. Consider chemoradiation before salvage surgery.

■ FOLLOW-UP

Rectal villous adenomas are particularly prone to recurrence. The rates are so high that there has been some question of a field change in the rectal mucosa. For this reason, follow-up must be careful and thorough. Proctoscopy every 3 months for a year, then every 6 months for 2 years, then yearly, is reasonable.

Keck and coworkers have authored a helpful article about the treatment of rectal villous tumors. They reported on 12 patients treated with rectal mucosectomy, 26 with transanal excision, and 23 with snare/fulguration. They report persistence rates (17%, 20%, and 40%, respectively) and recurrence rates (8%, 36%, and 44%, respectively). The data obviously favor mucosectomy, despite the observation that tumors treated in this way were larger (8.5 cm) than those treated by transanal excision (4.5 cm) or snare (4.2 cm). However, mucosectomy did result in minor incontinence in 17% of patients.

■ CONCLUSION

Rectal villous tumors can be treated successfully by transanal excision, snare excision, or mucosectomy in the majority of cases. Keys to successful management are a careful assessment including ultrasound to exclude invasive cancer, appropriate surgery based on tumor size and location, and close follow-up to detect and treat recurrence and persistence.

Suggested Readings

Keck JO, Schoetz DJ, Roberts PL, et al: Rectal mucosectomy in the treatment of giant rectal villous tumors. Dis Colon Rectum 1995;38: 233–238.

Older J, Older P, Colker J, Brown R: Secretory villous adenomas that cause depletion syndrome. Arch Int Med 1999;159:879–880.

Pikarsky A, Wexner S, Lebensart P, et al: The use of rectal ultrasound for the correct diagnosis and treatment of rectal villous tumors. Am J Surg 2000;179:261–265.

Said S, Stippel D: Transanal endoscopic microsurgery in large sessile adenomas of the rectum. A 10-year experience. Surg Endosc 1995;9:1106–1112.

Whitlow CB, Beck DE, Gathright JB: Surgical excision of large rectal villous adenomas. Surg Oncol Clin North Am 1996;5:723–734.

Winburn GB: Surgical resection of villous adenomas of the rectum. Am Surg 1998;64:1170–1173.

30

PREOPERATIVE EVALUATION OF THE RECTAL CANCER PATIENT: ASSESSMENT OF OPERATIVE RISK AND STRATEGY

P. Terry Phang, MD
W. Douglas Wong, MD, FACS, FRCS

The goal of preoperative evaluation of the patient who has rectal cancer is to allow individualized management based on the extent of disease with consideration of cancer management principles, operative risk, and postoperative functional outcome. Management of rectal cancer is different from management of colon cancer because of narrow confines of the pelvis, adjacent genitourinary nerves and organs, and proximity to the anal sphincter. Preservation of the anal sphincter with avoidance of a permanent colostomy is an important consideration for the patient. Although nonindividualized therapy could mandate abdominoperineal resection regardless of tumor stage or comorbid status, preoperative staging provides the opportunity to select patients suitable for sphincter-preserving therapy.

Preoperative staging of rectal cancer is mandatory in order to achieve optimal cancer management outcomes. The 1990 National Institute of Health (NIH) consensus recommended postoperative adjuvant chemoradiation for stages 2 and 3 rectal cancers, but the current trend favors recommendation of preoperative adjuvant chemoradiation to decrease local recurrence as well as to improve survival. Because preoperative adjuvant chemoradiation is now recommended, preoperative staging is mandatory.

In this chapter we discuss our approach to preoperative evaluation of rectal cancer, including clinical assessment, diagnosis by endoscopy and biopsy, and preoperative imaging with endorectal ultrasound, magnetic resonance imaging (MRI), and computed tomography (CT). The goal is to identify features that affect recommendations for local therapy versus segmental resection as well as selection of patients for preoperative adjuvant chemoradiation. Preoperative evaluation may reveal incurable metastases, in which case management strategy would change to that best for palliation. Preoperative evaluation of operative risk is necessary to optimize perioperative patient safety. Preoperative assessment of expected postoperative anorectal function is important to provide opti-

mal bowel function for the highest postoperative quality of life. Finally, preoperative evaluation should exclude synchronous lesions and provide a basis for comparison to postoperative surveillance studies. We present our management strategy individualized by preoperative staging and operative risk.

■ CLINICAL ASSESSMENT

By history, patients who have rectal cancer may be asymptomatic or may present with altered bowel habits—new onset of constipation or diarrhea, decreased stool caliber, or intermittent bright red rectal bleeding. Perianal pain may mean invasion of the anal sphincter; tenesmus is an indication of decreased rectal capacity from a large tumor; and abdominal distention and cramps may occur from circumferential narrowing of the rectosigmoid or anal canal.

Physical examination may be unremarkable or may demonstrate findings of anorectal or pelvic mass, hepatomegaly, or enlarged Virchow's or inguinal nodes. Digital rectal examination should evaluate tumor size, position (anterior, posterior, lateral), and distance of the tumor relative to the anorectal ring, which marks the upper border of the anal sphincter. Fixity of the lesion to the underlying rectal wall and to perirectal fat and pelvic structures should be noted. On occasion, enlarged perirectal lymph nodes can be palpated separate from the primary rectal cancer. Distance of the lesion from the anal sphincter, tumor size, and depth of invasion as determined by physical examination are key determinants of management strategy.

Physical examination provides information on tumor stage. Lesions less than 3 cm in diameter, superficial depth of invasion, and exophytic morphology have more favorable prognosis than larger, ulcerating lesions with invasion of muscularis and perirectal fat. The likelihood of lymph node metastasis is increased with larger and more deeply penetrating lesions. Superficial tumors less than 3 cm in diameter which occupy a single quadrant of the rectal circumference and have favorable histologic features have cure rates of 89 to 96%. Similarly, polypoid lesions have a cure rate of 90% compared to 33% for ulcerating lesions. Thus, local excision may be recommended for superficially invasive, small, histologically favorable (moderate differentiation and absence of lymphovascular invasion) distal rectal lesions. However, clinical staging has variable accuracy of 40 to 80%. Accuracy of clinical staging is greater for tumors invasive of perirectal fat than for tumors invasive of partial thickness of the bowel wall. Therefore, preoperative imaging is mandatory for the most accurate staging assessment.

Preoperative consideration of functional circumstances is important for recommending management strategy. Blindness and severe arthritis are conditions that make stoma care very difficult. Quality of life considerations for such patients with a stoma may require finding caregivers for the stoma or even preclude curative abdominoperineal resection. Compromised oncologic management may be recommended in such cases, including local excision and chemoradiation rather than curative segmental resection. On the other hand, patients who are incontinent or paralyzed may be best served with abdominoperineal resection rather than suffering from diarrhea or urgency that results from low anterior resection. Previous radiation for urogenital or reproductive organ cancer precludes perioperative radiation for rectal cancer. Consideration of these special circumstances is important to functional outcome.

■ ENDOSCOPIC EVALUATION AND BIOPSY

Diagnosis is confirmed by endoscopy and biopsy. Endoscopic evaluation determines distance of the lesion from the anal verge, size and percentage of circumference of the lumen occupied by the lesion, and whether the lesion is polypoid or ulcerating. Although rigid proctoscopy and flexible sigmoidoscopy are useful for assessment of the rectal lesion, examination of the colon should be performed for detection of synchronous colon neoplasms. Synchronous colon polyps may occur in 20 to 33% and synchronous colon cancer in 4 to 8% of patients with rectal cancer. We prefer colonoscopy for examination of the colon because of the ability to remove synchronous polyps. However, barium enema or CT colonography can also be used to detect synchronous neoplasms of the colon. Barium enema and CT colonography are likely to be as accurate as colonoscopy for detection of polyps larger than 1 cm.

Histologic characteristics on biopsy have prognostic value that can affect management strategy. Histologic characteristics that confer a worse prognosis include poor differentiation and vascular and lymphatic invasion. Because of increased risk of nodal metastases, segmental resection is recommended for these histologically advanced lesions rather than local therapy. However, correlation of degree of differentiation on biopsy compared to the final pathologic examination is only 40%, owing to significant sampling error. DNA ploidy status of the biopsy sample has been related to risk of local recurrence, distant metastases, and survival, but overall prognostic significance remains controversial.

■ PREOPERATIVE STAGING WITH IMAGING MODALITIES

Local-Regional Workup

Preoperative assessment of local-regional stage is important to management strategy. Endorectal ultrasound, CT, and MRI are currently used to assess for extent of invasion and for regional node metastasis.

Endorectal ultrasound (Figs. 30-1 to 30-3) has excellent correlation with histopathologic stage for detecting depth of invasion, with accuracy of 81 to 95%. Overstaging is reported in 0 to 12% and understaging in 1 to 9% of cases. Overstaging results from desmoplastic inflammation at the deepest invasion point, hemorrhage in the rectal wall from biopsy, preoperative radiation, tangential scanning rather than scanning perpendicular to the rectal wall, or a

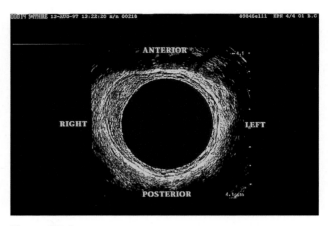

Figure 30-1
Endorectal ultrasound demonstrating superficially invasive uT1 (ultrasound stage T1) lesion. The innermost black ring of the rectal wall is the mucosa. The middle white ring is the submucosa. The outer black ring is the muscularis propria. In this image irregularity of the middle white ring indicates tumor involvement confined to the submucosa.

tendency of the observer to fear understaging depth of invasion. Understaging results from incomplete examination of stenotic tumors and difficulty of staging minimally invasive tumors and lymph nodes.

Endorectal ultrasound has only fair correlation with pathologic staging for detecting lymph node metastases. Accuracy of endorectal ultrasound for detecting lymph node metastases is reported as 58 to 87% in comparison to histopathologic staging. At the University of Minnesota, our accuracy for diagnosis of lymph node metastasis using endorectal ultrasound was 77% in 106 patients who had rectal cancer. Failure of endorectal ultrasound to detect lymph node metastasis may be attributed to presence of

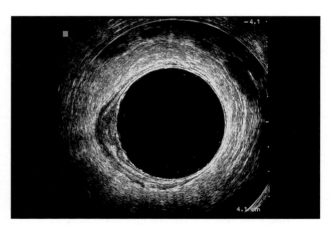

Figure 30-2
Endorectal ultrasound demonstrating a uT2 (ultrasound stage T2) lesion. Here, the tumor penetrates the middle white ring of the submucosa into the muscularis propria.

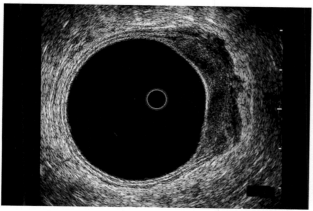

Figure 30-3

Endorectal ultrasound demonstrating a uT3 (ultrasound stage T3) lesion. Here, the tumor penetrates the outer black ring of the muscularis propria into the perirectal fat.

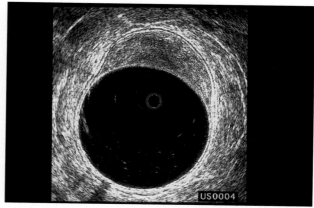

Figure 30-4

Endorectal ultrasound of a villous adenoma. The lesion is confined by the intact middle white ring of the submucosa.

micrometastases that are undetectable by current technology. In addition, size and shape characteristics for definitive diagnosis of lymph node metastasis have not been validated. Furthermore, transrectal biopsy of lymph nodes is not performed preoperatively because of difficulty in accessing the node without transgressing the primary tumor in the rectal wall. The experience of the observer is critical for accurate preoperative staging of rectal cancer using endorectal ultrasound.

Endorectal ultrasound is useful for assessment of malignant transformation in villous neoplasms. Malignant change occurs in 10% of "clinically benign" villous neoplasms. Biopsy does not reliably detect malignant change because random sampling results in poor negative predictive value. Malignant change is diagnosed on endorectal ultrasound by transgression of the submucosal plane (Fig. 30-4). However, the accuracy of endorectal ultrasound to assess malignant change is hampered in villous lesions close to the anal verge and in those with large, exophytic morphologic appearance. In one study, positive predictive value was 67% and negative predictive value was 89%. The high negative predictive value by endorectal ultrasound of the absence of invasive cancer in villous neoplasms has been confirmed by others. Therefore, villous lesions not transgressing the submucosal plane can be treated by submucosal excision with confidence that the lesion will be adequately excised even if in situ carcinoma is present. Full-thickness wall excision is recommended for lesions that clearly transgress or ambiguously border the submucosal plane.

Preoperative endorectal ultrasound has been used to assess tumor downstaging after chemoradiation. Here, accuracy is decreased because of overstaging due to inflammation after radiation. In our experience, positive predictive value of endorectal ultrasound was 72% for wall penetration and 56% for lymph node status after chemoradiation. Although negative predictive value by endorectal ultrasound for residual cancer has been reported as high as 100%, segmental resection remains the recommended treatment following chemoradiation.

At this time, endorectal ultrasound has greater accuracy than CT and MRI for assessing depth of invasion of rectal cancer and perirectal lymph node status (Table 30-1). CT and conventional MRI have relatively poor accuracy for distinguishing T1 and T2 staging because of inability to define layers in the bowel wall. Accuracy of CT and MRI to stage T3 and T4 lesions invading the perirectal fat and adjacent organs is much better than endorectal ultrasound for staging superficially invasive lesions owing to the contrast provided by perirectal fat. MRI technology is evolving for local staging of rectal cancer with the development of sequenced phase array, endorectal surface coils, and contrast-enhancing agents such as gadolinium. MRI has a potential advantage over endorectal ultrasound of being operative-independent. However, MRI is more expensive and less available than endorectal ultrasound.

MRI and CT are indicated for preoperative staging of advanced rectal cancer for assessment of proximity of radial margins of the cancer and perirectal lymph nodes

Table 30-1 Accuracy by Histopathologic Correlation

ASSESSMENT MODALITY	DEPTH OF INVASION	LYMPH NODE STATUS
Endorectal ultrasound	85% (67–95)	80% (67–88)
Computed tomography	70% (61–84)	55% (50–60)
Magnetic resonance imaging	79% (40–88)	72% (56–90)

*Results are mean (range) of reported series.

to the mesorectal fascia and for invasion of adjacent pelvic organs and the sacrum. The mesorectal fascia appears hypointense on T1-weighted images (Fig. 30-5). A margin of 5 mm between the nearest tumor and the mesorectal fascia has been shown to predict clear resection margins after total mesorectal excision. Ability to predict clear resection margins affects recommendation for choice of preoperative short-course radiation versus long-course chemoradiation. Further, preoperative MRI provides the surgeon with identification of the nearest margin of the tumor to the mesorectal fascia during TME (total mesorectal excision) dissection. In the distal rectum, preservation of anterior mesorectal fat and tumor encroachment of anterior organs (vagina, seminal vesicles, prostate) is assessed using endorectal ultrasound and MRI. For this reason, MRI surgical mapping is a necessary preoperative imaging study before undertaking TME.

Distant Metastatic Workup

Chest radiography is routinely obtained for preoperative staging as well as abdominal CT or liver ultrasound. Accuracy of CT and ultrasound for detection of liver metastases is 95%. Cystic characterization of small liver

lesions may be best assessed using ultrasound. Other metastatic screening tests, such as bone and brain scans, are obtained only if indicated by presenting symptoms. Detection of metastases at the time of initial presentation affects management strategy (discussed subsequently).

Serum Tumor Markers

Carcinoembryonic antigen (CEA) can be measured preoperatively with comparative serial postoperative measurements for early detection and cure of recurrent rectal cancer. Although cost-effectiveness of its use is questionable, it is reasonable to consider CEA measurement in selected patients who are candidates for curative resection of isolated recurrent pelvic cancer or isolated liver or lung metastases.

■ ASSESSMENT OF OPERATIVE RISK

Assessment of anesthetic and perioperative risk is necessary to minimize the chance of perioperative morbidity and death. It is most important that ischemic heart disease, congestive heart failure, hypertension, bronchoconstriction, and diabetes mellitus be optimized prior to surgery. Although warfarin and aspirin need to be stopped preoperatively, prophylaxis for perioperative thrombosis is indicated for all rectal cancer surgery. The American Society of Anesthesiologists Physical Status of Classification is standard for simple assignment of perioperative risk. The risk status encompasses the healthy patient (Class I), mild systemic disease with no functional limitation (Class II), severe systemic disease with definite functional limitation (Class III), severe systemic disease that is a constant threat to life (Class IV), and the moribund patient not expected to survive 24 hours with or without operation (Class V). Invasive perioperative monitoring is indicated for high-risk patients.

Perioperative risk is less for transanal local excision of distal rectal cancer than for transabdominal segmental rectal resection. Transanal excision is associated with less cardiopulmonary stress from blood loss, fluid shift, decreased chest wall and diaphragmatic excursion, and pain. Pain is minimal from local excision in relation to transabdominal resection. High perioperative risk status may influence the decision of whether the patient should be treated with curative or palliative intent.

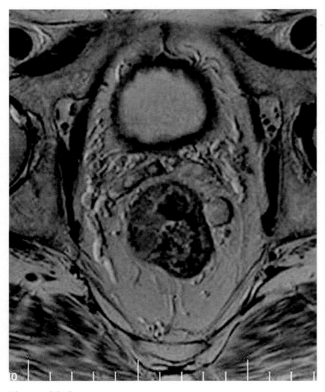

Figure 30-5
Magnetic resonance image (MRI) of a T3N1 rectal cancer. The cancer is nearly circumferential. An enlarged lymph node is seen adjacent to the left anterior rectal wall and is separated from the left anterior mesorectal fascia and left seminal vesicle. The mesorectal fascia marks the radial surgical excision margin relative to the nearest tumor encroachment.

■ PRACTICAL APPLICATION OF PREOPERATIVE STAGING

When preoperative staging identifies an early confined rectal cancer, local therapy can be considered. We favor local excision for cure of appropriate superficially invasive cancers of the distal rectum. Criteria of tumor characteristics for local excision are well to moderate differentiation, absence of vascular and lymphatic invasion, size less than 3 cm, absence of fixation of the lesion, endorectal ultrasound confirmed depth of invasion confined to the submucosa, uT1 (ultrasound stage T1, see Fig. 30-1), and absence of palpable or ultrasound-detected perirectal lymph nodes. We do not recommend local excision for lesions that penetrate into the muscularis propria, are uT2 (see Fig. 30-2), extend into the perirectal fat, or are uT3 (see Fig. 30-3) as assessed using preoperative endorectal ultrasound. Histopathologic characteristics obtained from initial biopsy or after local excision which portend risk of tumor recurrence are poorly differentiated histologic picture, vascular or lymphatic invasion, or involvement of resection margins by tumor. Presence of unfavorable histopathologic characteristics warrants adjuvant preoperative chemoradiation and segmental resection.

Preoperative adjuvant chemoradiation and segmental resection are recommended for preoperatively staged lesions penetrating the muscularis propria or presence of enlarged perirectal lymph nodes. Trials from Sweden and the Netherlands have shown good oncologic results from short-course preoperative radiation without preoperative chemotherapy for mobile rectal cancers. Cancers of the rectosigmoid and perhaps upper rectum more than 11 cm from the anal verge may not benefit from preoperative adjuvant chemoradiation. Segmental resection consists of TME (total mesorectal excision) in order to consistently achieve clear radial excision margins and to remove all perirectal lymph nodes within an intact fascial envelope. As well, TME spares pelvic autonomic nerve function. Subtotal TME with a distal 5 cm mesorectal margin suffices for rectosigmoid and upper rectal cancers. Subtotal TME with preserved rectal stump permits slightly improved anorectal function compared to the coloanal anastomosis required for TME. Abdominoperineal resection with TME is indicated for deeply invasive lesions encroaching on or invading the anal sphincter. Preoperative chemoradiation is recommended for low rectal cancers that require abdominoperineal resection. Tumor shrinkage after preoperative chemoradiation may permit sphincter-preserving low anterior resection; however, tumor cells can persist distal to the palpable receded distal tumor margin so that a distal mural margin of 1 to 2 cm is still recommended.

Preoperative evaluation may identify patients with incurable disease. In the presence of distant metastases, palliative local excision, segmental resection, and chemoradiation may be considered. For patients with severe comorbid disease in whom a general anesthetic, regional anesthesia, or chemoradiation is relatively contraindicated, endocavitary radiation may offer palliation. Chemoradiation as adjuvant for prevention of local recurrence is not recommended in the presence of extensive distant metastases.

■ SUMMARY

Preoperative assessment of the patient who has rectal cancer allows for an individualized management strategy.

Preoperative endorectal ultrasound, MRI, and CT are mandatory to determine suitability for local therapy and for preoperative adjuvant chemoradiation. Functional outcome, cancer management principles, and operative risk are important considerations in the management strategy individualized by use of preoperative assessment of the rectal cancer patient.

Suggested Readings

Adam IJ, Mohamdee MO, Martin IG, et al: Role of circumferential margin involvement in the local recurrence of rectal cancer. Lancet 1994;344:707–711.

Chari RS, Tyler DS, Anscher MS, et al: Preoperative radiation and chemotherapy in the treatment of adenocarcinoma of the rectum. Ann Surg 1995;221:778–787.

Deen KI, Madoff RD, Belmonte C, Wong WD: Preoperative staging of rectal neoplasms with endorectal ultrasonography. Semin Colon Rectal Surg 1995;6:78–85.

Gastrointestinal Tumor Study Group: Prolongation of the disease-free interval in surgically treated rectal carcinoma. N Engl J Med 1985;312:1465–1472.

Golfieri R, Giampalma E, Leo P, et al: Comparison of magnetic resonance, computed tomography, and endorectal ultrasonography in the preoperative staging of neoplasms of the rectum-sigma. Correlation with surgical and anatomopathologic findings. Radiol Med 1993;85:773–783.

Greaney MG, Irvin TT: Criteria for selection of rectal cancers for local treatment. Dis Colon Rectum 1977;20:462–466.

Heald RJ, Moran BJ, Ryall RDH, et al: Rectal cancer, the Basingstoke experience of total mesorectal excision, 1978–1997. Arch Surg 1998;133:894–899.

Huddy SPJ, Husband EM, Cook MG, et al: Lymph node metastases in early rectal cancer. Br J Surg 1993;30:1456–1458.

Jones DJ, Moore M, Schofield PF: Prognostic significance of DNA ploidy in colorectal cancer: A prospective flow cytometric study. Br J Surg 1988;202:740–744.

Kapiteijn E, Marijnen CAM, Nagtegall ID, et al: Preoperative radiotherapy combined with total mesorectal excision for resectable rectal cancer. N Engl J Med 2001;345:638–646.

Krook JE, Moertel CG, Gunderson LL, et al: Effective surgical adjuvant therapy for high-risk rectal carcinoma. N Engl J Med 1991;324:709–715.

Martling AL, Holm T, Rutqvist LE, et al: Effect of a surgical training programme on outcome of rectal cancer in the County of Stockholm. Lancet 2000;356:93–96.

Merchant NB, Guillem JG, Paty PB, et al: T3N0 Rectal cancer: Results following sharp mesorectal excision and no adjuvant therapy. J Gastrointest Surg 1999;3:642–647.

Michelassi F, Vannucci L, Montag A, et al: Importance of tumor morphology for the long term prognosis of rectal adenocarcinoma. Am Surg 1988;54:376–379.

Minsky G, Rich T, Recht A, et al: Selection criteria for local excision with or without adjuvant radiation therapy for rectal cancer. Cancer 1989;63:1421–1429.

Morson BC: Factors influencing the prognosis of early cancer of the rectum. Proc R Soc Med 1966;59:607–608.

NIH Consensus Conference. Adjuvant therapy for patients with colon and rectal cancer. JAMA 1990;264:1444–1450.

Phang PT, MacFarlane J, Taylor RH, et al: Effects of positive resection margin and tumor distance from anus on rectal cancer treatment outcomes. Am J Surg 2002;183:504–508.

Quirke P, Durdey P, Dixon MF, Williams NS: The prediction of local recurrence of rectal adenocarcinoma due to inadequate surgical resection. Histopathological study of lateral tumour spread and surgical excision. Lancet 1986;2:996–999.

Rothenberger DA, Wong WD: Preoperative assessment of patients with rectal cancer. Semin Colon Rectal Surg 1990;1:2–10.

Stryker SJ, Kiel KD, Rademaker A, et al: Preoperative chemoradiation for stages II and III rectal carcinoma. Arch Surg 1996;131:514–519.

Swedish Rectal Cancer Trial: Improved survival with preoperative radiotherapy in resectable rectal cancer. N Engl J Med 1997;336:980–987.

Zaheer S, Pemberton JH, Farouk R, et al: Surgical treatment of adenocarcinoma of the rectum. Ann Surg 1998;227:800–811.

31

CANCER OF THE RECTUM: OPERATIVE MANAGEMENT AND ADJUVANT THERAPY

Josephine van Helmond, MD
Robert W. Beart, Jr., MD

As a discipline, the surgical management of rectal cancer is at an exciting stage. Resection of the primary tumor, sphincter preservation, and the retention of sexual function has received a great deal of attention. Refinements in knowledge of pelvic anatomy and physiology have brought us to a critical point in our understanding of rectal cancer and the functional consequences of its operative management. Also ongoing are refinements in adjuvant therapy for rectal cancer.

■ PREOPERATIVE EVALUATION AND STAGING

Digital examination and rigid proctoscopy remain the best means of evaluating a rectal cancer for resectability, potential for sphincter preservation, appropriateness of local excision, and abdominoperineal invasion. The size, location, and mobility of the tumor, as well as the possibility of adjacent organ involvement, also influence therapeutic decisions. Rigid proctosigmoidoscopy is the most accurate means of determining the distance of the cancer from the anal verge.

Computed tomographic (CT) scanning has been extensively used to evaluate the extent of the primary tumor. Accuracy rates have been reported as approximately 60 to 80% for staging of the primary tumor, and 55 to 85% for determination of nodal status. CT scan is used mostly to evaluate recurrent pelvic disease and metastatic sites.

Rectal magnetic resonance imaging (MRI) can delineate bowel wall layers with accuracy similar to endorectal ultrasound. Contrast-enhanced MRI and MRI endoscopy may improve tumor staging, but the accuracy of lymph node evaluation remains uncertain. General figures for accuracy of tumor staging range from 55 to 95%, with nodal staging accuracy from 72 to 95%.

Endorectal ultrasonography is currently the most promising method for evaluating the extent of the primary tumor. In selected cases, such as when planning local excision, endorectal ultrasound is of supplemental benefit to digital rectal examination. Ascertaining nodal involvement, by any means, is considerably limited. Overall accuracy of endorectal ultrasound for tumor staging ranges from 82 to 100%, and for staging nodal disease it ranges from 80 to 89%. Problems remain for stricturing tumors through which it is not possible to pass the ultrasound probe.

Fluorodeoxyglucose–positron emission tomography (FDG-PET) scanning is based on the high affinity of cancer cells for FDG. PET scanning may prove to be more accurate than CT scanning in detecting metastases. It can also help differentiate between postsurgical scar and recurrent disease. Currently, PET scanning is not used in preoperative staging.

■ SELECTION OF OPERATION

In 85 to 90% of patients with rectal cancer, the choice is between a low anterior resection and an abdominoperineal resection (APR) of the rectum. Tumors situated more than 5 cm from the anal verge or whose lowest edge does not impinge upon the puborectalis muscle are suitable for sphincter-preserving operations. Size, location, degree of tethering, mobility, and dimensions of the pelvis may influence the decision.

Patients with small (< 3 cm), mobile, sessile, or polypoid (as opposed to ulcerating) tumors with favorable histology (moderate to well-differentiated without lymphovascular or perineural invasion) (T1) may be candidates for local treatment. Endorectal ultrasonography is recommended preoperatively to assess mural penetration and lymph node status.

Minsky recommends postoperative radiation therapy after local excision for T1 tumors with poor pathologic features and all T2 tumors. T3 tumors have a high local recurrence rate of 25% after local excision and require radical resection with pre- or postoperative radiation therapy. Further principles and surgical options of local treatment for rectal cancer are discussed in Chapter 32.

■ PRINCIPLES OF OPERATION

Total Clearance of Tumor and Its Potential Spread

The goal of each operation is complete resection of that portion of the rectum containing the primary tumor en bloc with a complete mesenteric lymphadenectomy.

The fascia propria of the rectum is the minimum radial margin. The key to an adequate pelvic dissection is to ensure an intact rectal fascial envelope, including the mesorectum. Violating the fascia propria may allow tumor spillage and an increased possibility of recurrence.

Complete Mobilization of the Rectum

Inadequate mobilization of the rectum results in frequent compromise of the distal margin. Appropriate determination of the point of transection of the rectum requires its complete mobilization. This includes exposure of Denonvilliers' fascia and Waldeyer's fascia to the levator ani muscles and division of both lateral ligaments. With total mobilization, posterior or lateral rectal tumors rise up out of the deep pelvis, making sphincter preservation possible. Sympathetic and parasympathetic nerve preservation is possible with this dissection.

■ CONDUCT OF THE OPERATION

Examination under anesthesia is performed to confirm the location of the tumor and is frequently influential in planning treatment. Any changes in plans are best made at this time.

The patient is positioned in the perineal lithotomy position on stirrups. A lower midline incision is performed. The lowest end of the incision is at the mons pubis. Adequacy of the proximal extent of the incision is assessed by seeing the stomach in the operative field. The liver is evaluated for metastases, as well as the small bowel and its mesentery. The left colon and its mesentery are dissected from the retroperitoneum and the left ureter identified. The inferior mesenteric artery is divided as recommended by Miles and doubly ligated. The colon may be divided at this point or after the pelvic dissection, the latter method allowing for a "handle" on the left colon during the pelvic dissection. The colon is generally divided at the descending-sigmoid junction.

Before embarking on a description of the various modes of pelvic dissection, a definition of terms is warranted. *Mesorectal dissection* transects the pelvic fat along the fascia propria of the rectum, which encases the formal mesentery of the rectum. *Radical dissection* transects the fat of the pelvis adjacent and medial to the common iliac and hypogastric vessels. *Superradical dissection* removes the lymphatics lateral to the hypogastric vessels. Dissections that transgress the rectal mesentery are not recommended because of the increased risk of local recurrence.

Total Mesorectal Dissection
Dissection is along and including the fascia propria of the rectum, separating the mesorectum from the surrounding somatic structures. In this procedure, the hypogastric sympathetic nerves are seen and preserved. Slight tension should be applied to the specimen to identify and thus preserve these nerves. They are identified where they cross the aortic bifurcation and the sacral promontory. They can usually be followed as they course along the lateral aspects of the pelvis, medial to the hypogastric vessels.

Identification of the parasympathetic branches from sacral nerve roots 2 through 4 is more difficult, but these, too, often are seen passing lateral to the sacrum and distal to the pyriformis muscles, and posterior to the lateral ligaments, bilaterally.

Radical Dissection
Dissection involves the plane of the endopelvic fascia, at least below the level of the iliac bifurcation and the hypogastric nerves. This approach accomplishes the en bloc dissection of the mesorectum and of the endopelvic fascia, leaving a small amount of areolar tissue adjacent to the fascia propria. The dissection is performed along the medial margins of the vascular structures, the internal iliac vessels. Nerves can be preserved with this technique and urinary retention and impotence are minimized.

As the pelvic dissection progresses distally, the lateral ligaments are divided. Rarely are ligatures or clips required when dividing the lateral ligaments. Inferiorly, only the fascia propria and attachments and Waldeyer's fascia confluence hold the rectum posteriorly. The mesorectum thins out so significantly that after division of the rectum, little if any cleaning of the mesorectum is required for anastomosis. Anteriorly, Denonvilliers' fascia or the rectovaginal septum may be used as the standard plane for dissection, unless an anterior or circumferential tumor dictates a wider margin, such as resection of the posterior vaginal wall. Dissection is performed until the levator muscles are visible posteriorly and laterally to the rectum. Occasionally, the most anterior distribution is not visible.

Abdominoperineal Resection
If at this point in the operation it is determined that an APR must be performed, the perineal dissection is begun. A synchronous two-team APR can be performed in those patients in which it is clearly indicated from the outset.

The landmarks for the cutaneous incision in the perineum are (1) the perineal body anteriorly (midway between the anal midpoint and the base of the scrotum or the introitus), (2) the coccyx posteriorly, and (3) the ischial tuberosities laterally.

In the case of posterior vaginectomy, the skin incision is begun at the right and left anterior positions along the vaginal orifice. Dissection is performed with cautery throughout. The skin and subcutaneous tissues are incised for 360 degrees. The medial skin edges are approximated with Kocher clamps. The ischiorectal space is entered. The individual branches of the pudendal nerves and arteries can be identified coursing radially through the ischial rectal space at the right and left anterior positions. These are identified, clamped, cut, and suture ligated. When this has been accomplished on both sides of the rectum, the posterior dissection approaching the coccyx may be completed. The levators are divided just anterior to the coccyx until the retrorectal space is entered from below.

With the surgeon using two fingers in the pelvis for traction, the levators are divided as close to the ischial tuberosities as possible using cautery current. The specimen is then delivered to the perineal operator. At this point the puborectalis muscles are intact, and only the anterior dissection remains to be completed. In the male, the lower extent of the genitorectal septum can be appreciated by inserting one's "traction hand" ventral to the rectum with the prostatic capsule behind one's fingers.

Gentle dissection with a clamp allows one to develop the appropriate plane between the rectum and the remaining genital structures. If Denonvilliers' fascia has been adequately dissected from above, the prostate should be free or nearly free at this time.

The puborectalis muscle is cut and the specimen is amputated and removed from the field. Hemostasis in the prostatic capsule and adjacent tissues is best accomplished at this time.

Primary closure of the subcutaneous fat and skin is performed. The levators have been resected and cannot be closed. A significant posterior vaginectomy precludes primary closure of the vagina.

Closed suction drains are placed from above or from below. The use of polyglycolic acid mesh, omentum, or other methods of small bowel elevation may be considered prior to abdominal closure.

Low Anterior Resection

If a sphincter-preserving operation is possible after complete pelvic dissection to the levator ani muscles, the totally mobilized rectum containing the primary tumor is amputated. The rectum is held tautly while the distal 30-TA stapler and proximal bowel clamp are applied at right angles to the longitudinal axis of the rectum, approximately 5 cm below the lowest palpable edge of tumor. After placement of the TA stapler and bowel clamp the rectum is divided, ensuring the remaining rectal stump will allow the head of the circular EEA stapler. After adequate mobilization of the left colon, which may involve splenic flexure mobilization, an end-to-end anastomosis is then performed, employing a circular 29-EEA stapler, with the anvil purse-stringed into the proximal colon. Complete proximal and distal anastomotic donuts are identified.

Closed suction drains are placed posterolaterally between the sacrum and the rectum, reaching to the levators. These drains are placed to eliminate serosanguineous fluid that could contribute to abscess formation and are not intended to eliminate dead space. They are removed on the fourth or fifth postoperative day, after the patient is tolerating any oral diet. If an anastomotic leak occurs, they will control the leak in 50% of patients.

The colonic segment must lie flush against the hollow of the sacrum. This positioning is accomplished only by complete mobilization of the colonic segment of the resection. If the distal segment of rectum cannot allow the head of the circular EEA stapler after resection, continuity is re-established and sphincter preservation accomplished by the coloanal technique.

Given adequate vascular supply and no tension on the anastomosis, a diverting colostomy is not necessary. Instead, a colostomy mainly provides relief from the discomfort associated with poor anal function during the immediate postoperative period.

■ COLOANAL ANASTOMOSIS

The coloanal anastomosis is reserved for a highly defined group of patients. If the tumor is felt to impinge on the puborectalis muscle, the patient is not a candidate for a sphincter-preserving operation. In addition, in some cases a conventional intrapelvic low anterior resection is not technically feasible, even though a cancer is located in the midrectum. Generally, this situation occurs when the rectal remnant is no longer visible from above despite firm upward perineal pressure. Two thirds of such cases occur in male patients, commonly in those with enlarged prostates. In other cases there is little if any rectal remnant after a suitable

distal margin has been obtained. In these cases, the *perianal coloanal anastomosis* has been employed with success.

The operation consists of a primary hand-sewn anastomosis at the dentate line. The complete lymphadenectomy has already been accomplished transabdominally. If any rectal mucosa is present, it should be saved, but the operation should be classified as a low colorectal anastomosis performed transanally, as opposed to a true coloanal anastomosis. The anastomosis is performed with interrupted sutures of 2-0 or 3-0 vicryl. The distal "bites" include the internal anal sphincter. A diverting colostomy is employed in all cases of coloanal anastomosis in anticipation of poor immediate functional results with severe perineal irritation and excoriation.

Functional results are assessed approximately 9 to 12 months after closure of the diverting colostomy, which may be performed about 6 weeks after the initial surgery. In general, a low rectal anastomosis employing any length of distal cuff yields better functional results than any coloanal anastomosis. At least 85% of patients are fully continent, at rest and at night, and are aware of the need to defecate. But for up to 1 year bowel habits are erratic, and patients are heavily dependent on a high-fiber diet and the use of medication.

Long-term results of coloanal anastamoses were published in 1995 from the Mayo Clinic. We looked at 177 patients with coloanal anastomoses, of which 15% received J-pouch anastomoses. Locoregional recurrence was 7% and 5-year survival rate was 69%. Fecal continence was noted in 78% of patients, and no J-pouch patients reported fecal incontinence.

J-Pouch Anal Anastomosis

The benefits of a J-pouch anal anastomosis, when compared to a straight coloanal anastomosis, include decreases in stool frequency, urgency, and nocturnal bowel movements. Physiologically, the J-pouch functions as a reservoir with increased compliance. When possible, the descending colon or transverse colon should be used because it is less muscular than the sigmoid colon.

■ THE LATERAL PLANES OF PELVIC DISSECTION

One of the most difficult questions in pelvic surgery for rectal cancer is how to obtain the best lateral margins of dissection. Operations for rectal cancer are generally based on the presumed degree of mural penetration and on the patterns of potential lymph node spread. The classic zones of spread have been upward along the superior hemorrhoidal artery to the inferior mesenteric artery and laterally along the internal iliac or hypogastric lymph nodes.

More recently, we have become increasingly aware of the role played by direct lateral spread of the primary tumor in causing local recurrences, posteriorly and laterally. The extent of resection, that is, the planes of pelvic dissection, play a material role in preventing such recurrences. *Failure to circumvent radial spread of disease is the primary reason for surgical failure.* Arguments exist concerning the correct planes of dissection, with few surgeons actually comparing standardized procedures.

Reports from this country and from Japan reviewing radical pelvic dissections have produced strikingly similar results, with 5-year survival rates with Dukes' stage C rectal cancer exceeding 50%, without added therapy. The Japanese, however, advocate dissection lateral to the internal iliac vessels in the obturator spaces, even where gross nodal disease is not evident. This technique is not practiced in the United States, where supporters of radical dissection advocate sharp pelvic dissection along or medial to the vascular or musculoskeletal boundaries of the pelvic side walls.

Critics of the superradical pelvic dissection have raised questions: Which patients benefit from this operation, in view of the low incidence of involved lateral lymph nodes? What is the benefit of hypogastric node dissection when few patients with involved hypogastric lymph nodes survive despite hypogastric lymph node dissection?

One may anticipate that 10 to 20% of patients will have lymph node involvement along the iliac and hypogastric arteries. However, these nodes may indicate a high likelihood of systemic spread and a low cure rate, despite extensive surgery. Most would agree that the superradical dissection, lateral to the iliac and hypogastric vessels, is more difficult and time-consuming with an attendant higher morbidity rate (as high as 80% urinary retention and 76% impotence). It is not the standard procedure for treatment of rectal cancer in the United States.

Heald, who advocates dissection along the fascia propria of the rectum, total mesorectal excision, reports an extraordinarily low rate of pelvic recurrence of 5% and a high rate of sphincter preservation. It remains for a multi-institutional controlled prospective trial to determine the value of wider pelvic dissections.

■ DISTAL MARGINS OF RESECTION

Traditionally, the 5-cm distal margin of resection has been the gold standard of sphincter-preserving operations. A significant problem arises when choosing a point of transection less than 5 cm from the lowest edge of tumor. Many surgeons narrow their margins of dissection as they head toward the selected point of transection. And many surgeons confuse the distal margin of *dissection* with the distal margin of *resection*.

The major cause of pelvic recurrence is not inadequate distal clearance as much as the narrow lateral margins partially adopted in planning the point of transection. Williams and coworkers have elegantly demonstrated that the downward extension of tumor beyond 2 cm is rare and is generally present only in patients with poorly differentiated tumors.

The key to the proper selection of a point of transection of the rectum is *total mobilization of the rectum* prior to selecting a point for its division. The margins of dissection must not be compromised because total mobilization of the rectum ensues. Although one strives for a 5-cm distal margin, it will frequently be shorter, in the range of 3 to 4 cm. The elasticity of the low rectum ensures that the patho-

logic margin is much shorter than the surgical margin. Under these circumstances, the shorter distal margin offers no compromise whatsoever to the survival of the patient.

■ RESULTS OF SPHINCTER-PRESERVING OPERATIONS

Sphincter-preserving operations for rectal cancer are the accepted standard for cancers of the midrectum, between 6 to 12 cm from the anal verge. However, sphincter complex involvement is an absolute contraindication to sphincter-preserving procedures. Limited preoperative sphincter function, pelvic fixation and tumors less than 2 cm from the anorectal ring are relative contraindications to sphincter-preserving procedures. Cancers above 10 to 12 cm from the anal verge behave like colonic cancers and cannot legitimately be included with rectal cancers when reporting survival and local recurrence statistics.

It has been well demonstrated in the literature that sphincter-preserving operations for cancers of the midrectum are associated with a higher 5-year survival rate than that afforded by APR.

Five-year survival rates for Dukes' stage C rectal cancer treatable by low anterior resection with pelvic lymphadenectomy approach 60 to 65% without adjuvant radiation. Similarly, reductions in local recurrence rates have accompanied the improved survival rates reported in most series. Dramatic reductions in local recurrence rates have been observed in Dukes' stage B as well as Dukes' stage C disease, practically eliminating the need for adjuvant radiation therapy in the majority of those with Dukes' stage B tumors.

Reducing the leak rate after intrapelvic colorectal anastomosis has been an ongoing effort. Two decades ago, the anastomotic leak rate averaged 20% nationwide in various surgical series and surveys. With the introduction of the anastomotic circular stapling devices, these immediate leak rates declined first to the range of 7 to 8% and more recently to the range of 5%. Most credit this reduction in morbidity rate to the technique of anastomosis. In reality, along with improvements in the anastomotic technique have come improvements in the entire technique for low anterior resection. These involve proper mobilization of the colon and complete mobilization of the rectum prior to performing the anastomosis.

With the absence of tension on the colorectal anastomosis, at any level, the individual method of colonic apposition or anastomosis becomes less important. The circular anastomotic stapling device is the best method available for ease of use, technical excellence of the anastomosis when properly performed, and the technical advantages the instrument offers.

■ PRESERVATION OF SEXUAL AND URINARY FUNCTIONS

Sexual dysfunction can be a consequence of pelvic surgery, as the median age of patients with rectal cancer is 62 years old. The hypogastric nerves (sympathetic fibers) are at greatest risk as they pass over the sacral promontory. Other sympathetic fibers forming the pelvic plexus may be injured during lateral dissection and division of the lateral ligaments of the rectum. The parasympathetic fibers of S2 to S4, which are responsible for erection, are not nearly as visible as the hypogastric nerves. These generally emerge distal to the pyriformis muscles.

The sacral parasympathetic nerves join the sympathetic fibers within the pelvic plexus. The latter are responsible for emission and ejaculation. Sites of potential injury occupy the entire field of pelvic dissection for rectal cancer, from the sacral promontory superiorly to the pelvic plexus to the distal course of the hypogastric nerves over the lateral ligaments, and to Denonvilliers' fascia.

When a dilemma exists between preservation of autonomic function and determining a negative margin of resection, one must choose in favor of complete eradication of the tumor. Currently, individual surgeons have embarked upon efforts to design operations that combine adequate pelvic resection and nerve preservation. This can only be accomplished with an exquisitely detailed knowledge of pelvic anatomy and mastery of pelvic dissection.

■ ADJUVANT RADIATION THERAPY

Most data regarding the role of radiation therapy in rectal cancer are based on the poor results of conservative surgery. Adjuvant radiation therapy is currently divided into preoperative, postoperative, or both ("sandwich therapy") and is combined with techniques to minimize toxicity.

Preoperative Radiation Therapy

Potential advantages to preoperative radiation therapy include decreased seeding of tumor in the pelvis, increased radiosensitivity, and possible conversion from an APR to a sphincter-preserving procedure. Patients may have fewer side effects when receiving preoperative versus adjuvant radiation therapy. The reason may be the reduction of exposure to the small bowel with neoadjuvant radiation therapy.

Preoperative radiation therapy has been shown to downstage tumors and reduce the bulk of the primary tumor, thereby allowing for a sphincter-preserving procedure. However, most studies have not shown improvements in survival.

Randomized studies of preoperative radiation exist. Many have involved relatively low doses of irradiation and demonstrated local control of pelvic recurrence. The European Organization for Research and Treatment of Cancer reports that with 3450 rads of preoperative radiation therapy, recurrence has been reduced from 30 to 15% at 5 years, with an overall 5-year survival rate of 70%. This rate is not significantly better when compared with a rate of 60% accomplished with surgery alone.

The Swedish Rectal Cancer Trial published their results in 1997. They reported that 1168 patients with resectable rectal cancer were randomized to receive 25-Gy preoperative radiation therapy versus no neoadjuvant radiation. Local recurrence was 11% in the irradiated group versus 27% in the surgery-alone group. Overall 5-year survival rate was 58% in the radiation-surgery group versus 48% in the surgery-alone group. The paper contends that a short-term regimen of high-dose preoperative radiotherapy reduces local recurrence rates and improves survival among patients with resectable rectal cancer.

The high 27% recurrence rate in the surgery-alone group calls into question the surgical technique utilized. The reported 5% recurrence rate after total mesorectal excision also calls into question whether preoperative radiation therapy may be necessary if an adequate resection and lymphadenectomy are performed. The multicenter Dutch study reported recently addressed this question and showed a significant reduction in local recurrence after preoperative patients undergoing total mesorectal excision. This was especially notable in tumors of the lower and middle rectum.

Postoperative Radiation Therapy

Postoperative irradiation has the major advantage that it is employed for a known stage and extent of disease. In addition to stage, other factors, such as delay in surgery, sphincter preservation, and the elimination of patients with distant metastases, support the use of postoperative irradiation in the view of others. Postoperative radiation therapy does have the disadvantage of acute toxicity rates as high as 20 to 30%, mostly secondary to small bowel involvement. Numerous techniques can be used to minimize the toxicity of treatment, including elevation of the small bowel out of the pelvis by the use of polyglycolic acid mesh, tissue expanders, and omental pedicles. Small bowel x-ray studies, treatment of the patient in the prone position, four-field techniques, treatment of the patient with the bladder distended, and anterior blocking have been employed effectively in order to reduce the small bowel toxicity of postoperative irradiation therapy.

Among randomized studies of postoperative irradiation therapy, three reports stand out. These studies include a randomized surgery-only control compared with postoperative irradiation. Reports from the Gastrointestinal Tumor Study Group demonstrated no difference in the overall rate of local recurrence (24% versus 20% with radiation therapy) and a minor increase in survival with radiation therapy (52% versus 43%). This minor increase in survival must be weighed against an 18% incidence of severe or life-threatening toxicity due to enteritis.

In the National Surgical Adjuvant Breast Program (NSABP) and Denmark trials, no differences in survival have been seen at 5 years. However, the latter trials show a smaller incidence of severe complications. Thus, a decrease in local recurrence rates in nonrandomized studies has been confirmed, but to a much lesser extent in randomized studies. This finding has not yet translated into any increase in overall 5-year survival rates.

Sandwich Radiation Therapy

Sandwich techniques have been employed in order to utilize the maximum dose of irradiation while reducing the morbidity. Effective local control by surgery combined with irradiation has been reported by Shank and coworkers, Mohiuddin and associates, and Brenner.

COMBINED CHEMOTHERAPY AND RADIATION THERAPY

Currently, adjuvant therapy focuses on the combined use of chemotherapy and irradiation. Beginning with the GI Tumor Study Group (GITSG Trial #7175), several trials involving postoperative irradiation, chemotherapy, or combined irradiation and chemotherapy have been completed in the United States. In the GITSG study at an 80-month median follow-up, patients receiving combined radiation and chemotherapy had a 33% rate of recurrence compared with 55% in patients undergoing surgery alone ($p < 0.010$). Local recurrence, although evident in 14 of 32 control patients, was observed in only 5 of 46 patients receiving combined therapy.

At 8 years of follow-up, the benefit of treatment persisted; in addition to a disease-free survival advantage, an overall survival advantage was evident. However, severe or life-threatening toxicity occurred in 18% of patients receiving radiation therapy and in 60% of those undergoing combined radiation and chemotherapy. Toxicity consisted mainly of radiation enteritis and acute nonlymphocytic leukemia in one patient undergoing chemotherapy. Subsequent studies have been designed to minimize the toxicity while still capturing the benefit of treatment.

The second major study was reported by the North Central Cancer Treatment Group (NCCTG). First initiated in 1979, a total of 204 patients with Dukes' stages B and C rectal cancer received either irradiation alone (4500 to 5040 cGy) or in combination with methyl-CCNU and 5-fluorouracil (5-FU). After a median follow-up of more than 7 years, the combined therapy reduced the rate of recurrence by 34%. In addition, combined therapy reduced the rate of cancer-related deaths by 36% and the overall death rate by 29%. Severe treatment-related reactions, usually small bowel complications, occurred in 6.7% of all patients receiving radiation. Complication rates were comparable in both groups. The study concludes that a combined adjuvant treatment of 5-FU-based chemotherapy and radiation improves the outcome of patients with Dukes' stage B and C rectal cancers, as compared with postoperative radiation therapy alone.

The NSABP has performed a trial of postoperative observation, pelvic irradiation of up to 5300 cGy or chemotherapy with 5-FU, methyl-CCNU, and vincristine. With a 54-month follow-up time, there is a statistically significant survival advantage for patients receiving chemotherapy. Patients who received irradiation alone had no apparent benefit, with the exception of a mild reduction in local recurrence rates from 25 to 15%. Treatment was well tolerated and without long-term side effects.

Based on the NIH Consensus Conference published in 1990, combined modality treatments for stages II and III rectal cancer include six cycles of 5-FU-based chemotherapy with concurrent pelvic irradiation. Overall, adjuvant chemoradiation reduces locoregional recurrence by 50% and improves survival by 10 to 15%.

Current adjuvant therapy trials are testing different chemotherapy regimens with regard to dose, timing, drug selection, and method of delivery. In addition are ongoing clinical trials comparing preoperative and postoperative chemoradiation in order to clarify whether neoadjuvant chemoradiation confers decreased toxicity and better sphincter function as well as comparable locoregional recurrence rates and survival.

Three randomized trials comparing preoperative and postoperative combined therapy are ongoing (two in the United States and one in Germany). However, they suffer from lack of accrual.

Suggested Readings

Beart R, Melton L, Maruta M, et al: Trends in right and left-sided colon cancer. Dis Colon Rectum 1983;26:393–398.

Beart RW, Steele GD, Menck HR, et al: Management and survival of patients with adenocarcinoma of the colon and rectum: A national survey of the commission on cancer. J Am Coll Surg 1995;181:A225–A236.

Beart RW Jr, Moertel CG, Weiland HS, et al: Adjuvant therapy for resectable colorectal carcinoma with fluorouracil administered by portal vein infusion. Arch Surg 1990;125:897–901.

Cavaliere F, Pemberton JH, Cosimelli M, et al: Coloanal anastomosis for rectal cancer: Long-term results at the Mayo and Cleveland Clinics. Dis Colon Rectum 1995;38:807–812.

Enker WE, Pilipshen SG, Heilweil ML, et al: En bloc pelvic lymphadenectomy and sphincter-preservation in the surgical management of rectal cancer. Ann Surg 1986;203:426–433.

Giovannucci E, Rimm EB, Stampfer MJ, et al: A prospective study of cigarette smoking and risk of colorectal adenoma and colorectal cancer in U.S. men. J Nat Cancer Inst 1994;86:183–191.

Gunderson LL, Beart RW, O'Connell MJ: Current issues in the treatment of colorectal cancer. Crit Rev Oncol Hematol 1988;6:223–260.

Heald R, Husband E, Ryall R: The mesorectum in rectal cancer surgery–The clue to pelvic recurrence? Br J Surg 1982;69:613–618.

Hizawa K, Suekane H, Aoyagi K, et al: Use of endosonographic evaluation of colorectal tumor depth in determining the appropriateness of endoscopic mucosal resection. Am J Gastroenterol 1996; 91(4):768–771.

Kahn H: Preoperative staging of irradiated rectal cancers using digital rectal examination, computed tomography, endorectal ultrasound, and magnetic resonance imaging does not accurately predict TO, NO pathology. Dis Colon Rectum 1997;40(2):140–144.

Köckerling F, Raymond MA, Altendorf-Hofmann A, et al: Influence of surgery on metachronous distant metastases and survival in rectal cancer. J Clin Oncol 1998;16(1):324–329.

Minsky BD: Adjuvant therapy for rectal cancer: Results and controversies. Oncology 1998;12(8):1129–1146.

Nivatvongs S, Rojanasakul A, Reiman H, et al: The risk of lymph node metastasis in colorectal polyps with invasive adenocarcinoma. Dis Colon Rectum 1991;34:323–328.

Porter GA: Surgeon-related factors and outcome in rectal cancer. Ann Surg 1998;227(2):157–167.

Quirke P, Durdey P, Dickson MF, William NS: Local recurrence of rectal adenocarcinoma due to inadequate surgical resection: Histopathological study of lateral tumor spread and surgical excision. Lancet 1986;2:996–999.

Richard JH: Rectal cancer: The Basingstoke experience of total mesorectal excision, 1978–1997. Arch Surg 1998;133:894–898.

Rosen M, Chan L, Beart RW Jr, et al: Follow-up of colorectal cancer: A meta-analysis. Dis Colon Rectum 1998;41(9):1116–1126.

Senagore A, Lavery, DeVos W, Pickleman J: Chances of cure are not compromised with sphincter-saving procedures for cancer of the lower third of the rectum–Discussion. Surgery 1997;122(4):784–785.

Sentovich SM: Accuracy and reliability of transanal ultrasound for anterior anal sphincter injury. Dis Colon Rectum 1998;41:1000–1004.

Steele G, Augenlicht L, Begg C, et al: National Institutes of Health Consensus Development Conference Statement: Adjuvant therapy for patients with colon and rectum cancer. JAMA 1990;244:1444–1450.

Tavani A, Fioretti F, Franceschi S, et al: Education, socioeconomic status and risk of cancer of the colon and rectum. Int J Epidemiol 1999;28(3):380–385.

Walsh PC, Schlegel PN: Radical pelvic surgery with preservation of sexual function. Ann Surg 1988;208:391–399.

Williams NS, Dixon MF, Johnston D: Reappraisal of the 5-centimetre rule of distal excision for carcinoma of the rectum: A study of distal intramural spread and of patients' survival. Br J Surg 1983; 70:150–154.

Winawer SJ, Zauber AG, Ho MN, et al: Prevention of colorectal cancer by colonoscopic polypectomy. N Engl J Med 1993;329:1977–1981.

32

RECTAL CANCER: LOCAL TREATMENT

David Rothenberger, MD
Julio Garcia-Aguilar, MD, PhD

Surgical treatment of rectal cancer is based on the oncologic principles established by Halsted more than a century ago. Cancer was believed to be a local disease that disseminated in an orderly fashion from the site of origin to the regional lymph nodes and from there to the bloodstream to establish distant metastases. Accordingly, operations were developed to treat rectal cancer by excising the rectum as well as its lymphatic drainage. Abdominoperineal resection and low anterior resection have remained the gold standard in the surgical management of rectal cancer for decades. Unfortunately, these operations are accompanied by significant mortality, morbidity, and distressing functional consequences. Urinary and sexual dysfunction are frequent complications of these operations, and even patients who can be spared from a permanent colostomy frequently complain of urgency, tenesmus, and incontinence. In addition, a significant number of rectal cancer patients do not benefit from the potential advantages of such radical surgery. Some individuals are diagnosed when their cancer is still localized in the bowel wall and can be cured by local treatment. Other patients with seemingly localized tumors will die of disseminated distant metastasis despite extensive resections. Both groups undergo an unnecessarily radical procedure if a standard resection is performed. Thus, it is not surprising that surgeons are increasingly interested in determining the appropriate role of therapeutic alternatives to radical resection such as local excision, endocavitary radiation, and electrocoagulation. In properly selected patients, these types of local therapy result in tumor control equivalent to that observed after radical surgery.

■ PATIENT EVALUATION

Preoperative evaluation of patients with rectal cancer should include a medical history and general physical examination. A digital rectal examination is performed to assess anal sphincter function and the location, size, and fixity of a distal tumor. Diagnosis should be confirmed by endoscopy and biopsy. A complete colonoscopy is performed to exclude synchronous colon cancer or polyps, but the rigid proctoscope is preferred to assess the clinical characteristics of the tumor such as the distance from the dentate line, size, and macroscopic appearance. A large

biopsy can be obtained through the rigid proctoscope. A chest x-ray and abdominal and pelvic computed tomographic (CT) scan are obtained to exclude pulmonary and liver metastases and check for the presence of extrarectal pelvic spread. Except in clinically advanced tumors with a stricture, an endorectal ultrasound examination is performed.

■ SELECTION CRITERIA FOR LOCAL TREATMENT

Optimal treatment of rectal cancer requires consideration of the tumor characteristics including size, location, depth of invasion, nodal status, and histology, and patient factors including operative risk, functional status, and the patient's wishes.

Tumor Criteria

Only anatomically accessible tumors that are localized to the bowel wall are candidates for curative local therapy. Once the tumor has spread to the perirectal fat or the regional lymph nodes, it can almost never be cured by local therapy alone. Therefore, the main selection criteria are depth of invasion and nodal status.

The depth of invasion is particularly important because it is directly related to the incidence of lymph node involvement, local recurrence, and 5-year survival. Depth of invasion can be assessed both clinically and with the help of special diagnostic tests. Clinical assessment by digital rectal examination is useful only for tumors located in the distal portion of the rectum and permits only a gross estimation of depth of invasion. Its accuracy varies significantly with the experience of the examiner and the stage of the tumor. Clinical staging by digital examination identifies the presence of extrarectal invasion with reasonable accuracy but fails to discriminate the degree of intramural invasion and fails to identify more than 50% of the pathologically proved involved nodes. Therefore, clinical examination is more accurate in staging locally advanced tumors than early tumors, and thus its value in selecting patients for local therapy is limited.

Endorectal ultrasonography has been the most useful technique available for preoperative staging of rectal cancer. Although the resolution decreases in the mobile upper third of the rectum, ultrasonography is usually reliable and technically possible to perform for most lesions up to 12 cm from the anal verge. When compared with histopathologic staging, its accuracy at predicting depth of mural invasion ranges between 81 and 95% and at detecting lymph node metastasis between 58 and 87%. A modification of the TNM staging, with degrees of invasion that correspond very closely to the pathologic stages, is currently used for the preoperative ultrasonographic staging of rectal tumors. We use this information in our decision making to select tumors suitable for local therapy.

CT scanning demonstrates extrarectal invasion but cannot distinguish the individual layers of the bowel wall and is thus less useful in the selection of patients for local therapy. The accuracy of CT scan in the diagnosis of lymph node metastasis, based exclusively on size criteria, is less than that of endorectal ultrasonography.

Magnetic resonance imaging (MRI) is equivalent to endorectal ultrasonography in demonstrating extrarectal invasion but has not been as reliable in distinguishing individual layers of the bowel wall. The use of an endorectal coil may enhance the resolution of the MRI and allow better discrimination of the different layers of the rectal wall. Preliminary studies using new MRI technologies suggest that its accuracy in predicting depth of invasion and lymph node involvement is similar to that of endorectal ultrasonography. The technique is expensive and currently is available only at selected centers.

Several studies have demonstrated that poorly differentiated and mucinous cancers and tumors with vascular and lymphatic invasion have a high incidence of lymph node metastasis and are associated with poor outcome. Local therapy as the sole form of treatment is generally contraindicated in patients with such unfavorable histology.

Macroscopic tumor characteristics provide additional information about the behavior of the tumor. Ulcerated tumors tend to have more advanced locoregional disease and worse prognosis than do exophytic tumors. However, current data suggest that exophytic and ulcerated tumors with the same depth of rectal wall invasion carry the same risk of lymph node metastasis. Therefore, local therapy is not contraindicated based on macroscopic tumor characteristics alone.

For many years only tumors smaller than 3 cm in diameter were considered for curative local therapy. Larger tumors tend to be more advanced, but several studies have demonstrated that when corrected for histologic grade and depth of invasion, tumor size is not an independent risk factor for lymph node metastasis and overall prognosis and is not, in itself, a contraindication to local therapy.

In recent years, most surgeons have restricted the use of local therapy for rectal cancer to T1 or T2, node-negative, histologically favorable adenocarcinomas if they are accessible and small enough to be completely excised with clear margins or encompassed within the field of endocavitary radiation.

Patient Criteria

Every patient with a rectal cancer who meets the preceding selection criteria is a candidate for local treatment. However, local therapy is especially advantageous in medically unfit patients and in patients with significant distant metastases who are unlikely to survive long but have troublesome symptoms from their rectal cancer. In such patients, the tumor criteria are often liberalized to allow local treatment of more advanced cancers. Additionally, some patients refuse radical surgery, especially if a colostomy is likely. To accommodate the patient's demands, the curative intent of therapy may be compromised. Conversely, the benefits of local therapy may be negated in patients with underlying fecal incontinence or with a rectal cancer invading the anal sphincter.

■ CHOICE OF LOCAL THERAPY

In patients with identical stage tumors, tumor recurrence and patient survival appear to be similar with different forms of local therapy. Local excision either by traditional endoanal exposure or by a transanal endoscopic microsurgery (TEM) technique has the advantage over other forms of local therapy of providing a specimen. Analysis of the specimen allows the surgeon to confirm the diagnosis, assess the completeness of the excision, stage the depth of tumor penetration in the rectal wall, and identify unfavorable histopathologic features. Endocavitary radiation has the advantage of being an outpatient treatment done without anesthesia. Even frail patients can tolerate this treatment. Electrocoagulation can be used for palliation to control local symptoms, but we do not use it with curative intent.

■ FOLLOW-UP

Regardless of which modality of local therapy is used, early diagnosis of local recurrence is important because it appears that radical surgery can effectively control many recurrences. Therefore, every patient undergoing curative local therapy for rectal cancer is closely monitored postoperatively for local recurrence. After surgery, we perform baseline digital rectal, proctoscopic, and endorectal ultrasonography examinations every 4 months for 3 years and every 6 months for 2 additional years. An area suspicious for recurrence should be biopsied.

■ LOCAL EXCISION: TECHNIQUE

Most local excisions for rectal cancer can be done through a transanal approach. A preoperative bowel preparation including oral antibiotics is routinely administered to minimize the risk of intraoperative contamination. We use perioperative prophylactic intravenous antibiotics and prophylaxis for deep venous thrombosis. A bladder catheter is routinely inserted.

The procedure is usually performed under general or regional anesthesia, but in selected circumstances, it can be done under local anesthesia and intravenous sedation. Adequate exposure is essential. We perform most local excisions in the prone jack-knife position. The need for good illumination cannot be overemphasized, and, therefore, we always use headlights. The perianal area is exposed by taping the buttocks apart, and the Lone Star retractor (Lone Star Medical Products, Inc., Houston, TX) is used to efface the anus and facilitate exposure of the distal anal canal. To expose the rectum, we use the Pratt,[Au] Sawyer, Hill-Ferguson, or Ferguson Mon retractors because they expose approximately 50% of the circumference of the rectum and anal canal. More proximal lesions may require longer retractors such as malleables, Wylie renal vein, or narrow Deavers.

We use the electrocautery unit to mark the intended incision line, leaving a 1-cm margin of normal mucosa around the tumor. For lesions located proximally, we place traction sutures distal and lateral to the tumor to bring the lesion closer to the anal orifice. Using the electrocautery unit, a full-thickness incision is started in the distal border of the line of resection. To ensure a full-thickness incision, the perirectal fat should be identified clearly. As the incision is extended proximally, traction sutures should be placed sequentially around the area of excision to maintain control of the rectal wall. In anteriorly located lesions, care is taken to avoid injury of adjacent structures, such as vagina, prostate, or urethra. An accidental opening of the peritoneal cavity can be safely closed.

The specimen should be pinned down with orientation marks and transferred to pathology for fixation and evaluation by permanent sections. Resection margins should be inked. The rectal wall defect is closed often in a transverse fashion with a single layer of full-thickness absorbable sutures. A proctoscopic examination at the end of the procedure is performed in order to be certain that the rectal lumen was not inadvertently closed or narrowed.

Prophylactic antibiotics are administered preoperatively and for two doses after the operation. Pain control is usually not a problem. Clear liquids may be started on the same evening of the operation, and the diet is advanced as tolerated. Most patients are discharged within 48 hours of operation.

The transsacral posterior proctotomy originally described by Kraske adds minimally to the exposure offered by the transanal approach and carries the potential risk of fistula formation. The posterior transsphincteric approach popularized by York-Mason requires division of the sphincter complex and carries the risk of wound dehiscence and postoperative incontinence. In the past, these techniques were used occasionally for anterior, proximally based lesions. Today, both approaches are rarely used. Transanal endoscopic microsurgery (TEM) is a new technical alternative that is very useful for proximal rectal tumors that cannot be easily excised by standard transanal techniques. Although some have advocated using this approach for all local excisions, we have not found that to be necessary.

■ LOCAL EXCISION: RESULTS

Local recurrence after transanal excision ranges from 0 to 18% for T1 lesions and from 11 to 47% for T2 lesions. Radical resection for local recurrence that follows transanal excision may salvage between 25 and 100% of patients, with overall survival rates ranging from 73 to 100%. In our own recent series of 82 patients treated by local excision for cure and followed for an average of 54 months, local recurrence developed in 10 of 55 patients (18%) with T1 lesions and 10 of 27 patients (37%) with T2 lesions. The incidence of distant failure was 5%, and 17 of 20 patients with local recurrence underwent salvage surgery. Although most patients were disease-free after the salvage procedure, it was unclear whether delayed radical

surgery after failure of local excision was therapeutically equivalent to radical surgery alone performed at the time of initial diagnosis.

We compared 108 patients with T1 and T2 rectal cancers treated by transanal excision with 153 patients with T1N0 and T2N0 rectal cancers treated with radical surgery. Neither group received chemoradiation. Mean follow-up period was 4.4 years after local excision and 4.8 years after radical surgery. The estimated 5-year local recurrence rate was 28% (18% for T1 tumors and 47% for T2 tumors) after local excision versus 4% (0% for T1 tumors and 6% for T2 tumors) after radical surgery. The estimated 5-year overall survival rate was 69% after local excision (72% for T1 tumors and 65% for T2 tumors) and 82% after radical surgery (80% for T1 tumors and 81% for T2 tumors). Differences in survival rates between local excision and radical surgery were statistically significant in patients with T2 tumors. We concluded that local excision as the only form of treatment for T2 rectal cancers may compromise overall survival when compared to radical resection.

In our most recent review of this subject, we reported the course of 29 patients who underwent salvage radical surgery for local recurrence after a full-thickness transanal excision for stage 1 rectal cancer. Recurrence involved the rectal wall in 26 patients (90%) and was purely extrarectal in only 3 (10%). The radical resection was considered curative in 23 patients (79%). At a mean follow-up period of 39 months (range, 2 to 147 months) after radical surgery, 17 patients (59%) remained free of disease. The disease-free survival rate was 68% for patients with tumors with favorable histology. We concluded that salvage surgery for recurrence after local excision of rectal cancer may not provide results equivalent to those achieved following radical treatment performed at the time of initial diagnosis.

■ ENDOCAVITARY RADIATION: TECHNIQUE

Cancer of the rectum is a radiosensitive tumor, and early rectal cancer can be controlled by irradiation alone. Papillon has popularized contact x-ray therapy as the sole form of treatment in early rectal cancer. With this form of treatment, the tumor receives six applications of high-dose (20 to 30 Gy), low-voltage (50 kV) irradiation over the course of 6 weeks. The radiation is delivered through a special proctoscope with a 3-cm-diameter field and an effective depth of 6 mm, thereby maximizing tumor exposure and minimizing irradiation to the surrounding normal tissues. Each application produces a rapid shrinkage of the tumor, and, therefore, the operator can adjust the dose and the focus at every session. Each application lasts no more than 2 minutes and can be delivered in an outpatient setting. A booster dose of 20 to 30 Gy to the tumor bed in 24 hours using iridium-192 wire implants is frequently used in France, where doctors have the most experience with this treatment modality.

ENDOCAVITARY RADIATION: RESULTS

Local control with endocavitary radiation for T1 and T2 rectal cancer, with 192-iridium boost in selected patients, ranges from 71 to 89%, but these results improve to 82 to 99% after surgical salvage of local recurrences. Overall survival and tumor-specific survival rates of 83 to 94% have been reported, and most of these patients maintain a functionally competent rectum. In our own series of 83 patients with T1 (49) or T2 (34) cancers treated for cure by endocavitary radiation, the local recurrence rate was 16% for T1 and 29% for T2 tumors. When endocavitary radiation was used for curative intent treatment of seven T3 cancers and one T4 cancer, local recurrence developed in all but one patient.

Our current policy is to recommend endocavitary radiation with curative intent for small, appropriately located T1 and highly selected T2 rectal cancers. The selection criteria are similar to our criteria now used for local excision. The main disadvantage of endocavitary radiation therapy is that it does not provide a specimen to confirm the level of invasion. This technique is a useful alternative for patients medically unfit for anesthesia and for those who refuse an operation.

ELECTROCOAGULATION

The use of electrocoagulation to treat cancer was introduced by Byrne more than a century ago. Although this technique has never gained widespread acceptance, it has been used with good results at some institutions. Advocates claim that electrocoagulation is less likely to seed viable tumor cells than is local excision, but the disadvantages include the lack of pathology specimen for staging, the reliance on visual and tactile information to confirm tumor eradication, the morbidity of postoperative fever and hemorrhage, and the frequent need for repeated operations.

Electrocoagulation can be used with curative or palliative intent, although we limit its use to palliation. When intended for cure, patient selection is critical. The preoperative workup, the indications for the procedure and the selection criteria are very similar to those described for local excision. Tumors should be mobile, exophytic, less than 4 cm in diameter, and located below the peritoneal reflection. Preoperative endorectal ultrasound helps determine the depth of invasion and the presence of metastatic pararectal lymph nodes. Anteriorly located tumors are less suitable for electrocoagulation because of the proximity of the peritoneal reflection and the prostatic capsule or the rectovaginal septum.

Patients receive a phosphate enema the same morning of the operation. Prophylactic antibiotics are not routinely used. The operation is performed under general or regional anesthesia in the lithotomy or prone position, depending on the location of the tumor. A large operating proctoscope with a built-in suction channel to eliminate the smoke is commonly used. Perianal block helps to dilate the anal canal and minimize the amount of general anesthesia. Different groups used different treatment modalities. Salvati and associates use bipolar electrocautery with a large ball tip to coagulate the tumor surface. Madden combed away the tumor with a wire loop connected to a low-intensity cutting current. Crile and Turnbull claimed to achieve greater heat penetration and better tactile discrimination with a needlepoint electrode connected to an electrocuatery unit with a spark-gap generator. The coagulated tissue is removed with uterine curettes and tissue forceps until normal tissue is exposed. Postoperative fever is common. Patients can usually be discharged within 48 hours of the operation, tolerating regular diet and with minimal discomfort. Complications include bleeding, stricture, urinary retention, electrical burns, perianal abscess, and perforation.

Close follow-up with monthly proctoscopic examination is recommended during the first year. Any indurated area should be biopsied. Repeated electrocoagulation is indicated in recurrences localized to the bowel, but recurrences that involve the perirectal fat or perirectal lymph nodes should be treated by radical excision.

The 5-year survival rate after electrocoagulation for rectal cancer varies between 47 and 67%, but comparison between these series and with other forms of local therapy are limited by differences in selection criteria.

CURRENT POLICY FOR LOCAL THERAPY

To achieve optimal function and maximum patient survival, the surgeon must balance the predicted biologic behavior and other characteristics of the patient's cancer, the morbidity of the proposed treatment, and the patient's operative risk factors and personal needs. It is disappointing that despite decades of work and refinements of sophisticated imaging techniques, we continue to both overcall and undercall the stage of rectal cancer in a significant percentage of patients. The appropriate selection of patients with cancers ideally treated by curative local therapy remains problematic. Our high local recurrence rate and potential for compromising survival have convinced the authors to restrict the use of curative-intent local therapy in good-risk patients to only the most favorable rectal cancers. For high-risk operative patients and for patients with metastatic disease or those who refuse recommended radical resection, local therapy sometimes followed by chemoradiation is a viable alternative. (Our current approach is outlined in Figure 32-1).

For accessible, small, or well or moderately differentiated rectal cancers unequivocally staged as uT1N0 without evidence of distant spread, curative local therapy can be safely recommended even in good-risk patients. We favor local excision either by traditional endoanal exposure or by transanal endoscopic microsurgery (TEM) because it provides a specimen. If the margins after local excision are not clear of cancer, re-excision or more aggressive treatment by radical resection is recommended. If the permanent histologic examination after

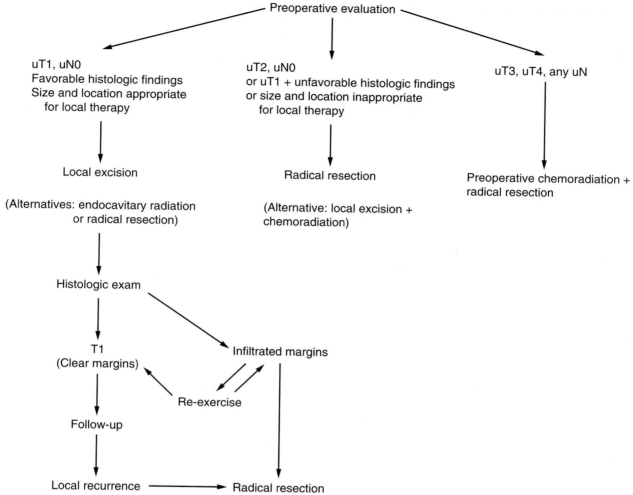

Figure 32-1
Curative management of rectal cancer.

local excision reveals a more advanced tumor stage (T2 or T3) or unfavorable histologic features (poorly differentiated, mucinous, or lymphovascular invasion), a radical resection is recommended, especially if sphincter preservation is possible.

For a uT2N0 histologically favorable rectal cancer in a good-risk patient without distant metastasis, radical resection without adjuvant chemoradiation is recommended. For distal uT2N0 rectal cancers which would require an abdominoperineal resection and permanent colostomy, patients often seek alternative options. Local excision coupled with chemoradiation is recommended by many surgeons in this setting, but its therapeutic equivalency to radical surgery has not yet been proved. When patients with such a tumor refuse our advice for radical resection or are at increased risk for death from a radical resection, we discuss the pros and cons of local therapy ± chemoradiation and proceed accordingly. The need for close post-treatment follow-up is stressed because it is often possible

to salvage such patients should local recurrence develop after the initial local therapy.

For any T3 or N+ rectal tumor, local therapy is considered palliative. In general, palliation is best achieved when the primary lesion can be totally excised or destroyed. Follow-up to control regrowth is essential to minimize symptoms.

Suggested Readings

Bleday R, Breen E, Jessup JM, et al: Prospective evaluation of local excision for small rectal cancers. Dis Colon Rectum 1997;40:388–392.

Brodsky JT, Richard GU, Cohen AM, et al: Variables correlated with the risk of lymph node metastasis in early rectal cancer. Cancer 1992;69:322–326.

Buess G, Mentges B, Manncke K, et al: Technique and results of transanal endoscopic microsurgery in early rectal cancer. Am J Surg 1992;163:63–65.

Enker WE, Havenga K, Polyak T, et al: Abdominoperineal resection via total mesorectal excision and autonomic nerve preservation for low rectal cancer. World J Surg 1997;21:715–720.

Garcia-Aguilar J, Mellgren A, Sirivongs P, et al: Local excision of rectal cancer without adjuvant therapy: A word of caution. Ann Surg 2000; 231:345–351.

Garcia-Aguilar J, Pollack J, Lee S-H, et al: Accuracy of endorectal ultrasonography in preoperative staging of rectal tumors. Dis Colon Rectum 2002;45:10–15.

Kim NK, Kim MJ, Yun SH, et al: Comparative study of transrectal ultrasonography, pelvic computerized tomography, and magnetic resonance imaging in preoperative staging of rectal cancer. Dis Colon Rectum 1999;42:770–775.

Mellgren A, Sirivongs P, Rothenberger DA, et al: Is local excision adequate therapy for early rectal cancer? Dis Colon Rectum 2000;43: 1064–1074.

Ott DJ: Staging rectal carcinoma with MR imaging: Improving accuracy with newer techniques. Am J Gastroenterol 2000;95:1359–1360.

Rothenberger DA, Garcia-Aguilar J: Role of local excision in the treatment of rectal cancer. Semin Surg Oncol 2000;19:367–375.

Zenni GC, Abraham K, Harford FT, et al: Characteristics of rectal carcinoma that predict the presence of lymph node metastasis: Implications for patient selection for local therapy. J Surg Oncol 1998;67:99–103.

33

CANCER OF THE RECTUM: FOLLOW-UP AND MANAGEMENT OF LOCAL RECURRENCE

Harvey G. Moore, MD
Lawrence E. Harrison, MD
José G. Guillem, MD, MPH

More than 40,000 cases of rectal cancer occur annually in the United States, and approximately 5 to 30% of these patients will go on to manifest pelvic recurrence after curative resection. These patients often experience uncontrollable pelvic pain, dysesthesia, tenesmus, and other local complications that severely impair quality of life. Because control of local recurrence can palliate these problems and, in select cases, may prolong disease-free and overall survival time, early diagnosis and aggressive treatment of locally recurrent rectal cancer in carefully selected patients is justified.

■ NOMENCLATURE OF PELVIC RECURRENCE

A useful nomenclature for describing pelvic recurrence is based on the anatomic region(s) of the pelvis involved with disease (Fig. 33-1). We have found that this system facilitates a standardized treatment approach for this heterogeneous population, as well as subsequent meaningful comparisons of outcome.

Pelvic recurrence is classified as involving the axial, anterior, posterior, or lateral regions. The axial region includes both mucosal and perirectal soft tissue recurrences. This type of recurrence can occur following a transanal or trans-sphincteric excision. Similarly, an anastomotic recurrence after a low anterior resection (LAR) with primary reconstruction is also included in this category. The axial region also encompasses recurrences in the mesorectum, as well as the relatively uncommon perineal recurrence following abdominoperineal resection (APR). Anterior recurrences involve the genitourinary tract. In females this region includes the vagina, uterus, urinary bladder, and distal ureters, and in males, it includes the seminal vesicles, prostate, urinary bladder, and distal ureters. Posterior region recurrences include tumors involving the sacrum, and lateral recurrences involve the soft tissues of the pelvic sidewall (iliac vessels, middle third of the ureters, lymph nodes, nerves, and muscle) and lateral bony pelvis.

■ CLINICAL EVALUATION FOR SUSPECTED PELVIC RECURRENCE

Complaints such as changes in bowel habits, blood per rectum, and obstipation may herald a local recurrence after transanal excision or an LAR. Vaginal bleeding or urinary symptoms may reflect involvement of the genitourinary tract, and perineal pain or a persistent fistula following APR may reflect a perineal recurrence or disease involving the sacrum. Leg edema or neurogenic pain in the sciatic distribution are ominous findings and suggest extensive pelvic sidewall involvement.

Physical examination should include a thorough examination of the abdomen, including palpation for an enlarged liver or tumor mass. A digital rectal examination is essential for any patient status after LAR or local

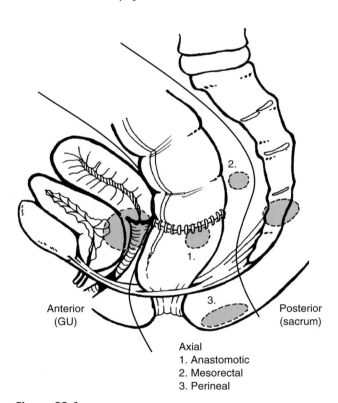

Figure 33-1
Regions of rectal cancer pelvic recurrence. Pelvic recurrence can be classified based upon the anatomic region(s) of the pelvis involved with disease. Axial recurrences can involve the (1) anastomosis, (2) mesorectum or perirectal soft tissue, or (3) the perineum following abdominoperineal resection. Anterior recurrences involve the genitourinary tract including the bladder, vagina, uterus, seminal vesicles, and prostate. Posterior recurrences involve the sacrum and presacral fascia. Lateral recurrences (not shown) involve the soft tissues of the pelvic sidewall and lateral bony pelvis.

excision to detect occult blood or an anastomotic recurrence. Examination of the groin and supraclavicular region is required to exclude adenopathy. Assessment of neuromuscular function in the lower extremities can identify deficits resulting from peripheral nerve involvement by lateral tumor recurrence. In females, a bimanual pelvic examination may reveal disease involving the rectovaginal septum, vagina, uterus, and adnexal structures. Close examination of the perineal region after APR should also be performed to detect tenderness, a mass, or a fistula. In females following APR, a pelvic examination helps detect early pelvic recurrences as well as assessment of extent of disease involvement.

Rigid proctosigmoidoscopy is useful in the workup of a recurrence because it can document the most distal extent of disease relative to the uppermost part of the anorectal ring. Palpation with the tip of the sigmoidoscope to assess the extent of pelvic sidewall involvement can help distinguish recurrence with sidewall involvement from a true anastomotic recurrence. In patients with pelvic recurrence being considered for radical surgery, a complete colonoscopy should be performed preoperatively to rule out synchronous proximal disease.

Although highly operator-dependent, endorectal ultrasound (ERUS) can detect pelvic masses and enlarged lymph nodes, and can be used for ERUS-directed biopsy for pathologic confirmation. In addition, it may be used via the vagina to assess status in female patients after APR. Although differentiation of fibrosis from recurrence remains a problem, the addition of color Doppler may help distinguish viable tumor from fibrosis because of the relatively increased vascularity of neoplastic tissue. In addition, serial examinations over time may detect the presence of recurrence in the setting of stable postoperative fibrosis.

Computed tomographic (CT) scan is extremely useful for the detection and staging of locally recurrent rectal cancer. CT evidence of local recurrence may include asymmetric thickening of the bowel wall, obliteration of perianastomotic fascial or fat planes, a presacral or lateral sidewall mass, or enlarged regional lymph nodes. Postoperative or postradiation changes may lead to fibrosis and linear streaks in the perirectal fat, indistinguishable from a true recurrence. It is often useful to obtain a CT scan 2 to 4 months after completion of therapy to establish a baseline for future comparison. Although false-negative results are not uncommon, the sensitivity and specificity of CT scan to detect pelvic recurrence range from 60 to 71% and 72 to 85%, respectively.

Magnetic resonance imaging (MRI) often complements CT findings by adding further anatomic detail pertaining to the extent of local pelvic structure involvement in up to 40% of patients. Indeed, MRI appears to be superior to CT scan at detecting tumor infiltration of surrounding structures for locally advanced primary and recurrent rectal cancer. This additional information may be useful in the preoperative planning of the extent of an en bloc resection. Dynamic contrast-enhanced subtraction (DCES) MRI with gadolinium (Gd-DPTA) may be more accurate than traditional T2-weighted spin-echo images in differentiating fibrosis from pelvic recurrence.

Positron emission tomography (PET) is one of the more promising nuclear imaging modalities for detecting pelvic recurrence of rectal cancer. PET imaging with the glucose analog [18F]fluorodeoxyglucose (FDG) has been highly successful at imaging a variety of human tumors, including colorectal cancer that is avid for FDG. This success is due, in large part, to the ability of FDG-PET to distinguish postoperative fibrosis and radiation changes from viable, recurrent tumor. FDG-PET may also identify hepatic metastases as well as extrahepatic disease that may preclude an attempt at curative resection. Using current digital technology, PET scan images can be superimposed on CT scan images (PET/CT fusion images), thus generating both anatomic and metabolic information.

■ MANAGEMENT OF PELVIC RECURRENCE

Approximately 30 to 50% of local recurrences will be confined to the pelvis and therefore will be amenable to potentially curative resection. An algorithm for the management of local recurrence is shown in Figure 33-2. After the diagnosis of pelvic recurrence is confirmed, patients will fall into one of four categories (see following paragraphs) based on the presence of extrapelvic disease, local resectability, and symptoms. Other important considerations with regard to operative strategy include patient age and presence of comorbid disease.

Category I: Asymptomatic Local and Distant Recurrence
Curative options for patients with concomitant local and distant recurrences are few, so treatment should be offered judiciously, particularly for asymptomatic patients. A small, highly select group may benefit from resection of two sites of isolated disease (i.e., pelvis and lung or liver). However, data supporting the efficacy of this approach are just beginning to emerge. Data from our institution suggest that a highly select group of patients with locally recurrent and distant metastatic disease may be rendered disease-free with synchronous or staged resection, resulting in an overall median survival time of 23 months.[1]

Category II: Symptomatic Local Recurrence in the Presence of Distant Disease
The goal for treating symptomatic local recurrence in the presence of distant, unresectable metastases should be to minimize morbidity and maximize palliation. Treatment options for patients with bleeding per rectum secondary to local recurrence include fulguration, radiation, or palliative surgical resection. Radiation is an effective modality for the palliative treatment of pain, bleeding, neurologic symptoms, and symptoms related to mass effect. Patients with bowel obstruction due to a recurrence within 10 to 12 cm of the anal verge may be safely palliated with fulguration, laser ablation, or endoscopic stenting. Palliation for a more proximal colon obstruc-

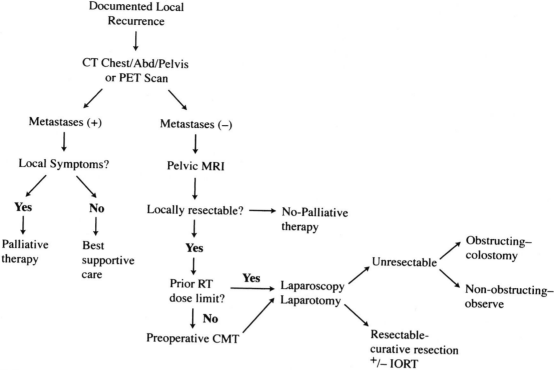

Figure 33-2

Strategy in management of locally recurrent rectal cancer. Initial evaluation generally includes a computed tomographic (CT) scan of the abdomen and pelvis performed with both intravenous and oral contrast media in order to exclude distant metastatic disease. Fluorodeoxyglucose positron emission tomography (FDG-PET) scanning is an alternative. Symptomatic recurrence in patients with disseminated disease may benefit from palliative therapies (fulguration, laser ablation, radiation, endoscopic stenting, colostomy, or palliative resection). A highly selected subset of patients may benefit from resection of multiple sites of isolated disease (pelvis and lung or liver). Pelvic magnetic resonance imaging (MRI) may add additional information to CT scan regarding adjacent organ involvement and extent of required en bloc resection. In patients who have not received a full course of pelvic radiation therapy, preoperative combined modality therapy (CMT) may be given. Diagnostic laparoscopy may identify intra-abdominal disease and thus could avoid an unnecessary laparotomy in unresectable patients. A laparoscopically assisted loop colostomy or ileostomy may be created in cases of impending obstruction.

tion may be achieved with either a resection or diverting colostomy. Patients with a near-obstructing recurrence are at significant risk for progression to complete obstruction secondary to swelling and edema from external beam radiation. In these cases, a lumen of at least 1 cm should be maintained.

Category III: Unresectable Isolated Local Recurrence

Treatment options for patients with isolated, unresectable pelvic recurrence that has not received large doses of external beam radiation include preoperative combined modality therapy (CMT). A trial of external beam radiation with a radiosensitizing agent such as 5-fluorouracil (5-FU) may result in a sufficient response to allow a resection with negative histologic margins. Limitations include entrapment of small bowel in the pelvis following the initial resection, or a compromise in luminal diameter with impending obstruction. In these individuals, a laparo-

scopically assisted loop colostomy or ileostomy will prevent the development of clinical obstruction while the patient receives CMT. For the symptomatic patient, bypass, colostomy, stent, or fulguration may palliate symptoms until chemoradiation produces an effect. Another recently described palliative option is CT-guided radiofrequency ablation, which shows promise for recurrent tumors larger than 4 cm.

Category IV: Resectable Isolated Local Recurrence

Surgical resection offers the only known curative option for patients with isolated pelvic recurrence. The probability of resection and surgical options for these patients are dictated, in part, by their primary procedure and region of recurrence.

Cystoscopy with bilateral stent placement is recommended for all patients with a pelvic recurrence, especially when bladder involvement is suspected. The operative approach begins with exploratory laparotomy, at which time 25 to 50% are found to be unresectable. When technically feasible, a diagnostic laparoscopy is a reasonable initial approach to rule out involvement of peritoneum, omentum, periaortic lymph nodes, and the liver. Laparoscopically directed intraoperative ultrasound may also be used to exclude liver metastases. If unresectable extrapelvic disease or locally recurrent disease is detected and confirmed on frozen section, a laparoscopically assisted loop colostomy or ileostomy is an option in cases of impending obstruction. Overall, between 29 and 54% of patients with locally recurrent rectal cancer are able to undergo a curative resection (generally defined as complete resection with negative microscopic margins). Reported 5-year survival rates for patients undergoing R0 resection ranges between 20 and 41%.

Axial Recurrences

These recurrences most likely represent a failure to obtain adequate distal margins during LAR, tumor implantation into the mesorectum during local excision, or perineal tumor implantation during APR. Sphincter preservation may be an option for high axial anastomotic recurrences. However, the quality of life of individuals undergoing a resection of locally recurrent disease with sphincter preservation may be diminished. Furthermore, significant lateral extension often requires a combined abdominoperineal approach to ensure negative circumferential margins of resection (CMR). Wide local excision of a perineal soft tissue recurrence following APR may render the patient free of disease. However, perineal recurrence is often a harbinger of disease deeper in the pelvis, thereby necessitating a combined abdominoperineal approach to assure a curative resection. The outcome for patients with recurrent disease limited to the bowel wall is markedly superior.

Anterior Recurrences

Recurrences involving the genitourinary tract require en bloc removal of involved pelvic viscera to achieve negative histologic margins. A posterior exenteration (APR with total abdominal hysterectomy, bilateral salpingo-oophorectomy, and posterior vaginectomy) is indicated for anterior pelvic recurrence in women with isolated uterine/vaginal involvement and no bladder involvement. A partial cystectomy or total exenteration is required when tumor involves the bladder. In women who have had an abdominal hysterectomy, an anterior recurrence generally mandates a total exenteration as there is usually no plane between the recurrence and the bladder. After cystectomy, urinary drainage is provided by either a simple ileal conduit or a more complex continent pouch. Although resection of the anterior structures including the uterus or bladder may facilitate negative resection margins anteriorly, obliteration of anatomic planes by previous surgery (especially APR) and radiation limits the ability to ensure negative posterior and lateral resection margins.

Pelvic exenteration is a technically challenging and potentially morbid procedure and should therefore not be attempted unless an R0 resection (histologic and gross negative margins) is anticipated. Complication rates following total pelvic exenteration range between 22 and 78% with an in-house hospital mortality rate of 0 to 10%. In carefully selected patients, pelvic exenteration may be associated with a median survival time of 20 to 56 months and a 5-year survival rate of up to 50%. In a series of 55 patients from our institution with advanced primary or locally recurrent colorectal cancer undergoing total pelvic exenteration, an R0 resection was achieved in 73%, and median disease-specific survival time for all patients was 49 months at a median follow-up of 26 months. A history of prior APR was an independent predictor of poor outcome. Although results for patients with recurrent disease may not be as good as for those with primary tumors, 5-year survival rates of 23 to 28% have been reported for patients with locally recurrent rectal cancer requiring pelvic exenteration.

Posterior Recurrences

In select posterior recurrences when sacral invasion is limited to the sacral fascia or superficial periosteum, an en bloc resection by periosteal elevation may achieve negative margins. When bony invasion of the sacrum is present, R0 resection may still be achieved using a combined abdominosacral resection. A sacrectomy may be performed in combination with an APR or pelvic exenteration, depending on the extent of pelvic disease. These formidable resections take from 6 to 12 hours and may involve significant blood loss. The most potentially morbid aspect of an abdominosacral resection is the bony sacral transsection due to the risk of significant hemorrhage and sacral nerve root damage. Major morbidities associated with this procedure include intestinal and urinary fistula, wound complications, pulmonary embolus, and bladder dysfunction.

Bladder dysfunction is related to the level of sacral transsection, with sacral transsections below S3 usually not affecting urinary continence. Mild urinary dysfunction occurs with unilateral division of S2 or S1. If both S2 nerve roots are resected, bladder dysfunction occurs, whereas bilateral division of the S1 nerve roots results in complete bladder denervation. The feasibility and safety of sacral resection has been demonstrated by several centers, with recent operative mortality rates ranging from 0 to 9%.

Lateral Recurrences

Lateral recurrences along the pelvic sidewall are the least likely to be salvaged with surgical resection. These tumors often adhere to the bony pelvis or invade the sciatic nerve. Patients may present with disabling pain radiating to the buttocks, perineum, and posterior thighs. Like sciatic nerve involvement, ureteral obstruction due to recurrent disease is associated with a low likelihood of R0 resection. Iliac nodal disease can be removed en bloc with a local soft tissue resection. This operation may entail partial ureterectomy, as well as partial resection of major arteries and veins, including the iliac vessels.

■ THE ROLE OF CHEMORADIATION FOR PELVIC RECURRENCE

The use of radiation therapy alone for the treatment of locally recurrent rectal cancer results in a reported 5-year survival rate of 5 to 10%. However, radiation may be an effective means of palliation for patients with unresectable pelvic recurrence. The role of radiation in the setting of locally resectable recurrent disease may be limited by previous treatment. Preoperative external beam radiation, often in combination with 5-FU-based chemotherapy, can help salvage fixed, inoperable, or borderline resectable recurrences. In addition, preoperative chemoradiation may facilitate less extensive resections, increasing the rate of sphincter preservation. In a recent study of 35 previously nonirradiated rectal cancer patients with pelvic recurrence from rectal cancer and deemed unresectable (based on involvement of adjacent pelvic organs), the use of preoperative radiation and 5-FU-based chemotherapy resulted in a resection with negative histologic margins in 61% of cases. Others have reported similar results. The use of preoperative chemoradiation prior to pelvic exenteration for recurrent and locally advanced rectal cancer has also been shown to be an independent predictor of improved survival versus surgery alone.

Intraoperative radiation therapy (IORT) allows the delivery of a large fraction of radiation directly to the bed of resection while avoiding exposure of normal, surrounding tissues. IORT can be delivered to areas of questionable or microscopically positive resection margins either at the time of resection via electron beams from a linear accelerator or after surgery by implantation of radioactive sources (brachytherapy). An alternative means for delivering IORT utilized at Memorial Sloan-Kettering Cancer Center (MSKCC) involves a flexible, high-dose rate (HDR) remote afterloader called the Harrison-Anderson-Mick (HAM) applicator. The HAM applicator conforms well to the tumor bed and is capable of delivering the maximum dose to the proposed target area while sparing the surrounding normal tissues. The procedure is performed in a dedicated, shielded operating room to avoid moving the patient during the operation.

IORT is generally combined with neoadjuvant or adjuvant chemoradiation for locally recurrent rectal cancer. In the MSKCC experience, 100 patients with locally recurrent rectal cancer were treated with HDR-IORT following resection. Thirty-seven previously nonirradiated patients received preoperative pelvic radiation in combination with 5-FU-based chemotherapy. All patients received surgery plus IORT (12.5 to 17.5 Gy). At a median follow-up of 23 months, actuarial 5-year disease-free survival (DFS) and disease-specific survival (DSS) rates were 22% and 39%, respectively. Independent predictors of improved DFS, DSS, and local control were R0 resection and absence of vascular invasion in the recurrent specimen.

Despite using lead shields to protect adjacent soft tissues such as the ureter, iliac vessels, and sciatic nerve, these structures nevertheless may be damaged secondary to extensive surgery compounded by the effects of radiation therapy. Peripheral neuropathy occurs in up to 16% of patients.

■ RECONSTRUCTION OPTIONS FOR PERINEAL DEFECTS

Healing of the perineal defect following APR for recurrent rectal cancer may be limited, especially in patients receiving preoperative CMT. In selected patients, optimal healing potential may be achieved with a variety of myocutaneous flaps. These flaps, based on a nonirradiated vascular pedicle, provide sufficient bulk to fill the dead space following a wide pelvic resection and may improve function in women undergoing posterior vaginectomy.

Traditional options include the gracilis flap (unilateral or bilateral), the gluteus muscle flap, and the inferiorly based transverse rectus abdominis (TRAM) flap. Advantages of the gracilis flap, based on the medial circumflex femoral branch of the profunda femoris artery, include proximity and lack of donor-site morbidity. Disadvantages, however, include a tenuous vascular pedicle and often insufficient muscle bulk to fill a large pelvic defect. The TRAM flap is similar to that used for breast reconstruction, except that it is based inferiorly on the deep inferior epigastric vessels. Advantages include a durable vascular pedicle, good muscle bulk, and ease of creation, resulting in minimal prolongation of operating time. Use of the rectus abdominis muscle may, however, result in significant abdominal wall morbidity and may limit potential stoma sites should colostomy resiting become necessary.

■ SUMMARY

Patients with recurrent rectal cancer represent a complex challenge. Because nearly 50% of rectal cancer pelvic recurrences are isolated, and therefore potentially amenable to curative resection, aggressive surveillance appears to be justified. Radical re-resection for selected patients with pelvic recurrence offers excellent palliation, and in combination with CMT (including IORT) results in long-term survival in up to one third of carefully selected patients. Improvements in conventional imaging modalities including PET, CT scan, and MRI may facilitate early diagnosis of local recurrence as well as accurate assessment of extent of local involvement leading to improved patient selection and likelihood of a curative resection.

Suggested Readings

Akhurst T, Larson S: Positron emission tomography imaging of colorectal cancer. Semin Oncol 1999;26:577–583.

Guillem JG, Ruo L: Strategies in operative therapy for locally recurrent rectal cancer. Semin Colon Rectal Surg 1998;9(4):259–268.

Hartley JE, Guillem J, Lopez RA, et al: Resection of locally recurrent colorectal cancer in the presence of distant metastases: Can it be justified? Ann Surg Oncol 2003;10(3):227–233.

Jimenez R, Shoup M, Cohen AM, et al: Contemporary outcomes of total pelvic exenteration in the treatment of colorectal cancer. Dis Colon Rectum 2003;46;1619–1625.

Moore HG, Akhurst T, Larson S, et al: A case-controlled study of 18-F fluorodeoxyglucose positron emission tomography in previously irradiated rectal cancer patients. J Am Coll Surg 2003;197(1):22–28.

Pearlman NW: Surgery for pelvic recurrences. In Cohen AM, Winawer SJ (Eds.). Cancer of the Colon, Rectum, and Anus. New York, McGraw-Hill, 1995, pp 863–872.

Pilipshen SJ, Heilweil M, Quan SH, et al: Patterns of pelvic recurrence following definitive resections of rectal cancer. Cancer 1984; 53(6):1354–1362.

Salo JC, Paty PB, Guillem J, et al: Surgical salvage of recurrent rectal carcinoma after curative resection: A 10-year experience. Ann Surg Oncol 1999;6(2):171–177.

Shibata D, Guillem JG, Lanouette N, et al: Functional and quality-of-life outcomes in patients with rectal cancer after combined modality therapy, intraoperative radiation therapy, and sphincter preservation. Dis Colon Rectum 2000;43(6):752–758.

Shibata D, Hyland W, Busse P, et al: Immediate reconstruction of the perineal wound with gracilis muscle flaps following abdominoperineal resection and intraoperative radiation therapy for recurrent carcinoma of the rectum. Ann Surg Oncol 1999;6(1):33–37.

Shoup M, Guillem JG, Alektiar KM, et al: Predictors of survival in recurrent rectal cancer after resection and intraoperative radiotherapy. Dis Colon Rectum 2002;45(5):585–592.

34

PERINEAL HERNIA

David E. Beck, MD

Abdominal perineal resection and pelvic exenteration are regularly performed for advanced rectal cancer. During follow-up, many of these patients will demonstrate a perineal bulging, which increases with increased abdominal pressure (as during coughing, straining, or a Valsalva maneuver). This perineal hernia develops because a large portion of the pelvic floor is removed. The absent pelvic floor allows the small bowel to descend through the pelvis into the perineum. Although the presence of a postoperative perineal hernia is common, it is unusual for the hernia to cause symptoms. Reported symptoms have included pain, bowel or urinary tract obstruction, and perineal skin breakdown. The incidence of patients requiring repair has been estimated at 1% of abdominal perineal resections (APRs) and 3 to 10% of pelvic exenterations. This low incidence is confirmed by the relative paucity of cases reported (<75 cases). This chapter will discuss patient evaluation and methods of treatment.

■ PATIENT SELECTION

Repair of a perineal hernia is major surgery and should be reserved for the symptomatic patient who is a reasonable operative candidate. Patients are evaluated preoperatively for operative risks and to exclude the possibility of recurrent tumors. This evaluation includes a complete history and physical examination, as well as routine blood studies. Contrast radiologic studies of the intestine and urinary tract or endoscopy as well as ultrasound or computed tomographic (CT) scans of the abdomen and pelvis complete the workup. Upright anteroposterior and lateral films of the pelvis during a small bowel follow-through study demonstrate the loops of small bowel herniating into the pelvis. As with all procedures, the potential benefits of relieving symptoms must be balanced against the risks of surgery. A history of pelvic irradiation increases the potential risks of hernia repair.

■ PREOPERATIVE PREPARATION

The patient is prepared with an oral mechanical bowel preparation (polyethylene glycol electrolyte lavage solution) and receives systemic prophylactic antibiotics (e.g., cefotetan). Oral antibiotics may also be administered after completion of the mechanical preparation.

■ PROCEDURE

The patient is placed in a modified Lloyd-Davies position, which allows access to the perineum if a combined approach is required and room for a second assistant to provide retraction in the pelvis. In addition, this position allows easy preoperative placement of ureteric stents if desired. The pelvis is explored through a lower midline incision. If no recurrent tumor is present, the loops of small bowel in the pelvic hernial sac (Fig. 34-1) are freed by division of their adhesions. Care is taken to identify and protect the ureters.

The pelvic floor is reconstructed using a single or double layer of prosthetic material. Although several types of material have been described, most authors have used a double layer of polypropylene mesh. This material is permanent and allows for good tissue ingrowth. Other materials that have been used include absorbable mesh (e.g., Vicryl) and expanded PTFE. The edges of the mesh are sutured to the edges of the pelvic outlet with interrupted nonabsorbable suture (e.g., 2-0 Ethibond). Posteriorly, the mesh is attached to Waldeyer's fascia and sacral periosteum at or below the level of S3; anteriorly, it is sutured to the vagina or prostatic capsule (Fig. 34-2). The bladder base is avoided because posterior fixation may cause urinary retention. Laterally, the fasciae of the pelvic side wall and ligamentous structures are used to anchor the mesh (Fig. 34-3). In placing these sutures care is taken to avoid the large pelvic vessels. The attachment of the mesh is below the level of the ureters. An obturator may be placed into the vagina via the perineum to aid in operative identification of the vaginal cuff. The edges of the mesh are marked with small metallic clips that allow easy documentation of the mesh position on a plain abdominal x-ray film postoperatively. If sufficient omentum is present

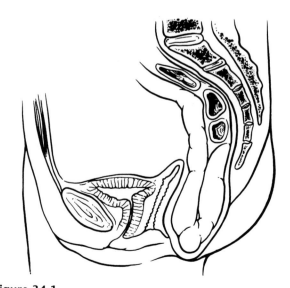

Figure 34-1
Sagittal section of the pelvis demonstrating a perineal hernia with incarcerated small bowel.

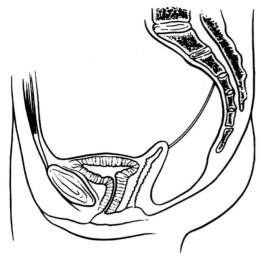

Figure 34-2
Sagittal section of the pelvis with mesh in place.

in the abdomen, a pedicle flap is constructed and placed between the mesh and the small bowel. This reduces the chance of bowel adhering to or being eroded by the mesh. If a significant dead space is created below the mesh, a closed suction Silastic drain is placed below the mesh to aid in obliteration of the space. It is brought out the abdomen through a separate incision.

■ ALTERNATIVE METHODS

Earlier reports recommended a perineal approach for repair of these hernias. Although this method was believed to reduce morbidity, it had several disadvantages. First, if the genitourinary structures are present, the pelvic inlet cannot reached from the perineum and the mesh must be sutured to the perineal diaphragm (the weak point in such a repair). Second, it is difficult to separate the adherent small bowel loops in the hernia sac. If bowel or a vascular structure is injured, it is very difficult to repair because the exposure is limited from the perineum. Finally, the ability to exclude recurrent tumor is limited with such an approach.

The abdominal approach allows confirmation of the absence of recurrent tumor and mobilization of the small bowel under direct vision. The mesh can be attached at an appropriate level in the pelvis, and the chance of injury to other pelvic structures is reduced. A combined approach (abdomen and perineal) provides the advantages of the abdominal method and the ability to resect the attenuated skin of the perineum. For patients with large defects or to avoid the use of prosthetic material, a gracilis myocutaneous flap can be used to repair the hernia defect. Although prepared to use these methods, the author has thus far not found them necessary.

For patients with minimal symptoms or for those in whom the risks of operation are thought to be prohibitive, a support garment (girdle or Jobst pantyhose) may provide palliation.

■ POSTOPERATIVE CARE

Postoperative care is similar to that of other patients undergoing a laparotomy. Diet is advanced when bowel function returns and the antibiotics are stopped within 24 hours postoperatively. If a drain is used, it is removed when the output has diminished to approximately 50 mL per day.

■ COMPLICATIONS

In addition to the usual complications that might attend any laparotomy, the placement of the prosthetic material to reconstruct the perineal diaphragm carries the poten-

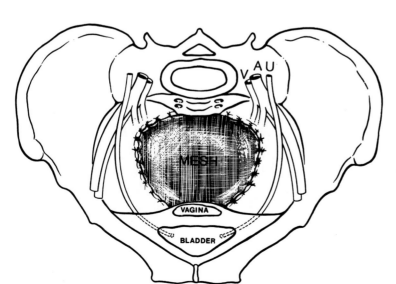

Figure 34-3
View of the pelvis from above with mesh in place. (A = common iliac artery, U = ureter, V = common iliac vein.)

tial risk of detachment of the mesh from the pelvic wall, leading to recurrence. The resulting defect around the mesh is likely to be smaller and more prone to strangulate the herniating viscus. This situation demands urgent re-exploration and repair of the defect.

A second and potentially more serious complication is a pelvic infection. An infection in or near the mesh requires its removal. The most common site of contamination is spillage from the bowel. If multiple enterotomies, significant spillage of intestinal content, or contamination of the mesh occurs, it is safer to abandon the planned repair and terminate the operation. After the patient recovers, a hernia repair may be rescheduled.

Suggested Readings

Beck DE, Fazio VW, Jagelman DG: Postoperative perineal hernia. Dis Colon Rectum 1987;30:21–24.

Hansen MT, Bell JL, Chun JT: Perineal hernia repair using gracilis myocutaneous flap. South Med J 1997;90:75–77.

Pearl RK: Perineal hernia. In Nyhus LM, Condon RE (Eds.): Hernia. Philadelphia, JB Lippincott, 1989, p 442.

Singer AA: Ultrasonographic diagnosis of perineal hernia. J Ultrasound Med 1994;13:987–988.

35

PREOPERATIVE PREPARATION OF THE COLON AND RECTAL SURGICAL PATIENT

Terry C. Hicks, MD, MS

Once the surgeon has confirmed the need to perform an operation, he or she must focus on the physiologic and psychological preoperative preparation of the patient. Advances in preoperative preparation have reduced the morbidity and mortality rates from colon and rectal surgery. However, the surgeon must still identify serious medical problems that can be adequately treated prior to surgery and address factors such as bowel preparation, preoperative antibiotic utilization, anesthesia, analgesia, deep venous thrombosis prevention, and informed consent. This approach requires a thorough knowledge of the disease process and an ability to evaluate the surgical risk.

■ PREOPERATIVE COMMUNICATION

The doctor/patient relationship is integral in the preoperative preparation of colon and rectal surgery patients. This relationship provides patient confidence and lays a risk-prevention foundation against medical malpractice complaints. Adequate time must be devoted so that the patient and the family understand clearly the indications for surgery, the proposed procedure, the potential risks and alternatives, and expectations of future lifestyle needs.

■ ASSESSING OPERATIVE RISKS

Operative risk assessment includes an accurate medical history and a thorough physical examination combined with appropriate biochemical and technologic testing.

Major factors to consider include the cardiac, pulmonary, renal, hepatic, hematologic, and nutritional status of the patient. A classification system proposed by the American Society of Anesthesiologists (ASA) is summarized in Table 35-1. When ordering "routine" preoperative investigations, it should be remembered that most have not been shown to change management unless symptoms have been present.

Cardiovascular Evaluation

To assess myocardial function, the results of a thorough cardiovascular history and examination should be correlated with the results of basic tests such as electrocardiogram and chest x-ray. A recent myocardial infarction is the most important risk factor for a perioperative infarction. Historically, patients undergoing general anesthesia following a myocardial infarction have a perioperative reinfarction risk of 27 to 36% for the initial 3 months, 11% between 3 and 6 months, and approximately 5% after 6 months. Therefore, most surgeons postpone purely elective colon and rectal surgery for up to 6 months following an acute myocardial infarction. More urgent operations, such as for a potentially resectable malignant tumor, are undertaken 4 to 6 weeks after an uncomplicated infarction or a favorable exercise tolerance test (see Table 35-2).

Pulmonary Evaluation

Postoperative respiratory complications occur in approximately 5 to 7% of abdominal operations. Patients with normal preoperative pulmonary function may develop

Table 35-1	The American Society of Anesthesiologists (ASA) Physical Status Classification
CLASS	**DESCRIPTION**
P1	A normal healthy patient
P2	A patient with mild systemic disease
P3	A patient with severe systemic disease
P4	A patient with severe systemic disease that is a constant threat to life
P5	A moribund patient who is not expected to survive without the operation
P6	A declared brain-dead patient whose organs are being removed for donor purposes

Source: Excerpted from Manual for Anesthesia Department Organization and Management. 2003–2004. A copy of the full text can be obtained from ASA, 520 N. Northwest Highway, Park Ridge, Illinois, 60068-2573.

Table 35-2 Weighting of Cardiac Risk Factors

CRITERIA	POINTS
Historical	
Age over 70 years	5
Myocardial infarction during previous 6 months	10
Examination	
S₃ gallop/jugular venous distention	11
Significant aortic valvular stenosis	3
Electrocardiogram	
Premature atrial contractions or rhythm other than sinus	7
More than 5 premature ventricular contractions per minute	7
General Status	3
Abnormal blood gases	
K⁺/HCO₃⁻ abnormalities	
Liver disease/bedridden	
Operation	
Emergency	4
Intraperitoneal/intrathoracic/aortic	3
Total possible points	53

Source: Modified from Goldman L, Caldera DL, Nussbaum SR, et al: Multifactorial index of cardiac risk in noncardiac surgical procedures. N Engl J Med 297:845, 1977.

Table 35-3 Risk Factors for Postoperative Pulmonary Complications

Thoracic and upper abdominal surgery
Preoperative history of chronic obstructive pulmonary disease (COPD)
Preoperative purulent productive cough
Anesthesia time greater than 3 hours
History of cigarette smoking
Age greater than 60 years
Obesity
Poor preoperative state of nutrition
Symptoms of respiratory disease
Abnormal findings on physical examination
Abnormal chest film findings

Source: Houston MC, Ratcliff DG, Hays JT, Gluck FW: Preoperative medical consultation and evaluation of surgical risk. South Med J 80:1385, 1987.

complications secondary to the anesthetic agents or the operation, and other factors may add risk (Table 35-3). The operative risk is four times higher in elderly patients with chronic lung disease. Cigarette smokers have pulmonary complication rates up to 20% owing to their decreased mucociliary clearance in the respiratory tract. This rate may be reduced if these patients can cease smoking for 4 to 6 weeks before the operation. Perioperative pulmonary complications are also seen in obese patients undergoing prolonged procedures.

A preoperative chest film is often part of routine screening for those over 40 years of age, although increasingly this is reserved for patients with specific symptoms. For those with questionable lung function, pulmonary function tests (including arterial blood gases) are helpful in assessing postoperative risks from pulmonary problems. If the respiratory system is significantly compromised, preoperative intervention with ventilation therapy using mucolytic agents, postural drainage, and possibly the administration of corticosteroids may be needed to optimize their preoperative respiratory status.

Renal Status

Renal abnormalities are less common than pre-existing cardiovascular or respiratory disease. However, patients with renal disease are more susceptible to intra- and postoperative complications. Renal disorders can be associated with electrolyte imbalances, anemia, or hypertension. Preoperative screening measures include blood urea nitrogen, creatinine determination, and a urinalysis, which also includes β-hCG (human chorionic gonadotropin) testing for women of childbearing age. Patients with renal insufficiency may require perioperative alterations in their fluid

and electrolyte balance. This knowledge of the renal status is also helpful for those situations that arise in the operating room in which potentially renal toxic contrast materials may be needed for investigative purposes.

Blood Volume Status

Blood volumes may be decreased secondary to bleeding from inflammatory bowel disease or colorectal carcinoma. Low hemoglobin concentrations decrease oxygen transport capacity and increase the risk for perioperative complications. The surgeon and the anesthesiologist must find a consensus on the management of preoperative anemia. Historically, preoperative hemoglobin concentrations below 10 g/dL were transfused until restored to this level. However, the National Institutes of Health's Red Cell Conference found that patients without other existing comorbidities would tolerate values as low as 7 g/dL without postoperative sequelae. Therefore, the potential benefits of transfusion must be weighed against the risks. Current risks include a 1% risk for allergic reaction and transmission of communicable diseases such as hepatitis and HIV missed by screening.

In evaluating the risk of bleeding, the physician should determine whether a family member has had a prior bleeding or thromboembolic episode. The patient should also be questioned about prior transfusions; heavy menstrual bleeding; easy bruising; nosebleeds; coexistent liver or kidney disease; excessive ingestion of alcohol, aspirin, or other nonsteroidal anti-inflammatory drugs; and utilization of lipid-lowering drugs or anticoagulants such as warfarin. With a negative history for these risk factors, the cost-effectiveness of routine coagulation screening tests is extremely low.

Nutritional Status

Nutritional status is an important preoperative consideration because poor nutrition is associated with adverse perioperative effects. A negative nitrogen balance leads to the depletion of serum proteins, causing sodium retention, water retention, edema, and poor wound healing. Malnutrition is also associated with a reduced immune competence, leading to a greater risk of postoperative infection. Although nutritional science has improved over time, no universally accepted method for nutritional assessment exists. The clinician's approach may include history, anthropometric measurements, and biochemical measurements. The weight history is a useful tool for assessing nutritional status and includes an assessment of current weight, how that weight relates to ideal body weight (obtained from standard tables), and any recent weight loss. The dietary and medical history should not be overlooked, as they may correlate with the weight history.

Anthropometric measurements include the triceps skinfold and midarm circumference. These values are helpful in assessing fat stores and skeletal muscle mass. Biochemical measurements of plasma protein such as albumin, transferrin, prealbumin, and retinol-binding protein are reasonable indicators of protein status. In an attempt to quantify nutritional status, Mullen and colleagues devised a prognostic nutritional index (PNI):

$$PNI = 150 - 16.6 \, (ALB) - 0.78 \, (TSF) \\ - 0.2 \, (TFN) - 5.8 \, (DH)$$

where ALB is serum albumin reported in g/dL, TSF is the triceps skinfold measured in mm, TFN is the serum transferrin level measured in mg/dL, and DH is the greatest skin reaction to injected antigens (mumps and dermatophytin). Mullen and associates noted that a high PNI seemed to indicate more complications. Although this cumbersome formula is not easy for the busy clinician to utilize, such an evaluation often can be obtained by a hospital nutritional support team. Total lymphocyte counts and delayed cutaneous hypersensitivity are other measures of the body's ability to respond to infection, but they are compromised only with severe malnutrition. A single, more clinically useful method is the subjective global assessment described by Detsky and associates. As summarized in Table 35-4, it divides nutritional status into three categories: well nourished, moderately malnourished, and severely malnourished.

■ BOWEL PREPARATION

Bowel preparation before elective colon and rectal surgery is standard practice. Mechanical bowel cleansing and the administration of perioperative antibiotics along with blood banking practices and careful surgical techniques have lowered the perioperative mortality rate to less than 4% and the morbidity rate due to infectious complications to less than 9%.

With a preoperative bowel preparation, the surgeon attempts to simplify the colonic surgery and prevent infectious sequelae. These sequelae include infections of the wound and the abdominal wall, intra-abdominal sepsis (anastomotic disruption), and secondary septicemia. The perfect bowel preparation would be safe, provide good cleansing, have minimal side effects, be compatible for inpatient and outpatient utilization, and be cost effective. When studies of the various methods of preoperative bowel preparation are reviewed, it becomes apparent that there is no satisfactory scientific basis for a rational choice. As a result of this confusing body of literature, clinicians must settle for some uncertainty in choosing a preoperative bowel preparation regimen, keeping an open mind as more valid data become available.

The colon is an organ that holds varied and concentrated amounts of bacteria. These bacteria are potentially fatal if exposed to other tissue. Beginning at the distal ileum, the concentration of bacteria increases as stool solidifies and reaches the distal colon. Intraluminal bacteria are a mixture of aerobic coliforms and anaerobic, nonsporulating gram-negative rods, numbering 10^6 to 10^8 organisms per gram of feces for aerobic bacteria and 10^9 to 10^{11} organisms per gram of feces for anaerobic bacteria. Mechanical bowel cleansing and prophylactic antibiotics

Table 35-4 Subjective Global Assessment			
CRITERIA	**WELL-NOURISHED STATUS**	**MODERATELY MALNOURISHED STATUS**	**SEVERELY MALNOURISHED STATUS**
Medical history			
Body weight change in last 6 months	Loss <5%	Loss 5–10%	Loss >10%
Dietary intake	Balanced diet that meets requirements	70–90% of requirements	<70% of requirements
Gastrointestinal symptoms (vomiting, diarrhea)	None	Intermittent	Daily for >2 weeks
Functional capacity	Full capacity	Reduced	Bedridden
Physical examination			
Subcutaneous fat	Normal	↓	↓↓
Muscle mass (quadriceps, deltoids)	Normal	↓	↓↓
Edema (ankle, sacral)	None	+	++
Ascites	None	+	++
Serum albumin	>4.0 g/dL	3.0–4.0 g/dL	<3.0 g/dL

Source: Modified from Beck DE: Preoperative preparation. In Handbook of Colorectal Surgery. St. Louis, Quality Medical Publishing, 1997, pp 129–145.

reduce the bacterial concentration in the colon lumen in an attempt to prevent infectious sequelae.

■ MECHANICAL PREPARATION

Mechanical cleansing of the colon can be accomplished by enemas, cathartics, or lavage. Whatever cleansing modality is used, it will reduce the quantity of stool but will not significantly reduce the concentration of bacteria remaining in the colon lumen.

Cathartics

Traditionally, most techniques of emptying the colon use irritant-type purgatives and enemas to move feces, combined with dietary restrictions so as not to add to the fecal bulk. Unfortunately, the cathartic and enema cleansing method requires 2 to 3 days to complete and is often associated with significant physiologic side effects, such as dehydration and electrolyte alterations. This technique has been reported to produce adequate and acceptable cleansing in approximately 70% of patients. Although lavage preparations (see lavage section) are presently the most commonly used mechanical preparation, there is a growing patient dissatisfaction with this technique because of the volume that needs to be drunk. Recent prospective randomized trials comparing sodium phosphate and polyethylene glycol (PEG)–based oral lavage solutions have shown both solutions to be equally effective and safe, but patient tolerance of the sodium phosphate is better than the traditional PEG solution. Although both sodium phosphate and PEG solutions produce significant decreases in serum calcium levels, sodium phosphate has also been reported to produce dehydration and hyperphosphatemia. The physiologic alterations associated with sodium phosphate may limit its usefulness when renal function is impaired, and the physician should always be aware of these side effects when utilizing sodium phosphate as a mechanical preparation.

Enemas

Enema preparations work by irritation of the colon or by dilution. Preparations may contain tap water, soapsuds, saline, or chemicals such as mineral oil or phosphate mixtures. As a single agent for preparation, enemas are usually unsuccessful and may be associated with physiologic complications such as dehydration, increase in body fluid, electrolyte abnormalities, and hypothermia. This problem specifically restricts enema utilization in the patient with renal impairment. Enema use may also result in mechanical complications such as perforation in high-risk patients with inflammation or obstruction of the colon or rectum.

Oral Lavage

Oral lavage has resulted in two distinct improvements: the quality of the preparation and the decreased time required for mechanical cleansing. Normal saline was used in initial trials with the oral lavage technique. After the passage of a nasogastric tube, the patient received 1 L of fluid per hour. Adequate cleansing required 7 to 10 L of normal saline and was often associated with significant complications, such as fluid and electrolyte changes and subsequent weight gain. If the solution was not administered at body temperature, hypothermia could result. Because this technique required the insertion of a nasogastric (NG) tube, was skill- and labor-intensive, and was associated with physiologic complications that restricted its use in patients with impaired renal or cardiovascular status, its use was short lived.

Mannitol

In concentrations of 10 to 15% this nonabsorbed osmotic agent has proved to be successful in cleansing the bowel with volumes as small as 1 L, although it does cause dehydration. Mannitol is metabolized by colonic bacterial flora, which produce potentially explosive gas. Electrocautery-induced colonic explosions have been reported in endoscopic and surgical patients given mannitol. Because of such potential catastrophic sequelae, oral mannitol lavage is rarely used in current clinical practice.

Polyethylene Glycol Lavage

This solution is polyethylene glycol (PEG) 3350 and an electrolyte solution containing sodium 125 mmol/L, sulfate 40 mmol/L, fluoride 35 mmol/L, bicarbonate 20 mmol/L, and potassium 10 mmol/L. This solution presently is produced as GoLytely and CoLyte. These lavage solutions have become the primary choice for colonoscopy and elective colon surgery. Ingestion of 2 to 4 L (8 oz every 10 minutes) of the solution produces an excellent bowel preparation in 90 to 100% of patients, usually in less than 4 hours, without electrolyte or metabolic complications. A slightly modified lavage solution (increased PEG and decreased sodium sulfate) has recently been marketed as NuLytely.

Unfortunately, some patients experience symptoms of nausea and fullness with polyethylene glycol preparation. Metoclopramide to alleviate these symptoms has been tried, but several studies failed to document usefulness.

Special Situations

When a patient has a partially obstructed colon and does not have an inflammatory bowel process, preparation with small increments of Fleet's Phospho-Soda, GoLytely, or mineral oil solutions can be considered. Balloon dilatation, laser recannulation, and intraluminal stent placement have also been described.

Intraoperative Lavage

During emergency surgery or operations in which the patient has an inadequate bowel preparation, an intraoperative lavage may be considered. This allows the surgeon to perform a resection with a primary anastomosis. Two major techniques are used: The transabdominal technique (Fig. 35-1) involves the insertion of a catheter (20 Fr Foley) into the cecum through a stab incision in the terminal ileum at the appendix. After inflation of the catheter balloon, it is pulled flush against the ileocecal valve or the base of the appendix. The distal end of the mobilized

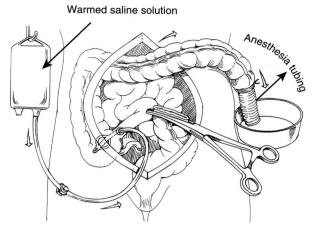

Figure 35-1
Intraoperative lavage.

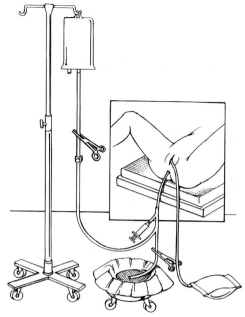

Figure 35-2
Appropriate patient positioning for performing the low anterior resection or abdominal perineal resection or abdominal perineal resection (Lloyd-Davies stirrups not shown). Rectal irrigation system and Foley catheter insertion completed.

colon is intubated with a sterile, large-bore tubing (i.e., ribbed anesthesia tubing), which is secured in place with umbilical or vascular tape. After the drainage tube is directed into a bucket or closed collection system placed on the floor, the Foley catheter is connected to a warm saline solution and the colon is irrigated with 2 to 4 L of fluid or until clear (Fig. 35-2).

The transrectal approach utilizes a large Foley or Malecot catheter (32 Fr). After careful placement in the rectum, the balloon is inflated if it is the Foley type. A Y-connector is attached to the catheter to provide ingress and egress sides. Warm saline is passed through the ingress as the egress side is clamped until the bowel segment is filled and then the ingress is occluded while the egress tube is open to allow the fluid mix to drain into a collection system on the floor. The process is continued until the bowel is clean. Some surgeons choose to conduct the final irrigation with an antimicrobial solution, such as dilute povidone-iodine.

■ ANTIBIOTICS

In current practice and in the absence of obstruction, a mechanical preparation is routinely combined with antibiotics as part of a preoperative bowel preparation prior to colon surgery. Although mechanical cleansing reduces residual fecal mass, it does not affect the number of organisms present per gram of residual stool. To attack these residual bacteria, antimicrobial agents have been added to the preoperative bowel preparation regimen. Many clinical series have confirmed that infection rates were significantly higher with mechanical preparations alone compared to the combination of mechanical preparations and prophylactic antibiotics. Although most surgeons now use a combined mechanical and antibiotic preparation, discussion continues as to whether the antibiotics should be administered enterally and selected primarily for their intraluminal activity, or administered parenterally and selected for their systemic effects, or both.

Oral Antibiotics

Selection criteria for an appropriate oral antibiotic regimen are based on knowledge of the normal bowel flora, the bacteriology of the infections following colon operations, any synergies among bacteria found in postoperative infections, and the antibiotic sensitivity of the bacteria.

The normal colonic flora is composed of approximately 20 species of aerobic bacteria and greater than 50 species of anaerobic bacteria. In postoperative infections in colon and rectal surgery, *Bacteroides fragilis* is the most commonly cultured species, followed by *Clostridium* and *Peptostreptococcus*. The most common cultured aerobic bacterium from colon and rectal surgical infections is *Escherichia coli*. Because colon and rectal infections are caused by endogenous bacteria that have violated the colonic mucosal barrier, prophylactic antibiotics should be effective against these bacteria. Nichols and colleagues introduced neomycin and erythromycin base as the oral prophylactic antibiotic combination for colon operations. These antibiotics were chosen because they were well tolerated, inexpensive, and remained in the bowel lumen (although oral erythromycin does produce measurable serum concentrations). Development of resistant bacteria was not found to be a significant problem if these agents were used for less than 24 hours. The authors gave 1 g of each antibiotic orally at 1:00 PM, 2:00 PM, and 11:00 PM on the day prior to surgery, anticipating an 8:00 AM operating time the following day. If the surgery was planned for later than 8:00 AM, the timing of these doses was adjusted appropriately. Neomycin was selected because of its activity against aerobic coliforms, whereas the erythromycin base was chosen because of its activity against anaerobic bacteria. Some surgeons have substituted metronidazole (250 to 500 mg) in place of the erythromycin to prevent gastrointestinal symptoms associated with erythromycin.

Parenteral Antibiotics

Systemic antibiotic use in elective colon and rectal surgery is prophylactic rather than therapeutic in design. Prophylactic antibiotic use is directed at preventing potential infectious sequelae. Unfortunately, many studies of prophylactic parenteral antibiotics in colon and rectal surgery have yielded conflicting results. Because of this lack of consistency, antibiotic bowel preparation remains one of the more controversial issues in surgical care. Administration of intravenous antibiotics without oral antibiotics has shown success in some trials but has failed in others. Parenteral agents that have shown efficacy independently or in combination with an aminoglycoside include cefoxitin, cefotetan, metronidazole, and doxycycline. Cefotetan in a single dose has been as effective as multiple-dose cefoxitin in preventing infectious sequelae after colon and rectal surgery.

Oral and Parenteral Antibiotics Combined

Studies comparing oral antibiotic with parenteral antibiotics suggest no significant difference in infectious complications. However, under select circumstances, the use of oral antibiotic agents in combination with parenteral antibiotics may still represent a valid choice. In two surveys of colon and rectal surgeons, more than 88% used both oral and systemic antibiotics before elective colon resection. The most commonly utilized combination was oral neomycin and erythromycin and a parenterally administered second-generation cephalosporin that possessed aerobic and anaerobic activity. The combination of oral and parenteral antibiotics produced a low incidence of infection and may be helpful in cases in which the oral antibiotics have been administered in an inappropriate time sequence or the operation has been delayed.

Topical Prophylaxis

The use of topical prophylactic antibiotics in elective colon surgery has not been widely adopted. Although early studies indicated that topical ampicillin was associated with only a 3% wound infection rate, these studies were flawed because some patients received either oral or parenteral antibiotics while others underwent emergency resection without mechanical bowel preparation. Controlled studies of topical ampicillin used in conjunction with oral and parenteral antibiotics showed no statistical reduction in infection. Experimental studies of

povidone-iodine irrigation solutions confirmed a reduction in luminal bacteria, but the number of mucosal bacteria were not significantly affected. This technique has not gained general acceptance among colon and rectal surgeons.

The author's preferred bowel preparation is summarized in Table 35-5.

■ PREVENTION OF VENOUS THROMBOEMBOLISM

Venous thromboembolism continues to be a serious and occasionally fatal complication of major surgical procedures. It is estimated that pulmonary embolism causes death in more than 100,000 hospitalized patients each year. The actual incidence of venous thromboembolism is much greater than reported because many deaths due to pulmonary embolism may go undetected in hospitals because of their low autopsy rates (7%). Studies in academic medical centers have confirmed that only approximately 30% of patients who have had a fatal pulmonary embolism had a correct diagnosis prior to autopsy. Because of these factors, pulmonary embolism may represent the most common preventable cause of hospital death.

Prophylaxis for venous thromboembolism is supported by the fact that the clinical diagnosis is unreliable and insensitive and potentially exposes the susceptible patients to higher risks. Another consideration is the fact that most deaths from pulmonary embolism usually occur within 30 minutes of the acute event so that therapeutic anticoagulation would not be effective. Patients who develop unrecognized and untreated deep vein thrombosis (DVT) have the potential for long-term morbidity secondary to future episodes of recurrent venous thromboembolism and postphlebitic syndrome.

Despite the widespread literature supporting the efficacy of prophylaxis, some surveys indicate that the majority of surgeons do not routinely prescribe prophylaxis for high-risk patients. These studies indicate that academic teaching hospitals utilized DVT prophylaxis in 44% of high-risk patients and nonteaching hospitals had a rate of less than 20%.

The failure of physicians to use prophylaxis more widely is multifactorial. Physicians often cite the low overall incidence of significant venous thromboembolism. Another reason is the concern about bleeding complications from anticoagulants. Multiple double-blind randomized trials, however, have demonstrated no significant increase in major bleeding with the use of low-dose unfractionated heparin (LDUH) and low-molecular-weight heparin (LMWH). With these agents, however, there is a documented increase in wound hematomas that is associated with sequelae such as wound infection and dehiscence. Heparin-induced thrombocytopenia has also been cited as a potential risk of heparin preparations, but clinical reviews suggest that this complication occurs in only approximately 3% of cases. In this age of cost containment, nonsupporters

Table 35-5 Bowel Preparation Regimen

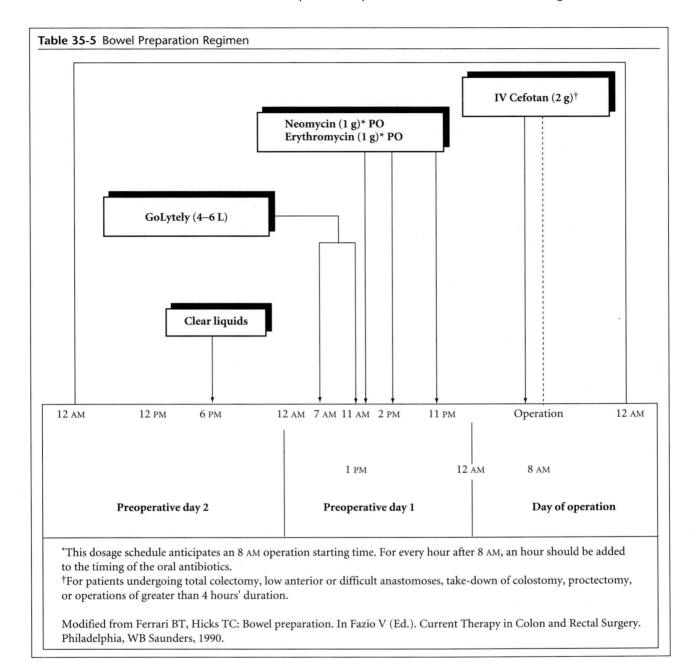

*This dosage schedule anticipates an 8 AM operation starting time. For every hour after 8 AM, an hour should be added to the timing of the oral antibiotics.

†For patients undergoing total colectomy, low anterior or difficult anastomoses, take-down of colostomy, proctectomy, or operations of greater than 4 hours' duration.

Modified from Ferrari BT, Hicks TC: Bowel preparation. In Fazio V (Ed.). Current Therapy in Colon and Rectal Surgery. Philadelphia, WB Saunders, 1990.

of prophylaxis have also argued that the cost benefit ratio of DVT prophylaxis does not support its use. However, multiple studies evaluating this concern have found that prophylaxis is highly cost effective. The last factor for surgeons not utilizing prophylaxis is their failure to recognize the magnitude of the problem. Because DVT often goes clinically undetected, the physicians' perception may become their reality.

Hospitals with educational programs directed at DVT prophylaxis noted a 20% increase in prophylaxis use. These programs provided both clinical practice updates and hospital-specific data indicating the need for the implementation of DVT prophylaxis guidelines.

Risk Consideration

The appropriate use of DVT prophylaxis is dependent upon the clinician's knowledge and identification of specific clinical risk factors in individual patients. The definitions of patients at risk for venous thrombosis and pulmonary embolism are not precise but serve as a useful tool for identifying those patients who may benefit from prophylaxis. Patients are routinely divided into low, moderate, high risk, and very high risk, depending upon the number of risk factors present. Identified risk factors (Table 35-6) include advanced age (40 years and greater), prior venous thromboembolism, cancer, major abdominal and pelvic surgery, obesity, varicose veins, congestive heart failure, myocardial infarction, stroke, and prolonged immobility or paralysis. Hypercoagulable states and hemostatic abnormalities also are considered risks.

Prevention

Prevention of DVT includes pharmacologic and nonpharmacologic means. Pharmacologic agents presently include subcutaneous heparin, low-dose aspirin, warfarin, and low-molecular-weight heparin. The most frequent nonpharmacologic measures include elastic stockings and sequential compression stockings. Sequential compression stockings have been shown to be effective in patients at low and moderate risk but require attention by the clinician because noncompliance and improper use can be a problem. Sequential compression stockings may be contraindicated in the presence of significant peripheral vascular disease. Graduated elastic stockings are appropriate only for low-risk procedures or patients at low risk who are undergoing moderate risk procedures.

In the United States, subcutaneous heparin at a dose of 5000[Au] U twice a day has gained widespread use because of its efficacy and low morbidity rate. The complications of subcutaneous heparin include minor bleeding (wound hematomas) at a rate of less than 3% and the rare occurrence of thrombocytopenia. Platelet counts of less than $100 \times 10^9/L$ should alert the clinician to this potential complication. Low-molecular-weight heparin and other heparin admixtures are gaining popularity in the United States and have proved to be equivalent to heparin therapy for prophylaxis of venous thromboembolism following general surgery. Unfortunately, these agents are presently relatively cost-prohibitive despite their enhanced safety profile and efficacy. Patients who are in the very high risk group are candidates for warfarin therapy, although some authors believe dextran may be equally efficacious. Many clinicians have found low-dose heparin combined with sequential compression stockings to be efficacious in the very high risk group.

In summary, attention to preoperative preparation is essential to obtaining consistently good results in colorectal patients. Knowledge and use of the information discussed in this chapter will minimize patient risk and improve outcomes.

Suggested Readings

Beck DE: Mechanical cleansing for surgery. Perspect Colon Rectal Surg 1994;7(1):97–114.

Clagett GP, Anderson FA Jr, Heit J, et al: Prevention of venous thromboembolism. Chest 1995;108:312S–334S.

Dudrick SJ: Parenteral nutrition. In Dudrick SJ, Baue AE, Eiseman B, et al (Eds.). Manual of Preoperative and Postoperative Care, 3rd ed. Philadelphia, WB Saunders, 1983, pp 86–105.

Ferrari BT, Hicks TC: Preoperative bowel preparation. In Fazio V (Ed.). Current Therapy in Colon and Rectal Surgery. Philadelphia, WB Saunders, 1990.

Gay CF Jr: Medicolegal issues. In Hicks TC, Beck DE, Opelka FG, Timmcke AE (Eds.). Complications of Colon and Rectal Surgery. Baltimore, Williams & Wilkins, 1996, pp 468–477.

Koruth NM, Krukowski ZH, Youngson GG, et al: Intraoperative colonic irrigation in the management of left-sided large bowel emergencies. Br J Surg 1985;72:708–711.

LaFrance RJ, Miyagawa CI: Pharmaceutical considerations in total parenteral nutrition. In Fischer JE (Ed.). Total Parenteral Nutrition. Boston, Little Brown, 1991, pp 87–97.

Levine GM. Nutritional support in gastrointestinal disease. Surg Clin North Am 1981;61:701–708.

Miller TA, Duke JH: Fluid and electrolyte management. In Dudrick SJ, Baue AE, Eiseman B, et al (Eds.). Manual of Preoperative and Postoperative Care, 3rd ed. Philadelphia, WB Saunders, 1983, pp 38–67.

Mullen JL, Buzby GP, Waldman MT, et al: Prediction of operative morbidity by preoperative nutritional assessment. Surg Forum 1979;30:80–82.

Nichols RL, Holmes JWC: Antibiotics in colon surgery. In Zuidema GD, Yeo CJ (Eds.). Shackelford's Surgery of the Alimentary Tract, vol 4. Philadelphia, WB Saunders, 2002, pp 150–163.

Oliveira L, Wexner S, Daniel N, et al: Mechanical bowel preparation for elective colorectal surgery. A prospective, randomized, surgeon-blinded trial comparing sodium phosphate and polyethylene glycol-based oral lavage solutions. Dis Colon Rectum 1997;40:585–591.

Shires GT, Shires GT III, Lowry SF: Fluid, electrolyte, and nutritional management of the surgical patient. In Schwartz SI, Shires GT, Spencer FC, et al (Eds.). Principles of Surgery, 6th ed. New York, McGraw-Hill, 1994, pp 61–94.

Stamos MJ, Theuer CP, Headrick CN: General postoperative complications. In Hicks TC, Beck DE, Opelka FG, Timmcke AE (Eds.). Complications of Colon and Rectal Surgery. Baltimore, Williams & Wilkins, 1996, pp 118–142.

Wexner SD, Beck DE: Sepsis prevention in colorectal surgery. In Fielding LP, Goldberg SM (Eds.). Operative Surgery, 5th ed. London, Butterworth-Heinemann, 1993, pp 41–46.

Wilson SE, Sokol T: Antimicrobials in elective colon surgery. Infect Surg 1985;10:609–611.

Table 35-6 Risk Factors for Deep Vein Thrombosis

CLINICAL RISK FACTORS	OPERATIVE RISK FACTORS
Age >40 years	Duration of surgery >1 hr
Prior DVT or pulmonary emboli	Pelvic surgery
Malignancy	Major orthopedic surgery
Obesity	General (versus regional) anesthesia
Congestive heart failure/ cardiomyopathy	Use of stirrups (lithotomy position)
History of stroke or myocardial infarction	
Estrogen use (high dose)	
Pelvic/hip fracture	
Paraplegia/quadriplegia	
Prolonged immobility	
Hypercoagulable state	
Varicose veins	
Sepsis	
Polycythemia rubra vera	
Inflammatory bowel disease	
Dehydration	
Postpartum state	
Preoperative hospitalization >5 days	

Source: Stamos MJ, Theuer CP, Headrick CN. General postoperative complications. In Hicks TC, Beck DE, Opelka FG, Timmcke AE (Eds.). Complications of Colon and Rectal Surgery. Baltimore, Williams & Wilkins, 1996.

36

MEDICAL TREATMENT OF ULCERATIVE COLITIS AND OTHER COLITIDES

Bret A. Lashner, MD, MPH
Aaron Brzezinski, MD, FRCP(C)

■ ULCERATIVE COLITIS

Clinical Features Related to Treatment

The most typical presenting features in ulcerative colitis patients are rectal bleeding and diarrhea, but tenesmus, abdominal pain, and extraintestinal manifestations are common. The inflammatory process in ulcerative colitis typically begins in the rectum and extends proximally with continuous disease. The extent of disease is the single most important determinant of both prognosis and response to medical therapy. From a series of 1116 patients followed for at least 5 years, at presentation 46% of patients had proctosigmoiditis, 17% had left-sided disease (to the splenic flexure), and 37% had pancolitis (Farmer and associates, 1993). Patients with pancolitis were more likely to develop toxic megacolon, refractory symptoms, malignancy, and extraintestinal manifestations and to require surgery. Of note, disease extent often changed during the course of the disease, with 56% of patients having limited disease extending proximally. About 15% of ulcerative colitis patients will demonstrate a mild inflammatory process of the terminal ileum, termed "backwash ileitis."

Medical therapy is most often determined by severity of symptoms and the most time-honored and reliable criteria to assess disease severity was developed in 1955 by Truelove and Witts to categorize disease activity into mild, moderate, and severe (Truelove and Witts, 1955, Table 36-1). Patients can be further classified as having fulminant or toxic colitis by having with more than 10 bowel movements per day, continuous bleeding, transfusion requirement, hypoalbuminemia, abdominal distention and tenderness, fever or leukocytosis, and radiologic evidence of colonic wall edema and possibly dilatation.

The diagnosis of ulcerative colitis can be made with typical endoscopic features (superficial ulcerations, granularity, and distorted mucosal vascular pattern extending from the rectum proximally) with negative stool cultures, and exclusion of all reasonable alternatives in the differential diagnosis. Principal alternative diagnoses include Crohn's colitis, infectious colitis, antibiotic-associated colitis, ischemic bowel disease, and diverticulitis. Ischemic bowel disease and diverticulitis are especially important diagnoses to exclude in the ulcerative colitis patient initially diagnosed when over 50 years old (Lashner and Kirsner, 1991).

Extraintestinal manifestations of ulcerative colitis can be as troubling as the colonic disease. The most common manifestation is arthritis, either mono- or asymmetric pauci-articular, involving the large joints with no synovial destruction. Patients with arthritis more often are female, are seronegative, exhibit no subcutaneous nodules, and have arthritis that correlates with disease activity. This type of arthritis responds to treatment of active bowel disease. Axial arthritis, related to human leukocyte antigen (HLA)-B27, does not correlate with disease activity and may be progressive and severe.

Erythema nodosum, seen in up to 3% of patients, and the ulcerating, purulent, necrotic skin lesion of pyoderma gangrenosum, seen less commonly, represent vasculitic extraintestinal manifestations of ulcerative colitis. Healing of pyoderma is prolonged and usually requires immunosuppression therapy with corticosteroids, immunosuppressive drugs (azathioprine, dapsone, or cyclosporine), and oral antibiotics for superinfection. Occasionally in severe and progressive cases, colectomy is required to promote healing.

Symptoms and signs of ocular manifestations of inflammatory bowel disease include blurred vision, eye pain, photophobia, inflammatory cells in the anterior chamber, and keratitic precipitates. Patients with uveitis often exhibit an association with HLA-B27, but patients with episcleritis and iritis usually do not have such an association. Once again, anti-inflammatory treatment of bowel disease is the recommended therapy.

Cholestatic liver disease, either pericholangitis or primary sclerosing cholangitis, is the most common hepatic abnormality of inflammatory bowel disease, seen in up to 5% of patients, and is more common in ulcerative colitis than in Crohn's disease. Patients with primary sclerosing cholangitis can develop worsening biliary obstruction and secondary biliary cirrhosis requiring consideration for liver transplantation. Extremely rarely, primary sclerosing cholangitis will progress to cholangiocarcinoma. Cholestatic liver disease in ulcerative colitis appears to be a risk factor for the development of cancer and dysplasia of the colon. Neither colectomy nor anti-inflammatory therapy are effective for treatment of primary sclerosing cholangitis.

Table 36-1 Truelove and Witts' Criteria for Disease Severity in Ulcerative Colitis

CRITERIA*	MILD ACTIVITY	SEVERE ACTIVITY
Daily bowel movements	≤5	>5
Hematochezia	Small amounts	Large amounts
Temperature	<37.5°C	≥37.5°C
Pulse	<90 bpm	≥90 bpm
Sedimentation rate	<30 mm/hr	≥30 mm/hr
Hemoglobin	>10 g/100 mL	≤10 g/100 mL

*Patients with some, but not all six, of the above criteria for severe activity have moderately active disease.

Medical Treatment Options

Medical treatment options for ulcerative colitis may be divided into conventional and alternative. Conventional agents are approved in the United States for use in ulcerative colitis. Alternative therapies are used for ulcerative colitis patients but are approved for other indications.

Conventional Therapies

Supportive measures are important initial therapy for patients with an inflammatory bowel disease flare. Fluids, anticholinergics, antidiarrheals, and some form of stress management, possibly psychiatric counseling, will ameliorate symptoms in some patients. Such treatment occasionally allows for the naturally remitting feature of the disease to manifest before more specific therapies are instituted.

In general, patients with active ulcerative colitis best tolerate a diet low in fiber. Complete bowel rest with total parenteral nutrition is not effective in ulcerative colitis patients, possibly due to low levels of luminal short-chain fatty acids (SCFAs) in fasting patients. SCFAs are produced from colonic bacterial fermentation of undigested dietary fiber and are preferred as fuel sources to glucose or ketone bodies by colonocytes in vitro. Unless ulcerative colitis patients are being prepared for surgery, it is best to allow enteral nutrition during a flare.

Enema preparations of concentrated SCFAs given twice daily have been used successfully to treat patients with active ulcerative proctosigmoiditis. Isosmotic, pH-neutral enemas of butyrate or a mixture of acetate, butyrate, and proprionate have been mostly successful for the topical treatment of left-sided disease refractory to conventional therapies. Eicosapentaenoic acid (fish oil) acts by competing with arachidonic acid for metabolism by lipoxygenase to produce leukotriene B5, a much less potent proinflammatory agent than the arachidonic acid metabolite leukotriene B4. High doses of orally administered fish oil have been shown to treat ulcerative colitis successfully and to allow steroids to be tapered, but the high doses necessary for an effect produce an unfortunate smell.

Salicylates

Sulfasalazine was first used in the 1940s for treatment of rheumatoid arthritis, but its effectiveness in ulcerative colitis was discovered soon after. Sulfasalazine is composed of a molecule of 5-aminosalicylic acid (5-ASA) linked by a diazo bond to sulfapyridine. 5-ASA, the active moiety for treating ulcerative colitis, is released in the colon when bacterial azo reductases cleave the diazo bond. The action of 5-ASA is mostly local and involves both interference with the cyclooxygenase and lipoxygenase pathways of arachidonic acid metabolism, as well as free radical scavenging. Sulfasalazine, up to 8 g per day, is useful in treating active disease, and at 2 g per day is used for maintaining remission for a year or more. Unfortunately, usefulness is limited by toxicity in approximately 40% of patients. Side effects include allergy, nausea, headaches, anorexia, hemolysis, neutropenia, hepatitis, pancreatitis, and azoospermia, and are mostly attributed to the sulfapyridine moiety of the molecule. Sulfasalazine is a competitive inhibitor of folic acid absorption; thus, folate-binding proteins should be overwhelmed with an oral supplement of folic acid.

Newer 5-ASA agents have improved on the adverse effect profile of sulfasalazine by eliminating the need for the carrier sulfapyridine. All these drugs are more costly, and none appear to be more effective than sulfasalazine. Alternative agents available in the United States approved for treatment in active ulcerative colitis patients are olsalazine (Dipentum), Asacol, balsalazide (Colazol), and Pentasa (Table 36-2). Olsalazine is composed of two 5-ASA molecules linked by a diazo bond. Colonic bacterial azo reductases are required for release of the active agents. Although olsalazine is effective, a profound secretory diarrhea occurs in more than 10% of patients and limits usefulness. Asacol consists of 5-ASA protected in a pH-sensitive eudragit-S capsule. When the pH approaches 7 in the terminal ileum, the compound dissolves and 5-ASA is released. Balsalazide is 5-ASA linked by a diazo bond to an inert carrier molecule. Colonic bacterial cleavage of the diazo bond is required for 5-ASA release. Therefore, balsalazide is effective only for colonic inflammation. Pentasa consists of 5-ASA packaged in a time-release ethylcellulose compound, releasing 5-ASA evenly throughout the small and large bowel. Even though it is approved for ulcerative colitis treatment only, the advantage of Pentasa over other 5-ASA preparations would be its potential value for treatment of small bowel inflammation of Crohn's disease.

Topical 5-ASA, Canasa, or Rowasa enemas or suppositories given once or twice per day are effective for treating distal disease. Even in patients with more proximal disease who are receiving oral 5-ASA therapy, topical therapy often will help the troubling symptoms of tenesmus, urgency, frequency, and bleeding. Occasionally, a patient with active pancolitis is completely asymptomatic once the rectal inflammation is controlled with topical 5-ASA therapy.

Corticosteroids

Corticosteroids, administered orally, intravenously, or topically, are highly effective for treatment of active ulcerative colitis. The mode of action is through inhibition of phospholipase A$_2$ and the subsequent decrease in levels of prostaglandins and leukotrienes. Long-term use of corticosteroids, though, is limited by adverse effects, and, therefore, corticosteroids cannot be used for disease that is slow to respond (refractory disease) or for maintenance therapy. The usual dose of prednisone where maximal effect is achieved with the fewest adverse effects is 40 mg per day. Doses higher than 40 mg per day are not more effective and have worse side effects. Intravenous corticosteroids are useful for severely active disease, but once again, doses need not exceed the prednisone equivalence of 40 mg per day. For left-sided disease, 100 mg hydrocortisone enemas delivered twice or three times per day are often effective. As with 5-ASA enemas, treatment of rectal disease often will greatly improve symptoms without controlling more proximal inflammation. Approximately 40% of a hydrocortisone enema is absorbed. Principal adverse effects of short-term corticosteroid use include glucose intolerance, acne, moon facies, insomnia, hyperphagia, psychosis,

Table 36-2 5-Aminosalicylic Acid Preparations Available in the United States and the Sites of Maximal Effect in the Gastrointestinal Tract

MEDICATION	UNIT DOSE	DOSAGE	COLON THERAPEUTIC ACTIVITY	SMALL BOWEL THERAPEUTIC ACTIVITY
Sulfasalazine	500 mg	2–4 g/day	+++	−
Olsalazine	250 mg	1–3 g/day	+++	−
Pentasa	250 mg	2–4 g/day	++	++
Asacol	400 mg	1.6–4.8 g/day	+++	+
Balsalazide	750 mg	6.75 g/day	+++	−
Rowasa enemas	4 g	4 g/day	+++	−
Rowasa suppositories	1 g	2 g/day	+++	−

Activity of agent: − = none/minimal, + = minor, ++ = moderate, +++ = good

headache, and peptic ulcer disease, and for long-term use side effects include hypertension, hyperlipidemia, hirsutism, cataracts, glaucoma, osteopenia, avascular necrosis, myopathy, and, possibly, pancreatitis.

Alternative Therapy. There has been much interest in producing steroid analogs that act as well as steroids but have fewer adverse effects. Such steroid analogs need to be protected from proximal absorption so they can act locally in areas of inflammation. Once absorbed, these drugs are metabolized and inactivated during the first pass in the liver. Of the three steroid analogs studied in ulcerative colitis—tixocortol, fluticasone, and budesonide—only budesonide has shown much promise. Budesonide is a potent, water-soluble analog of hydrocortisone and has been approved to treat active Crohn's disease of the distal small bowel and proximal colon. An enema preparation is available in Canada but not in the United States. In a randomized clinical trial with both extensive and limited ulcerative colitis patients, 10 mg budesonide given orally was equivalent in effectiveness, but with much less adrenal suppression, to 40 mg of prednisolone. For left-sided ulcerative colitis, 2-g budesonide enemas were as effective as prednisolone enemas or 5-ASA enemas.

Cyclosporine

Cyclosporin A is an 11–amino acid cyclic polypeptide derived from two types of fungi and is in widespread use as an immunosuppressant in organ transplantation. It reversibly inhibits interleukin-2 (IL-2) gene transcription, which in turn reduces the activation of lymphocytes, mostly T-helper lymphocytes; T-suppressor lymphocytes, B lymphocytes, and macrophages are mostly spared. Cyclosporine is 80% bound to lipoproteins and, because it is secreted in the bile, requires an intact enterohepatic circulation to maintain levels. It is metabolized and inactivated by the hepatic cytochrome p450 system, and levels will be affected by drugs that induce cytochrome p450. Nephrotoxicity, hepatotoxicity, hypertrichosis, gingival hyperplasia, tremors, paresthesias, seizures, and lymphoproliferative disorders are the most common adverse effects. Cyclosporine, apparently, does not adversely influence the safety of urgent colectomy for ulcerative colitis. From a series of 14 patients unsuccessfully treated with cyclosporine, the complication rate following colectomy

was not unusually high and the length of postoperative stay was not inordinately long.

A randomized clinical trial of 4 mg/kg/day of intravenous cyclosporine for 20 severely active ulcerative colitis patients showed complete clinical response within a mean of 7 days in 9 of 11 (82%) patients treated with cyclosporine and in none of 9 patients treated with placebo. The trial was terminated early due to the ethical considerations. Long-term response on oral cyclosporine of at least 6 months with avoidance of colectomy was seen in only 5 of the original 11 patients (45%). Of note, 5 of the 9 placebo-treated patients were well enough to receive cyclosporine rather than have colectomy, and all 5 responded in the short and long term. Experience throughout the United States has not demonstrated such overwhelming success. A review of experience in the Seattle community showed a 57% short-term response and 33% long-term response. Enemas of 350 mg cyclosporine are not more effective than placebo for left-sided ulcerative colitis.

Azathioprine and 6-Mercaptopurine

6-Mercaptopurine (6-MP), a purine analog, and its S-imidazole precursor azathioprine are immunosuppressive agents that act by causing chromosome breaks and blunting the proliferation of rapidly dividing cells, such as lymphocytes. There is preferential suppression of T cells over B cells. Both medications are metabolized by the xanthine oxidase system and should be used with caution and at low doses with allopurinol. Azathioprine and 6-MP have a more favorable adverse effect profile than corticosteroids. Approximately 2% of patients will require discontinuation due to reversible marrow suppression, 3% will develop acute pancreatitis, and 2% will develop allergy characterized by abdominal pain, fever, and rash. A histiocytic lymphoma of the brain has been reported in a patient taking 6-MP.

For ulcerative colitis patients refractory to 5-ASA and steroids, 6-MP can induce a remission and allow steroids to be tapered or minimized in more than half of patients. Hence, these medications have been termed *steroid-sparing*. Furthermore, azathioprine or 6-MP can maintain a remission induced by steroids or cyclosporine for at least 2 years. The duration of therapy most often required for effectiveness is at least 3 months, and delayed therapeutic responses have been demonstrated after 1 year of therapy.

Because of the delay, adjusting the dose according to response, as in most clinical situations, may not be feasible. It has been suggested that the dose of these immunosuppressants be increased until mild leukopenia develops. Crohn's disease patients treated for leukopenia have a faster and more complete response. It has yet to be shown that measuring the 6-MP metabolites, 6-thioguanine and 6-methylmercaptopurine, can guide clinicians to find the very narrow window between effectiveness and toxicity.

Alternative Therapies

Nicotine. Interesting case reports and remarkably consistent epidemiologic studies have shown that cigarette smoking confers protection from the development of ulcerative colitis. Current adult smokers are less likely than community-based control subjects to develop ulcerative colitis; former smokers are more likely than control subjects to develop ulcerative colitis. At the time of diagnosis, less than 20% of ulcerative colitis patients are smokers, compared to upward of 35% in the U.S. adult population. Exposure to passive smoking increases, not decreases, the risk in children of developing ulcerative colitis. The mechanism of the protective effect of cigarette smoking on ulcerative colitis in adults is not known but could be related to the potentiation of colonic mucus among smokers.

Randomized clinical trials have shown that treating mildly to moderately active ulcerative colitis patients with either nicotine gum at 20 mg per day or nicotine patches up to 25 mg per day is successful, especially in former smokers. Compared to 15 mg of prednisolone, the beneficial effect of nicotine patches is not as great. Typical side effects (parched throat, tachycardia, headache, and nausea) of the "nicotine rush" are minimized with the use of the patch instead of the gum. Nicotine addiction is not a problem if therapy lasts less than 8 weeks. Maintenance therapy with nicotine patches is not effective.

Heparin. It was found serendipitously that a patient with active ulcerative colitis who required heparin for deep venous thrombosis went into complete remission.

Treatment of an additional nine patients with active ulcerative colitis refractory to corticosteroids with 10,000 units of heparin subcutaneously twice daily showed a complete remission in eight patients and a partial response in the other patient. Another report showed that heparin administration induced a rapid resolution of chronically active symptoms of ulcerative colitis, arthralgia, and pyoderma gangrenosum. If the pathogenesis of ulcerative colitis includes microthrombosis in the intestinal circulation, then the counterintuitive use of heparin may be a therapeutic advance. Prospective clinical trials are awaited.

Clinical Scenarios

Various common clinical scenarios for ulcerative colitis patients suggests different treatment options using the above-mentioned medications. Table 36-3 summarizes some of these options, which are discussed in the following sections.

Quiescent Disease

Remission may be maintained in ulcerative colitis patients with long-term use of a 5-ASA product or azathioprine. These drugs are effective for at least 2 years.

Mildly or Moderately Active Disease

Many treatment options are available for patients with mildly to moderately active disease. An oral or topical 5-ASA product is the usual first-line agent and often is effective. Both oral and topical agents may be given in patients with extensive disease to treat the rectal and proximal disease separately. For patients who do not respond to 5-ASA, prednisone use of up to 40 mg per day often is effective. Other alternative therapeutic options that may be used instead of or in conjunction with steroids are nicotine patches, short-chain fatty acid enemas, or heparin.

Severely Active Disease

Patients with severely active disease most often will require hospital admission and the use of intravenous steroids. 5-ASA agents are not effective in this setting. If symptoms do not resolve within 7 days, consideration should be

---

Table 36-3 Clinical Scenarios of Ulcerative Colitis and Recommended Medical Options

CLINICAL SCENARIO	RECOMMENDED MEDICAL OPTIONS
Quiescent disease	5-Aminosalicylic acid Azathioprine or 6-mercaptopurine
Mildly or moderately active disease	5-Aminosalicylic acid, corticosteroids Alternative therapies: nicotine, short-chain fatty acid enemas, heparin
Severely active colitis	Intravenous corticosteroids Intravenous cyclosporine
Fulminant or toxic colitis	Intravenous corticosteroids
Refractory disease and steroid dependence	Azathioprine or 6-mercaptopurine, methotrexate Alternative therapies: nicotine, short-chain fatty acid enemas, heparin
Pregnancy	5-Aminosalicylic acid and/or corticosteroids
Cancer risk	Surveillance colonoscopy with colectomy for the detection of any dysplasia Folic acid supplementation

given for either the addition of intravenous cyclosporine or surgery. If cyclosporine fails within 14 days (response is usually within the first 7 days), then surgery should be recommended. If cyclosporine induces a remission, this remission may be maintained with azathioprine.

Fulminant or Toxic Colitis

The medical options for patients with fulminant or toxic colitis are limited. Intravenous corticosteroids are the only presurgical option, and a response must be rapid for the patient to avoid surgery. Intravenous antibiotics are often used but have been shown to be ineffective and, in fact, could exacerbate symptoms if an antibiotic-associated colitis develops.

Refractory Disease and Steroid Dependence

Persistent symptoms of mildly to moderately active disease despite 5-ASA agents and steroids will require additional medical therapy. Symptoms that recur soon after prednisone is tapered also will require additional therapy. The principal additional agents in these settings are either azathioprine or 6-MP. Maximal doses, up to 6-MP 1.5 mg/kg/day or azathioprine 2.5 mg/kg/day, should be given if tolerated for a minimum of 1 year prior to abandoning therapy and resorting to surgery. Other possible alternative therapeutic agents for refractory disease or steroid dependence include nicotine patches, short-chain fatty acid enemas, or heparin.

Pregnancy

Treating the mother is the most important watchword of medical therapy in ulcerative colitis patients. If the mother's disease is under control, the chance for premature labor or spontaneous abortion is no different from that for an unaffected mother. The activity of inflammatory bowel disease in the mother during pregnancy is dependent on the disease activity at the time of conception. If the disease is inactive at conception, the probability of a serious flare developing during pregnancy is low. Conversely, if conception occurs during relapse, there is a 30% chance of further worsening of symptoms during pregnancy.

Prednisone and the 5-ASA agents are very safe during pregnancy and should be used if the mother requires these medications to maintain remission or control symptoms. Low-birth-weight infants, once believed to be due to corticosteroid use during pregnancy, are now believed to be related to disease activity and nutritional deficiencies. Even though sulfasalazine has a sulfa moiety, sulfasalazine does not cause kernicterus. Azathioprine and 6-MP have been used often in uneventful pregnancies. However, these medications are not recommended during pregnancy and extreme caution as well as frank discussions with the patient are necessary when prescribing these therapies. Methotrexate is contraindicated during pregnancy.

Cancer Risk

Over the course of the disease, colorectal cancer will occur in approximately 6% and be the cause of death in 3% of ulcerative colitis patients with extensive disease, rates that are much higher than for the general population (Lashner, 1992; Connell et al, 1994). The risk for colorectal cancer is known to increase with increasing extent and duration of disease, with older age at symptom onset, and with primary sclerosing cholangitis. High-risk patients, those with extensive disease for at least 7 years, should be advised to enroll in surveillance programs in which colonoscopies with frequent biopsies are performed every 1 to 3 years, depending on the patient's individual risk. In the early years of disease (7 to 20 years) colonoscopy every 3 years is recommended, in the middle years (20 to 30 years) colonoscopy every 2 years is recommended, and beyond 30 years, when the risk is highest, annual colonoscopy is recommended (Lashner, 1992). Patients with primary sclerosing cholangitis should be surveyed annually. Total proctocolectomy is recommended if either low-grade or high-grade dysplasia or asymptomatic cancer is detected (Riddell et al, 1983; Bernstein et al, 1994). Additional indications for colectomy include a stricture or extensive pseudopolyposis that cannot be adequately surveyed. Although these recommendations have not been demonstrated to reduce the cancer-related mortality rate compared to an unscreened population, cancer surveillance for ulcerative colitis patients has become the standard of care and must be offered to eligible patients.

The only medical therapy that may prevent the development of cancer or dysplasia is folic acid supplementation. Patients with ulcerative colitis are especially prone to develop folic acid deficiency due to intestinal losses from active disease, inadequate intake, and competitive inhibition of absorption by sulfasalazine. Folic acid supplementation with 0.4 mg in a multivitamin or 1 mg in a sole supplement should be given routinely to ulcerative colitis patients.

■ OTHER COLITIDES

Interestingly, some of the therapies typically used for ulcerative colitis have been used successfully for treating other colitides.

Collagenous and Lymphocytic Colitis

Collagenous and lymphocytic colitis account for approximately 5% of chronic secretory diarrheas. Typically, patients with collagenous or lymphocytic colitis are females who present in the sixth decade of life with chronic watery diarrhea, usually greater than 500 mL per day, that does not improve with fasting and, on electrolyte analysis, does not have an osmolar gap. Diarrhea may be intermittent and may include a mucous discharge, but there usually is no hematochezia. These diseases are associated with rheumatoid arthritis, scleroderma, atrophic gastritis, chronic active hepatitis, primary biliary cirrhosis, hypothyroidism, hyperthyroidism, Hodgkin's disease, and non-Hodgkin's lymphoma. The diagnosis can be confirmed by documenting a secretory diarrhea, normal-appearing colonic mucosa at colonoscopy, and abnormal histologic appearance. Specimens from collagenous colitis patients have a band of eosinophilic deposits, composed of type III collagen and fibronectin, under the surface epithelium. The band measures between 7 and 100 μm in thickness. Other findings include a thickened basement membrane and an excess of lymphocytes, plasma cells, eosinophils, and mast cells in the lamina propria. Patients with lymphocytic colitis have no subepithelial eosinophilic deposit. Histologic abnormalities may be limited to the proximal colon, spare the rectum, and be discontinuous, making colonoscopy with extensive biopsy of the right and left side necessary.

The natural history of collagenous and lymphocytic colitis is usually self-limited. The diarrhea may resolve even without resolution of the eosinophilic deposition. There appears to be no malignant potential and no risk of development of inflammatory bowel disease. Histologic regression of the collagen deposits and improvement of diarrhea have been reported with prednisolone or sulfasalazine. Bismuth subsalicylate and loperamide also can control symptoms, but histologic improvement has not been documented with these agents.

Diversion Colitis

Diversion colitis, bypass colitis, exclusion colitis, and disuse colitis are synonyms for the colonic inflammatory process that invariably occurs when the fecal stream is diverted from a colonic segment. Symptoms completely resolve with reanastomosis. Except with inflammatory bowel disease patients, there is no evidence for inflammation in the distal segment prior to surgery. Hematochezia and mucous discharge from the rectum or mucous fistula are the primary symptoms that may occur as early as 1 month following diversion but have been reported as much as 3 years later. Patients with diversion colitis may be asymptomatic with only pathologic or endoscopic findings. Typical histologic findings include mucin depletion, mucosal edema, decreased number and depths of crypts, superficial ulcerations, expansion of cellular elements of the lamina propria, granulocyte infiltration, and fibrosis of the lamina propria. The colonoscopic appearance of a diverted segment may show typical features of colitis such as narrowing, erythema, ulceration, friability, exudate, or a distorted mucosal vascular pattern.

The three proposed pathogenetic hypotheses of diversion colitis include stasis of enteric succus, colonization from pathogenic bacteria, and loss of luminal nutrients. Saline enemas are ineffective treatment for diversion colitis, making stasis an unlikely cause. The anaerobic bacteria count in the diverted colon drops by 100-fold following diversion, a number which is too small to increase breath hydrogen following glucose enema administration. Furthermore, antibiotic treatment designed to restore presurgical proportions of bacterial species have not improved colonoscopic findings. However, replacement of luminal nutrients markedly improves symptoms and findings, making this purported etiology the most likely.

Colonocytes are nourished from the bloodstream as well as from luminal contents. Unabsorbed carbohydrates are metabolized by colonic bacteria to synthesize short chain fatty acids (SCFAs). In vitro studies have shown that SCFAs are a preferred fuel source over glucose or ketone bodies. The most favored nutrient source for colonocytes is butyrate, but proprionate and acetate also are utilized effi-

ciently. Blood concentrations of SCFAs are negligible. From a normal diet in an intact colon, a concentration of 100 to 200 mM/L of SCFAs is recovered in stool, while a diverted segment has less than 5 mM/L. Twice-daily 60-mL SCFA enemas delivered into the diverted segment completely resolved symptoms and endoscopic or histologic inflammation. One formulation that works well is a combination of 60 mM acetate, 30 mM proprionate, and 40 mM butyrate with sufficient sodium chloride and sodium hydroxide to bring the osmolality to 280 mOsm and the pH to 7.0; 100 mM butyrate enemas at the same osmolality and pH should also be successful. Responses also have been seen with 5-aminosalicylic acid enemas (Tripodi and associates, 1992). The best therapy for diversion colitis is reanastomosis. However, enemas given daily or even every other day can be used to maintain remission until reanastomosis becomes feasible.

Radiation Colopathy

Radiation therapy delivered to organs adjacent to the colon or rectum often induces a radiation colopathy in 5 to 10% of patients. With newer concentrating techniques, the dose-limiting organ capable of tolerating ionizing radiation has changed from the skin to the gastrointestinal tract. The most common malignancies that are usually treated with radiation and that cause radiation colitis are transitional cell carcinoma of the bladder, squamous cell carcinoma of the cervix, endometrial cancer, and adenocarcinoma of the prostate or rectum.

Early radiation injury is caused by direct damage to the crypt cells of the epithelium, and late injury is caused by damage to the vascular endothelium and connective tissue; 6000 cGy delivered to a region of the colon or 8000 cGy delivered to the rectum will induce early or late radiation colopathy in approximately 50% of patients. Apparently, the margin of safety is very narrow because these doses are close to those required for treatment of the tumor.

Early radiation colopathy often occurs within the first month of therapy. With epithelial disruption, diarrhea, hematochezia, tenesmus, and mucous discharge are the most common presenting symptoms. Colonoscopically, the mucosa is edematous, with a loss of mucosal vascular pattern, friable, and with superficial ulcerations, all findings similar to ulcerative colitis. The extent of involvement, though, is confined to the radiated part, and not continuous as in ulcerative colitis. Histologic findings include a decrease in the height of the epithelial cells, mucin depletion, ulceration, and crypt abscesses. Anterior rectal ulcerations, luminal narrowing, radiologic "thumbprinting," and loss of haustrations are additional signs of early toxicity.

Therapy of early radiation toxicity includes symptomatic treatment such as antispasmodics, antidiarrheals, bulking agents, and topical anesthetics. Steroid enemas may help but 5-aminosalicylic acid agents are not effective. Attempts to minimize the risk of developing early radiation injury include surgical fixation of bowel away from the anticipated port, administration of free radical scavengers such as diallyl sulfide (garlic), use of cyclooxygenase inhibitors such as aspirin, hyperbaric oxygen, or glutamine-supplemented diets.

Late injury from radiation therapy often occurs within 5 years but may not occur for several decades after therapy. Symptoms are slowly progressive and are related to changes in the submucosal layers. Common presenting complaints include abdominal pain and diarrhea related to the development of fibrous strictures and partial obstruction. Fistulas, perforation, and impaired motility may also occur. For late radiation proctopathy, tenesmus, mucous discharge, change in stool caliber, and hematochezia are other presenting complaints. Endoscopically, telangiectasias, granularity, friability, discrete ulcers in the anterior rectum, and strictures are often found. Late radiation injury resembles ischemia with submucosal fibrosis, telangiectasias of small vessels, hyalinized endothelium of larger blood vessel walls, fistulas, and fissures.

Treatment of late complications of radiation therapy is often not effective. Steroid enemas or other medical therapies are of marginal benefit. Nd:YAG (neodymium: yttrium-aluminum-garnet) laser or bipolar electrocoagulation of bleeding telangiectases may help with hematochezia. Occasionally, strictures can be dilated manually or with endoscopically placed balloon dilators. Because of the brittle nature of radiated bowel, perforation is a frequent complication of bowel dilation. Surgery for obstruction, bleeding, fistulas, or perforation is high risk because of frequent delayed healing of the wound and surgical anastomosis.

Drug-Induced Colitis

Certain drugs may cause inflammation of the colon indistinguishable endoscopically from inflammatory bowel disease. The distinction, though, is most important because drug-induced colitis is best treated by withdrawal of the medication, and inflammatory bowel disease often requires the institution of potentially toxic medications. Mucosal inflammation of the colon is a rare adverse effect from some commonly used medications such as oral contraceptives and nonsteroidal anti-inflammatory drugs (NSAIDs). Even if the incidence of colitis is exceedingly low, the common use of these medications makes drug-induced colitis potentially a more important problem than inflammatory bowel disease. Other medications that may cause a drug-induced colitis include methyldopa, penicillamine, potassium supplements, 5-fluorouracil, oral gold, and isotretinoin.

The colitis from oral contraceptives can be indistinguishable from Crohn's colitis, with patients presenting with chronic diarrhea and having aphthoid ulcers throughout the colon (Tedesco and associates, 1982). Symptoms and signs of oral contraceptive colitis completely resolve without sequelae upon discontinuation of the hormone. The pathogenesis is believed to be due to an occlusive vascular phenomenon.

The colitis from oral NSAIDs mimics ulcerative colitis in symptoms and colonoscopic appearance. The inflammation is diffuse with superficial ulcerations. The pathogenesis of NSAID-induced colitis involves cyclooxygenase inhibition and the loss of cytoprotective prostaglandins.

The differentiation between inflammatory bowel disease and NSAID-induced colitis is further complicated because arthritis, a condition usually treated with NSAIDs, may or may not be related to inflammatory bowel disease. A patient who is being treated for arthritis and who develops symptoms and signs suggestive of ulcerative colitis should have drug-induced colitis ruled out by observing symptoms after NSAID discontinuation prior to confirming a diagnosis of inflammatory bowel disease. NSAIDs also may induce a flare of ulcerative colitis in remission. Severe complications besides bleeding include stricture from submucosal fibrosis, perforation from deep ulceration, and diaphragmatic-like narrowing in the small bowel or the colon.

Suggested Readings

Adler DJ, Korelitz BI: The therapeutic efficacy of 6-mercaptopurine in refractory ulcerative colitis. Am J Gastroenterol 1990;85:717–722.

Bernstein CN, Shanahan F, Weinstein WM: Are we telling patients the truth about surveillance colonoscopy in ulcerative colitis? Lancet 1994;343:71–74.

Bjarnason I, Zanelli G, Smith T, et al: Nonsteroidal anti-inflammatory drug-induced intestinal inflammation in humans. Gastroenterology 1987;93:480–489.

Boyko EJ, Koepsell TD, Perera DR, Inui TS: Risk of ulcerative colitis among former and current cigarette smokers. N Engl J Med 1987;316:707–710.

Breuer RI, Soergel KH, Lashner BA, et al: Short chain fatty acid rectal irrigation for left-sided ulcerative colitis: A randomized, placebo-controlled trial. Gut 1997;40:485–491.

Brzezinski A, Rankin GB, Seidner DL, Lashner BA: Use of old and new oral 5-aminosalicylic acid formulations in inflammatory bowel disease. Cleve Clin J Med 1995;62:317–323.

Cabrere GE, Scopelitis E, Cuellar ML, et al: Pneumatosis cystoides intestinalis in systemic lupus erythematosus with intestinal vasculitis: Treatment with high dose prednisone. Clin Rheumatol 1994;13:312–316.

Colonna T, Korelitz BI: The role of leukopenia in the 6-mercaptopurine-induced remission of refractory Crohn's disease. Am J Gastroenterol 1994;89:362–366.

Connell WR, Lennard-Jones JE, Williams CB, et al: Factors affecting the outcome of endoscopic surveillance for cancer in ulcerative colitis. Gastroenterology 1994;107:934–944.

Dwarakanath AD, Yu LG, Brooks C, Pryce D, Rhodes JM: "Sticky" neutrophils, pathergic arthritis, and response to heparin in pyoderma gangrenosum complicating ulcerative colitis. Gut 1995;37:585–588.

Ernest DL, Trier JS: Radiation enteritis and colitis. In Sleisenger MH, Fordtran JS (Eds.). Gastrointestinal Disease, 5th ed. Philadelphia, WB Saunders, 1993.

Farmer RG, Easley KA, Rankin GB: Clinical patterns, natural history, and progression of ulcerative colitis: A long-term follow-up of 1,116 patients. Dig Dis Sci 1993;38:1137–1146.

Fernandez-Banares F, Bertran X, Esteve-Comas M, et al: Azathioprine is useful in maintaining long-term remission induced by intravenous cyclosporine in steroid-refractory severe ulcerative colitis. Am J Gastroenterol 1996;91:2498–2499.

Fleshner PR, Michelassi F, Rubin M, et al: Morbidity of subtotal colectomy in patients with severe ulcerative colitis unresponsive to cyclosporine. Dis Colon Rectum 1995;38:1241–1245.

Gaffney PR, Doyle CT, Gaffney A, et al: Paradoxical response to heparin in 10 patients with ulcerative colitis. Am J Gastroenterol 1995;90:220–223.

Galandiuk S, Fazio V: Pneumatosis cystoides intestinalis: A review of the literature. Dis Colon Rectum 1986;29:358–363.

Guest CB, Reznick RK: Colitis cystica profunda: Review of the literature. Dis Colon Rectum 1989;32:983–988.

Harig JM, Soergel KH, Komorowski RA, Wood CM: Treatment of diversion colitis with short-chain fatty acid irrigation. N Engl J Med 1989;320:23–28.

Hawthorne AB, Logan RFA, Hawkey CJ: Randomized controlled trial of azathioprine withdrawal in ulcerative colitis. Br Med J 1992;305:20–22.

Kobayashi T, Kobayashi M, Naka M, et al: Response to octreotide of intestinal pseudoobstruction and pneumatosis cystoides intestinalis associated with progressive systemic sclerosis. Intern Med 1993;32:607–609.

Kozarek R, Bedard C, Patterson D, et al: Cyclosporine use in the precolectomy chronic ulcerative colitis patient: A community experience and its relationship to prospective and controlled clinical trials. Am J Gastroenterol 1995;90:2093–2096.

Lashner BA: Recommendations for colorectal cancer surveillance in ulcerative colitis: A review of research from a single university-based surveillance program. Am J Gastroenterol 1992;87:168–175.

Lashner BA: Red blood cell folate is associated with the development of dysplasia and cancer in ulcerative colitis. J Cancer Res Clin Oncol 1993;119:549–554.

Lashner BA, Hanauer SB, Silverstein MD: Testing nicotine gum for ulcerative colitis patients: Experience with single patient trials. Dig Dis Sci 1990;35:827–832.

Lashner BA, Heidenreich PA, Su GL, et al: Effect of folate supplementation on the incidence of dysplasia and cancer in chronic ulcerative colitis. Gastroenterology 1989;97:255–259.

Lashner BA, Kirsner JB: Inflammatory bowel disease in older people. Clin Geriatr Med 1991;7(2):287–299.

Lashner BA, Provencher KS, Seidner DL, et al: The effect of folic acid supplementation on the risk for cancer or dysplasia in ulcerative colitis. Gastroenterology 1997;112:29–32.

Lashner BA, Shaheen MJ, Hanauer SB, Kirschner BS: Passive smoking is associated with an increased risk of developing inflammatory bowel disease in children. Am J Gastroenterol 1993;88:336–359.

Lemann M, Galian A, Rutgeerts P, et al: Comparison of budesonide and 5-aminosalicylic acid enemas in active distal ulcerative colitis. Aliment Pharmacol Ther 1995;9:557–562.

Lichtiger S, Present DH, Kornbluth A, et al: Cyclosporine in severe ulcerative colitis refractory to steroid therapy. N Engl J Med 1994;330:1841–1845.

Lofberg R, Danielsson A, Suhr O, et al: Oral budesonide versus prednisolone in patients with active extensive and left-sided ulcerative colitis. Gastroenterology 1996;110:1713–1718.

Lofberg R, Ostergaard Thomsen O, et al: Budesonide versus prednisolone retention enemas in active distal ulcerative colitis. Aliment Pharmacol Ther 1994;8:623–629.

Mantzaris GJ, Hatzis A, Kontogiannis P, Treadaphyllou G: Intravenous tobramycin and metronidazole as an adjunct to corticosteroids in acute, severe ulcerative colitis. Am J Gastroenterol 1994;89:43–46.

Meyers S, Sachar DB, Present DH, Janowitz HD: Olsalazine sodium in the treatment of ulcerative colitis among patients intolerant of sulfasalazine: A prospective, randomized, placebo-controlled, double-blind, dose-ranging clinical trial. Gastroenterology 1987;93:1255–1262.

Nakada T, Kubota Y, Sasagawa I, et al: Therapeutic experience of hyperbaric oxygenation in radiation colitis: Report of a case. Dis Colon Rectum 1993;36:962–965.

Present DH: 6-Mercaptopurine and other immunosuppressive agents in the treatment of Crohn's disease and ulcerative colitis. Gastroenterol Clin North Am 1989;18:57–72.

Present DH, Meltzer SJ, Krumholz MP, et al: 6-Mercaptopurine in the management of inflammatory bowel disease: Short- and long-term toxicity. Ann Intern Med 1989;111:641–649.

Pullan RD, Rhodes J, Ganesh S, et al: Transdermal nicotine for active ulcerative colitis. N Engl J Med 1994;330:811–815.

Retsky JE, Kraft SC: The extraintestinal manifestations of inflammatory bowel disease. In Kirsner JB, Shorter RG (Eds.): Inflammatory Bowel Disease, 4th ed. Baltimore, Williams & Wilkins, 1995.

Riddell RH, Goldman H, Ransohoff DF, et al: Dysplasia in inflammatory bowel disease: Standardized classification with provisional clinical applications. Hum Pathol 1983;14:931–968.

Rokkas T, Filipe MI, Sladen GE: Collagenous colitis with rapid response to sulfasalazine. Postgrad Med J 1988;64:74–76.

Sandborn WJ, Tremaine WJ, Offord KP, et al: Transdermal nicotine for mildly to moderately active ulcerative colitis. Ann Intern Med 1997;126:364–371.

Sandborn WJ, Tremaine WJ, Schroeder KW, et al: A placebo-controlled trial of cyclosporine enemas for mildly to moderately active left-sided ulcerative colitis. Gastroenterology 1994;106:1429–1435.

Selhub J, Dhar GJ, Rosenberg IH: Inhibition of folate enzymes by sulfasalazine. J Clin Invest 1978;61:221–224.

Sheppach W, Sommer H, Kirchner T, et al: Effect of butyrate enemas on the colonic mucosa in distal ulcerative colitis. Gastroenterology 1992;103:51–56.

Shetty K, Rybicki L, Brzezinski A, et al: The risk of cancer or dysplasia in ulcerative colitis patients with primary sclerosing cholangitis. Am J Gastroenterol 1999;94:1643–1649.

Silverstein MD, Lashner BA, Hanauer SB: Cigarette smoking and ulcerative colitis: A case-control study. Mayo Clin Proc 1994;69:425–429.

Sloth H, Bisgaard C, Grove A: Collagenous colitis: A prospective trial of prednisolone in six patients. J Intern Med 1991;229:443–446.

Souba WW, Klimberg VS, Copeland EM: Glutamine nutrition in the management of radiation enteritis. J Parent Enteral Nutr 1990;14:106S–108S.

Stampfl DA, Friedman LS: Collagenous colitis: Pathophysiologic considerations. Dig Dis Sci 1991;36:705–711.

Steinhart AH, Brzezinski A, Baker JP: Treatment of refractory ulcerative proctosigmoiditis with butyrate enemas. Am J Gastroenterol 1994;89:179–183.

Stenson WF, Cort D, Rodgers J, et al: Dietary supplementation with fish oil in ulcerative colitis. Ann Intern Med 1992;116:609–614.

Tedesco FJ, Volpicelli NA, Moore FS: Estrogen- and progesterone-associated colitis: A disorder with clinical and endoscopic features mimicking Crohn's colitis. Gastrointest Endosc 1982;28:247–249.

Thomas GA, Rhodes J, Ragunath K, et al: Transdermal nicotine compared with oral prednisolone therapy for active ulcerative colitis. Eur J Gastroenterol Hepatol 1996;8:769–776.

Thomas GAO, Rhodes J, Mani V, et al: Transdermal nicotine as maintenance therapy for ulcerative colitis. N Engl J Med 1995;332:988–992.

Tripodi J, Gorcey S, Burakoff R: A case of diversion colitis treated with 5-aminosalicylic acid enemas. Am J Gastroenterol 1992;87:645–647.

Truelove SC, Witts LJ: Cortisone in ulcerative colitis: Final report on a therapeutic trial. BMJ 1955;2:1041–1048.

Valenzuela M, Martin-Ruiz JL, Alvarez-Cienfuegos E, et al: Colitis cystica profunda: Imaging diagnosis and conservative treatment: Report of two cases. Dis Colon Rectum 1996;39:587–590.

Zala L, Hunziker T, Braathen LR: Pigmentation following long-term bismuth therapy for pneumatosis cystoides intestinalis. Dermatology 1993;187:288–289.

37

CHRONIC ULCERATIVE COLITIS: SURGICAL OPTIONS

P. J. McMurrick, MBBS (Hon), FRACS
R. R. Dozois, MD, MS, FACS, FRCS (Glas) (Hon), DSC

Prior to the late 1960s, surgical options for patients with chronic ulcerative colitis (CUC) were limited to total proctocolectomy with permanent Brooke ileostomy or colectomy with ileorectal anastomosis. Retaining the rectum avoided a permanent stoma, but left a substantive focus of disease, with its potential for recurrent disease or cancer. Two other surgical options were subsequently developed: the continent reservoir ileostomy, or Kock pouch, and the ileal pouch–anal anastomosis (IPAA). The latter has become firmly established as the operation preferred by most patients, because of the advantages of complete eradication of disease, avoidance of a permanent stoma, and excellent long-term outcome. More recently, some surgeons have abandoned mucosectomy to simplify the procedure and improve nighttime continence. It is the purpose of this chapter to clarify the indications for surgery in patients with CUC, to define the current role of the various surgical options, to discuss technical aspects of each operation, and to highlight the recognition and management of special difficulties.

■ INDICATIONS FOR OPERATION IN CHRONIC ULCERATIVE COLITIS

Chronic Ulcerative Colitis Refractory to Medical Management

This group includes patients whose symptoms cannot be controlled with maximal medications or who require continuous or frequent courses of steroids and other immunosuppressives.

Onset of Complications of Medical Management

In those patients for whom medical control of ulcerative colitis requires chronic use of steroids or immunosuppressive agents, morbidity relating to these medications is common. In this setting the "cost" of morbidity of ongoing medications needs to be carefully weighed against the likely favorable outcome of surgery.

Elevated Risk or Diagnosis of Colonic Carcinoma

The risk of colonic carcinoma in ulcerative colitis is significantly elevated after approximately 8 to 10 years of disease, particularly in those patients with pancolonic involvement. This risk is particularly high in patients with epithelial dysplasia and DALM (dysplasia-associated lesion or mass), which is associated with a 40 to 50% rate of occult malignancy. Although colectomy is mandated in patients with high-grade dysplasia, increasing evidence of a significant risk of clinically silent carcinoma in low-grade dysplasia has seen a broadening of the indications for surgery. This risk of carcinoma in patients with low-grade dysplasia is not clearly established, but is in the order of 10 to 20% at the time of colonic resection. This group of patients should be fully informed of the elevated risk of developing carcinoma, and offered the opportunity to discuss the risks and benefits of proctocolectomy, even if the clinical course of their disease may have been stable. Finally, the diagnosis of an established carcinoma obviously mandates surgical resection, but may not preclude the restorative proctocolectomy.

Patient Choice

Many patients with incapacitating disease, when fully informed of the expected outcome of the ileoanal pouch procedure, will opt for surgery. All patients with CUC that demonstrates frequent clinical flares or has proved difficult to control with medical therapy should be offered this option. The discussion entails full disclosure of expected morbidity, and the option of resection should be weighed against the option of ongoing medical therapy, which has its own related morbidity. It has been our experience that close cooperation between the physician and the surgeon managing patients with CUC promotes rational and informed decision making by the patient.

A treatment algorithm aimed at guiding decision-making in patients with CUC is presented in Figure 37-1.

■ PREPARATION FOR SURGERY

To optimize the outcome of surgery, patients should be taken to surgery in good general condition. Specifically, significantly malnourished patients should undergo a pre-

CUC refractory to medical management
    Steroid dependent
    Multiple flares
Onset of complications of medical management
Increased risk of carcinoma
    Duration > 10 years
    Dysplasia or "DALM"
Patient choice

Figure 37-1
Treatment decision making in chronic ulcerative colitis.

operative period of nutritional support, which may entail either nasogastric hyperalimentation or parenteral nutrition. Patients with an albumin level of less than 2.5 g/dL have an increased rate of postoperative morbidity. Preoperative parenteral nutrition should be considered in those patients who have been admitted with an acute flare of disease, and in whom surgery is a likely prospect. The hemoglobin level should be corrected to within normal limits. Patients with current or recent steroid use will require perioperative steroid coverage with gradual postoperative taper.

■ ILEAL POUCH–ANAL ANASTOMOSIS

Rationale
This procedure entails resection of the cecum, colon, proximal rectum, and distal rectal mucosa, thus fully eradicating all colonic and rectal manifestations of the disease and its cancer risk. The addition of an ileal reservoir anastomosed to the anal canal allows re-establishment of intestinal continuity and preservation of fecal continence. Because the distal rectal mucosa is excised endoanally, the risk of damage to the nerve supply of the pelvic organs is reduced, and there is no potentially troublesome perineal wound.

Patient Selection
Prior to consenting to undergoing restorative proctocolectomy, the patient must have reasonable expectations of outcome after the procedure. In our experience, patients will average six bowel movements per day, with reasonable ability to discriminate gas from stool. Genuine preoperative incontinence is a strong contraindication to pouch surgery (see later discussion). In addition, a variable degree of nocturnal minor incontinence must be expected, and the patient must be prepared and healthy enough to undergo a two-stage procedure. Patients whose lifestyle or profession would not permit such limitations must be considered for alternative procedures.

Technique of Operation
The operation of IPAA, when performed for CUC, is most commonly performed in two stages. Restorative proctocolectomy protected by a diverting ileostomy is the first stage, and takedown of the ileostomy is the second. The anesthetized patient is positioned on the operating table in the modified Trendelenburg position, permitting ready access to the abdomen and the perineum, reducing operating time, and avoiding the potential risk of prematurely removing the rectum in a patient who at laparotomy may be found to have Crohn's colitis and in whom rectal preservation might have been feasible. Given that the procedure usually takes more than 3 hours to perform, meticulous attention is paid to protecting potential pressure areas on the patient's wrists, elbows, and calves. After the cecum, colon, and proximal two thirds of the rectum have been mobilized and their blood supply ligated, the distal ileum is divided and secured with the GIA stapler, and the distal rectum is severed just above the levators with a TA-35 stapler. Great care is taken to preserve the distal portion of the ileocolic artery and its anastomosis to the marginal arterial arcade. The entire specimen is then submitted for immediate frozen section examination by an experienced pathologist to exclude unsuspected Crohn's colitis. The small intestinal mesentery is then mobilized to ensure that the apex of the future reservoir (15 to 20 cm proximal to the cut end of the ileum) will reach 2 to 3 cm beyond the inferior margin of the pubis, a reliable indication that the reservoir itself will easily be brought down to the dentate line without undue tension (Fig. 37-2). Should the apex of the future reservoir not comfortably reach this point, a number of operative techniques may be employed to improve the mobility of the distal ileum.

Stages of the procedure are as follows:

1. Mobilization of the small bowel mesentery to the third part of the duodenum is a maneuver that should be routine in any IPAA operation. The mesentery of the distal ileum is lifted out of the abdomen, and all peritoneal attachments other than those surrounding the vascular mesentery are divided to the most superior point possible, the third part of the duodenum.
2. Transverse incision of the peritoneal layers of the small bowel mesentery is performed next. A small advantage in length may be gained by placing a series of transverse peritoneal incisions. Care must be taken not to excessively skeletonize the blood vessels by removing too much of the peritoneal and fatty tissue, as this may result in weakening of the tissue bridge containing these blood vessels, and subsequent tearing.
3. When the mesentery is fully mobilized, it may be held in position with an operative light opposite the surgeon to allow transillumination of the mesentery, confirming the position of the major vessels. Division of either the distal ileocolic or branches of the superior mesen-

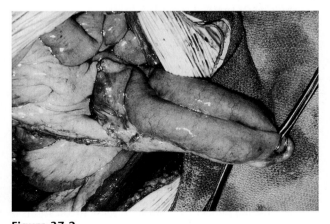

Figure 37-2
Operative site for ileal pouch–anal anastomosis showing reach of small intestine mesentery.

teric arteries may be permissible, provided an adequate anastomosis between the two systems can be confirmed in the marginal vessels (Fig. 37-3). This anastomosis may be confirmed by placement of a vascular bulldog clip across either vessel and subsequently assessing the presence of adequate pulsation in the remaining system. Any tethering areas of mesentery that can be demonstrated not to include blood vessels may also be divided. These techniques must be tailored to the individual patient on the basis of the length required, and the pattern of blood vessels present.

4. In patients who are particularly tall or obese, extreme difficulty in gaining sufficient length may be anticipated. A maneuver recently has been described which may aid in gaining significant mesenteric length in such cases. During ligation of the vascular pedicles of the colon, the middle colic artery and its right branch can be preserved and the left branch ligated (Fig. 37-4). The mesentery of the colon with its marginal artery proximal to this point is then preserved, and the colon is removed by division of the tissue between the marginal artery and the mesenteric wall of the colon. In this fashion the arcade of the right colon, as well as its supply from the right branch of the middle colic artery, are preserved. With this maneuver both the ileocolic artery and distal superior mesenteric artery can be fully divided while allowing potential for significant extra mobilization of the apex of the pouch. Application of bulldog clips to these vessels to ensure adequate flow through the marginal arcade should be performed prior to dividing these arteries. Finally, should

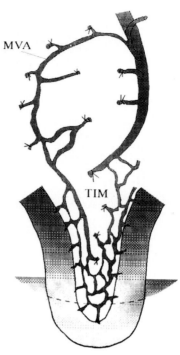

Figure 37-4
Retention of the right colonic vascular arcade to aid in lengthening of the small bowel mesentery.

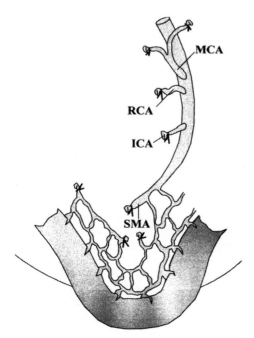

Figure 37-3
Sites for ligation of major vessels. ICA = ileocolic artery, MCA = middle colic artery, RCA = right colic artery, SMA = superior mesenteric artery.

there not be sufficient length to allow anastomosis to be achieved, an alternative pouch configuration should be considered, specifically either an S- or W-shaped pouch.

Otherwise, we favor the J-pouch configuration for its simplicity, speed of formation, its excellent fit into the concavity of the sacrum, excellent emptying, and its reservoir capacity, usually nearing 400 mL. The J-shaped pouch is constructed by stapling two 15- to 20-cm limbs of ileum together with the GIA anastomotic stapler. The anus is then gently dilated and effaced with either two Gelpi retractors placed at a right angle, or a Lone Star retractor to expose the dentate line clearly. Infiltration of the external sphincter with local anesthetic may provide maximal dilation. Infiltration of the submucosa with a dilute solution of epinephrine (1:100,000) reduces bleeding and facilitates mucosal stripping. The mucosa is excised with electrocautery, commencing at the dentate line and extending cephalad and circumferentially from a distance not exceeding 2 to 4 cm. The full thickness of the remaining rectum is then transected proximal to the row of staples, and an intact tube of anal canal and rectal mucosa and remaining rectum are removed en bloc and delivered transanally. The shorter mucosectomy reduces operating time, minimizes contamination and the risk of infection, favors full expansion of the ileal reservoir, and decreases the possibility of leaving behind potentially premalignant mucosal cells. The ileal reservoir is then pulled down endoanally through the muscular cuff (Fig. 37-5) and

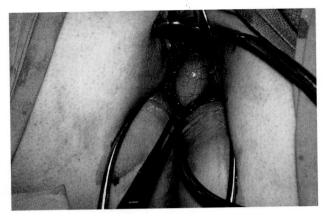

Figure 37-5
Apex of reservoir pulled through mucosa-denuded anal canal with Babcock clamp.

anchored in place with four corner sutures of 2-0 chromic catgut, and its most distal portion is opened transversely and anastomosed at the dentate line using interrupted sutures of 3-0 polyglycolic acid placed intraluminally. A soft Silastic drain is positioned in the presacral space behind the reservoir and brought out through a left-sided abdominal stab wound to drain the retropouch space. The pelvic floor is reconstructed around the reservoir. Finally, a loop ileostomy is established in the lower portion of the right abdominal wall. On average, patients leave the hospital 8 to 20 days after the operation and return 2 months later, at which time a "pouchogram" is performed to ensure complete healing of the reservoir as well as of the anastomosis. If complete healing is confirmed, intestinal continuity can be restored.

Ileal Pouch–Anal Canal Anastomosis Without Mucosectomy

Some authors prefer a technique of double stapling of the anastomosis, transecting with a stapler the very distal rectum or proximal anal canal, avoiding a mucosectomy and anastomosing the pouch by means of a circular end-to-end stapler. This technique is touted as being faster, and of having the proposed advantage of maintaining the transitional zone of anal mucosa, which may improve neorectal sensation and continence.

In most patients, we prefer complete removal of the diseased rectal mucosa. We believe that complete removal of the transitional zone mucosa ensures maximal reduction of risk of future disease flares and carcinoma and reduction of extraintestinal manifestations of CUC. This premise is supported by the finding of inflamed rectal mucosa in transitional zone of the majority of patients undergoing proctocolectomy for CUC. This rectal mucosa has been demonstrated in a Mayo Clinic series to extend to within 1 cm of the dentate line in 89% of patients. Moreover, randomized prospective trials from Finland, Sweden, England, and the Mayo Clinic, comparing IPAA with mucosectomy, with ileal pouch–distal rectal anastomosis without mucosectomy, have failed to demonstrate any functional advantage

of the technique retaining transitional zone mucosa. Hence, we still favor the technique of mucosectomy with direct anastomosis between the pouch and the dentate line.

Immediate Results of IPAA: Postoperative Morbidity

Since 1981, more than 1900 IPAAs have been constructed at the Mayo Clinic. Nearly 90% of these patients suffered from ulcerative colitis, and 96% had a J-pouch formed. In more than 200 patients, no mucosectomy was done and the anastomosis was stapled. A review was recently undertaken of 1310 CUC patients who had undergone formation of an IPAA in a J-pouch configuration with mucosectomy and hand-sewn anastomosis at the Mayo Clinic. Diverting ileostomy was performed in 96% of these patients. The perioperative mortality rate was 0.2%, and 19% suffered complications in the immediate postoperative period. The risk of *pelvic sepsis* (abscess or phlegmon) has gradually diminished from 7% in our early experience (1981 to 1985) to 3% more recently (1990 to 1993). Of those patients with pelvic sepsis, 36% could be managed with a combination of antibiotic therapy or CT-guided percutaneous drainage, and 64% required operative drainage. Overall, 15% developed perioperative *small bowel obstruction*, with nearly one quarter of those patients needing laparotomy. These figures increased with longer follow-up (see later discussion). The requirement for laparotomy in this series, although apparently high, has fallen from the figures for earlier experience, and does not differ greatly from series of patients undergoing proctocolectomy and Brooke ileostomy or Kock pouch formation.

■ INTERMEDIATE AND LATE RESULTS

In the same series, the risk of clinical *pouchitis* continued to increase with time, with a cumulative risk of 48% at 10 years. In patients suffering one attack, the incidence of a second attack within 2 years was 64%. Most patients respond favorably to a short course of antibiotics, usually metronidazole or ciprofloxacin, but some patients experience recalcitrant chronic pouchitis that may ultimately lead to pouch excision. This result is particularly true in patients whose colitis is complicated by primary sclerosing cholangitis (see Contraindications). *Bowel obstruction* is also a progressive problem, and its incidence increases with time. At 5 years follow-up, the incidence was 14.5%, and at 10 years it was 22.3%. Approximately half of these patients responded to conservative therapy. *Anastomotic stricture* is common after the procedure, but usually resolves with one dilation, under either sedation or general anesthesia. This occurred in 14% of patients in earlier Mayo Clinic series, but recurred in only 4%. *Pouch failure* is defined as removal of the pouch or inability to reverse the diverting stoma. In the Mayo Clinic series, the cumulative risk of pouch failure at 10 years was 8.9%. Almost always, failure was due to the subsequent diagnosis of Crohn's disease, insurmountable pelvic sepsis, or fistula; poor function; and pouchitis.

Functional Results

All patients could evacuate their neorectum spontaneously. The mean number of stools per day is 6 ($\pm$2) with 1 ($\pm$1) nocturnal stool. The need for stool bulking agents and antidiarrheal agents decreases with time. Eighty-nine percent of patients had excellent daytime continence, but more than 30% had minor leakage at night (defined as leakage on straining, twice or less per week). Overall, 94% regarded their result as satisfactory, and only 6% indicated that they would prefer a change. The vast majority had improvement of their daytime activities compared to the time prior to the operation. We believe that this series confirms earlier data suggesting that a J-shaped IPAA with mucosectomy for CUC is safe and effective and provides patients with a good quality of life.

Contraindications

Absolute contraindications include the presence of true incontinence prior to colectomy, findings of Crohn's disease, and the presence of rectal carcinoma, especially in the distal half of the rectum. Relative contraindications include age (>55 years), certain occupations that keep patients away from toilet facilities, gross obesity, or general health factors that make this intricate, multistaged operation more risky. Obese or tall body habitus, although not precluding IPAA, should alert the surgeon to the possibility of technical difficulties in pulling the small bowel down to the dentate line. Such patients should be warned of that risk and the possible need for a permanent stoma.

Indeterminate Colitis or Crohn's Disease

Crohn's disease remains an absolute contraindication to IPAA formation. For some time now, it has been the practice of the colorectal service at the Mayo Clinic to resect the colonic specimen at the level of the pelvic brim, and to submit the specimen for frozen section examination to exclude Crohn's disease before resecting the rectum. This information allows conversion of the operation from IPAA to ileorectostomy should the specimen confirm the presence of Crohn's disease and should the rectum be only mildly or moderately involved. In addition, all precautions are taken to exclude Crohn's disease prior to operation. All patients undergo colonoscopy and biopsy with review by an experienced pathologist. Patients who have previously presented with suggestive perianal disease, especially anal tags, abscess, or fistula, are treated with particular suspicion.

Despite all efforts to identify patients with Crohn's disease prior to operation, a small number will be identified only at the time of colonic resection or at some time after formation of IPAA. If such patients undergo IPAA, it is important to reassure them that the results may not be necessarily disastrous. Indeed, it is important to recognize that these patients are not representative of the general pool of patients with Crohn's disease, as they include only those patients who have not manifested clinical features suggestive of Crohn's disease, or even histologic features of Crohn's disease at the time of the initial colonic resection.

A recent Mayo Clinic series examined the outcome of patients who underwent IPAA and in whom a subsequent postoperative diagnosis of Crohn's disease was later confirmed. From a total of 1509 patients who underwent IPAA for the apparent indication of ulcerative colitis, 37 patients were subsequently identified as having Crohn's disease (2.5%). Thirty percent developed complex fistulas and Crohn's disease recurred in the pouch in 54%. The early postoperative complication rate was 30%. Twenty patients (55%) still have a pouch with an acceptable functional outcome an average of 10 years postoperatively. Similarly, some controversy remains regarding the role of IPAA in patients with so-called "indeterminate colitis"; that is, histologic features of both ulcerative colitis and Crohn's disease are present in the operative specimen, but the patient does not manifest any clinical features of Crohn's disease. Clearly, the pathologic diagnosis will vary among centers, or even among individual pathologists. At the Mayo Clinic, the outcome of 71 IPAAs performed in patients with indeterminate colitis and followed a mean of 57 months was compared to a control group of more than 1200 patients who had undergone IPAA for CUC. The functional outcome was found to be essentially identical between the two groups. The pouch failure rate, however, was much higher in the indeterminate colitis group (19%) compared with the CUC group (8%) ($P < 0.03$). Hence, our policy has remained that of proceeding with IPAA in the setting of a diagnosis of indeterminate colitis, with full disclosure of likely outcome to the patient. We believe that a one-stage procedure without diversion is contraindicated in this setting.

Primary Sclerosing Cholangitis

A recent series from the Mayo Clinic addressed the issue of outcome after IPAA in CUC patients suffering from primary sclerosing cholangitis (PSC). Of a total of 1097 patients who had undergone IPAA, 54 (5%) also had documented PSC. The two groups were otherwise well matched. The rate of pouchitis in those patients with PSC was 63%, compared with a rate of 32% in the control group. The incidence was not related to the severity of liver disease. This series strongly suggests a common link in their pathogenesis. A further series demonstrated that orthotopic liver transplantation does not alter the disease course for pouchitis in most of these patients.

Although these figures remain a concern, we still regard IPAA as the operation of choice for patients with PSC and CUC. Proctocolectomy and Brooke ileostomy is associated with development of peristomal varices in more than 50% of patients. Thus far, no patients in the Mayo Clinic series have developed anastomotic varices after IPAA.

The Grossly Malnourished Patient

Some patients at presentation for consideration for surgery will exhibit clinical and laboratory features consistent with marked malnourishment, specifically significant weight loss, hypoalbuminemia, and edema. In this group of patients, consideration should be given to performing a three-stage procedure: (1) abdominal colectomy and Brooke ileostomy, leaving the rectum intact; (2) completion proctectomy, IPAA, and loop ileostomy formation; and (3) closure of loop ileostomy. The rectal stump may be brought to the anterior abdominal wall as a mucous fistula if the rectum appears to be severely diseased at initial laparotomy.

Sexual Function, Pregnancy, and Delivery in Women with Ileal Pouch–Anal Anastomosis

Given that the majority of patients who develop ulcerative colitis will do so either during or before their prime reproductive years, the impact of IPAA on sexual function, pregnancy, and delivery is a most important consideration. In our group, 1% of men became impotent after IPAA and 2% developed absent or retrograde ejaculation. In women undergoing IPAA, dyspareunia was reported in 7%; this incidence compares favorably with that reported after ileorectostomy (53%). The fear of leakage of stool inhibited sexual relations in 3% of women. A further review of women undergoing proctocolectomy and formation of Kock pouch reported a significantly higher rate of dyspareunia and sexual dysfunction than those having an IPAA. These results again confirm the favorable effect of leaving the anal sphincter mechanism and pelvic floor intact, and a physiologic reservoir in the presacral space between the sacrum and the vagina.

Finally, we found that the IPAA is compatible with safe pregnancy and normal vaginal delivery. Pregnancy did not adversely affect pouch function. The number of daily bowel movements increased only modestly, the increase noted in the last trimester of pregnancy and persisting for about 3 months after delivery. The type of delivery did not affect pouch function postpartum. We believe that the presence of an ileal pouch does not mandate cesarean section, and such a decision should be based on obstetric indications. If necessary, a mediolateral episiotomy can be performed safely.

Cancer and the Ileal Pouch

The presence of a cancer complicating ulcerative colitis found either preoperatively or unexpectedly at the time of proctocolectomy may mandate an alteration in the procedure performed. If a colonic carcinoma carries a relatively good prognosis, it is reasonable to perform an IPAA. If a carcinoma has a poor prognosis, ileorectostomy may be a preferable operation. This procedure would combine the advantages of removing the vast majority of large bowel, while avoiding a stoma in a patient with a limited prognosis. If the carcinoma involves the proximal rectum, and frozen section reveals a T3 or node-positive lesion that will need chemoradiation postoperatively, an IPAA may still be reasonable but will require an oncologic type of proctectomy. In such patients, the pouch failure rate is greater than 15%, whether the malignant lesion recurs or not. If the tumor is located in the lower half of the rectum, rectal amputation and permanent ileostomy are indicated.

■ CURRENT ROLE OF OTHER SURGICAL ALTERNATIVES

The Continent Ileostomy of Kock

After proctocolectomy, an ileal reservoir can be constructed from approximately 45 cm of terminal ileum. A nipple valve is created by intussuscepting a portion of the ileum back into the pouch and anchoring the intussusceptum into place with three rows of staples. The end of the efferent limb of ileum is brought to the surface as a flush stoma. The nipple valve is continent, and the pouch is drained by insertion of a catheter through the stoma and nipple valve. Hence, no stoma bag need be worn in between intubations, thus rendering the arrangement far more convenient to the patient than a conventional Brooke ileostomy.

This procedure has not enjoyed widespread acceptance because of its intricate construction and the relatively high risk of valvular dysfunction, requiring one or more revisional operations. The concept, however, is most ingenious and attractive and is largely responsible for the resurgent interest in the ileoanal anastomosis with the addition of a reservoir. Despite extensive experience with the procedure and multiple technical modifications, a valve revision rate of about 20% continues to plague patients. No doubt, experience, improved technique, and careful selection of patients can minimize this risk. Thin, young, female patients, especially those who have not previously had a proctocolectomy, tend to fare best. Moreover, nonspecific reservoir ileitis believed to be due to bacterial overgrowth and characterized by low-grade fever, bleeding, diarrhea, and even arthralgia is seen in approximately 10% of patients but generally responds favorably to oral antibiotics. Surgical excision of the reservoir due to recurrent pouchitis is seldom necessary. In the extensive experience of Kock in Sweden, as well as our own experience with more than 500 such operations, the procedure can be performed safely, and ultimately 95% of the patients achieve satisfactory continence and do not wear an external appliance. Moreover, the quality of life of such patients appears to surpass that of patients with a Brooke ileostomy. The Kock pouch can be a useful alternative for certain categories of patients: (1) those who already have a Brooke ileostomy and wish to improve their quality of life further; (2) those who are not good candidates for IPAA because of poor sphincter tone; and (3) those in whom an IPAA has failed, but who wish to attempt Kock pouch formation. In this situation, the existing reservoir may be usable to create the continent ileostomy. The operation should be discouraged in those patients older than 50 years of age, those with significant obesity, or those believed to be psychologically incapable of dealing with multiple revisions and possible failure.

Proctocolectomy and Brooke Ileostomy

Twenty-five years ago, this combination was the most commonly performed operation for CUC in most centers. For the majority of patients, however, it is clearly no longer the operation of choice. However, in some clearly defined patient groups, formation of a permanent stoma has a place. The procedure has the advantage of technical simplicity, and is thus highly reproducible at centers that do not have a core interest in colorectal surgery. The obvious disadvantages are those of a permanent stoma and the inherent problems associated with the appliance, and a perineal wound that may be bothersome if healing is delayed or fails to occur.

Situations in which a permanent ileostomy may be considered appropriate include the following:

1. The older patient. Patients older than 60 years of age are generally not good candidates for IPAA formation or for a Kock pouch.
2. Work-related contraindication. Some types of work make it difficult to pass stool up to eight times per day, and the patient may thus prefer the certainty of an ileostomy bag.
3. The patient whose general condition mandates a short, single-stage procedure. The grossly malnourished patient or the patient with severe intercurrent comorbidities may not tolerate a long operative procedure or the increased likelihood of complications.
4. The obese patient or the patient in whom the small bowel will not reach the pelvic floor.
5. The incontinent patient. Some patients coming to surgery for IPAA will have had a degree of incontinence prior to operation, relating principally to the severity of their diarrhea, the presence of a nondistensible rectum, and urgency. Many of these patients could have adequate continence if their disease were controlled or after IPAA formation. Although true incontinence is a contraindication to IPAA, any patient being considered for surgery for CUC with a history of loss of control of stool should be carefully assessed by digital examination and manometry to ascertain whether there is true sphincter malfunction, or whether the problem is secondary to poor disease control, prior to being denied the option of IPAA.
6. Patients with Crohn's disease.

Colectomy with Ileorectal Anastomosis

Colectomy with ileorectostomy has numerous advantages over IPAA, but remains in our opinion a more limited option. Clearly, this operation has the advantages of surgical simplicity, avoids a two-stage operation, and should avoid the risk of loss of sexual function that may occur with proctectomy. Results of the operation are highly reproducible due to the lack of technical difficulty.

Failing to remove the rectum fails to remove the seat of disease in CUC and leaves behind a possible focus of malignancy, necessitating lifelong surveillance. In addition, CUC often renders the rectum nondistensible, thus reducing its physiologic function as a compliant organ. Hence, bowel frequency and continence after ileorectostomy may be less than desirable.

It is indeed argued that although a focus of disease is left behind after ileorectal anastomosis (IRA), the disease is often relatively easy to control after surgery, as the entire focus of disease can be medicated by means of enema with steroids or 5-ASA derivatives. Unfortunately, this treatment is not universally effective, and there may be an ongoing need for oral medication, including steroids, after IRA. Proponents of IRA also argue that with proper endoscopic surveillance, the risk of developing incurable malignancy after IRA should be minimal. Colectomy with IRA has a clear role in the following patient subgroups:

1. Patients with advanced PSC. Patients with PSC and portal hypertension may benefit from IRA, thus avoiding the problems of parastomal varices with procto-colectomy and ileostomy or of pouchitis after IPAA, especially if an IPAA proves to be technically difficult.
2. Patients with uncontrolled CUC and shortened life span. In those patients in whom an advanced colonic carcinoma is discovered at laparotomy or in whom life expectancy is reduced for reasons of other comorbidity, the concern of future neoplastic transformation of the rectal mucosa is of lesser importance, and hence an IRA becomes an attractive option and possibly the operation of choice in this setting.

■ CONCLUDING REMARKS

We firmly believe that, at the present time, IPAA represents the operation of choice for the vast majority of patients with CUC in whom surgery is indicated. It is crucial, however, that surgeons treating this disease are aware of the alternative surgical options, all of which maintain an important role for specified subsets of patients. Recent large series of IPAA with long-term follow-up confirm the excellent functional results and low morbidity rate that can be expected in the vast majority of patients, after operation in a center of interest. Results clearly improve with experience, and it is of pivotal importance that surgeons undertaking IPAA be adequately trained in the alternative techniques and the specific difficulties of the operations.

Suggested Readings

Goes RN, Nguyen P, Huang D, Beart RW Jr: Lengthening of the mesentery using the marginal vascular arcade of the right colon as the blood supply to the ileal pouch. Dis Colon Rectum 1995;38(8):893–895.

McIntyre PB, Pemberton JH, Wolff BG, et al: Indeterminate colitis: Long-term outcome in patients after ileal pouch-anal anastomosis. Dis Colon Rectum 1995;38:51–54.

Meagher AP, Farouk R, Dozois RR, et al: J ileal pouch-anal anastomosis for chronic ulcerative colitis: Complications and long-term outcomes in 1310 patients. Br J Surg 1998;85:800–803.

Penna C, Dozois RR, Tremaine W, et al: Pouchitis after ileal pouch-anal anastomosis for ulcerative colitis occurs with increased frequency in patients with associated primary sclerosing cholangitis. Gut 1996;38:234–239.

Sagar, PM, Dozois RR, Wolff BG: Long-term results of ileal pouch-anal anastomosis in patients with Crohn's disease. Dis Colon Rectum 1996;39(8):893–898.

Zins BJ, Sandborn WJ, Penna CR, et al: Pouchitis disease course after orthotopic liver transplantation in patients with primary sclerosing cholangitis and an ileal pouch-anal anastomosis. Am J Gastroenterol 1995;90(12):2177–2181.

38

MANAGEMENT OF TOXIC ULCERATIVE COLITIS

John R. Oakley, MBBS, FRACS

Episodes of severe ulcerative colitis may occur as the first manifestation of the disease or during the course of a protracted illness. Although in ulcerative colitis the attacks tend to occur after a longer duration of disease and at an older age than with Crohn's colitis, and fewer patients present initially with a severe attack or with toxic megacolon, in general, the manner of presentation and the management differ little in the two conditions.

Historically, severe or toxic colitis has carried a high mortality rate. Happily, this situation has dramatically improved in recent years because of the earlier recognition of severe attacks, more aggressive and effective medical management, and the realization (and somewhat belated acceptance) that early surgery performed on those patients who do not respond rapidly saves lives and reduces morbidity. The relatively recent development of pelvic pouch surgery, which provides an alternative to permanent ileostomy for many of these patients, almost certainly has led to earlier referral and earlier acceptance of surgery.

■ RECOGNITION OF THE TOXIC PATIENT

The terms *acute, severe, toxic,* and *fulminant* have all been used to describe seriously ill patients with ulcerative or Crohn's colitis. In the order listed here they could be regarded as describing a progressive spectrum of severity of disease, but in practice the terms are almost synonymous and tend to be used almost interchangeably. Although attempts have been made to more accurately define these terms (especially toxic colitis), such definitions, while useful for reporting and comparing series of cases, carry the danger of being too rigid and thereby potentially exclude patients who do not comply with all the necessary criteria, but who are no less ill and require the same aggressive management.

Toxicity is manifest clinically by tachycardia, fever, pallor, lethargy, or shock secondary to dehydration or sepsis. Other features commonly present include abdominal tenderness, hypotension, electrolyte imbalance, anemia, dehydration, mental changes, and stool frequency of greater than eight per day. Anorexia, nausea, and abdominal pain may provide a clue to otherwise unrecognized severe disease. A persistent tachycardia may also alert the physician to more severe disease in a patient with few other manifestations of serious illness. Worsening diarrhea or bleeding often indicates more severe disease, but fewer bowel movements can be misleading, as the stool frequency often decreases with the development of toxic dilatation. Abdominal tenderness or diminished bowel sounds usually imply severe disease. However, in some patients the severity of the attack can be underestimated, as they may actually appear quite well. In those receiving oral or systemic steroids, or other immunosuppressive drugs, abdominal pain and many of the telltale signs of toxicity may be reduced or masked. Abdominal distention usually indicates the presence of development of toxic colonic dilatation or megacolon. In this setting, localized or generalized tenderness may indicate impending or free perforation, but it is important to realize that either can occur in the absence of colonic dilatation or abdominal distention. Profound anemia, hypoproteinemia, hypokalemia, and biochemical evidence of dehydration and renal or hepatic impairment may also reflect the severity of the attack.

■ MEDICAL MANAGEMENT

Initial Diagnosis and Investigation

Patients with the manifestations of severe or toxic colitis are admitted to the hospital. Initial investigations include a complete blood cell count, a serum electrolyte and biochemical profile, blood cultures, blood coagulation studies, and C-reactive protein. A plain abdominal radiograph to rule out toxic megacolon and to detect sealed or unsuspected free perforation is performed and if clinically indicated, a chest radiograph and electrocardiogram are also obtained.

In the patient in whom the diagnosis of primary inflammatory bowel disease has not yet been clearly established, stool cultures are obtained to look for infective agents, including *Salmonella, Campylobacter, Yersinia,* and *Clostridium difficile,* and stool is examined for amebas. A limited proctoscopic examination, with minimal insufflation of air, is also performed in this group of previously undiagnosed patients to help exclude pseudomembranous colitis, or ischemic colitis in the older age group. Rectal biopsies may occasionally be helpful.

Colonoscopy is usually contraindicated in the assessment of these patients. It rarely contributes to their management and (along with the necessary prior preparation) carries a risk of perforation and of precipitating toxic megacolon.

Resuscitation

Intravenous fluids are required, with correction of electrolyte disturbances (particularly hypokalemia and hyponatremia). In the anemic or bleeding patient, blood is given. Hypoprothrombinemia is treated with vitamin K.

A central venous cannula is often inserted early in the patient's hospital stay. This is useful in the early resuscitation of hypovolemic patients, but more often serves as a route for hyperalimentation during the intensive medical treatment that follows, and in the early postoperative period if the patient requires surgery. Nasogastric suction is not used routinely but is employed if there is vomiting or the development of colonic dilatation.

Antibiotics

The routine use of antibiotics is controversial. There is little evidence that they alter the course of the colitis itself, but they may reduce any serious consequences from infection secondary to the inflamed and ulcerated bowel, or from small sealed-off perforations. For this reason antibiotics effective against aerobic and anaerobic organisms are frequently used. One suitable combination is an aminoglycoside such as gentamicin or tobramycin, together with metronidazole, both given intravenously. Ampicillin or amoxicillin may be added in some patients. Other satisfactory alternatives are a second-generation cephalosporin, possibly combined with metronidazole, or one of the third-generation cephalosporins.

Corticosteroids and Immunosuppressive Drugs

Corticosteroids have clearly been shown to be effective in treating acute colitis and are normally given intravenously. Most commonly, hydrocortisone, 50 to 100 mg intravenously, is given every 6 hours by bolus or by continuous infusion. A total dose of 400 mg per day is rarely exceeded, as the additional benefit of any higher dose is minimal. The physician must be conscious of the possibility, especially in treating the long-term corticosteroid-dependent patient, that the steroids may make the signs of toxicity less severe or less apparent. In those patients in whom a satisfactory response is obtained (the majority), the intravenous steroid dose is reduced after 5 to 7 days to approximately 200 mg of hydrocortisone per day (or its equivalent) and is changed to oral prednisone, 30 to 40 mg per day in divided doses, once the gastrointestinal tract is able to be used. Lengthy periods during which the equivalent of 40 to 50 mg of prednisone is used daily are also to be avoided. The policy should be one of an initial short course of high-dose intravenous steroids, with fairly rapid tapering if a satisfactory result is obtained. If the patient does not show clear evidence of improvement, surgery, rather than an increase in the steroid dosage or its duration, is indicated.

Immunosuppressive drugs such as azathioprine and 6-mercaptopurine have little place in the treatment of acute or toxic colitis, even for their steroid-sparing effect. This is largely because of the long delay in achieving any therapeutic effect after commencing the medication. In patients who have been receiving long-term immunosuppressive agents and for whom surgery seems likely or inevitable, these medications are ceased and an attempt is made, when possible, to taper the steroid dosage before surgery as much as the patient's underlying condition and the steroid requirements for surgery will allow.

High-dose intravenous cyclosporine may induce remission in some patients unresponsive to corticosteroids, but any improvement is usually not apparent for 5 to 7 days and the margin between benefit and toxicity is narrow. Furthermore, the majority of patients who do respond will relapse within 6 months and require colectomy. Hence, the role of high-dose cyclosporine in the management of severe colitis has yet to be precisely defined. The concern about an increased postoperative complication rate in patients treated with cyclosporine prior to surgery appears to be unfounded.

Diet and Nutrition

Evidence to support bowel rest (with strictly nothing taken by mouth) for patients with toxic colitis is scanty. One policy is to allow only ice chips or sips of water or clear liquids and not to use nasogastric suction routinely. Patients with a less severe attack of colitis may be permitted a low-residue diet and oral medications where appropriate.

In many patients, hyperalimentation is instituted early in the course of treatment, but usually not until the initial hypovolemia, electrolyte abnormalities, and anemia have been corrected. Many patients with toxic colitis are chronically ill and nutritionally depleted, or will rapidly become so during a severe attack. Although there is little evidence to suggest that hyperalimentation per se reduces the activity of the disease, it does help to restore the nutritionally depleted patient and probably reduces the complications and morbidity if surgery is eventually required.

Other General Measures

Strict bed rest is not necessary and when possible the patient is encouraged to maintain a level of activity compatible with his or her general condition and feeling of well-being. Some toxic or confused patients require sedation, but this is kept to a minimum to avoid masking alterations in the patient's condition. Narcotics are used with caution because of the possibility of obscuring signs of peritonitis, and because of the potential for precipitating or aggravating toxic megacolon. Anticholinergics and antidiarrheal agents are avoided for the same reason, and because they can confuse the clinical assessment of disease severity.

■ ASSESSMENT OF THERAPEUTIC EFFECT

Unless the patient requires immediate surgery because of free perforation, generalized peritonitis, endotoxic shock, massive colonic hemorrhage, or dramatic deterioration over the 12 to 24 hours immediately preceding admission, he or she is observed very closely for the next 24 to 72 hours to assess the response to medical management. Diminishing toxicity, reduced fever, a reduced pulse rate and white blood cell count, and a rising serum albumin level are encouraging, but a persistent high or increasing pulse rate or falling blood pressure is an ominous sign. Increasing abdominal pain, tenderness, and distention all signal deterioration. Of particular importance is a daily (sometimes twice daily) plain radiograph of the abdomen (with erect views if possible) to detect the early signs of toxic megacolon. The patient is examined several times each day and the possibility of surgery is discussed early, as well as with the family, especially if the patient's mental status is altered by the toxicity from the colitis.

■ INDICATIONS FOR SURGERY

An indication for surgery may be present at the time of presentation or may arise at any time during treatment and observation. Evidence of generalized peritonitis or free perforation with pneumoperitoneum or generalized abdominal tenderness, severe localized abdominal tenderness, endotoxic shock, or massive colonic hemorrhage indicates the need for emergency surgery. Development of toxic megacolon is usually, but not always, an indication for early surgery, and its management is further discussed later in this chapter.

If evidence of deterioration in the patient is seen at any time after adequate medical management has been instituted, or if clear improvement is not evident within 24 to 72 hours, surgery should be advised. There must be good objective evidence that the patient is getting better. If, after 5 to 7 days, the patient has shown only minor improvement and still has a persistent tachycardia, fever, elevated white blood cell count, abdominal tenderness, or frequent stools or bleeding, the chances of obtaining a remission are slight and the risk of operative fatality and morbidity increase significantly. In most such cases, surgery is advisable. Patients still having eight or more bowel movements per day after 3 days of intensive therapy, and those with three to eight bowel movements a day and a C-reactive protein level greater than 45 mg/L, will almost always require colectomy during that admission.

A more difficult group of patients are those who respond reasonably well, but incompletely, to medical treatment and continue to feel slightly unwell or have manifestations of low-grade smoldering disease. Switching to oral medication and a normal diet frequently produces a flare-up of symptoms and convinces a reluctant patient (and/or surgeon) that surgery is indicated.

■ SURGICAL MANAGEMENT

Preparation of the Patient for Surgery

The patient and family are told the reasons for advising surgery and given a broad outline of the surgical alternatives, both immediate and long term, without necessarily going into a detailed discussion of future options. The possibility of a permanent ileostomy does need to be discussed, but with a reassuring explanation that these days some sort of alternative is usually possible. However, some patients will not be suitable for later sphincter-preserving operations because of Crohn's disease or other anorectal or anatomic problems.

Stoma marking is always performed preoperatively. The preferred site is through the rectus muscle, usually just below and to the right (but clear) of the umbilicus, avoiding previous scars, skin folds, and bony prominences. A mechanical bowel preparation is not used.

Steroids are continued, and intravenous antibiotics are given perioperatively and continued postoperatively for 1 to 5 days, depending on the findings at surgery.

Choice of Operation

In the setting of severe or toxic colitis the two principal alternatives are (1) subtotal (abdominal) colectomy with end-ileostomy and (usually) rectosigmoid mucous fistula, and less commonly (2) proctocolectomy with either end-ileostomy or (very rarely) ileoanal pouch anastomosis with temporary loop ileostomy.

Ileostomy alone has no place in the treatment of these patients, but when combined with a decompression "blowhole" colostomy, may still have a role in some patients with toxic megacolon. This option will be discussed later in more detail. In rare circumstances, subtotal colectomy with an ileorectal anastomosis and temporary diverting loop ileostomy is performed, but only if the patient is not severely ill and if the rectal disease is relatively mild.

The choice of operation will depend very largely on the severity of the colitis, the overall condition of the patient, and the dosage and duration of previous steroid and immunosuppressive therapy. However, in practical terms subtotal colectomy and ileostomy will be the operation of choice for the vast majority of patients with severe or toxic colitis, especially if there is uncertainty about whether the patient has ulcerative colitis or Crohn's disease. Each of the procedures is discussed separately.

Subtotal Colectomy and Ileostomy

Subtotal colectomy and ileostomy is the most widely used and safest procedure in these patients requiring surgery for severe or toxic colitis. It normally allows the patients to recover their good health, usually without major troublesome symptoms from the retained rectum. It also has the major advantage of allowing subsequent surgery (be it ileorectal anastomosis, ileoanal pouch anastomosis, or completion proctectomy) to be performed in healthy, nontoxic, well-nourished patients on minimal or no steroid or immunosuppressive maintenance. However, the requirement for a second or even third operation in most patients is a disadvantage. Subtotal colectomy with ileostomy is the procedure of choice if free perforation is already present or if it should occur during mobilization of the bowel.

In those few patients in whom the principal indication for surgery is massive colonic hemorrhage, there is a potential danger of the bleeding continuing from the retained rectum. However, there are very few patients in whom such severe bleeding occurs that proctectomy becomes necessary during the postoperative period. If proctectomy is required, a low Hartmann's closure of the rectum, leaving the sphincters, is preferable to a total proctectomy.

The operation of subtotal colectomy is performed with the patient supine. The abdomen is opened through a long midline incision. Paramedian incisions compromise the sites of future stomas, which are frequently required in patients with inflammatory bowel disease.

During mobilization of the bowel, care is taken to preserve the main ileocolic vessels, with their branches being divided close to the cecum, thereby preserving the main trunk of both the ileocolic and superior mesenteric vessels for any future pouch construction. The terminal ileum is mobilized only enough to allow the bowel to easily reach the anterior abdominal wall for the ileostomy construction. Dissection near the root of the mesentery close to the origin of the superior mesenteric artery at the level of the duodenum and pancreas is avoided, because the resulting scarring and adhesions may make difficult any subsequent attempts to obtain sufficient mesenteric length to allow a pouch to reach to the anal canal. The individual sigmoid branches, rather than the main trunk, of the inferior mesenteric vessels are divided. This procedure reduces bunching of the tissues and facilitates the distal sigmoid reaching the anterior abdominal wall. It also reduces the risk of damage to the pelvic autonomic nerves.

Three different techniques can be used to create the rectosigmoid mucous fistula. The preferred method, if possible, is to divide and close the bowel with staples or sutures at a level so that the staple line lies without tension in the subcutaneous plane. The muscle of the bowel wall is then sutured circumferentially to the surrounding abdominal wall muscle or fascia, and the skin is closed over the bowel end. This technique effectively quarantines the end of the bowel from the peritoneal cavity so that in the event of the closure breaking down, an intraperitoneal abscess is avoided and drainage can easily occur through the skin incision. Although rectosigmoid stump suture breakdown does occur in a number of patients, the majority are able to avoid the nuisance of a separately constructed mucous fistula. This subcutaneous implantation of the bowel should be located toward the lower end of the incision, above the pubic hairline if possible, and should be sufficiently separated from the ileostomy site so that it will not interfere with pouching should the stump subsequently discharge.

In some patients a formal primary maturation of the mucous fistula to the skin is preferred, but in very severe colitis, the bowel wall may be so friable that it will not hold staples or sutures. In this case, the sigmoid stump is left protruding 2 to 3 inches beyond the level of the skin and wrapped snugly with a 2-inch gauze roll, thereby anchoring it to the abdominal wall until it becomes sufficiently adherent for the bowel to be amputated at skin level and the mucous fistula matures. This stage can normally be performed under local anesthesia after 7 to 10 days.

When there is a perforation in the rectum, or when the rectosigmoid is so friable that none of these techniques can be employed safely, the rectum can be divided just above the anterior peritoneal reflection. A Foley or similar catheter is placed into the rectal stump and brought out through the lower end of the abdominal incision, along with several Penrose drains, which are sutured around the upper end of the stump using absorbable chromic catgut sutures. A wide-bore catheter is also placed transanally into the rectum for counter drainage.

Whichever of the techniques to manage the rectosigmoid stump is chosen, it should not be done until just before the abdomen is closed, in order to avoid tearing out any sutures or otherwise traumatizing the rectosigmoid stump during other intra-abdominal manipulation.

Proctocolectomy and Ileostomy

Although once advocated as the operation of choice for acute ulcerative colitis, there is now little place for proctocolectomy and ileostomy in the acute setting. This is partly because the development of pelvic pouch surgery for ulcerative colitis and its acceptance as a good alternative to permanent ileostomy has resulted in the sphincters being preserved in most patients having surgery for severe or toxic colitis, as well as in those in whom the exact diagnosis is uncertain. Furthermore, proctocolectomy is technically more demanding and carries higher mortality and morbidity rates than subtotal colectomy, especially in these severely ill patients. The pelvic dissection is often more vascular and the risk of postoperative pelvic and intra-abdominal sepsis, small bowel obstruction, and enterocutaneous fistula is increased, as is the risk of damage to the pelvic autonomic nerves. However, the operation may have a place in the rare patient with profuse colonic bleeding, or in the less severely ill patient who is not considered suitable for later sphincter-saving procedures, or who does not want to have this form of surgery.

Proctocolectomy with immediate ileoanal pouch reconstruction has the potential for the same complications as proctocolectomy with end-ileostomy, but also has the added morbidity of pouch construction and anastomosis. It cannot therefore be recommended in the patient with a very severe or toxic colitis, but may have a rare place in the less severely ill patient with acute colitis, who has not been on high doses of steroids or immunosuppressive drugs. To avoid damage to the autonomic nerves, the rectal dissection is conducted in a plane close to the wall of the bowel, with the perineal dissection starting at the intersphincteric groove and proceeding in the intersphincteric plane.

■ TOXIC MEGACOLON

The development of toxic colonic dilatation is perhaps the most serious and life-threatening complication that can occur in patients with severe acute colitis. It should, however, be regarded as part of the spectrum of disease in severe attacks of colitis rather than as a separate entity. Fulminant colitis, without megacolon, can be just as devastating and can be followed by the same complications (including perforation) that occur with megacolon. Furthermore, the megacolon can occasionally resolve, still leaving the patient very ill from toxic colitis.

These patients therefore present in a manner similar to those without megacolon, but in addition, colonic dilatation and usually abdominal distention occur either by the time of presentation or during subsequent treatment. Historically, toxic megacolon was defined as being present if, in a patient with toxic colitis, the colon measures 5 cm or more in diameter on a plain radiograph of the abdomen. However, rigid adherence to such a definition may be unhelpful or even dangerous, because some patients who do not comply strictly with this definition can have just as adverse an outcome as those who do. No minimal diameter should be regarded as a requirement for the diagnosis of toxic megacolon.

Pathogenesis, Prevention, and Diagnosis

Although toxic megacolon is more common with pancolitis, it can occur in left-sided disease. When occurring in a patient with previously undiagnosed colitis, other causes such as amebic colitis, ischemic colitis, and pseudomembranous colitis must be excluded.

The pathogenesis is unclear, but the most accepted explanation is that the transmural inflammatory response that occurs in severe colitis produces paralysis of the smooth muscle of the colon wall, either by a direct effect or by interfering with the myenteric plexus. Hypokalemia, narcotics, anticholinergics, antidiarrheal medications, and even steroids have been implicated as predisposing factors, but the association is probably coincidental or temporal rather than causal. Nevertheless, it is customary and wise to avoid the use of these agents in patients with severe colitis. Barium enema has also been implicated as a precipitating cause and should also be avoided, not only for this reason, but also because it adds little or nothing to the management of the patient with a severe attack and may lead to, or complicate, perforation. Colonoscopy is avoided for the same reasons.

The diagnosis of toxic megacolon should be suspected in any patient with severe colitis, especially if abdominal distention develops, with or without an increase in tenderness. A reduction in stool frequency or bowel sounds resulting from the progressive paralysis of the bowel wall may herald the development of megacolon rather than an overall improvement. It is preferable, however, not to wait for these clinical signs, but to obtain daily or twice-daily plain radiographs of the abdomen. Radiologically, in addition to the colonic dilatation (usually found in the transverse colon and splenic flexure, but sometimes in the sigmoid or right colon), there may be a disturbed or absent haustral pattern, outlined "islands" of residual mucosa surrounded by extensive ulceration, and occasionally evidence of gas outside the normal lumen of the bowel, suggesting sealed-off perforations. The appearance (and sometimes the disappearance) of the dilatation can be quite sudden, possibly without many other obvious changes in the patient's condition, but a rapid increase in dilatation is a sinister event and should be regarded as an indication for surgery.

Medical Management and Indications for Surgery

The medical treatment of toxic megacolon is similar to that already described for toxic or fulminant colitis, except that a nasogastric tube to continuous suction is usually employed, and serial radiographs are obtained more frequently to assess progress.

Evidence of free perforation or generalized peritonitis is an indication for immediate surgery. Septicemia, significant deterioration of the patient's condition, and major associated colonic hemorrhage are also indications for urgent operation. In the absence of these indications,

there has been debate as to how long it is safe to wait before operating on a patient with toxic megacolon. Some surgeons believe that the diagnosis itself is an indication for urgent surgery because of the dramatic increase in mortality rate that occurs in the event of a perforation, but there has been a recent trend to observe patients very carefully for a limited time (24 to 72 hours at the most), provided that there is no other evidence of deterioration in their condition. Nevertheless, many of these patients continue to be toxic and still require surgery, and of the small number who do go rapidly into remission, the majority undergo colectomy within a few months. A sensible and safe policy is therefore to advise early (but not necessarily immediate) surgery for toxic megacolon, except in those patients whose toxicity and dilatation is clearly lessening rapidly during the early observation period.

Choice of Operation

The three most commonly performed procedures are (1) subtotal colectomy and end-ileostomy, (2) total proctocolectomy and ileostomy, and (3) diverting loop ileostomy accompanied by a decompressing skin-level "blowhole" colostomy.

Subtotal Colectomy with End-Ileostomy and Mucous Fistula

Subtotal colectomy with end-ileostomy and mucous fistula is preferred in the vast majority of patients, and is clearly the operation of choice in the event of free colonic perforation. The operative technique is essentially the same as that described for acute colitis without megacolon. The distended colon can be decompressed safely using a wide-bore needle attached to the suction tubing, after quarantining the rest of the abdominal cavity with packs to reduce the potential for contamination during the decompression maneuver and during mobilization of the splenic flexure, where perforation is most likely to occur. For this reason, the splenic flexure is approached after the remainder of the colon has been mobilized, allowing rapid control of an intraoperative perforation, if it occurs.

Proctocolectomy

In the presence of toxic megacolon, proctocolectomy is a technically demanding procedure with increased mortality and morbidity rates. It therefore has little, if any, place in the treatment of these patients, except perhaps in patients with associated profuse bleeding, or with a perforation very low in the rectum.

Diverting Loop Ileostomy and Decompressive "Blowhole" Colostomy

The diverting loop ileostomy and decompressive "blowhole" colostomy technique described by Turnbull and colleagues from the Cleveland Clinic has not gained wide acceptance. The operation was initially developed during the 1960s because it had been recognized that the mortality rate after colectomy for toxic megacolon remained high if the colon was perforated during its removal, a situation that was particularly prone to happen, even with the gentlest handling, if the omentum or adjacent small bowel loops had sealed off any small perforations. Iatrogenic free perforations were thereby avoided with this operation, which was simple and could be performed quickly with minimal operative trauma. Detoxification was rapid in the vast majority of patients, and the mortality rate was considerably lower than that for subtotal colectomy. However, the operation was only a staging procedure to allow the patient to be prepared for later colectomy after 4 to 6 months, and was not suitable when there was prior perforation or profuse bleeding.

These days, with better and more effective medical management (including an increased awareness and earlier diagnosis of toxic megacolon) and the recognition of the need for early surgery, far fewer patients with advanced disease and walled-off perforations are presenting for surgery. This, together with the advent of better antibiotics and more sophisticated postoperative supportive measures has led many surgeons to feel that colectomy can and should be performed in most patients. However, there remains a small group of patients in whom multiple sealed-off perforations are found at laparotomy or whose general condition is so poor that the lesser procedure should be considered. However, free perforation or generalized peritonitis are contraindications to this operation. The abdomen is explored through a small lower midline incision. A loop of terminal ileum 35 to 40 cm above the ileocecal valve (above the area of any possible future pouch) is selected and brought through a transrectus incision for creation of the loop ileostomy. The location of the dilated transverse colon is noted and marked (if this has not already been done preoperatively with a plain radiograph, using a small coin in the umbilicus as a marker). The main incision is closed and a smaller, usually vertical, incision 4 to 6 cm in length is then made over the dilated transverse colon through or on either side of the midline and extended down through the parietal peritoneum. The seromuscular layer of the underlying colon is then sutured to the parietal peritoneum with continuous fine absorbable sutures, sealing off the incision from the main peritoneal cavity. The colon is then deflated with a large-bore needle and suction before the bowel is opened in the line of incision and the edges are everted and sutured to the surrounding skin or to the subcutaneous fat or muscle, depending on the mobility of the edges of the bowel. The loop ileostomy is then opened eccentrically and everted and sutured to the skin.

Suggested Readings

Goligher JC, Hoffman DC, De Dombal FT: Surgical treatment of severe attacks of ulcerative colitis with special reference to the advantage of early operation. Br Med J 1970;4:203.

Fazio VW: Toxic megacolon in ulcerative colitis and Crohn's colitis. Clin Gastroenteral 1980;9:389–407.

Oakley JR, Fazio VW, Lavery IC: Toxic colitis and toxic megacolon: Results of surgery. In Goebell H (Ed.). Inflammatory Bowel Diseases. Progress in Basic Research and Clinical. UK, Kluwer Academic, 1991. Proceedings of the 60th Falk Symposium, Freiburg-im-Breisgau, Germany, Oct. 18–20, 1990.

Sartor RB: Cyclosporine therapy for inflammatory bowel disease. N Engl J Med 1994;330:1897–1898.

Travis SP, Farrant JM, Richets C, et al: Predicting outcome in severe ulcerative colitis. Gut 1996;38:905–910.

39

PELVIC POUCH ANASTOMOTIC COMPLICATIONS AND MANAGEMENT

Kutt Sing Wong, MD, MBBS, FRCS (Ed), FRCS (Glas), FAMS

Feza H. Remzi, MD, FACS, FASCRS

Since its introduction by Parks in 1978, restorative proctocolectomy (RP) with ileal pouch–anal anastomosis (IPAA) has become the preferred surgical option for treatment of mucosal ulcerative colitis (MUC) and familial adenomatous polyposis (FAP). It restores gastrointestinal continuity, re-establishes transanal defecation, and avoids a permanent stoma. While there is a high degree of patient satisfaction with this procedure, it has a significant incidence of anastomotic complications, ranging between 24 and 32%. Poor bowel function and sometimes pouch loss are potential outcomes of such complications, which undermine the merits of this operation.

Anastomotic complications after RP are classified as follows:

1. Anastomotic leaks
2. Pouch fistulas
3. Anastomotic strictures
4. Leaks from the tip of the J-pouch

■ ANASTOMOTIC LEAKS

Pouch-anal anastomotic leaks may be clinically overt or detectable radiologically only by a Gastrografin enema performed before ileostomy closure. Depending on the diagnostic criteria, the incidence varies between 4.5% and 10%.

Risk Factors

Risk factors for anastomotic leakage are prolonged steroid usage, hypoalbuminemia, anemia, hypoxemia from cardiac or respiratory insufficiency, ischemia of bowel ends, and tension on the anastomosis. Whether the anastomotic technique (hand-sewn with mucosectomy versus stapled without mucosectomy) contributes to any differences in anastomotic complications is debatable. Two prospective randomized studies found no differences in anastomotic complications. However, a large nonrandomized series from the Cleveland Clinic, comparing 238 hand-sewn with 454 stapled IPAAs, found significantly fewer anastomotic complications in the stapled group, leading to the conclusion that stapled anastomoses are safer than hand-sewn. Conceivably, a higher level of the anastomosis in stapled IPAA exerts less tension on the anastomosis than the hand-sewn technique.

A temporary defunctioning loop ileostomy has traditionally been used because of the risks of anastomotic leak and the fact that many patients with MUC frequently are on steroids and malnourished. In contrast to a defunctioning loop ileostomy after a low anterior resection and a colonic J-pouch, RP involves a more proximal loop ileostomy with high stoma output, predisposing to dehydration and electrolyte abnormalities. Furthermore, there is the issue of a second operation to close the stoma, which incurs additional cost and significant operative morbidity in some series. For these reasons, some surgeons have advocated a single-stage procedure in good-risk patients.

Although a diverting loop ileostomy does not prevent anastomotic leaks, the sepsis associated with a leak is considerably reduced. Moreover, in the presence of an anastomotic leak, there is a lower relaparotomy rate and a lower likelihood of pouch failure in diverted patients. In a recent large series of 1504 cases of ileostomy closure after RP, operative morbidity is acceptable when compared to the risk of an anastomotic leak. The most common complication of ileostomy closure after RP is small bowel obstruction, which responds to conservative therapy in the majority of cases. Therefore, the decision to perform RP without temporary diversion should be carefully considered.

A one-stage procedure may be considered only in the absence of risk factors endangering anastomotic healing such as anemia, malnutrition, and steroid usage. Equally important in making that decision is the conduct of the operation with good hemostasis, minimal contamination, lack of tension on the anastomosis, and complete tissue donuts. Our recent experience with omission of temporary diversion in RP showed that, in the presence of stringent selection criteria, quality of life at intervals of 3 months, 1 year, 3 years, 5 years, and 10 years is similar between diverted and nondiverted patients. In addition, the incidence of septic complications such as pelvic abscesses, anastomotic leaks, and fistulas is similar between both groups. However, it must be cautioned that failure to meet these criteria made diversion necessary to minimize postoperative septic sequelae and the prospect of pouch loss.

Diagnosis

Clinical presentation of a pouch-anal anastomotic leak ranges from persistent lower abdominal pain and tenderness to generalized peritonitis and pouch-cutaneous fistulas. Occasionally, ileus with associated abdominal distention and absent bowel sounds may be the main presenting feature. Other "telltale" signs include persistent postoperative fever, profuse vomiting, anorexia, and frequent loose stools. Varying degrees of systemic sepsis may be found. Subtlety of clinical manifestations often requires the clinician to have a high index of suspicion in order to rule out the likelihood of an anastomotic leak.

Typically, there is leukocytosis with a preponderance of neutrophils. However, in patients who had been on prolonged steroid therapy, white blood cell count may be normal. Dilated bowel loops or free intraperitoneal air may be evident on a plain abdominal radiograph. A computed tomographic (CT) scan of the abdomen and pelvis with triple contrast (oral, intravenous, and perianal) is the preferred radiologic imaging study. Besides providing radiologic evidence of a leak, a CT scan allows percutaneous drainage of a localized pelvic collection, which may prevent a relaparotomy.

In some asymptomatic patients, a leak is detected only by a Gastrografin enema prior to ileostomy closure.

Management

Fortunately, most IPAA leaks are not life threatening. When a leak is detected in an asymptomatic patient by a preileostomy closure Gastrografin enema, no further treatment is required, except to defer ileostomy closure. A repeat Gastrografin enema should be performed 3 months later. If no abscess cavities are present and the sinus track leading from the anastomosis is narrowed or obliterated, then ileostomy closure can be performed, provided the patient remains stable and asymptomatic.

In a symptomatic patient who is stable, is not septic, and has no peritonitis, initial treatment should include intravenous antibiotics, drainage, and bowel rest. Antibiotic coverage should include both aerobic gram-negative and anaerobic organisms. In the presence of a sizable *pelvic abscess* with no definite leak, percutaneous drainage under CT guidance may avert a relaparotomy. When drain output decreases to less than 100 mL over 24 hours, a tube sinogram provides useful information in terms of the decision to remove the drainage tube.

In some instances, a leak results in a presacral collection. Examination under anesthesia (EUA) allows evaluation of the abscess collection and passage of a transanal catheter through the anastomotic defect into the cavity. The catheter is changed for a smaller one when sinogram demonstrates shrinkage and resolution of the abscess cavity. Removal of the catheter can be carried out safely when there is clinical and radiologic evidence of resolution of the abscess cavity/presacral sinus tract.

Bowel rest is instituted initially in all symptomatic cases. When there are signs of clinical improvement, the patient may be advanced to oral liquids and eventually resumption of diet.

Worsening signs and symptoms after EUA and transanal drainage through the defect or generalized peritonitis are indications for emergent laparotomy. This procedure should be preceded by immediate fluid resuscitation and administration of intravenous broad-spectrum antibiotics.

In patients with a diverting ileostomy, thorough peritoneal lavage with copious amounts of warm saline followed by placement of wide-bore drains would be the cornerstone of surgical therapy. In nondiverted patients, adding a diverting loop ileostomy after peritoneal lavage and drainage is appropriate. Except when the pouch is nonviable, rarely will pouch disconnection or excision be necessary.

■ POUCH FISTULAS

Pouch fistulas are defined as connections from the pouch to the vagina, bladder, or perineal skin. They were first reported in 1985 and rates have ranged from 4 to 16%. The development of pouch fistulas occurs more commonly in patients with inflammatory bowel disease than patients with FAP. Underlying factors for development of pouch fistulas include presence of sepsis, anastomotic leaks, type of pouch constructed, and a postoperative diagnosis of Crohn's disease. Technical risk factors include local pouch ischemia and, in the case of a pouch-vaginal fistula (PVF), entrapment of the posterior vaginal wall in a stapled anastomosis. The higher incidence of PVF after an ileal J-pouch compared with an S-pouch could well be a reflection of the use of staplers in the anastomosis. From a technical perspective, a key point to note is that when the circular stapler is introduced transanally, the trocar should emerge posterior to the stapler line before "marrying" with the anvil so that the risk of vaginal wall entrapment is minimized.

Signs and symptoms of pouch fistulas are dependent on the location and size of the fistula. They include perineal discharge and sepsis, poor bowel function, pneumaturia, and fecal discharge per vagina. Diagnosis of a fistula can generally be made clinically. Imaging studies such as a Gastrografin enema and CT scanning may be necessary to define its exact anatomy. In order to delineate its origin from the ileoanal anastomotic site, careful inspection of the anastomosis and use of a small catheter placed distally so as not to exclude the anastomosis are essential.

Pouch-Vaginal Fisulas

Development of a PVF can lead to a poor functional result and is one of the main causes of pouch failure. The majority of patients with PVF can be managed initially by local procedures. More commonly, the transanal ileal advancement flap is employed. The technique of this advancement flap is similar to that for a transanal advancement flap for anal fistulas. The tenets of a successful transanal ileal advancement flap repair are control of sepsis, careful hemostasis, excision of concurrent strictures, and a tension-free closure. This approach may involve the use of draining setons and drainage of any associated abscess before repair.

Transvaginal repair is preferred by some surgeons, however. Advantages cited are a cleaner surgical field, avoidance of sphincter injury with consequent fecal incontinence, and easier access compared with a transanal approach, especially when there is some degree of stricturing in the anal canal.

It is our belief that success rates are higher with closure of the fistula on the high-pressure side, using the transanal approach. In a large series of 60 patients with PVF from the Cleveland Clinic, success rates were better with transanal repair.

Repeat IPAA (R-IPAA) for pouch salvage, either as primary treatment or for recurrent PVF, is another option. This procedure was performed in 16 patients from the same series, with eventual healing in 10. Promising results were reported from other series, too, thus lending credence to R-IPAA as a viable option for pouch salvage.

The overall success rate for PVF repair is 52%. Recurrence and pouch failure rates are high, portending a substantial risk of pouch excision and a permanent ileostomy. Temporary fecal diversion at the time of local repair procedures may augment healing rates.

The success of primary healing appears to be related to the timing of occurrence of a PVF following RP. A better outcome is obtained with fistulas occurring within 6 months of RP than with those occurring later. This difference may be related to a delayed diagnosis of Crohn's disease. The majority of patients (up to 40%) with a late diagnosis of Crohn's disease and PVF ultimately underwent pouch excision. Therefore, patients with a known diagnosis of Crohn's disease should not undergo RP because of the high failure rates.

Pouch-Vesical Fistulas

Patients with pouch-vesical fistulas present with pneumaturia and recurrent urinary tract infections. This complication is rare. Most frequently, the bladder dome is involved. Surgical treatment consists of disconnection of the fistula and closure of defects of the bladder and ileal pouch, preferably with omental interposition. Temporary fecal diversion should also be performed.

Pouch-Anal Fistulas

These fistulas should be treated in a manner similar to cryptoglandular anal fistulas. Thus, the options would include simple fistulotomy for low inter- or trans-sphincteric anal fistulas and setons for high fistulas involving a substantial portion of the anal sphincter complex. A transanal mucosal advancement flap can be considered for patients with more complex fistulas after control of any associated sepsis.

Fibrin Glue

The use of fibrin glue for pouch-anal fistulas is controversial as the only reports in the literature describe its use in complex cryptoglandular anal fistulas.

Infliximab

Experience with infliximab, the anti–tumor necrosis factor monoclonal antibody, has been limited. Ricart and associates treated seven ileoanal pouch patients with pouch fistulas and a subsequent diagnosis of Crohn's disease with infliximab. Of the three patients who had PVF, two had complete healing and one sustained a recurrence after initial healing. It may be worthwhile to implement a trial of infliximab in patients with a revised diagnosis of Crohn's and subsequent fistulas.

■ ANASTOMOTIC STRICTURES

The incidence of an ileoanal anastomotic stricture varies between 5% and 38%. The variability in the incidence can be explained by the inconsistent definition of an ileoanal stricture. Strictly speaking, an anastomotic stricture should be defined as a symptomatic narrowing of the ileoanal anastomosis requiring either two or more outpatient dilatations or at least one dilatation under anesthesia.

Symptoms of an ileoanal anastomotic stricture include frequent watery stools, urgency of defecation, abdominal cramping, feeling of incomplete evacuation, and minor fecal leakage. Digital examination not only confirms the diagnosis but also allows assessment of the severity of stenosis as well as digital dilatation. Many patients will have a fibrous web at the anastomosis prior to ileostomy closure which can be disrupted by digital or proctoscopic dilatation. For this reason, at the time of ileostomy closure, it has been our practice to perform a routine digital and proctoscopic assessment and dilatation when the patient is under general anesthesia. We believe that this practice will prevent progression of these fibrous webs to subsequent stricture development.

Significant predisposing factors to stricture formation are use of a temporary defunctioning ileostomy and previous anastomotic complications such as a pelvic abscess or a leak.

In the presence of a defunctioning loop ileostomy, the dilating effect of an uninterrupted fecal stream in the anastomosis is lost, which may account for the higher incidence of stricture formation in diverted patients.

Evidence for the type of anastomosis (hand-sewn versus stapled) that might predispose to stricture development is variable. However, because stapled anastomoses result in fewer septic complications than hand-sewn ones, it may well be that uncomplicated stapled anastomoses result in a lower number of strictures.

Postoperative septic complications are the main contributing factor in the development of a stricture. Strictures resulting from postoperative sepsis are the most difficult to treat, requiring repeated dilatation or other revisional procedures.

The majority of patients with anastomotic strictures are successfully treated with dilatation. Recurring strictures may need excision of the fibrotic ring and ileal mucosa advancement to bridge the mucosal gap. In a small percentage of patients in whom all these measures have failed, especially when the strictures are the result of septic complications, R-IPAA may be necessary. In a series of 141 strictures in 1005 IPAAs, only 3 patients underwent relaparotomy.

The failure rate of IPAA as a result of a stricture alone with no sepsis is low (0.5%). Key technical maneuvers to avoid stricture formation are avoidance of tension on the anastomosis and meticulous surgical technique so as to avoid postoperative septic complications.

■ LEAK FROM THE TIP OF THE J-POUCH

A leak from the tip of the J-pouch is a rare complication following RP and is defined as a leak from the blind limb of the ileal J-pouch. In a study describing 14 patients with a documented leak from the tip of the J-pouch, steroid dependency and a high body surface area were found to be significant predisposing factors for this complication.

The majority of these patients usually present in the late postoperative period (>30 days after RP). Symptoms include fever, purulent wound discharge, and abdominal pain. The diagnosis can often be confirmed radiologically by a CT scan with triple contrast or a contrast enema.

Choice of treatment depends on whether a diverting loop ileostomy is present. In a stable patient who presents before ileostomy closure and with no peritonitis, CT-guided drainage is all that is required as the initial treatment. Surgical repair of the leak is performed at a later date and involves suturing or restapling of the J-pouch tip. The ileostomy may be closed at the time of the repair, or closure may be deferred.

In a nondiverted patient or in patients presenting after ileostomy closure, laparotomy, drainage, and a diverting ileostomy should be performed in the first instance. Surgical repair of the leak should be attempted at least 3 months later and ileostomy closure performed either concurrently or at a subsequent setting.

■ REPEAT ILEAL POUCH–ANAL ANASTOMOSIS (R-IPAA)

When local procedures fail in patients with pouch-related anastomotic complications, R-IPAA may be needed to salvage the pouch. Surgery for R-IPAA is performed with the patient in the modified Trendelenberg position with Lloyd-Davis stirrups. Ureteric stents are inserted to minimize the risk of inadvertent ureteric injury. Local (transanal) repair of pouch anastomotic complications should always be attempted if the following conditions are present:

1. Absence of gross sepsis and tissue edema.
2. Granulation tissue associated with abscess cavities is minimal and easily curetted.
3. Fistulas are close to the anal verge and easily accessible locally.
4. Short stricture.

If local repair is not feasible, a laparotomy and complete pouch mobilization should then be carried out.

Pelvic dissection begins laterally where tissue planes are least distorted and continues caudally. Posterior dissection proceeds cranially and caudally after entering the presacral space behind the superior mesenteric vessels. Pouch mobilization is completed by anterior mobilization and when all-around dissection is carried out caudally to the level of the levators. Injury to the nervi erigentes must be carefully avoided in the course of dissection so as to reduce the incidence of postoperative sexual dysfunction. After disconnection of the ileoanal anastomosis, the small bowel is carefully lifted out of the pelvis and adhesions are divided sharply. Enterotomies and serosal tears are identified and repaired. At this stage, all granulation tissue should be thoroughly curetted, fibrotic scars excised, and pouch defects repaired under direct vision. Anal mucosectomy is then performed.

The pelvic pouch is then resewn to the anal canal at the level of the dentate line using interrupted 2-0 polyglycolic acid sutures. If the original pouch cannot be salvaged, then a new J-pouch is created. However, the decision to excise the original pouch and create a new one must be weighed carefully because loss of small intestinal length may result in a permanent ileostomy if the new pouch were to fail. A defunctioning loop ileostomy is constructed at the end of the operation.

In a series of 35 patients from the Cleveland Clinic who underwent R-IPAA for septic complications, 86% had a functioning pouch. Although functional problems such as seepage and pad use are reported after R-IPAA, patients with successful R-IPAA would still choose to undergo the operation again. Thus, for prevention of pouch failure, aggressive surgical therapy such as R-IPAA is justified because of the high incidence of pouch salvage with this operation.

Suggested Readings

Breen EM, Schoetz DJ, Marcello PW, et al: Functional results after perineal complications of ileal pouch–anal anastomosis. Dis Colon Rectum 1998;41:691–695.

Burke D, van Laarhoven CJ, Herbst F, et al: Transvaginal repair of pouch-vaginal fistula. Br J Surg 2001;88:241–245.

Fazio VW, Wu JS, Lavery IC: Repeat ileal pouch-anal anastomosis to salvage septic complications of pelvic pouches: Clinical outcome and quality of life assessment. Ann Surg 1998;228(4):588–597.

Fazio VW, Ziv Y, Church JM, et al: Ileal pouch-anal anastomoses: Complications and function in 1005 patients. Ann Surg 1995;222(2):120–127.

Lewis WG, Kuzu A, Sagar PM, et al: Stricture at the pouch-anal anastomosis after restorative proctocolectomy. Dis Colon Rectum 1994;37:120–125.

Oncel M, Remzi FH, Church JM, et al: Leak from the tip of the J-pouch: Risk factors, presentation, management and outcome. Dis Colon Rectum (in press). (Presented at the meeting of the American Society of Colon and Rectal Surgeons, New Orleans, LA, June 21–26, 2003.)

Remzi FH, Fazio VW, Preen M, et al: Omission of temporary diversion after restorative proctocolectomy and ileal pouch–anal anastomosis: Surgical complications, functional outcome and quality of life analysis. Dis Colon Rectum (in press). (Presented at the meeting of the American Society of Colon and Rectal Surgeons, Chicago, IL, June 3–7, 2002.)

Shah NS, Remzi FH, Massmann A, et al: Management and treatment outcome of pouch-vaginal fistulas following restorative proctocolectomy. Dis Colon Rectum 2003;46:911–917.

Tjandra JJ, Fazio VW, Milsom JW, et al: Omission of temporary diversion in restorative proctocolectomy—Is it safe? Dis Colon Rectum 1993;36:1007–1014.

Wong KS, Remzi FH, Church JM, et al: Loop ileostomy closure after restorative proctocolectomy: Outcome in 1504 patients. Dis Colon Rectum (in press). (Presented at the meeting of the American Society of Colon and Rectal Surgeons, New Orleans, LA, June 21–26, 2003.)

Ziv Y, Fazio VW, Church JM, et al: Stapled ileal pouch anal anastomoses are safer than handsewn anastomoses in patients with ulcerative colitis. Am J Surg 1996:171:320–323.

40

POUCHITIS AND FUNCTIONAL COMPLICATIONS OF THE PELVIC POUCH

William J. Sandborn, MD

The ideal outcome following colectomy with ileal pouch–anal anastomosis (IPAA) for ulcerative colitis or familial polyposis is five to six semiformed bowel movements occurring during daytime hours, no nocturnal stools, no incontinence, no need for bowel-related medications, and no other bowel symptoms. Unfortunately, many patients fall short of the ideal. The goal of this chapter is to review the diagnosis and treatment of pouchitis and pouch dysfunction following IPAA.

■ EVALUATION ACCORDING TO THE PRESENTING SYMPTOMS

Pouch dysfunction following IPAA may manifest symptomatically as increased stool frequency, difficulty evacuating the pouch, or abdominal pain or bloating. The differential diagnosis for each of these symptomatic presentations is shown in Table 40-1. An algorithm for approaching the evaluation of pouch dysfunction according to the presenting symptoms is shown in Figure 40-1 and discussed in the following sections.

Increased Stool Frequency

Patients with increased stool frequency should undergo pouch endoscopy with examination of both the pouch and the neoterminal ileum above the pouch, and biopsy of the pouch mucosa. Endoscopic findings of inflammation in the pouch can presumptively be called pouchitis and treated with antibiotics (see later discussion). A wide spectrum of endoscopic and histologic findings within the pouch are compatible with pouchitis, including diffuse inflammation, aphthous ulcers, deep linear ulcers, stellate ulcers, patchy inflammation, acute (neutrophil) inflammation, and even granulomas on biopsy. All patients with an IPAA have chronic (lymphocyte) inflammation and villous atrophy on biopsy, and these findings in isolation do not mean the patient has pouchitis. A change in the diagnosis to Crohn's disease should be entertained only if there is evidence of Crohn's disease outside the pouch, such as demonstration of Crohn's disease in the colectomy specimen; fistulas at sites other than the anastomosis of the pouch to the anus; or endoscopic or radiographic evi-

dence of inflammation in the small bowel above the pouch. In some cases, patients will only have inflammation distal to the anastomosis in residual rectal mucosa. This condition, which has been called "strip pouchitis," or "cuffitis," is really persistent ulcerative colitis. Patients with pouch inflammation who fail to respond to antibiotic therapy for pouchitis should be evaluated for specific bacterial infections with *Salmonella*, *Shigella*, *Escherichia coli*, *Campylobacter*, or *Clostridium difficile*, and for specific viral infection with cytomegalovirus, all of which have been reported as causes of pouchitis in patients with an IPAA.

Patients with increased stool frequency who do not have endoscopic or histologic evidence of inflammation do not have pouchitis. Such patients should be evaluated for decreased pouch compliance with rectal balloon distention/manometry studies. If decreased pouch compliance is found, then transrectal ultrasound, pelvic computed tomographic (CT) scan, or magnetic resonance imaging (MRI) should be performed to exclude peripouch sepsis.

Difficulty Evacuating the Pouch

Patients with difficulty evacuating the pouch should be examined for anastomotic stricture. It is important to fully insert the examining index finder. The remaining anal canal often elongates in IPAA patients, and the anastomosis may in reality be positioned 3 to 5 cm proximal to the anus. Incomplete digital examination may miss a significant anastomotic stricture. If the digital examination is normal, a pouchogram x-ray should be performed to evaluate for evidence of pouch stricture, obstruction, and dilation. In patients with either S-pouch or lateral reservoir pouch construction, careful radiographic evaluation for kinking of the afferent ileal limb should be undertaken. In patients with a dilated pouch without concomitant stricture or obstruction on pouchogram x-ray, as well as in patients with a normal pouchogram x-ray but severe symptomatic difficulty in evacuating the pouch, nuclear scintigraphic emptying studies may be useful to quantitate pouch evacuation.

Abdominal Pain or Bloating

Patients with cramping abdominal pain, bloating, and abdominal distention should be evaluated with small bowel x-ray to exclude Crohn's disease and partial small bowel obstruction due to adhesions or stricture. Patients with pouchitis may also experience symptoms of cramping abdominal pain prior to defecation, and thus patients with these symptoms should undergo pouch endoscopy.

■ TREATMENT OF SPECIFIC CONDITIONS

The treatment for specific conditions resulting in pouch dysfunction are shown in Table 40-2 and discussed next.

Pouchitis

Medical treatments reported to be of benefit in patients with pouchitis are shown in Table 40-3, and an algorithm

Table 40-1 Differential Diagnosis for Pouch Dysfunction by Symptoms

SYMPTOM	DIFFERENTIAL DIAGNOSIS
Increased stool frequency	Pouchitis
	Bacterial infection with *Salmonella*, *Shigella*, *Escherichia coli*, or *Campylobacter*
	Specific bacterial infections with *Clostridium difficile*
	Viral infection with cytomegalovirus
	Decreased pouch compliance
	Idiopathic
	Secondary to peripouch abscess/sepsis
	Irritable bowel syndrome
	Crohn's disease
Difficulty evacuating	Anastomotic stricture
	Long efferent limb (S-pouch or lateral reservoir)
	Pouch stricture or obstruction
	Idiopathic decreased pouch evacuation, with or without dilated atonic pouch
Abdominal pain/bloating	Crohn's disease
	Adhesions
	Irritable bowel syndrome

of the approach to medical treatment of pouchitis is shown in Figure 40-2. Treatment is initiated with metronidazole 250 mg three times a day for 10 days. Both a distant recurrence and an early recurrence shortly after discontinuing metronidazole would be treated similarly. If pouchitis recurs a third time over a short period, then maintenance therapy with metronidazole at the lowest effective dose is warranted. For patients who develop side effects to metronidazole, and for patients who fail to respond, treatment with other types of antibiotics such as ciprofloxacin is often the next step. The strategy is again one or two trials of a short course of therapy with the initiation of maintenance therapy for a third recurrence. In patients who appear to develop bacterial resistance after prolonged suppressive antibiotic treatment, cycling of three or four antibiotics in 1-week intervals may be useful, and probiotic therapy with V5L #3 can be used to maintain remission. Those patients who do not respond to

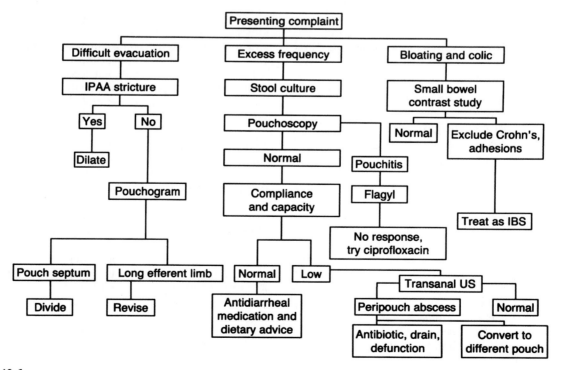

Figure 40-1
Investigation of pouch dysfunction. (IBS = irritable bowel syndrome; IPAA = ileal pouch–anal anastomosis; US = ultrasound.) (From Sagar PM, Pemberton JH: Ileo-anal pouch function and dysfunction. Dig Dis 1997;15:172–188.)

Table 40-2 Treatment of Specific Conditions Resulting in Pouch Dysfunction

CONDITION	TREATMENT
Pouchitis	Antibiotics/probiotics
Specific infection	Antimicrobial therapy
Idiopathic decreased pouch compliance	Diet, antidiarrheal agents
Peripouch abscess/sepsis	Antibiotics, drainage, diversion
Crohn's disease	Medical therapy
Anastomotic stricture	Dilation
Long efferent limb	Shorten limb or revise pouch
Idiopathic decreased pouch evacuation enemas	Biofeedback, catherization, tapwater
Irritable bowel syndrome	Antispasmodics, antidiarrheal agents, fiber

metronidazole, other antibiotics, or probiotics should be treated with 5-aminosalicylate or corticosteroid agents. Topical pouch treatment with 5-aminosalicylate enemas or suppositories, or with corticosteroid enemas, is often tried initially. Sulfasalazine, Pentasa, or oral steroids may also be useful. There is no information about whether Asacol dissolves in the pouch. Some patients may require combination therapy with multiple agents, similar to treatment for inflammatory bowel disease (IBD). Therapy with short-chain fatty acid (SCFA) enemas, glutamine suppositories, and allopurinol has been reported, but the data are unconvincing, and these agents are not widely utilized for pouchitis. Approximately 3% of patients will be refractory to medical therapy and will require an operative approach with permanent ileostomy and either pouch exclusion or excision.

Table 40-3 Treatments Reported to be Efficacious for Pouchitis

CLASS	EXAMPLE
1. Antibiotics	Metronidazole
	Ciprofloxacin
	Amoxicillin/clavulanic acid
	Erythromycin
	Tetracycline
2. Probiotics	VSL #3
3. 5-Aminosalicylates	Mesalamine enemas
	Sulfasalazine
	Oral mesalamine
4. Corticosteroids	Conventional corticosteroid enemas
	Oral corticosteroids
5. Nutritional agents	SCFA* enemas or suppositories
	Glutamine suppositories
6. Immune modifier agents	Cyclosporine enemas
	Azathioprine
7. Other agents	Allopurinol
	Bismuth carbomer enemas
8. Surgical options	Ileal pouch exclusion
	Ileal pouch excision

*SCFA = short-chain fatty acids.
Source: Modified from Sandborn WJ: Pouchitis following ileal pouch–anal anastomosis: Definition, pathogenesis, and treatment. Gastroenterology 1994;107:1856–1860.

At the Mayo Clinic, in patients with IPAA for ulcerative colitis, the cumulative risk of developing at least one episode of pouchitis is 32%. Of those patients who develop pouchitis, 36% have one or two acute pouchitis episodes that respond to treatment with antibiotics, 49% relapse more frequently (at least three acute episodes) but respond to antibiotics, and 15% require maintenance suppressive therapy and have been labeled as having "chronic pouchitis." Of this latter group with chronic pouchitis, almost 50% require surgical exclusion or excision of the pouch. An algorithm showing the clinical course of pouchitis in Mayo Clinic IPAA patients is shown in Figure 40-3.

Specific Pouch Infections

Specific infections of the ileoanal pouch may require treatment with antimicrobial agents. *Campylobacter* infection is treated with oral erythromycin 250 to 500 mg four times a day or ciprofloxacin 500 mg twice a day for 7 days. *Shigella* infection is treated with oral ciprofloxacin 500 mg twice a day or trimethoprim-sulfamethoxazole DS twice a day for 5 days. *Salmonella* infection is generally self-limited and treatment is usually not recommended; if treatment is necessary, the regimen is the same as that for *Shigella* infection. Enteroinvasive *E. coli* is a self-limited infection, and treatment is usually not recommended. *Clostridium difficile* is treated with oral vancomycin 125 to 500 mg four times a day or metronidazole 250 mg four times a day for 10 days. Cytomegalovirus infection is treated with intravenous ganciclovir 5 mg/kg twice a day for 14 to 21 days.

Decreased Pouch Compliance

Patients with decreased pouch compliance secondary to peripouch sepsis should be treated with antibiotics, surgical or radiologic drainage of associated abscesses, and often defunctioning of the pouch. Patients with idiopathic decreased pouch compliance should be treated symptomatically with frequent small-volume meals and antidiarrheal medications.

Crohn's Disease

Crohn's disease of the pouch is treated similarly to Crohn's disease in other settings. Patients with inflammatory Crohn's disease involving the pouch or the small bowel above the pouch will usually benefit from treatment with

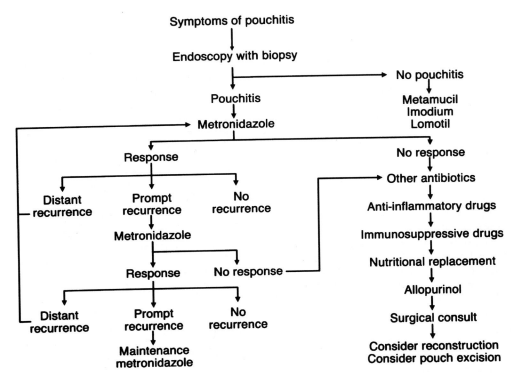

Figure 40-2
Treatment algorithm for pouchitis. Other antibiotics include ciprofloxacin, amoxicillin/clavulanate, erythromycin, tetracycline, and cycling of multiple antibiotics. Anti-inflammatory drugs indicate mesalamine enemas; sulfasalazine; and oral mesalamine. Immunosuppressive drugs refer to steroid enemas, oral steroids, azathioprine, and cyclosporine enemas. Nutritional replacement refers to short-chain fatty acid enemas and glutamine suppositories. (From Sandborn WJ: Pouchitis following ileal pouch–anal anastomosis: Definition, pathogenesis, and treatment. Gastroenterology 1994;107:1856–1860.)

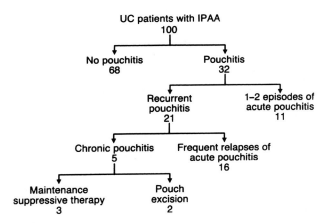

Figure 40-3
Clinical outcome with regard to pouchitis in 100 ulcerative colitis (UC) patients undergoing abdominal colectomy with ileal pouch–anal anastomosis (IPAA). (From Sandborn WJ. Pouchitis: Definition; risk factors; frequency; natural history; classification; and public health perspective. In McLeod RS, Martin F, Sutherland LR, et al (Eds.): Trends in Inflammatory Bowel Disease Therapy 1996. Lancaster, UK, Kluwer Academic Publishers, 1997, pp 51–63.)

an antibiotic such as metronidazole or ciprofloxacin. Pentasa at doses of 3 to 4 g per day may also be tried. For patients with more severe symptoms, treatment with oral corticosteroids, and in some cases azathioprine, 6-mercaptopurine, or methotrexate may be required. For patients with perianal or fistulizing Crohn's disease, antibiotics and immune modifier therapy with cyclosporine, tacrolimus, azathioprine, or 6-mercaptopurine and infliximab may be required.

Anastomotic Stricture

Anastomotic strictures may occur in up to 38% of patients with IPAA. Strictures may be complicated by pouch stasis and secondary pouchitis. Anastomotic strictures should be dilated under anesthesia. Repeated dilations may be required in some patients. In patients with multiple episodes of recurrent anastomotic stricture, self-dilation may be useful.

Long Efferent Limb

Patients with S-pouches and lateral reservoir pouch construction may develop kinking of the efferent limb or "spout" with subsequent difficulty in evacuating the pouch. The treatment for this problem is surgical with either shortening of the efferent limb or pouch revision.

Idiopathic Decreased Pouch Evacuation

Patients may develop a dilated atonic pouch or may have decreased efficiency of pouch evacuation in the absence of an anastomotic stricture or other stricture or obstruction in the pouch. Idiopathic decreased pouch evacuation may be complicated by pouch stasis and secondary pouchitis. Treatment approaches can include biofeedback, intermittent transanal catherization to drain the pouch, tap-water enemas, and treatment of secondary pouchitis. In severe cases, permanent ileostomy with pouch exclusion or excision may be required.

Irritable Bowel Syndrome

The diagnosis of irritable bowel syndrome in patients with IPAA should be made only when all the other possible diagnoses outlined here have been excluded. Treatment of irritable bowel syndrome should be symptomatic. Cramping symptoms can be treated with antispasmodic agents. Increased stool frequency can be treated with fiber and antidiarrheal medications.

■ CONCLUSION

Pouch dysfunction following colectomy with IPAA requires diagnostic evaluation based on the patient's symptoms. Emphasis should be placed on making a specific diagnosis as to the cause of the pouch dysfunction, and then instituting specific treatment for that diagnosis. This approach will be successful in restoring most patients to an acceptable level of pouch function.

Suggested Readings

Colombel JF, Ricart E, Loftus EV Jr, et al: Management of Crohn's disease of the ileoanal pouch with infliximab. Am J Gastroenterol 2003;98: 2239–2344.

Di Febo G, Miglioli M, Lauri A, et al: Endoscopic assessment of acute inflammation of the reservoir after restorative ileo-anal anastomosis. Gastrointest Endosc 1990;36:6–9.

Hurst RD, Molinari M, Chung TP, et al: Prospective study of the incidence, timing and treatment of pouchitis in 104 consecutive patients after proctocolectomy. Arch Surg 1996;131:497–500.

Mahadevan U, Sandborn WJ: Diagnosis and management of pouchitis. Gastroenterology 2003;124:1636–1650.

Penna C, Dozois R, Tremaine W, et al: Pouchitis after ileal pouch-anal anastomosis for ulcerative colitis occurs with increased frequency in patients with associated primary sclerosing cholangitis. Gut 1996;38:234–239.

Sagar PM, Pemberton JH: Ileo-anal pouch function and dysfunction. Dig Dis 1997;15:172–188.

Sandborn WJ: Pouchitis following ileal pouch-anal anastomosis: Definition, pathogenesis, and treatment. Gastroenterology 1994;107:1856–1860.

41

THE CONTINENT ILEOSTOMY—MANAGEMENT OF COMPLICATIONS

Leif Hultén, MD, PhD, FACS

Despite keen advocates for the continent ileostomy over the years, many surgeons have been reluctant to adopt the procedure. It has been marred by a high postoperative morbidity rate, and many modifications in surgical technique and postoperative management have been made over the years to remedy these problems. The early septic complications, such as anastomotic leaks with peritonitis and intra-abdominal abscess, fistulas, and wound sepsis and dehiscence, which were initially a discouraging factor of major concern, have been markedly reduced. Major complications, mostly intestinal obstruction, local abscess, necrosis of the nipple valve, and fistula, are reported to occur in about 10% of cases. The late complications are almost entirely related to the nipple valve. The success of the operation stands with the competence and stability of this intussusception, which remains its Achilles heel. Sliding or prolapse of the valve renders the pouch incontinent. An internal fistula, often developing through the base of the nipple valve, will also result in leakage of intestinal contents, bypassing the valve.

Since the advent of the pelvic pouch procedure, there are today even fewer advocates for the continent ileostomy. However, the technique still has a definite place in surgery. Many conventional ileostomy patients may wish to undergo a conversion to a continent ileostomy owing to ileostomy problems, and certain patients will be unsuitable for sphincter-saving procedures. Moreover, it appears that the excision rate for pelvic pouches increases with the passage of time, and a failing pelvic pouch may well be converted to a continent ileostomy rather than being excised. Therefore, surgeons in specialist clinics offering patients a pelvic pouch should also be familiar with the continent ileostomy technique.

The central problem in regard to the Kock pouch construction has been how to make the valve stable, and a number of technical modifications have been introduced with that objective in mind. The collective results imply that the incidence of revisional surgery due to any of the above-mentioned defects has decreased from 40 to 50% with the early techniques to about 20 to 25% with the introduction of the currently most popular method of mesenteric stripping and stapling of the nipple valve. The results reported by the experts are encouraging, with a revision rate of about 10%.

The current most popular method of formation of the ileal pouch and creation of the nipple valve emphasizes four important measures contributing to valve stability. Stripping of the peritoneal leaves of the valve mesentery and the mesenteric fat of the nipple valve segment to reduce the bulk of tissue interposed in the intussusception, and stabilization of the intussuscepted valve by means of staplers are the two most important steps. To avoid necrosis of the tip of the valve it has been recommended to remove 10 staples near the hinge of the loading unit. A firm side-to-side fixation of the nipple valve to the reservoir wall for prevention of sliding or prolapse was originally suggested by Kock and more recently by Fazio and Tjandra (1992). Moreover, Barnett uses a segment of intestine with its lumen in continuity with the pouch as a collar to wrap around the base of the nipple, creating a valve similar to Nissen fundoplication. Another interesting modification has recently been described by Kaiser and associates (2002). The value of these modifications are still scientifically unproved.

Careful and correct formation of the exit conduit channel with firm anchoring of the reservoir to the abdominal wall and strict routines in the postoperative management of the pouch—extending the drainage interval in a gradual fashion—are the two other measures supposed to favor stabilization of the nipple valve. Although detailed instructions on the aftercare have been given extensive space in many recent articles on the subject, the importance of this last point has often been neglected in the past.

The importance of a defunctioning ileostomy for reducing the early morbidity rate, or at least minimizing the consequences of any complication developing during the early postoperative phase, is controversial, but such a safety measure should probably be recommended for the beginner before experience has been gained.

However, the continent ileostomy is a demanding procedure with a high potential for complications, and special skill and experience are required for their recognition and management.

■ EARLY COMPLICATIONS

Septic complications, such as local or diffuse peritonitis due to suture leakage or abscess, require immediate and proper treatment. A local peritonitis with or without abscess should be drained and a proximal loop ileostomy established. A fistula either may heal spontaneously on this treatment or could be subject to revision by another operation 2 or 3 months later. Ischemic necrosis of the outlet may also occasionally develop in the early postoperative phase. Depending in its extent, it may either be treated conservatively by prolonged tube drainage of the pouch. When more extensive as judged by ileoscopy, it is managed by establishment of a loop ileostomy. In both situations revisional surgery can then be performed at a convenient time a few months later.

Bleeding from the pouch during the first postoperative days is common. The irrigation fluid will sometimes be heavily bloody. The stapling technique has proved to be particularly likely to cause bleeding, and some surgeons advise against its use. Profuse bleeding may sometimes occur even after a careful suturing technique with clots accumulating in the pouch blocking the draining catheter. Too little attention has been directed to the importance of the postoperative catheter drainage. With strict irrigation routines and the use of a proper draining system, in most cases this complication can be managed conservatively.

■ LATE COMPLICATIONS

Despite increased surgical experience, improvements in technique, and strict routines in the postoperative management, there remains a tendency for slippage or prolapse of the nipple valve in the long run and for fistula to develop at its base with resulting loss of continence.

Slippage of the Nipple Valve

Difficulties in intubation of the reservoir because of angulated course of the outlet and later on leakage of gas and feces are indications of valve slippage. Patients may sometimes attend acutely with an overdistended reservoir due to inability to insert the catheter. By means of a pediatric sigmoidoscope it is possible to follow the typically angulated course into the reservoir. Once the reservoir has been emptied, an indwelling catheter should be passed through the sigmoidoscope, which is then removed. Surgical revision by formal laparotomy is required for re-establishment of continence, however. The surgical approach to be employed depends on the precise findings at laparotomy.

The stoma and outlet is first dissected free and the reservoir mobilized into the wound. It may occasionally be possible without damage to "deinvaginate" the intussusception completely by careful dissection of the walls forming the nipple valve. Provided that the outlet is sufficiently long to reach skin level, the reservoir is simply opened and a 5-cm-long nipple valve is created again and fixed in position.

In other cases complete deinvagination of the nipple valve may be impossible or the afferent segment is damaged by the dissection or proves to be insufficient in length. The segment then has to be sacrificed and a new nipple valve and outlet constructed. This can be done by two different procedures.

The most common technique is to divide the entrance conduit 15 to 20 cm from the reservoir (Fig. 41-1). The intestinal segment still attached to the pouch is carefully prepared by peritoneal stripping and defatting of the mesentery, and a new nipple valve is fashioned and stabilized according to the stapling techniques described. The reservoir is rotated to enable the new outlet to be passed through the abdominal channel and a new stoma has to be formed. Special attention should be directed to firm anchoring of the pouch. The channel through the abdominal wall should be narrowed if necessary to fit the outlet properly or a new trephine wound should be created.

The alternative procedure is to provide a new exit conduit and nipple valve by incising a 15- to 20-cm segment of ileum at a convenient level above the reservoir (Fig. 41-2), and inserting it between the reservoir and the abdominal wall.

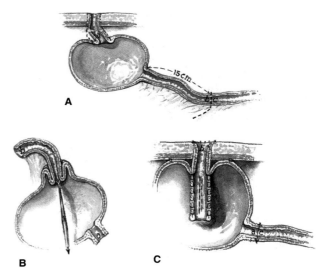

Figure 41-1
Rotation of the pouch A, The outlet and nipple valve resected and 15 to 20 cm of the entrance conduit prepared for intussusception. B and C, A new nipple valve and outlet created.

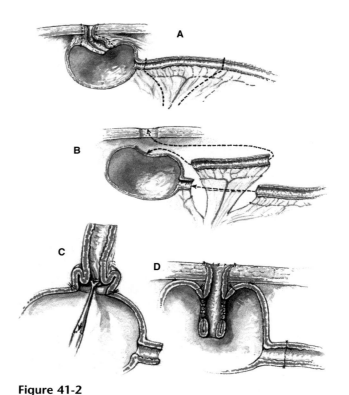

Figure 41-2
A new outlet and nipple valve created by means of an interposed ileal segment. A, A 15- to 20-cm length of terminal ileum is prepared. B, The bowel is divided and mobilized with preservation of blood supply. The old outlet and valve are excised. C, The new outlet is anastomotosed to the pouch and a nipple valve inserted. D, The terminal ileum is re-anastomotosed to the pouch.

Prolapse of Nipple Valve

A prolapse can often be easily reduced manually but requires surgical connection by laparotomy for lasting cure. An overly wide channel through the abdominal wall is one of the causes underlying this condition. This complication has also been observed during pregnancy. The stoma and exit conduit should therefore be dissected free, with complete mobilization of the reservoir. The channel should be narrowed by suturing the rectal muscle and the fascia, allowing the exit conduit to fit snugly. Another alternative is to select another site for the ileostomy and create a new trephine wound through intact abdominal wall. Anchoring the nipple valve side-to-side to the reservoir wall is a recent technical modification introduced by Kock to prevent nipple valve dislocation (Fig. 41-3).

Fistula Through the Nipple Valve

A fistula at the base of the valve was formerly a common complication caused by silk sutures and has also been seen frequently following the use of synthetic material (Marlex or Mersilene mesh) to stabilize the intussusception. Most authors advise against the use of these products, so the complication has now become rare. Repair of the fistula may be accomplished by local sutures after excision of its edges, sometimes without a formal laparotomy. In more complicated cases and in those in which such a repair has been unsuccessful, resection of the nipple valve with its outlet and pouch rotation with construction of a new valve as described for sliding is required.

Miscellaneous Complications

Perforation of the reservoir is a very rare complication that might be caused by too vigorous insertion of the catheter or by penetration of a sharp object such as a fishbone. The closure of a perforation should be protected by a loop ileostomy. Volvulus of the reservoir has been reported but should not occur if the fixation of the reservoir is performed according to current principles. Fibrosis of the tip of the nipple valve is another complication that may require dilatation and occasionally reconstruction. Skin stricture around the stoma is common but is easily dealt with by local revision.

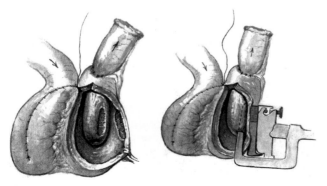

Figure 41-3
Stapling the nipple to the pouch wall.

Necrosis of the Exit Conduit or the Nipple Valve

This vascular complication is due to faulty technique employed for preparing and stabilizing the nipple valve. Rough handling during peritoneal stripping and defattening of mesentery, improper positioning of stapler rows, or strangulation of nipple valve or exit conduit mesentery by sutures or in a narrow abdominal aperture may each or in combination compromise vascular supply. Great care should be taken to avoid these errors.

Recurrent Nipple Valve Complications

The policy in our institution has always been to recommend the patient to have revisional surgery to re-establish continence in case of nipple dysfunction. Only occasionally is it necessary to remove the pouch owing to any of these complications.

In this context it must be emphasized that surgical revision of nipple dysfunction, although requiring another laparotomy, is not necessarily a major undertaking. Even if such a reconstruction is again followed by sliding or any other defect of the nipple valve function, a further operation for restoration of continence is usually justified and will be successful eventually. It also appears that once a patient has experienced the benefits of a continent ileostomy, such a patient usually insists on further revisional surgery and refuses to have the reservoir removed. An indwelling ileostomy valve device has been described to deal with an incontinent valve but should only occasionally be a permanent measure, being restricted mainly to patients who are physically unfit to withstand another laparotomy.

Relaparotomy

The time when a relaparotomy should be done varies with the type and severity of the complication and with the patient's general condition. For many of the complications occurring during the immediate postoperative phase, such as profuse bleeding or suture leakage with local or diffuse peritonitis, the need for acute laparotomy is obvious. In less threatening situations (a fistula or nipple valve necrosis) relaparotomy can be delayed and performed at a more convenient time when the patient has recovered and the inflammatory reaction has subsided. Most surgeons agree that a delay of about 2 to 3 months before relaparotomy is best. During the delay, the patient may be obliged to drain the pouch with an indwelling catheter or use an ileostomy bag.

Ileitis (Pouchitis)

The cause of the nonspecific inflammatory reaction that sometimes develops in the reservoir or the afferent intestinal loop is still unknown (Svaninger et al, 1993). It may be mild or asymptomatic, being apparent endoscopically as a reddened, edematous mucosa. In more severe cases the patients suffer from colicky pain and diarrhea with liquid, bloody feces. It is often readily reversed by oral antibiotics (metronidazole), although continuous drainage may be required in severe cases. A loop ileostomy may be justified as an alternative measure, when other treatment has failed, and before removal of the pouch. It has been suggested that pouchitis is bacterial; however, because the condition appears to be connected exclusively to patients operated upon for ulcerative colitis, the cause is more likely to be inherent in the original disease. As compared to the other complications, which can all be managed surgically, pouchitis was therefore considered a particularly distressing and ominous complication. When looked upon in a longer perspective, however, such fears appear to be unfounded. Although the overall failure rate of the Kock pouch may approach 10 to 15%, pouchitis appears only occasionally to be the reason for pouch excision. Moreover, there is a general impression that the episodes of pouchitis become milder or may even disappear with the passage of time

Epithelial Dysplasia and Cancer Risk

Sporadic reports of dysplasia and the occasional adenocarcinoma in the ileal pouch mucosa have been published (Cox et al, 1997), demonstrating a further complication of the ileal pouch.

Some reports suggest that dysplastic transformation in pelvic pouches is a rare phenomenon, and, therefore, the risk of further progression to cancer should be small (Sarigol et al, 1999). Others (Gullberg et al, 1997) claim the opposite view. Common to these studies is that the observation time is relatively short, and, therefore, there are doubts as to the reliability of these statements. The long-term results presented recently from a study on patients with a continent ileostomy are more reliable and reassuring. With an average follow-up of 30 years, the incidence of mucosal dysplasia in the ileal pouch mucosa in a comparatively large series of patients kept under close supervision proved to be low, and no case of carcinoma or high-grade dysplasia was observed (see Duff et al, 2002; Hultén et al, 2002).

Ileal Pouch Adenomas in Patients with Familial Polyposis

The tendency of small bowel adenomas to develop many years after colectomy for familial polyposis may be another problem in patients with a continent ileostomy. Adenomas with the potential to progress to adenocarcinoma can develop in the mucosa of the continent ileostomy. The risk of developing one or more adenomas over a 10-year period has been calculated to be about 35%, and patients with adenomas appear more likely to have duodenal and ampullary adenomas. Regular endoscopic surveillance of patients with a Kock pouch is therefore recommended, with a frequency similar to that of upper gastrointestinal endoscopy.

■ CRITERIA OF SELECTION

The main indications for a continent ileostomy are ulcerative colitis and familial polyposis, but the procedure has also been used in patients with multiple colorectal carcinoma, aganglionosis coli, anal incontinence, and severe constipation. In patients with Crohn's disease the operation has been marred by a very high rate of immediate and late complications, and most surgeons therefore consider Crohn's disease a contraindication. However, in very selected cases, patients who have had proctocolectomy for Crohn's colitis without involvement of the distal ileum, who are disease free for at least 5 years, may be offered a Kock pouch. In our institution older age does not preclude the Kock pouch provided that the patient is mentally fit. In fact, the patient's manual skill, which will be inevitably reduced with time, is less demanding in the management of the reservoir than that necessary to change the appliance used for the conventional ileostomy.

■ CONTINENT ILEOSTOMY OR PELVIC POUCH

The pelvic pouch procedure has become the most popular method today for curative treatment of ulcerative colitis and familial polyposis. The failure rate after construction of a pelvic pouch in patients with ulcerative colitis (UC) varies. Tulchinsky and associates reported a failure rate of 9% on 635 patients with an average follow-up of 3 years, but Korsgen and associates reported a 19% failure rate in 154 patients. It is interesting that most pouch failures seem to occur late. Pelvic sepsis, poor function, pouchitis, and overlooked Crohn's disease seem to be the main reasons for failures. The failure rate when calculated and expressed in crude figures is often unreliable, and actuarial methods should be a more correct statistical method to determine this cumulative risk. A life table calculation based on figures presented so far would imply that the cumulative risk for pouch failure in a UC patient would be up to 15% over 10 years (Setti-Carraro et al, 1994) and 30 to 40% in patients who develop septic complications (Heuschen et al, 2002). So the long-term results imply that the ileoanal pouch may not be the panacea it was initially thought to be.

Three options most readily come to mind for patients with a failing pouch. It may be defunctioned with an ileostomy proximal to the pouch, it may be revised, or it may be excised. Clearly, the first option is usually a temporary measure, while refashioning of the pouch or the ileoanal anastomosis—which may well be tried—is often associated with an unsuccessful result. According to reports in the literature, pouch excision with construction of a conventional ileostomy appears to the most common measure employed for these patients. This may be a very unfortunate decision, however, as such an operation will unevitably be associated with loss of a significant length of terminal ileum. Apart from the practical problems of a "high-flow" ileostomy, saltwater imbalance and malabsorption of bile acids and vitamin B_{12} will develop. Kusunoki and coworkers (1990) and Hultén and coworkers (1992, 2001) therefore recommend conversion of the failed ileal pouch–anal anastomosis to a continent ileostomy as a fourth alternative.

The foregoing would imply that a surgical team adopting the pelvic pouch procedure should also be conversant with the continent ileostomy technique and be prepared to offer patients this operation as a second alternative—a

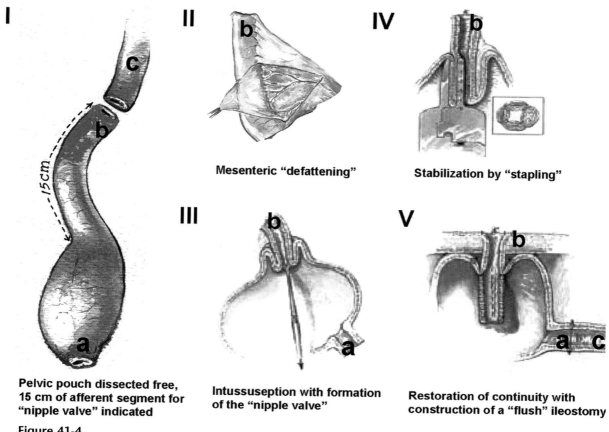

Figure 41-4
Conversion of a pelvic pouch to a continent ileostomy.

technically demanding but often beneficial procedure worthwhile for motivated patients (Fig. 41-4).

Thus, primary candidates for a continent ileostomy will still be patients who have a standard ileostomy and have had a proctectomy, those who prefer this pouch to a pelvic ileal reservoir, and patients with irreparable rectal incontinence, including those with a failed ileal pouch–anal anastomosis. It seems reasonable to assume that during the next decade there may well be a great revival of interest in the continent ileostomy technique.

■ CONCLUDING REMARKS

It appears reasonable to assume that anyone with a keen interest in colorectal surgery should be able to adopt the continent ileostomy technique in its present fashion and put it into practice with a good prospect of success. In many patients complications will occur requiring reintervention before the ideal functional stage is reached.

Experience and surgical skill are needed to maximize the success rate, but competence is also required for proper management of the complications. A sufficiently large patient flow is important to achieve and maintain expertise, and the continent ileostomy should therefore be done in specialized surgical units where a team of surgeons must be prepared to accept a long-term commitment to these patients.

Suggested Readings

Barnett WO: New approaches for continent ostomy construction. J Miss State Med Assoc 1987;28:1–3.

Behrens DT, Paris M, Luttrell JN: Conversion of failed ileal pouch–anal anastomosis to continent ileostomy. Dis Colon Rectum 1999;42:490–496.

Cox CL, Butts DR, Roberts MP, et al: Development of invasive adenocarcinoma in a long-standing Kock continent ileostomy: Report of a case. Dis Colon Rectum 1997;40(4):500–503.

Duff SE, O'Dwyer ST, Hultén L, et al: Dysplasia in the ileoanal pouch. Colorect Dis 2002;4:420–426.

Fazio VW, Tjandra JJ: Technique for nipple valve fixation to prevent valve slippage in continent ileostomy. Dis Colon Rectum 1992;35:1177–1179.

Gullberg K, Stahlberg D, Liljeqvist L, et al: Neoplastic transformation of the pelvic pouch mucosa in patients with ulcerative colitis. Gastroenterology 1997;112(5):1487–1492.

Heuschen UA, Hinz U, Allemeyer EH, et al: Risk factors for ileoanal J pouch-related septic complications in ulcerative colitis and familial adenomatous polyposis. Ann Surg 2002;235(2):207–216.

Hultén L: Conversion of a failing pelvic pouch to a continent ileostomy—"Last images." Tech Coloproctol 2001;5:190.

Hultén L: Proctocolectomy and ileostomy to pouch surgery for ulcerative colitis. World J Surg 1998;22:335–341.

Hultén L: Continent ileostomy (Kock's pouch) vs restorative procto-colectomy. World J Surg 1985;9:952–959.

Hultén L, Fasth S, Hallgren T, Öresland T: The failing pelvic pouch conversion to continent ileostomy. Int J Colorect Dis 1992;7:119–121.

Hultén L, Willén R, Nilsson O, et al: Mucosal assessment for dysplasia and cancer in the ileal pouch mucosa in patients operated on for ulcerative colitis—A 30 year follow-up study. Dis Colon Rectum 2002;45:448–452.

Kaiser AM, Stein JP, Beart RW Jr: T-pouch: A new valve design for a continent ileostomy. Dis Colon Rectum 2002;45:411–415.

Korsgen S, Nikiteas N, Ogunbiyi OA, Keighley MR: Results from pouch salvage. Br J Surg 1996;83:372–374.

Kusunoki M, Sakanoue Y, Shoji Y, et al: Conversion of malfunctioning J-pouch to Kock pouch. Acta Chir Scand 1990;156;179–181.

Parc YR, Olschwang S, Desaint B, et al: Familial adenomatous polyposis: Prevalence of adenomas in the ileal pouch after restorative proctocolectomy. Ann Surg 2001;233:360–364.

Sarigol S, Wyllie R, Gramlich T, et al: Incidence of dysplasia in pelvic pouches in paediatric patients after ileal pouch–anal anastomosis for ulcerative colitis. J Pediatr Gastroenterol Nutr 1999;28(4):429–434.

Setti-Carraro P, Ritchie JK, Wilkinson KH, et al: The first 10 years' experience of restorative proctocolectomy for ulcerative colitis. Gut 1994;35(8):1070–1075.

Stryker SJ, Carney JA, Dozois RR: Multiple adenomatous polyps arising in a continent reservoir ileostomy. Int J Colorect Dis 1987;2;43–45.

Svaninger G, Nordgren S, Öresland T, Hultén L: Incidence and characteristics of pouchitis in the Kock continent ileostomy and in the pelvic pouch. Scand J Gastroenterol 1993;28:695–700.

Tulchinsky H, Hawley RR, Nicholls J: Long-term failure after restorative proctocolectomy for ulcerative colitis. Ann Surg 2003;238:229–234.

42

UNHEALED PERINEAL WOUND

Neil H. Hyman, MD

Throughout the 20th century, rectal excision via a combined abdominal and perineal approach has been a mainstay of surgical treatment for rectal cancer and inflammatory bowel disease. Dealing with the perineal wound after these procedures has been problematic, and much has been debated about the ideal method to achieve complete healing of the perineum. Most recently, with the emphasis on sphincter-saving techniques to treat rectal cancer and inflammatory disease, this issue has received much less attention. Nonetheless, an unhealed perineal wound remains a major source of frustration for patients and surgeons alike. There is still disagreement regarding the optimal method of preventing this troublesome complication and how to treat it once it has occurred. An unhealed perineal wound can be arbitrarily defined as unhealed 6 months after proctectomy.

An understanding of how the pelvis and perineum heal after proctectomy is essential to both prevention and treatment of the unhealed perineal wound. After excision of the rectum, a large pelvic cavity is created. Clearly, posterior migration of the anterior genitourinary structures and descent of the peritoneal floor assist in narrowing this space. However, the posterior and lateral aspects of the pelvis are bordered by bony structures, and it seems unlikely that they are capable of substantially contributing to closure of this space. As such, there will always remain the potential for a large space that will become a rigid, fibrotic cavity and the source of a chronic unhealed perineal wound. It is simply too large a space to "granulate" in. As such, open packing of the pelvis and perineum to allow for such ingrowth is a technique that virtually assures a high failure rate.

Successful techniques will allow this space to become filled by healthy, well vascularized tissue. One may fill the pelvis with omentum or simply leave the pelvic parietal peritoneum open and allow small bowel to obliterate the space.

■ CAUSES

Perineal wounds may not heal because of technical factors, patient factors, or disease-specific factors. The importance of filling the pelvic dead space with healthy soft tissue has been emphasized. Excessive bleeding during proctectomy with hematoma formation or contamination of the pelvis with fecal contents will adversely affect postoperative healing. The resulting pelvic collection will result in a rigid, fibrotic cavity that will be slow to heal, or will remain unhealed. A recent series noted that all patients developing a perineal hematoma or infection after surgery developed nonhealing perineal sinuses. Nonabsorbable sutures may serve as foreign bodies and may impair healing.

Patient-specific factors such as malnutrition, diabetes, or obesity may contribute to poor healing. The underlying indication for rectal excision is also clearly a major issue. It has been widely noted that perineal wounds are most likely to remain unhealed after proctectomy for inflammatory bowel disease. Unhealed perineal wounds are more common after proctectomy for Crohn's disease than ulcerative colitis. Rectal resection for cancer seems to yield the lowest rate of a nonhealing perineal wound. The reason for this is likely multifactorial. Patients with Crohn's disease will commonly have considerable perirectal fibrosis or fistulization, making proctectomy technically more difficult. As such, the chance of inadvertent rectal perforation with contamination of the pelvis is higher, and there is even the opportunity to leave residual rectal wall with its secretory mucosa in the pelvis.

In addition, the subset of Crohn's disease patients with extensive perianal fistulas and sepsis create special problems in perineal wound healing. Further, many patients with inflammatory bowel disease are on potent immunomodulatory agents and may have poor nutritional status. It has been shown that rectal cancer patients who have undergone preoperative radiation therapy have a higher probability of wound breakdown. Pelvic irradiation causes local ischemia and fibrosis, which may be exacerbated by the effects of concomitant chemotherapy.

■ PREVENTION

Obviously, it is far preferable to prevent an unhealed perineal wound than to treat one. Surgical technique is of paramount importance. Filling the pelvis with well-vascularized omentum or small bowel without closure of the pelvic peritoneum is advised. Meticulous hemostasis and the use of a closed suction drain to prevent seroma or hematoma formation seems prudent. However, these drains may serve as a nidus for infection, and should be removed within the first few postoperative days.

A thorough knowledge of pelvic anatomy and appropriate tissue planes is invaluable in performing the difficult proctectomy. For example, in the patient with advanced pelvic fibrosis due to Crohn's disease, avoidance of rectal perforation and pelvic contamination may be difficult even for the experienced surgeon. The technique of intersphincteric proctectomy with preservation and closure of the levator ani muscles and external sphincters allows for secure closure of the pelvic floor. Further, this dissection is done in a relatively avascular plane, which avoids hematoma creation and excessive blood loss.

Patient-specific factors should be corrected as far as possible. A period of nutritional support may be indicated preoperatively, and any specific nutrient deficiencies should be corrected. Patients with a so-called "watering can" perineum present special problems in postoperative wound healing. A very high percentage of these patients will develop unhealed perineal wounds, and the ideal method of treating these patients has yet to be defined. A variety of strategies have been devised or advocated. This particular situation bears special comment, as it is the source of a high percentage of unhealed perineal wounds in a modern surgical practice. Some of the methods described to deal with this include the following: (1) Preliminary stoma formation with the intent of diminishing local perianal sepsis prior to a later definitive proctectomy. (2) Near total proctocolectomy, leaving a very short anorectal stump, avoiding the perineal dissection altogether. (3) Preliminary unroofing of fistulous tracks, intending to eliminate local sepsis prior to definitive proctectomy at a later date. (4) Debridement and unroofing of fistulous tracks can be done at the time of definitive proctectomy. The levators are closed, and the skin and subcutaneous tissue are left open to heal by secondary intention. Skin coverage may be achieved at a later date as necessary.

Based on experience with all these approaches we are happiest with the fourth option. Preliminary ileostomy does not reliably reduce perianal disease activity and only seems to add an additional, unhelpful step in most patients. Near total proctectomy with ultra-low Hartmann stump, thereby avoiding any incisions in the septic perineum, seems appealing. However, this approach has been disappointing, as most patients continue to have symptoms from purulent drainage even with a very short stump. Routine preliminary unroofing prior to a later proctectomy has not been particularly helpful.

Rather, at FAHC, unroofing and thorough debridement of thickened, inflamed skin combined with intersphincteric proctectomy appears to yield the best results. A solid pelvic floor muscle closure is employed and only the skin and subcutaneous tissue are left open. Sometimes skin grafts are required to speed healing if extensive skin excision has been required.

■ DIAGNOSIS

Unhealed perineal wounds are clinically evident from the history and physical examination. Patients in whom surgical intervention is being considered require thoughtful diagnostic evaluation. Superficial sinuses, involving only the skin and soft tissue, are relatively straightforward to treat and do not generally need extensive diagnostic testing. However, patients with extension into the pelvis and associated large, fibrotic cavities will require a whole different level of intervention and planning.

After history taking, the first step is always a careful physical examination. The volume and nature of the drainage may be a clue to the extent of the problem. For example, a previously unsuspected enteroperineal fistula, rather than an unhealed perineal wound, may be present. A sinogram can be especially helpful, particularly if communication with the small bowel is suspected. In other cases the sinogram can demonstrate the size and nature of an associated cavity. If recurrent Crohn's disease is suspected, a small bowel series will be helpful. When a complex cavity seems to be present with extension into the pelvis, a computed tomographic (CT) scan or magnetic resonance image (MRI) will generally be helpful in delineating anatomy and planning treatment. An examination under anesthesia may be all that is needed in many patients. Foreign bodies, such as pieces of an old pelvic drain or suture material, need to be removed. In some cases, residual rectal mucosa may be present. Transvaginal ultrasound may be helpful in selected cases and can be used intraoperatively to help define anatomic relationships.

■ TREATMENT

Despite apparent advances in surgical techniques, unhealed perineal wounds remain a substantial problem. A recent series using intersphincteric proctectomy still reported a 38% incidence of perineal wound problems. The first step is generally patience. Some wounds may be slow to heal, but will ultimately close. Attention to proper hygiene and periodic follow-up may lead to a healed wound. Some wounds may take a full year to completely heal. As long as there is progress, there is hope. Further, many patients have relatively low output wounds that they can easily manage and do not particularly bother them. These patients do not necessarily need any treatment at all.

■ OPERATIVE MANAGEMENT

In terms of planning operative treatment, it can be helpful to divide unhealed wounds into superficial sinuses versus those that are associated with a chronic pelvic cavity (Fig. 42-1). Symptomatic superficial sinuses can be effectively treated with curettage. The patient is examined under anesthesia to confirm that there is no undiagnosed chronic pelvic collection. A curette is used to remove chronically infected granulation tissue, and skin bridges are unroofed. A wound is created so that there is an adequate opening in the skin to allow for healing "from the bottom up." Particularly for larger wounds, the curettage may have to be repeated to encourage shrinkage of the space.

Although it is reasonable to expect a subcutaneous space to fill in with soft tissue, it is not a reasonable expectation for a large, chronic, fibrotic pelvic cavity. As such, curettage does not suffice in this situation. After excision and debridement of the fibrotic rind, there will remain a chronic cavity requiring placement of healthy, well-vascularized tissue. Gracilis muscle interposition is our procedure of choice to fill this space. The coccyx often must be excised and the lower two segments of the sacrum may be safely resected as needed to provide for wound closure without tension. Although the gracilis is harvested initially in the lithotomy position, the prone jack-knife position always seems to provide the most comfortable exposure for debridement and muscle fixation in this

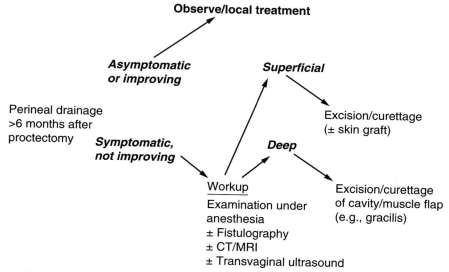

Figure 42-1
Proposed algorithm for treatment of patients with unhealed perineal wound.

setting. Although other muscles have been proposed for use in filling this space, the gracilis muscle has probably been utilized most widely. The gracilis muscle is divided distally at its insertion and tunneled into the perineal wound. It is important that the pelvic cavity be properly assessed and that careful attention is given to avoiding injury of surrounding pelvic structures prior to fixing the gracilis into position. Other techniques, such as fibrin glue or nitrogen mustard injection, have been described. We have had no luck with fibrin glue in this setting and do not offer this procedure.

■ SUMMARY

Sphincter-saving techniques have diminished the number of proctectomies being performed both for inflammatory bowel disease and for malignancy. However, the unhealed perineal wound remains a major source of chronic morbidity following proctectomy. The incidence is highest after proctectomy for Crohn's disease and lowest after excision for cancer. Good surgical technique is the key to minimizing the incidence of this complication. The parietal peritoneum should be left open and small bowel or omentum allowed to fill the pelvic space. Open packing is generally to be condemned. Closed suction drains, removed relatively early in the postoperative period, may decrease the possibility of hematoma or seroma formation. Infection or hematoma seem to contribute to the problem of unhealed perineal wounds.

Asymptomatic patients do not necessarily require any treatment. Superficial sinuses may be treated with curettage. Deep, chronically fibrotic pelvic cavities require debridement and placement of well-vascularized, healthy tissue such as gracilis muscle.

Suggested Readings

McLeod RS: Chronic ulcerative colitis. Traditional surgical techniques. Surg Clin North Am 1993;73(5):891–908.

Mikkola K, Luukkonen P, Jarvinen HJ: Restorative compared with conventional proctocolectomy for the treatment of ulcerative colitis. Eur J Surg 1996:162(4):315–319.

Oakley JR, Fazio YW, Jagelman DG, et al: Management of the perineal wound after rectal excision for ulcerative colitis. Dis Colon Rectum 1985;28:885–888.

Ryan JA: Gracilis muscle flap for the persistent perineal sinus of inflammatory bowel disease. Am J Surg 1984;148:64–70.

Silen W, Glotzer DJ: The prevention and treatment of the persistent perineal sinus. Surgery 1974;75(4):535–542.

Tompkins RG, Warshaw AL: Improved management of the perineal wound after proctectomy. Ann Surg 1985;202(6):760–765.

43

MEDICAL TREATMENT OF CROHN'S DISEASE

Aaron Brzezinski, MD, FRCP(C)
Bret A. Lashner, MD, MPH

Crohn's disease is a chronic, recurrent, inflammatory disease of unknown etiology that affects the gastrointestinal tract. Its distinct clinical and pathologic features make treatment challenging. Crohn's disease is characterized by skip lesions and transmural inflammation, and it can affect any segment of the gastrointestinal tract. Furthermore, the disease has protean presentations including inflammation, fistula, stricture, or a combination of these. Its course is characterized by episodes of remission and exacerbation.

The medical treatment of Crohn's disease is largely determined by a combination of site of involvement, disease severity, and disease behavior. Patients may need treatment to induce remission, maintain remission, or treat complications. The most common pattern of involvement in patients with Crohn's disease is ileocolonic. At presentation, this pattern occurs in about 40% of patients. The second most common anatomic pattern is small intestinal involvement (35% of patients), while isolated colonic disease is found in 25%. Gastroduodenal involvement occurs in approximately 5% of patients. The least common pattern is esophageal disease. The treatment of patients with Crohn's disease can be divided into treatment for acute disease and maintenance of remission.

■ MEDICATIONS FOR TREATMENT OF CROHN'S DISEASE

Azo Bond Compounds

5-Aminosalicylic Acid and Sulfasalazine

5-Aminosalicylic acid (5-ASA) was first used for treating patients with ulcerative colitis in 1942. A Swedish physician, Dr. Nana Swartz, was studying the use of sulfasalazine in patients with arthritis. It was believed that the combination of an anti-inflammatory, 5-ASA, and an antibiotic, sulfapyridine, would be beneficial for patients with some forms of arthritis. In the study group were patients with ulcerative colitis and enteropathic arthritis, whose colitis improved with the use of sulfasalazine. Since then, sulfasalazine has played a major role in the treatment of patients with inflammatory bowel disease, both ulcerative colitis and Crohn's disease.

Sulfasalazine has two molecules bound by a diazo bond, 5-ASA and sulfapyridine. After oral ingestion, sulfasalazine arrives intact into the colon, where the 5-ASA is cleaved from the sulfapyridine by bacterial action. 5-ASA is the active anti-inflammatory compound, acting directly on the diseased mucosa rather than by a systemic effect. This concept is of vital importance in choosing which 5-ASA compound to give to patients with Crohn's disease. For example, a patient with jejunal disease will not have a therapeutic benefit from a preparation releasing 5-ASA in the colon, and a patient with colonic disease needs a compound that primarily releases 5-ASA in the colon. Approximately 30% of patients are either intolerant or allergic to sulfapyridine (Table 43-1). For these individuals, newer 5-ASA compounds are available.

Sulfasalazine is available in a 500-mg tablet and in an enteric-coated delayed-release tablet. The enteric-coated form causes fewer symptoms of gastric intolerance such as anorexia, nausea, and vomiting. Sulfasalazine interferes with folic acid absorption; therefore, it is advisable to prescribe supplemental folic acid at a dose of 0.4 to 1.0 mg per day to patients on this medication. For induction of remission we use a dose of 4 to 6 g per day divided in four doses; 2 to 4 g per day is used for maintenance of remission.

Olsalazine

Olsalazine (Dipentum) is composed of two molecules of 5-ASA linked by an azo bond. Like sulfasalazine, it requires colonic bacteria producing azo-reductase to cleave both molecules. It is therefore easy to understand

Table 43-1 Side Effects of Sulfasalazine
COMMON SIDE EFFECTS (30 TO 35%)
Headache
Anorexia
Nausea, vomiting, dyspepsia
Oligospermia (reversible upon discontinuation)
LESS COMMON (3 TO 4%)
Hemolytic anemia
Rash
Pruritus
Urticaria
UNCOMMON (<1.5%)
Transverse myelitis, seizures, peripheral neuropathy, hearing loss, tinnitus
Hepatitis, pancreatitis
Abdominal pain, bloody diarrhea
Aplastic anemia, agranulocytosis, megaloblastic anemia, methemoglobinemia
Epidermal necrolysis, alopecia
Anaphylaxis
Arthralgia
Interstitial nephritis, nephrotic syndrome, hematuria, proteinuria
Pneumonitis with or without eosinophilia, fibrosing alveolitis, pleuritis

why olsalazine is effective only in the colon. Olsalazine can be used in patients with colonic disease who are allergic to or intolerant of sulfasalazine. The main side effect of olsalazine is a secretory diarrhea, which occurs in up to 17% of patients taking the medication. The diarrhea can be minimized by taking olsalazine with food. Olsalazine is available in capsules containing 250 mg of olsalazine sodium. For induction of remission, we use a dose of 2 g per day in two divided doses, and for maintenance of remission, 1 g per day is recommended.

pH-Sensitive Preparations

Several pH-sensitive formulations have been developed. The basic principle is to encapsulate 5-ASA in a pH-sensitive resin, which dissolves at a specific pH. Because there is a pH gradient in the gastrointestinal system, the 5-ASA is released at a specific site. The pH in the proximal gastrointestinal tract is acidic, and the distal segments are more alkaline. The only pH-sensitive preparation available for clinical use in the United States is Asacol. In Canada and Europe, other preparations are available. Claversal, Mesasal, and Salofalk are 5-ASA coated with an acrylic resin, Eudragit-L. This resin dissolves at pH 6, and so these preparations release 5-ASA in the distal ileum and colon.

Asacol

Asacol is 5-ASA in a capsule coated with an acrylic resin, Eudragit-S. This resin dissolves at pH 7. Asacol begins to dissolve in the terminal ileum, but releases most of its 5-ASA in the colon. Asacol is available in 400-mg capsules. It has proved to be safe and effective in patients who are intolerant or allergic to sulfasalazine. For induction of remission, the dose ranges from 2.4 g per day to as high as 6.4 g per day, in four to six divided doses. For maintenance of remission, the dose that we use is 2.4 g per day or greater, if needed.

Slow-Release Preparation: Pentasa

The azo compounds and the pH-dependent preparations release most of their 5-ASA in the colon, with only very small amounts of 5-ASA released in the small bowel. Pentasa (methalamine) is an ethylcellulose-coated, controlled-release formulation of 5-ASA that releases approximately 50% of the 5-ASA in the small intestine and 50% in the colon. For this reason, Pentasa should be the 5-ASA preparation of choice for patients with Crohn's disease of the small intestine or for those with ileocolitis. In the United States, the FDA has approved Pentasa for patients with ulcerative colitis, but has not approved it yet for patients with Crohn's disease. For induction of remission, we use a dose of 4 g per day in four divided doses, and for maintenance of remission, 2 to 4 g per day in divided doses.

Antibiotics

The way antibiotics work in treating patients with Crohn's disease is unknown. Some antibiotics, like metronidazole, affect lymphocyte function in vitro, but whether this occurs in vivo is unclear. Another possible mechanism of antibiotic action in patients with Crohn's disease is to decrease intestinal microbial flora leading to a decreased antigenic load.

Metronidazole

Metronidazole is an oral synthetic antimicrobial and antiprotozoal agent. It is particularly effective in patients with colonic and perianal Crohn's disease. The usual dose is 10 to 20 mg/kg/day divided in three doses. Duration of treatment varies from weeks to months. Patients should be warned about the Antabuse effect (a tendency to develop nausea and vomiting after drinking alcohol), the risk of peripheral neuropathy, usually beginning as paresthesias, and the potential for teratogenicity. Other common side effects include a metallic taste and nausea.

Ciprofloxacin

Ciprofloxacin is a fluoroquinolone antibiotic with broad-spectrum antibacterial coverage. It has been used for treating a variety of gastrointestinal infections, and empirically in patients with perianal Crohn's disease. In uncontrolled trials, ciprofloxacin was effective in patients with severe perianal Crohn's disease at doses of 1000 to 1500 mg for 3 to 12 months.

Ciprofloxacin has been used in combination with metronidazole with good results in healing perianal Crohn's disease. However, the beneficial effects are seen only during treatment; the symptoms recur upon discontinuation of the antibiotics.

Corticosteroids

Corticosteroids are the most potent anti-inflammatory medications used to induce remission of Crohn's disease. Depending on the site of involvement and severity of disease, they can be used orally, parenterally, or topically. The corticosteroids used to treat patients with Crohn's disease are the glucocorticoids. These drugs have significant effects on protein synthesis; glucose, fat, and calcium metabolism; and electrolyte balance. They also have immunosuppressive effects by affecting humoral and cellular immune responses.

Prednisone is the most commonly used oral corticosteroid for Crohn's disease. It is a synthetic glucocorticoid requiring hepatic hydroxylation to prednisolone to be effective. Absorption after oral administration is not affected by the presence of small bowel disease. Prednisone has four times the anti-inflammatory potency of cortisone, with less sodium retention. It is best to start with a high dose and taper slowly, for example, starting at 40 to 60 mg per day and tapering by 5 mg every 5 to 7 days. The entire amount can be given as a single dose in the morning.

For intravenous use, the two most common drugs used are hydrocortisone and methylprednisolone. Hydrocortisone is given at a dose of 300 mg per day. Although there are no controlled data, hydrocortisone seems to be more effective when administered as a continuous infusion. Methylprednisolone is slightly more potent than prednisolone, and it can be used orally or intravenously. The intravenous dose is 40 to 60 mg per day.

Budesonide is a fluorinated glucocorticoid with a high first-pass liver metabolism and very potent anti-inflammatory effects. In Canada and Europe, budesonide is available as an enema and as an oral preparation. Clinical trials with a controlled ileal release preparation suggested that the optimal dose to induce remission is 9 mg per day. Side effects are greatly diminished because of its rapid metabolism. It is effective in inducing remission in patients with Crohn's ileocolitis, however, it is not effective in maintenance of remission.

ACTH

ACTH (adrenocorticotropic hormone) is almost never used today. It may have a slight therapeutic advantage in patients who have not received corticosteroids, but it is expensive, has to be given by intramuscular injection, and in patients previously treated with steroids, the adrenal response is unpredictable.

Immunosuppressive Agents

The two immunosuppressive medications commonly used in treating Crohn's disease are 6-mercaptopurine (6-MP) and azathioprine, which is an S-imidazole-substituted form of 6-MP. 6-MP and azathioprine are antimetabolites, and, to date, it is unclear whether they are equally effective. However, toxicity is similar for both, and if a patient has side effects or an allergic reaction to one of these medications, the same reaction will occur with the other. The most common side effects are listed in Table 43-2. The dosages of azathioprine and 6-MP are adjusted according to the white blood cell count. Azathioprine can be given up to 2.5 mg/kg/day, whereas the dose of 6-MP is up to 1.5 mg/kg/day, as long as the white blood cell count remains above 3000 per mm^3.

Patients should be advised of the potential side effects of the immunosuppressive drugs and the need to monitor the complete blood cell (CBC) count with differential and liver tests. For women, it may be advisable to do a Papanicolaou smear to monitor for cervical dysplasia, because there is an increased frequency of cervical cancer in patients on these medications. There is no agreement on the optimal method to monitor blood tests. We recommend a CBC/differential count on a weekly basis for the first 4 weeks, then every second week for 2 months, and then on a monthly basis for the duration of treatment. Liver tests should be done every 3 to 6 months. Ideally the total leukocyte count should be 3000 to 4000 cells per mm^3, and the total polymorphonuclear (PMN) count should be greater than 1000 cells per mm^3. If the transaminases are greater than three times normal, the medication should be discontinued. An important drug interaction to remember is with allopurinol, since this is an inhibitor of xanthine oxidase and delays the metabolism of azathioprine and 6-MP. 6-Thioguanine (6-TG) is a breakdown product of 6-MP and can now be measured. Evidence is increasing that adjusting 6-MP doses based on 6-TG levels may improve clinical outcome, but the test is relatively expensive and further work is needed before this can be recommended routinely.

After starting immunosuppressive drugs, a clinical benefit is usually noted by the fourth month, but some patients can take as long as 1 year. The slow onset of action may be responsible for negative results in short-term trials, such as the National Cooperative Crohn's Disease Study (NCCDS). Patients with Crohn's colitis and ileocolitis appear to have a better response than patients with ileitis alone. About 55% of patients on immunosuppressive drugs can discontinue oral steroids, and another 20% can decrease the dose of oral steroids. Fistula improvement or healing occurs in 30 to 40% of patients.

More than 90% of patients who achieve remission on 6-MP or azathioprine maintain remission while on the drug, whereas about 80% relapse when the drug is discontinued. The optimal duration of treatment is unclear, but patients derive benefits while taking the medication for at least 4 years. These drugs appear to be safe during pregnancy. Alstead and coworkers reported on the use of azathioprine in 14 inflammatory bowel disease patients during 16 pregnancies with no adverse effects. There is experience in more than 1000 renal transplant patients, without an increase in adverse outcomes compared to the general population.

Infliximab

Infliximab is a monoclonal anti-tumor necrosis factor (anti-TNF) antibody that was designed to block the TNF receptor in an effort to downregulate autoimmune responses. Over the last 5 years, it has been used increasingly for patients with Crohn's disease. The initial description showed a significant benefit for patients with Crohn's disease, including fistulous disease; however, in some cases this is a reduction from three to one perianal fistula. Nevertheless, the medication is becoming widely used in an effort to reduce need for surgery. General indications include complex perianal fistulous disease that may otherwise be likely to require a defunctioning or permanent stoma. Patients who are on immunosuppressive drugs and who are nonsmokers have better responses than others.

Issues such as the overall cost-benefit ratio, and whether long-term administration is effective or cost-efficient remain unproved, and some concern remains over potential long-term complications. Longer term follow-up has suggested that infliximab may maintain remission, but lymphoma, tuberculosis, and lupus may occur. Furthermore, although many patients respond initially, recurrences can be frequent, particularly for fistulous disease.

Table 43-2 Side Effects of 6-Mercaptopurine and Azathioprine

Common side effects (2 to 10%)
Allergic reactions (fever, rash, arthralgia, myalgia)
Nausea
Pancreatitis
Bone marrow suppression
Infections
Rare side effects
Hepatitis
Non-Hodgkin's lymphoma (controversial)
Carcinoma of the cervix
Diarrhea

■ TREATMENT OF ACUTE DISEASE

In order to adequately treat a patient with an acute exacerbation of Crohn's disease, it is important to determine sites of involvement and disease severity. Sites of involvement are best determined by endoscopy and radiology. Disease severity can be determined by using the Crohn's disease activity index (CDAI), or simply by using common sense and determining how ill a patient is. Those patients with mild exacerbations can be treated as outpatients with either 5-ASA medications, antibiotics, or corticosteroids. Patients with severe exacerbations or those who are toxic are best treated as inpatients with intravenous corticosteroids while under close supervision by experienced gastroenterologists and surgeons.

The choice of 5-ASA medication should be dictated by site of involvement. For patients with ileitis, or ileocolitis, Pentasa (mesalamine) is more appropriate. Patients should be cautioned that Pentasa has a slow onset of action. The importance of compliance must be emphasized; patients have to take four 250-mg capsules four times per day, and the medication is expensive. For patients with colonic disease, any one of the 5-ASA medications with a diazo bond (sulfasalazine or olsalazine) or Asacol is appropriate. For patients with more severe disease, the next step for those with ileocolitis is corticosteroids. For patients with colonic disease alone or perianal disease, antibiotics such as metronidazole or ciprofloxacin can be used prior to initiation of corticosteroid.

When using a corticosteroid, our preference is to prescribe prednisone at a starting dose between 40 and 60 mg per day. Patients have less sleep disturbance when the drug is given as a single dose. We usually taper by 5 mg a week until a daily dose of 15 mg is reached, at which time 5-ASA is introduced, or an antibiotic is prescribed for those with perianal disease. The steroid taper is continued. Severely ill patients require hospitalization. Our preference for these patients is to use hydrocortisone at a dose of 300 mg per day by continuous infusion. If there is evidence of strictures or fistulas, then an antibiotic should be added to the regimen. If there is no significant improvement within 1 week, the patient will probably require surgery. In the absence of contraindications, intravenous cyclosporin A can be tried in patients with fistulous disease.

If there is no need for immediate surgery, patients with severe exacerbation admitted for medical treatment should have serum cholesterol measured. These patients might require treatment with cyclosporin A, which is contraindicated in patients with a serum cholesterol less than 120 mg/dL because of the risk of seizures. Prior to using cyclosporin A, patients should be informed of the potential for side effects, including seizures, paresthesia, hypertension, nephrotoxicity, hypertrichosis, and even death from opportunistic infections. If the patient consents, then cyclosporine is prescribed at a dose of 4 to 5 mg/kg/day by continuous infusion. The response to cyclosporine is rapid, usually within 4 days, but at times it can be delayed for as long as 7 to 10 days.

Patients who achieve remission on cyclosporin A can be started on oral cyclosporine. We usually also start another immunosuppressive agent, such as azathioprine or 6-mercaptopurine, for maintenance of remission. Cyclosporine does not maintain remission, and should not be continued for more than 4 months. We routinely prescribe trimethoprim/sulfamethoxazole for *Pneumocystis carinii* pneumonia (PCP) prophylaxis, and for those allergic to sulfamethoxazole, another PCP prophylaxis regimen should be used.

Stricturing Disease

Patients with strictures, without significant obstructive symptoms, are prescribed intermittent courses of antibiotics to decrease bacterial overgrowth. If a patient has a significant stricture, with obstructive symptoms, then surgery will be required eventually and patients should not be subjected to the long-term toxicity of a corticosteroid. These patients are better treated with timely surgery, followed by either metronidazole, 20 mg/kg/day in three divided doses for 3 months; a 5-ASA medication; or azathioprine or 6-mercaptopurine to delay disease recurrence, depending on the patient's prior history and the extent of the disease.

Symptomatic Treatment

Even though all treatments for Crohn's disease are directed at symptoms, some treatments do not directly affect inflammation. The judicious use of anticholinergics is recommended to improve quality of life in patients with Crohn's disease. It is best to reserve these agents for patients in remission, but as long as the patient does not have a severe exacerbation, they are safe. Most patients benefit from antidiarrheal agents, such as loperamide or diphenoxylate. We recommend patients to take these medications every 4 to 6 hours, rather than after every loose stool. Some patients benefit from codeine sulfate at a dose of 30 to 60 mg three or four times per day.

When patients have choleraic diarrhea, cholestyramine is indicated. The dose of cholestyramine varies. Most patients respond to two or three 4-g doses per day. Cholestyramine binds other medications and nutrients, and for this reason, it should not be ingested within 2 hours of taking other medications. Choleraic diarrhea occurs when less than 100 cm of terminal ileum are either diseased or resected. When more than 100 cm are involved, patients develop steatorrhea due to bile salt depletion. The latter patients do not benefit from cholestyramine, and are best treated by referring the patient to a dietitian, prescribing a low-fat diet and medium chain triglycerides (MCT oil).

Reducing Postoperative Recurrences

As a broad generalization, 50% of patients who undergo resection of active Crohn's disease will require further surgery within 10 years. Sympotic recurrence rates and endoscopic recurrence rates are far higher. Thus, a discussion as to whether "prophylaxis" is required is important. Mesalamine significantly reduced recurrence from 41 to 31%, was not very effective for small bowel disease, and requires the patient to take 12 pills per day or more. Immunosuppression with 6-MP is becoming more accepted, and is becoming more frequently used in our practice. Suitable candidates are those undergoing a second operation (or more), and those with diffuse jejunoileal disease. Perhaps the most important advice is for patients who smoke to cease smoking tobacco.

Nutrition

One of the more common concerns of patients with Crohn's disease relates to diet. Most patients will ask, "what can I eat?" For a patient in clinical remission without significant strictures, no specific dietary restrictions are indicated. For those patients with significant strictures, avoidance of foods containing large nonabsorbable fibers, such as popcorn, corn, peanuts, carrots and celery is indicated. Patients should also be advised to eat small frequent meals, rather than large meals.

For patients who have undergone ileal resections, the diet depends on the extent of the resection. Patients having less than 100 cm of terminal ileum diseased or resected develop bile salt malabsorption but do not deplete their bile salt pool. The bile salts enter the colon, causing a choleraic diarrhea. These patients usually respond to bile salt sequestrants such as cholestyramine. When more than 100 cm of terminal ileum is diseased or resected, the liver cannot compensate for the bile salt losses, and patients develop fat malabsorption. These patients should be treated with a low-fat diet supplemented with medium chain triglycerides (MCT oil). These patients should also undergo a Schilling test, as they may have vitamin B_{12} malabsorption, requiring parenteral replacement with 1000 µg IM once a month. Other vitamins that are poorly absorbed in patients with steatorrhea are the fat-soluble vitamins A, D, and E. They should be measured and supplemented to avoid further morbidity. Vitamin K status can be inferred by measuring the prothrombin time.

Patients with Crohn's disease and diarrhea are at risk of developing zinc deficiency, and patients with a significant small bowel resection can also develop chromium and selenium deficiency. These essential metals are measurable and should be replenished accordingly. Many patients with Crohn's disease develop anemia. Anemia is usually multifactorial, with the most common etiologies including iron deficiency, vitamin B_{12} deficiency, and anemia of chronic disease. The administration of erythropoietin may be indicated in selected patients.

With regard to elemental and enteral formulations, patients with Crohn's disease frequently have weight loss and are malnourished. Reasons are multiple including decreased oral intake because of anorexia or other symptoms, protein losses, malabsorption, increased energy requirements, and drug-nutrient interactions. Elemental diets, polymeric diets, and diets based on tripeptides and dipeptides have been used as primary treatment for patients with Crohn's disease. The studies are difficult to interpret because of small numbers, dropouts, and group heterogeneity. However, elemental and enteral formulations seem to be helpful for improving the nutritional status of patients with Crohn's disease. For certain other groups of patients, such as those with small bowel disease alone, these dietary manipulations may induce remission.

Psychosocial Aspects

The peak age for presentation of Crohn's disease is in the teens and early adulthood. Crohn's disease is a chronic illness, frequently with an unpredictable course, and requiring medical and surgical treatments with physical and functional side effects. We find it very useful to have an open discussion with patients for educational purposes, while discussing their concerns about prognosis, medications and side effects, pregnancy, and other matters. Patients have to develop coping mechanisms, and frequently, referral to a psychologist or assistance from a social worker is invaluable. We routinely provide patients with information about the Crohn's and Colitis Foundation, and encourage them to become members. Most patients have a normal life expectancy, are employed, and lead a normal life.

Suggested Readings

Brzezinski A, Rankin GB, Seidner DL, Lashner BA: Use of old and new oral 5-aminosalicylic acid formulations in inflammatory bowel disease. Clev Clin J Med 1995;62:317–323.

Connell WR, Kamm MA, Dickson M, et al: Long-term neoplasia risk after azathioprine treatment in inflammatory bowel disease. Lancet 1994;334:1249–1252.

Cuillerier E, Lemann M, Bouhnik Y, et al: Azathioprine for prevention of postoperative recurrence in Crohn's disease: a retrospective study. Eur J Gastroenterol Hepatol 2001;13(11):1291–1296.

Dubinsky MC, Lamothe S, Yang HY, et al: Pharmacogenomics and metabolite measurement for 6-mercaptopurine therapy in inflammatory bowel disease. Gastroenterology 2000;118(4):705–713.

Feagan BG, Rochon J, Fedorak RN, et al: Methotrexate for the treatment of Crohn's disease. N Engl J Med 1995;332:292–297.

Greenberg GR, Feagan BG, Martin F, et al: Oral budesonide for active Crohn's disease. N Engl J Med 1994;331:836–841.

Hanauer SB: Drug therapy. Inflammatory bowel disease. N Engl J Med 1996;334:841–848.

McCleod RS, Wolff BG, Steinhart AH, et al: Prophylactic mesalamine treatment decreases postoperative recurrence of Crohn's disease. Gastroenterology 1995;109:404–413.

Parsi MA, Achkar JP, Richardson S, et al: Predictors of response to infliximab in patients with Crohn's disease. Gastroenterology 2002;123(3):707–713.

Pearson DC, May GR, Fick GH, Sutherland LR: Azathioprine and 6-mercaptopurine in Crohn's disease. Ann Intern Med 1995;122:132–142.

Poritz LS, Rowe WA, Koltun WA: Remicade does not abolish the need for surgery in fistulizing Crohn's disease. Dis Colon Rectum 2002;45(6):771–775.

Prantera C, Zannoni F, Scribano ML, et al: An antibiotic regimen for the treatment of active Crohn's disease: A randomized, controlled clinical trial of metronidazole plus ciprofloxacin. Am J Med 1996;91:328–332.

Present DH, Rutgeerts P, Targan S, et al: Infliximab for the treatment of fistulas in patients with Crohn's disease. N Engl J Med 1999;340:1398–1405.

Rutgeerts P, D'Haens G, Targan S, et al: Efficacy and safety of retreatment with anti-tumor necrosis factor antibody (infliximab) to maintain remission in Crohn's disease. Gastroenterology 1999;117(8543):761–769.

Singleton JW, Hanauer SB, Gitnick GL, et al: Mesalamine capsules for the treatment of active Crohn's disease: Results of a 16-week trial. Gastroenterology 1993;104:1293–1301.

Targan SR, Hanauer SB, van Deventer SJ, et al: A short-term study of chimeric monoclonal antibody cA2 to tumor necrosis factor α for Crohn's disease. Crohn's Disease cA2 Study Group. N Engl J Med 1997;337:1029–1035.

44

CROHN'S COLITIS

Lawrence P. Prabhakar, MD
Bruce G. Wolff, MD

Isolated Crohn's colitis is a fairly frequent presentation of Crohn's disease. Although Crohn himself initially did not think that regional enteritis occurred in the colon, it is now widely recognized as a continuum of the same pathologic process. Crohn's disease can occur from mouth to anus with the same pathologic features of linear ulceration, skip areas, a tendency to fistulize, full-thickness involvement, rake or bear claw ulcers, and aphthous ulceration with cleanly demarcated edges. Although rectal or colonic biopsy may be helpful, the diagnosis is most often based on endoscopic or radiologic findings. Granulomas are found in only 15% of tissue specimens. Anorectal manifestations of Crohn's disease are more likely to be associated with Crohn's colitis than with ileocolitis or small bowel Crohn's disease. Crohn's disease confined to the lower rectum or anus occurs in 5% or less of all patients with the disease, although the disorder may be first diagnosed by the presence, particularly in a young patient, of a complex anal fistula or an anal fissure with atypically shaggy edges and a bluish tint to the surrounding anoderm. Any child or teenager with unusual anorectal pathology should receive a workup of the entire GI tract to rule out Crohn's disease before proceeding with surgery.

Between 70 and 90% of patients with Crohn's disease undergo surgery. Although the operation rate for Crohn's colitis in several series is less than that for ileocolitis, surgical intervention is common. Crohn's colitis can frequently be differentiated from chronic ulcerative colitis preoperatively, but even after a colectomy and detailed pathologic examination, a misdiagnosis between the two entities can approach 10% of cases in long-term follow-up. Indications for elective surgical intervention in Crohn's colitis are similar to those for Crohn's disease of the small intestine: stricture, chronic obstruction, abscess or fistula, bleeding (which occurs rarely), and extracolonic complications that may respond to surgery such as pyoderma gangrenosum, periarteritis nodosa, and uveitis. In general, such complications occur less frequently with Crohn's colitis than with ileocolitis or small bowel disease only. Emergency indications include toxic megacolon or fulminant colitis, acute obstruction, rarely massive hemorrhage, perforation, and undrained abscess. A common indication in our practice is disease intractability. In children, growth retardation is another indication for considering surgery.

■ THE APPENDIX

Fewer than 100 cases of isolated Crohn's disease of the appendix have been reported in the world literature. Operative management of this very rare presentation is simple appendectomy, if the cecal wall is not involved. *Yersinia* infection is sometimes difficult to differentiate from Crohn's disease of the appendix.

A more controversial decision is that of incidental appendectomy when a patient is found to have terminal ileitis or ileocolitis instead of appendicitis. Most surgeons would perform an incidental appendectomy if the base of the appendix and surrounding cecum do not appear to be involved in the acute inflammatory process. If a patient has had abdominal symptoms for more than a week prior to operation, the risk from complications of fistulization and abscess formation is apparently increased. If there is a severe inflammatory process, with phlegmon of the terminal ileum and cecum, or if the cecum is involved, the appendix should not be removed if it is not inflamed. Occasionally, a situation is encountered in which the entire ileum, appendix, and cecum are involved in an inflammatory process with ischemic segments or obstruction. In this situation, a resection of the terminal ileum, cecum, and a portion of the ascending colon with ileostomy and mucous fistula would be desirable.

■ CROHN'S COLITIS

Crohn's colitis, which occurs more commonly in males and in older persons, may be treated surgically. The three surgical options are segmental resection, subtotal colectomy with either ileorectostomy or ileosigmoidostomy, and proctocolectomy and Brooke ileostomy. It has not been our practice to knowingly perform a continent ileostomy or ileoanal pouch operation in patients with Crohn's colitis, although this happens 2 to 3% of the time. In our series, 45% of these patients developed complications and eventually required pouch removal, but the remainder had an acceptable result. However, we still feel that the ileoanal pouch procedure should not be performed if the diagnosis of Crohn's colitis is known at the time of the procedure.

Patients with colonic Crohn's disease without obstruction or stricture and who are not frail or elderly, receive an outpatient bowel preparation, once their workup, including laboratory tests, has been performed. A lavage preparation using polyethylene glycol iso-osmotic solution, frequently chilled and flavored with artificially sweetened lemonade drink, is given to the patient over 4 to 5 hours, until the effluent is clear. Almost all patients are able to drink the 2 to 4 L with encouragement by the nursing staff, but a few may require placement of a nasogastric tube with constant infusion of the solution. Once this preparation is completed, 2 g of metronidazole and 2 g of neomycin are given orally, and this dose is repeated in 4 hours. This approach has replaced the standard 2-day cathartic enema preparation owing to better patient tolerance. However, in patients with some element of obstruction or stricture the cathartic enema preparation with erythromycin and neomycin antibiotics given orally, as described by Nichols and Condon, may be more appropriate. Perioperative intravenous antibiotics may also be used in place of the oral antibiotic preparation. If a patient has been on steroids within 3 months prior to operation, we would administer a steroid preparation. In patients with anal fissures or fistulas, we give metronidazole in the perioperative period, usually 0.5 g in three divided doses per day. Although the reason for the efficacy of metronidazole in treating anorectal Crohn's disease is not known, several studies have confirmed its usefulness. Most likely the drug reduces secondary bacterial opportunistic infection. Prior to surgery, our practice is to have the patient marked for an ileostomy after examining the patient both supine and sitting to determine appropriate and comfortable placement of the ileostomy. This evaluation is especially important in overweight individuals. Occasionally, patients may be shown to have an abundance of inflammation in the pelvic region that may obscure identification of the ureters. In this subset of patients, we use preoperative placement of ureteric stents to aid intraoperative identification and preservation of these structures.

The best surgical option for those patients with limited or segmental colonic Crohn's disease has been much debated. Segmental colectomy with colocolostomy or abdominal colectomy with ileosigmoid or ileorectal anastomosis has occasionally been performed at our institution for patients with localized Crohn's colitis. We recently reported our experience to determine the risk of recurrence requiring medical or surgical treatment and permanent stoma formation. We identified 49 patients who had undergone either segmental colectomy or abdominal colectomy with ileosigmoid or ileorectal anastomosis and were available for follow-up. Those patients with primary anorectal or primary ileal disease or who had undergone a total proctocolectomy were excluded. Thirty-nine patients had a segmental colectomy and 10 underwent an abdominal colectomy. Following surgery, 22 patients (45%) required no further treatment whatsoever during the follow-up period. Of the 27 patients who experienced a recurrence, 11 (23%) were treated medically and 16 (33%) required another operation. If we consider the patients requiring another operation, 10 patients had another limited resection and 6 required completion proctocolectomy. A third procedure for recurrence was required in 6 patients, only 1 of whom underwent completion proctocolectomy and ileostomy for control of disease. Thus, 86% of the patients in our study remained stoma-free. Yet, even in those 7 patients requiring a stoma, the mean stoma-free interval was 23 months. Factors such as extent of resection, margins of resection, disease location, and extent of disease did not predict recurrence. Segmental colectomy did have a greater recurrence rate than abdominal colectomy and ileosigmoid or ileorectal anastomosis, but the rate of stoma formation did not differ between the two groups. Therefore, although there is a clear and definite risk of recurrent colorectal disease, segmental and abdominal colectomy are both viable options for patients with limited colonic Crohn's disease.

If severe anorectal Crohn's disease is present in conjunction with Crohn's colitis, proctocolectomy with Brooke ileostomy is the procedure of choice. If a patient has severe lower colonic and anorectal disease, something short of a proctocolectomy may be performed, with a descending or sigmoid colostomy. In all cases of Crohn's disease, we attempt to obtain gross and histologic confirmation of uninvolved bowel. If a margin is histologically involved, we will resect an additional few centimeters, but if this portion is also involved, we accept a higher recurrence rate and perform either an anastomosis or a stoma at that point. If additional Crohn's disease is present more proximally in the bowel, then we attempt to obtain only grossly free margins. Experience with strictureplasty has supported the assertion that anastomoses with histologically involved margins heal as well as those with completely normal tissue.

The major postoperative complications that can occur are anastomotic leak and fistulization, so obviously grossly normal-appearing or histologically normal tissue is preferable for anastomosis. If left-sided colonic Crohn's disease extends all the way to the transverse colon, most of the absorptive capacity of the colon resides in the resected specimen. Therefore, we would resect the right hemicolon as well and perform a Brooke ileostomy. We feel that with the removal of so much storage capacity the patient is not able to irrigate an end-transverse colostomy because the stool at this level resembles small intestinal chyme. Therefore, a well-made Brooke ileostomy is preferable to a wet transverse colostomy.

Proctocolectomy offers perhaps the lowest risk of recurrence for any surgical procedure performed for Crohn's disease of the colon and anorectum. The recurrence rate of 10 to 25% compares favorably with the usual 50% recurrence rate quoted for Crohn's disease elsewhere in the bowel. One significant problem is that only 50 to 60% of the perineal wounds heal promptly. Thirty percent may exhibit delayed healing for up to 1 year, and 15 to 20% may still have persistent perineal sinus after 1 year. We customarily close the pelvic peritoneum after the rectum and anus have been removed and insert round Silastic drains through the perineal skin and ischiorectal area up into the presacral space, under the pelvic peritoneum. These drains should be placed more anteriorly on the perineum so that the patient is able to sit without discomfort. We feel that this dependent drainage is preferable to transperitoneal drainage, although transperitoneal drainage has also shown to be effective in several studies. The perineum is then carefully closed in multiple layers with interrupted absorbable sutures and then the skin is closed with a running subcuticular absorbable stitch. Postoperatively, a dilute Betadine (povidone-iodine) solution is infused through one of the two drains at a rate of 50 mL per hour for 24 hours, while the other drain is left to suction. Then, for the next 48 hours, the Betadine solution is discontinued and a normal saline solution is substituted. Both drains are then left to suction for an additional 48 hours, after which they can be removed if the drainage is less than 50 to 75 mL per day. The perineal skin may be cleansed with Betadine solution periodically and an attempt to keep moisture from collecting over the incision should be made by inserting dry gauze in the intergluteal and perineal clefts. The irrigation and aspiration should be meticulously charted, and if the nursing staff reports a net loss of fluid greater than 100 mL, the irrigation is promptly discontinued and the drains are aspirated. Further loss of fluid is prevented by placing both drains to low intermittent suction and complete discontinuation of irrigation.

ADDITIONAL ASPECTS OF CROHN'S COLITIS

Anorectal Crohn's Disease

Proximal Resection

A question frequently arises concerning the efficacy of resection of active proximal Crohn's disease in a patient with active anorectal Crohn's disease. What might we expect as far as improvement of the anorectal Crohn's disease? We have found that such resection may be beneficial if all the proximal bowel disease can be removed. However, if there is a recurrence in the proximal bowel, the anorectal Crohn's disease usually worsens. This relief of anorectal Crohn's disease is often limited to 6 to 24 months. Because of current trends toward conservative surgery, proximal resection can be attempted, if the patient is counseled that a second major operative procedure may be necessary, because there is only a 30% success rate for improvement in anorectal disease. Obviously, if proximal disease is contiguous with the anorectum, then complete removal of all disease is desirable.

Proximal Diversion

In patients with severe anorectal Crohn's disease, there has been a tendency in the past to perform proximal diversion of the fecal stream in the hopes that disease would improve to the point where re-establishment of intestinal continuity would be feasible. Several studies have shown that few patients have gone on to re-establishment of intestinal continuity with good results. Perhaps the only place for complete proximal diversion is prior to repair of a rectovaginal or rectourethral fistula, although even this is controversial.

Toxic Megacolon

As many as 20% of patients with Crohn's colitis may present with toxic megacolon. Once the diagnosis has been established, delay in treatment can result in mortality rates up to 30% and as high as 80 to 85% if there is associated perforation. A recurrence rate of 20% has been reported in patients who have undergone medical management, and we have found that 90% of patients with toxic megacolon eventually require an operation. Therefore, medical management should be viewed only as preoperative management. This treatment should consist of fluid resuscitation, intravenous broad-spectrum antibiotics, and correction of electrolyte abnormalities. If the colitis is indeterminate, the patient should undergo subtotal colectomy and over-

sewing of the rectal stump. This procedure allows the option for an ileoanal pouch procedure at a later date if the disease proves to be ulcerative colitis. If there is *no doubt* as to the diagnosis of Crohn's disease, even in the urgent setting, proctocolectomy can be safely undertaken if care is taken to avoid perforation with subsequent peritonitis. If the bowel is very friable, if perforation and spillage have occurred or if the patient is hemodynamically unstable, a lesser procedure should be performed as quickly as possible. In this setting, the associated mortality rate is about 5%.

Urinary Tract and Crohn's Colitis

Ureterolysis for retroperitoneal compression of the ureter due to inflammation from Crohn's disease was once a frequently used option. Simonovitch and Fazio have suggested that removal of the intra-abdominal source of inflammation results in relief of the ureteric obstruction, obviating the need for ureterolysis.

Colovesical fistulas can occur, with common presenting symptoms of pneumaturia or, more commonly, chronic pyuria. Crohn's disease may or may not be suspected preoperatively. Ileosigmoid fistula with an enterovesical fistula occasionaly found in patients with Crohn's disease. Cystoscopy is the most useful diagnostic procedure for confirming this complication of Crohn's colitis. Resection of the fistulizing segment of colon with closure of the bladder is the procedure of choice. Postoperatively, Foley catheter drainage is maintained for 10 days.

Ileosigmoid Fistula

Ileosigmoid fistula is a frequent phenomenon seen with primary ileocolitis. The fistulizing segment is almost always the terminal ileum, and only rarely does the sigmoid contain prima facie evidence of Crohn's disease. Preoperatively or intraoperatively this segment can be examined with a flexible sigmoidoscope and a determination made. If there is no evidence of Crohn's disease in the sigmoid colon, other than the site of fistulization, then formal sigmoid resection can be avoided. Only ileal resection should be performed with division of the fistula, freshening of the colonic edges, excision of the fistulous colonic orifice, and primary closure. Results using this conservative procedure are equal to en bloc sigmoid and ileal resection.

Rectovaginal Fistula

As mentioned previously, rectovaginal fistulas can be repaired with or without proximal diversion of the fecal stream. Diversion alone does not result in spontaneous closure of the fistula in the vast majority of cases. Once a repair of the rectovaginal fistula has been performed, the ultimate test of healing is re-establishment of intestinal continuity. Unfortunately, many patients have recurrence of their fistula and require proctectomy. Of the techniques of rectovaginal fistula repair available, we prefer a transanal repair for low fistulas, with excision of the fistula and a mucosal-submucosal flap advancement with the vaginal side being left open for drainage. High fistulas require an anterior resection, low anterior resection, or even a coloanal procedure.

Colonic Crohn's Disease and Carcinoma

The incidence of adenocarcinoma associated with chronic colonic Crohn's disease is much lower than that associated with chronic ulcerative colitis. Unfortunately, carcinoma has occurred in bypassed segments of colon, which are not available for surveillance, as well as rectal remnants, which may not be as closely scrutinized as the more active segments of the intestinal tract of inflammatory bowel disease patients. Carcinoma is often not diagnosed preoperatively in these patients because tumor symptoms can mimic those of the underlying disease. Nevertheless, patients who have longer than a 7-year history of Crohn's colitis are at increased risk for developing carcinoma (up to 20-fold). These cancers tend to have a similar prognosis to spontaneous large bowel cancers, although there may be a higher rate of synchronous lesions.

Suggested Readings

Andersson P, Olaison G, Hallbook O, Sjodahl R: Segmental resection or subtotal colectomy in Crohn's colitis? Dis Colon Rectum 2002;45:47–53.

Agrez MV, Valente RM, Pierce W, et al: Surgical history of Crohn's disease in a well-defined population. Mayo Clin Proc 1982;57:747–752.

Farnell MB, van Heerden JA, Beart RW Jr, Weiland LH: Rectal preservation in nonspecific inflammatory disease of the colon. Ann Surg 1980;192:249–253.

Goligher JC: The long-term results of excisional surgery for primary and recurrent Crohn's disease of the large intestine. Dis Colon Rectum 1985;28:51–55.

Grant CS, Dozois RR: Toxic megacolon: Ultimate fate of patients after successful medical management. Am J Surg 1984;147:106–610.

Prabhakar LP, Laramee C, Nelson H, Dozois RR: Avoiding a stoma: Role for segmental or abdominal colectomy in Crohn's colitis. Dis Colon Rectum 1997;40:71–78.

Ribero MB, Greenstein AJ, Sachar DB, et al: Colorectal adenocarcinoma in Crohn's disease. Ann Surg 1996;223:186–193.

Simonovitch J, Fazio VW: Ureteral obstruction secondary to Crohn's disease. Am J Surg 1980;139:95.

Tjandra JJ, Fazio VW: Surgery for Crohn's colitis. Int Surg 1992;77:9–14.

Gordon PH, Nivatvongs S (Eds.). Principles and Practice of Surgery for the Colon, Rectum and Anus. St. Louis, Quality Medical Publishing, 1992.

Wolff BG: Crohn's disease: The role of surgical treatment. Mayo Clin Proc 1986;61:292–295.

Wolff BG: Surgical management of Crohn's disease. Probl Gen Surg 1984;1:51–59.

Wolff BG, Beart RW Jr, Frydenburg HB, et al: The importance of disease-free margins in resections for Crohn's disease. Dis Colon Rectum 1983;26:239–243.

Wolff BG, Culp CE, Beart RW Jr, et al: Anorectal Crohn's disease. Dis Colon Rectum 1985;28:709–711.

Young-Fadok, TM, Wolff BG, Meagher A, et al: Surgical management of ileosigmoid fistulas in Crohn's disease. Dis Colon Rectum 1997;40:558–561.

45

PERIANAL CROHN'S DISEASE

Peter A. Cataldo, MD
Douglas Yoder, MD

Perianal Crohn's disease was first recognized by Bissell in 1934, 2 years after the original description of regional enteritis by Crohn, Ginzburg, and Oppenheimer. It has been reported to occur in 25 to 75% of patients with Crohn's disease. Perianal disease may be present prior to (5 to 10%), concomitant with (20 to 30%), or after (60 to 70%) the diagnosis of intestinal Crohn's disease. It is most commonly associated with large bowel disease (40 to 50%) but also occurs with ileocolic (30 to 35%) and small bowel disease (15 to 20%). If perianal disease is the presenting complaint almost all patients will develop intestinal disease within 5 years, most commonly of the large bowel.

Lesions associated with perianal Crohn's disease include edematous skin tags, fissures, perianal fistulas, anovaginal fistulas, abscesses, ulcers, and strictures. Microscopic confirmation is possible if granulomas are present but they occur in less than 30% of patients. The diagnosis is usually made on clinical grounds in a patient with suspicious lesions and an established diagnosis. In the absence of a diagnosis of regional enteritis, a presumptive diagnosis can be made when other lesions with a similar appearance have been ruled out. Differential diagnoses include cryptoglandular sepsis, tuberculosis, hidradenitis suppurativa (hidradenitis suppurativa and Crohn's disease may coexist), actinomycosis, anal neoplasia, and anal venereal diseases.

An unusual-appearing perianal lesion should generate a high index of suspicion for the presence of perianal Crohn's disease. When possible the gastrointestinal (GI) tract should be completely evaluated prior to any surgical therapy. An upper GI series with small bowel follow-through combined with a colonoscopy will diagnose any synchronous intestinal disease. In patients with an established diagnosis of Crohn's disease the degree of intestinal activity should be assessed, particularly the presence or absence of rectal involvement.

■ TREATMENT

Treatment depends upon the type and extent of perianal disease. Patients often present with undrained or inadequately drained sepsis, making examination in the office too uncomfortable. An examination under anesthesia is usually needed to define the exact nature of the problem and to ensure adequate drainage. A conservative philosophy is warranted when treating perianal Crohn's disease. Healing may be poor, and even minimal damage to a perhaps compromised anal sphincter in the face of chronic diarrhea may leave a patient permanently incontinent. It is essential to identify the patient's complaint and its effect on quality of life. Once this has been done, goals of therapy should be established, and an appropriate therapeutic plan developed.

■ PERIANAL ABSCESSES

Abscesses require incision and drainage. Crohn's abscesses tend to be more complex and generally require examination and drainage under anesthesia. Perioperative magnetic resonance imaging (MRI) studies may be helpful in identifying occult abscesses. Transanal ultrasound, either preoperatively or intraoperatively, has been beneficial in identifying abscesses missed on clinical evaluation. Its sensitivity is low, however, in defining fistulous tracts.

MRI provides excellent anatomic detail, showing abscesses, and fistulous tracts, and their relationships with the anal sphincters. It has been shown to be superior to examination under anesthesia in several small series, with sensitivities and specificities as high as 97 and 100%. In most cases, however, careful examination under anesthesia will identify all pathologic changes and dictate appropriate care.

■ ANAL FISSURE

Patients suffering from Crohn's disease may develop two types of fissures. Standard anal fissures, generally appearing in the anterior or posterior midline, are associated with sphincter hypertonia and are very painful. Crohn's fissures occur off the midline, are broad-based, are not associated with increased sphincter pressures, and are usually painless. If significant pain is present, an underlying abscess should be suspected.

An initial conservative approach is warranted. Anal ointments, warm soaks, and normalization of bowel movements has resulted in healing in 65 to 80% of patients at 6 months. Topical agents such as nitroglycerine ointment have been employed in the treatment of acute and chronic fissures. It releases nitrous oxide and lowers sphincter pressures. No reports of nitroglycerine use in Crohn's fissures have been published, but healing rates of 60 to 80% have been reported in the general population. In addition, 0.2% nifedipine ointment is now proven efficacious in the treatment of anal fissures with fewer side effects than nitroglycerine.

Surgical treatment should be considered only in patients with painful fissures who fail conservative therapy. If the fissure or ulcer is broad-based, off the midline, and associated with low anal tone, then a sphincterotomy should not be performed because it will not heal the ulcer and will lead to incontinence. Instead, a careful examination under anesthesia should be performed, anal sepsis searched for and drained appropriately, and the edges of the fissure débrided.

Painful, midline fissures, associated with increased sphincter pressures and refractory to conservative management, will respond well to sphincterotomy, particularly in the absence of active rectal Crohn's disease. The Lahey-Hitchcock Clinic reported their experience in treating 56 patients with Crohn's disease and anal fissures. Half were treated with medical therapy. Eighty-eight percent of patients who underwent sphincterotomy healed compared to only 43% who underwent proximal intestinal resection.

■ FISTULA-IN-ANO

In planning therapy for anal fistulas three factors should be considered: (1) whether or not the lesions are symptomatic, (2) the presence or absence of rectal involvement with Crohn's disease, and (3) the anatomy of the fistulous tracts (high versus low; simple versus complex; single versus multiple).

Asymptomatic fistulas require no treatment. Optimal medical control of rectal disease ensures maximal success rates in any surgical procedure. Preoperative MRI or ultrasound (possibly with the addition of hydrogen peroxide into the fistulous tracts) may help to define fistulous anatomy. In most cases examination under anesthesia with careful probing of the tracks is sufficient, but instillation of hydrogen peroxide or methylene blue into fistulas will help identify all extensions.

Therapy should be tailored to relief of symptoms and preservation of anal sphincters. Superficial fistulas in patients with normal rectums respond very well to simple fistulotomy with low complication rates. In high fistulas the two therapeutic options are long-term seton placement and endoanal advancement flaps. Setons are simple to place, applicable to even very involved situations with a diseased rectum, disrupt no musculature, and are associated with high success rates. Silastic setons are nonirritating and are well tolerated for even long periods of time. Several series have reported 70 to 80% relief of symptoms, no incontinence, and low recurrence rates after seton removal.

Endoanal advancement flaps are more complex procedures and, therefore, associated with higher morbidity rates. However, they offer the opportunity for complete healing. Some have added a protective stoma during the healing period. The Cleveland Clinic has reported 101 cases with a healing rate of 70%. Crohn's fistulas healed as well as those not associated with Crohn's disease. Asymptomatic fistulas require no treatment; low-lying fistulas can be safely treated with simple fistulotomy. Complex fistulas in patients with quiescent rectal disease arising from a single internal opening respond well to anal advancement flaps. Fistulas with multiple internal openings and ongoing suppuration, or those associated with active rectal disease, are best treated with multiple setons.

■ HEMORRHOIDS AND SKIN TAGS

Edematous skin tags are the most common anal manifestation of Crohn's disease, are rarely symptomatic, and should not be excised. Concomitant Crohn's disease and significant hemorrhoidal disease is rare. Conservative therapy with emphasis on controlling diarrhea or constipation should give adequate symptom relief in most circumstances. Surgeons at St. Mark's Hospital reported very poor results in 20 patients with perianal Crohn's disease who underwent hemorrhoidectomy. The complication rate was greater than 50% and six patients eventually required proctectomy for complications related to hemorrhoidectomy. In contrast, Wolkomir and Luchtefeld reported uncomplicated healing in 15 of 17 patients with a 3% proctectomy rate at 11 years (none related to complications of hemorrhoid surgery). Despite these encouraging results, hemorrhoidectomy should be considered only when all other measures fail.

■ ANOVAGINAL FISTULAS

Anovaginal fistulas associated with Crohn's disease are either secondary to cryptoglandular infection that drains into the vagina or are direct extensions of active intestinal disease. In the latter case fistulas are large, the rectum is severely involved, and proctectomy is often required. For small anterior fistulas that cause minimal or no symptoms, no treatment is needed. However, symptomatic anovaginal fistulas can be successfully treated with anal advancement flaps. Hull and Fazio reported surgical treatment of anovaginal fistula in 48 patients with Crohn's disease. Nine patients underwent total proctocolectomy, and four patients had setons placed. Thirty-five patients underwent repair with anal advancement flaps. Primary healing occurred in 19 (54%), and with secondary procedures a total of 68% of patients achieved complete healing. Limited series have reported good results with transvaginal approaches for repair as well as the use of anocutaneous advancement flaps.

■ EPIDERMOID ANAL CARCINOMA

Several small series have reported the development of epidermoid carcinoma in cases of long-standing perianal Crohn's disease, occurring after the disease has been present longer than 10 years. Malignancy is difficult to distinguish from chronic inflammation, and any nonhealing lesions should be biopsied. Once the diagnosis has been made, treatment must be individualized. Results of primary chemoradiation have not been reported. Proctectomy is almost universally necessary. It is essential to maintain a high index of suspicion because anal malignancy in association with Crohn's disease often presents at an advanced stage and cure rates are poor.

■ MEDICAL THERAPY

Medical therapy for perianal Crohn's disease includes antibiotics, anti-inflammatory medications, and immunosuppressive drugs. Few placebo controlled trials exist and spontaneous improvement in perianal symptoms is well recognized. Therefore, it is difficult to interpret the efficacy of various medical treatments. Healing rates of 50 to 100% have been reported, but relapse rates are very high once therapy has been discontinued.

Metronidazole has both antibacterial and immunosuppressive activity and has been reported to improve symptoms in 75 to 100% of patients. It can achieve healing in 50% of patients with chronic fistulas. Doses of 1000 to 1500 mg daily are recommended. Unfortunately, side effects commonly develop, and fistula recurrence rates are high once medication is discontinued. Some advocate metronidazole postoperatively after abscess drainage or fistulotomy to improve healing rates, but no controlled trials exist.

Recently, ciprofloxacin has been shown to be beneficial in several noncontrolled trials. Side effects seem to be lower than for metronidazole, but recurrence rates are high. Corticosteroids have been used systemically, topically, and intralesionally. In small series intralesional depo-methylprednisolone resulted in excellent relief of symptoms in five of seven patients. However, no controlled trials have proved steroid therapy to be effective.

Immunosuppressive drugs including imuran, 6-mercaptopurine (6-MP), and cyclosporin A have been reported to be effective in several small trials. Delay to response is prolonged, complications are high, and recurrence upon cessation is common. The anti–tumor necrosis factor (anti-TNF) antibody infliximab has proved effective in bringing about initial healing of Crohn's fistulas in 45% of patients. Without repeated infusions of infliximab, recurrence is common. The strategy of using an immunosuppressive agent to maintain the early healing recently has been shown to be successful in 75% of patients. Most of these patients had perianal disease.

In summary, medical therapy plays an important role in treatment of perianal Crohn's disease, especially for patients in whom rectal or anal disease makes fistula repair impossible. It should not supplant drainage of infection collections, but it may be effective in patients with a difficult, painful, draining perineum without identifiable abscess cavities. It may also be used as an adjunct to surgical therapy.

Least toxic medications such as metronidazole or ciprofloxacin should be employed first. Infliximab and immunosuppressive drugs should be reserved for patients with severe disease, those who are unsuitable for surgery, or those who fail surgical therapy.

■ INTESTINAL RESECTION/ PROXIMAL DIVERSION

Intestinal surgery in association with perianal disease consists of either proximal diversion (with or without resection), proximal resection with re-establishment of continuity, or proctectomy with creation of permanent stoma. Proximal intestinal resection in order to improve perianal symptoms has met with mixed results. Heuman and coworkers from Sweden identified a close association between proximal intestinal disease and anal symptoms.

Resection of proximal disease without intestinal recurrence resulted in a complete perineal healing in 80% of patients, but all patients with recurrent intestinal disease had persistent perianal disease. Long-term follow-up of patients with perianal disease treated at the Mayo Clinic revealed a similar phenomenon. The majority of patients who underwent intestinal resection showed a significant improvement in perianal disease. This improvement, however, was long standing only in patients whose proximal disease did not recur. Orkin and Telander, however, failed to identify any significant benefit from proximal intestinal resection in a pediatric population.

Proximal diversion is also employed in the management of perianal manifestations of Crohn's disease. In many series it has been associated with high rates of improvement. Harper and coworkers found improvement or healing in 72% of patients after creation of split ileostomies. Williamson and Hughes, however, identified worsening of distal intestinal disease after diversion and urged caution because of distal anal obstruction of the diverted segment. Fecal diversion appears most beneficial in patients with significant perianal sepsis and uninvolved rectums. However, relapses are common, and likelihood of requiring a permanent stoma is high.

Proctectomy is performed less often than in the past. In most cases it is required for refractory perianal disease combined with a severely involved rectum. The Mayo Clinic reported that 20% of patients required proctectomy over a 20-year period. When proctectomy is performed in association with significant perianal suppuration, perineal wound complications are common. Active anal infection should be controlled prior to proctectomy if at all possible. Intersphincteric proctectomy is recommended, and perineal wounds should be left open.

In summary, intestinal surgery is rarely required for perianal disease. Proximal intestinal resections do not reliably cure perianal disease and should not be performed unless necessary for intestinal symptoms.

Fecal diversion is occasionally beneficial but not associated with long-term success. Diversion is best reserved for ongoing perianal sepsis when local measures fail and the rectum is minimally involved. Proctectomy should be reserved for severe disease with both perianal and rectal involvement.

■ MISCELLANEOUS APPROACHES TO THERAPY

Alternative treatment strategies have arisen for patients with refractory perianal problems. Hyperbaric oxygen therapy is reported to be beneficial. Lavy and coworkers reported healing of perianal lesions in 7 of 10 patients after 20 daily sessions at 2.5 atmospheres. In addition, fibrin glue instillation has been used for complex fistulas. Others have reported healing in 6 of 10 patients with complex perianal fistulas, three of whom had Crohn's disease. These modalities, however, have not gained widespread acceptance and should be considered experimental.

■ CONCLUSIONS

Perianal manifestations of Crohn's disease are varied, ranging from asymptomatic skin tags to complex abscesses or fistulas. In treating these patients it is essential to understand their troubling symptoms and to institute directed therapy. Unwarranted or overaggressive procedures, particularly those involving the anal sphincters, can have disastrous results. However, well-planned surgery with defined goals can significantly improve patients' quality of life, often with minimal morbidity. Medical therapy may relieve symptoms in selected circumstances and may be of benefit in association with surgery in order to improve healing.

Suggested Readings

Abcarian H: Perianal Crohn's disease. Semin Colon Rectal Surg 1994;5(3):210–215.

Arseneau KO, Cohn SM, Cominelli F, Connors AF Jr: Cost-utility of initial medical management for Crohn's disease perianal fistulae. Gastroenterology 2001;120:1640–1656.

Dietrich A, Schonfelder M: Crohn's disease: Bowel resection to protect the proctium in severe perianal disease? Langenbecks Arch Surg 2001;386:38–41.

Fleshner PR, Schoetz DJ Jr, Roberts PL, et al: Anal fissure in Crohn's disease: A plea for aggressive management. Dis Colon Rectum 1995;38:1137–1143.

Harper PH, Kettlewell MG, Lee EC: The effect of split ileostomy on perianal Crohn's disease. Br J Surg 1982;69:608–610.

Heuman R, Boeryd B, Bolin T, Sjodahl R: The influence of disease at the margin of resection on the outcome of Crohn's disease. Br J Surg 1983;70:519–521.

Hull TL, Fazio VW: Surgical approaches to low anovaginal fistula in Crohn's disease. Am J Surg 1997;173:95–98.

Hyman N: Endoanal advancement flap repair for complex anorectal fistulas. Am J Surg 1999;178:337–340.

Lavy A, Weisz G, Adir Y, Ramon Y, Melamed Y, Eidelman S: Hyperbaric oxygen for perianal Crohn's disease. J Clin Gastroenterol 1996;19:202–205.

McClane SJ, Rombeau JL: Anorectal Crohn's disease. Surg Clin North Am 2001;81:169–183.

Ochsenkuhn T, Goke B, Sackmann M: Combining infliximab with 6-mercaptopurine/azathioprine for fistula therapy in Crohn's disease. Am J Gastroenterol 2002;97(8):2022–2025.

Orkin BA, Telander RL: The effect of intra-abdominal resection or fecal diversion on perianal disease in pediatric Crohn's disease. J Pediatr Surg 1985;20:343–347.

Ozuner G, Hull TL, Cartmill J, Fazio VW: Long-term analysis of the use of transanal rectal advancement flaps for complicated anorectal/vaginal fistulas. Dis Colon Rectum 1996;39:10–14.

Penninckx F, D'Hoore A, Filez L: Advancement flap plasty for the closure of anal and recto-vaginal fistulas in Crohn's disease. Acta Gastroenterol Belg 2001;64:223–226.

Present DH, Rutgeerts P, Targan S, et al: Infliximab for the treatment of fistulas in patients with Crohn's disease. N Engl J Med 1999;340:1398–1405.

Poritz LS, Rowe WA, Koltun WA: Remicade does not abolish the need for surgery in fistulizing Crohn's disease. Dis Colon Rectum 2002;45:771–775.

Ramzan NN, Leighton JA, Heigh RI, Shapiro MS: Clinical significance of granuloma in Crohn's disease. Inflamm Bowel Dis 2002;8:168–173.

Rutgeerts P; Management of perianal Crohn's disease. Can J Gastroenterol 2000;14(suppl C):7C–12C.

Schwartz DA, Wiersema MJ, Dudiak KM, et al: A comparison of endoscopic ultrasound, magnetic resonance imaging, and exam under anesthesia for evaluation of Crohn's perianal fistulas. Gastroenterology 2001;121:1064–1072.

Sloots CE, Felt-Bersma RJ, Poen AC, et al: Assessment and classification of fistula-in-ano in patients with Crohn's disease by hydrogen peroxide enhanced transanal ultrasound. Int J Colorectal Dis 2001;16:292–297.

Williamson ME, Hughes LE: Bowel diversion should be used with caution in stenosing anal Crohn's disease. Gut 1994;35:1139–1140.

Wolkomir AF, Luchtefeld MA: Surgery for symptomatic hemorrhoids and anal fissures in Crohn's disease. Dis Colon Rectum 1993;36:545–547.

46

ACUTE APPENDICITIS

Elliot Prager, MD

Although the incidence of acute appendicitis appears to have been waning slightly over the past few decades, it remains a frequent cause of acute abdominal pain and urgent operative intervention. If untreated, acute appendicitis will progress from inflammation to perforation with abscess formation or diffuse peritonitis, making timely operative intervention imperative.

Even though it has been 120 years since the initial elucidation of the pathophysiology of appendicitis by Dr. Reginald Fitz, making the diagnosis with confidence still remains a challenge today. For many years a 15 to 20% rate of pathologically normal appendices in any appendectomy series was acceptable, the reasoning being that it is far more preferable to intervene unnecessarily rather than risk perforation. Many factors in the medical environment have seemed to place pressure on this tenet, however, and now a host of diagnostic techniques can be used to minimize uncertainty. There is some question as to the propriety of this goal, especially in light of recent pathologic evaluation, which measured cytokine expression, in appendiceal tissue (tumor necrosis factor α and interleukin-2), suggesting that a substantial portion of the appendices considered normal by traditional microscopic evaluation are, in fact, inflamed. This finding would certainly be consistent with many surgeons' experience that patients with histologically normal appendices are often rendered asymptomatic by appendectomy.

Equally interesting are the results of a contemporary Canadian study involving over 125,000 appendectomies in hundreds of hospitals. The study demonstrated that for each 10% increase in the diagnostic accuracy rate, the perforation rate increased 14%. Last, a study comparing patients submitted for evaluation and appendectomy prior to 1984 with a similar number treated after 1988 found no difference in the rate of perforation, rate of "normal" appendectomy, or the length of hospitalization despite heavy use of ultrasonography, laparoscopy, and computed tomography (CT) in the latter groups. They conclude, and this author heartily concurs, that employment of more sophisticated diagnostic techniques is usually not warranted.

■ DIAGNOSIS

The analysis of the patient with possible appendicitis can be divided into three parts: history, physical examination, and routine laboratory and x-ray tests (complete blood cell count, urinalysis, and abdominal flat plate). The history is the most variable of these assessments but classically should be 5 to 10 hours in duration, consisting of the onset of periumbilical or epigastric pain followed by nausea and possible emesis, followed then by localization of the pain to the right lower quadrant. All the foregoing is accompanied by anorexia. Such a classical history can be markedly altered, even to the final location of pain (a long retrocecal appendix may produce right upper quadrant pain), but most components will be present in a majority of the patients.

Physical examination should disclose pain in the right lower quadrant, most often McBurney's point (one third of the way medially between the anterior superior iliac spine and the umbilicus), right lower quadrant direct tenderness with the possibility of rebound, and referred direct or rebound tenderness. Obturator or psoas signs may be positive and, if so, will provide a clue as to the location of the inflamed appendix. Tenderness may be felt on rectal examination; if the appendix has ruptured and a pelvic abscess has formed, it might be felt on digital rectal examination also. The temperature will be elevated, usually in the range of 100 to 101° F.

Laboratory examination should disclose an elevated white blood cell count usually in the range of 12,000 to 15,000 cells/mm^3, associated with a shift to the left. Urinalysis may show a few white or red blood cells, but significant numbers of either might suggest ureteral calculus, pyelonephritis, or urinary bladder infection. Abdominal radiograph will occasionally demonstrate an appendicolith, and a pattern of small bowel obstruction might be associated with perforation and abscess. Free air would be extremely rare and suggests diverticulitis or perforated ulcer. A pregnancy test should be obtained on all female patients in the reproductive years with intact pelvic organs.

If all three components—history, physical examination, and laboratory findings—are consistent with appendicitis, that is sufficient to proceed to the operating room. If two of the three components are strongly supportive of the diagnosis, one might still proceed in most patients. If there is less concurrence and for females in whom ovarian or tubo-ovarian pathology is a possibility, one should use additional diagnostic measures or observe over a period of hours. When dealing with the very young and the elderly, in whom the omentum may not be well developed and who therefore cannot readily wall off a perforation, however, one might operate earlier and with less rigorous criteria.

■ ADDITIONAL DIAGNOSTIC TOOLS

Ultrasonography

The specificity and sensitivity of ultrasonography for the diagnosis of acute appendicitis is in the 60% range in most patients but is improved in a thin patient. The classic positive findings are a target sign in the transverse projection demonstrating an appendix at least 1 cm thick.

Ultrasonography is also helpful in elucidating tubo-ovarian disease when that is a significant consideration. A negative study however, cannot rule out appendicitis.

Tagged White Blood Cell Imaging
This study has a high specificity and sensitivity but will take at least 60 to 90 minutes to accomplish and often takes longer to initiate; in addition, it is not readily available in many institutions.

Computed Tomography
This study, even without oral contrast material, has a sensitivity and specificity approaching 90%. It is three times as expensive as ultrasound, however, and requires considerable more time to arrange and accomplish. CT is an excellent study for the patient with a right lower quadrant mass in whom it is necessary to differentiate between a phlegmon and perforation with abscess. In the latter clinical situation the radiologist may not only make the diagnosis but also drain the abscess percutaneously at the time

of the study, often obviating the need for any future operative intervention.

Laparoscopy
Laparoscopy usually involves using a general anesthetic and considerable expense as well as inherent morbidity and is therefore not justified as a purely diagnostic method in the acute setting. The author has attempted examination under local anesthesia in the emergency room using a 3 mm laparoscope and found it less than satisfactory, but other more experienced laparoscopists might feel otherwise.

The evaluation of the patient with suspected appendicitis is summarized in Figure 46-1.

■ THERAPY

Acute appendicitis requires surgical treatment, with the previously mentioned exception of percutaneous CT-guided drainage of an abscess associated with perforation.

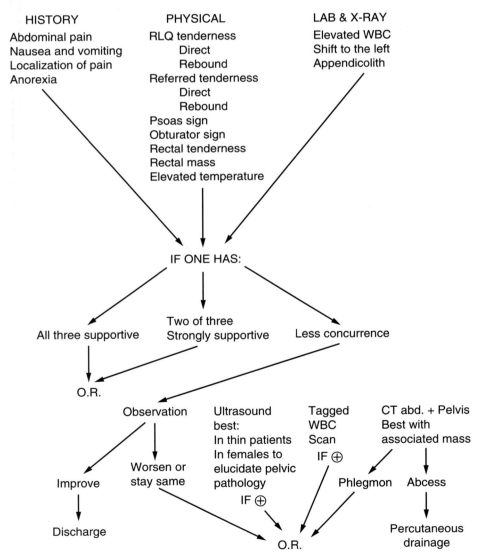

Figure 46-1
Algorithm for the evaluation of the patient with suspected appendicitis.

If CT demonstrates a phlegmon without abscess, there is controversy regarding whether such a patient should be treated conservatively with bowel rest, antibiotics, and an interval appendectomy 6 to 12 weeks after resolution, or should undergo immediate operation. The complication rate appears to be essentially the same with either approach. Initial conservative treatment does necessitate an additional hospitalization and surgery, and should therefore be second choice in the absence of significant comorbid factors.

For all other patients with appendicitis, the major question currently is whether surgery should be performed laparoscopically or through an incision. Proponents of the laparoscopic approach claim shorter hospitalization times and quicker recovery, but detractors maintain the advantages to be marginal at best and the technique is considerably more expensive. This author favors an incision in the majority of cases but would utilize laparoscopy if there was sufficient doubt regarding the diagnosis but no doubt that surgical intervention was necessary. In either case, the patient should be given a single preoperative dose of a broad-spectrum antibiotic, which should not be continued postoperatively in any case of nonperforated or nongangrenous appendicitis.

Incisional Technique
Even after more than 100 years, the incision first described by Dr. Charles McBurney, Chief of Surgery at Roosevelt Hospital in New York City, remains the most desirable. Made obliquely over McBurney's point, it serially divides in the direction of their fibers the external oblique, internal oblique, and transversus fascia, thus exposing the peritoneum. It will facilitate locating the cecum and appendix if the loose lateral attachments of the peritoneum are bluntly separated with the forefinger, enabling the peritoneum to "pooch" upward. After entering the peritoneal cavity, obtain a culture if there is turbid fluid, and grasp the cecum in order to trace the taenia to the appendix. Once located, the appendix can be delivered into the wound. Blunt finger dissection usually suffices to free it from surrounding adhesions, but occasionally appendectomy must be accomplished in a retrograde fashion. Once mobilized the meso-appendix should be divided between clamps and ligated. All that is then necessary is to ligate the appendix at its base, clamp with a straight clamp 2 to 3 mm distal to one's tie, and then divide between tie and clamp, flush on the clamp. The exposed mucosal surface can be directly cauterized (an interposed clamp is not necessary), and the procedure is complete. Inversion is not required. If the operation is done in a retrograde fashion, the first step is ligation of the appendix at its base and division on a straight clamp. The clamp then allows the surgeon to gently draw up and serially clamp and divide the meso-appendix.

If there is a phlegmon of the appendix at the base of the cecum, it is advisable to perform a partial cecectomy along with appendectomy. This is easily effected with a stapling device utilizing heavy staples. There is usually no need to reinforce the staple line with sutures.

If there is an abscess cavity, it should be cultured and thoroughly irrigated with sterile saline. A soft Silastic closed drain should be placed through a separate inferior stab wound, the peritoneum closed, and the muscle layers closed serially with interrupted absorbable sutures. In this instance, as well as with perforated appendices, the skin and subcutaneous tissue should be left open. In the absence of perforation, the entire wound may be closed and no drainage is necessary.

Laparoscopic Appendectomy
If the laparoscopic technique is employed, three ports should be used, a 10-mm camera port in the subumbilical location, a 12-mm port to accommodate a stapler in the left lower quadrant and a 5-mm port in the right mid to upper abdomen. If needed, an additional 5-mm port can be placed in the suprapubic position. Division of the meso-appendix and closure of the appendiceal base can be accomplished with either linear staples or ligatures. This technique can be more trouble than necessary and offers no advantage in any patient with prior surgery to the abdomen or pelvis, who is less than 5 feet tall or 100 lb, or under 15 years of age.

■ SPECIAL CONSIDERATIONS

A number of clinical situations may be encountered while operating for what had been thought to be acute appendicitis. These entities might be unexpected but should not be unanticipated.

Sigmoid Diverticulitis
For the patient having the usual sigmoid phlegmon without free perforation or abscess associated, the appendix should be removed, the wound closed, and the patient treated medically for diverticulitis. If there is free perforation or contained perforation with abscess, a Hartmann resection in addition to appendectomy is indicated. In most cases this is best done through a separate midline incision.

Cecal Diverticulitis
Even in the face of an unprepared bowel, this situation is best served by partial colectomy and primary anastomosis, which is often easily accomplished through an extension of the existing incision.

Crohn's Disease
Very simply, the appendix should be removed in the absence of gross involvement of the cecum and appendiceal base with Crohn's disease. Nothing should be done operatively to the small bowel unless there is a perforation. Postoperatively, the patient should be started on appropriate medical therapy.

Carcinoid
Most carcinoids associated with appendicitis will be significantly smaller than 2 cm and therefore require nothing more than appendectomy for adequate treatment. In the rare instance of a lesion 2 cm or greater, right hemicolectomy should be performed.

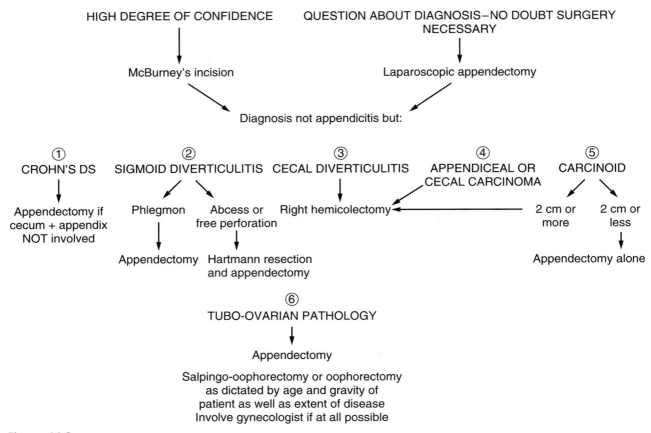

Figure 46-2
Algorithm for the surgical treatment of other conditions found at the time of surgery for suspected appendicitis.

Cancer

The presence of adenocarcinoma either of the appendix or more usually the base of the cecum dictates a right hemicolectomy.

Tubo-ovarian Pathology

A gynecologist, if available, should be summoned immediately to take over care of the patient following appendectomy. If consultation is not feasible, a conservative approach, especially in a premenopausal patient, is indicated. Ruptured corpus luteum cysts can be wedged out. Unilateral tubo-ovarian abscess may be excised and drained, but bilateral disease in women in the child-bearing years should be treated with antibiotics initially.

Figure 46-2 summarizes the surgical treatments for appendicitis discussed here.

Suggested Readings

Bonanni F, Reed J 3rd, Hartzell G, et al: Laparoscopic versus conventional appendectomy. J Am Coll Surg 1994;179(3):273–278.

McCahill LE, Pellegrini CA, Wiggins T, Helton WS: A clinical outcome and cost analysis of laparoscopic versus open appendectomy. Am J Surg 1996;171(5):533–537.

Sarfati MR, Hunter GC, Witzke DB, et al: Impact of adjunctive testing on the diagnosis and clinical course of patients with acute appendicitis. Am J Surg 1993;166(6):660–664; discussion 664–665.

Wen SW, Naylor CD: Diagnostic accuracy and short-term surgical outcomes in cases of suspected acute appendicitis. Can Med Assoc J 1995;152(10):1617–1626.

Wuang Y, Reen DJ, Puri P: Is a histologically normal appendix following emergency appendectomy always normal? Lancet 1996;347(9008):1076–1079.

47

CECAL ULCER

Anthony J. Senagore, MD, MS, MBA, FACS

Nonspecific solitary ulcer of the cecum is an uncommon lesion initially reported by Cruveilhier in 1832. Subsequent descriptions of this entity, consisting mainly of case reports or small case series, have revealed an entity that requires a high index of suspicion and a variety of diagnostic modalities to confirm the diagnosis. This unusual clinical entity has also been termed *isolated cecal ulcer, simple cecal ulcer,* or *acute cecal ulcer.* In fact, cecal ulcer is frequently a diagnosis of exclusion because of the need to rule out more serious clinical entities such as cancer or inflammatory bowel disease.

■ ETIOLOGY

The etiology of cecal ulcer remains unclear; however, there appears to be a growing association of this entity and cytomegalovirus (CMV) infection, particularly in transplant patients. The reputed etiologies supported by individual case reports include genetic, infectious, mechanical, vascular, neurogenic, drug-induced, and chemical. Cytomegalovirus infection accounts for the most frequently described etiologic agent for reported cases of cecal ulcer and appears to be increasingly more frequent in transplant patients. Sutherland and coworkers (1979) reported the single largest series of CMV-induced cecal ulcers in renal transplant patients. The majority of these patients had accompanying organ rejection or systemic sepsis. CMV infection occurs frequently in this patient population; however, a subgroup with primary infection after transplant appears prone to develop more aggressive infections. Although CMV-induced cecal ulcer is typically associated with significant immunosuppression, it has also been reported after prolonged use of a left ventricular assist device. Therefore, isolated cecal ulcer should be considered when lower gastrointestinal (GI) bleeding occurs in patients with any potential for immunosuppression.

Kaufman and coworkers presented a series of three patients with solitary cecal ulcers associated with the use of nonsteroidal anti-inflammatory drugs (NSAIDs). These cases presented with much larger areas of ulceration in the cecum and ascending colon with an abrupt cutoff of the lesion and an associated weblike deformity. The mechanism of cellular injury with these agents is unclear; however, the occasional tight stricture makes the exclusion of malignancy difficult and may necessitate surgery.

Another putative cause of cecal ulcer is isolated cecal diverticulitis as supported by a series of 10 patients reported by Anscombe and associates. Cecal diverticulitis shares the relatively younger age associated with cecal ulcer and is presumed to occur as a result of inflammation which destroys the diverticulum, leaving only an ulcer. This inflammation may become transmural, as evidenced by the fact that all the patients reported by Anscombe required laparotomy for presumed appendicitis or perforated cecal cancer.

Cecal ulcer has also been reported to be the result of microvascular thrombi or chemical irritation from acidic ileal effluent. However, consistent documentation of thrombi or significant alterations of the composition of ileal content in cases of cecal ulcer have substantiated neither of these theories. Similarly, steroids and oral contraceptives have been implicated in cecal ulcer because of an association with the induction of hypercoagulable states. The fact that so many theories exist with respect to the etiology of cecal ulcer indicates that the real mechanism for the disease has remained elusive.

■ CLINICAL FEATURES

Cecal ulcers constitute 50% of all isolated colonic ulcers and occur with a 2:1 male predominance. Although the typical patient is in the fifth decade of life, reports have noted patients ranging from 12 to 80 years old. The most frequent presentation of cecal ulcer is nonspecific right lower quadrant pain, often mimicking appendicitis. In fact, in several early series peritonitis or localized abscess in the cecal area was a frequent operative finding. Lower GI bleeding is another common presentation for this entity, particularly in recent years. Other less frequently seen symptoms include diarrhea, constipation, and intestinal obstruction. Laparotomy may reveal a cecal mass that is indistinguishable from carcinoma.

■ PATHOLOGY

The cecum is the most frequent location for colonic ulcers, and the lesions range in size from 5 mm to 10 cm. The ulcers typically develop on the anterior wall of the cecum along with a significant circumferential edema, which may give the appearance of tumor on contrast enema. Histologic evaluation of the lesion reveals fibrous necrotic granulation tissue, associated with a chronic inflammatory reaction with lymphocyte and fibroblast infiltrates. The lesions have discrete borders adjacent to completely normal anatomy. Reports of microvascular thrombosis within the submucosal vessels, without similar findings in larger mesenteric vessels, have implicated localized ischemia as an etiology. In cases associated with CMV, the typical finding is of viral inclusions within endothelial cells and fibroblasts in the lamina propria.

■ DIAGNOSIS

Many of the early reports of cecal ulcer relied on operative findings in patients who presented with an acute abdomen. However, more recent reports have indicated that a variety of studies may aid in the diagnosis, although the disease should be a diagnosis of exclusion. Contrast studies may be helpful to rule out more common disease such as Crohn's or ulcerative colitis. As a rule, however, barium enema is not very helpful. Computed tomographic (CT) scan may demonstrate thickening of the cecal wall and some pericolonic fat stranding, but these findings are nonspecific. In cases of suspected CMV infection, urine cultures for the virus should be performed. Colonoscopy has offered a more accurate means of identifying this lesion and, even more important, ruling out a carcinoma. Prior to the availability of endoscopic evaluation, the diagnosis required laparotomy. Colonoscopy should be considered in patients with unusual complaints or evidence of chronic or acute lower GI bleeding. Colonoscopy also offers the ability to perform biopsy, which may allow conservative management of the lesion. In cases of massive lower GI bleeding, angiography is an important modality. Angiography will frequently identify the site of bleeding and may allow for control of hemorrhage by the infusion of intra-arterial vasopressin. There are no specific angiographic findings of a cecal ulcer.

■ MANAGEMENT

History is an important aspect of the decision-making process for diagnostic intervention in any patient with lower GI bleeding. This importance is particularly true for cecal ulcer because of the common association with use of NSAIDs or chronic immunosuppression. Obviously, these clinical scenarios should be easily determined prior to any intervention. In the case of immunosuppression, the significant potential for CMV infection in the cecum should be evaluated with appropriate serologic tests and endoscopic biopsy. Conversely, the retrospective diagnosis of an NSAID-induced cecal ulcer should lead one to discontinue the use of these medications for that patient. However, the majority of cecal ulcers are not associated with any underlying acute or chronic disease process, and, therefore, the cause frequently is identified at the time of endoscopy. Endoscopy allows direct visualization and localization of the lesion as well as histologic confirmation of the underlying pathology and potential pathogens. Endoscopic cauterization or injection of these bleeding lesions may be necessary at the time of endoscopy, and the physician should be prepared to perform such procedures.

Once the lesion is identified and resuscitation of the patient is complete in the face of ongoing bleeding in a hemodynamically stable patient, the next diagnostic and potential therapeutic modality is angiography. A number of case reports have demonstrated the effectiveness of angiographic localization of the hemorrhage coupled with vascular embolization as needed. Although some reports attest to the high degree of success with this approach, it does carry the risk of cecal perforation. Another alternative is selective intra-arterial infusion of vasopressin for the management of ongoing bleeding. This approach is usually successful in stopping the bleeding, but is associated with frequent rebleeding when the drug is terminated. Therefore, this choice appears to be helpful in allowing stabilization of the patient but would not appear to offer definitive management of the lesion. Unfortunately, this technique also carries a risk for perforation of the ulcerated cecum. These modalities, although somewhat risky, should be strongly considered in immunosuppressed patients with CMV infection because the mortality rate due to the associated immunosuppression and sepsis is very high.

In the rare patient who presents with right lower quadrant pain or hemorrhage uncontrolled by any of the nonoperative techniques, cecectomy should be considered. This formidable operation carries a high perioperative morbidity/mortality rate in the immunosuppressed patient but is highly successful in the nonimmunosuppressed patient. Laparoscopic techniques have been applied to this entity as an alternative to open celiotomy.

■ SUMMARY

Isolated cecal ulcer is a rare entity, which frequently presents as lower GI hemorrhage. Occasionally, the lesion can be confused with a carcinoma. Because of the high mortality rate associated with such lesions in immunosuppressed patients, therapy should be conservative. Endoscopy should be considered early with either endoscopic or angiographic control of hemorrhage. Failing nonoperative modalities for the control of hemorrhage or when faced with an underlying neoplasm, open or laparoscopic resection of the cecum should be performed.

Suggested Readings

Anscombe AR, Keddie NC, Schofield PF: Solitary ulcers and diverticulitis of the caecum. Br J Surg 1967;54:553–557.

Cruveilhier J: Un beau cas de cicatrisation d'un ulcere de l'intestin gae le clatant d'une douzaine d'armels. Bull Soc Anat 1893;7:1–2.

Delamarre J, Capron JP, Fievet P, et al: Bleeding cecal typhoid ulcer. Value of emergency angiography for selective surgical hemostasis. Hepatogastroenterology 1983;30:266–267.

Fenoglio-Preiser CM, Lantz PE, Listrom MB, et al: Gastrointestinal Pathology: An Atlas and Text. New York, Raven Press, 1989, p 691.

Himal HS: Benign cecal ulcer. Surg Endosc 1989;3:170–172.

Icenogle TB, Peterson E, Ray G, et al: DHPG effectively treats CMV infection in heart and heart-lung transplant patients: A preliminary report. J Heart Transplant 1987;6:199–203.

Kaufman HL, Fischer AH, Carroll M, Becker JM: Colonic ulceration associated with nonsteroidal anti-inflammatory drugs: Report of three cases. Dis Colon Rectum 1996;39:705–710.

Last MD, Lavery IC: Major hemorrhage and perforation due to a solitary cecal ulcer in a patient with end-stage renal failure. Dis Colon Rectum 1983;26:495–498.

Marn CS, Vu BF, Nostrant TT, Ellis JH: Idiopathic cecal ulcer: CT findings. Am J Roentgenol 1989;153:761–763.

Pfau P, Rothstein RD: Cytomegalovirus cecal ulcer in a patient awaiting cardiac transplantation. Am J Gastroenterol 1996;91:2435–2436.

Phillips WS, Burton NA, Macmanus Q, Lefrak EA: Surgical complications in bridging to transplantation: The Thermo Cardiosystems LVAD. Ann Thorac Surg 1992;53:482–486.

Rex, DK, Broadie TA, Hull MT: Endoscopic detection of a tiny cecal ulcer containing carcinoma in situ. Indiana Med 1991;84:692–694.

Roby R IV, Montgmery M IV, Scoggin SD, Jew A: Laparoscopic-assisted excision of a solitary cecal ulcer. J Laparoendosc Surg 1993;3: 405–409.

Rosen-Levin EM, Schwartz IS: Solitary cecal ulcer due to cytomegalovirus in a leukemic patient. Mt Sinai J Med 1985;52:138–141.

Shallman RW, Kuehner M, Williams GH, et al: Benign cecal ulcers. Spectrum of disease and selective management. Dis Colon Rectum 1985;28:732–737.

Sutherland DE, Chan FY, Fourcar E, et al: The bleeding cecal ulcer in transplant patients. Surgery 1979;86:386–398.

Sutherland D, Frech RS, Weil R, et al: The bleeding cecal ulcer: Pathogenesis, angiographic diagnosis, and nonoperative control. Surgery 1972;71:290–294.

48

PSEUDOMEMBRANOUS COLITIS

James P. Celebrezze, Jr., MD
David S. Medich, MD

Pseudomembranous colitis (PMC) is usually a diarrheal illness associated with the gram-positive anaerobic bacterium *Clostridrium difficile*. It has also been termed *Clostridium difficile* colitis or antibiotic-associated colitis. Widespread use of broad-spectrum antibiotics, both for surgical prophylaxis and treatment of infectious disease, as well as increased use of immunosuppressive agents accompanying organ transplantation, has led to an increased incidence of PMC. Additionally, as the complexity and severity of illnesses treated in intensive care units increases, more severely ill patients may require treatment for PMC. Although PMC is mostly a disease requiring medical management, surgery may be warranted in rare instances.

■ HISTORY

The first case of PMC was reported over 100 years ago. Initially, the disease was described as an enterocolitis and its cause was attributed to heavy metal poisoning, ischemic heart disease, uremia, or intestinal obstruction associated with carcinoma. In the 1950s and 1960s, *Staphylococcus aureus* was implicated as the causative agent and PMC was described as *staphylococcal enteritis*. When PMC was associated with the use of clindamycin, an effective antistaphylococcal agent, it became clear that *S. aureus* was not the cause. Pioneering work by Bartlett and associates identified *C. difficile* as the toxin-producing causative agent.

■ ETIOLOGY

PMC is almost invariably associated with prior antibiotic use. Virtually all antibiotics, with the exception of oral vancomycin, have been implicated in the development of PMC (Table 48-1). Antibiotics suppress the normal colonic flora, allowing selective growth of *C. difficile* and the production of its toxin.

C. difficile may be an endogenous resident of the human colon or may be acquired by the fecal-oral route. It is estimated that 1 to 3% of the healthy adult population are asymptomatic carriers of *C. difficile*. These carriers can excrete *C. difficile* spores but rarely excrete the cytotoxin.

In contrast, asymptomatic carrier rates in infants who have not received antibiotics are as high as 64%, and these infants excrete toxin in 55% of cases. These healthy infants carry the toxigenic form of *C. difficile* but are resistant to symptoms in the first year of life owing to the immaturity of their enterocyte toxin-receptor site.

By the fecal-oral route, asymptomatic carriers and symptomatic patients alike provide a vector for transmission. The spores may survive for weeks or months on inanimate objects such as rings and stethoscopes and can be passed by caregivers to patients. This type of transmission may account for the clustering of PMC cases and the variable incidence among different institutions.

Other risk factors for the development of PMC include age greater than 60 years, prolonged antibiotic treatment, irradiation, obstructive pulmonary disease, malignancy (especially hematologic), mechanical bowel preparation, enteral feedings, care in the intensive care unit, and immunosuppression. Immunosuppressed patients may account for up to 20% of PMC cases, and PMC can occur in these patients without the prior use of antibiotics. Causes of immunosuppression include human immunodeficiency virus (HIV) disease, malnutrition, immunosuppressive medications used by transplantation services, and chemotherapy for malignancies.

■ PATHOPHYSIOLOGY

The exact cause of the diarrhea associated with *C. difficile* is unclear. The organism produces at least two toxins that are of clinical importance. Toxin A is an enterotoxin and cytotoxin and is responsible for the inflammatory colitis that allows toxin B to enter the colonic cells. Toxin B is a potent cytotoxin and is the toxin readily detectable in diagnostic assays. The organism also synthesizes collagenase, which may facilitate mucosal breakdown. Toxin and bacterial translocation occurs across the disrupted colonic epithelial barrier and may enter the portal circulation. Hepatic macrophages phagocytize the toxin causing the release of tumor necrosis factor (TNF) and interleukins 1 and 6. The release of these chemical mediators is then responsible for the systemic septic response seen with PMC.

Pathologic findings tend to be limited to the colon. However, the jejunum has been implicated as a reservoir for *C. difficile*, and a syndrome virtually identical to PMC

Table 48-1 Antibiotics Associated with *Clostridium difficile* Colitis

Higher incidence
  Cephalosporins
  Penicillins
  Clindamycin
Lower incidence
  Aminoglycosides
  Quinolones
  Ureidopenicillins
  Trimethoprim

has occurred in patients with pelvic ileal pouches or with ileostomies. The small bowel may become susceptible to *C. difficile* infection owing to the morphologic changes that occur in the small intestine after colectomy.

DIAGNOSIS

The typical clinical presentation of PMC occurs 7 days after the initiation of antibiotic therapy (range, 2 to 21 days after cessation of antibiotics). The tetrad of common symptoms includes profuse, watery diarrhea (90 to 95%), fever (80%), cramping abdominal pain (80 to 90%), and leukocytosis (80%). Physical examination findings may be mild and nonspecific, especially in the postoperative period, or more pronounced when toxic colitis has developed. Up to 5% of patients may present with an "acute surgical abdomen," making the diagnosis more difficult, as will be discussed.

The gold standard for diagnosis is the detection of *C. difficile*–associated toxin in the stool. This detection is most commonly done by enzyme-linked immunosorbent assay (ELISA), which has a sensitivity of 70 to 95% and a specificity of 99 to 100%. Results are generally available in a matter of hours. Repetitive specimen collection on the same day does not increase the sensitivity of testing. Cultures for *C. difficile* are more sensitive but also are more expensive and time-consuming, and as many as 3% of healthy asymptomatic adults may be carriers. For these reasons, culturing is usually reserved for epidemiologic studies.

Sigmoidoscopy and colonoscopy are particularly useful in differentiating PMC from other colitides (Table 48-2). Typical macroscopic findings of PMC consist of multiple, raised, adherent, yellow to white plaques 2 to 5 mm in size. The intervening mucosa may appear edematous and inflamed or conversely normal. Not all patients with toxin-positive *C. difficile* colitis will have abnormal mucosa or pseudomembranes; some patients with mild disease may have normal mucosa. In addition, the disease may have a patchy distribution. It may spare the rectum completely in up to 70% of cases, or typical findings of pseudomembranes may be beyond the limits of flexible sigmoidoscopy (10% of patients). This finding has led many to recommend colonoscopy for patients with suspected PMC and normal sigmoidoscopy or for patients in whom the diagnosis is in question.

Biopsy of the pseudomembranes reveals them to consist primarily of polymorphonuclear cells, fibrin, mucus, and epithelial debris. Histologically, PMC is difficult to differentiate from ischemic colitis, but the two diseases are readily distinguishable endoscopically.

Radiologic imaging has a less well defined role. In the past double contrast barium enema was advocated, but more recent experience would suggest that it may worsen the colitis, and therefore it is not recommended. Conversely, computed tomography (CT) may have an increasing role in the diagnosis and management of PMC. Findings typical of PMC include diffuse colonic wall thickening, doughnut-like appearance of the ascending and descending colon, and colonic dilatation. In the small percentage of patients who present with toxic symptoms or an acute surgical abdomen but with an appropriate history for PMC, these characteristic CT findings may influence the treating physician to initiate medical therapy and avoid "unnecessary" laparotomy. In addition, CT may be useful in excluding other diagnoses in patients not responding to medical therapy.

THERAPY

The initial therapy for suspected PMC is the cessation of the offending antibiotic therapy. Supportive measures such as bowel rest and intravenous hydration may be useful, but the administration of antidiarrheal agents is contraindicated. Most patients will have resolution of their symptoms without additional therapy, but the diarrheal state may be protracted, lasting up to 5 weeks. Additionally, patients will excrete *C. difficile* even after resolution of diarrhea, posing a risk of colonization or illness to other people. For these reasons, antibiotic therapy directed at *C. difficile* is recommended for patients with PMC.

Current antibiotics effective for the elimination of *C. difficile* from the gastrointestinal tract include vancomycin and metronidazole. Vancomycin is poorly absorbed from the gastrointestinal tract and therefore achieves adequate concentrations for the eradication of *C. difficile* when given orally in doses of 125 mg four times daily for 7 days. Higher doses are not more effective, nor do they decrease relapse rates. Vancomycin can also be administered via enema or directly through an ostomy in appropriate circumstances (500 mg in 1 L normal saline administered three times daily). Parenteral administration of vancomycin is ineffective in the treatment of PMC. Metronidazole is a good alternative to vancomycin and has the advantages of being effective in oral or parenteral forms and is generally less expensive. The typical dosing

Table 48-2 Differential Diagnosis of Pseudomembranous Colitis	
OTHER COLITIDES	**CHARACTERISTICS**
Ulcerative colitis	Bloody diarrhea; typically chronic or long-standing symptoms or disease; endoscopic appearance with friability, increased vascularity, pseudopolyps
Crohn's disease	Chronic symptoms of disease; characteristic endoscopic appearance with inflamed, edematous mucosa with linear ulcers
Ischemic colitis	Bleeding dominant symptom; risk factors present; distinctive endoscopic appearance
Amebic dysentery	Bloody diarrhea; history of foreign travel; characteristic finding on microscopic examination of stool

regimen is 500 mg administered three times daily for 10 to 14 days.

Other medical therapies include bacitracin administered orally, anion-exchange resins such as cholestyramine, and the administration of fecal enemas. Bacitracin is no more effective than vancomycin but can be used in patients with drug sensitivities to both vancomycin and metronidazole. Exchange resins have been used effectively in patients with resistant PMC after a failed course of vancomycin.

Restoration of normal fecal flora with the administration of fecal enemas is an effective therapy for mild cases of PMC, either as initial therapy or for recurrent disease. Not surprisingly, patient acceptance issues and concern for transmission of other infectious diseases substantially reduce this modality's usefulness.

Although symptoms are initially resolved with specific anticlostridial antibiotics in 95% of patients, relapse rates of 10 to 20% occur with medical management. These relapses usually occur within 2 weeks of cessation of therapy. A high risk of relapse occurs in patients with chronic renal failure, those with previous episodes of PMC, and patients continuing other antibiotic therapy. It is estimated that one half of "relapses" are really due to reinfection. Relapses may be treated with a repeat course of vancomycin or metronidazole with 95% response rates. However, the relapse rate after an initial recurrence is as high as 65%. No randomized, controlled, prospective trial for the therapy of multiple relapse of PMC exists. However, a tapering course of vancomycin over 4 to 6 weeks may be effective (Table 48-3). Further relapses may be treated with additional vancomycin with the addition of rifampin, cholestyramine, probiotics, or intravenous immunoglobulin.

■ SURGICAL THERAPY

Although the vast majority of cases of pseudomembranous colitis will respond to the preceding medical therapies, 3 to 20% will progress to a toxic state. In these patients with toxic colitis, 65 to 100% will require surgical intervention. Additionally, some patients with PMC may present as a surgical emergency. These patients often will have atypical symptoms such as obstipation, making differentiating the condition from intestinal obstruction or ischemia difficult. Patients operated upon for a diagnosis other than PMC present difficult intraoperative decisions to the treating surgeon.

When PMC progresses to fulminant disease, surgical intervention becomes indicated in cases of colonic perforation, toxic megacolon, or disease refractory to medical management. Operative intervention carries an overall 25 to 67% mortality rate. Increased mortality rates are seen in the elderly, with the use of immunosuppressive drugs, in patients with underlying malignancy, in patients receiving antibiotic therapy for more than 7 days, and when diagnosis is delayed. Delay in diagnosis may be the single most important predictor of fatality. Jobe and associates reported that patients who succumbed to fulminant PMC despite operative intervention had a delay in therapy of 10.7 days versus 5.4 days for those who survived.

Typical laboratory findings in fulminant colitis include profound leukocytosis, often exceeding 30×10^9 cells/L. Endoscopic findings, while diagnostic for PMC, do not predict the severity of disease or prognosis for success with medical management. However, in patients operated upon for a surgical emergency, intraoperative sigmoidoscopy or colonoscopy may aid in decision making by allowing examination of the colonic mucosa. Plain film radiologic evaluation is nonspecific, but CT has demonstrated itself to be useful in the management of severe to fulminant PMC. Typical findings of severe PMC on CT include a thickened, edematous colon with pancolonic involvement and free intraperitoneal fluid.

The management of a patient with fulminant antibiotic-associated colitis is similar to the management of other toxic colitides. If no absolute indication for operative intervention exists, such as no evidence of perforation or diffuse peritonitis, then aggressive medical management is instituted. If after 48 to 72 hours there is no significant improvement, surgery is warranted. Also, if the patient's condition worsens during the initial 48 hours, despite medical management, surgery is warranted.

Upon laparotomy, typical findings include purulent ascites with multiple polymorphonuclear neutrophils on Gram's stain and a diffusely thickened, edematous colon. External inspection of the colon can be misleading in judging extent of disease and therefore should not influence the limits of resection. As in any case of toxic colitis, subtotal colectomy with end-ileostomy should be performed as the surgical treatment for toxic PMC. Other options include nontherapeutic laparotomy, creation of an ileostomy or colostomy alone, cecostomy with trans-stomal instillation of vancomycin, segmental resection, or "blowhole" colostomy with defunctioning loop ileostomy and trans-stomal instillation of vancomycin. Procedures less than subtotal colectomy are generally associated with higher mortality rates (Table 48-4). Subtotal colectomy with ileostomy has many other advantages over lesser procedures. It avoids an intra-abdominal anastomosis, removes the organ responsible for ongoing sepsis, diverts stool away from the rectum, allows for good symptomatic relief, and avoids pelvic dissection with its corresponding morbidity. Ileorectal anastomosis can be accomplished 3 to 6 months after recovery.

Table 48-3 Treatment of Recurrent *Clostridrium difficile* Colitis

First recurrence
Repeat 10–14 days of metronidazole or vancomycin
Second recurrence
Vancomycin taper:
  125 mg every 6 hours for 7 days
  125 mg every 12 hours for 7 days
  125 mg every day for 7 days
  125 mg every other day for 7 days
  125 mg every third day for 7 days

Table 48-4 Operative Treatment of *Clostridium difficile* Colitis

AUTHORS	NUMBER OF PATIENTS	OPERATION (NUMBER OF PATIENTS)	OPERATIVE MORTALITY RATE (%)
Jobe et al.	10	Colectomy (type not stated) (7)	43
		Laparotomy (3)	0
Lipsett et al.	13	Overall mortality rate	38.5
		Left hemicolectomy (4)	100
		Subtotal colectomy/ileostomy (9)	14
Medich et al.	14	Laparotomy (7)	28
		Segmental colectomy (3)	67
		Subtotal colectomy/ileostomy (4)	0
Morris et al.	23	Subtotal colectomy or "colectomy" (17)	24
		Ileostomy, cecostomy, or decompressive (6)	26
Grundfest-Broniatowski et al.	12	Ileostomy and blowhole colostomy (3)	66
		Laparotomy (4)	25
		Subtotal colectomy/ileostomy (5)	43
Trudel et al.	7	Subtotal colectomy/ileostomy (7)	72

In cases in which PMC is not suspected preoperatively but is discovered when a laparotomy is undertaken for an acute abdomen, treatment recommendations are less clearly defined. No prospective study exists on the subject, and retrospective reviews often have widely divergent results. This lack of specificity is likely due to variability in defining an acute abdomen, and therefore variability in disease severity. Drapkin and coworkers reported five cases of nontherapeutic laparotomy in patients who had postoperative confirmation of *C. difficile*–associated colitis. All five recovered with medical management. Conversely, in a previous publication from one of the authors (DSM), six of nine patients operated upon for acute abdomen underwent nontherapeutic procedures. Three of these patients improved with medical management, two recovered only after subsequent subtotal colectomy, and one succumbed to multisystem organ failure. If the correct diagnosis of PMC is not made preoperatively but is discovered intraoperatively, our current approach is based on disease severity. Patients who have preoperatively required vasopressors, who have required mechanical ventilation, or who have developed other organ dysfunction or failure are treated with subtotal colectomy and end-ileostomy. In less ill patients, however, it would seem reasonable to institute medical management after a nontherapeutic laparotomy. If medical management should fail, subtotal colectomy should be employed as a salvage technique. It should be emphasized, however, that intraoperative diagnosis should be an uncommon event when modern imaging and endoscopic technologies are utilized in conjunction with appropriate clinical suspicion.

■ SUMMARY

PMC requires appropriate clinical suspicion and adequate laboratory and endoscopic evaluation to establish diagnosis. When treated expeditiously with cessation of the offending antibiotics, supportive care, and anti–*C. difficile* antibiotics, medical management is largely successful. Despite resolution of symptoms, recurrence of disease is common. PMC can progress to a fulminant disease requiring timely surgical intervention and mature clinical judgment. When surgery is deemed necessary, subtotal colectomy with ileostomy is the procedure of choice, but mortality rates remain high owing to the critically ill nature of these patients.

Suggested Readings

Altemeier WA, Hummel RD, Hill EO: Staphylococcal enterocolitis following antibiotic therapy. Ann Surg 1963;157:847–858.

Bartlett JG: *Clostridium difficile* infection: Pathophysiology and diagnosis. Semin Gastrointest Dis 1997;8:12–21.

Bartlett JG, Chang TW, Gurwith M, et al: Antibiotic associated pseudomembranous colitis due to toxin-producing clostridia. N Engl J Med 1978;296:531–534.

Cleary RK: *Clostridium difficile*-associated diarrhea and colitis: Clinical manifestations, diagnosis, and treatment. Dis Colon Rectum 1998;41:1435–1449.

Drapkin MS, Worthington MG, Chang TW, Razvi SA: *Clostridium difficile* colitis mimicking acute peritonitis. Arch Surg 1985;120:1321–1322.

Fekety R: Guidelines for the diagnosis and management of *Clostridium difficile*-associated diarrhea and colitis. Am J Gastroenterol 1997;92:739–750.

Finney JMT: Gastro-enterostomy for cicatrizing ulcer of the pylorus. Bull Johns Hopkins Hosp 1893;4:53–55.

Grundfest-Broniatowski S, Quader M, Alexander F, et al: *Clostridium difficile* colitis in the critically ill. Dis Colon Rectum 1996;39:619–623.

Jobe BA, Grasley A, Deveney KE, et al: *Clostridium difficile* colitis: An increasing hospital-acquired illness. Am J Surg 1995;169:480–483.

Kyne L, Kelly CP: Recurrent *Clostridium difficile* diarrhoea. Gut 2001;49:152–153.

Lipsett PA, Samantaray DK, Tam ML, et al: Pseudomembranous colitis: A surgical disease? Surgery 1994;116:491–496.

Medich DS, Lee KKW, Simmons RL, et al: Laparotomy for fulminant pseudomembranous colitis. Arch Surg 1992;127:847–853.

Morris JB, Zollinger RM, Stellato TA: Role of surgery in antibiotic-induced pseudomembranous enterocolitis. Am J Surg 1990;160:535–539.

Rubin MS, Bodenstien LE, Kent KC: Severe *Clostridium difficile* colitis. Dis Colon Rectum 1995;38:350–354.

Tedesco FJ: Pseudomembranous colitis: Pathogenesis and therapy. Med Clin North Am 1982;66:655–665.

Trudel JL, Deschenes M, Mayrand S, Barkun AN: Toxic megacolon complicating pseudomembranous enterocolitis. Dis Colon Rectum 1995;38:1033–1038.

Vesoulis Z, Williams G, Matthews B: Pseudomembranous enteritis after proctocolectomy: Report of a case. Dis Colon Rectum 2000;43:551–554.

49

CYTOMEGALOVIRUS ILEOCOLITIS AND KAPOSI'S SARCOMA IN AIDS

Robert Gilliland, MD, FRCS (Gen)
Mirza Khurrum Baig, MBBS, FRCS
Steven D. Wexner, MD, FACS, FASCRS

In 1981, the Centers for Disease Control (CDC) in the United States reported an outbreak of *Pneumocystis carinii* pneumonia and Kaposi's sarcoma associated with an acquired immunodeficiency in young unmarried men. By the end of 1981, 316 patients diagnosed with what became known as acquired immune deficiency syndrome (AIDS) had been reported. The transmissible agent, a retrovirus, was identified first by Barre-Sinoussi and colleagues in 1983. Initially designated as HTLV-III, it was renamed as the human immunodeficiency virus (HIV) in 1986.

AIDS has now reached worldwide epidemic proportions. According to the estimates from the Joint United Nations Programme on HIV/AIDS (UNAIDS) and the World Health Organization (WHO), 36.1 million adults and 1.4 million children were living with HIV at the end of 2000. During 2000, approximately 5.3 million people became infected with HIV. As of December 31, 2000, 774,467 AIDS cases in the United States had been reported to the Centers for Disease Control and Prevention (CDC). In addition, this year also saw 3 million deaths from HIV/AIDS, a higher global total than in any year since the beginning of the epidemic, despite antiretroviral therapy that staved off AIDS and AIDS-related deaths in the richer countries (CDC, 2001). In less developed countries heterosexual spread is the usual method of transmission, but in the Western world homosexual males are the most frequently affected. In the United States, homosexual and bisexual men previously accounted for 75% of the reported cases of AIDS, but this percentage has decreased as the incidence among heterosexual patients and intravenous drug abusers rises. Although affected men outnumber affected women, approximately 41% (12.1 million) of the overall documented cases are in women. The overall proportion of women with this disease has risen as a result of intravenous drug abuse either directly or via affected sexual partners.

HIV is transmitted via direct contact with infected body fluids, of which blood, semen, and vaginal secretions have the highest concentration of the virus. Direct inoculation into the bloodstream via infected needles or blood products is the most efficient method of transmission. A single act of sexual intercourse with an infected partner carries a 1% probability of becoming infected. Different sexual acts carry different degrees of risk, receptive anal intercourse with ejaculation having the highest. The rectal mucosa is fragile and has an excellent blood supply. Small tears during intercourse may allow direct transmission of the virus into the bloodstream. Unprotected vaginal sex is also a high-risk activity. Sexually transmitted diseases, such as syphilis, HPV, and chancroid, that result in open sores, will facilitate the transmission of the disease.

After entering the body, HIV preferentially attacks T lymphocytes, which carry the CD4 marker eventually leading to their destruction. These lymphocytes are also known as helper T cells and play a central role in cell-mediated immunity as well as a facilitative role in humoral immunity. Infection results not only in a decrease in their number but also in a decrease in their ability to recognize antigens. Macrophages also become less responsive, and B cells produce fewer specific antibodies. These changes render the patient increasingly susceptible to infections and tumor development.

Infection with HIV is usually accompanied by a short viral-like illness lasting 3 to 14 days. HIV has a long latency period, and some patients may remain healthy for many years. Stress, poor nutrition, drug abuse, and other sexually transmitted diseases may act as cofactors to accelerate the onset of the disease. When symptoms from HIV infection eventually appear, they are similar to those of many other common viral illnesses. However, the resultant pyrexia, malaise, weight loss, night sweats, and lymphadenopathy do not resolve.

HIV infection cannot be detected until antibodies to it have been produced by the body's immune system, a process known as seroconversion. Although this usually occurs within 2 to 6 weeks of initial exposure, some early studies indicated that 5% of patients had not seroconverted by 6 months. The improved sensitivity of HIV antibody tests have demonstrated that such delayed seroconversion is unlikely. An enzyme-linked immunosorbent assay (ELISA) against HIV antibody is the initial screening test. If a positive result is obtained, it is repeated and positivity is confirmed by Western blotting. In combination, these tests are 99% specific and sensitive.

Prior to 1992 a diagnosis of AIDS was made only in HIV-infected individuals who developed one or more indicator conditions specified by the CDC. This list initially contained only the most common clinical conditions associated with end-stage disease, such as *Pneumocystis carinii* pneumonia. However, as experience has grown, the catalogue of indicator conditions has expanded considerably. In 1993, the CDC also expanded the definition of AIDS to include those asymptomatic patients with CD4 counts <200 cells/mm^3, indicating the importance of CD4 monitoring in the staging and management of the disease.

High-risk homosexual males and AIDS patients regularly present to colorectal surgeons because the lower gastrointestinal tract is the most frequently affected system in these patients. As a consequence, colorectal surgeons are frequently the first physicians to see these patients, often before the diagnosis of AIDS is confirmed. The reason for the increased risk of colorectal disease in homosexual and bisexual men with AIDS is unknown. However, there is evidence that the intestinal mucosa of these patients contains decreased numbers of CD4 cells and increased numbers of suppressor T cells (CD8), changes which are not noted in healthy homosexual control subjects. Some evidence suggests that sperm alloantigens are the direct cause of this immune dysregulation, as only those males who participate in anoreceptive intercourse exhibit these changes. Thus, anoreceptive intercourse may not only predispose these patients to HIV infection but also to the colorectal manifestations of AIDS.

In patients with AIDS, highly active antiretroviral therapy (HAART) improves outcomes; patients live longer and have more sustained viral load suppression, and costs of care are lower. HAART medications are presently divided into three categories: protease inhibitors, nonnucleoside reverse transcriptase inhibitors, and nucleoside reverse transcriptase inhibitors. These antiviral drugs carry their own risk for causing adverse reactions, as well as drug interactions. HAART, involving treatment with three or four antiretroviral agents, has greatly improved the effectiveness of therapy for HIV infection. It has also extended the number of possible drug interactions that may occur in treated patients. There are 105 possible two-drug interactions among the 15 currently approved antiretroviral agents. Well-characterized interactions involving inhibition of drug metabolism have been exploited to reduce dose size or frequency and to simplify treatment regimens. Many additional interactions are possible with other drugs used to treat or prevent complications of HIV infection. In industrialized countries HAART has changed the natural history of HIV/AIDS, although the long-term effectiveness of HAART is unknown. The HIV may develop resistance to these drugs in the future. However, there is no question that prevention works and remains the best and most cost-effective approach for bringing the HIV/AIDS epidemic under control and saving lives.

■ CYTOMEGALOVIRUS COLITIS

Although cytomegalovirus (CMV) infection is almost ubiquitous among the male homosexual population, CMV colitis is thought to occur almost exclusively in immunosuppressed patients. Risk of exposure to CMV increases with age and geographic location. Approximately 60% of the general adult population in the United States has serologic evidence of prior infection with CMV. Comparatively, in China more than 90% of adults are seropositive for CMV. The incidence of CMV disease, one of the most prevalent infections in HIV-infected persons in the early 1990s, has decreased by more than 80% since the introduction of HAART. The rare cases of CMV disease still observed in the Western countries occur mainly in profoundly immunosuppressed patients who have failed to respond to HAART. About one third of AIDS patients have gastrointestinal CMV disease, and the entire tract can be involved from the mouth to the anus. The colon is involved

in approximately 10% of all AIDS patients, and the clinical disease usually occurs when CD4 counts have fallen below 100 cells/mm^3. CMV infection has been demonstrated in up to a quarter of AIDS patients who required abdominal surgery. The development of symptomatic colitis has serious prognostic implications, with an average survival time of 4 months in some studies.

The role of CMV in the development of colitis remains unclear. Most authors believe that infection with this agent produces a vasculitis affecting mainly the submucosal capillaries and arterioles leading to thrombosis, focal ischemia, and ulceration. However, it is possible that the virus may act as a promotor or cofactor for opportunistic organisms that often coexist. These organisms include *Salmonella, Shigella, Campylobacter, Clostridium difficile, Cryptosporidium, Microsporidium, Entamoeba,* and *Giardia.* Corticosteroids have been implicated as a risk factor in the development of CMV disease.

Diarrhea and abdominal pain are the cardinal symptoms of CMV enterocolitis but are often associated with fever and weight loss. The diarrhea is sometimes bloody and can be profuse. Diarrhea, however, is a common symptom in AIDS patients and may be caused by one of the opportunistic agents already mentioned. Therefore, stool cultures should performed routinely. Perianal ulceration may occur and must be distinguished from herpes simplex virus ulcers. The disease may progress rapidly to severe hemorrhagic colitis, toxic megacolon, and perforation.

Patients presenting with the preceding symptoms and an unremarkable abdominal examination will often undergo a barium enema. The appearances are nonspecific and include diffuse mucosal ulceration, granularity, skip areas, thumbprinting, linear ulceration, and thickening of the terminal ileum. The computed tomographic findings in CMV colitis include marked colonic wall thickening, mural ulceration and edema, and pericolonic stranding. Although some of these features are suggestive of CMV colitis, none are pathognomonic.

The diagnosis is also suggested by the endoscopic identification of submucosal hemorrhage and diffuse mucosal ulceration in the colon. Grossly, these lesions range from erythematous patches with or without shallow punctate ulcers, to multiple wide coalescing ulceration, occasionally reminiscent of ulcerative colitis (Fig. 49-1). Colonic ulcers tend to have smooth edges, and a whitish membrane similar to that seen in pseudomembraneous colitis may be present. Ulcers commonly occur diffusely throughout the colon but may occasionally cluster in the right hemicolon. Rectal ulcers have a tendency to be deeper than colonic ulcers and have irregular edges.

The diagnosis is confirmed by the histologic appearance and culture of biopsies, which should be obtained from multiple areas within the colon because of the multifocal nature of the disease. The diagnostic yield from the right colon tends to be higher than the remainder of the colon. Furthermore, because up to 25% of patients with histologically proved CMV colitis have normal-looking mucosa on endoscopy, random biopsies from several areas of the colon are recommended in any AIDS patient undergoing evaluation of a diarrheal illness. The pathogno-

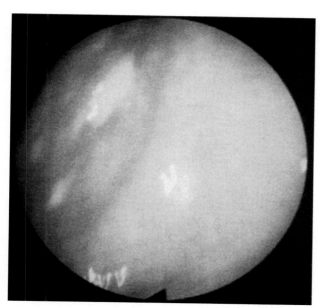

Figure 49-1
This typical colonoscopic appearance of cytomegalovirus ulcers shows the fibrin-covered, shallow, smooth-edged ovoid ulcers.

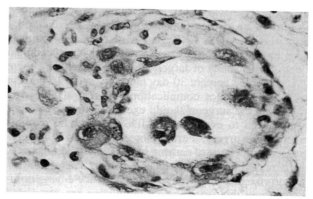

Figure 49-2
Intranuclear inclusion bodies are diagnostic of cytomegalovirus infection.

monic histologic features are large basophilic, intranuclear cytomegalic viral inclusion bodies and granular cytoplasmic inclusions (Fig. 49-2). These inclusions are often noted within endothelial cells in areas of inflammation or ulceration. As the infected cytomegalic cells undergo necrosis, the inclusion bodies become less clear, and the cell takes on a blurred purple-red appearance (Fig. 49-3). These smudge cells, although not pathognomonic of CMV colitis, are highly suggestive of this diagnosis. CMV culture of the biopsied tissue is not routinely done because it requires several weeks to yield results. Serologic tests are not helpful for the diagnosis of acute CMV because of the high prevalence of seropositivity and the need for a four-fold increase in titer during a 4-week interval to establish a diagnosis. New tools for CMV viremia detection have been developed, including the use of polymerase chain reaction (PCR) technology, and detection of antigen pp65 by the antigenemia test in the peripheral blood polymorphonuclear cells. These tests are more sensitive than cultures and correlate with clinical CMV in AIDS patients.

Ganciclovir is a nucleoside analog of guanosine that inhibits viral DNA polymerases by competitively inhibiting the incorporation of deoxyguanosine triphosphate into elongating viral DNA. Both randomized and sequential studies have shown it to be effective in the treatment of symptomatic patients with biopsy-proved CMV colitis; 5 mg/kg is administered by intravenous infusion (10 mg/mL) over 1 hour, repeated every 12 hours for 14 to 21 days.

Multiple complications may occur with this regimen, of which the most frequent and potentially hazardous is myelosuppression with resultant neutropenia and thrombocytopenia. The complete blood cell count (CBC)

should be monitored regularly during treatment. In the event of a neutropenia below 1000 cells/μL, the dose should be reduced to 3 mg/kg every 12 hours until the count is above 1000 cells/μL. Simultaneous administration of zidovudine (AZT) often induces profound myelosuppression and should be avoided. Less frequent side effects include dyspepsia, malaise, hepatic and renal impairment, and mood disturbance.

Patients frequently require maintenance therapy, which can be given either as a 14-day intravenous course every 4 to 6 weeks or as an oral preparation, 1 g three times a day continuously. As maintenance may be needed lifelong, careful counseling as to the benefits or otherwise of medication should be undertaken prior to commencement of therapy.

Foscarnet is a pyrophosphate analog active against herpesviruses and CMV. It has activity against most ganciclovir-resistant strains of CMV; 60 mg/kg is given by intravenous infusion (12 mg/mL) over 1 hour three times a day for 14 to 21 days. Maintenance with 60 mg/kg/day can be continued, increasing to 90 to 120 mg/kg if

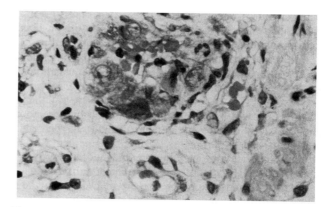

Figure 49-3
The cytomegalic "smudge" cell suggests cytomegalovirus proctocolitis.

required and tolerated. Renal impairment, which can occur in up to 50% of patients, may limit its use. Combination use of ganciclovir and foscarnet has shown no improvement in efficacy compared to monotherapy.

Other drug treatments include cidofovir and more recently, valganciclovir, an orally administered prodrug of ganciclovir. There is evidence to suggest that it is as effective as intravenous ganciclovir for the treatment of CMV retinitis and is currently being studied as a preemptive therapy in patients at high risk of CMV disease. Other promising new drugs for CMV treatment include methylenecyclopropane nucleoside analogs and benzimidazole. The most novel compound is the antisense oligonucleotide fomivirsen that has principally been evaluated in CMV retinitis. The role of immunotherapy with either immunoglobin prophylaxis or the novel adoptive immunotherapy needs further evaluation. However, the widespread introduction of HAART in patients with AIDS has been associated with a very significant reduction in the incidence of all opportunistic infections, including CMV disease.

Surgery is usually reserved for patients presenting with life-threatening hemorrhage or perforation and is associated with a poor outcome. The 30-day mortality rate following emergency surgery is approximately 60%, with death usually the result of hemorrhage, anastomotic complications, fulminant sepsis, or multisystem organ failure. Because of the proclivity for metachronous bleeding or perforation with this condition and the inability of these patients to withstand anastomotic complications, total abdominal colectomy with end-ileostomy is the operation of choice in the emergent situation. Should patients survive the perioperative period, the long-term outlook is bleak, with few patients surviving beyond 6 months.

The high mortality rate associated with emergency surgery has led some authors to operate a policy of elective resection for proved CMV colitis, especially if medical treatment has failed to induce remission. Söderlund and associates report their results in eight patients who had failed medial therapy and had elective right-sided colonic resections with anastomosis. Only two minor postoperative complications were encountered and only one patient died within 30 days of surgery. The overall mean survival was 13 months, and six patients experienced complete or partial palliation for a median period of 14 months. These encouraging results led the authors to recommend early surgical intervention for those patients with localized but pronounced CMV enterocolitis before hemorrhage or perforation has occurred.

■ KAPOSI'S SARCOMA

Kaposi's sarcoma (KS) is an angioproliferative disease occurring in several different clinical-epidemiologic forms that share the same histologic traits and are all associated with infection by the human herpesvirus. Until recently, KS was thought of as an endothelial tumor in elderly Mediterranean males, in whom it had a relatively benign course. However, presently it is more commonly encountered in AIDS patients, in whom it is the most common malignant tumor. In contrast to the 10:1 to 15:1 male-female ratio seen in the classic variant, AIDS-associated KS occurs with a male-female ratio of 50:1, most commonly in patients aged between 20 and 40 years. Among homosexual and bisexual men with AIDS, 43% have KS and indeed the condition often prompts diagnosis of the underlying syndrome. The incidence of KS is several times higher in patients who acquire AIDS by sexual transmission rather than via the intravenous route. Furthermore, the geographic distribution of AIDS-related KS is similar to the prevalence of sexually acquired AIDS. Thus, although the exact etiology of KS in AIDS patients remains uncertain, sexual transmission seems likely, with anal-oral contact being the main route of transference in homosexual men.

The pathogenesis, histologic origin, and behavior of these lesions remain uncertain. They were previously thought to be of endothelial origin, as factor VIII antigen had been identified by immunoperoxidase staining in the spindle cells. However, smooth muscle–specific α actin has been identified, raising the possibility of a mesenchymal origin. It has been suggested that the activation of cytokines such as tumor necrosis factor-α, interleukins 1 and 6, transforming growth factor-β, and basic fibroblast growth factor in conjunction with the already present HIV-induced immune function abnormalities may induce proliferation of the mesenchymal progenitor cells. This proliferation may be further modulated by HIV gene products such as the HIV tat protein. The biologic behavior of KS, whether hyperplastic or neoplastic, is still under debate. Some authors have identified different grades of histologic and immunophenotypic differentiation. As these grades correlate with the extent of invasion and differentiation, they suggest that KS lesions have the fundamental behavioral characteristics of malignant tumors.

KS lesions may involve skin, mucosal surfaces, lymph nodes, or visceral organs. Indeed 25 to 75% of all AIDS patients have disseminated KS. Gastrointestinal lesions occur in almost half of those who have cutaneous lesions. Indeed, the likelihood of gastrointestinal lesions being present correlates with the number of cutaneous lesions. One study reported gastrointestinal tumors in 33% of those with fewer than 10 cutaneous lesions compared with 80% of those with 11 or more lesions. The lesions may develop anywhere between mouth and anus but are more common in the upper alimentary tract than in the colon. They are usually asymptomatic but may present with bleeding, obstruction, perforation, or a protein-losing enteropathy. Rectal KS may present with diarrhea, tenesmus, and bleeding, and patients often have other associated anorectal conditions.

Radiographically, intestinal KS may be difficult to distinguish from Crohn's disease or adenocarcinoma because of the presence of plaques, nodules, strictures, and skip areas. However, the diagnosis is made by endoscopic recognition and histologic verification where possible. The lesions are raised, round, sessile, red nodules ranging between 2 mm and 2 cm in diameter, with the larger lesions having central umbilication (Fig. 49-4). The color

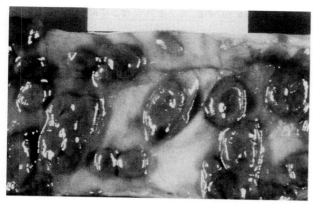

Figure 49-4
The gross appearance of typical nodular colorectal Kaposi's sarcoma.

is due to extravasated blood cells and hemosiderin deposits. In addition to this macular form, they may appear as submucosal ecchymoses or granulation tissue. Owing to the submucosal nature of the lesion, histopathologic confirmation is often difficult. Superficial biopsy is unhelpful, and the use of an 8-mm biopsy forceps is recommended. If a biopsy of sufficient depth is obtained, histologic examination reveals spindle-shaped cells with central hemorrhage, extravasated red blood cells, and hemosiderin-laden macrophages (Fig. 49-5).

With the exception of pulmonary KS, these lesions are rarely the immediate cause of death in AIDS patients. However, the diagnosis of gastrointestinal KS has significant prognostic implications. One study reported a 24-month mortality rate of 89% for patients with gastrointestinal KS compared with a mortality rate of 12% for those without alimentary involvement.

Radiation has been used successfully to treat rectal tumors but is of little value in treating more disseminated lesions. Chemotherapy with single agents, multiple agents, and interferon has been examined. High-dose subcutaneous interferon-α (10 to 18 MU daily) has been used, but the dose-dependent side effects such as nausea, flulike symptoms, lethargy, and depression can limit its usefulness. Although AZT has no specific antitumor activity, it is often given in combination with interferon-α for its anti-HIV action. The myelosuppression often encountered with this combination can be ameliorated using recombinant human granulocyte colony-stimulating factors. Combination chemotherapy using different combinations of bleomycin, vincristine, vinblastine, cyclophosphamide, doxyrubicin, and etoposide have been used for disseminated KS. Some combinations have been found to be more effective than single agents alone, but it should be remembered that the immunosuppressive effects of chemotherapy may lead to an increased incidence of opportunistic infections, so no improvement in overall survival is likely. Thus, these agents should be reserved for symptomatic patients only. Other drugs used for treatment of KS include dapsone, Doxil (liposomal anthracyclines), paclitaxel, thalidomide, IM-862, and retinoids. Surgery is indicated only for complications such as uncontrolled hemorrhage, perforation, or obstruction, and resection should be limited to the diseased segment. Alternatively, if obstruction secondary to a rectosigmoid KS lesion is imminent, then proximal fecal diversion may be useful. In this setting, laparoscopy may be considered to limit direct exposure of the operating team to the peritoneal cavity.

Suggested Readings

Cheung TW, Teich SA: Cytomegalovirus infection in patients with HIV infection. Mt Sinai J Med 1999;66:113–124.

Ensoli B, Sgadari C, Barillari G, et al: Biology of Kaposi's sarcoma. Eur J Cancer 2001;37(10):1251–1269.

Holkova B, Takeshita K, Cheng DM, et al: Effect of highly active antiretroviral therapy on survival in patients with AIDS associated pulmonary Kaposi's sarcoma treated with chemotherapy. J Clin Oncol 2001;19(18):3848–3851.

Joint United Nations Programme on HIV/AIDS: www.CDC.gov. 2001.

Karakozis S, Gongora E, Cacers M, et al: Life threatening cytomegalovirus colitis in the immunocompetent patient. Report of a case and review of literature. Dis Colon Rectum 2001;44:1716–1720.

Kearns AM, Turner AJ, Eltringham GJ, Freeman R: Rapid detection and quantification of CMV DNA in urine using LightCycler-based real time PCR. J Clin Virol 2002;24(1–2):131–134.

Khare MD, Sharland M: Cytomegalovirus treatment options in immunocompromised patients. Expert Opin Pharmacother 2001;2(8):1247–1257.

Levine AM, Tulpule A. Clinical aspects and management of AIDS related Kaposi's sarcoma. Eur J Cancer 2001;37(10):1288–1295.

Mentec H, Leport C, Leport J, et al: Cytomegalovirus colitis in HIV-1-infected patients: A prospective research in 55 patients. AIDS 1994;8:461–467.

Salmon-Ceron D: Cytomegalovirus infection: The point in 2001. HIV Med 2001;2(4):255–259.

Sebastian JJ, Uribarrena R: Cytomegalovirus ileocolitis: Different manifestations of the same illness in the terminal ileum and colon. Endoscopy 1996;28:729.

Söderlund C, Bratt GA, Engström L, et al: Surgical treatment of cytomegalovirus enterocolitis in severe immunodeficiency virus infection. Report of 8 cases. Dis Colon Rectum 1994;37:63–72.

Tirelli U, Franceschi S, Carbone A: Malignant tumours in patients with HIV infection. BMJ 1994;108:1148–1153.

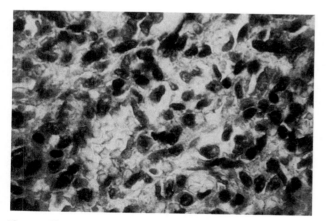

Figure 49-5
Microscopic examination of Kaposi's sarcoma identifies spindle cells, extravasated red blood cells, and lymphovascular "slits."

Wang CY, Schroeter AL, Su WP: Acquired immunodeficiency syndrome-related Kaposi's sarcoma. Mayo Clin Proceed 1995;70:869–879.

Wexner SD, Smithy WB, Trillo C, et al: Emergency colectomy for cytomegalovirus ileocolitis in patient s with the Acquired Immune Deficiency Syndrome. Dis Colon Rectum 1988;31:755–761.

Whitley RJ, Jacobson MA, Freidberg DN, et al: Guidelines for the treatment of cytomegalovirus disease in patients with AIDS in the era of patent antiretroviral therapy: Recommendations of an international panel. International AIDS Society—USA. Arch Intern Med 1998;158:(9):957–969.

50

DIAGNOSIS AND MEDICAL MANAGEMENT OF ACUTE COLONIC DIVERTICULITIS

James S. Wu, MD, PhD
David M. Einstein, MD

Colonic diverticula are mucosal/submucosal herniations that protrude through points of weakness in the colonic wall, where intramural vasa recta penetrate the circular muscle of the bowel between the taenia coli (Fig. 50-1A to C). Diverticulitis occurs when inflammatory changes have occurred in and around the diverticula, and is usually caused by microperforation of a diverticulum. Diverticulitis provokes adhesion of structures and organs in the area of the inflammation that often seals the perforation and results in a localized inflammatory process or phlegmon. When this localized inflammation subsequently resolves, the diverticulitis is uncomplicated. Complications of diverticulitis happen when the process of sealing the perforation is ineffective or only partially effective, when the inflammatory adhesions cause kinking of adjacent small bowel, when the infection perforates into adjacent organs, or when edema of the colonic wall causes obstruction. The complications are listed in Table 50-1. Although some patients who develop diverticulitis require surgery, many recover with medical therapy alone. This discussion will focus on the following aspects of diverticulitis: presentation, differential diagnosis, diagnostic tests, and recommendations regarding medical management.

■ PRESENTATION

Although diverticulitis can sometimes be relatively asymptomatic (especially when the infected diverticulum is posterior and the inflammation is within the colonic mesentery), it is usually heralded by the abrupt onset of severe, persistent abdominal pain at the site of inflammation. The severity of the presentation may range from mild to life-threatening, depending upon the extent of inflammation and peritoneal contamination. Although diverticulitis most commonly involves the sigmoid colon, it may occur at other colonic sites. The pain of sigmoid diverticulitis is usually felt in the left lower quadrant of the abdomen. However, right lower quadrant or suprapubic pain may occur when there is displacement of redundant sigmoid colon to the middle or right side of the lower abdomen. Nonspecific symptoms such as anorexia, nau-

sea, vomiting, constipation, fever, or diarrhea also may be present. Dysuria may be reported if the inflamed colon abuts the bladder. Complaints seen in fistulous disease include pneumaturia or fecaluria for colovesical fistula; feculent discharge from the vagina for colovaginal fistula; diarrhea for colon–small intestinal fistula; and a draining sinus for cutaneous fistula.

Examination typically reveals a febrile patient, distressed by pain, with tenderness in the lower abdomen. Localized signs of peritoneal irritation with guarding and rebound tenderness are often seen. A phlegmon or fluid collection may be palpable as a mass on abdominal, rectal, or pelvic examination. Psoas and obturator signs may be present if the inflammatory process is located next to these muscles and erosion of the inflamed colon into an adjacent hollow viscus results in the discharge of gas and feces into the affected organ. Generalized peritonitis is an indication of a free perforation.

■ DIAGNOSTIC TESTS

Tests may be ordered to establish the diagnosis of diverticulitis and to exclude disorders that can present with features similar to diverticulitis such as those shown in Table 50-2. The white blood cell count is typically elevated with a predominance of polymorphonuclear leukocytes. Urinalysis may reveal pyuria if the inflammatory process is adjacent to the urinary collecting system. Plain abdominal films are often normal but may show evidence of ileus, obstruction, or pneumoperitoneum. In the acute setting, computed tomography (CT) is the preferred test to establish the diagnosis of diverticulitis. A CT examination of the abdomen and pelvis with oral, rectal, and intravenous contrast defines both the colonic and extracolonic anatomy. Four CT criteria are commonly used to diagnose diverticulitis: (1) diverticula, (2) infiltration of the pericolic fat, (3) thickness of the colonic wall, (4) and abscess formation (Fig. 50-2). CT can detect an associated abscess located either adjacent to the primary inflammatory process or elsewhere in the pelvis or abdomen (Fig. 50-3). Complications such as ureteral obstruction and fistulas also can be seen (Fig. 50-4A and B). CT scan is not only diagnostic but can also be therapeutic. For example, CT-guided percutaneous drainage of a pericolic abscess may avert an emergency colonic resection with colostomy and allow a subsequent one-stage resection and primary anastomosis (Fig. 50-5). Finally, CT is an excellent way to follow the course of disease toward resolution or increased severity.

Water-soluble contrast enema and abdominal ultrasound also have roles in the diagnosis of acute diverticulitis. Barium is avoided in the acute setting because of the possibility of a leak. Advantages of early water-soluble contrast enema include the detection of a colorectal cancer, or a perforation with extravasation of contrast. Both of these findings would alert the clinician to the need for timely surgery. Classic contrast enema features of diverticulitis include a long, gradually tapering area of narrowing containing diverticula, some of which may show

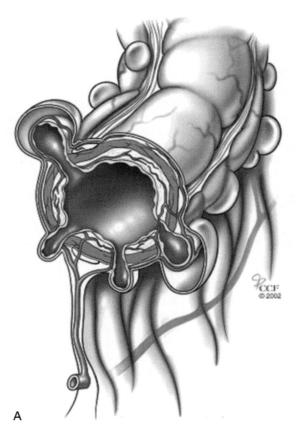

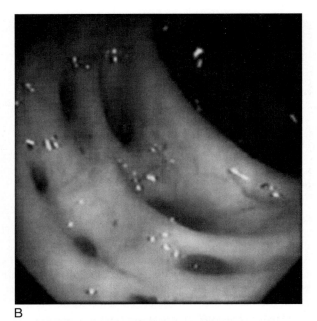

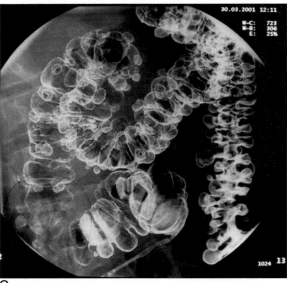

Figure 50-1

A, Colonic diverticulosis seen in cross section shows mucosa/submucosa protruding through openings in the muscular bowel wall where vasa recta penetrate. *B,* Numerous diverticula seen on colonoscopy. *C,* Multiple diverticula seen on air contrast barium enema.

spiculation or extravasation (Fig. 50-6). An intramucosal fistula tract will result in the "double-tracking" sign with a tract of contrast seen parallel to the lumen (Fig. 50-7). Despite these benefits, physicians tend to be reluctant to use

contrast enemas early in the course of suspected perforated diverticulitis because of the fear of extending a contained perforation into a free intra-abdominal perforation. In addition, the true extent of the extracolonic inflammatory

Table 50-1 Complications of Colonic Diverticulitis
Free perforation
Abscess
Sepsis
Intestinal obstruction
Ureteral obstruction
Hemorrhage
Fistula

Table 50-2 Diverticulitis: Differential Diagnosis
Colon cancer
Appendicitis
Irritable bowel syndrome
Inflammatory bowel disease
Ischemic colitis
Bowel obstruction
Gynecologic disease
Urologic disease

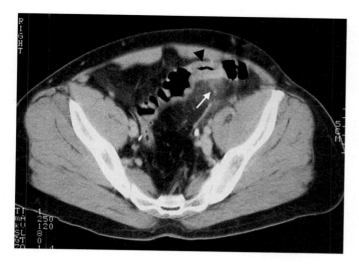

Figure 50-2
Computed tomographic findings of acute sigmoid diverticulitis include mesenteric fat infiltration (*white arrow*) and bowel wall thickening (*black arrowhead*).

process cannot be estimated by this test. Barium contrast studies can be used to establish the presence of fistulous connections between the colon and small intestine, urinary bladder, or other pelvic organs after the acute process has resolved (Fig. 50-8*A* to *C*).

Abdominal ultrasound can establish the diagnosis of diverticulitis by revealing a thickened colonic wall. Ultrasound has found the most utility in establishing the presence of an abscess and guiding abscess drainage. Although the role of contrast enema and ultrasound has diminished since the introduction of CT, both may prove invaluable if CT is unavailable or if CT findings are equivocal.

Flexible endoscopy is not usually performed in a patient with acute diverticulitis, because of the chance of unsealing a contained perforation. Gentle proctoscopy can still be done, however, to make sure the rectum is normal and to settle unresolved questions of diagnosis before surgery. After inflammation has subsided, a full colon evaluation either by colonoscopy or by the combination of flexible sigmoidoscopy combined with air contrast barium enema is done to exclude carcinoma and inflammatory bowel disease.

■ MEDICAL MANAGEMENT OF DIVERTICULITIS

If the symptoms and findings are mild and the patient is able to eat, a low-residue diet and oral antibiotics can be prescribed with follow-up in the outpatient setting. Patients needing fluid resuscitation, intravenous antibiotic therapy, immediate diagnostic testing, or radiologic/surgical intervention must be admitted to a hospital. Once the disease is diagnosed, its severity is assessed. In 1963, Hughes, Cuthbertson, and Carden proposed a four-stage classification scheme based on severity of peritoneal contamination found at surgery (Table 50-3). In 1978, Hinchey and associates proposed a similar system (Table 50-3). Presently, diverticulitis can be staged without surgery using a CT staging system proposed by Neff and colleagues in 1989 (Table 50-3). Their system is based on the four stages originally outlined by Hughes and Hinchey plus a fifth stage (0), which is used to describe diverticular inflammation contained within the serosa, resulting in cellulitis of the colon wall. This CT staging system describes the extent of diverticulitis in terms that are

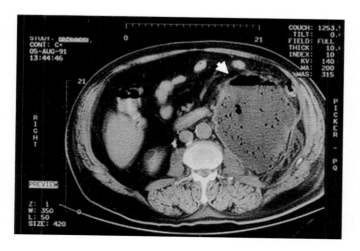

Figure 50-3
Computed tomographic scan showing a large abscess with air-fluid level (*white arrow*).

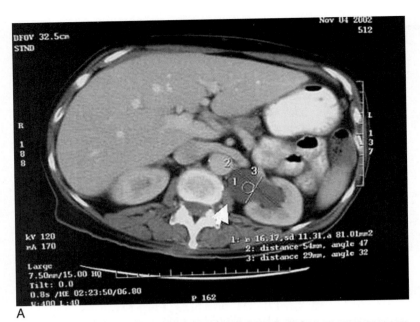

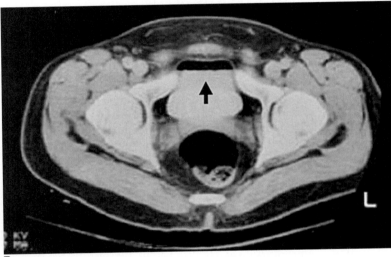

Figure 50-4
A, Ureteral obstruction due to diverticulitis causing hydronephrosis *(white arrow).* *B,* Computed tomographic scan shows air in bladder due to colovesical fistula *(black arrow).*

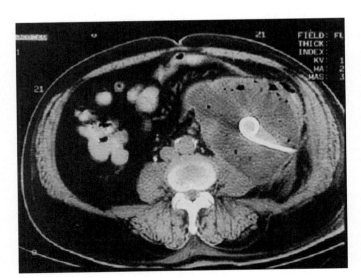

Figure 50-5
Percutaneous drainage of diverticular abscess.

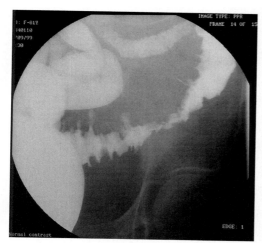

Figure 50-6
Water-soluble contrast enema demonstrates characteristic findings of diverticulitis: a long segment of narrowing with gradual tapering margins and several abnormal-appearing diverticula.

readily understood by surgeons, and helps guide treatment. For uncomplicated diverticulitis (stages 0 and I), nonoperative treatment is preferred because most patients will recover and not have a second attack of diverticulitis in the long term. Patients with mild symptoms who are able to tolerate a diet may be treated as outpatients with a low-residue diet and oral antibiotics. Immunosuppressed and elderly patients with mild uncomplicated disease require close monitoring in the hospital because their presentation can be deceptively benign. The threshold for surgery in such patients is lower than that for patients with a healthy immune system. Systemically ill patients are hospitalized.

The cornerstones of medical treatment of acute uncomplicated diverticulitis are strict bowel rest (with gastrointestinal decompression if necessary), fluid resuscitation, and intravenous antibiotic therapy directed at colonic flora. Infections due to diverticulitis are often polymicrobial and include both aerobic gram-negative and anaerobic organisms. Antibiotic coverage against *Bacteroides fragilis* is included because this organism may be important in abscess formation.

Percutaneous drainage is considered if an abscess is found on initial testing or on follow-up (Neff stage II) (see Table 50-3 and Fig. 50-5). Initial drainage of abscesses may allow resection and primary anastomosis to be done at future surgery and allow the patient to avoid staged procedures that would include creation of a colostomy. Drainage of small (<3 cm) abscesses is not usually necessary because they may resolve spontaneously by draining back into the colonic lumen. If there is a large abscess that is not amenable to drainage because of its location or other factors, surgery is indicated.

Surgery is the recommended treatment for complicated diverticulitis and for additional indications such as those listed in Table 50-4. The role and timing of surgery in patients whose first attack of uncomplicated diverticulitis occurs at a young age are controversial. If an abscess is successfully drained, elective surgery can be done after 6 weeks. Some patients with a drained abscess avoid surgery altogether, although the presence of a clinically obvious perforation carries a poor prognosis for avoiding surgery.

Patients are assessed by frequent abdominal examinations and reviews of vital signs. Nonoperative therapy can be continued as long as clinical findings do not worsen. Meperidine is an appropriate analgesic because it decreases intraluminal pressure, while morphine is usually avoided because it increases intracolonic pressure. Most patients improve over several days. With resolution of fever and decrease in pain, a low-residue diet is resumed and patients are released on oral antibiotics. Invasive studies are delayed for 4 to 6 weeks. The colon is then evaluated by colonoscopy or flexible sigmoidoscopy combined with barium enema to exclude colorectal cancer. After recovery from an initial episode of diverticulitis, patients are advised to eat an appropriate amount of dietary fiber

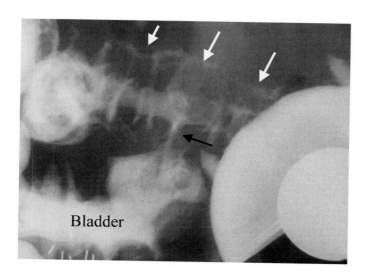

Figure 50-7
Water-soluble contrast enema demonstrates "double tracking" sign (*white arrows*). A colovesical fistula is also present (*black arrow*).

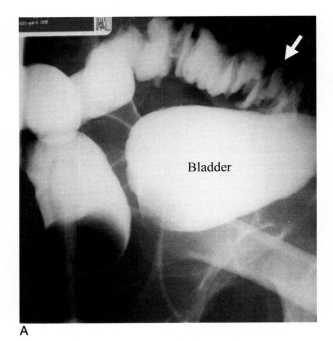

Bladder

A

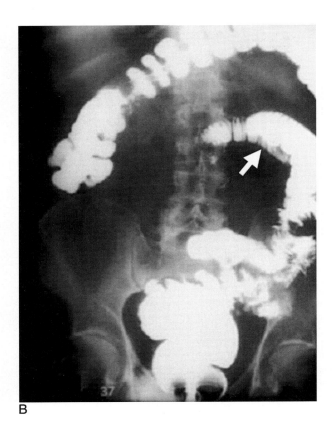

B

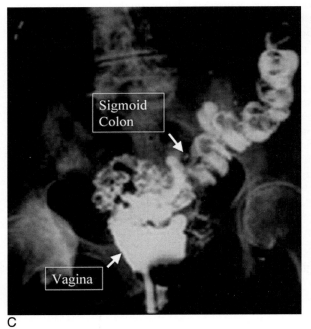

Sigmoid
Colon

Vagina

C

Figure 50-8
A, Water-soluble contrast enema in this patient with acute diverticulitis demonstrates opacification of the bladder due to a colovesical fistula. A Foley catheter is in place. *B*, Coloenteric fistula causing diarrhea diagnosed by barium enema. Note small intestine filling with contrast medium from the sigmoid colon. *C*, Vaginogram showing a fistula between the sigmoid colon and the vaginal cuff after hysterectomy. (Courtesy of Mark Baker, MD.)

and avoid overindulgence in foods that may cause trauma to the diverticula (e.g., seeds and popcorn). Long-term fiber supplementation may protect from recurrence.

If fever or pain does not resolve, a follow-up CT scan can be requested to look for an abscess that may have developed or become more apparent since admission. Ultimately, failure to improve prompts surgery.

■ SUMMARY

Colonic diverticulitis is diagnosed by history, physical findings, and imaging studies, mainly CT scan. The severity of symptoms and signs ranges from mild to life-threatening.

Patients with minimal findings who are able to eat can be managed as outpatients with oral antibiotics. Patients who are toxic or systemically ill are admitted to a hospital for intravenous antibiotics, and those with a drainable abscess seen on scanning have it drained. Patients with compromised immune status, sepsis, peritonitis, or advanced age should be considered for early surgery. Currently, CT examination is the preferred diagnostic test for acute diverticulitis because it provides information on colonic and extracolonic anatomy. This information can be used to stage the disease and can influence management decisions regarding surgery and interventions such as percutaneous abscess drainage. Most patients recover without the need for surgery.

Table 50-3 Classifications of Diverticulitis

STAGE	HUGHES, CUTHBERTSON, CARDEN	HINCHEY	DORINGER/NEFF CT SCAN	TREATMENT
0			Diverticula Pericolonic infiltration Thickening of colonic wall (pericolonic phlegmon)	Conservative
1 / I	Local peritonitis	Pericolic abscess confined by the mesentery	Pericolonic abscess (up to 3 cm, limited to mesentery)	Conservative
2 / II	Local paracolic or pelvic abscess	Pelvic abscess resulting from local perforation of a pericolic abscess	Pelvic abscess (perforation of the mesentery)	Percutaneous drainage, one-stage resection
3 / III	General peritonitis due to ruptured paracolic or pelvic abscess	Generalized peritonitis resulting from the rupture of either a pericolic abscess or a pelvic abscess into the general peritoneal cavity	Extrapelvic abscess	Surgery Eventual percutaneous drainage with surgery followed electively
4 / IV	General peritonitis due to free perforation of the colon	Fecal peritonitis resulting from free perforation of a diverticulum	Large diverticular penetration with spread of fecal material into the abdominal cavity	Urgent surgery

Table 50-4 Diverticulitis: Indications for Surgery

One attack of complicated diverticulitis
Lack of improvement with medical therapy
Recurrent attacks of diverticulitis (two or more)
Inability to exclude carcinoma
Fistula formation
Generalized peritonitis
Undrainable abscess
High-grade bowel obstruction

Acknowledgments. The authors wish to thank Ms. Amy Moore of the Cleveland Clinic Editorial Department for her thoughtful review of this manuscript and Mr. Joe Pangrace of the Cleveland Clinic Medical Illustration Department for his excellent art work.

Suggested Readings

Ambrosetti P, Becker C, Terrier F: Colonic diverticulitis: Impact of imaging on surgical management—A prospective study of 542 patients. Europ Radiol 2002;12:1145–1149.

Ambrosetti P, Jenny A, Becker C, et al: Acute left colonic diverticulitis—Compared performance of computed tomography and water-soluble contrast enema: Prospective evaluation of 420 patients. Dis Colon Rectum 2000;43:1363–1367.

Chautems RC, Ambrosetti P, Ludwig A, et al: Long-term follow-up after first acute episode of sigmoid diverticulitis: Is surgery mandatory? A prospective study of 118 patients. Dis Colon Rectum 2002;45:962–966.

Cheskin LJ, Bohlman M, Schuster MM: Diverticular disease in the elderly. Gastroenterol Clin North Am 1990;19:391–403.

Cunningham MA, Davis JW, Kaups KL: Medical versus surgical management of diverticulitis in patients under age 40. Am J Surg 1997;174:733–736.

Detry R, Jamez J, Kartheuser A, et al: Acute localized diverticulitis: Optimum management requires accurate staging. Int J Colorect Dis 1992;7:38–42.

Doringer E: Computed tomography of colonic diverticulitis. Crit Rev Diagn Imag 1992;33:421–435.

Drummond H: Sacculi of the large intestine, with special reference to their relations to the blood vessels of the bowel wall. Br J Surg 1916;4:407–413.

Elsakr R, Johnson DA, Younes Z, Oldfield EC III: Antimicrobial treatment of intra-abdominal infections. Dig Dis 1998;16:47–60.

Haglund U, Hellberg R, Johnsén C, Hultén L: Complicated diverticular disease of the sigmoid colon. An analysis of short and long term outcome in 392 patients. Ann Chir Gynaecol 1979;68:41–46.

Hiltunen KM, Kolehmainen H, Vuorinen T, Matikainen M: Early water-soluble contrast enema in the diagnosis of acute colonic diverticulitis. Int J Colorect Dis 1991;6:190–192.

Hinchey EJ, Schaal PGH, Richards GK: Treatment of perforated diverticular disease of the colon. Adv Surg 1978;12:85–109.

Hughes ESR, Cutherbertson AM, Carden ABC: The surgical management of acute diverticulitis. Med J Aust 1963;1:780–782.

Hulnick DH, Megibow AJ, Balthazar EJ, et al: Computed tomography in the evaluation of diverticulitis. Radiology 1984;152:491–495.

Jasper DR, Weinstock LB, Balfe DM, et al: Transverse colon diverticulitis: Successful nonoperative management in four patients. Report of four cases. Dis Colon Rectum 1999;42:955–958.

Kellum JM, Sugerman HJ, Coppa GF, et al: Randomized, prospective comparison of cefoxitin and gentamicin-clindamycin in the treatment of acute colon diverticulitis. Clin Ther 1992;14:376–384.

Köhler L, Sauerland S, Neugebauer E: Diagnosis and treatment of diverticular disease. Results of a consensus development conference. Surg Endosc 1999;13:430–436.

Konvolinka CW: Acute diverticulitis under age forty. Am J Surg 1994;167:562–565.

Kourtesis GJ, Williams RA, Wilson SE: Acute diverticulitis: Safety and value of contrast studies in predicting need for operation. Aust NZ J Surg 1988;58:801–804.

Larson DM, Masters SS, Spiro HM: Medical and surgical therapy in diverticular disease: A comparative study. Gastroenterology 1976;71:734–737.

Lo CY, Chu KW: Acute diverticulitis of the right colon. Am J Surg 1996;171:244–246.

Neff CC, van Sonnenberg E: CT of diverticulitis: Diagnosis and treatment. Radiol Clin North Am 1989;27:743–752.

Oliver G, Peters W, Ross T, et al: Practice parameters for the treatment of sigmoid diverticulitis—Supporting documentation. Dis Colon Rectum 2000:43:289–297.

Painter NS: Diverticular disease of the colon: The first of the Western diseases shown to be due to a deficiency in dietary fiber. S Afr Med J 1982;61:1016–1020.

Parks TG, Connell AM: The outcome in 455 patients admitted for treatment of diverticular disease of the colon. Br J Surg 1970;57:775–778.

Perkins JD, Shield CF III, Chang FC, Farha GJ: Acute diverticulitis. Comparison of treatment in immunocompromised and nonimmunocompromised patients. Am J Surg 1984;148:745–748.

Schwerk WB, Schwarz S, Rothmund M: Sonography in acute colonic diverticulitis: A prospective study. Dis Colon Rectum 1992; 35:1077–1084.

Slack WW: The anatomy, pathology, and some clinical features of diverticulitis of the colon. Br J Surg 1962;50:185–190.

Spivak H, Weinrauch S, Harvey JC, et al: Acute colonic diverticulitis in the young. Dis Colon Rectum 1997;40:570–574.

Taylor KJW, Wasson JF, de Graaff C, et al: Accuracy of grey-scale ultrasound diagnosis of abdominal and pelvic abscesses in 220 patients. Lancet 1978;I:83–84.

Verbanck J, Lambrecht S, Rutgeerts L, et al: Can sonography diagnose acute colonic diverticulitis in patients with acute intestinal inflammation? A prospective study. J Clin Ultrasound 1989;17:661–666.

Vignati PV, Welch JP, Cohen JL: Long-term managment of diverticulitis in young patients. Dis Colon Rectum 1995;38:627–629.

Wong WD, Wexner SD, Lowry A, et al: Practice parameters for the treatment of sigmoid diverticulitis—Supporting documentation. The Standards Task Force. The American Society of Colon and Rectal Surgeons. Dis Colon Rectum 2000;43:290–297.

51

SURGICAL TREATMENT OF DIVERTICULITIS

Mark Killingback, AM, MS (Hon),
FACS (Hon), FRACS, FRCS, FRCS (Ed)

■ ACUTE DIVERTICULITIS

Krukowski and coworkers reviewed 725 emergency operations performed in Aberdeen between 1977 and 1983 and found that 21 (2.9%) were operations for acute diverticulitis. It is not, therefore, a common surgical emergency in any one hospital. Despite advances in resuscitation, anesthesia, surgical technique, intensive care, and antibiotics the mortality rate remains high in those hospitals admitting a broad spectrum of patients as emergencies. Between 1983 and 1992, 233 patients were operated on as emergencies at seven teaching hospitals in Sydney. There were 45 postoperative deaths, giving a mortality rate of 19.3%. Most deaths were due to abdominal sepsis, comorbidity, or a combination of these factors.

Specific Investigations

A plain x-ray of the abdomen may show evidence of free peritoneal or retroperitoneal gas, but lack of free gas does not exclude a perforated colon. Pelvic ultrasound examination can achieve a high level of accuracy in the diagnosis of acute diverticulitis and associated abscess. Similarly, computed tomographic (CT) examination is now established as an important examination in these patients. It may demonstrate free gas not seen on a plain x-ray, an inflammatory mass, or a paracolic abscess. The latter, if unilocular, is now an indication for radiologically guided catheter drainage, which can be very successful in experienced departments. In a combined series of 65 patients in whom such abscesses were treated by catheter drainage 45 patients (69%) were converted to elective operations (Table 51-1). Limited water-soluble contrast enema can also be a useful investigation and may complement other findings. It may exclude or confirm the presence of colon perforation or reveal an alternative diagnosis, such as carcinoma.

Indication for Laparotomy

Clinical signs of peritonitis, septic shock, and free gas on x-ray will indicate the need for early laparotomy. In some patients signs of small or large bowel obstruction may be the dominant clinical parameters guiding the decision for surgical treatment. Careful clinical judgment is needed if managing an immunosuppressed patient, for example, on steroid therapy, as the clinical response may be minimal and expressed only as continuing pain without fever, abdominal signs, or leukocytosis. Delay in diagnosis may therefore occur unless specific investigations are undertaken with a high index of suspicion that occult perforation of the colon may be present. Prompt surgical treatment is necessary in most of these patients if fatality is to be avoided. Some patients not treated immediately by operation will fail to improve on antibiotic therapy, indicating the need for operative intervention. If radiologically guided catheter drainage of an abscess is unsuccessful, then surgery is indicated.

Preoperative Preparation

Specific requirements will include the insertion of a nasogastric tube, as 20% of these patients have associated small bowel obstruction. A urinary catheter is important to assess urine output during the preoperative resuscitation period. Although not all patients require intensive resuscitation, the elderly or patients with fecal peritonitis may be in extremis and require a critical period of metabolic correction prior to surgical treatment. In such patients with an unstable circulation and previous cardiovascular disease, rapid fluid replacement may be required, and a Swan-Ganz catheter may be necessary to monitor fluid levels. Broad-spectrum antibiotics should be administered in maximum doses. In these patients it is important that a team approach is quickly instituted with anesthetist and intensivist. The period of resuscitation must be carefully judged, as improvement will occur up to a certain point, beyond which the critical factor is the surgical removal of pus or feces from the peritoneal cavity. Attention must be given to marking appropriate stoma sites on each side of the abdomen.

Principles of Management

Patients admitted with acute diverticulitis are often elderly, and many will also be suffering significant comorbidity. Most of these patients (approximately 65%) will be presenting with their first attack of diverticulitis (Royal Australasian College of Surgeons survey on acute diverticulitis, 1967–1970). The experience of the surgical, anesthetic, and nursing team is an important consideration and must affect decisions taken for surgical treatment. The aim of treatment is to effectively deal with abdominal sepsis and not to consider definitive treatment of diverticular disease. Therefore, limited resections are appropriate. The source of the infection is best removed from the abdominal cavity by resection, which is essential if there is a free perforation present. If, however, a nonperforated phlegmon is found at laparotomy and there is concern about the risks of extending the operation by resection, then resolution by antibiotics alone can sometimes be achieved. A proximal transverse colostomy will not prevent continuing infection in the presence of perforation if there is still stool present in the left colon. The clinical and operative findings do not usually exclude the possibility that the primary pathology is carcinoma, which must be considered.

Table 51-1 Percutaneous Drainage* of Abscess

AUTHOR	DRAINAGE	CONVERSION TO ELECTIVE SURGERY
Neff, Van Sonnenberg, and Casola (1987)	16	11
Mueller, Saini, and Wittenberg (1987)	20	12
Stabile, Puccio, Van Sonnenberg, and Neff (1990)	19	14
Hemming, Davis, and Robins (1991)	6	4
Hachigian, Honickman, Eisenstat, et al. (1992)	4	4
Totals	65	45 (69%)

*Guided by computed tomography.

Laparotomy

If diverticulitis is suspected as the cause of the patient's abdominal sepsis, then the Lloyd-Davies position is preferable for the laparotomy. This position is not often employed for emergency abdominal surgery but can be extremely helpful in the management of acute complicated disease of the left colon. An adequate midline incision is preferred. Small bowel, if obstructed, should be decompressed, preferably by "milking" the fluid and gas back into the stomach, where it is aspirated with a large nasogastric tube. The inflamed segment of sigmoid colon may be mobile with obvious access to the diseased segment. Alternatively, a large inflammatory mass may be adherent to the pelvis (obscuring a deep pelvic abscess). The perforation may be obvious or it may be within the epicolic or mesenteric fat. Blunt digital dissection is often the safest method of mobilizing the colon, and such dissection should reveal the details of the disease. Lateral paracolic gutter and interloop and subphrenic abscesses must be looked for as they may already be established at the time of the laparotomy. The type of disease causing peritoneal infection must now be carefully assessed, as it will affect surgical treatment. Acute diverticulitis causing peritonitis occurs in three principal forms.

1. Nonperforated phlegmon
2. Abscess
3. Free (or concealed) perforation

The peritoneal cavity may contain turbid fluid associated with a nonperforated phlegmon. There may be a localized or generalized purulent peritonitis. Fecal peritonitis is present in 15% of patients. Surgical treatment must take into account the general condition of the patient, the type of pathologic condition, and its potential for continuing abdominal sepsis. The type and extent of peritonitis should also be considered when deciding the operation to be performed.

Acute Phlegmonous Diverticulitis (31%)

When a perforation is not present there may be no obligation to resect the inflamed segment of colon as many of these patients will respond to antibiotics. This pathology should not be managed by a proximal stoma, which would in most instances commit the patient to resection at a later stage or leave an elderly patient "stranded" with a stoma. Under ideal circumstances with a fit patient and possibly in

a patient with previous attacks, a resection with primary anastomosis may be undertaken. Patients managed without resection should have a soft Penrose rubber drain placed near the phlegmon for 5 or 6 days to anticipate a delayed perforation. In a RACS survey 6% of patients with a non-perforated phlegmon formed a fistula after laparotomy.

Pelvic or Paracolic Abscess (31%)

If a perforation in the colon is found in association with an abscess, the colon should be resected. Alternatively, a perforation may be indirect and associated with a tortuous track from a diverticulum via the mesentery. Although such a perforation is unlikely to leak fecal material into the peritoneal cavity, purulent infection will continue and a delayed fistula may occur. Resection of the inflamed segment is the preferred treatment. If previous inflammation has produced a fixed inflammatory mass in the pelvis which cannot be mobilized without unwarranted tissue dissection and bleeding, and if no free perforation can be detected, then drainage of this abscess without resection might be considered. The drainage should be an active one with irrigation suction drains placed into the abscess and maintained for 10 to 11 days to induce the cavity to shrink. Passive drainage of such abscesses is not satisfactory, as the infected space will only reduce in size at a much slower rate. It is in this circumstance that a proximal defunctioned stoma may have a role. It may be possible to perform on-table irrigation from the colostomy site to the rectum and thus empty the colon between the colostomy and the anus. When the patient has recovered from this operation, elective resection should be undertaken because closure of the proximal stoma without resection will in most instances be followed by a recurrence of the inflammatory disease.

Free Perforation (38%)

Although in the past a number of alternatives have been practiced current surgical treatment is to remove the perforation from the peritoneal cavity. The excision of the perforated segment of colon can be restricted to a short segment of colon ("perforectomy"), but the excision must be beyond the inflamed mass; otherwise, it will be impossible to construct an appropriate and effective stoma, or unsafe to perform an anastomosis. It is reasonable to mobilize the colon sufficiently to achieve operative requirements, but deep dissection of the presacral space and proximal mobilization of the splenic flexure are unwarranted if a Hartmann operation is to be performed and should be minimized in those patients in whom immediate anastomosis is intended.

Hartmann Operation

For many patients the safest procedure is a Hartmann operation. It may be modified with an end-colostomy and a distal mucous "fistula." The proximal end of the colon should be brought through the left rectus muscle as an end-colostomy sutured to the skin of the abdomen. The distal colon is brought out through the lower end of the midline wound and attached to the skin and aponeurosis.

Care must be taken with the proximal colostomy that the "tunnel" in the abdominal wall does not constrict the bowel and a sufficient amount of colon protrudes beyond the skin so that there is no possibility of retraction after operation. In the unprepared colon axial shortening of the colon stimulated by the presence of feces may cause retraction with serious consequences. For this reason sutures are inserted between the peritoneum and the emerging colon at the colostomy site. The paracolostomy space is not closed, as the colostomy emerging through the left rectus muscle will leave a large lateral space which is rarely associated with postoperative obstruction.

Conservative resection will allow the lower segment in many instances to reach the abdominal wall without tension. In one third of the patients the perforation is located in the distal part of the sigmoid colon, and, therefore, the distal segment is too low to form a safe mucous fistula without tension. Full presacral dissection to elevate the distal segment also creates problems as the subsequent reconstructive operation will be more difficult. Closure of the rectum (classical Hartmann operation) is by hand suture or transverse stapling, which is then attached to the promontory of the sacrum by nonabsorbable sutures so that it does not retract into the pelvis.

Resection and Immediate Anastomosis

Immediate anastomosis (with or without a proximal stoma) avoids a second major procedure to reverse the Hartmann operation, which may entail a difficult pelvic dissection. Not all patients are fit enough for this second stage and some may be left with a permanent stoma. Immediate anastomosis will require more dissection, further blood loss, and more time, and probably should not be undertaken without on-table irrigation of the colon. The anastomosis must be made through normal tissue with minimal involvement by diverticulosis, and, therefore, more proximal and distal mobilization may be required.

This procedure has been performed with good results but careful selection of patients is necessary. If the patient is generally fit and stable during the operation and the peritonitis is limited to the region of the inflamed colon, then immediate anastomosis can be an appropriate operation if the surgeon is experienced in colorectal surgery. The postoperative mortality rate of acute diverticulitis with peritonitis is still significant, and fatalities are mainly due to abdominal sepsis and the patient's comorbidity. The surgeon must be confident that a longer and more technically demanding operation is as safe as resection without immediate anastomosis.

Proximal Stoma Without Resection

A proximal transverse colostomy with or without suture repair of the perforation has currently been superseded by resection to remove the source of infection. It is of interest, however, that a prospective randomized trial in Denmark has found no statistical difference in the mortality and morbidity rates when comparing this technique to the Hartmann operation.

Management of the Abdominal Cavity

At the time of laparotomy copious irrigation of the abdominal cavity must be undertaken with warm saline. Any particulate matter must be thoroughly cleansed from the abdomen, and any inflammatory nest debrided as far as possible. Topical peritoneal antibiotic therapy is not used. Postoperative antibiotic lavage of the peritoneal cavity, although advocated by some, is not practiced by the author. If the area of the resected sigmoid colon is "clean," then no drain is required. Alternatively, if there is an inflammatory nest which has been associated with an abscess, then suction irrigation drains should be placed next to it, and this drainage maintained over a period of some days (Table 51-2).

Reversal: Hartmann Operation

There is an advantage in delaying this operation for 6 months after surgery, as patients can develop reactive phlegmonous adhesions, which can make the second-stage operation more difficult. At 6 months these adhesions have usually become atrophic and are easier to dissect. Recent publications have criticized this rationale for delaying the reversal procedure, suggesting that there is no difference in operative difficulty and morbidity if the operation is performed a few weeks after the initial resection. Difficulties of the pelvic dissection can be minimized at the initial procedure, by avoiding dissection in the presacral space, hitching the stump to the sacral promontory, and achieving a careful closure of the rectal stump which does not subsequently leak and cause pelvic infection. The defunctioned segment may become contracted and thickened (a disadvantage of a prolonged period between operations), and the pelvic peritoneum may be considerably affected by fibrosis subsequent to the abdominal infection. Not all patients will have

Table 51-2 Irrigation and Suction Drainage for Inflammatory Nest or Abscess		
DAY	**IRRIGATION**	**SUCTION**
1	6 L normal saline	−80 mm Hg
2–10	1 L normal saline	−80 mm Hg
11	Remove drains, replace with No. 16 F Nelaton catheter: sinogram	
11–16	Shorten drain daily until removed	

the Hartmann operation reversed (usually related to comorbidity), and this is a potential disadvantage compared with resection and anastomosis.

For the distal dissection, the author prefers to mobilize and identify the distal stump, reaching a level of healthy rectal wall for anastomosis. This dissection can be assisted by the insertion of a sigmoidoscope to identify the closed rectal stump. Once the distal segment has been properly prepared with healthy, supple rectum, the circular staple technique for anastomosis is preferred, although if the rectal wall is contracted and thickened, hand suture technique may be preferable. The alternative of "stabbing" the staple rod through the anterior wall of the rectum without full mobilization has been advocated and is apparently successful, but some significant anastomotic complications have occurred (personal communications) and this technique is not preferred.

Prognosis Subsequent to Acute Diverticulitis

If a patient admitted to a hospital with a first attack makes a satisfactory recovery without operation, should elective resection of the diverticular disease be advised? If subsequent clinical, endoscopic, and radiologic assessment show resolution of the inflammatory process, most surgeons would not advise surgical treatment. This view is supported by Sarin and Boulous, who prospectively followed 144 patients for a median of 48 months after admission with acute complications of diverticular disease. There was a readmission rate of only 9.0% with recurrent disease. A prospective audit in the United Kingdom by Farmakis and associates, however, came to a different conclusion after a 5-year follow-up of 120 patients previously admitted to a hospital with acute complications of diverticular disease. Of the 43 patients originally managed without operation, 37 (86%) developed serious complications of diverticular disease, and 9 (21%) died as a result of those complications. The authors therefore recommended that if the patient is fit for an interval resection, surgical treatment should be advised. Ambrosetti and coworkers have related prognosis of an acute attack to the computed tomographic (CT) examination and have recommended subsequent elective resection for those patients whose CT examination during admission showed features of "severe" diverticulitis. Severe diverticulitis was defined as extraluminal air, extravasation of contrast material, and abscess formation. Acute diverticulitis (requiring hospital admission) in patients under 50 years of age may carry a greater risk of long-term complications, but studies in the literature do not clarify this contention as conclusions differ.

■ ELECTIVE SURGERY FOR DIVERTICULAR DISEASE

The basis for the recommendations of the elective management of diverticular disease is a series of patients treated between 1962 and 1997 by one surgeon for which the clinical, operative, and postoperative details have almost entirely been audited prospectively. Table 51-3 refers to these patients in two groups. Primary resection

(i.e., initial resection) of the left colon was performed in 227 patients with immediate anastomosis in 225 (one patient underwent elective Hartmann operation and one patient was resected subsequent to an abdominoperineal resection for carcinoma of the rectum).

Classification of Pathology

Noninflammatory Diverticular Disease

In 1963 Morson drew attention to the absence of inflammation in 35.3% of electively resected specimens of diverticular disease at St. Mark's Hospital, London. These patients were treated surgically for symptoms that were believed to be inflammatory in origin. Although inflammation of diverticular disease can resolve remarkably between exacerbations, such findings indicated that dysfunction of the left colon without inflammation can be responsible for symptoms. In the author's series of 227 patients, 35 (15.4%) have been classified as having noninflammatory diverticular disease. In patients 1 to 100 the incidence was 21%, and for patients 101 to 200, it was 11%. These findings were usually unexpected at operation, because many of the patients had presented with typical features of recurrent diverticulitis.

Diverticulitis is often classified in the literature as uncomplicated and complicated, but these terms do not emphasise the differences between types of diverticulitis which relate to the extent of spread of the inflammatory process.

Localized Diverticulitis

It is not known whether diverticulitis commences within an intact diverticulum or is initiated by a microperforation, but clinical manifestations can be due to inflammation confined to the vicinity of the diverticulum. The inflammatory process may track into the mesentery to form a phlegmonous reaction without pus formation (phlegmonous diverticulitis described by Pheils and associates) or a chronic abscess confined to the mesentery by its peritoneal covering (Fig. 51-1). The findings at operation may vary from a slight thickening of the pericolic area and mesentery to an extensive and complex intramesenteric process. The abscess, while still localized by the peritoneum of the mesentery, can track along the colon or encircle it (Fig. 51-2), a process of "dissecting diverticulitis." These

Table 51-3 Elective Surgery, for Diverticular Disease, 1962–1997

RESECTION	NO. OF PATIENTS
Primary Resection	
Left colon	227
Colectomy IRA	3
Secondary Resection	
Reversal Hartmann operation	15
Referred complications of primary resection	12
Total	257

LOCALIZED DIVERTICULITIS

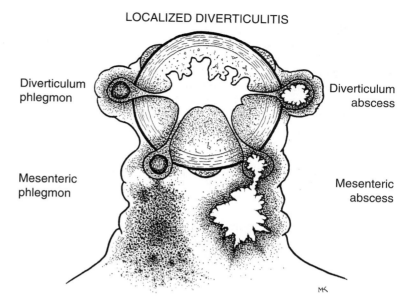

Diverticulum phlegmon

Diverticulum abscess

Mesenteric phlegmon

Mesenteric abscess

Figure 51-1
Localized diverticulitis is contained within the peritoneum covering the colon and mesentery and may be a small focus of infection or more complex.

localized forms of diverticulitis, however, can be removed with minimal involvement of adjacent structures, in contrast to more complicated disease that extends beyond the anatomic compartment of the colon and mesentery. Localized diverticulitis was present in 80 patients (35.2%).

Extracolic Diverticulitis

Once the peritoneums of the colon and mesentery have been breached by the inflammatory process, adjacent structures (visceral or parietal) will become involved. This involvement will manifest as abscess or fistula formation (Fig. 51-3), which now has the potential to produce complex pathology involving adjacent structures and posing significant technical problems for surgical management. Extracolic diverticulitis was present in 112 patients (49.3%).

Either variety of inflammatory diverticulitis may result in stricture formation owing to a combination of muscle thickening, compression by an adjacent inflammatory

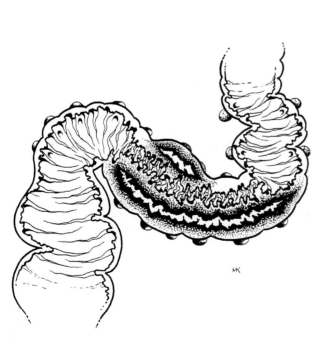

Figure 51-2
An abscess still localized to the anatomic compartment of colon and mesentery may track along or encircle the colon as "dissecting diverticulitis."

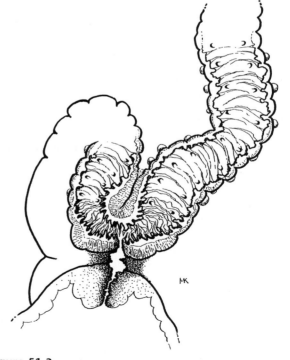

Figure 51-3
Extracolic diverticulitis forming a pelvic inflammatory mass with stricture, a pelvic abscess, and fistula.

focus, edema of the bowel wall, redundancy of the mucosa due to axial shortening of the colon, fibrosis affecting the bowel wall, and distortion by angulation. These changes will often produce a mass, which may be detected clinically, radiologically, and certainly at operation. The pathologic changes may cause acute or chronic colon obstruction and may involve the left ureter and large vessels on the left pelvic brim. Diverticulitis was found as a single focus in 87% of resected specimens, whereas multiple foci were present in 25 patients (13.8%).

Investigation

Flexible endoscopy is mandatory to assess diverticular disease to be treated by operation. Ideally, the colon should be assessed by colonoscopy to exclude multiple pathologic processes, as well as excluding carcinoma in the pathologic section of colon. The thin-caliber gastroscope or pediatric colonoscope may be necessary to negotiate a sigmoid stricture that prevents assessment with a standard colonoscope.

Contrast enema is still a useful investigation that can be complementary to endoscopy. It may distinguish between diverticulitis and carcinoma, demonstrate an extravasation into an abscess or fistula usually not seen on colonoscopy, and map the distribution of diverticula, which can assist in selecting the distal and proximal limits of the resection. It will usually negotiate a stricture to assess the colon, although caution is necessary as the barium proximal to the stricture may precipitate colon obstruction. CT scan, while appropriate for assessing the presence of an acute abscess, is not so helpful in elective investigation of a patient with chronic symptoms. CT surveillance of a patient with an inflammatory mass subsequent to an acute diverticulitis can be useful in assessing its resolution. Pelvic ultrasound examination has the advantage of a simpler and more convenient technique for organ imaging but is usually not preferred to CT. It can be useful in the diagnosis of colovesical fistula.

An intravenous pyelogram (IVP) is not recommended in all patients being treated by operation and may be unnecessary if a CT examination is available. Assessment of the urinary tracts is important if there is an abdominal or pelvic mass present, a stricture close to the brim of the pelvis on the left side, a colovesical fistula, or previous pelvic surgery.

Indications for Resection

Chronic Abdominal Pain

Pain in the left iliac fossa with or without bowel symptoms is frequently diagnosed as symptomatic diverticular disease. Symptoms can be indistinguishable from the spastic type of irritable bowel syndrome. Local tenderness or a mass in the abdominal or pelvic colon would favor (but not confirm) the diagnosis of diverticulitis. Radiologic assessment is often unhelpful in this group of patients in detecting minimal inflammatory changes. There is no direct relationship between the extent of diverticular disease on barium enema and the likelihood of its causing symptoms. Such patients therefore will be advised to undergo surgical treatment on the basis of clinical findings. There is frequently a poor relationship between the severity of symptoms and the extent of inflammatory changes found at operation. Of the 227 patients, 30 were operated on for chronic abdominal pain. The pathology found was noninflammatory diverticular disease in 63% and localized diverticulitis in 37%. One patient with localized diverticular disease had been regarded as a morphine addict rather than suffering real symptoms. At operation a grossly thickened mesenteric abscess was found undoubtedly responsible for the symptoms.

It is, however, the group of patients with noninflammatory diverticular disease who are more likely to complain of recurrence of pain after operation and be considered as having "recurrent diverticulitis." This may be due to the fact that diverticular disease was not originally responsible for the symptoms. Caution in advising surgical treatment is therefore appropriate. In the 15-year period 1966–1980, 24 of 30 patients were resected for chronic abdominal pain, whereas in the subsequent 16-year period 1981–1996, only 6 of 30 such patients were managed by operation.

Recurrent Attacks

The severity of recurrent diverticulitis may vary from a few days of pain in the left iliac fossa with or without systemic symptoms to a major illness requiring hospital care. The patient's age and comorbidity, as well as the number and severity of attacks, will influence the decision to advise surgical treatment. Generally, a fit patient suffering a severe episode of diverticulitis could be considered for surgery, more so if the patient suffers a second attack of significance. An elderly patient suffering less severe clinical manifestations would be managed without operation if investigations revealed uncomplicated diverticular disease. Didactic advice on the number of attacks requiring operation is therefore not appropriate. Fifty-three of 227 patients were treated by resection for recurrent attacks. The pathology found at operation was noninflammatory diverticular disease, 22%; localized diverticulitis, 68%; and extracolic diverticulitis, 10%.

Complications

Stricture. Soon after an acute attack a stricture may be diagnosed but is not necessarily a case for surgical treatment. Such "hot" strictures can resolve but should be closely followed to ensure that resolution occurs and that there is no possibility of carcinoma. A chronic stricture, however, is unlikely to resolve and is usually an indication for operation. Careful examination of barium enema films may reveal continuity of mucosal pattern throughout the stricture. The stricture should be examined by colonoscopy when a thin-diameter gastroscope is often necessary to negotiate the narrow lumen and exclude the presence of carcinoma. If the stricture cannot be negotiated by endoscopy and carcinoma is not seen, the stricture is usually due to diverticulitis.

Fistula. The presence of a fistula is an indication for surgical treatment in most patients. Its presence may be clinically quiescent and well tolerated if there is no intervening abscess and the fistula track is of a small diameter. In frail elderly patients, therefore, surgery may be avoidable.

Inflammatory Mass. Clinically, a mass in the pelvis may be due to extensive noninflammatory diverticular disease, but tenderness on rectal examination may indicate inflammatory changes have occurred. The mass may be recognized by palpation as localized diverticulitis. If the pelvic floor is indurated or rigid, this usually indicates a chronic pelvic abscess. A palpable mass in the left iliac fossa (as distinct from a palpable colon) invariably means inflammatory complications. Such a mass may be a phlegmonous inflammatory reaction only or may be associated with an abscess. If the abscess has a patent communication with the causal diverticulum, a contrast enema may demonstrate extravasation into it.

Possible Carcinoma. The patient's symptoms can begin insidiously, rather than the more typical symptoms of an inflammatory process in the abdomen. Physical examination rarely assists in distinguishing diverticulitis and carcinoma. Despite investigations, some doubts may exist that carcinoma has been excluded. This was so in 41 of 227 patients (18.1%) and was therefore an additional indication for surgical treatment. Three patients (1.3%) were found to have coexistent carcinoma of the resected colon.

Colonic Obstruction. Chronic obstruction may occur in advanced noninflammatory diverticular disease without inflammatory complications owing to the shortening of the colon, thickened muscle, and redundant mucosa. It usually manifests as intermittent left iliac fossa pain and constipation. The tips of the redundant mucosa will often be intensely hyperemic, forming pseudopolyps caused by the "milking" effect of the stool through the narrow and rigid colon. Colon obstruction, however, is more likely to be due to a chronic inflammatory stricture, and surgical treatment is the obvious option.

Ureteric Obstruction. It is unlikely that this complication would be present without associated and recognized inflammatory complications of the colon. It may be caused by periureteric fibrosis or pressure from a sigmoid mass impacted in the pelvis. Siminovitch and Fazio have reported an incidence of ureteric obstruction of 5% in patients whose diverticular disease was treated by operation.

Giant Diverticulum. This rare complication of diverticular disease may be diagnosed on x-ray as a large gas-filled "cyst" in the lower abdomen or may be demonstrated by contrast enema. It is a condition prone to complications and therefore best managed by resection.

Preparation for Operation

Stoma siting is essential prior to the patient's leaving for the operating room. The operation is best performed with the patient in the modified lithotomy (Lloyd-Davies) position. Ureteric catheters should be used selectively if involvement of the ureters is a possibility. The author has employed them in 17 of 227 patients (7.5%).

Operation

Technique of Dissection

If there is attachment of the colon to strategic structures, the surgeon must decide the optimal perimeter of the resection. The operative assessment of the pathology may not distinguish between diverticulitis and carcinoma. The preoperative investigations of endoscopy, barium enema, and CT need to be reconsidered to assist in coming to a decision. Intraoperative colonoscopy may be helpful. Needle biopsy of the mass with immediate histologic reporting has been advocated, but there would be a risk of contaminating the operative field with malignant cells if carcinoma was present. If there is still doubt at operation as to the presence of carcinoma, then the operation should be performed as for malignant disease.

The initial dissection should aim to free the pelvic loop from the pelvis to which it may be firmly attached. A trial by digital dissection is often helpful, as this technique will reduce the risk of damaging pelvic structures. If sharp dissection of the pelvis is necessary, the plane of dissection should be through white scar tissue, which will minimize structural damage. This mobilization may be assisted by early transection of the proximal colon so that the colon below this level can be displaced forward, allowing better access to the posterior plane of dissection. After identification the ureter should be traced to the pelvis and sometimes beyond, but this can be difficult as it may disappear under a sheet of dense fibrous tissue. Ureterolysis is rarely necessary but may be indicated if there is dilatation of the ureter due to encasement in scar tissue. This procedure should be approached with caution, as there is a risk of devascularization of the ureter. Not infrequently, the inflammatory mass is intimately adherent to the left pelvic brim where the ureter and large vessels are at risk. If the surgeon is satisfied that carcinoma is not present, the plane of dissection can be intramural through the muscle wall of the colon even exposing the mucosa, leaving a plaque of bowel wall attached to the left pelvic brim (Fig. 51-4). Vascular ligation should be below the left colic artery where possible and appropriate, because it may have a critical role in the blood supply of the left colon.

Distal Level of Resection

The usual point of distal resection is through the upper third of the rectum if the bowel wall at that level is normal. In the presence of a pelvic abscess, the upper third of the rectum may still be satisfactory, even though there is an inflammatory nest on the pelvic floor. In other instances there are secondary inflammatory changes of edema, inflammation, and rigidity in the upper third of the rectum which will not allow safe anastomosis at this level, which then needs to be extraperitoneal, well distal to the inflammatory reaction. The distal level of 225 anastomoses is shown in Figure 51-5.

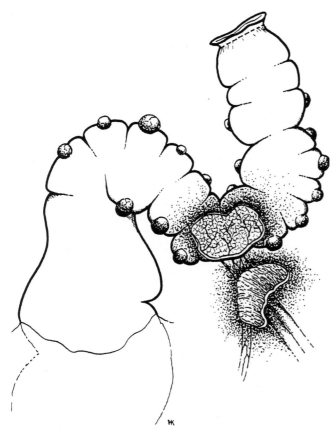

Figure 51-4
Intramural dissection leaving a "patch" of colon attached to the pelvic brim can protect strategic structures.

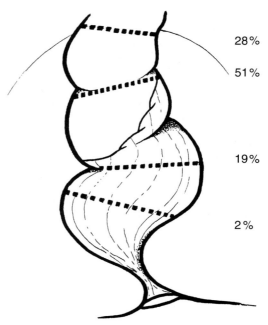

Figure 51-5
Distal levels of resection for anastomosis in author's series are shown here, indicating that some anastomoses were extraperitoneal.

Proximal Level of Resection

No evidence suggests that extensive left colon resections reduce the risk of recurrent diverticulitis, but in some patients the population of diverticula is so concentrated that it is common sense to resect above such disease. Although the occasional diverticulum near an anastomosis can be inverted without difficulty, a number of diverticula adjacent to an anastomosis may be a risk, particularly with the stapling technique. The proximal level of resection, therefore, will vary between the sigmoid descending junction and the vicinity of the splenic flexure. It can be difficult at operation to identify the extent of diverticula in the left colon, and a preoperative barium enema may be helpful. The maneuver of "milking" contents of the colon into the left colon will create pressure and identify diverticula as they expand, indicating the optimal level of resection. The colon for anastomosis must be supple without muscle thickening or inflammatory changes.

Anastomosis When Abscess Is Present

There is a prevalent opinion that in the presence of an abscess immediate anastomosis should not be performed and that a Hartmann procedure is preferable. The author

does not agree with this viewpoint, having performed an elective Hartmann operation in only 1 patient in 227 patients who were resected (0.4%). The presence of an abscess at operation does not affect the anastomosis if prolonged pelvic drainage is used, preventing the reforming of pelvic suppuration.

Colovesical Fistula

This may be a relatively simple surgical problem in which the inflamed colon is closely adherent to the bladder wall without an intervening abscess and with a small defect in the vault of the bladder. It may, however, be associated with an intervening abscess eroding the bladder wall and a large fistula associated with a significant inflammatory reaction. The fistula is usually near the vault of the bladder but occasionally may be closer to the trigone. In most patients repair of the bladder wall is not required. A large defect in the bladder wall can be closed by suture with excision of the inflammatory edges, if appropriate. The colon disease is treated on its own merits, and the need for a proximal stoma is related only to the integrity of the anastomosis and not to the presence of the fistula. Where feasible, interposition of the mobilized greater omentum is advised to prevent the recurrence of a colovesical fistula if an anastomotic leak occurs.

Anastomotic Technique

Although various techniques can prove satisfactory, the author prefers single circular stapling, which has been used in 158 patients. The double-stapling technique preferred by some surgeons has been used only once to perform an anastomosis in the lower third of the rectum. The muscle wall of the rectum for anastomosis must not be affected by inflammatory disease.

Specific difficulties may occur when stapling anastomoses after resection of diverticular disease. Spasm in the upper third of the rectum (otherwise normal) may be a feature and can be reduced by an antispasmodic. The muscle wall of the rectum can be thicker than usual, and there is a tendency for the longitudinal layer of muscle to evert during apposition of the stapler. If a proximal stoma has been present for some prolonged period, the defunctioned colon may be thick-walled with fragile muscle and a markedly contracted lumen unsuitable for the stapling technique. Fibrosis due to a chronic abscess on the pelvic floor may produce fixation of the tissues, impeding the safe passage of the stapler along the rectal stump. The techniques of anastomosis used in 225 patients are shown in Table 51-4.

Proximal Stoma

Of 205 patients undergoing primary resection and anastomosis of the left colon without a pre-existing stoma, 29 (14.2%) were managed with a synchronous proximal stoma. The use of loop ileostomy as a defunctioning stoma began in 1976 and has been preferred to a loop transverse colostomy since 1989. The indications for a proximal stoma are related to disease in the bowel wall, technical aspects of the anastomosis, the overall extent of the procedure (blood loss, duration), and the general condition of the patient. These indications are set out in Table 51-5.

The use of a proximal stoma is directly related to the extent of inflammatory process found at operation. It was necessary in 1 patient (2.9%) resected with noninflammatory diverticular disease, 5 patients (6.3%) with localized diverticulitis, and 23 patients (25.6%) with extracolic diverticulitis.

Drains

Drainage of the anastomosis per se is not advocated after resection of diverticulitis. It remains traditional, however, to drain the presacral space if this is fully dissected. Presacral drains have not been proved to reduce the incidence of anastomotic defects, however. If hemostasis in the pelvis is not satisfactory, then drains certainly have a role. Turnbull was convinced that a residual inflammatory "nest" (chronic abscess wall) left in the pelvis after resection and anastomosis would cause subsequent suppuration and potentially damage the anastomosis. He used a "21-day" drain of Penrose rubber to prevent this compli-

Table 51-4 Technique for Anastomosis	
TECHNIQUE	**NO. OF PATIENTS**
Two-layer suture	33
One-layer suture	34
Circular stapling	158
Total	225

Table 51-5 Indications for a Synchronous Proximal Stoma	
INDICATIONS	**PATIENTS (29)***
Rectal wall pathology Inflammation/distal fistula	10
Colon pathology Obstruction/vascular	10
Extensive pelvic sepsis	3
Anastomosis: technical problems	4
Patient Frail/immunosuppressed patient/complex operation	13

*More than one indication in some patients.

cation. Passive drainage, however, may result in a large infected space, which may not heal for weeks or even months.

Balanced irrigation-suction drainage (prolonged pelvic drainage) has been found preferable to passive drains in the preceding circumstances, resulting in a drain track closely fitting the caliber of the drain at 11 to 12 days. The drain is then removed by progressive withdrawal over 4 to 5 days. This technique used in the presence of an abscess has allowed anastomoses to be performed and obviated the need for the Hartmann operation. The regimen for management of the drain is shown in Table 51-2. In addition to drainage, the inflammatory "nest" should be débrided by curettage and excision.

■ LAPAROSCOPIC SURGERY

Laparoscopic techniques for colon surgery are now established, and various centers report early recovery and discharge from the hospital after colon resection. With experience, conversion rates are low and operation time is comparable to open surgery. Further reports are needed to evaluate its role dealing specifically with the more complex inflammatory situation encountered in many elective resections of diverticular disease. The mortality and morbidity rates must be demonstrated to be comparable to open resection, particularly in complicated disease.

■ POSTOPERATIVE MORTALITY RATE

Surgeons know well that diverticulitis can present a major technical challenge for surgery and carries a significant risk for the patients, particularly if they are elderly and suffering comorbid disease. There were 4 deaths following 227 resections (1.8%) in the series discussed in this chapter. The causes of death were unrecognized leukemia, anaphylaxis during platelet transfusion, cardiac syncope, and stroke. Large series of elective surgery without postoperative deaths have been published by Moreaux and Vons (177 patients) and Veidenheimer (133 patients).

■ POSTOPERATIVE MORBIDITY RATE

In 227 patients postoperative intra-abdominal complications occurred in 31 patients (13.6%), including 5 of 35 patients (14.3%) who were resected for noninflammatory diverticular disease, 4 of 80 patients (5.0%) who were resected for localized diverticulitis, and 22 of 112 patients (19.6%) who were resected for extracolic diverticulitis. The incidence of intra-abdominal sepsis and clinical anastomotic leak was significantly higher in the patients resected for extracolic diverticulitis. Postoperative sepsis has been reduced by parenteral antibiotics and progress in minimizing anastomotic leak. In the author's view this improvement has been due to better selection of the distal level of anastomosis, a safe technique of bowel apposition (stapling), débridement of the inflammatory "nest," and selected use of prolonged irrigation drains.

Anastomotic Leak

This complication may threaten the patient's life, produce prolonged septic morbidity, and initiate or prolong the need for a stoma, and in some patients this leak can leave them with a failed anastomosis. A clinical leak may be overtly manifest by peritonitis, pelvic abscess, or a fecal fistula. It may also be obvious clinically but the consequences obscured by the presence of a stoma (occult clinical leak).

Limited contrast enema studies performed after operation will reveal otherwise undetected anastomotic leaks, and this finding may have an impact on management (for example, delay in closing a proximal stoma). Table 51-6 indicates the incidence and types of anastomotic leak in 222 patients, of whom 220 were investigated radiologically.

The majority of anastomoses have been in the upper third of the rectum and rectosigmoid junction (171), and although anastomotic leak has virtually been eliminated when operating for carcinoma at this level, there were 9 anastomotic leaks (clinical and radiologic) in these patients operated on for diverticular disease. In most of these 9 patients incorrect selection (before 1979) of the level of anastomosis was the most likely cause of the anastomotic complication. This complication could have been significantly reduced if normal rectum had been selected for anastomosis. It is very important, therefore, to recognize that inflammatory changes on the wall of the upper third of the rectum secondary to a loop

of sigmoid diverticulitis lying in the pelvis may jeopardize the healing of an anastomosis at that level. Not surprisingly, the total leak rate (clinical and radiologic) varied with the disease at operation. After resection of noninflammatory diverticular disease, the leak rate was nil; for localized diverticulitis it was 1.3%, and for extracolic diverticulitis it was 11.4%.

Since 1979 circular stapling has been the preferred technique of anastomosis (157 single and 1 double stapling). There have been one clinical leak (clinically occult leak in the presence of a stoma 0.6%) and two radiologic leaks (1.3%). This improvement does not establish that stapling is superior to suturing but indicates that it has been a satisfactory technique.

■ RELATIONSHIP OF PATHOLOGY CLASSIFICATION TO MANAGEMENT AND OUTCOME

Noninflammatory diverticular disease and localized diverticulitis can usually be managed in a similar way and with a similar outcome. Once the inflammatory process has violated the anatomic compartment by perforation (extracolic diverticulitis) and formed a pericolic abscess or fistula, the technical problems have the potential to become complex. It is in this group of patients that a proximal stoma is more likely and abdominal drains may be required. Mortality and intra-abdominal morbidity rates are higher after resection of extracolic diverticulitis.

■ RECURRENT DIVERTICULITIS AFTER RESECTION

Recurrent diverticulitis after resection is generally regarded as uncommon and few studies have addressed it. Benn and coworkers from the Mayo Clinic found an incidence of 6.7% if the anastomosis was performed in the upper part of the rectum and a significantly higher incidence (12.5%) if the anastomosis was in the lower sigmoid colon. This report supports the view that the anastomosis should be made in the rectum. In a review by letter and telephone, 112 patients have been followed up to assess possible recurrence of diverticulitis. It was difficult to make an objective diagnosis as the description of symptoms were analyzed to assess recurrent diverticulitis. Eleven patients (9.8%) complained of recurrent abdominal pain, but only one patient (0.9%) had documented evidence (x-ray) of recurrent disease. Some patients with no diverticula on barium enema were diagnosed erroneously by themselves or their family physician as suffering from diverticulitis. It is probably significant that the highest incidence of recurrent pain occurred in 3 of 16 patients (8.8%) in whom the original disease was noninflammatory, suggesting the possibility that the initial symptoms were due to an alternative diagnosis, such as spastic colon. If all 11 patients with pain after resection are included as "recurrence," the maximum possible incidence is 9.8%. It seems likely, however, that the true recurrence

Table 51-6 Anastomotic Leak*		
TYPE OF LEAK	**NUMBER**	**INCIDENCE (%)**
Overt clinical leak	1	0.5
Occult clinical leak (obscured by proximal stoma)	4	1.8
Radiologic leak (limited contrast enema)	8	3.6
Total	13	5.2

*In 222 patients, of whom 220 underwent radiologic examination.

of diverticulitis after resection in those 112 patients was significantly less. In the 32 patients in whom the anastomosis was made at the level of the promontory of the sacrum (rectosigmoid) the incidence of recurrence of pain was 12.5%. In 54 patients followed up in whom the anastomosis was in the upper rectum, the incidence of recurrence of pain was 11.1%, which is not significantly different. This finding suggests that the rectosigmoid level can be used for anastomosis if the bowel wall appears normal, but careful assessment of the barium enema and the pathology at operation is essential.

Suggested Readings

Ambrosetti P, Grossholz M, Becker C, et al: Computed tomography in acute left colonic diverticulitis. Br J Surg 1997;84:532–534.

Benn PL, Wolff BG, Ilstrup DM: Level of anastomosis and recurrent diverticulitis. Am J Surg 1986;151:269–271.

Church JM: Surgical treatment of sigmoid diverticulitis. Schweiz Med Wschr 1991;121:744–748.

Elliott TB, Yego S, Irvin TT: Five-year audit of the acute complications of diverticular disease. Br J Surg 1997;84:535–539.

Farmakis N, Tudor RG, Keighley MRB: The 5-year natural history of complicated diverticular disease. Br J Surg 1994;81:733–735.

Hachigian MP, Honickman S, Eisenstat TE, et al: Computed tomography in the initial management of acute left-sided diverticulitis. Dis Colon Rectum 1992;35:1123–1134.

Hackford AW, Veidenheimer MC: Diverticular disease of the colon. Current concepts and management. Surg Clin North Am 1985;65:347–363.

Hemming A, Davis N, Robins RE: Surgical versus percutaneous drainage of intra-abdominal abscesses. Am J Surg 1991;161:593–595.

Killingback MJ: Elective surgery for sigmoid diverticular disease. In Fielding LP, Goldberg SM (Eds.): Rob and Smith's Operative Surgery: Surgery of the Colon, Rectum and Anus, 5th ed. Oxford, Butterworth-Heinemann, 1993, pp 369–386.

Killingback MJ: Management of perforative diverticulitis. Surg Clin North Am 1983;63:97–115.

Kronborg O: Treatment of perforated sigmoid diverticulitis: A prospective randomized trial. Br J Surg 1993;80:505–507.

Krukowski ZH, Koruth NM, Matheson NA: Evolving practice in acute diverticulitis. Br J Surg 1985;72:684–686.

Moreaux J, Vons C: Elective resection for diverticular disease of the sigmoid colon. Br J Surg 1990;77:1036–1038.

Morson BC: The muscle abnormality in diverticular disease of the colon. Proc Royal Soc Med 1963;56:798–800.

Mueller PR, Saini S, Wittenberg J: Sigmoid diverticular abscess: Percutaneous drainage as an adjunct to surgical resection in 24 cases. Radiology 1987;164:321–325.

Neff CC, Van Sonnenberg E, Casola G: Diverticular abscesses: Percutaneous drainage. Radiology 1987;163:15–18.

Pheils MT, Duraiappah B, Newland RC: Chronic phlegmonous diverticulitis. Aust NZ J Surg 1973;42:337–341.

Rodkey GV, Welch CE: Changing patterns in the surgical treatment of diverticular disease. Ann Surg 1984;466–478.

Roberts P, Abel M, Rosen L: Practice parameters for sigmoid diverticulitis—Supporting documentation. Dis Colon Rectum 1995;38:126–132.

Roberts PL, Veidenheimer MC: Current management of diverticulitis. Adv Surg 1994;27:189–208.

Rothenberger DA, Wiltz O: Surgery for complicated diverticulitis. Surg Clin North Am 1993;73:975–992.

Sarin S, Boulos PB: Long-term outcome of patients presenting with acute complications of diverticular disease. Ann R Coll Surg Eng 1994;76:117–120.

Siminovitch JMP, Fazio VW: Obstructive uropathy secondary to sigmoid diverticulitis. Dis Colon Rectum 1980;23:504–507.

Stabile BE, Puccio E, Van Sonnenberg E, Neff C: Preoperative percutaneous drainage of diverticular abscess. Am J Surg 1990;159:99–105.

Tudor RG, Farmakis N, Keighley MR: National audit of complicated diverticular disease: Analysis of index cases. Br J Surg 1994;81:730–732.

Veidenheimer MC: Clinical presentation and surgical treatment of complicated diverticular disease. In Allan RN, Keighley MR, Alexander-Williams J, et al (Eds.): Inflammatory Bowel Diseases. Edinburgh, Churchill Livingstone, 1983, pp 519–528.

52

DIVERTICULITIS AND FISTULA

Rodney J. Woods, MBBS, FRACS

Fistulas arising in association with diverticular disease are uncommon, and may be internal fistulas or external colocutaneous fistulas. Internal fistulas can be colovesical (65%), colovaginal (25%), coloenteric (7%), or colouterine (3%). These fistulas may be multiple, and even rarer types of internal fistulas have been reported. Spontaneous fistulas result from a localized sigmoid perforation that has resolved, or has partially resolved, by decompression into an adjacent organ. Fistulas may also be secondary to a previous surgical procedure, ranging from a simple percutaneous drainage of an abscess to a resection complicated by an anastomotic dehiscence. Internal fistulas may be spontaneous or follow previous surgical procedures. Colocutaneous fistulas, however, nearly always follow previous surgical procedures.

■ INTERNAL FISTULAS

Presentation and Diagnosis

Most patients present electively with a mature fistula without evidence of significant sepsis. At times, however, critically ill patients present with undrained sepsis, malnutrition, and immunosuppression associated with colocutaneous fistulas. These conditions often develop following a number of recent surgical endeavors. These patients can present a serious surgical challenge.

Colovesical fistulas are more common in men (2:1) because of the protection given by the broad ligament and uterus in females. Fifty percent of women with this type of fistula have had a hysterectomy. Symptoms are primarily urologic, including cystitis (90%), pneumaturia (75%), and fecaluria (50%). Patients with colovaginal fistulas commonly have a vaginal discharge (95%) and an opening seen at the apex of the vagina (87%). High output of colocutaneous fistulas suggest an associated enteric fistula (Table 52-1).

Investigations

Specific investigations depend on the clinical presentation. Investigations assist in outlining the fistulous tract and, more important, in determining the pathologic cause of the fistula. Colon cancer and Crohn's disease must be excluded. A colon cancer will change the surgical technique considerably, requiring an en bloc excision of the surrounding organs, compared to blunt dissection, the method of choice of diverticulitis. Crohn's disease, both of the colon and the ileum, can masquerade as complicated diverticulitis, and preoperative diagnosis will usually alter the surgical management.

Rigid Proctoscopy and Flexible Endoscopy

All patients require endoscopic evaluation of the rectum and sigmoid colon. The rectosigmoid usually cannot be traversed with the proctoscope when there is complicated diverticular disease. Associated anal disease should be noted, as this may suggest inflammatory bowel disease. Flexible endoscopy is more accurate than contrast studies in assessing the mucosa of the sigmoid colon. The procedure can be difficult because of sigmoid loop tethering in the pelvis in addition to associated spasm and edema. Sedation may be required. Stricturing may prevent complete endoscopic evaluation. In these cases a narrow flexible endoscope can be of value. In patients who have had a previous resection, it is important to note the level of the anastomosis and the presence of any residual diverticular disease above or below the anastomosis. CT colonography is a new investigative means that may assist in the exclusion of malignancy when conventional endoscopy fails.

Contrast Studies

Contrast studies can complement flexible endoscopy, although they are not indicated in all cases. The diverticular disease can be confirmed and other lesions are excluded. An internal fistula can be outlined in 40 to 50% of cases. If a previous anastomosis is present, its level, as well as any residual diverticular disease, can be assessed. The main value of the contrast studies is in the evaluation of fistula disease in postoperative patients.

Fistulogram

In patients with colocutaneous fistulas a fistulogram will confirm the presence of a fistula and delineate any other organ involvement, particularly the small bowel.

Intravenous Pyelogram

An intravenous pyelogram (IVP) has traditionally been performed to assess the function of both kidneys and to

Table 52-1 Evaluation and Treatment of Internal Fistulas

FISTULA	SYMPTOMS	INVESTIGATIONS	TREATMENT
Colovesical	Cystitis, 90% Pneumaturia, 75% Fecaluria, 50%	Cystoscopy + in 90% of cases Endoscopy (exclude carcinoma/Crohn's disease)	Resection/anastomosis Bladder drainage, 7 days
Colovaginal	Discharge, 90%	Vaginoscopy + in 90% of cases Endoscopy	Resection/anastomosis Close vaginal defect

delineate the anatomy of the ureters, although it is not helpful in demonstrating the fistula track in colovesical fistulas. A computed tomographic (CT) scan has replaced the IVP as the investigation of choice in this setting (see following section).

Abdominopelvic Computed Tomographic Scan

If there is evidence of persistent, undrained, intra-abdominal sepsis or an abdominal mass, an abdomino-pelvic CT scan is performed. This procedure is often indicated in postoperative fistulas. If an abscess is found, it may be accessible to the radiologist for percutaneous drainage with possible downstaging of the patient's future surgical course.

Cystoscopy and Urine Culture

In patients with a colovesical fistula, a urine culture will often show mixed organisms and cystoscopy will show an abnormality suggestive of, or proof of, a fistula in 92% of cases. Carcinomatous invasion of the bladder can be excluded if there is intraluminal extension.

Ureteric Stents

Ureteric stents are placed routinely in patients whose dissections may prove to be difficult. These patients include those with abdominal or pelvic masses and those who have had previous surgery for diverticulitis.

Medical Treatment

Patients require the usual medical workup for any major abdominal surgery, including antibiotics and correction of any nutritional deficiencies. An enterostomal therapist sees the patient preoperatively to pouch any fistula, for preoperative discussion, and to mark the site of a possible stoma.

Indications and Timing of Surgical Treatment

Surgery is indicated for both symptomatic relief and to eradicate any septic focus that might lead to septic episodes. Virtually all patients with fistulas are candidates for surgery unless they have severe concomitant medical disease making the hazards of surgery too great.

Patients with spontaneous internal fistulas and colocutaneous fistulas following simple drainage of abscesses can undergo surgery on a semielective basis once they are declared medically fit. Uncommonly the fistula may be associated with more urgent pathology (e.g., perforation, abscess) that is the primary problem. In these cases management is obviously determined by the more urgent pathology. Colocutaneous and postoperative internal fistulas are discussed later.

Surgical Treatment

All patients require mechanical bowel preparation and antibiotic prophylaxis. Anti–venous thrombosis prophylaxis is also administered. The patient is placed in the Lloyd-Davies position and a cystoscopy with placement of stents is performed if indicated.

The essentials of the operation are the same as for any operation for diverticular disease and include the following:

1. A long midline incision
2. Splenic flexure mobilization
3. Adequate resection
4. A good, tension-free, viable anastomosis
5. Diversion in selected patients
6. No anastomosis in selected patients
7. Removal of any inflammatory focus or at least ensuring that it is quarantined from the anastomosis

A long midline incision allows mobilization of the splenic flexure safely. The splenic flexure must be mobilized to achieve a tension-free anastomosis because the sigmoid colon and its mesentery are usually shortened and thickened, and the anastomosis must be between the descending colon (or more proximal) and the rectum.

A resection, if technically possible, should always be performed to remove the septic focus. Proximal diversion may not improve the patient's symptoms and, in fact, fistulas can develop in the presence of a proximal stoma. The sigmoid colon is usually pinched off the attached organ, although if a carcinomatous fistula cannot be excluded, then an en bloc resection with an adequate a margin of the attached organ is mandatory. The left colon is mobilized, taking down the splenic flexure with a high ligation of the inferior mesenteric vessels, allowing better mobilization of the left colon. The proximal line of transection must be not only above any obvious inflammatory disease but also above any obvious muscle hypertrophy gauged by palpation. Sometimes this thickening extends to the transverse colon. Not all diverticular disease must be removed, but muscle hypertrophy must be resected. The distal line of transection is at an area of supple upper rectum, or occasionally in the lower rectum if the upper rectum is secondarily inflamed.

The anastomosis can be performed by hand or by stapling technique. Stapling should not be used if the bowel ends are not supple and easily inverted. There should be no tension at the anastomosis. Occasionally, the inferior mesenteric vein needs to be divided for a second time just below the pancreas to reduce any tension. An anastomosis should not be performed if there is a loaded obstructed colon. In these cases, a resection and endcolostomy with implantation of the rectosigmoid stump into the wound are preferable. This procedure is preferable to a Hartmann's resection because the stump is easy to find and it can usually be brought to the surface—in 75% of cases, the perforative disease is in the middle and upper sigmoid colon. The appropriate resection is then performed at the second stage. Indications for diverting stomas must be individualized, usually performed when there is some concern with the anastomosis, when there is a significant degree of remaining inflammatory tissue adjacent to the anastomosis, or when the bowel preparation is suboptimal. Any adjacent inflammatory tissue is managed by curettage and drainage. In large areas with big abscess cavities, wide drainage is needed and may be achieved with multiple Penrose drains. These drains can later be replaced with a mushroom drain. Drainage must be continued for at least 3 weeks. If the omentum can reach this area, it is used to quarantine the inflammatory focus from the anastomosis.

The fistularized organs are managed as follows: In colovesical fistulas, the bladder defect is closed if identified. At least 7 days of urethral catheter drainage is required and sometimes a cystogram can be performed before removing the catheter. Vaginal defects, if identified, are repaired. An omental plug can be sutured to bladder or vaginal defect to separate them from the colorectal anastomosis. Small bowel resection is required in coloenteric fistulas, although in colouterine fistulas, a hysterectomy is not mandatory.

Results

In a review of 84 patients treated solely at the Cleveland Clinic Foundation for internal fistulas from January 1962 to April 1986, it was concluded that a primary resection with anastomosis was the operation of choice. In the latter half of the series, 76% of patients had one-stage procedures. During this same period, no diverting stoma without resection was performed. It was found that the pathology was localized and usually not urgent (only two urgent operations were performed in the series), which allowed for this high rate of one-stage procedures. There were three deaths; two were immediate postoperative cardiac deaths and the other was caused by a pulmonary embolus on the fifth day. There were two clinical anastomotic leaks, one of which required surgery.

■ COLOCUTANEOUS AND POSTOPERATIVE INTERNAL FISTULAS

Management of these fistulas is similar to that for spontaneous internal fistulas, although some important differences exist (Fig. 52-1). Such fistulas may follow simple abscess drainage diversion without resection, resection with anastomosis, or even develop from a defunctioned rectosigmoid stump. Fecal diversion does not prevent fistula formation, but it does reduce morbidity. Patients need to be resuscitated with attention to their nutritional profile and treatment of sepsis. Patients with high-output fistulas may have an associated enteric fistula and are more likely to have nutritional deficiencies. Total parental nutrition does not close the fistula but improves the patient's condition. Persisting abscesses can sometimes be drained percutaneously using CT or ultrasonographic guidance. This may downstage the future surgical course of the patient. The timing of surgery in these patients with respect to previous abdominal surgery is important. In general, the longer the delay, the easier it is to successfully accomplish the next operation. If possible, delay further surgery for at least 6 weeks, and preferably for 12 weeks, following a recent laparotomy. In patients without previous resectional surgery, a resection as outlined earlier is performed. The decision of whether to perform an anastomosis, and if so, whether to create a diverting stoma, must be individualized.

Not all patients having had a previous resection do not require further surgery, although patients with postoperative internal fistulas usually do require further resection. In patients with mature postoperative colocutaneous fistulas it is possible that the fistula will close with conservative measures, when they have previously had an adequate resection with a true colorectal anastomosis. Factors that predispose to failure of the conservative approach are persisting sepsis; residual diverticular disease following an inadequate resection, particularly if there is remaining distal sigmoid producing functional obstruction; fistulas to other organs; and Crohn's disease. Certainly in a tertiary referral practice as demonstrated by the experience of the Cleveland Clinic Foundation discussed later, nearly all patients require further surgery because they usually have already failed to improve following conservative

COLOCUTANEOUS AND POSTOPERATIVE INTERNAL FISTULAS

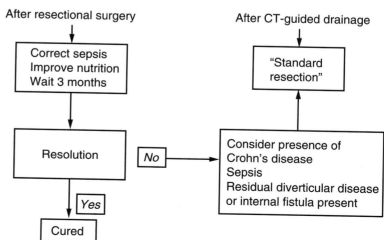

Figure 52-1
This algorithm shows the important differences in the management of internal fistulas.

management. Management of each case, however, must be individualized. If any of the detrimental factors mentioned previously are present, further resection is needed.

Results

In a review of 93 patients with colocutaneous fistulas complicating diverticulitis treated at the Cleveland Clinic Foundation between 1965 and 1983, the authors made the following observations. Diverting stomas do not prevent fistula formation but reduce morbidity. Thirty percent of such patients have associated internal fistulas, most of them being coloenteric. Sixty-six percent of patients with a presumed colorectal anastomosis actually had a colosigmoid anastomosis. Following surgery at the Cleveland Clinic Foundation, there was one postoperative death, and 48% of patients had complications. There were 5 recurrent fistulas and 14 new fistulas. Five of these 19 patients were found to have Crohn's disease. This study suggested that the number of these complicated postoperative cases and the resultant high morbidity following surgical management could be reduced significantly if an adequate resection was done initially with anastomosis to the rectum, and if Crohn's disease, if present, was diagnosed initially and the appropriate treatment initiated.

Suggested Readings

Fazio VW, Church JM, Jagelman DJ, et al: Colocutaneous fistulas complicating diverticulitis. Dis Colon Rectum 1987;30:89–94.

Gall FP, Tonak, Altendorf A: Multivisceral resections in colorectal cancer. Dis Colon Rectum 1987;30:337–341.

Grissom R, Snyder TE: Colovaginal fistula secondary to diverticular disease. Dis Colon Rectum 1991;34:1043–1049.

Vasilevsky CA, Belliveau P, Trudel JL, et al: Fistulas complicating diverticulitis. Int J Colorectal Dis 1998;13:57–60.

Woods RJ, Lavery IC, Fazio VW, et al: Internal fistulas in diverticular disease. Dis Colon Rectum 1988;31:591–596.

53

LOWER GASTROINTESTINAL BLEEDING

Jeffrey L. Cohen, MD, FACS, FASCRS

Massive lower gastrointestinal bleeding represents a serious and potentially life-threatening situation. Although rectal bleeding can be seen in any age group, the vast majority of patients requiring admission to the hospital are elderly and have coexistent medical problems. Most of these patients will cease bleeding early in their hospital course, but as many as 25 to 30% will rebleed during or after their hospitalization. In the adult population, diverticulosis and vascular ectasias account for greater than 90% of the causes of colonic hemorrhage. Other less common causes of lower gastrointestinal bleeding are included in Table 53-1. Although the focus of this chapter will be on the general evaluation and management of lower gastrointestinal hemorrhage, it is worthwhile to briefly examine and contrast the two most common causes.

■ ETIOLOGY

In Western society, as much as 65% of the population will have diverticulosis by age 85. Twenty percent of patients with diverticulosis coli will present with bleeding during their lifetime, and 5% will have severe hemorrhage. Although 80 to 90% of these patients will cease bleeding spontaneously, it can be expected that bleeding will recur in 25%. Most diverticula are located in the sigmoid and descending colon; however, diverticular bleeding is distributed fairly equally between the right and left sides of the colon. Regardless of location, the pathogenesis is felt to be injury to the submucosal branch of the vasa recta. It has been speculated that the wider necks of right-sided diverticula allow for a greater length of artery to be exposed to injury, thus increasing the percentage of bleeding from proximal diverticulosis.

Vascular ectasias of the colon are also felt to be acquired lesions because they are rarely observed in patients under the age of 40. Also known as angiodysplasia or arteriovenous malformations, these lesions are predominantly located on the right side of the colon. It is likely that the increased wall tension of the cecum accounts for the distribution of these lesions. As described by Boley, repeated low-grade obstruction of the submucosal veins over many years leads to the characteristic tortuous, dilated, thin-walled vessels, which can be identified both grossly and histologically. Arteriovenous connections are a relatively late finding in

this process, resulting from increased pressure leading to disruption of the precapillary sphincters. A high incidence of cardiac disease, especially aortic stenosis, has been observed in patients with vascular ectasias. As many as 25% of patients presenting with bleeding arteriovenous malformations have been noted to have aortic stenosis. Although bleeding has been reported to cease with aortic valve replacement, gastrointestinal hemorrhage is not an indication for open heart surgery. Rather, the decision to perform aortic valve replacement should be made on the basis of traditional indications, with surgery for lower gastrointestinal bleeding proceeding first if critical aortic stenosis is not present.

Bleeding from vascular ectasias tends to be venous in origin and, therefore, is not usually as brisk as that seen with diverticulosis. In more than 90% of patients, bleeding will stop spontaneously, but unlike diverticulosis, repeated episodes of bleeding are common and their incidence approaches 85%.

■ INITIAL EVALUATION AND RESUSCITATION

Because many patients who present with lower gastrointestinal hemorrhage have associated hemodynamic changes, resuscitation must accompany the initial evaluation. Despite the varied etiologies for lower gastrointestinal hemorrhage, the initial approach is standard.

While trying to quantify the degree and characteristics of a patient's bleeding, it is important to realize that even small amounts of blood in the toilet can appear massive to the patient who is unfamiliar with this symptom. Because blood is a potent cathartic, more importance can be attached to the frequency of bloody bowel movements prior to presentation than trying to quantify the exact amount. As noted previously, hemodynamic instability is frequently associated with significant lower gastrointestinal bleeding, and it is much easier to focus on and treat while evaluating underlying causes. It should be pointed out that a lack of hemodynamic instability does not necessary imply a minor bleed. A recent study from our institution revealed that 90% of patients with a positive arteriogram for bleeding presented as normotensive or hypotensive, and only 30% were tachycardic.

Table 53-1 Etiology of Colonic Hemorrhage
Diverticular disease
Vascular ectasias
Colonic neoplasms
Ischemic colitis
Radiation colitis
Inflammatory bowel disease
Trauma
Hematologic disorders
Rectal varices
Hemorrhoids
Anal pathology

As the initial evaluation progresses, the basics of cardiopulmonary resuscitation must be followed. Large-bore intravenous catheters should be placed with infusion of a balanced salt solution. Laboratory studies of blood are drawn and must include hemoglobin, hematocrit, coagulation studies, and a blood typing and crossmatch. Attempts should be made to keep the patient normothermic with a warm room environment and fluid warmers. Placement of a Foley catheter will allow for accurate assessment of urinary output and assist in fluid replacement. Patients with massive hemorrhage, severe cardiac disease, or multiple comorbid diseases will benefit from intensive monitoring, which may include systemic arterial, pulmonary arterial, electrocardiographic, and oximetric monitors.

Early in the evaluation a nasogastric tube should be placed. In many studies of lower gastrointestinal bleeding, as many as 10% of patients initially felt to be bleeding from a colonic source were ultimately determined to be bleeding from an upper gastrointestinal lesion. If clear bile is not returned on nasogastric aspiration, upper endoscopy should be performed as part of the evaluation. Even if clear bile is noted on gastric lavage, upper gastrointestinal bleeding can be seen in up to 16% of patients. The nasogastric tube may be left in place to use as access for a rapid mechanical bowel preparation to perform early colonoscopy.

While the resuscitation effort is proceeding, important information should be obtained from the patient's history in relation to risk for continued or recurrent bleeding. Eliciting a history of alcohol or aspirin ingestion, a prior history of gastrointestinal bleeding, or the presence of any bleeding diathesis, as well as finding comorbid diseases, is extremely important to the overall management of the patient.

On physical examination, particular attention should be paid to identifying stigmata of advanced liver disease. In addition, the presence of an abdominal mass may indicate an unsuspected colon carcinoma. Although diverticulitis is not usually seen with bleeding diverticulosis, a finding of abdominal tenderness may suggest that possibility. More likely, however, would be the diagnosis of ischemic colitis or inflammatory bowel disease when a patient presents with abdominal pain, tenderness, and lower gastrointestinal hemorrhage.

Finally, rigid sigmoidoscopy is essential early in the evaluation of patients with lower gastrointestinal bleeding. It is generally performed in the emergency room while the resuscitation effort is proceeding to rule out an anorectal source of bleeding. Hemorrhoids associated with portal hypertension can bleed massively, and other low rectal or anal sources of bleeding may be treatable in the acute setting. Additionally, observation of the rectal mucosa may suggest a possible source of bleeding, such as infectious, inflammatory, or ischemic proctocolitis.

■ DIAGNOSTIC INVESTIGATIONS

The diagnostic phase of lower gastrointestinal bleeding usually proceeds once the patient has been stabilized in the emergency room. However, owing to the dynamic nature of colonic hemorrhage, diagnostic testing occasionally must be initiated while the patient is still being resuscitated. In fact, aggressive diagnostic maneuvers can have the benefit of localizing bleeding that will otherwise cease and be impossible to localize if expectant management is initiated. It has been argued that most bleeding (90%) will stop spontaneously, thereby negating the need for an aggressive workup, but studies have shown that as many as 25 to 30% of patients will suffer from a significant rebleeding episode. Identifying the bleeding source is especially important in these patients, and early aggressive diagnostic procedures may achieve this goal and may allow for nonoperative therapeutic maneuvers as well.

The three most commonly utilized diagnostic studies performed for lower gastrointestinal bleeding are radionuclide scanning, angiography, and colonoscopy. In many patients, a combination of these tests will be indicated, and occasionally, because of recurrent bleeding, it will be necessary to repeat them. Both angiography and colonoscopy can be of potential therapeutic benefit, and this advantage adds to their attraction as diagnostic modalities.

Scintigraphy

Two radionuclide scans are available to image gastrointestinal bleeding. Initially, sulfur colloid was employed as an intravascular marker that could not return to the vascular compartment once bleeding into the intestine had taken place. However, its rapid clearance by the reticuloendothelial system leads to two distinct disadvantages of its use. First of all, the patient must be actively bleeding at the time of injection because over 90% of the trace is cleared within 7 minutes. Second, accumulation of activity by the liver and spleen effectively obscures the two flexures from visualization of bleeding.

A second technique, technetium-labeled red blood cells, has supplanted sulfur colloid scanning as the nuclear medicine technique of choice. It is equally safe and effective, and its only disadvantage is the 30 to 40 minutes required to label the red blood cells. Technetium-labeled red blood cell scans are reported to be sensitive to bleeding at rates as low as 0.05 to 0.1 mL per minute. The tagged red blood cells have an extended half-life, and scanning can take place for 24 hours after injection.

Although tagged red blood cell scanning has gained wide acceptance as a modality to detect gastrointestinal bleeding, it is arguable whether scintigraphy can localize a bleeding site reliably. In a recent review of 72 technetium-labeled red blood cell scans performed at our institution, 71% of the positive scans accurately localized the site of bleeding as confirmed by surgery, angiography, or endoscopy. This finding is supported by other studies in the literature which average a false localization rate of 25%. Recently, it has been reported that the accuracy of scanning can be enhanced by performing dynamic scintigraphy with stratification of results based on early radionuclide blushing. Thus, the early positive results may more accurately indicate localization of the bleeding site. Given the rapid movement of extravasated blood both antegrade and retrograde within the intestine, the relatively high false localization rate is not surprising. Therefore, basing an operative procedure on the results of red blood cell scintigraphy alone should be discouraged, and supplemental confirmation should be obtained prior to surgery if possible.

Radionuclide scanning has also been suggested as a cost-effective screening tool prior to angiography. Given its increased sensitivity, relative safety, and decreased cost as compared with angiography, scintigraphy should be an ideal test to perform to increase the yield of positive angiograms. Unfortunately, it has been difficult to support this in practice, possibly because the delay in obtaining an angiogram while performing scintigraphy has allowed the "window of opportunity" to pass. In reviewing our experience with angiography, a prior positive nuclear scan did not increase the percentage of positive angiograms as compared with patients who underwent angiography as the initial diagnostic procedure.

In conclusion, the exact role of radionuclide scanning remains unclear. The examinations are minimally invasive and inexpensive, have low complication rates, and may alert physicians to those patients who are likely to require surgical intervention. However, at this point, it is not safe to limit a workup to and base treatment on a radionuclide scan alone. Furthermore, its value as a screening modality for the cost-effective use of angiography remains questionable, and many institutions are now using angiography as a "first-line" diagnostic tool.

Angiography

Selective mesenteric angiography has become widely used for lower gastrointestinal hemorrhage because it has the benefit of being not only diagnostic, but frequently therapeutic. By localizing bleeding to a specific vessel, angiography tremendously facilitates surgery. Furthermore, transcatheter therapy, either pharmacologically or through embolization, can successfully treat the source of bleeding while avoiding a surgical procedure.

Minimal preparation is necessary for angiography, but because it must be assumed that the patient is actively bleeding, continuous monitoring is necessary in the radiology suite. Resuscitation should be continued while a Foley catheter prevents a bladder full of contrast material. Selective injection is performed first through the superior mesenteric artery because bleeding is most likely in this distribution. Injections of the inferior mesenteric and celiac axes follow because in up to 10% of patients with presumed lower gastrointestinal bleeding, the ultimate source is proximal to the ligament of Treitz. Bleeding can be detected at rates as low as 0.5 to 1.0 mL per minute. Although extravasation of contrast material is unequivocal evidence for a bleeding source, angiography can also detect other lesions such as tumor blush or angiodysplasia. Extravasation may be seen in less than 15% of patients with vascular ectasias; however, angiographic signs of their presence include a prominent early filling vein, a vascular tuft, or a late draining vein.

When angiography documents a bleeding site, transcatheter therapy can be instituted in an attempt to stop the bleeding. The two alternatives that are available are intra-arterial infusion of vasopressin or transcatheter embolization of the vessel. Superior mesenteric arterial infusion of vasopressin reduces splanchnic blood flow by up to 65%, hopefully allowing a hemostatic plug to form in the bleeding vessel. Vasopressin infusion is initiated at 0.2 U per minute with repeat angiography performed 20 minutes later to document the effectiveness of the infusion. The rate can be increased to 0.4 U per minute, after which the marginal benefit is outweighed by its side effects. Because of a cardiac complication reportedly as high as 43%, these patients require continuous cardiac monitoring, preferably in an intensive care setting. While success rates have been reported as high as 90%, up to 50% of patients will rebleed upon cessation of therapy. Our experience of a 41% rebleeding rate has led us to conclude that the major benefit of vasopressin is in stabilizing a patient's clinical situation, allowing for a semielective resection to be performed.

An alternative to vasopressin infusion is transcatheter embolization of the affected vessel. This technique has been proposed as having permanent control of the bleeding vessel as well as avoidance of the troublesome side effects of vasopressin. Early techniques employed temporary agents placed in a fairly central location so as to spare distal communicating vessels and allow for their eventual recanalization. Although theoretically transcatheter embolization was expected to reduce the complication of intestinal ischemia, ischemia still occurred in up to 20% of cases.

More recently, the development of small-caliber angiographic catheters has allowed for superselective catheterization of peripheral vessels. This advance has permitted a more selective therapeutic intervention and limited the potential for widespread intestinal ischemia. Platinum-fibered coils or polyvinyl alcohol particles are used as permanent embolic agents. To date, we have used this approach in 65 patients with angiographically proved lower gastrointestinal bleeding. Only one patient has rebled during the hospitalization and this bleeding was from a second angiodysplastic lesion. Four patients developed signs and symptoms of ischemia requiring urgent surgical intervention. These data seem to suggest that superselective embolization has lower risks of rebleeding and fewer complications than vasopressin infusion. There is a possibility that transcatheter embolization carries a higher risk if used after vasopressin therapy has failed and, therefore, probably should be avoided in this setting.

Colonoscopy

Colonoscopy is an extremely valuable diagnostic tool in the evaluation of lower gastrointestinal bleeding. With few exceptions, it should be performed at some time in the evaluation of any patient presenting with acute rectal bleeding. The major issue relates to timing of colonoscopy during the patient's hospitalization. Many are proponents of immediate colonoscopy upon admission to the hospital without utilization of a colonic preparation. Because blood is an excellent cathartic, many feel that early colonoscopy with "jet" irrigation of the colon has a high likelihood of determining the site of bleeding. Success rates as high as 80% have been reported with this approach, but we emphasize that this examination is technically very difficult to perform, and it has several drawbacks. Even with highly skilled endoscopists performing "emergent" colonoscopy, the cecal intubation rate is less than that for elective procedures. Furthermore, patient instability can severely limit the ability to administer sedatives and analgesics. Finally, residual blood markedly reduces the ability to visualize mucosal detail, which is critical in the diagnosis of angiodysplasia.

A preferable approach is to attempt to predict whether a patient has already stopped bleeding early in the evaluation period. If the patient is hemodynamically stable and not passing fresh blood per rectum, the patient is prepared for "urgent" colonoscopy. Polyethylene glycol is administered over 4 to 6 hours, preferably through a nasogastric tube if it has been left in place. Colonoscopy can be performed in a much more controlled setting. The patient, at this point, has been determined to be hemodynamically stable and can be sedated, allowing for a safer procedure. Mucosal detail is usually comparable to that of elective procedures, although the ability to perform high-pressure irrigation to remove adherent clot must be available.

It is unusual to detect an actively bleeding lesion during colonoscopy performed in this setting. However, suspicious lesions other than diverticula have been reported in up to 50% of patients. Neoplastic lesions can be removed or biopsied at the time of colonoscopy. Areas of ulceration or active colitis can also be biopsied. There is some controversy as to whether angiodysplastic lesions which are not actively bleeding should be treated "prophylactically" if detected. Our approach is to treat if there are no other potential bleeding sources found during the patient's evaluation and if there is a high degree of suspicion that the vascular ectasia had recently bled. If there are numerous, nonbleeding angiodysplastic lesions, their distribution is noted and no active therapeutic intervention is undertaken. The method of coagulation that is preferred in our gastrointestinal unit is the heater probe to surround the lesion and finally to cauterize the central area. Care is taken to use low-power settings, especially in the right colon, which is relatively thin-walled. Other methods of coagulation that can be utilized are bicap electrocautery, needle injection, or Nd:YAG (neodymium: yttrium-aluminum-garnet) laser therapy.

It is important to perform colonoscopy in all patients who have undergone therapeutic angiography. Although the patient may have stopped bleeding with either vasopressin or embolization, there is a 5 to 30% incidence of neoplastic lesions in this setting. Furthermore, the mucosa can be evaluated for evidence of ischemia, especially if the patient develops abdominal pain or tenderness.

■ SURGERY

The majority of patients with lower gastrointestinal bleeding stop spontaneously and never need surgery. Surgery is reserved for the 10 to 25% of patients who continue hemorrhaging despite nonoperative attempts to control bleeding or who develop massive repeated episodes of bleeding. It has been shown that patients requiring four or more units of blood in the first 24 hours of treatment have a 50% chance of requiring operation. However, because there are no absolute predictors of who will require surgery for lower gastrointestinal bleeding on admission, all patients with massive hemorrhage should be evaluated and treated as though they may eventually require operative exploration and bowel resection.

Every effort should be made to localize the bleeding source preoperatively. If the stability of the patient allows, as many diagnostic modalities as necessary should be utilized to accurately localize the source of bleeding and guide surgical treatment. Not only is blind exploration of the bleeding patient a frustrating and often futile exercise, it is also dangerous. Emergency colectomies for nonlocalized bleeding are associated with a mortality rate of 10 to 30% and, if a segmental resection is performed in this setting, a recurrence rate of bleeding of 33%. Although subtotal colectomy has become the preferred option for nonlocalized bleeding to minimize the risks of rebleeding, this procedure should still be avoided if at all possible. A total abdominal colectomy with ileorectostomy can be a debilitating procedure in the older population, for whom it is frequently necessary. Frequent diarrheal bowel movements associated with varying degrees of incontinence can severely affect quality of life in this group of patients. Over the past 15 to 20 years, our ability to preoperatively localize sites of lower gastrointestinal hemorrhage has improved considerably, thereby obviating the need for this procedure in most patients. Subtotal colectomy should be reserved for patients with significant recurrent bleeding in whom repeated attempts at localization have failed and in whom gastric, small bowel, and rectal sources have been ruled out. Patients in this situation may benefit from intraoperative enteroscopy prior to resection.

When the bleeding site has been localized, segmental resections are the preferred treatment option. Mortality rate in this setting is under 10%, and studies have demonstrated rates of rebleeding ranging from 0 to 14%. The decision to perform an anastomosis depends on intraoperative conditions, as well as the patient's stability and comorbid conditions. Of these factors, continued hemodynamic instability remains the most important determinate in performing a diverting ostomy at the time of operation. Because many of these patients are older and have coexistent disease, prolonging the operation and placing an anastomosis at risk is not wise. Should the situation be equivocal, performing a primary anastomosis with a temporary proximal diverting ileostomy is a useful alternative. Finally, despite blood's being an excellent cathartic, in the urgent or emergency situation bowel preparation is often not adequate to safely perform a primary anastomosis. As long as the patient is hemodynamically stable, intraoperative on-table colonic lavage is an appropriate adjunct to diminish the consequences of anastomotic leak.

The surgeon is occasionally faced with the dilemma of the patient who has had bleeding localized to the right colon. However, extensive left-sided diverticulosis is also present and the question arises as to the performance of a subtotal colectomy. The most appropriate procedure in this setting remains a right hemicolectomy. Multiple studies have shown that the rebleeding rate from left-sided diverticulosis is quite low.

■ THE PROBLEM PATIENT: INTERMITTENT RECURRENT GASTROINTESTINAL BLEEDING

Occasionally, patients will develop acute, self-limited gastrointestinal bleeding and fail to localize on multiple diagnostic studies. It must be emphasized that as long as the patient remains hemodynamically stable, continued diagnostic evaluation is indicated. Blind exploration has virtually no role in this setting. Bleeding scans, angiography, or endoscopic procedures may need to be repeated several times. For patients who do not bleed massively and have significant comorbidities, conservative treatment with intermittent transfusions may ultimately be the most appropriate course.

Aggressive attempts have been made to increase the diagnostic sensitivity of angiography in this setting. Performing "semielective" or "provocative" angiography with the use of agents such as heparin, urokinase, or tolazoline has been demonstrated to increase the yield of positive angiograms from 32 to 65%. Caution must be used with this technique, with the patient understanding that immediate surgical exploration may be required.

The development of small bowel enteroscopy, using both video-endoscopes and the capsule camera, has allowed for identification of obscure bleeding sites that have been hard to detect by other means. This evaluation has been especially beneficial in identifying small bowel ectasias, which are the most common source of bleeding in the small bowel when other tests have been negative. Although video-enteroscopy is somewhat difficult to perform and time-consuming, reported rates of positive findings are as high as 80%. Most important, if diffuse small bowel ectasias are discovered, surgery can be avoided because the rebleeding rate following segmental small bowel resection in this setting approaches 50%. Proximal small bowel lesions may be successfully treated nonoperatively via endoscopic cauterization with the push enteroscope.

As a last resort, intraoperative enteroscopy can be performed. Though technically enteroscopy is a difficult procedure, success rates of greater than 50% have been reported. Unlike conventional colonoscopy, the bowel mucosa should be inspected in an antegrade fashion because significant trauma can occur to the bowel wall, thereby obscuring visualization of potential lesions. One advantage of this technique is the ability to transilluminate the bowel, potentially demonstrating vascular lesions in this way.

Suggested Readings

Boley SJ, Brandt LF: Vascular ectasias of the colon—1986. Dig Dis Sci 1986;31(suppl):265–425.

Browder W, Cerise EJ, Litwin MS: Impact of emergency angiography in massive lower gastrointestinal bleeding. Ann Surg 1986;204:530–536.

Lewis BS, Wenger JS, Waye JD: Small bowel enteroscopy and intraoperative enteroscopy for obscure gastrointestinal bleeding. Am J Gastroenterol 1991;86: 171–174.

Pennoyer WP, Vignati PV, Cohen JL: Management of angiogram positive lower gastrointestinal hemorrhage: Long-term follow-up of nonoperative treatments. Int J Colorectal Dis 1996;11:279–282.

Zuckerman DA, Bocchini TP, Birnbaum EH: Massive hemorrhage in the lower gastrointestinal tract in adults: Diagnostic imaging and interventions. Am J Roentgenol 1993;161:703–711.

54

LARGE BOWEL OBSTRUCTION

L. Peter Fielding, MB, FRCS, FACS

Under normal conditions, stool traverses the gut in liquid, semiliquid, or solid states from the ileocecal valve to the anal verge. Any process that interferes with this orderly progression of bowel content may appear clinically as large bowel obstruction.

Large bowel obstruction is common and remains a challenging clinical problem. Expertise in the areas of clinical evaluation, anatomy, physiology, operative techniques, and critical care is required. There is no substitute for clinical experience for successful treatment in these often very sick patients. In this area of clinical medicine even experienced surgeons should consult with colleagues to discuss clinical options. For the less experienced, such consultations seem mandatory.

Bowel obstruction may be classified in terms of anatomy (see Table 54-1), physiology (see Table 54-2), or diagnosis (see Tables 54-3 and 54-4). However, treatment for an individual patient depends on assessing all the information derived from all these classifications and integrating it into a management plan. This integration of data into a therapeutic strategy calls for considerable experience and clinical judgment. Nevertheless, two basic philosophies underlie all management strategies for patients with large bowel obstruction: first, supportive measures followed by minimal surgery, and second, resuscitation and then resective surgery.

This chapter describes the classifications of large bowel obstruction and provides some insight into the decision-making issues that help to determine management suited to the needs of the patient.

■ ANATOMIC CLASSIFICATION

Although the anatomic features of large bowel obstruction vary, they may be simplified into four groups, as outlined in Table 54-1.

Lesions Extrinsic to the Bowel Wall
Compression of the gut by extrinsic intra-abdominal tumor or abscess sufficient to cause large bowel obstruction is not common. However, simple external pressure caused by bowel angulation in a hernia may be sufficient to obstruct the flow of bowel contents and give rise to a change in bowel habit and eventually the clinical features of obstruction.

The most common lesion in this category is postoperative band adhesion, which although more common in the small bowel, can affect the colon. Furthermore, the site of such adhesive obstruction may form the fulcrum around which a volvulus may occur.

Lesions Intrinsic to the Bowel Wall
These lesions are the most common cause of large bowel obstruction. Not only do conditions of the bowel wall itself cause narrowing, but they also interfere with peristalsis, thus acting as a physiologic "brake" on peristalsis. This effect compounds any bowel narrowing that may be present. Inflammatory bowel disease (particularly Crohn's disease), tumor, and ischemia (acute or chronic) are all quite common etiologies. Other lesions such as endometriosis or postirradiation stricture are rare and may be found to be the cause of obstruction only at laparotomy.

Bowel Obstruction Causes from within the Lumen
The majority of cases in this group are caused by fecal impaction in the rectum, particularly in elderly patients without obvious intrinsic disease. However, it should be noted that the final event that transforms a bowel stricture into full obstruction is probably the impaction of stool in the segment of bowel narrowing. In the presence of a known etiology for bowel narrowing, such stool impaction is, by convention, not used in any classification because it adds little to the description or understanding of the subject.

Although gallstone ileus usually occurs by obturation of a gallstone (which has fistulized into the gut) in the terminal ileum, the stone can travel to the distal sigmoid colon and is a rare cause of large bowel obstruction. Similarly,

---

Table 54-1 Anatomic Classification of Large Bowel Obstruction

1. Lesions extrinsic to the bowel wall
   Compression (tumor, abscess)
   Hernia
   Postoperative adhesion
2. Lesions intrinsic to the bowel wall
   Tumor
   Inflammatory bowel disease
   Diverticular disease
   Endometriosis
   Ischemia
   Postirradiation stricture
3. Lesions within bowel lumen
   Foreign body
   Gallstone obstruction
   Intussusception
      Ileocolic
      Colocolic
      Colorectal
   Fecal impaction
4. Bowel torsion
   Volvulus
      Cecal
      Transverse colon
      Sigmoid colon

foreign bodies passed per anum may become lost and can cause a bowel blockage or even local perforation.

Intussusception of the ileocolic, colocolic, or colorectal type may rarely present as bowel obstruction. The usual focal lesions that form the nidus for the intussusception are a Peyer's patch of the ileum in children and a tumor (benign or malignant) in adults.

Torsion of the Bowel

This condition has special problems of presentation and management. Volvulus may affect the right, transverse, or sigmoid colon, the last being most common. Not only does volvulus cause an obstruction of the proximal bowel, but more importantly, it gives rise to a closed-loop segment of bowel. The closed loop rapidly distends with fluid and gas, and once torsion is complete, becomes ischemic within a few hours. Perforation of the bowel may occur if treatment is delayed for more than 6 to 8 hours and may be seen in the loop itself or at the site of the "bowel twist" because of local ischemic pressure necrosis.

■ PATHOPHYSIOLOGIC CLASSIFICATION

Patients with large bowel obstruction vary greatly in their severity of illness at the time of presentation. Some have simple colicky abdominal pain and distention, with little else. At the other end of the spectrum, some patients have severe systemic decompensation as a consequence of fluid sequestration in the gut and endotoxemia.

Identification of the best treatment for patients with large bowel obstruction has, in recent years, been hampered by the absence of a clear definition of these conditions in relation to the degree of illness of the patient. Table 54-2 presents a simple and clinically useful guide to the degree of obstruction, which helps to determine both preoperative management and intraoperative techniques.

Mild Obstruction—Bowel Stenosis

Stool can accumulate proximal to a bowel stenosis for a long time without any significant systemic effect. However, if the stool exerts local pressure on the bowel wall, mucosal ulceration or even frank perforation may occur. In the absence of these local effects, mild obstruction can be treated as an elective case except for the problem of bowel preparation. Stenotic lesions of the right (or transverse) colon can be treated with right (or extended right) hemicolectomy if care is taken to keep the stool within the bowel lumen. Gut continuity can be established by a standard anastomosis between the ileum and distal colon, which has usually been adequately prepared by enemas. If the distal bowel is not empty, it can be washed out during surgery. Some surgeons believe that this approach should be followed for lesions down to and including the sigmoid colon, with subtotal or total colectomy followed by immediate gut reconstruction. However, others consider that such an extensive bowel resection leads to excessive stool frequency, particularly if anal sphincter function is diminished.

If the proximal colon needs to be retained but there has been poor bowel preparation because of a stenotic lesion, "on table" gut irrigation is a useful technique (see later discussion).

Moderate Bowel Obstruction—Stenotic Lesion with Proximal Accumulation of Fluid and Gas

The presence of fluid and gas proximal to a site of obstruction is a common and very important event in the overall pathophysiology of large bowel obstruction. Such accumulation is a universal finding in both large and small bowel once complete obstruction has been present for a few days. This clinical entity has been reproduced in subacute and chronic forms in animal models.

In the early stages of gas and fluid accumulation, there is progressive bacterial overgrowth (especially *Bacteroides* species), an increase in bowel wall thickness due to edema, and an increase in blood flow to the bowel. As a very late event, in massively dilated proximal bowel or in the closed-loop obstruction, the bowel eventually becomes ischemic and may undergo necrosis.

A full pathophysiologic explanation of these observations is not yet available, but a coherent picture that explains the clinical features found in patients who have the most severe type of bowel obstruction associated with systemic change is emerging.

Severe Obstruction—Gas and Fluid Accumulation Together with Systemic Changes

Some patients with bowel obstruction not only have advanced changes in the gut but also exhibit cardiorespiratory and venomotor tone problems. These features may be explained by a combination of events: sequestration of fluid and electrolytes into the bowel lumen, increased blood flow to the obstructed segment, migration of endotoxin from the bowel lumen into the portal circulation, and translocation of bacteria through the bowel wall into the peritoneal cavity and portal circulation.

These events are often played out against a background of cardiorespiratory disease or other metabolic conditions such as hypothyroidism or diabetes. Thus, it is not sur-

Table 54-2 Classification of Large Bowel Obstruction Based on Physiologic Effects			
DEGREE OF OBSTRUCTION	**SOLIDS ONLY**	**SOLIDS + GAS**	**SOLIDS/GAS ± SYSTEMIC SIGNS**
Mild	+	−	−
Moderate	+	+	−
Severe	+	+	+

prising that some of these patients can be severely compromised because of both local and systemic effects of obstruction. It is clear that they require very special management, and if the clinical relevance of the findings described earlier are accepted, certain conclusions may be drawn.

Protection and maintenance of optimal cardiopulmonary function is of prime importance. The usual cause of early death in these patients is cardiopulmonary failure, and elaborate preventive measures must be taken in order to reduce the high mortality and morbidity rates. For example, there appears to be a somewhat cavalier approach to resuscitation by giving large amounts of fluid and electrolyte solutions, assuming that the patient has adequate cardiac, pulmonary, venomotor, and renal reserves. In a "normal" younger patient, the physiologic reserves in these functions would help compensate for any inappropriately high or low resuscitative volume measures. However, in the more frail elderly patient, these reserve functions may not be present, and very careful and repeated evaluations are required to determine the effects of treatment as the treatment is being given.

These patients should be monitored in an intensive care unit. In the more difficult cases, a Swan-Ganz catheter should be inserted, and mechanical ventilation and full parenteral nutritional support should be instituted early in clinical management.

None of these recommendations are new. It is necessary to support these patients vigorously and to remove the source of the problem. In the past, the source was thought to be the obstructing lesion itself. We now understand that the problem is caused by physiologic changes in the whole length of the dilated and edematous bowel; the blood flow to this dilated segment is greatly increased, and there is leakage of fermenting luminal contents into the portal circulation with translocation of bacteria. In patients who are systemically compromised, the removal of the dilated plethoric bowel, as well as the cause of the obstruction itself, may provide significant clinical advantage.

Whatever the eventual explanation of the pathophysiologic events, it is clear that these patients require very careful and comprehensive management, with treatment directed to the relief of the obstruction, removal of intraluminal fluid, and excision of physiologically compromised bowel, while supporting the principal organ systems during the initial recovery period.

■ DIAGNOSES ASSOCIATED WITH LARGE BOWEL OBSTRUCTION

The most common causes of large bowel obstruction have been mentioned in Table 54-1. Inhibition of peristalsis may occur secondary to other systemic regional or organ-based conditions (Table 54-3); of greater rarity are those conditions in which there is a primary abnormality of peristaltic activity (Table 54-4). These comprehensive and rather diverse diagnostic lists cover a vast field of medicine, and the conditions listed in Tables 54-3 and 54-4 are presented for completeness but are all rare.

Table 54-3 Causes of Inhibition of Intestinal Peristaltic Activity
Peritoneal causes
Sepsis (local or generalized)
Irritation from foreign body or chemical agent
Infarcted bowel
Intraperitoneal blood
Extraperitoneal intra-abdominal causes
Extra- or retroperitoneal
Bleeding
Spinal injury
Pelvic fracture
Aortic aneurysm
Pancreatitis
Severe pain, e.g., renal or biliary colic
Extra-abdominal causes
Myocardial infarction
Pneumonia
Intracranial hemorrhage or thrombosis
Neurosurgical procedure
Thoracic injury
Immobilization with plaster casts
Systemic causes
Electrolyte problems: hypokalemia, hypomagnesemia
Metabolic problems: alkalosis, uremia, diabetes
Drugs: anticholinergics, narcotics, ganglion-blocking agents

Source: Sykes P: Management of postoperative bowel distension and obstruction. In Fielding LP, Welch J (Eds.). Intestinal Obstruction. London, Churchill Livingstone, 1987, p 164.

However, the conditions listed in Table 54-1 are the principal causes of large bowel obstruction and may present different degrees of clinical problems, as classified in Table 54-2. After investigation, some patients are found to have an apparent (pseudo-) mechanical type of bowel distention; they are considered later as a separate group.

■ MANAGEMENT

All these patients require management that is divided into three distinct phases: resuscitation, preoperative management, and operative strategy.

Resuscitation
The tests that should be considered for all patients presenting with bowel obstruction are listed in Table 54-5. All patients require intravenous hydration. Vomiting indicates the need for nasogastric intubation. Pre-existing cardiac disease suggests that central venous pressure monitoring should be established, whereas a history of congestive heart failure with cardiac insufficiency or frank failure indicates the need for a Swan-Ganz catheter to take the appropriate measurements, to calculate cardiac output, and to assess fluid requirements.

Preoperative Management
Once the patient has been resuscitated, operation is necessary in the great majority unless (1) an enema has disimpacted the obstruction sufficiently to allow decompression,

Table 54-4 Diseases that Cause Gastrointestinal Motility Disturbance

SMOOTH MUSCLE DISEASES	NEUROLOGIC DISEASE
Visceral myopathy	Visceral neuropathy
Familial	Familial
Nonfamilial	Nonfamilial
Collagen disease	Parkinson's disease
Scleroderma	Hirschsprung's disease
Dermatomyositis	Chagas' disease
Systemic lupus erythematosus	Ganglioneuroma of intestine
Muscular dystrophies	Diabetes mellitus
Myotonic dystrophy	Pheochromocytoma
Duchenne's muscular dystrophy	Pharmacologic causes
Metabolic disturbances	Phenothiazines
Myxedema	Tricyclic antidepressants
Hypoparathyroidism	Antiparkinsonian medications
Porphyria	Ganglionic blockers
Miscellaneous	Clonidine
Eosinophilic gastroenteritis	*Amanita* (mushroom) poisoning
Chronic radiation enteritis	
Amyloidosis	

Source: Anuras S, Shirazi SS: Severe gastrointestinal motility disturbance mimicking bowel obstruction. In Fielding LP, Welch J (Eds.). Intestinal Obstruction. London, Churchill Livingstone, 1987, p 154.

(2) a volvulus has been decompressed by intubation, or (3) a pseudomechanical obstruction has been identified and successfully treated by endoscopy. Quite recently, a new technique of "stenting" neoplastic obstructing lesions has been described, and this technique may be a useful new method to treat such acute obstructions and allow for elective investigation and treatment to take place. (See Suggested Readings at the end of this chapter.)

Perioperative antibiotics should be administered. All patients undergoing large bowel surgery, with the exception of those with a confirmed diagnosis of lesions on the right side of the colon (proximal to the splenic flexure), should be placed in the extended lithotomy position.

Operative Strategy

In all operative plans, even before exploration is undertaken, the colon should be decompressed by removing accumulated gas. The technique is simple; a 21-gauge needle is attached to a sucker and passed obliquely through a tenia into the transverse colon. Pressure is applied in both flanks to force gas from the ascending and descending colon segments to the transverse colon. The needle point must be kept in the gas bubble, or it will soon become blocked with liquid feces. The colon collapses rapidly with this maneuver. In the unusual circumstance that the small bowel is also distended in such a way as to hamper exploration and surgery, it is emptied by retrograde "stripping" of its liquid contents into the stomach which are then withdrawn through a wide-bore nasogastric tube.

Once these general measures have been achieved, the strategy of surgical management depends on the cause of the bowel obstruction.

■ LARGE BOWEL CANCER

Choice of Operation

The practice of surgery is a process of evolution rather than revolution. It evolves with increased understanding of surgical physiology and of the general principles of patient management. From the earliest years, the problems of large bowel surgery in the presence of obstruction have centered on (1) the prevention and treatment of sepsis if the obstructed bowel content contaminates the peritoneal cavity, (2) the difficulty of handling grossly distended bowel, and (3) the questions of primary versus delayed anastomosis. To deal with these impediments, the standard procedure has been to overcome the obstructing element by proximal decompression without contamination and then to return later to undertake a definitive procedure. This approach greatly prolongs total hospital stay and is associated with considerable risk of death. Furthermore, some patients who originally intended to have their tumor resected never complete the three-stage procedure. Thus, there is an a priori case for considering resection at the first laparotomy—a fact that was intuitively realized by Paul and Mickulicz when they introduced their extraperitoneal operation with a double-barreled colostomy. However, this procedure does not include an adequate lymph node and mesenteric clearance and thus is an unsatisfactory cancer operation today.

Until quite recently the three-stage method—proximal colostomy, tumor resection, and colostomy closure—was standard. Progress has since come from two sources: (1) extension of the colectomy to a subtotal removal and (2) methods for decompression and preparation of the bowel on the operating table that permit primary anastomosis.

Table 54-5 Investigations to Be Considered for Patients with Bowel Obstruction
BLOOD
Hemoglobin
White blood cell count
Blood smear
Platelets
Blood group
BIOCHEMISTRY
Urea
Electrolytes
Creatinine
Osmolality
Glucose level
Blood cultures
Clotting screen
LUNGS
Chest x-ray film
Blood gases
Lung function tests
Sputum culture
HEART
Electrocardiogram
Central venous pressure
Pulmonary artery wedge pressure
KIDNEYS/URINE
Volume
Glucose
Urea
Electrolytes
Osmolality
Culture
ABDOMEN
Plain x-ray films
Intravenous pylorogram
Barium/Gastrografin enema
Computed tomographic scan

In 1966, Hughes reported on the use of extended right hemicolectomy with primary ileocolic anastomosis in the treatment of obstructing colonic cancer. In most instances the ileocecal valve is competent in malignant colonic obstruction and the small bowel is essentially normal; consequently, it is suitable for anastomosis. If the large bowel is removed completely down to the usual level beyond the growth, an ileocolic anastomosis can be performed safely. Because many obstructing growths are in the descending or sigmoid colon, a subtotal colectomy with ileosigmoid or ileorectal anastomosis is necessary.

This operation is a well-conceived and satisfactory procedure in many instances but has two potential disadvantages: (1) the water-absorbing surface of the colon is quite drastically reduced and bowel motions tend to be semiformed or loose and occur with increased frequency, and (2) if the patient is elderly and there has been some loss of sphincter activity, he or she may have difficulty in controlling the altered fecal load. Radical subtotal colectomy should therefore be reserved for patients who are young or have good sphincter function. The operation, which is not much greater in magnitude than a regional colectomy, has the additional advantage of reducing the area of colonic mucosa at risk from metachronous cancer and simplifies follow-up. It is certainly the procedure of choice for lesions that extend down to the distal aspect of the splenic flexure.

Beyond this point many surgeons will feel more comfortable if the proximal large bowel can be preserved. Two methods other than formal three-stage management are available. The first is radical resection with an end-colostomy and mucous fistula or, for a more distal growth, a Hartmann's procedure; the second is resection and primary anastmosis.

Many surgeons are choosing these options, as evidenced by the spontaneous increase in primary resections during the course of the Large Bowel Cancer Study, in which the figures for this procedure have changed from about 50% in 1976 to 80% 4 years later.

Operative Details

For all resections a medial-to-lateral dissection should be done (vascular pedicle first followed by tumor isolation and then resection). Although Turnbull's personal results did not establish this as the treatment of choice, more recent work has suggested that the burden of proof that Turnbull's "no touch" technique is inappropriate now lies with those who oppose it.

If the surgeon chooses to perform a primary resection without anastomosis, the rest of the technique is conventional and does not require further description except to emphasize the need to mobilize the splenic flexure thoroughly so that redissection is not required at the time of restoration of bowel continuity.

Resection with immediate anastomosis should take place only if the bowel is emptied at operation. Numerous series attest to the importance of fecal loading in the genesis of anastomostic complications. Some surgeons have reported small series of "instant preparation" using intraluminal antibiotics or antiseptics, but this approach tempts fate. Antegrade "on-table" irrigation is the most favored method of intraoperative bowel preparation described elsewhere. In summary, a large-bore (No. 20 Fr) Foley catheter is inserted into the cecum either via the appendix stump, if that organ is present, or within a purse-string suture in the cecum. A soft clamp is applied before the incision is made. Corrugated anesthetic tubing is inserted into the distal colon and secured. About 4 L of warm, physiologically balanced saline solution are now run into the bowel from proximal to distal end with bowel contents being "encouraged" to pass through the anesthetic scavenging tubing and into a closed-circuit receptacle on the operating room floor. When the effluent is clear, the cecum and ascending colon usually contain a pool of saline solution, which is quite easy to expel if the 3-L bag reservoir is placed on the operating room floor with the clamp open; the fluid will siphon out of the colon.

Once the colon has been irrigated and then emptied in both directions, the Foley catheter is removed and the appendix stump or cecum is closed in the usual way. The distal colon is trimmed back to undamaged bowel in preparation for a one-layer end-to-end anastomosis, which is carried out after the distal bowel has been washed per rectum.

One of the criticisms of this technique for primary anastomosis is that the proximal bowel is dilated, edematous, and flaccid and is therefore unsuitable for an anastomosis. However, after operative decompression and "on-table" lavage, we have not found this to be true; the bowel immediately reverts to near-normal size and edema diminishes, leaving a bowel suitable for an anastomosis.

Gastrostomy is less popular now than it was in the last 2 decades; moreover, its efficacy has never been conclusively confirmed or refuted by a prospective randomized trial. Nevertheless, it is a rational method to drain the stomach effectively in patients over the age of 50 who have had a major operation as an emergency and in whom unequivocal recovery of bowel function may be delayed. These views are supported by a recent review. In addition, although the serious complication rate should be kept low, a gastrostomy can make the management of patients with intra-abdominal sepsis with temporary intestinal failure much easier.

If the patient presents with substantial systemic problems caused by very advanced intestinal obstruction, it seems prudent to decompress the bowel thoroughly at the time of surgery but to bring the proximal colon out as a colostomy and distal end as a mucous fistula or, if there is inadequate bowel length, to oversew the distal end as a Hartmann-type procedure.

It should be mentioned that a substantial number of surgeons feel uncomfortable about this activist approach for left-sided colonic obstruction caused by tumor. These surgeons may prefer fashioning a so-called "defunctioning" transverse loop colostomy and performing a definitive resection at a later date. However, review of this particular policy demonstrates that the overall mortality and morbidity rates for all operations associated with the management of the obstruction are approximately the same as those for the more activist approach of immediate tumor resection.

DIVERTICULAR DISEASE

Diverticulitis may give rise to bowel stenosis, but the subsequent obstruction is usually slow in onset. The descending colon does not dilate because of muscular hypertrophy, and most of the distention occurs in the right and transverse parts of the colon. These patients can usually be prepared with a few days of intravenous fluids, preoperative antibiotics, and absence of all oral intake and enemas. A one-stage resection and anastomosis are then possible.

By contrast, some patients are systemically sick and have a dramatic increase in the size of the cecum. These patients require urgent surgical treatment and bowel decompression by transverse loop colostomy through a right upper transverse abdominal incision.

However, obstruction of the sigmoid colon in patients with diverticular disease may be secondary to a large abscess located in the left lower quadrant with bowel perforation. Today, the trend in these patients is to drain the abscess and carry out bowel resection at a later date. Immediate bowel reconstruction is controversial. The concept of on-table bowel irrigation is applicable in the management of such patients and has already been described.

VOLVULUS

Volvulus of the sigmoid colon with minimal proximal distention may be treated in low-risk patients by immediate resection and anastomosis. In most cases, however, the patients are elderly and debilitated. Decompression with rigid sigmoidoscopy and a long rectal tube or by a colonoscope can serve as the first procedure and should be attempted gently in every patient. If rectal tube or colonoscopic detorsion is not successful, a laparotomy is needed. In the past, simple detorsion has been practiced, but surgeons need to be aware that once the contained bowel content is released into the proximal and distal colons, a sudden deterioration of cardiopulmonary function may occur. Furthermore, the site of torsion may have undergone ischemic necrosis and would need to be inspected extremely carefully to assess the possibility of delayed perforation. This author's preference is *not to untwist* the volvulus but to resect the area and carry out a delayed anastomosis or to utilize the "on-table" irrigation methods already described to achieve a primary anastomosis in patients who are generally fit.

Torsion of the cecum is often followed very rapidly by the onset of bowel necrosis, and immediate operation is indicated. A one-stage resection and anastomosis is the best procedure because simple detorsion is likely to be followed by recurrence at an early date. Consequently, if resection does not seem feasible, a cecostomy should be performed to fix the cecum in its proper position.

Volvulus of the transverse colon is rare. It is best treated by transverse colectomy or extended right hemicolectomy, depending on the state of the proximal bowel. A delayed anastomosis may be wise in a systemically debilitated patient for the reasons already discussed.

INFLAMMATORY DISEASES OF THE BOWEL

Inflammatory bowel disease may give rise to bowel obstruction by the onset of either toxic megacolon or stricture. The most common forms of inflammatory bowel disease in the United States are mucosal ulcerative colitis, Crohn's disease, and antibiotic-associated colitis. Amebiasis is quite frequent in the tropics.

Toxic megacolon is initially treated by fluid replacement, appropriate antibiotics, and high doses of steroids. In the absence of substantial and clear-cut improvement within 48 hours, surgical treatment is mandatory. The operative approach is controversial. Many surgeons advocate total colectomy, ileostomy, and distal mucous fistula. An anastomosis is contraindicated. Others follow the teaching of Turnbull and create a loop ileostomy to defunction the colon and "blow-hole" stomas in the most dilated segments, usually the transverse colon. Both techniques require considerable expertise to make them successful, and the author prefers a policy of early surgery and bowel resection.

Benign strictures can occur in patients with inflammatory bowel disease because of an inflammatory phlegmon or postinflammatory fibrosis. The former may settle with aggressive treatment, but the latter, if symptomatic, requires resection. On histologic examination, some fibrotic strictures are shown to be tumors, and thus, preoperative biopsy is necessary to help guide management.

■ COLONIC ILEUS

This group of conditions is characterized by failure of peristalsis in the absence of mechanical bowel obstruction.

Postoperative Ileus
Nasogastric sump suction instituted before an operative procedure and continued for a few days thereafter will prevent most cases of postoperative ileus. However, when it occurs, paralytic ileus may be manifested in the entire colon. It is closely related to toxic megacolon but can be treated with much greater safety by colonoscopy.

Ogilvie's Syndrome
This condition is common, particularly in the elderly and in those with psychiatric problems or laxative abuse. In these patients, there appears to be a mechanical obstruction distal to the splenic flexure, but on investigation, no organic stenotic lesion can be found. Colonic decompression by colonoscopy is the simplest and most effective therapy, but it may need to be repeated. If this method is not available or is unsuccessful, a cecostomy performed under local anesthesia can be a lifesaving measure.

Other Colonic Motility Disturbances
Although they are rare, these conditions may be extremely difficult to treat. They may occur in the presence of some other systemic disease, such as scleroderma, Chagas' disease, or diabetes. Furthermore, there is a group of ill-defined diseases that seem to merge with the problems of chronic constipation and appear to be due to motility disturbances of the colon (see Table 54-4). Such patients all appear to have increased transit times through the colon; for some, this may become intolerable. Obviously, every attempt should be made to treat these problems with medical methods such as laxatives and enemas; however, medical therapy tends to become progressively less effective.

In a few instances it may be necessary to resort to an ileostomy or colostomy or even a colectomy to relieve obstructive colicky abdominal pain and distention. Obviously, this measure should be used only as a method of last resort, but it can bring complete relief to a small group of patients.

■ INTUSSUSCEPTION

Bowel intussusception is most common in children and is nearly always of the ileocecal type. In many instances it can be treated by a carefully administered barium enema and in others by operative reduction. Resection is necessary only when the intussusception is irreducible, which is quite unusual.

By contrast, in adults idiopathic ileocolic intussusception is rare, and in most cases a tumor such as a lipoma, colonic polyp, or malignant tumor is the nidus at the apex of the lesion. Reduction of the intussusception is usually difficult and unsuccessful; thus, resection and anastomosis become the treatment of choice.

■ OBTURATION OBSTRUCTION

Obturation obstruction may be caused by a gallstone impacted in the sigmoid colon, a barium rock that will not pass through an area of stricture, or a large fecalith. Masses of agglutinated vegetable products can form bezoars that nearly always obstruct the small bowel rather than the colon. If a gallstone is suspected, its size on x-ray film may be misleading because it is often larger than the central calcification visible. Air in the biliary tract may be seen if looked for carefully, and a barium enema or colonoscopy can be helpful to establish a diagnosis. At the time of operation, if there is no distal obstruction, the foreign body may be pushed back into a normal segment and removed by colotomy.

The colon may become incarcerated in a hernia and become obstructed. At the time of operation the bowel must be carefully inspected for ischemia, particularly at the site of the internal hernial opening where a narrow band of necrosis may have occurred. In the absence of such local or segmental ischemia, the colon is returned to the abdominal cavity and no further procedure is necessary. Local ischemia to the segment often relents once the constricting ring is released and warm packs are placed around the bowel for some minutes. If the ischemia does not diminish or if there are bands of focal necrosis, segmental resection will be required, and the abdomen formally opened to manage this injury. A narrow band of questionable bowel may be imbricated with a series of musculoserosal sutures, making sure that a significant narrowing of the bowel is avoided.

■ IATROGENIC OBSTRUCTION

Strictures may occur after resection and anastomosis. Factors that increase the chances of postanastomotic stricture are an extraperitoneal location in the middle or low rectum, an anastomosis made in inflamed bowel, prolonged disuse of the anastomosed segment, and perianastomotic sepsis (which usually implies an anastomotic leak). Such strictures have been noted after both hand-sewn or stapled anastomoses but seem to be more common with the latter, particularly when an end-to-end stapler has been used. Early passage of fecal matter through an anastomosis has been shown to reduce the formation of strictures both experimentally and clinically. Thus, the largest-sized staple machine should be used, which usually mandates the mobilization of splenic flexure to obtain soft distensible bowel in order to receive the apparatus.

If some type of colonic decompression has been used in such patients, it is wise to be assured of the integrity of the anastomosis and to close the stoma within 1 month after the original operation to avoid this problem. Late strictures also may occur if a resection has been done in an area of active inflammation due to Crohn's disease.

Ischemic strictures are rare but may occur, for example, if the inferior mesenteric artery is ligated at the time of aortic aneurysmectomy (or after an episode of ischemic colitis). These strictures are preferably treated by resection and anastomosis, but if this is impossible, a proximal stoma is necessary.

Radiation strictures are very difficult to treat successfully because tissue healing, including suture lines, is impeded by lack of blood supply. Proximal stomas placed in the transverse colon may be the only option. In a few instances in which radiation therapy has spared the extraperitoneal rectum, the transverse or ascending colon can be used for anastomosis after a wide resection has been carried out.

■ OBSTRUCTION IN CHILDREN

Bowel distention in children is a specialist's subject and is not considered in this chapter. Intussusception, necrosing enterocolitis, Hirschsprung's disease, and imperforate anus are the most frequent causes, and all require treatment by a specialist.

Suggested Readings

Anuras S, Shirazi SS: Severe gastrointestinal motility disturbance mimicking bowel obstruction. In Fielding LP, Welch J (Eds.). Intestinal Obstruction. London, Churchill Livingstone, 1987, p 154.

Canon CL, Baron TH, Morgan DE, et al: Treatment of colonic obstruction with expandable metal stents: Radiologic features. Am J Roentgenol 1997;168:199.

Fielding LP: Colonic surgery for acute conditions: Obstruction. In Fielding LP, Goldberg SM (Eds.). Rob and Smith's Operative Surgery, 5th ed. London, Chapman & Hall Medical, 1996, pp 397–415.

Fielding LP, Welch J (Eds.): Intestinal Obstruction. London, Churchill Livingstone, 1987, pp 49–56, 127–138, 139–152.

Hughes ESR: Mortality of acute large bowel obstruction. Br J Surg 1966;53:593–594.

Kozarek RA, Brandabur JJ, Raltz SL: Expandable stents: Unusual locations. Am J Gastroenterol 1997;92:812.

Lowden AGR: Deflation of distended bowel at operation. Lancet 1951;1:1103–1104.

Paul FT: Personal experiences in the surgery of the large bowel. Lancet 1912;2:217–226.

Phillips RKS, Hittinger R, Fielding LP: Malignant large bowel obstruction. Br J Surg 1985;72:296–302.

Sykes P: Management of postoperative bowel distension and obstruction. In Fielding LP, Welch J (Eds.): Intestinal Obstruction. London, Churchill Livingstone, 1987, p 164.

Tejero E, Fernandez-Lobato R, Mainar A, et al: Initial results of a new procedure for treatment of malignant obstruction of the left colon. Dis Colon Rectum 1997;40:432.

Turnbull RB, Kyle K, Watson FR, Spratt J: Cancer of the colon: The influence of the no-touch isolation technic on survival rates. Ann Surg 1967;166:420–427.

Von Mickulicz J: Small contributions to the surgery of the intestinal tract. Boston Med Surg J 1903;148:608–611.

Welch CE: Obstruction and pseudo-obstruction of the gastrointestinal tract. In Malt RA, Moncure AC, Ottinger LW (Eds.): Complex Operations at the Massachusetts General Hospital. Philadelphia, WB Saunders, 1983, p 64.

Wiggers T, Arends JW, Jeekel J, et al: The "no-touch" isolation technique in colon cancer. A prospective controlled trial. J Exp Clin Cancer Res 1983;2(suppl):37.

55

VOLVULUS OF THE COLON

David N. Bimston, MD
Steven J. Stryker, MD

■ HISTORY

Volvulus of the colon was first recorded in ancient Egypt in the Ebers Papyrus, which describes the natural history of sigmoid volvulus. Hippocrates (about 400 BC) noted that certain bowel obstructions, possibly representing sigmoid volvulus, could be decompressed by the insertion of a long suppository. In the mid-19th century this lesson was once again proposed by Gay, who recognized that in cadavers a sigmoid volvulus could be detorsed by the insertion of a tube per rectum. However, because of high surgical mortality rates, the care of colonic volvulus remained noninterventional until the early 20th century, when improved operative techniques and perioperative care allowed surgical intervention to become standard. The last major therapeutic advance took place in 1947 when Bruusgaard heeded the lesson of Hippocrates and demonstrated a significantly reduced mortality rate in sigmoid volvulus treated acutely with endoscopic decompression.

■ INCIDENCE, ETIOLOGY, AND PATHOGENESIS

Sigmoid volvulus is the third most common cause of colon obstruction in developed Western countries after cancer and diverticulitis, and accounts for 2 to 4% of intestinal obstructions. In many third-world countries, however, sigmoid volvulus is the most common cause of large bowel obstruction and can account for up to 30% of intestinal obstructions. In developed countries the mean age of onset is between 60 and 70 years, whereas in third-world nations the mean age is between 40 and 50 years. This regional variation in age and incidence may be related to a difference in etiology. The basic anatomic abnormality noted in all patients with volvulus is a redundant loop of sigmoid colon with a narrow base of attachment of the mesosigmoid. Some hypothesize that the high-fiber diet common to third-world countries may somehow result in colonic redundancy and account for the regional variation in incidence and age. In the United States and Europe the usual patient is elderly and has a history of chronic constipation or cathartic/laxative abuse. Less often, they may be institutionalized secondary to a neuropsychiatric disorder. Colonic motility disorders may

cause the sigmoid redundancy found in this group of patients. Volvulus also has an increased incidence in patients with colonic motility disorders such as Hirschsprung's or Chagas' disease.

Cecal volvulus often complicates acute medical conditions. Patients present 10 to 20 years younger than those with sigmoid volvulus, and have different precipitating factors including pregnancy, recent surgery, obstructing lesions of the left colon, or congenital malrotation/bands. Cadaveric studies have demonstrated that between 11 and 22% of the U.S. population have a cecum with enough mobility to develop a volvulus. Like sigmoid volvulus, the pathogenesis of cecal volvulus involves an organoaxial rotation of the bowel, which leads to a closed-loop obstruction of the lumen and mesenteric blood flow obstruction. As intraluminal pressure and venous obstruction increase, arterial inflow becomes compromised, leading to bowel gangrene.

Cecal bascule, a condition in which the bowel folds anteriorly and superiorly over a fixed ascending colon, is often mistaken for a form of cecal volvulus. It presents as acute bowel obstruction, but unlike volvulus there is no axial rotation of the bowel and no concomitant mesenteric vascular obstruction. When it does occur, gangrene is caused solely by increased intraluminal tension.

■ DIAGNOSIS

Both sigmoid and cecal volvulus often present with abdominal pain and distention, nausea and vomiting, constipation or obstipation, and an empty rectum. Forty to 60 percent of patients with sigmoid volvulus have a history of previous similar attacks. Plain abdominal radiograms have been shown to be diagnostic in over 50% of cases of sigmoid volvulus and when combined with barium enemas are diagnostic in 90%. The classic plain radiographic finding of sigmoid volvulus is a markedly distended anhaustral loop of bowel extending from the left lower quadrant to the right upper quadrant and resembling a "bent inner tube" or "omega" (Fig. 55-1A and B). When barium is used to evaluate sigmoid volvulus, a tapering opacity reminiscent of a "bird's beak" is formed by the column of contrast (Fig. 55-1C). Radiographic studies are less successful in diagnosing cecal volvulus. Plain radiographs can lead to the correct diagnosis in as few as 20% of cases because the accompanying small bowel dilatation can result in a misdiagnosis of small bowel obstruction. The classic plain x-ray demonstrates a distended loop of bowel in the left upper quadrant, which has retained haustral marking, and a right lower quadrant void of the cecum (Fig. 55-2A and B). As with sigmoid volvulus, barium enema can increase the diagnostic accuracy of plain films to 50 to 90%. Computed tomographic (CT) scan technology can also be used to evaluate colonic volvulus. A "whirl" sign has been described to represent the tightly twisted mesentery of the afferent and efferent limbs of the volvulus (Fig. 55-3). Although a column of barium can act as both a diagnostic and therapeutic agent by identifying and detorsing a volvulus, most authors no

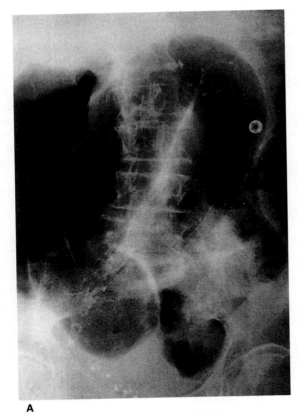

A

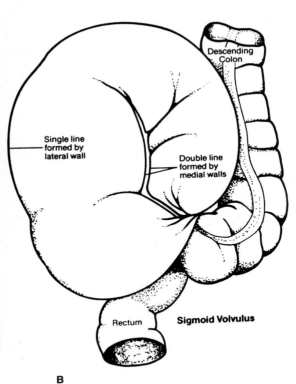

B

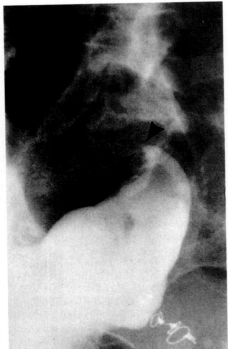

C

Figure 55-1

A, Supine abdominal radiograph of sigmoid volvulus. *B*, Diagram of sigmoid volvulus. *C*, Barium enema of the twisted colon of sigmoid volvulus represented as a "bird's beak." (*A* and *C* from Messmer JM: Gas and soft tissue abnormalities. In Gore RM, et al [Eds.]. Textbook of Gastrointestinal Radiology. Philadelphia, WB Saunders, 1994, pp 176, 1253; *B* from Rennell C, McCort JJ: Bowel gas and fluid. In McCort JJ [Ed.]. Abdominal Radiology. Baltimore, Williams & Wilkins, 1981, pp 97–180.)

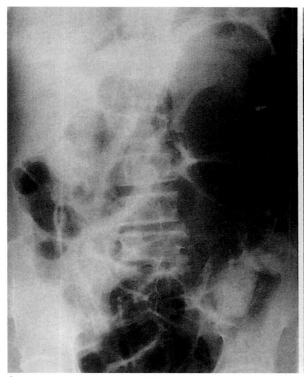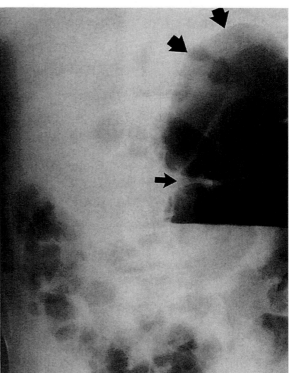

A

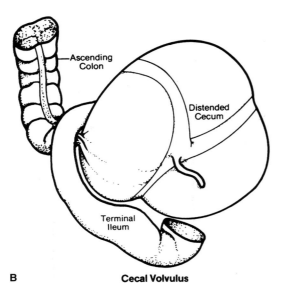

B   **Cecal Volvulus**

Figure 55-2
A, Supine abdominal radiograph of cecal volvulus demonstrating distended cecum, dilated terminal ileum, and a right lower quadrant devoid of colon. *B*, Diagram. (*A* from Gore RM, Eisenberg RL: In Gore RM, et al [Eds.]. Textbook of Gastrointestinal Radiology. Philadelphia, WB Saunders, 1994, pp 177, 1253; *B* from Rennell C, McCort JJ: Bowel gas and fluid. In McCort JJ [Ed.]. Abdominal Radiology. Baltimore, Williams & Wilkins, 1981, pp 97–180.)

longer use this method therapeutically because of the risk of bowel perforation and the inability to examine the colon for ischemic changes. Endoscopy is now the gold standard for both the diagnosis and therapy of sigmoid volvulus and plays an important role in the diagnosis of cecal volvulus.

■ OPERATIVE THERAPY

Timing of Surgery

The decision for operative intervention is based upon two criteria: (1) the possibility of colonic ischemia and (2) failure of endoscopic detorsion. When evaluating the patient

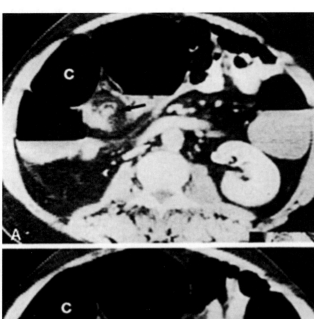

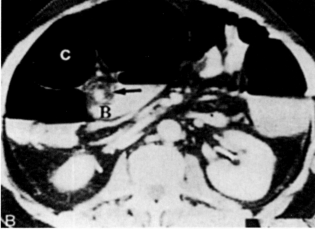

Figure 55-3
Computed tomographic scan images of colonic volvulus demonstrating a "whirl sign" (*arrow*). The distended proximal colon (C) and a "beak sign" (B) leading into the volvulus are also seen. (From Shaff MI, Himmelfarb E, Sacks GA, et al: The whirl sign: A CT finding in volvulus of the large bowel. J Comput Assist Tomogr 1985;9:410.)

with suspected volvulus the examiner must determine whether the patient has a viable colon and is a candidate for endoscopic therapy or has an ischemic colon and must go emergently to the operating room for resection. Fever, peritonitis, and leukocytosis are the findings most consistent with colon ischemia but are neither sensitive nor specific. Lactic acidosis is not a sensitive test for early colonic ischemia but is highly suggestive of bowel infarction. Patients with one or more of the foregoing findings should be considered for urgent operative intervention for suspected ischemic bowel. If endoscopic decompression is successful (75 to 90% of cases) and no ischemic changes or blood is noted in the colon, then elective colon resection is pursued. Elective resection is recommended during the same hospital admission because recurrence rates of 40 to 50% have been reported after endoscopic decompression alone. If endoscopic decompression fails or

ischemic changes are found in the colon, emergent operation is indicated.

Preoperative Preparation
Patients with volvulus, as with all forms of closed loop bowel obstruction, present with significant fluid and electrolyte imbalances. Preoperative optimization begins with intravascular fluid repletion (0.9% saline or lactated Ringer's solution) and correction of electrolyte abnormalities. Blood products may be required in patients with anemia and significant cardiac disease. In patients with a significant comorbid condition or cardiac disease, Swan-Ganz monitoring may be warranted.

Nasogastric decompression should be performed in all forms of colonic volvulus. Decompression is helpful in (1) differentiating volvulus from acute gastric distention, (2) relieving gastric dilation and minimizing further small bowel distention, and (3) preventing aspiration.

Sigmoid Volvulus
The surgical management of sigmoid volvulus is determined by the viability of the patient's colon. Colonic gangrene is seen in approximately 5 to 10% of cases of colonic volvulus. When gangrenous bowel is encountered at laparotomy, classic teaching suggests that sigmoid colectomy be performed, followed by the creation of an end-colostomy together with a mucous fistula or a Hartmann's procedure. Although in the presence of gangrene, colectomy is fraught with a 50 to 80% mortality rate, endoscopic or nonoperative therapy is associated with an almost 100% mortality rate. When gangrenous bowel is discovered or there are other unfavorable conditions, such as colonic perforation with peritoneal contamination, sepsis or hemodynamic instability, or the presence of significant comorbidity/malnutrition, we would invariably proceed with colonic resection and Hartmann's closure of the rectal stump.

When viable intestine is encountered at emergency laparotomy the surgeon is faced with a number of therapeutic choices: simple detorsion, colopexy, mesoplasty, tube cecostomy, colectomy with colostomy, and colectomy with primary anastomosis. Simple detorsion is the safest of these procedures. The intraoperative time is limited, the unprepared colon is not opened, and sutures are not placed in the thin or edematous colon wall. However, simple detorsion, like endoscopic decompression, is plagued by a 40 to 50% recurrence rate and must be followed by a second operative procedure. In order to limit recurrence, a number of alternative colonic fixation procedures have been developed: sigmoidopexy—suturing the sigmoid colon to the anterior abdominal wall or in an extraperitoneal pouch; mesoplasty—plicating and shortening the sigmoid mesocolon; and tube colostomy to fix the sigmoid to the abdominal wall. These techniques have never been examined in a large series or in a randomized fashion and have been noted in several reviews to have a high rate of recurrence. More recently, alternative methods to standard -pexy and -plasty procedures have been described. Miller reports laparoscopic fixation of the sigmoid colon to the anterior abdominal wall in several locations in an attempt to prevent recurrence and obviate the need for laparotomy. Other groups have demonstrated the ability to fix the sigmoid colon to the anterior abdominal wall via colonoscopy. Like their traditional counterparts, these newer nonresectional procedures for treating volvulus are anecdotal or small studies and have not provided adequate follow-up to judge long-term efficacy. Colectomy with either creation of a mucous fistula or Hartmann's procedure is a relatively quick technique and eliminates the risk of recurrence but must be followed by a second surgery if colonic continuity is to be restored. We find that conventional sigmoid resection and primary anastomosis can be performed safely in most patients, even in the urgent setting. In these healthier patients, primary anastomosis of the obstructed and unprepared bowel is an option but has not been universally accepted owing to its association with a low, but worrisome, risk of anastomotic leak. More recently, the use of intraoperative colonic irrigation in the management of unprepared large bowel emergencies has been described. This procedure diminishes the fecal load of the unprepared colon and theoretically decreases the risk of anastomosis breakdown. Other authors have described their limited experience with transcolonic tubes to stent and protect the anastomosis from the fecal stream during the process of healing. Both of these methods are relatively new and have not been examined in randomized trials but provide attractive options for future investigations. Our institutional experience suggests that primary anastomosis can be performed in most circumstances with minimal risk of anastomotic leak.

Endoscopic decompression of a sigmoid volvulus is the procedure of choice when bowel viability is not suspect. Numerous studies have reproduced Bruusgaard's high success and low mortality rates for sigmoidoscopic decompression of volvulus. More recent studies employing colonoscopy to reach twisted bowel above the reach of rigid sigmoidoscopy have demonstrated success rates as high as 95%. Because of the 40 to 50% recurrence rates seen after endoscopic decompression, early surgical intervention, usually within the same hospital stay, is recommended. The elective procedure typically performed after successful endoscopic therapy and following preoperative bowel preparation is sigmoid colon resection and primary anastomosis. This operation can be performed safely in most patients but can have mortality rates as high as 15 to 20% in patients when significant comorbidities are present.

Cecal Volvulus

Similar to sigmoid volvulus, the initial management of cecal volvulus is based upon whether or not ischemic bowel is suspected. If the patient appears to have compromised bowel, the appropriate treatment is fluid resuscitation followed by emergency laparotomy and colonic resection. Twenty to 30% of patients with cecal volvulus will be found to have gangrenous bowel on exploration. If bowel gangrene is not suspected, further endoscopic or radiographic examinations may be undertaken to secure a diagnosis. Unlike sigmoid volvulus, endoscopic decompression has not become the gold standard of treatment. Several reports in the literature have demonstrated that endoscopic detorsion of the cecum is technically feasible but demanding, not widely practiced, and often unsuccessful. Instead, operative therapy is recommended after a diagnosis of cecal volvulus has been confirmed.

Several intraoperative methods of treating cecal volvulus are available and include simple detorsion, cecopexy, tube cecostomy, cecopexy with tube cecostomy, and colonic resection. Simple detorsion is associated with a high recurrence rate (10 to 20%) and therefore is not recommended. The risks and benefits of cecopexy, cecostomy, and colonic resection are debated in the literature. Cecopexy does not require that the unprepared colon be opened and therefore is associated with a low rate of infection. However, the distended colon wall is thin and the risk of microperforation during suture placement is high. Several studies have demonstrated recurrence rates similar to detorsion alone. The proponents of this procedure argue that improper suture placement leads to such high recurrence rates. When multiple sutures are placed appropriately along the lateral border of the right colon and around the cecum the recurrence rate can be almost as low as with resection. Tube cecostomy requires that enterotomy be performed and is therefore associated with a higher infection rate than simple cecopexy. Cecostomy, however, allows for decompression of the colon and is associated with a low rate of recurrence (1 to 2%). Anderson and Welch have demonstrated that a combination of tube cecostomy and cecopexy was effective in preventing recurrence over a follow-up period of 9.8 years. Right hemicolectomy has no associated recurrence but is reported in numerous studies to have the highest rate of infection of the three procedures and can be complicated by anastomotic leak. Our institutional experience suggests that right hemicolectomy is the procedure of choice when either gangrenous or viable bowel is encountered. We have found that most patients tolerate colonic resection and primary anastomosis with low rates of infection and anastomotic leak. In unstable patients or those with delayed diagnosis of perforation complicated by fibrinous peritonitis, we recommend hemicolectomy with ileostomy and closure of the transverse colon stump. If a patient is unable to undergo colonic resection secondary to medical instability or significant comorbid illness, we favor tube cecostomy, performed under local anesthesia.

Transverse Colon and Splenic Flexure Volvulus

Isolated cases of both transverse colon and splenic flexure volvulus can be found in the literature. Transverse colon volvulus is associated with a high mortality rate secondary to failure to diagnose, but splenic flexure volvulus is associated with a low mortality rate for unclear reasons. Both are caused by abnormal fixation of the colon and its mesentery. Detorsion is associated with a high recurrence rate in both lesions, and most authors prefer resection with either primary or delayed anastomosis. As with both sigmoid and cecal volvulus, we believe that primary anastomosis can be performed in most circumstances when the patient is unstable or peritoneal soiling is evident.

■ CONCLUSION

Accurate preoperative diagnosis of colonic volvulus can be difficult, and diagnostic delay is associated with a high mortality rate. Although radiologic studies are often instrumental in making a correct diagnosis, prolonged diagnostic investigation can lead to poor outcome. A high level of suspicion and rapid endoscopic/surgical intervention is necessary for optimal treatment.

Acknowledgment. We thank Richard M. Gore, MD, for providing the radiographs, diagrams, and computed tomographic scan of the sigmoid and cecal volvulus. Figures in this chapter have been used with permission of Gore RM, Eisenberg RL: Large bowel obstruction. In Gore RM, Levine MS, Laufer I (Eds.). Textbook of Gastrointestinal Radiology. Philadelphia, WB Saunders, 1994, pp 1247–1260.

Suggested Readings

Anderson JR, Welch GH: Acute volvulus of the right colon: An analysis of 69 patients. World J Surg 1986;10:336–342.

Brothers TE, Strodel WE, Eckhausser FE: Endoscopy in colonic volvulus. Ann Surg 1987;206(1):1–4.

Gibney EJ: Volvulus of the sigmoid colon. Surg Gynecol Obstet 1991;173:243–255.

Miller R, Roe AM, Eltringham WK, Espiner HJ: Laparoscopic fixation of sigmoid volvulus. Br J Surg 1992;79:435.

Peoples JB, McCafferty JC, Scher KS: Operative therapy for sigmoid volvulus: Identification of risk factors affecting outcome. Dis Colon Rectum 1990;33:643–646.

Rabinovici R, Simansky DA, Kaplan O, et al: Cecal volvulus. Dis Colon Rectum 1990;33:765–769.

56

PSEUDO-OBSTRUCTION (OGILVIE'S SYNDROME)

Theodore J. Saclarides, MD
Jacqueline Harrison, MD

Acute colonic pseudo-obstruction (Ogilvie's syndrome) is a poorly understood clinical entity characterized by a non-mechanical, functional obstruction of the large intestine. Its diagnosis may be delayed in a patient who can ill afford the potential morbidity and death this entity carries if not promptly treated. Sir Heneage Ogilvie first described the condition in 1948 while caring for two patients with colonic dilatation without a demonstrable mechanical cause. Both patients had cancer with extensive involvement of the retroperitoneum near the celiac plexus. He hypothesized that this neural involvement produced a functional obstruction. Although little headway has been made in understanding the underlying pathophysiology of colonic pseudo-obstruction, innovations in medical, endoscopic, and minimally invasive surgical techniques may decrease the number of patients requiring laparotomy.

■ SIGNS AND SYMPTOMS

Ogilvie's syndrome may present similarly to a mechanical obstruction, with marked abdominal distention being the most consistent physical finding. Abdominal pain, nausea, vomiting, and constipation are frequent complaints, although the latter is not always present; 40% of patients have diarrhea. Abdominal pain may be colicky in nature, but is frequently a constant pain related to the intestinal distention. Fever can occur, and, if present, must raise suspicion of a perforation. Abdominal tenderness is not a consistent finding (found in only 50% of patients) and if present in the right lower quadrant, one should suspect cecal perforation or ischemia. Bowel sounds may be normal, hypoactive, or even hyperactive and high-pitched. The main diagnostic clue is the clinical setting at presentation. The patient is typically middle-aged or elderly, male (2:1 male-female ratio), and usually hospitalized with a serious systemic illness, an unrelated surgical problem (e.g., coronary bypass, orthopedic surgery), or traumatic injuries (e.g., pelvic fracture, burns) (Table 56-1).

■ LABORATORY AND RADIOLOGIC FINDINGS

Electrolyte derangements are the rule rather than the exception, with hypocalcemia, hyponatremia, and hypokalemia being the most common. Leukocytosis is a variable finding but is especially common in the presence of bowel perforation or necrosis.

Plain abdominal films are frequently diagnostic if interpreted in the context of the preceding clinical presentation. The proximal colon is dilated; the small bowel will be of normal caliber unless an incompetent ileocecal valve permits reflux of air into the ileum. Typically, the dilated colon is gas-filled, haustral markings are maintained, and a transition from proximal dilated to decompressed distal colon is seen at the splenic flexure. This transition point may also be seen at the hepatic flexure or rectosigmoid junction.

Cecal dilatation is marked, frequently in the range of 10 to 14 cm. LaPlace's law ($T = P \bullet R/2$, where T represents wall tension, P is the transmural pressure, and R is the radius of the cylinder) states that the pressure required to stretch the walls of a hollow viscus decreases inversely with radius. Because the cecum is the widest portion of the colon, it will be the area that will dilate the most in response to intraluminal pressure increases, and thus is the most vulnerable portion of the colon to massive dilatation. Perforation is unlikely with a diameter of less than 12 cm but the risk increases markedly at a diameter of 14 cm or higher. A 1986 review of 221 patients by Vanek and Al-Salti reported no cases of perforation or ischemia when cecal diameter was less than 12 cm. At a diameter of 12 to 14 cm, the rate of perforation rose to 7% and climbed to 23% if cecal dilatation was beyond 14 cm. The rate of dilatation may determine the likelihood of perforation as well. Chronically dilated colon is less likely to perforate than bowel that has become acutely dilated. Serial plain abdominal radiographs are very useful in monitoring the progress of therapy and guiding further management.

■ ETIOLOGY

Several hypotheses have been proposed regarding the etiology of pseudo-obstruction, but it is unlikely that any single theory can explain all cases. These theories have one common theme, a disturbance of the normal balance of parasympathetic (stimulation)/sympathetic (inhibition) tone. Parasympathetic activity from the foregut to the splenic flexure is supplied by the vagus nerve; the distal colon receives parasympathetic innervation from sacral nerves 2 through 4. One theory states that massive afferent stimuli to these sacral nerves as a result of pelvic or abdominal surgery or trauma causes a blockade of their efferent activity. In other instances, the anticholinergic activity of certain drugs will decrease parasympathetic activity, thereby creating an atonic segment of bowel. Other authors point to excess sympathetic activity, as with myocardial infarction, surgery, or trauma, as the precipitating cause. As diverse as the associated conditions are, it is likely that these theories overlap, the net result being an imbalance between parasympathetic and sympathetic activity.

Table 56-1 Underlying Conditions Associated with Ogilvie's Syndrome

Cardiovascular	Malignancy
Myocardial infarction	Disseminated metastases
Congestive heart failure	Leukemia
Peripheral vascular disease	Pelvic radiotherapy
Cardiovascular surgery	Retroperitoneal cancer
Aortic aneurysm	Small cell lung cancer
Pulmonary	**Infection/inflammation**
Pneumonia	Sepsis
Mechanical ventilation	Abdominal/pelvic abscess
Pulmonary embolus	Appendicitis
Chronic obstructive pulmonary disease	Cholecystitis
Thoracic surgery	Pancreatitis
	Herpes zoster
Neurologic	Pseudomembranous colitis
Cerebrovascular accident	**Metabolic**
Nerve root compression	
Multiple sclerosis	Electrolyte abnormalities
Subarachnoid hemorrhage	Liver failure
Parkinson's disease	Uremia
Dementia	Diabetes mellitus
	Alcoholism
Trauma	Hypothyroidism
Abdominal trauma	Lead toxicity
Pelvic fracture	**Drugs**
Spinal trauma	
Femoral fracture	Antidepressants
Burns	Phenothiazines
	Opiates
Surgery	Antiparkinsonian drugs
Abdominal surgery	Laxative abuse
Pelvic/gynecologic surgery	Anticholinergics
Cardiovascular surgery	Benzodiazepines
Thoracic surgery	Vincristine
Hip surgery	Interleukin
Craniotomy	Amphetamines
Spinal surgery	Calcium-channel blockers
Cesarean section	Clonidine
Renal transplantation	**Obstetric**
Liver transplantation	
	Postpartum
	Cesarean section

■ DIAGNOSIS

The diagnosis may be suspected based on plain x-ray of the abdomen. Confirmation of the diagnosis and exclusion of a mechanical obstruction can be made with either a water-soluble contrast enema or colonoscopy. These additional studies are contraindicated if the patient has peritonitis; however, in the absence of rebound and guarding, water-soluble contrast enemas may help decompress the colon through their osmotic effect. Colonoscopy serves the dual purpose of ruling out a mechanical obstruction and of evacuating air from the colon, but must be performed with extreme caution as the bowel wall is thin and edematous.

■ TREATMENT

Initial Management

If the diagnosis is suspected and no physical evidence suggests colonic ischemia or perforation, conservative management may be initiated. This approach consists of electrolyte correction, nasogastric decompression (to evacuate swallowed air), restricting oral intake, and withdrawal of possible inciting medications such as opiates or anticholinergics (Fig. 56-1). Some physicians recommend placing a rectal tube for decompression, but this has not proved useful. Serial abdominal physical examinations and x-rays every 12 to 24 hours should be obtained to determine response to the foregoing measures. Cecal

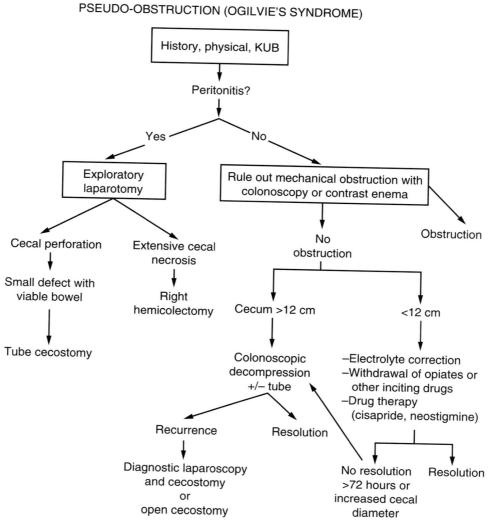

PSEUDO-OBSTRUCTION (OGILVIE'S SYNDROME)

Figure 56-1
Algorithm for the management of acute pseudo-obstruction.

diameter exceeding 12 cm or failure of the patient to improve within 48 to 72 hours is an indication for decompression.

Colonoscopy

The mainstay of decompressive therapy since 1977 has been colonoscopy. Gentle saline enemas can be administered to cleanse the colon of thick stool. Minimal sedation should be used and narcotics are to be avoided. Air should be insufflated in small amounts to prevent further increases in pressure, and the procedure should be aborted and laparotomy performed if there are signs of mucosal ischemia (bloody effluent or hemorrhagic mucosa).

To avoid the need for repeat colonoscopy, different techniques have been described for placing decompressive tubes during the initial endoscopy. A 480-cm guidewire is placed through the biopsy forceps channel, the colonoscope is removed with the wire held stationary, and then a vented enteroclysis tube is threaded over the guidewire. Harig and coworkers noted four of nine patients who had recurrent dilatation following an initially successful colonoscopy; however, no recurrence was seen in 10 patients when a long tube had been inserted. The tubes were left in place for 48 to 72 hours or until colonic motility returned.

A different method for tube placement that does not require a guidewire has been described that employs a Cantor tube with an emptied and cut balloon. The cut end of the balloon is grasped with a polypectomy snare and is positioned in the cecum using a colonoscope. Once the cecum is reached, the balloon is released from the snare and the colonoscope is carefully removed. A kidney, urinary, and bladder x-ray (KUB) is obtained after the procedure to confirm that the tube remained in the cecum, and then the tube is taped to the patient's buttocks and put to low intermittent wall suction. The risk that the tube will migrate during removal of the colonoscope should be greatly reduced if the instrument is removed carefully.

Colonic decompression is initially successful in 80% of cases; however, up to 20% of these patients will develop recurrent Ogilvie's syndrome (Table 56-2). For these cases, repeat decompressive colonoscopy is successful in over 85%, although Ogilvie's syndrome may continue to be a recurring problem. Colonic perforation occurs in 2% of endoscopic decompressions. Passage of the colonoscope to the cecum is not mandatory but, predictably, doing so is more likely to succeed in decompressing the colon. Jetmore and associates, in a series of 60 patients, had a 71% success rate when the colonoscope was advanced to the level of the ascending colon or cecum, compared to 37% when the colonoscope was passed to the hepatic flexure or distally. In that series, the colonoscope reached the cecum in approximately 50% of patients, to the right colon in another 20%, and to the transverse colon or lower in the remainder.

Cecostomy

Laparotomy has been traditionally indicated for failure of colonoscopic decompression, or for peritoneal signs indicating ischemia or perforation. If a cecal perforation is found at laparotomy but the bowel appears viable, tube cecostomy is performed frequently, using the perforation site as the site of tube entry. If the cecum is ischemic or if multiple tears are present, a right hemicolectomy is performed and either a primary anastomosis or ileostomy with a mucous fistula is carried out, depending on the degree of spillage and contamination. Limited cecal ischemia can be treated by excision of the nonviable portion and exteriorizing the colon via cecostomy.

For tube cecostomy, a limited right lower quadrant incision is used to gain access to the cecum, and three concentric purse-string sutures of 2-0 vicryl are placed in the seromuscular layers of the cecum centered around the proposed tube entry site. The cecum is opened and a 30 Fr Malekot catheter or large (22 to 24 Fr) Foley catheter is inserted into the lumen. The purse-string sutures are tied around the tube. The catheter is brought out through a separate stab wound in the abdominal wall, and multiple stitches of 2-0 vicryl are placed to anchor the seromuscular layer of the cecum to the parietal peritoneum of the abdominal wall. This procedure can be performed under local anesthesia. Meticulous care must be given postoperatively to maintain cecostomy tube patency. The tube should be put to gravity drainage and irrigated with 40 to 100 mL of saline every 2 to 4 hours. If cecal contents are viscid, a mixture of mineral oil and saline may more effectively cleanse the bowel. The volume of irrigant can be increased up to 500 mL on postoperative day 2 and the tube clamped for up to 2 hours after instillation to help soften thick contents.

A newer approach to failure of conservative management is laparoscopy to evaluate cecal viability and to place a cecostomy tube if the cecum is not compromised. A camera is placed just below the umbilicus; a port is then placed at the umbilical level in the right anterior axillary line for a grasper, which is used to move the cecum so that its entire intraperitoneal surface can be examined. Four T-fasteners are then placed into the cecum through the abdominal wall in a diamond configuration, with the proposed area of tube placement in the center of the diamond (Figs. 56-2 and 56-3). The T-fasteners are then used to

Table 56-2 Complication and Success Rates of Treatment Modalities

MODALITY	SUCCESS RATE	COMPLICATION RATE	RECURRENCE RATE
Endoscopic			
Colonoscopy	80%	Perforation (2%)	20%
Medical			
Neostigmine (n = 28)	89%	Bradycardia (7%)	4%
Epidural bupivacaine (n = 8)	63%	Urinary retention (12.5%)	—
Erythromycin*	—	None reported	
Surgical			
Open cecostomy	100%	Pericatheter leak (25%)	0%
		Skin excoriation (24%)	
		Catheter obstruction (5%)	
		Delayed closure (>2 weeks) after catheter removal (8%)	
		Fistula requiring secondary closure (3%)	
		Wound infection (31%)	
		Premature catheter dislodgment (3%)	
Laparoscopic cecostomy*	—	None reported	

*Case report only.

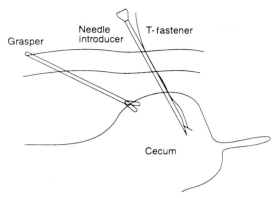

Figure 56-2
A slotted needle loaded with a T-fastener is placed through the abdominal wall and then through the cecal wall. Note the stabilization of the cecum with a grasper. The T-fastener is then released into the lumen of the cecum.

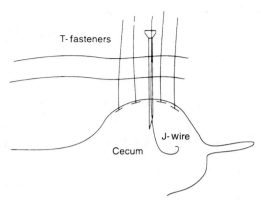

Figure 56-4
An 18-gauge needle is placed through the abdominal wall and cecum and a flexible J-wire is passed into the lumen.

hold the cecum against the abdominal wall and an 18-gauge needle is placed into the cecum (Fig. 56-4). A flexible J-tipped wire is placed into the cecum, and serial dilators are passed over the wire to create a tract. A Foley catheter, stiffened by a stylet introducer, is then placed over the wire and the balloon is inflated (Fig. 56-5). Placement of the catheter is confirmed radiographically, and contrast material is used to ensure there is no leakage around the tube. The T-fasteners are then secured to place the cecum against the abdominal wall, and 2 weeks later these sutures can be cut and the T-bars allowed to pass in the stool. Computed tomographic (CT)-guided tube cecostomy is another option, but viability of the colon cannot be assessed with this method. A comparison of this approach with open cecostomy in terms of morbidity and mortality rates has not been made.

Complications of tube cecostomy are similar to those seen with gastrostomy and jejunostomy tubes, including pericatheter leak, wound infection, incisional hernias, skin excoriation, premature catheter dislodgement, and problems with tube patency. These complications may affect up to 45% of patients. The perioperative mortality rate is high with cecostomy, but this figure reflects the patient's underlying medical condition and is usually not attributable directly to cecostomy.

Medical Therapy

Drug therapies aimed at correcting the underlying sympathetic/parasympathetic imbalance are gaining popularity. Intravenous neostigmine, which acts as a parasympathomimetic, has been used with some success in a number of patients, working within minutes to stimulate passage of flatus. Although apparently effective, neostigmine is not without morbidity, especially in elderly patients, who are precisely the ones at risk for pseudo-obstruction. The parasympathomimetic stimulation can lead to profound bradycardia, and atropine should be available when neostigmine is administered.

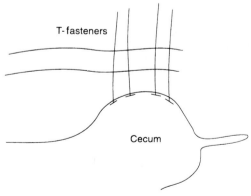

Figure 56-3
Four T-fasteners are placed into the cecum using the technique shown in Figure 56-2. The T-fasteners should be placed about 4 cm apart in a diamond configuration.

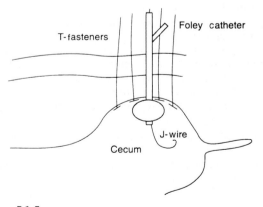

Figure 56-5
Serial dilators are passed over the flexible J-wire to enlarge the tract, and then a Malekot or Foley catheter is placed into the cecum.

Patients taking beta blockers, those with recent myocardial infarction, and those with metabolic acidosis should not be considered candidates for neostigmine because they are all at higher risk for dysrhythmias. Before neostigmine is administered, the presence of an obstructing colonic or rectal lesion must be ruled out. Thus, patients who have not undergone recent colonoscopy should be investigated by a water-soluble contrast enema prior to administration of neostigmine. Similarly, to minimize cardiac complications and allow early recognition of dysrhythmias, patients should have continuous electrocardiographic monitoring during the intravenous injection.

A 1995 study by Stephenson and coworkers showed resolution of pseudo-obstruction in 11 of 12 patients given neostigmine. The twelfth patient had initial resolution but a later recurrence and ultimately required a right hemicolectomy. A 1997 study by Turegano-Fuentes and coworkers showed resolution with one dose of neostigmine in 12 of 16 patients (75%), including one who had symptoms for 15 days. Another patient required two doses to achieve resolution, and the remaining three had only partial resolution of symptoms.

Epidural infusion of 0.25% bupivacaine has also been used, with a 62% success rate in a series of 18 patients by Lee and associates. The hypothesized mechanism of action is sympathetic blockade, thus eliminating sympathetic inhibition of colonic motility. Lee advises that epidural anesthesia should be instituted if conservative measures (NPO, correction of electrolytes, etc.) fail after 24 hours. The epidural infusion may be continued for up to 60 hours as long as improvement is seen and colonic dilatation doesn't worsen. If no improvement is seen after 24 hours, the epidural catheter is discontinued and colonoscopic decompression is performed.

The postoperative infusion of intravenous metoclopramide has been shown to have no effect on colonic motility in a study by Tollesson and coworkers. Motility was studied using radiopaque markers. Metoclopramide should not be used in patients with Ogilvie's syndrome, as it may increase small bowel motility, propelling more small bowel contents into the colon without a concomitant increase in colonic motility.

Other agents such as the motilin agonist erythromycin, intravenous cisapride, and somatostatin have had some success in sporadic case reports. However, no drug therapy for Ogilvie's syndrome has been evaluated in a prospective randomized trial, and the literature consists of only case reports and very small series of patients. Prospective randomized trials are necessary for evaluation of drug efficacy, as up to 85% of cases will resolve without colonoscopy or drug therapy within 3 days of onset. However, pharmacologic manipulation of the autonomic system has shown promise and, so far, no major adverse side effects when used with caution. Consideration should be given to adding pharmacotherapy to the initial management of pseudo-obstruction patients in an attempt to further decrease the number of these patients requiring surgical therapy.

■ SUMMARY

Ogilvie's syndrome remains a disease of uncertain etiology. For most patients, initial therapy with nasogastric decompression, fasting, and electrolyte correction will result in resolution with return of colonic motility. For those patients whose pseudo-obstruction does not resolve or who require decompression for a cecal diameter above 12 cm, colonoscopy is the initial treatment of choice. If colonoscopy is unsuccessful, tube cecostomy is indicated; this may be performed through either a limited right lower quadrant incision or a laparoscopic approach. Open laparotomy remains the standard of care for those patients with signs of ischemia or perforation. The use of drug therapy is increasing, but controlled randomized trials are needed to prove the efficacy of these various agents.

Suggested Readings

Benacci JC, Wolff BG: Cecostomy: Therapeutic indications and results. Dis Colon Rectum 1995;38:530–534.

Drudi S, Berry AR, Kettlewell GW: Acute colonic pseudo-obstruction. Br J Surg 1992;79:99–103.

Duh Q-Y, Way LW: Diagnostic laparoscopy and laparoscopic cecostomy for colonic pseudo-obstruction. Dis Colon Rectum 1993;36:65–70.

Harig JM, Fums DE, Loo FD, et al: Treatment of acute non-toxic megacolon during colonoscopy: Tube placement versus simple decompression. Gastrointest Endosc 1988;34:23–27.

Jetmore AB, Timmcke AE, Gathright JB Jr, et al: Ogilvie's syndrome: Colonoscopic decompression and analysis of predisposing factor. Dis Colon Rectum 1992;35:1135–1142.

Lee JT, Taylor BM, Singleton BC: Epidural anesthesia for acute pseudo-obstruction of the colon (Ogilvie's syndrome). Dis Colon Rectum 1988;31:686–691.

Martin FM, Robinson AM Jr, Thompson WR: Therapeutic colonoscopy in the treatment of colonic pseudo-obstruction. Am Surg 1988;54:519–522.

Nanni G, Garbini A, Luchetti P, et al: Ogilvie's syndrome (acute colonic pseudo-obstruction): Review of the literature (October 1948 to March 1980) and report of four additional cases. Dis Colon Rectum 1982;25:157–166.

Stephenson BM, Morgan AR, Salaman JR, Wheeler M: Ogilvie's syndrome: A new approach to an old problem. Dis Colon Rectum 1995;38:424–427.

Tollesson PO, Cassuto J, Faxen A, et al: Lack of effect of metoclopramide on colonic motility after cholecystectomy. Eur J Surg 1991;157:355–358.

Turegano-Fuentes F, Munoz-Jimenez F, Del Valle-Hernandez E, et al: Early resolution of Ogilvie's syndrome with intravenous neostigmine: A simple, effective treatment. Dis Colon Rectum 1997;40:1353–1357.

Vanek VW, Al-Salti M: Acute pseudo-obstruction of the colon (Ogilvie's syndrome): An analysis of 400 cases. Dis Colon Rectum 1986;29:203–210.

57

MANAGEMENT OF THE MALIGNANT POLYP

Robert Fry, MD

Endoscopic polypectomy is the preferred approach for most colorectal polyps; the majority of these lesions are benign and are cured if completely removed. It is now generally accepted that most malignant neoplasms of the large bowel arise from a preexisting benign polyp, by a process usually referred to as the "adenoma-carcinoma sequence." Greater understanding of the genetic abnormalities that lead to malignancy has enabled us to realize that there is a variable transition period during which a benign adenoma with no lethal potential may be transformed into an invasive cancer capable of metastasizing to distant organs.

■ ASSESSMENT OF POLYPS

Certain features of polyps are associated with malignancy, primarily size, shape, and histology. Polyps less than 1 cm in diameter have a small risk (<10%) of harboring malignancy. However, polyps larger than 2 cm in diameter have a risk of containing a cancer, a risk that is as high as 50% in some reports.

The polyp's shape is important in assessing the risk of associated cancer. Polyps on a stalk are less likely to contain cancer than flat, sessile lesions. The presence of ulceration, either in the head of a polyp on a stalk or in a sessile tumor, is highly suggestive of malignancy.

Finally, the histologic characteristics of the tumor can indicate whether there is a risk of malignancy. For example, tubular adenomas have a low risk and villous adenomas have a substantial risk of invasive cancer within the polyp.

Despite the fact that these signs can provide some indication as to the chances of a polyp's being malignant, most malignant polyps appear benign when resected during colonoscopy, and their malignant potential is recognized only after pathologic evaluation reveals the presence of cancerous cells invading the submucosa. The decision then must be made between no further treatment or surgical resection of the involved bowel and regional lymph nodes.

■ SURGERY OR ENDOSCOPIC RESECTION ALONE?

Surgical treatment considerations must weigh the chances of persistent or regional cancer being present against the morbidity and potential fatality associated with an abdominal operation. In some cases, the correct treatment is obvious. For example, partial colectomy could offer no benefit to an asymptomatic elderly patient with numerous liver metastases in whom a colonic polyp with invasive carcinoma has been completely excised. On the other hand, a healthy 45-year-old patient with a villous adenoma containing cancer that has been only partially excised from the cecum would obviously benefit from a resection of the right colon.

A number of outcome studies indicate that the risk of residual cancer after endoscopic resection of a malignant polyp is appreciably lower than the risk of abdominal surgery if certain criteria are met (Table 57-1): the endoscopist is confident that the polyp was completely resected, the histology of the cancer is not poorly differentiated, the cancer does not invade to the margin of resection, and there is no microscopic evidence of vascular or lymphatic invasion by the cancer. Patients with these favorable prognostic criteria should have another colonoscopic examination in 3 months to inspect the site of the polypectomy to verify complete excision.

If cancer is present at the margin of resection, the chances of local recurrence are obviously increased. Clinical experience has demonstrated the validity of this statement, but the circumstances may be more complicated than initially assumed. The obvious example is the case of a sessile villous adenoma that has been removed piecemeal. The endoscopist feels certain that the lesion has been completely excised, but one of the segments contains invasive carcinoma that involves a margin. If no other adverse prognostic factors are present, the decision for or against surgery becomes difficult indeed. Such circumstances require an explanation of the reason for uncertainty to the patient so that he or she can have an informed basis for participating in deciding the treatment. Certainly, factors such as the patient's age, general health, and willingness to have repeated colonoscopic examinations to inspect the site for recurrence must be considered in such circumstances.

The histologic differentiation of the cancer provides important prognostic information. Well-differentiated or

---

Table 57-1 Prognostic Factors of a Malignant Polyp

FAVORABLE CRITERIA

Complete endoscopic resection
Cancer confined to head of polyp
Margins not involved
Well-differentiated or moderately well-differentiated histologic features
No lymphatic or vascular invasion

UNFAVORABLE CRITERIA

Incomplete endoscopic resection
Cancer invades stalk of polyp
Cancer extends to margin of resection
Poorly differentiated, mucinous, or signet cell cancer
Lymphatic or vascular invasion

moderately well-differentiated lesions generally carry a good prognosis if other risk factors for metastases are not present. Conversely, poorly differentiated, mucinous, or signet-ring carcinomas tend to metastasize and carry a poor prognosis. A polyp containing a poorly differentiated carcinoma is not adequately treated by polypectomy alone.

Pedunculated polyps containing carcinoma should be evaluated carefully to determine the depth of invasion by the cancer. A pedunculated polyp consists of a head of neoplastic tissue connected to the colonic wall by a stalk covered with normal mucosa surrounding a core of submucosa. The junction at which the neoplastic head joins the stalk of normal mucosa is the neck of the polyp. Carcinoma confined to the head of a polyp seldom metastasizes. However, the incidence of lymphatic metastases is higher than 15% when the depth of invasion by the cancer reaches the neck or stalk of the polyp.

If a malignant polyp that has been resected has all the favorable prognostic criteria described here, the incidence of residual or nodal cancer is less than 0.5% for pedunculated polyps and less than 1.5% for sessile lesions. In contrast, if one or more unfavorable criteria are present, the incidence of lymph node metastases is approximately 8% for pedunculated polyps, and 15% for sessile polyps. The mortality rate associated with elective colonic resection is less than 0.2% for healthy young patients, but it may be appreciably higher for elderly patients with debility. The risk of surgery needs to be compared to the risk of residual cancer in making the appropriate therapeutic decision.

■ SURGICAL CONSIDERATIONS

Surgical treatment is usually indicated if a polyp cannot be excised with the colonoscope, or if the excised polyp is found to contain an invasive cancer with a significant potential for local recurrence or lymphatic metastases. In such circumstances the therapeutic goal is to resect the appropriate segment of colon and its mesentery. The nature of the operation obviously depends on the location of the cancer. Malignant polyps of the lower rectum are generally treated differently from similar polyps located in the more proximal large bowel. Bowel resection for such lesions usually requires abdominal perineal proctectomy with a permanent colostomy—a procedure that is difficult to accept for both patient and physician. The treatment of low rectal polyps containing invasive cancer is beyond the scope of this chapter, but local excision, endocavitary radiation, and local fulguration all play a role in therapy of such lesions. If such methods fail, the patient may still be salvaged by an abdominal perineal proctectomy. In general, there seems to be wisdom in the adage to "never excise the rectum for a cancer that cannot be seen or felt."

For lesions located elsewhere in the colon, the operation should include resection of the mesentery containing the lymphatic drainage from the site of the polyp. The risk from segmental colectomy generally pertains to the integrity of the anastomosis; there is little to be lost and much to be gained by including the lymphatic-bearing mesentery with the resected specimen.

A practical problem involving the extent of the colonic resection arises when a polyp has been completely excised, for the surgeon cannot rely upon the length of insertion of the colonoscope to reliably indicate the location of the polyp. A lesion located 50 cm from the anal verge on the colonoscope may be in the sigmoid or transverse colon. The appropriate operation for a transverse colon cancer requires ligation of the middle colic artery, whereas the inferior mesenteric artery should be divided for a sigmoid cancer. In such circumstances it is beneficial to mark the site of the polyp with 0.1 mL of India ink injected into the submucosa with a sclerosing needle at the time of polypectomy (Fig. 57-1). The India ink stains the serosa of the colon, exactly indicating the polyp site at the time of celiotomy.

A perplexing problem that occasionally arises is the young patient (<55 years old) who requires a celiotomy for treatment of an invasive colonic cancer and has several other benign neoplastic polyps scattered throughout the colon. In such circumstances—especially if the polyps number more than five and contain villous elements—

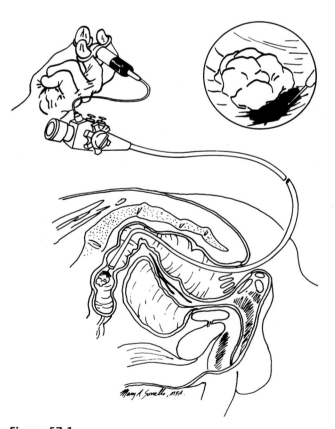

Figure 57-1
India ink is injected into the submucosa adjacent to the polyp. The ink stains the serosal surface of the colon, marking the location of the polyp for the surgeon.

consideration should be given to performing abdominal colectomy with an ileorectal anastomosis. It is reasonable to consider the colon with numerous polyps to be a pre-malignant organ. The patient's family history should be carefully assessed, and the patient should be considered for genetic counseling and testing. The minimal acceptable treatment program for such an individual would be yearly colonoscopic examinations, with the very real possibility that recurrent polyps may require further surgery. In this situation it is mandatory to present the patient with the therapeutic options as clearly as possible so that he or she can participate in arriving at an acceptable method of treatment.

Suggested Readings

Bond JH: Polyp guidelines: Diagnosis, treatment, and surveillance for patients with nonfamilial colorectal polyps. Ann Intern Med 1993;119:836–843.

Cranley JP, Petras RE, Cary WD, et al: When is endoscopic polypectomy adequate therapy for colonic polyps containing invasive carcinoma? Gastroenterology 1986;91:419–427.

Haggitt RC, Glotzbach RE, Soffer EE, Wrible LD: Prognostic factors in colorectal carcinomas arising in adenomas: Implications for lesions removed by endoscopic polypectomy. Gastroenterology 1985;89:328–336.

Richards WO, Webb WA, Morris SJ, et al: Patient management after endoscopic removal of the cancerous colon adenoma. Ann Surg 1987;205:665–672.

58

TREATMENT OF COLORECTAL ADENOMAS: SCREENING, FOLLOW-UP, AND SURVEILLANCE

Santhat Nivatvongs, MD, FACS

■ DEFINITIONS

A colorectal adenoma is an epithelial tumor composed of abnormal glands of the large bowel. These adenomas can be classified into three types according to the growth pattern of the glands (villous or tubular): If 0 to 25% of the glands are villous, they are classified as tubular adenomas; if 25 to 75% are villous, they are tubulovillous adenomas; and if 75 to 100% are villous, they are villous adenomas. Tubular adenomas account for 75% of all neoplastic polyps, villous adenomas 10%, and tubulovillous adenomas 15%. A villous growth pattern is most prominent in sessile large adenomas, particularly in those located distally in the rectum.

Dysplasia is the term describing the histologic abnormality of an adenoma according to the degree of atypical cells. The dysplasia is categorized as low grade (mild), moderate, or high grade (severe). Cells showing high-grade dysplasia are similar to cells found in a carcinoma but are limited to the epithelium. The frequency of high-grade dysplasia correlates with the size of the adenoma: Larger adenomas have a higher rate of high-grade dysplasia.

■ INCIDENCE

Neoplastic polyps are common in autopsy series. Adenomas are present in 34 to 52% of males and 29 to 45% of females over 50 years of age. Most adenomas (87 to 89%) are <1 cm in size. The National Polyp Study using colonoscopy showed the size distribution of colorectal polyps as follows: ≤0.5 cm, 38%; 0.6 to 1 cm, 37%, ≥1 cm, 25%. The study also noted that size, extent of villous component, and increasing age of the patient are independent risk factors for high-grade dysplasia. Invasive carcinomas are uncommon in adenomas <1 cm and the incidence increases with the size of the adenomas.

■ INDICATIONS FOR REMOVAL

It has generally been accepted that most colorectal carcinomas are derived from benign adenomas through the adenoma-carcinoma sequence. It takes about 5 years from a clean colon to the development of invasive carcinoma. Thus, removal of an adenoma prevents the development of colorectal carcinoma. In a case-control study, removal of rectal polyps in patients under surveillance with yearly rigid proctosigmoidoscopy resulted in a lower-than-expected incidence of rectal carcinoma. Similarly, the National Polyp Study showed that colonoscopic polypectomy results in a lower-than-expected incidence of colorectal carcinoma.

Most adenomatous polyps found on routine examination with rigid proctosigmoidectomy or flexible sigmoidoscopy are small and have minimal risk of harboring a carcinoma. Because we do not know whether these small polyps will continue to grow with eventual degeneration into an invasive carcinoma, their removal is logical, provided it can be performed with minimal or no risk of complications. This approach also gives the opportunity to clear the colon and rectum and, thus, extends the follow-up time to several years. Another concern is whether the patient has a synchronous polyp or polyps more proximally and, if so, whether it is important to have it removed. The incidence of synchronous polyps beyond the reach of the rigid proctoscope and flexible sigmoidoscope is about 50%. However, most of these polyps are small and have little clinical significance. Using death from carcinoma as the end point, the risk of development of carcinoma in the more proximal colon is significant if the polyp found in the rectum or sigmoid colon is >1 cm, if the polyp is a villous or tubulovillous adenoma, and if there are multiple adenomas. A single adenoma <1 cm without a villous component carries no significant risk of having a carcinoma more proximally.

There has been no randomized controlled study to discover whether a total colonoscopy should be performed if an adenoma is found in the rectum or sigmoid colon, but it is reasonable to individualize and tailor the practice to each patient. If the patient is young (e.g., <40 years old) or if the patient has a high risk of developing carcinoma more proximally (such as a >1 cm adenoma found in the rectum and sigmoid colon or a smaller adenoma with a villous component) a total colonoscopy along with removal of the adenoma should be the treatment of choice.

■ MANAGEMENT OF ADENOMAS OF THE COLON AND UPPER RECTUM

Polyps

Colonoscopy has revolutionized the management of large bowel polyps. Most polyps can be snared through the colonoscope with minimal adverse effects. At the present time, colonic resection or colotomy and polypectomy are reserved for cases in which colonoscopic polypectomy cannot be done, such as lesions that are too large or too flat, or when the colonoscope cannot be passed to the site of the polyp.

Clinically, the two morphologic types of polyps are pedunculated and sessile. The pedunculated polyp has a stem lined with normal mucosa, called a stalk or a pedicle, and has the appearance of a mushroom. A sessile polyp grows flat on the mucosa. A pedunculated polyp is rarely >4 cm in diameter, whereas a sessile polyp can be huge, encompassing the entire circumference of the large bowel. Most pedunculated polyps can be snared in one piece because the pedicles are rarely >2 cm in diameter. Sessile polyps <2 cm usually can be snared in one piece. Large sessile polyps should be snared piecemeal and in more than one session, if appropriate. For a large sessile or a flat adenoma, submucosal injection of saline to lift the polyp from the muscularis propria may make excision safer, although this technique is unproved. The excised polyps, particularly the sessile type, must be prepared properly and sectioned so that all the layers can be examined microscopically and invasive carcinoma ruled out. Flat adenomas are increasingly recognized with better magnification or the use of dye-spray techniques. These polyps may be more likely to harbor dysplasia than pedunculated polyps.

Transanal Excision of Rectal Adenoma

Adenomas of the rectum present a unique situation. Many of these lesions can be palpated with a finger, suction tube, or endoscope. Regardless of size, if the lesion is soft, it has a 90% chance of being benign. A large rectal adenoma can be removed in a number of ways, including snaring piecemeal through a rigid proctosigmoidoscope or a colonoscope, and formal transanal excision can be employed, depending on the site and size of the lesion.

Sessile Adenoma of Lower Rectum

A sessile adenoma with the proximal margin up to 7 cm from the anal verge can be excised in one piece. A Pratt anal speculum is used for exposure. Scissors or an electrocautery blade is used to dissect mucosa and submucosa from the underlying muscular wall of the rectum. A dilute epinephrine solution (1:200,000) is infiltrated into the submucosa to minimize bleeding and separate it from the muscle layer. An incision is made with a margin of about 1 cm of normal mucosa and submucosa. The distal margin of the adenoma is grasped with an Allis forceps for traction. A Hill-Ferguson retractor may work better at this point to allow prolapsing of the rectal wall. The entire lesion is then excised. The wound should be closed transversely to avoid tension and separation, using 3-0 synthetic braided sutures.

Sessile Adenoma of Midrectum

Transanal excision of a lesion in the rectum between 7 and 10 cm from the anal verge is difficult, if not impossible. The anal speculum cannot reach the adenoma for adequate exposure. However, if the lesion is smaller than 2.5 cm, it may still be excised. The operation described here employs a traction technique.

The anorectal submucosa is infiltrated with 0.25% bupivacaine containing 1:200,000 epinephrine to obtain complete relaxation of the anal canal and hemostasis. A Fansler anal speculum is used to expose the lesion. An elliptical excision is made with scissors, starting at the anal verge, similar to the technique of hemorrhoidectomy. The mucosa and the submucosa are dissected from the underlying internal sphincter muscle. With this submucosal pedicle used as traction, the dissection can be carried up to 10 cm from the anal verge without difficulty (Fig. 58-1A). When the upper margin of the polyp is reached, the dissection should encompass it with a 1-cm margin of normal mucosa. If the anorectal wall does not prolapse when the submucosal pedicle is pulled, the Fansler anal speculum should be replaced with a Hill-Ferguson retractor. The wound is closed longitudinally or transversely with 3-0 synthetic braided sutures (Fig. 58-1B). At completion, it is essential to make sure that the rectal lumen is patent. A proctosigmoidoscopy may be required.

For a large sessile lesion in the midrectum that cannot be removed by this technique, it can still be snared piecemeal with a colonoscope. Very seldom is a posterior approach of Kraske or York-Mason required. Transanal endoscopic microsurgery (TEM), which was first introduced by Buess and coworkers in Germany in 1983, is another technique that can be used for a midrectal lesion. The system uses a special rectal scope 4 cm in diameter and 20 cm long. The scope has a closed system of sealed caps with individual ports for forceps, suction, scissors, needle holder, and electrocautery. It is connected to a stereoscopic optical system for visualization and can be hooked up to a television screen. During the procedure, a continuous pressure-controlled insufflation of carbon dioxide keeps the rectum open for exposure. The patient is placed in a prone, lateral, or lithotomy position, according to the location of the polyp. Even a lesion high in the rectum can sometimes be removed this way. TEM is a complicated technique and is difficult to master. For a few medical centers and well-trained surgeons, TEM is an option that can obviate the need to perform a more radical operation, such as low anterior resection.

Circumferential Villous or Tubulovillous Adenoma of Low Rectum

A circumferential villous or tubulovillous adenoma with the lower margin in the lower rectum can be removed even if the proximal margin extends to the midrectum (Fig. 58-2A). Good exposure is essential for removal of a large polyp in the rectum. A Lone-Star self-retaining retractor helps the exposure tremendously. If it is not available, two Gelpi retractors placed at a right angle to each other at the anal verge can be used. The patient is placed in prone position with the buttocks taped apart. A circumferential incision is made around the dentate line to the submucosal plane using electrocautery. Diluted epinephrine 1:200,000 should be injected frequently to raise the submucosal plane. Using a Pratt anal speculum to stretch the anal canal up to about 7 cm will make the dissection in the submucosal plane easier all around. The submucosal tube is grasped with a ring forceps, and the submucosal dissection is carried as far proximally as needed (Fig. 58-2B). The circumferential dissection of the submucosa allows the rectum to prolapse during traction. A Pratt anal speculum, Hill-Ferguson retractor, and a small Deaver retractor should be used as appropriate.

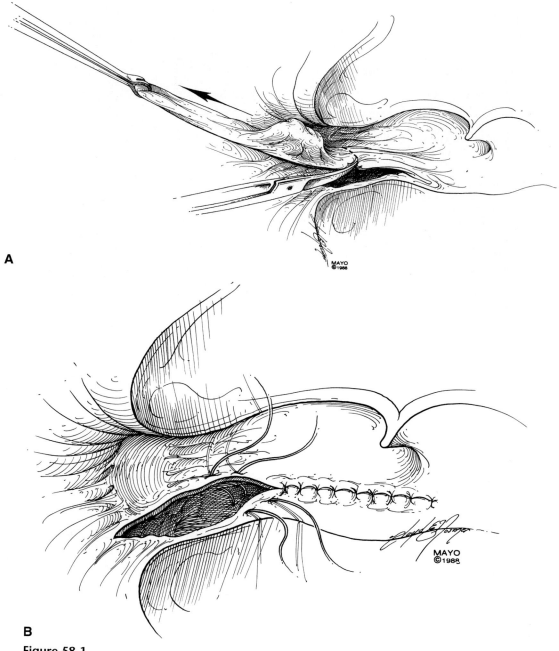

Figure 58-1
A, Sessile adenoma in the middle rectum. Elliptical excision starts at the dentate line or anal verge. *B*, Closure of the wound. For a large polyp, the wound should be closed transversely.

After the entire adenoma has been removed, the proximal cut end of the mucosa and submucosa can be brought down, along with the denuded muscle wall, to approximate circumferentially with the lower cut end at the dentate line using 3-0 synthetic braided sutures. At completion, the anorectal wall will be imbricated in the long longitudinal plane (Fig. 58-2C). Incontinence of gas and liquid stool may last for a few weeks. Circumferential submucosal dissection of the anorectum can be carried from the dentate line up to 10 cm from the anal verge, and occasionally up to 12 to 15 cm.

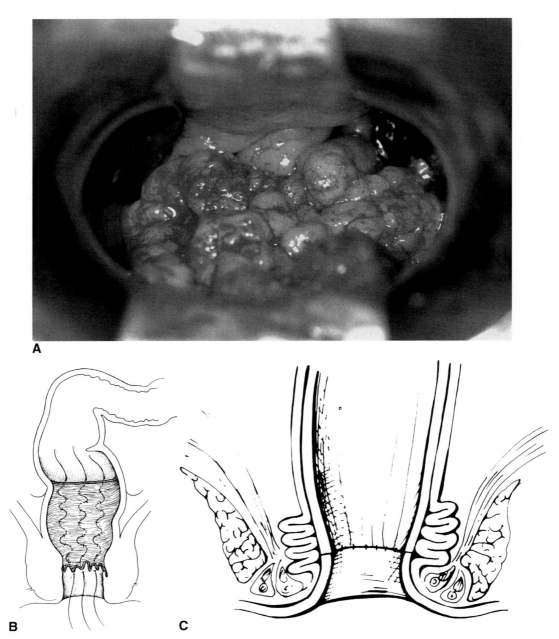

Figure 58-2
A, Circumferential villous adenoma of the lower rectum. *B,* Starting at the dentate line, the entire adenoma is excised circumferentially in the submucosal plane with electrocautery. The wound is brought down, incorporating the denuded muscle wall, to approximate the dentate line. *C,* At completion, the anorectal wall is pleated.

Natural History of Untreated Large Bowel Adenomas

A retrospective review of patients from the precolonoscopic era at the Mayo Clinic included 226 patients who had colonic polyps ≥1 cm in diameter in whom periodic radiographic examination of the colon was elected over excision. The risk of a ≥1 cm polyp's developing into an invasive carcinoma at 5, 10, and 20 years is 2.5%, 8%, and 24%, respectively. The cumulative probability of developing an invasive metachronous carcinoma at a site different from the index polyp is 2% at 5 years, 7% at 10 years, and 12% at 20 years. Over a median duration of polyp surveillance of 4.8 years (range 1 to 27 years), 5% of the index polyps (≥1 cm) disappeared, 57% have no growth noted, and 38%

demonstrate growth. These data further support the recommendation for excision of colorectal polyps ≥1 cm in diameter and a periodic examination of the entire colon.

■ SCREENING FOR COLORECTAL CARCINOMA

In 2003, United States cancer statistics predicted 147,500 new cases of colon and rectal cancer, of which 42,000 (28%) were cancers of the rectum. Of these, 57,100 will die from the cancer after treatment, a death rate of 39% or an overall survival rate of 61%. Death from colorectal cancers has declined for females during the past 50 years, but has not changed for males.

Survival of colorectal carcinoma (CRC) is closely related to the clinical and pathologic stage of the disease at diagnosis. Data from the German Multicenter Study in colorectal carcinoma showed 5-year survival rates in stages I, II, III, and IV as 76%, 65%, 42%, and 16%, respectively (surgical death is included).

Most CRCs are asymptomatic until they become advanced, when some partial obstruction occurs, causing abdominal pain or change in bowel habits. Although carcinoma of the colon and rectum bleeds occasionally and unpredictably, it may be possible to diagnose it at an early stage by examining occult blood in the stool. Through many observations and studies including the current knowledge of molecular genetics of CRC, the natural history of CRC starts with one crypt. The accumulation of mutations in several genes slowly gives rise to a small polyp, which may progress to an invasive carcinoma that eventually metastasizes. The National Polyp Study showed that it takes about 10 years for an invasive carcinoma to develop from a clean colon. This natural history provides a window of opportunity for detecting early carcinoma and removing precancerous polyps. Thus, screening strategies are directed toward detecting early carcinoma to reduce morbidity and fatality as well as removing premalignant polyps to reduce the incidence of CRC.

Colorectal carcinoma fulfills all the criteria for a justified screening. First, it is common and serious: It is the second leading cause of death from cancer in the United States, affecting males and females equally. Treatment of patients with advanced CRC is unsuccessful in many patients. Second, screening tests have been shown to achieve accurate detection of early-stage CRCs. Third, evidence from controlled trials and case-controlled studies suggests with various degrees of persuasiveness that removing adenomatous polyps reduces the incidence of CRC, and that detecting early-stage carcinomas reduces the chances of death from the disease. Finally, screening benefits outweigh its harms. The various ways of screening for CRC all have cost-effectiveness ratios comparable to those of other generally accepted screening tests.

Purposes of Screening
Screening identifies individuals who are more likely to have CRC or adenomatous polyps from among those without signs or symptoms of disease. It is the use of simple, affordable, and acceptable tests to identify a subgroup of the at-risk population more likely to have a clinically significant lesion or abnormality. *Screening,* which refers primarily to a population approach, has been used interchangeably with *early detection. Case finding* is another term that refers to early detection on an individual basis. All these terms refer to the identification of individuals with an increased probability of having colorectal neoplasia. The goal of screening for CRC is to reduce the mortality rate from the disease by detecting carcinomas at an early stage.

Once a screening test is positive, a complete workup of the entire colon and rectum is called for. It should be done with a total colonoscopy or alternatively a flexible sigmoidoscopy and a double-contrast barium enema.

Who Should Be Screened?
Most Americans are not currently screened for CRC. The National Health Interview Survey (NHIS) reported that between 1987 and 1992, 17.13% of people age 50 years or older had undergone fecal occult blood test (FOBT) in the previous year, and 9.4% had undergone sigmoidoscopy in the previous 3 years. In 1993, the telephone survey conducted through the Behavioral Risk Factor Surveillance System (BRFSS), of persons age 50 or older, found <40% reported having a sigmoidoscopy during the previous 5 years. In 1992, BRFSS found that <35% of respondents reported having had the FOBT. The situation may change because guidelines now recommend routine screening for those over 50 years of age.

About 75% of all new cases of CRC are found in people with no known predisposing factors for the disease. The incidence increases with age, beginning around age 40 years. People with no predisposing factors are considered to be at average risk of CRC. The remaining cases occur in people who are at higher-than-average risk of the disease: family history of CRC, previous adenomatous polyps or CRC, chronic ulcerative colitis (CUC), or Crohn's disease (CD). People with a family history of CRC (one or more parents, siblings, or children with the disease) but without any apparent defined genetic syndrome account for most of those at high risk (15 to 20%). Hereditary nonpolyposis colon cancer (HNPCC) accounts for 2 to 3% of all cases and familial adenomatous polyposis (FAP) about 1%. The remainder, about 1%, are attributed to a variety of uncommon conditions (CUC, CD, Peutz-Jeghers syndrome, juvenile polyposis) in which CRC risk is elevated but is not as high as in HNPCC and FAP. Other risk factors that should be kept in mind include older age, diet high in saturated fats, excessive alcohol, and sedentary lifestyle.

The screening of people at average risk is different from screening for people with high risk. The most recent important data on several aspects of screening have prompted some medical organizations and societies to change their guidelines. American Cancer Society guidelines advocate screening at age 50 unless increased risk factors mandate earlier screening. Recommended screening is a total colonoscopy or flexible sigmoidoscopy with hemoccult testing. Those with polyps undergo repeat surveillance after 3 years (Byers and associates). Such indications for screening have culminated in recent approval of screening for Medicare patients, and many other carriers are now following suit.

The algorithm for CRC screening and surveillance in average-risk and increased-risk populations is shown on Figure 58-3.

Screening Populations at Average Risk for Colorectal Carcinoma

The expert panel accepts five screening strategy options:

1. Fecal occult blood test (FOBT)
2. Flexible sigmoidoscopy
3. FOBT + flexible sigmoidoscopy
4. Double-contrast barium enema (DCBE)
5. Colonoscopy

Fecal Occult Blood Test

The Rationale. The concept of detecting carcinomas of the colon and rectum by testing for blood in the stool is based on the observation that carcinomas bleed more than normal mucosa. About two thirds of carcinomas bleed in the course of a week, and a higher proportion, perhaps more than 90%, will be detected with repeated testing over several years. However, bleeding tends to be intermittent, and blood is distributed unevenly in the stool. The amount of bleeding increases with the size of the polyp and the stage of the carcinoma. Testing for fecal occult blood will, therefore, lead to detection of some carcinomas; it will also lead to detection of polyps because they are much more common.

The Testing. A guaiac-based test for peroxidase activity is used for detecting blood in the stool. The one to which most of the available evidence relates is the Hemoccult II test. A more sensitive version, the Hemoccult II Sensa, is also available.

The Hemoccult test is not specific for cancer; nonneoplastic lesions, such as gum disease, gastritis, peptic ulcer disease, and hemorrhoids can also cause gastrointestinal bleeding. The test is not specific for blood per se, because other substances with peroxidase or pseudoperoxidase can cause a false positive reaction if they are present in the stool (red meat, some fruits and vegetables). Some commonly used drugs such as aspirin and nonsteroidal anti-inflammatory drugs (NSAIDs) can cause occult bleeding; therefore, these and other medications are gastric irritants and should be avoided. False negative tests may result because the cancer or polyps did not bleed while the sampled stool was being formed. Vitamin C and antioxidants can also interfere with the reaction and cause a false negative test result. Dietary iron supplements do not directly interfere with the test but by turning the stool dark, they can make it difficult to interpret the blue color change of a positive result.

Participants are asked to observe certain dietary restrictions, especially of red meat, certain vegetables, vitamin C, salicylates, NSAIDs, and iron for 2 days before the test and throughout the test period (3 consecutive days). The specimen should be taken from different parts of the stool and smeared on the Hemoccult slide. The slide should be kept at room temperature during the testing. A positive result is registered if a blue color appears upon adding the hydrogen peroxide to the stool on the card. The test is considered positive if any one of the six windows turns any degree of blue. Although a simple test, FOBT may be inaccurately interpreted, resulting in a false negative result. Proper training can easily improve the reading. Negative samples are usually read correctly.

Five prospective controlled trials of screening using FOBT have been reported (Table 58-1). All trials, except one pending final results, show that FOBT decreases the death rate from CRC. They also consistently show earlier stages of the cancers.

Participants who have positive FOBTs mostly have colonoscopy as their diagnostic workup. Disadvantages of this strategy are that currently available tests for fecal occult blood fail to detect many polyps and some cancers, and many people who test positive will undergo the discomfort and risk of full bowel preparation and examination to find that they do not have adenomatous polyps or cancers. Yearly hemoccult testing is recommended because the randomized trials show that yearly testing is more effective than testing every 2 years and because yearly testing may detect lesions that are missed on earlier rounds of screening but have not yet progressed to the stage in which they are less curable. Rehydration improves the sensitivity of the test at the expense of specificity, and a special diet can decrease the rate of false positive tests. Newer generation tests may increase sensitivity with minimal loss of specificity.

Criticism of the FOBT includes the issue of insufficient sensitivity for detecting colorectal neoplasia and that the mortality rate reduction in the trials is simply due to random colonoscopy, not the discriminating power of the FOBT itself. Some are concerned that the cost of screening is prohibitive or that this approach will not be cost effective. All this criticism, including the cost, has been refuted. The National Cancer Institute has come up with the figure that the cost per year of lives saved by CRC screening is about $25,000, well within the benchmark figure of $40,000 considered by the federal government to be cost effective.

Flexible Sigmoidoscopy

Although rigid sigmoidoscopy was used many years ago to screen for cancers of the rectum, flexible sigmoidoscopy has now largely replaced it because of better visualization and its higher reach and yield. The preparation is simply one or two packaged phosphosoda enemas 1 or 2 hours prior to the examination. A flexible sigmoidoscopy has three important advantages over FOBT: (1) it allows clinicians to visualize the bowel directly, (2) lesions can be biopsied as part of the procedure, and (3) it has high sensitivity and specificity for polyps in the part of the bowel examined. Thus, in addition to detecting early-stage cancers, it offers the possibility of reducing the incidence of CRC through the detection and subsequent removal of

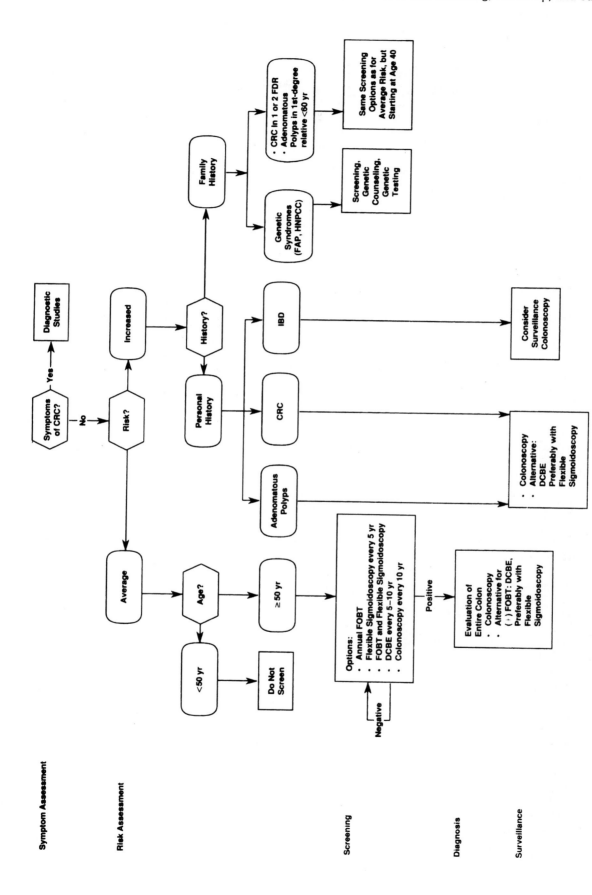

Figure 58-3

Algorithm for colorectal carcinoma screening. (CRC = colorectal carcinoma, DCBE = double-contrast barium enema, FAP = familial adenomatous polyposis, FOBT = fecal occult blood test, HNPCC = hereditary nonpolyposis colon cancer, IBD = inflammatory bowel disease.) (From Winawer SJ, Fletcher RH, Miller L, et al: Colorectal cancer screening: Clinical guidelines and rationale. Gastroenterology 1997;112:594–642, with permission from The American Gastroenterological Association.)

Table 58-1 Results of Fecal Occult Blood Test Trials (Hemoccult II)

TRIALS	COHORT SIZE	AGE	FOLLOW-UP (YR)	+RATE	FREQUENCY OF TEST (YR)	DUKES' STAGE	SCREEN (%)	CONTROL (%)	SENSITIVITY (%)	SPECIFICITY (%)	MORTALITY RATE REDUCTION
MN	46,551	50–80	13	9.8 *Rehydration*	1	A	30	22	92.2	90.4	33
						B	29	31			
						C	23	21			
						D	9	16			
						U*	9	10			
NY	21,756	40+	—	4	1	A	43	24	—	—	43 $p < 0.001$
						B	27	12			
						C	23	35			
						D	7	29			
Denmark	61,933	47–75	10	0.5–4.6	2	A	22 ($p < 0.01$)	11	—	—	18 $p = 0.03$
						B	34	37			
						C	19	23			
						D	20	24			
						U*	5	5			
England	150,251	45–74	7.8	1.2–2.7	2	A	20 ($p < 0.001$)	11	—	—	15 $p = 0.026$
						B	32	33			
						C	24	31			
						D	22	21			
						U*	2	4			
Sweden	68,308	60–64	3–7	4.4	1½–2	A	26 ($p < 0.03$)	9	88	—	Pending
						B	28	34			
						C	32	32			
						D	14 ($p < 0.04$)	25			

*U = unknown.

adenomatous polyps. However, flexible sigmoidoscopy has an important limitation. It can visualize only polyps and cancers in the left side of the colon. As with FOBT, evaluation of the entire colon is needed in patients in whom adenomatous polyps or cancers are found.

One advantage of flexible sigmoidoscopy is that it can be performed relatively quickly. The average procedure takes about 8 minutes. Biopsy specimens can be obtained during flexible sigmoidoscopy; however, polypectomy is not advised because of the possibility of explosion from an incomplete bowel preparation. In any case, a patient with a large polyp (>1 cm) should have a full colonoscopy followed by polypectomy.

Flexible sigmoidoscopy is considered to be positive if a carcinoma or any polyp >1 cm in diameter is found. More controversial is whether an adenoma smaller than 1 cm in diameter, especially tubular without high-grade dysplasia, constitutes a positive test requiring subsequent examination of the entire colon. The consequences of not following up small (<1 cm) adenomas by colonoscopy are described in several studies. In a study from the Mayo Clinic, people in whom polyps smaller than 1 cm were found on sigmoidoscopy have a risk of future cancer no greater than the general population. However, the polyps were electrocoagulated and the histologic characteristics are, therefore, not associated with an increased risk for CRC. A study from St. Mark's Hospital showed that if a polyp is a tubular adenoma and the size is smaller than 1 cm found on sigmoidoscopy, the risk of having carcinoma more proximally is not significant. However, if the tubular adenoma is larger than 1 cm, or if the small polyp is a villous or tubulovillous adenoma, the risk of having proximal carcinoma is significant. Two more recent randomized studies have shown that even hyperplastic polyps can be associated with more proximal lesions.

Studies that compare the number of polyps found in the first 60 cm of colonoscopy with the number found on full colonoscopy suggests that the 60-cm flexible sigmoidoscope would correctly identify 40 to 60% of all adenomas detected by colonoscopy. The characteristics of the proximal adenoma seem to correlate with the characteristics of the rectal and sigmoid adenoma; that is, when adenomas smaller than 1 cm in diameter are found in the rectum and sigmoid colon, it is unlikely that adenomas with advanced disease will be found more proximally. One should keep in mind that about a third of patients with proximal adenomatous polyps have no polyps in the distal colon and rectum. If these patients had undergone only flexible sigmoidoscopy, they would not have been identified as being at increased risk of CRC; that is, the sensitivity of the overall strategy of following up abnormal sigmoidoscopy with complete examination of the colon is about 67%.

No randomized controlled trial has yet addressed the effectiveness of screening sigmoidoscopy. The best available evidence on the effectiveness of rigid sigmoidoscopy in reducing death from CRC comes from the case-controlled studies. Rigid sigmoidoscopy is associated with a 59 to 80% reduction in mortality rate from carcinomas in that part of the colon and rectum reached by the rigid sigmoidoscope. Other indirect evidence comes from studies comparing the performance of rigid and flexible scopes. The flexible scopes detect more polyps and carcinomas. The case-controlled study of screening sigmoidoscopy also found that the effectiveness of screening is just as great for patients who have undergone the procedure 9 to 10 years before as for those who have undergone it more recently. In one study, 259 asymptomatic, average-risk persons (age ≥50 years) with negative flexible sigmoidoscopy underwent a second examination an average of 3.4 years after the first. The second examination found adenomas in only 6% of the subjects screened but found no carcinomas or large polyps.

The major complication of sigmoidoscopy is perforation of the colon and rectum. Data from large series of sigmoidoscopy show perforation rates ranging from 1 to 2 per 10,000 examinations. Slightly higher complication rates apply when biopsy or polypectomy is performed. No direct evidence of death from flexible sigmoidoscopy is found in the literature.

Combined Fecal Occult Blood Testing and Sigmoidoscopy

The combination of both screening methods may correct some of the limitations of each method used alone. Only one controlled trial from Sloan-Kettering Cancer Center, New York, has studied the additional benefit of adding FOBT to screening sigmoidoscopy. In this study, 12,479 people 40 years of age and older were allocated to annual screening either with rigid sigmoidoscopy combined with FOBT or with rigid sigmoidoscopy alone. After 5 to 11 years of follow-up, the mortality rate from CRC is lower in those receiving FOBT and sigmoidoscopy. This reduction in mortality is associated with earlier-stage cancers and longer survival in the FOBT group compared with the controlled group (70% versus 48%).

Barium Enema

Single-contrast barium enema is substantially less sensitive and less specific than double-contrast barium enema (DCBE) in detecting clinically important lesions. A complete colonic preparation with laxatives is essential. The examination takes 20 to 30 minutes. Studies showed that for 5 to 10% of barium enemas, the results are unsatisfactory, requiring another attempt or colonoscopy to visualize the entire colon. Sensitivity of DCBE is 50 to 80% for polyps <1 cm, 70 to 90% for polyps >1 cm, and 55 to 85% for Dukes' stages A and B carcinomas. Insensitivity is mainly related to inadequate visualization of parts of the bowel and to errors of interpretation. False positive findings are caused mainly by adherent stool and non-neoplastic mucosal irregularities, with rates ranging from <1% for cancers to 5 to 10% for large polyps and about 50% for small polyps. Most studies suggest that the success rate of DCBE, although lower than colonoscopy, is sufficient to detect the majority of clinically important lesions.

Traditionally, patients have undergone sigmoidoscopy before barium enema because barium enema is considered an especially inaccurate examination of the sigmoid colon and rectum. With improved DCBE techniques, the accuracy of the procedure in the rectosigmoid has been considered better, and some radiologists no longer recommend prior sigmoidoscopy. A randomized trial of DCBE and flexible sigmoidoscopy versus colonoscopy in 383 patients with gastrointestinal bleeding suspected to be from the colon found that colonoscopy detected more cases of polyps <9 mm than DCBE with sigmoidoscopy. However, there was no difference between groups in the number of patients detected with carcinomas or polyps ≥9 mm. DCBE and sigmoidoscopy together have been the first line of diagnostic evaluation for a large ongoing Swedish randomized, controlled trial of screening FOBT. In this study, DCBE alone missed 25% of carcinomas and a similar proportion of polyps >1 cm in the rectosigmoid colon. The flexible sigmoidoscope performed better than DCBE in this region, but this method overlooked 5% of carcinomas and 10% of adenomas >1 cm in the rectosigmoid (sensitivity of 95% and 90%, respectively). The combination of flexible sigmoidoscopy and DCBE has a sensitivity of 98% for carcinomas and 99% for adenomas.

No controlled comparisons have been made of the effectiveness of barium enema in screening for CRC in which death or any other adverse outcome from CRC is measured. Indirect evidence of the effectiveness of barium enema in screening comes from the fact that detecting polyps or early carcinomas by other screening tests reduces the incidence of and mortality rate from CRC and that DCBE detects many of these lesions. No studies directly address the question of how frequently barium enema should be performed in screening for indirect evidence reflecting current knowledge of the natural history of the disease and existing data on the performance and relative cost and safety of the procedure. The most serious complications of barium enema are bowel perforation, which occurs in 1 of 25,000, and cardiac complications, seen in 1 in 46,000.

Colonoscopy

Colonoscopy is the only technique currently available that offers the potential to both find and remove premalignant lesions throughout the colon and rectum. Screening for fecal occult blood detects only those polyps and cancers that bleed; sigmoidoscopy allows inspection of only the distal half of the large bowel; and DCBE, although it can image the entire large bowel, does not allow biopsy or polypectomy.

Colonoscopy requires a rather vigorous mechanical bowel preparation. Patients usually receive sedation that maintains consciousness. The cecum is reached in 80 to 95% of the procedures. Incomplete colonoscopies require either a repeat colonoscopy or supplemental barium enema. Colonoscopy can detect both carcinomas and polyps, although, like barium enema, it is less accurate when the polyps are small. Large polyps (≥1 cm) are rarely missed. Colonoscopy misses 25% of polyps <5 mm and 10% of polyps >1 cm.

No published studies directly examine the effectiveness of colonoscopy as a screening test for CRC in terms of

CRC deaths. However, it has been shown that detecting and removing polyps reduces the incidence of CRC, that detecting early-stage carcinomas lowers the mortality rate from the disease, and that colonoscopy detects most of these lesions.

Colonoscopy can be complicated by perforation, hemorrhage, respiratory depression due to sedation, arrhythmias, transient abdominal pain and ileus, and nosocomial infection. Approximately 1 in 1000 patients has perforation, 3 in 1000 have major hemorrhage, and 1 to 3 in 10,000 die as the result of the procedure. Complication rates may be higher if polypectomy is performed. About 5 in 1000 patients experience clinically significant respiratory depression.

No studies directly address the question of how frequently colonoscopy should be performed in screening for CRC. However, on the basis of the high accuracy of colonoscopy, the length of time needed for polyps to develop into carcinomas in the grossly normal colon, and estimates from a case-controlled study of proctosigmoidoscopy, screening colonoscopy every 10 years seems to be adequately protective, provided no polyps or carcinomas are detected.

Virtual colonoscopy, using high-resolution computed tomography (CT) with reconstruction of a two- or three-dimensional image of the colon, has the ability to visualize small polyps, but its role in screening remains undefined because of issues of cost, time to analyze the images, and the need to refer any polyps for subsequent colonoscopy.

When to Stop Screening

No direct evidence is available concerning the time at which screening should stop, but indirect evidence supports stopping screening in people nearing the end of life. Polyps take about 10 years to progress to cancer, and screening to detect polyps may not be in the patient's best interest if they are not expected to live at least that long. Also, screening and diagnostic tests are, in general, less well tolerated by elderly people. Therefore, there will come a time in most people's lives when the rigors of screening and diagnostic evaluation of positive tests are no longer justified by the potential to prolong life. The age at which to stop screening depends on the judgment of individual patients and their clinicians, taking into account the lead time between screening and its benefits and the patient's life expectancy.

Screening Populations at Increased Risk for Colorectal Carcinoma

Screening high-risk people could take several forms. Patients could begin screening at an earlier age if polyps and carcinomas might arise at an earlier age; they could be screened more frequently if the evolution from small polyps to carcinoma is more rapid; they could be screened by tests that reach the right colon if the carcinomas occur more proximally; or they could be screened with more sensitive methods such as colonoscopy or DCBE rather than FOBT or sigmoidoscopy, if the risk is high. Patients already found to have adenomatous polyps are at increased risk and are candidates for surveillance rather than screening.

Family History of Colorectal Carcinoma

This group is composed of individuals having one or more first-degree relatives with CRC; good evidence suggests that carcinomas arise at an earlier age in these people than in average-risk persons. In effect, the risk of a 40-year-old person with a family history of CRC is comparable to that of an average-risk 50-year-old person.

It is also clear that the incidence of CRC in this high-risk group is increased about twofold and that this increase seems to be greater in young adults than during later in life. Risk is higher if the relative developed CRC at a younger age. However, no evidence suggests that carcinomas develop more rapidly in people with a family history of CRC. Similarly, the distribution of carcinomas in the colon and rectum is apparently not substantially different in patients with a family history of CRC compared with average-risk people. In addition to the increased risk associated with having a family member with CRC, siblings and parents of patients with adenomatous polyps are also at increased risk for CRC. The risk is increased when the adenoma in the relative is diagnosed before age 60 or, in the case of siblings, when a parent has had CRC.

Genetic Syndromes

Genetic syndromes include familial adenomatous polyposis (FAP) and hereditary nonpolyposis colon cancer (HNPCC). In both cases, a specific genetic mutation has been found in the kindreds examined; more than 80% of affected individuals in FAP and HNPCC families are carriers of the known gene mutations. At present, it is not feasible or appropriate to screen the general population for these familial syndromes. However, if blood is available from a clinically affected relative in either syndrome and a genetic mutation has been identified, it is possible to determine if other members of the kindred are carriers because the genetic mutation is constant within kindreds and therefore more easily identified. A negative test in an individual from a family that has an affected member with a positive test essentially rules out the disease. A negative test in the absence of a positive test in the family does not rule out the disease. At present, HNPCC is being identified primarily by a family history that meets the Amsterdam criteria. For more details of these syndromes, please refer to the corresponding chapters.

■ SURVEILLANCE AFTER REMOVAL OF ADENOMATOUS POLYPS

The main options for surveillance are colonoscopy and DCBE. The best evidence of the effectiveness of surveillance is for colonoscopy. In the National Polyp Study (NPS), a cohort of 1418 patients who had undergone complete colonoscopy and removal of one or more adenomatous polyps from the colon or rectum are followed for an average of 5.9 years with periodic colonoscopy.

After adjusting for age, sex, and polyp size, rates of carcinoma are 76 to 90% lower than expected ($p < 0.0001$) from comparison with three reference groups who have not undergone surveillance. If the first surveillance colonoscopy is negative, subsequent examinations are highly unlikely to reveal further adenomatous polyps. Thereafter, follow-up at 3-year intervals is adequate.

No direct evidence is available concerning when to stop surveillance. As with screening, the age at which surveillance should stop will depend on the judgment of patients and their clinicians, taking into account the patient's medical history and comorbidity. The decision on when to stop will also depend on the characteristics of the polyps removed and the results of follow-up examinations.

People who have had a CRC are at increased risk of a second (metachronous) carcinoma, apart from their risk of recurrence of the original carcinoma; this statistic should be considered when making surveillance recommendations for these individuals. No controlled studies of the effectiveness of surveillance strategies in this situation exist. Available information suggests that the metachronous carcinomas have a biologic behavior that is not, on average, different from initial carcinomas, except in increased frequency of occurrence. Carcinomas are preceded by adenomatous polyps. Therefore, by analogy they should undergo surveillance comparable to that recommended after polypectomy. The choice of surveillance procedure (colonoscopy versus barium enema) might be affected by distortions of normal anatomy and the adhesions caused by the surgery and should be decided on an individual basis. Colonoscopy permits removal of polyps that occur with higher frequency in these patients. Flexible sigmoidoscopy increases the sensitivity of DCBE and can visualize the anastomosis in distal resections.

Suggested Readings

Atkin WS, Morson BC, Cuzick J: Long-term risk of colorectal cancer after excision of rectosigmoid adenomas. N Engl J Med 1992;326:658–662.

Bond JH: Screening for colorectal cancer: Confuting the refuters. Gastrointest Endosc 1997;45:105–109.

Buess GF, Raestrup H: Transanal endoscopic microsurgery. Surg Oncol Clin North Am 2001;10:709–731.

Byers T, Levin B, Rothenberger D, et al: American Cancer Society guidelines for screening and surveillance for early detection of colorectal polyps and cancer.

Fenlon HM, Nunes DP, Schroy PC III, et al: A comparison of virtual and conventional colonoscopy for the detection of colorectal polyps. N Engl J Med 1999;341:1496–1503.

Imperiale TF, Wagner DR, Lin CY, et al: Risk of advanced proximal neoplasms in asymptomatic adults according to the distal colorectal findings. N Engl J Med 2000;343:169–174.

Jemal A, Murray T, Samuels A, et al: Cancer statistics. CA Cancer J Clin 2003;53:5–26.

Otchy DP, Ransohoff DF, Wolff BG, et al: Metachronous colon cancer in persons who have had a large adenomatous polyp. Am J Gastroenterol 1996;91:448–454.

Rembachen BJ, Fujii T, Cairns A, et al: Flat and depressed colonic neoplasms: A prospective study of 1000 colonoscopies in the UK. Lancet 2000;355:1211–1214.

Selby JV, Friedman GD, Quesenberry CP Jr, Weiss NS: A case-control study of screening sigmoidoscopy and mortality from colorectal cancer. N Engl J Med 1992;326:653–657.

Stryker SJ, Wolff BG, Culp CE, et al: Natural history of untreated colonic polyps. Gastroenterology 1987;93:1009–1013.

Winawer SJ, Fletcher RH, Miller L, et al: Colorectal cancer screening: Clinical guidelines and rationale. Gastroenterology 1997;112:594–642.

Winawer SJ, Zauber AG, Hom N, et al: Prevention of colorectal cancer by colonoscopic polypectomy. The National Polyp Study Workshop. N Engl J Med 1993;329(6):1977–1981.

59

MOLECULAR GENETICS OF COLORECTAL CANCER

James M. Church, MBChB, M Med Sci, FRACS

Over the last 10 years there has been steady and sometimes spectacular progress in our knowledge and understanding of human genetics and the way it affects disease. The public is becoming increasingly aware of genetics, although their knowledge, obtained through the media, is often unsophisticated. Surgeons dealing with patients who have genetic diseases need to have a working knowledge of the topic themselves so that they are equipped to answer patients' questions and to recommend appropriate investigations and treatment. The aims of this chapter are to present the basics of human genetics in a simplified and understandable way, and to show how genetics are implicated in colorectal cancer development.

■ THE BASICS OF HUMAN GENETICS

Genetics is the study of genes. The word is derived from the Greek *gennan*, to produce. Genes are defined segments of deoxyribonucleic acid (DNA), and each one carries the code for (produces) a specific protein. Molecular genetics is the study of genes at a molecular level, and clinical genetics is concerned with the medical conditions caused by defective genes.

Deoxyribonucleic Acid

DNA is a complex molecule that is present in the nucleus of every cell in the body. It is composed of two strands, each with a phosphate sugar backbone to which a series of nucleotide bases is attached. The two strands are linked by bonds between complementary bases, adenine to thymine and cytosine to guanine. Physically, the molecule forms a double helix.

The Genetic Code

Each bonded pair of nucleotide bases is a base pair. A longitudinal sequence of three bases on one strand of DNA is a triplet, also known as a codon. A codon, or triplet, of nucleotide bases on one strand of DNA is the key to the genetic code; it codes for a specific amino acid. A gene comprises a series of codons that produce a sequence of amino acids constituting the polypeptide core of a specific protein. There are almost 3 billion base pairs in a molecule of DNA and about 50,000 genes. These genes represent only about 5% of the genetic material in the DNA.

Genes

When the DNA is dissolved in the nucleus an enzyme called ribonucleic acid (RNA) polymerase synthesizes a molecule of messenger (m) RNA from DNA. The nucleotide bases in the mRNA are complementary to those in the DNA, except that in RNA uracil replaces thymine. The noncoding sequences of the gene (introns) are then spliced out of the mRNA, leaving the coding sequence (exons). This sequence exits the nucleus. In a ribosome in the cytoplasm, transfer (t) RNA brings amino acids to the mRNA. One end of the tRNA unites with a nucleotide base and the other holds the amino acid. As the tRNA molecules line up according to how their nucleotides bond with complementary bases in the mRNA, their amino acids also line up and a polypeptide is formed.

Inactivation of Genes

Genes may lose their function in at least three ways. They may acquire a mutation, they may undergo loss or change of a segment (loss of heterozygosity), or they may be hypermethylated. Mutations and methylation can be inherited. Loss of heterozygosity occurs within a tumor.

Mutations

A mutation is a permanent structural change in a gene. A nucleotide base may change, may disappear, or may be added. Sometimes several bases may be deleted or added. When this happens, the gene may work normally (polymorphism) or it may not. When gene function is disturbed the protein coded for may not be made, may be shorter than normal, and may work partially or not at all.

Point mutations are changes in a single base pair. Substitution mutations, when a single base is changed, are generally mis-sense mutations, not associated with a truncated protein. Deletion or insertion of one or more bases will alter the reading frame of the genetic code: a frameshift mutation. Such mutations usually lead to a "stop" codon, which causes premature termination of protein transcription and leads to a truncated protein. Almost all *APC* gene mutations (causing familial adenomatous polyposis) are non-sense mutations, while there are a number of mis-sense mutations involving mismatch repair genes in hereditary nonpolyposis colorectal cancer (HNPCC). Without help from an associated disease phenotype, it is difficult to distinguish a mis-sense mutation from a polymorphism.

Polymorphisms

A polymorphism is a variation in the structure (and sometimes function) of a gene present in >1% of the population. Polymorphisms are responsible for the infinite variation in the human species. Polymorphisms in some genes may be associated with an increased risk of colorectal cancer. This would not be associated with an obvious inherited syndrome but a mild to moderate family history of the disease.

Recently, a polymorphism has been reported in codon I1307k in *APC*. Non-sense mutations in this codon cause severe polyposis, but this T-to-A polymorphism is associated with familial colorectal cancer in Ashkenazi Jews. It seems to cause hypermutability during translation in the surrounding gene and so indirectly produces truncated APC protein. Its role and that of other polymorphisms in familial colorectal cancer outside Ashkenazi Jews remain to be defined.

Mutations may be somatic (soma = body), occurring only in the cells of the organ concerned (e.g., in the colon to produce sporadic cancer or adenomas) or germ line (in the spermatocyte or oocyte). Only germ cell mutations are heritable, and only germ line mutations can be detected by genetic blood tests.

Mutations occur for a variety of reasons. Most are environmental, due to diet, nicotine, ultraviolet and other radiation, or factors in the workplace. Other mutations occur merely as the body ages—DNA escaping normal control and repair mechanisms. Some mutations are inherited.

Loss of Heterozygosity

When cells divide, the DNA condenses and forms chromosomes (chroma = color, soma = body). These chromosomes can be precipitated and stained, and displayed as a karyotype. Chromosomes are ordered by descending size. There are 46 chromosomes, 23 pairs, one of each pair coming from each parent. There are therefore two copies of each gene (alleles), one from each parent. These copies can be identical (the person is homozygous for that gene) or different (heterozygous). Genes are given a location according to the chromosome they are on, defined by number (1 to 22) and whether they are on the long arm (q) or short arm (p) of the chromosome. Normal alleles are usually not exactly identical from one person to another; they exist in different forms (polymorphisms). However, within a single individual each allele should be the same in every cell.

During mitosis, chromosome pairs are pulled apart, with one copy going to each daughter cell. Sometimes this process is faulty, leading to loss of a gene copy (allele) by nondisjunction (failure to separate), deletion, and translocation. Only one normal gene is left. Because the cell is originally heterozygous for the gene (one paternal copy and one maternal copy), loss of an allele makes the cell appear homozygous; the heterozygosity has been lost. Loss of heterozygosity (LOH) is seen in tumors and precipitates loss of gene function when the remaining normal allele is mutated.

Gene Methylation

Methylation is a way of controlling the expression of genes. It normally occurs at islands of high concentrations of CpG dinucleotides in the promoter region at the 5' (front) end of a gene. Promoter methylation silences the gene; it is not expressed; no protein is made. Abnormal promoter methylation has been implicated in colorectal carcinogenesis affecting at least *APC* and *hMLH$_1$*, among other genes.

Inheritance

Because we inherit one copy of each gene from each parent, we are at risk of inheriting any mutation that may be present in our parents' genes. If only one mutated allele is necessary to produce disease, the pattern of inheritance is dominant; each child has a 50-50 chance of inheriting the mutated gene and developing the disease. If inheritance of two mutated alleles is necessary to cause disease, the pattern is recessive. Each child has a 1:4 chance of inheriting the disease (assuming both parents are carriers).

DNA Repair

When cells divide, DNA polymerase replicates the DNA molecule. Errors occur during replication and are corrected by DNA polymerase, and by a system of proteins coded for by DNA mismatch repair genes. These DNA repair genes (*hMSH$_2$*, *hMSH$_3$*, *hMSH$_6$*, *hMLH$_1$*, *hPMS$_1$*, *hPMS$_2$*) are homologs of highly conserved genes found in lower species of organisms. When a DNA mismatch repair gene is mutated and loses function, the entire DNA molecule is subject to multiple errors. These errors can be assessed by examining DNA microsatellites, segments of repeated base pairs from 10 to 100 bases long that have a length specific for every individual. When the length of a satellite differs between tumor tissue and normal tissue in the same patient, microsatellite instability may be present. When a difference is seen in two or more (or >30%) of a panel of five microsatellites, instability is deemed to be present, and there is likely to be a problem with DNA repair. This instability is the basis for HNPCC. Genes that contain microsatellites within them are particular targets for mutations when DNA mismatch repair is deficient. Some examples of such genes are *TGFβIIR*, *BAX*, *Caspase*, *hMSH$_3$*, *hMSH$_6$*.

■ GENETICS AND COLORECTAL TUMORIGENESIS

Cancer is a genetic disease. It is due to loss of control of cell growth and differentiation, a control that is normally tightly maintained by a balance of growth-enhancing and growth-inhibiting factors. Normal cell growth is stimulated by proto-oncogenes. When proto-oncogenes are overactive or inappropriately expressed, control of cell growth is lost. Only one proto-oncogene allele needs to be overactive for cell growth to be enhanced. Tumor suppressor genes play an inhibitory role in normal cell growth. When tumor suppressor gene function is lost, cell growth is enhanced. Because there are two copies of each gene, both have to be inactivated for tumor suppressor gene function to be lost. With common colorectal cancer, inactivations of both alleles are sporadic events, and it takes 40 to 60 years for this to happen to enough genes to produce invasive neoplasia. In a dominantly inherited syndrome, however, an affected parent transmits one mutated copy of the gene (one "hit"), which is therefore present at birth in every cell in the child's body. These cells are now primed for neoplasia so that when the remaining normal (wild-type) allele is inactivated by another mutation, by LOH, or by methylation (second "hit"), neoplasia starts much earlier than when both "hits" are sporadic.

Tumor suppressor genes associated with colorectal cancer include *APC* (5q21) (inherited mutation is familial adenomatous polyposis) and *p53* (17p13) (inherited mutation is Li-Fraumeni syndrome).

Genetic Pathways to Colorectal Cancer

There are two main genetic mechanisms by which colorectal neoplasia occurs: by an accumulation of inactivated tumor suppressor genes and overactive proto-oncogenes (the chromosomal instability [CIN] pathway), or by loss of DNA mismatch repair (microsatellite instability [MIN] pathway). Each pathway involves abnormal gene function in key intracellular signaling cascades, where the abnormal genes interfere with the cascade and confer a growth advantage on the affected line of cells, allowing growth and differentiation to be increasingly uncontrolled. Genes affected by the MIN pathway contain microsatellites, making them natural targets for mutation in mismatch repair deficiency. In both pathways there is a progressive increase in genetic inactivation and over activation from normal tissue through adenomas to adenocarcinoma, paralleling the adenoma-carcinoma sequence. This genetic adenoma-carcinoma sequence, first described by Vogelstein at Johns Hopkins, is shown in Figure 59-1.

Cancer cells exhibit not only uncontrolled growth but an ability to escape normal senescence and death. Apoptosis, programmed cell death, occurs as a response to severe mutations or an accumulation of genetic damage. When such damage is detected, cells are directed either to cell repair or to apoptosis. Proteins produced by the genes *p53* (CIN pathway), *BAX* (MIN pathway), and *bcl₂* are among those regulating this mechanism. If *p53* is mutated and the protein has lost its function, cells with severely damaged DNA can escape apoptosis, and the genetic damage is transmitted to the next generation. Another mechanism by which cell death occurs is through loss of telomeres. Telomeres are "caps" on chromosomes that stabilize them during cell division. With each cell division, telomeres shorten until eventually their length is insufficient for stability and the cell self-destructs. This inbuilt senescence is avoided in 90% of cancer cells that, through an enzyme called telomerase, have acquired the ability to rebuild the stabilizing telomeres.

Genetic Testing

Some patients present with a family history suggestive of an inherited disorder, and others may be obviously so affected (e.g., a colon full of polyps). In such patients genetic testing must be considered in the proband (the first patient in a family to present) to confirm the diagnosis and to form the basis for management of the family. Genetic testing should be arranged in the context of an IRB-approved genetic program including pre- and post-test counseling.

Genetic testing seeks to identify the presence of a mutation in a specific gene. This identification can be done in several ways. DNA is usually obtained from blood lymphocytes. The DNA segment of interest can be amplified by the polymerase chain reaction (PCR) and the sequence of the DNA determined. Mutations are then detected by comparing the patient's DNA with the normal sequence. Once the mutation present in the family is known, screening of at-risk family members is quick and easy. Searching for the family mutation in the proband by DNA sequencing is laborious and time-consuming, however, and various "short cuts" are available. One such technique is the protein truncation test. Here patient RNA is used to produce complementary DNA (cDNA) which is amplified by PCR. The cDNA is used to make the protein normally produced by the gene in question. The protein products are then separated by gel electrophoresis. If proteins of different lengths are found, there must be a mutation affecting the length of the protein produced. This test doesn't identify the mutation but will diagnose its presence in an individual without the need for information about his or her family. Its value depends on the presence of a truncating mutation causing the disease in the family being tested.

Signaling pathway	*Wnt*/Wingless	EGF	TGFβ	*p53*	
Genetic event	LOH/mutation Hypermethylation	Activation	LOH/mutation Hypermethylation	LOH/mutation	
CIN pathway genes	*APC*	*K-ras*	*SMAD₄*/DCC	*p53*	
MIN pathway genes	Beta catenin	*K-ras*	TGFβIIR	BAX	
Histology	Hyperproliferation	Early adenoma	Intermediate adenoma	Late adenoma	Carcinoma

Figure 59-1
The adenoma-carcinoma sequence.

This is almost always true in familial adenomatous polyposis (FAP) but is not necessarily the case in HNPCC.

Linkage analysis is a test used when the location of the mutated gene is not known. It relies on finding a DNA marker close enough to the gene to be inherited with it. Then, if the marker is positive in a test patient, it is likely that the mutation is also present. This test relies on knowing the status (of both marker and disease) of sufficient affected family members to allow a confident prediction in someone whose status is not known.

Immunohistochemistry can be used to look for the expression of a gene in tissue. The tissue is stained with an antibody to the protein made by the gene. If the protein is not expressed, there will be no staining. This is presumptive evidence of an inactivating mutation, and is useful when looking for expression of any tumor suppressor gene (e.g., p53, mismatch repair genes $hMSH_2$, $hMSH_3$, $hMSH_6$, and $hMLH_1$).

Testing for microsatellite instability (MSI) may have a role in screening for HNPCC. A battery of microsatellites is used; for instability to be deemed present, two or more, or >30%, of the markers must be abnormal. About 15 to 17% of common colorectal cancers show MSI. Some show MSI to high levels and some to low levels. Almost all HNPCC tumors have high levels of MSI. Thus, a tumor that has high MSI in a patient with a strong family history of colorectal cancer is predictive of HNPCC.

■ THE IMPACT OF MOLECULAR GENETICS ON COLORECTAL SURGERY

Prevention
As the field of chemoprevention develops and matures, drugs capable of reversing or compensating for the molecular genetic events leading to colorectal cancer may be developed. Already evidence suggests that sulindac reverses p53 mutation and restores apoptosis in adenomatous polyps, and restores apoptosis in mismatch repair–deficient neoplasms. Newer COX-2 inhibitors such as celecoxib and rofecoxib also inhibit colorectal tumorigenesis, as does the COX-independent sulindac derivative exisulind (sulindac sulfone).

Diagnosis
As technology progresses and genetic testing becomes more affordable, a molecular genetic profile of a colorectal tumor will become part of routine diagnosis and staging. Such a profile will provide information over and above that derived from a clinicopathologic staging.

Prognosis
One "hot" area of research recently has been the search for ways to stage colorectal cancers genetically, allowing better selection of patients for adjuvant treatment based on the genetic "fingerprint" of the tumor. p53 mutation signifies a bad prognosis, and mismatch repair–deficient cancers have a better prognosis than predicted from histologic staging. The role of K-ras activation in formulating prognosis has yet to be defined, but mutations in other genes (e.g., beta catenin, E cadherin) may be associated with an increased risk of metastasis. Use of molecular genetic techniques to assess lymph node status may offer better prognostic information than histopathologic examination.

Selection of Treatment
The most common chemotherapeutic drug used in patients with colorectal cancer is 5-fluorouracil (5-FU). Evidence suggests that an intact DNA repair system is needed for 5-FU and related drugs to work. Mismatch repair–deficient tumors may therefore be relatively resistant to standard chemotherapy.

Mismatch repair–deficient tumors tend to be multiple, especially when they occur within the context of HNPCC. HNPCC patients undergoing surgery for a colon cancer or multiple adenomas should have a complete colectomy and ileorectal anastomosis (IRA) assuming sphincter function is normal and operative risk is low.

Screening
Screening for colorectal cancer may be revolutionized by molecular genetics, if current research into DNA stool analysis bears fruit. It is possible to recover DNA from stool and to search for mutations in genes associated with colorectal neoplasia. Preliminary results show sensitivity in the order of 70% and specificity over 90%. A stool DNA test for the microsatellite marker Bat-26 recently has been marketed as a test for mismatch repair–deficient neoplasia. If these tests can be cost-effective, they may prove much more specific and sensitive than any of the current occult blood tests.

Screening for colorectal neoplasia in members of high-risk kindreds can be refined by predictive testing for germline mutations. When a pathogenic mutation is found in a family, all at-risk members who do not have the mutation are excused from screening until they turn 50, at which age population-risk screening begins. Screening of the general population by DNA blood testing for cancer-predisposing polymorphisms is a distinct possibility. At least three polymorphisms associated with increased risk for colorectal cancer have been identified.

Surveillance
Surveillance protocols are designed according to risk of metachronous neoplasia. Molecular genetics may have an impact on these protocols by allowing better definition of the risks of metachronous lesions.

■ SUMMARY

Molecular genetics is likely to impact every aspect of colorectal cancer screening, surveillance, prevention, diagnosis, staging, and management. Knowledge of molecular genetics as applied to colorectal neoplasia is likely to be a prerequisite to caring for patients with colorectal neoplasia.

Suggested Readings

Burke W, Peterson G, Lynch P, et al: Recommendations for follow-up of individuals with an inherited predisposition to cancer. I. Hereditary nonpolyposis colon cancer. JAMA 1997;277:915–919.

Church JM, Williams BRG: Molecular Genetics and Colorectal Neoplasia: A Primer for the Clinician, 2nd ed. New York, Kluwer, 2003.

De Cosse JJ: Surgical prophylaxis of familial colon cancer: Prevention of death from familial colorectal cancer. J Natl Cancer Inst 1995;Monograph 17:31–33.

Fearon ER, Vogelstein B: A genetic model for colorectal tumorigenesis. Cell 1990;61:759–767.

Gradia S, Acharya S, Fishel R: The human mismatch recognition complex hMSH2-hMSH6 functions as a novel molecular switch. Cell 1997;91:995–1005.

Jarvinen HJ, Mecklin JP, Sistonene P: Screening reduces colorectal cancer rate in families with hereditary nonpolyposis colorectal cancer. Gastroenterology 1995;108:1405–1411.

Jorde LB, Carey JC, White, RL: Medical Genetics. St. Louis, Mosby-Year Book, 1995.

Laken SJ, Peterson GM, Gruber SB, et al: Familial colorectal cancer in Ashkenazim due to a hypermutable tract APC. Nat Genet 1997;17:79–83.

Leder P, Clayton DA, Rubenstein E (Eds.): Introduction to Molecular Medicine. New York, Scientific Medicine, 1994.

Lynch HT: Is there a role for prophylactic subtotal colectomy among hereditary nonpolyposis colorectal cancer germline mutation carriers? Dis Colon Rectum 1996;39:109–110.

Lynch HT, Smyrk T, Lynch J: Clinical and molecular genetic aspects of the Lynch syndromes. Semin Colon Rectal Surg 1995;6:38–47.

Madoff RD: Molecular biology of colorectal cancer. Semin Colon Rectal Surg 1998;9.

Rodriguez-Bigas MA, Boland CR, Hamilton SR, et al: A National Cancer Institute workshop on hereditary nonpolyposis colorectal cancer syndrome: Meeting highlights and Bethesda Guidelines. J Natl Cancer Inst 1997;89:1758–1762.

Rossi SC, Srivastava S: National Cancer Institute workshop on genetic screening for colorectal cancer. J Natl Cancer Inst 1996;88:331–339.

Vasen HFA, Nagengast FM, Khan PM: Interval cancers in hereditary nonpolyposis colorectal cancer. Lancet 1995;345:1183–1184.

Vogelstein B, Fearon ER, Hamilton SR, et al: Genetic alterations during colorectal-tumor development. N Engl J Med 1988;319:525–532.

Winde G, Schmid KW, Schlegel W, et al: Complete reversion and prevention of rectal adenomas in colectomized patients with familial adenomatous polyposis by rectal low-dose sulindac maintenance treatment. Dis Colon Rectum 1995;38:813–830.

60

FAMILIAL ADENOMATOUS POLYPOSIS

Claudio Soravia, MD, MSc
Zane Cohen, MD, FRCS(C), FACS

Familial adenomatous polyposis (FAP) is an inherited, autosomal dominant syndrome with complete penetrance, characterized by the development of multiple colorectal adenomatous polyps. The frequency at birth is estimated to be 1 in 10,000. In approximately 20% of FAP patients no family history can be traced owing to spontaneous mutations in the adenomatous polyposis coli (APC) gene or to illegitimacy. Important clinical features include variable age of onset (range, 10 to 40 years of age) and variable expression within and between families. If left untreated, one or more of the colorectal adenomas will progress to colorectal cancer (CRC). FAP accounts for only 1% of all CRCs. In addition to colorectal adenomas, other gastrointestinal lesions may occur, such as gastric and duodenal adenomas. Other benign and malignant extracolonic manifestations have been described, such as desmoid tumors, thyroid tumors, epidermoid cysts, osteomas, congenital hypertrophy of the retinal pigment epithelium (CHRPE), hepatobiliary tumors, adrenocortical tumors, and brain tumors.

This chapter stresses the role of predictive genetic testing and of particular genotype-phenotype correlations of the APC gene in the global management of affected patients and their families, and compares different surgical and medical options. The topic of desmoid tumors is discussed in Chapter 61.

■ GENETIC BACKGROUND

The genetic locus for FAP was mapped to chromosome 5q21 in 1987 and the responsible gene, APC, was cloned in 1991. APC is a tumor suppressor gene. Similar to the "two hit" theory proposed by Knudson for retinoblastoma, in FAP patients, a germline APC mutation (first hit) is followed by a somatic mutation or deletion (second hit) of the second APC allele. This series leads to a predisposition to malignant transformation. The normal APC protein plays important roles in cell-to-cell adhesion mechanisms, in cellular signal transduction, and in chromosomal separation during mitosis. Loss of APC function is one of the first abnormalities leading to abnormal cellular proliferation of the colonic epithelium. The APC protein may also participate in the regulation of cell cycle progression (leading to an epithelial hyperproliferative status) and may play a role in regulation of apoptosis or programmed cell death.

Genetic mutations of the APC gene have been studied extensively. Hot spots for germline mutations (where 20% of the mutations occur) are located at codons 1061 and 1309, whereas for somatic mutations, a cluster region has been determined between codons 1044 and 1554. Over 90% of the mutations result in truncated proteins. So far, genotype-phenotype correlative studies have shown a positive association of CHRPE with germline mutations spanning exons 9 to 15. A *profuse* colonic polyposis phenotype (more than 5000 adenomas), segregating with germline APC mutations in the region between codons 1250 and 1464, has been reported, whereas mutations between codons 213 and 1597 lead to a *sparse* FAP phenotype (up to 1000 to 2000 adenomas). Patients with few colonic adenomas and late onset of CRC show genetic alterations at the 5' end of the APC gene, at exon 9, and at the 3' (distal) end of the gene; this subgroup is named "attenuated" adenomatous polyposis coli (AAPC) phenotype. AAPC is a milder form of FAP. Phenotypically, AAPC differs from classical FAP in the number of colonic adenomas (less than 100), and the tendency for polyps to be located proximal to the splenic flexure. These adenomas may be flat rather than polypoid. Gastric fundic and duodenal polyps are also found; CHRPE is absent, and desmoid tumors have not yet been described in AAPC due to exon 3 or 4 mutations. Finally, the average age of onset of CRC is later in AAPC (on average, 55 years of age) than in classical FAP (on average, 39 years of age). More recently, germline APC mutations at codons 1924 and 1962 were shown to lead to the development of desmoid tumors, but with almost no colonic adenomas.

It has been suggested that the location of the APC mutation could guide the surgical choice between an ileorectal anastomosis (IRA) or ileal pouch–anal anastomosis (IPAA). It seems that the risk of rectal cancer in patients with a mutation beyond codon 1250 is indeed higher than that in patients with mutations preceding codon 1250. For the former group, an IPAA should be considered, provided that no other contraindication to this operation exists. For the latter group, an IRA might be sufficient. Such reports should, however, still be viewed with caution, and additional studies are needed to confirm these results. Specific APC mutation sites should rather be used for closer surveillance for extracolonic manifestations such as desmoid tumors. Our own experience with AAPC families with mutations at the proximal (exons 3 and 4) and distal ends of the APC gene suggests that the location of the colonic adenomas is, as expected, on the right side of the colon, and that the rectum seems to be spared. For such patients, IRA can be advised. Moreover, none of these patients with IRA has yet developed rectal cancer.

■ PREDICTIVE GENETIC TESTING

APC gene carriers and their at-risk relatives are best counseled and followed up in a polyposis registry in which a multidisciplinary team including colorectal surgeons, gastroenterologists, molecular biologists, and genetic counselors works with referring physicians. Figure 60-1 shows the algorithm that has been developed at the Familial Gastrointestinal Cancer Registry of the Mount Sinai Hospital in Toronto to assess these patients and families.

First, a clinical assessment is performed, looking for the presence of colorectal adenomas with or without CRC, gastroduodenal polyps, CHRPE, mandibular osteomas, and desmoid tumors. The second step consists of the genetic testing of these patients (RNA and DNA is extracted from white blood cells from fresh blood samples) using three strategies:

1. A simple, nonradioactive technique (the heteroduplex analysis, HA) is used for analysis of the two "hot spot" regions of the gene. HA is able to detect the presence of a DNA variant in the fragment analyzed, in this case, the unique five base pair deletions of codons 1061 (del ACAAA) and 1309 (del AAAGA). Its sensivity is 80%.
2. If HA is negative, the protein truncation test (PTT) assay is done. This technique is able to detect truncated proteins resulting from germline *APC* mutations (frameshift, splice-site, or nonsense mutations). The entire gene is analyzed in six overlapping segments. Briefly, we use a rabbit reticulocyte cell system for an in vitro transcription/translation of a fragment of *APC*

gene, with a radioactive isotope. A positive test gives the approximate location of the mutation. The PTT sensitivity is approximately 85%. The PTT assay requires significant levels of technical expertise as well as expertise in the interpretation of these results. Usually, direct sequencing is then undertaken to characterize the mutation.
3. In large kindreds, linkage analysis methodology can be used if the foregoing tests remain negative. Future prospects to improve mutation screening rates will include the enzyme mismatch cleavage methods and the use of artificial yeast assays to detect mis-sense mutations.

At our registry, predictive genetic testing is suggested to at-risk individuals from puberty. For children, flexible sigmoidoscopy is started at 10 years and repeated at intervals depending on the findings. Gene carriers are enrolled in surveillance programs and prophylactic surgery is recommended at an age suitable to the family and the surgeon. Almost all the positive gene carriers come to surgery within 2 years of clinical or molecular genetic diagnosis. Individuals from an FAP family with a known mutation who do not carry that mutation do not need any further surveillance. However, they still remain at the general pop-

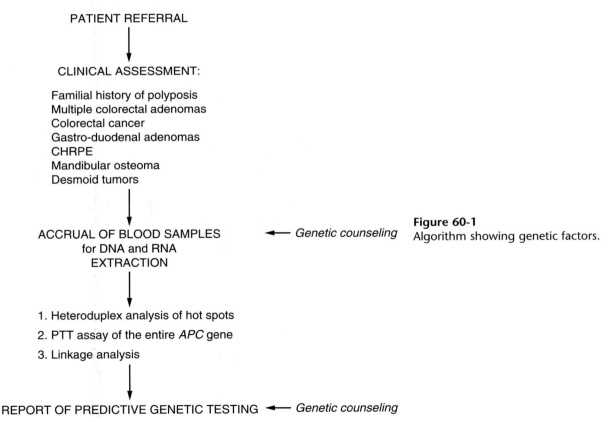

Figure 60-1
Algorithm showing genetic factors.

ulation risk level for CRC. The results of predictive genetic testing are given directly to the patient after appropriate pre- and post-genetic counseling. The patient then decides whether or not he or she wishes to forward them to his or her physician.

■ SURGICAL THERAPY

In 1919, Lockart Mummery performed the first colectomy with ileorectal anastomosis in an anemic FAP patient who presented with several episodes of lower gastrointestinal bleeding. Since that time, this procedure has gained widespread acceptance in the preventive treatment of FAP. However, controversy still exists as to whether colectomy with IRA or restorative proctocolectomy with IPAA and mucosectomy is the better procedure. Proctocolectomy with terminal ileostomy is now rarely performed. The advantages and limitations of each procedure are discussed in Table 60-1.

Once the molecular genetic diagnosis of FAP is confirmed, prophylactic surgery is required, whether or not patients are symptomatic. Preoperative evaluation should include full colonoscopy to evaluate the number and the distribution of the polyps, and to detect any cancer. Biopsies are taken in the rectal and anal mucosa to determine if any dysplasia is present.

Total Colectomy and IRA

This procedure consists of the removal of the entire colon, leaving approximately 15 cm of the rectum to which the ileum is anastomosed. The indication for this operation is patients with fewer than 10 rectal polyps, and those with the molecular diagnosis of AAPC. The main advantage of this procedure is its low postoperative morbidity rate (range, overall 16 to 21%), with small bowel obstruction being the most frequent complication. In the long term, these patients also show consistently good functional

results with little evidence of seepage, urgency, day- and nighttime incontinence, excessive stool frequency, and need for antidiarrheal medication. The IRA procedure can be performed laparoscopically.

The major concern after IRA is the risk of developing cancer in the retained rectum despite close follow-up. The risk is estimated to be 37% after 20 years. In the St. Mark's Hospital experience, a cumulative risk of 10% at 50 years of age and of 29% at 60 years of age reinforces the importance of endoscopic rectal surveillance and the need for rectal excision with conversion to either IPAA, permanent ileostomy, or Kock pouch. In our personal experience, 4 of 59 (6.7%) FAP patients developed rectal cancer despite close follow-up after colectomy and IRA. Patients with IRA should undergo yearly endoscopic surveillance of the rectum.

Restorative Proctocolectomy and IPAA with Mucosectomy

This operation is aimed at removing the colon and rectum down to the level of the dentate line. Therefore, the risk of CRC is theoretically eliminated. Specifically, the dissection stays close to the rectal wall in order to avoid injury to the pelvic nerves, thus preventing the complication of urinary and sexual dysfunction. Moreover, endoanal mucosal stripping must be performed carefully and completely. Residual mucosa left inadvertently may ultimately produce a cancer. Protracted stretching of the anus should also be avoided in order to minimize any injury to the sphincter. Our preference is to do this procedure in two stages. The first stage is IPAA with mucosectomy and diverting loop ileostomy. Colonic mobilization can be performed laparoscopically, with the IPAA performed via Pfannestiel incision. The second stage involves closure of the loop ileostomy approximately 3 months later. Postoperative morbidity rate is greater following IPAA than IRA, and although most of these complications are not life-threatening, they often require rehospitalization

Table 60-1 Prophylactic Surgery for FAP Patients (Excluding Propositus)			
FACTOR	**IRA**	**IPAA**	**PC WITH ILEOSTOMY/ KOCK POUCH**
Indications for surgery	< 10 rectal polyps AAPC	Most of FAP patients Rectal polyp carpeting Resectable rectal cancer Desmoids in family history	Older patients after IRA Poor anal sphincter tone Low rectal cancer nonresectable oncologically by IPAA
Age at surgery	Within 2 years of phenotypic expression and molecular diagnosis	Within 2 years of phenotypic expression and molecular diagnosis	At CRC diagnosis
Mortality rate	Very low	Very low	Very low
Morbidity rate	Low	High	Low (high with Kock pouch)
Functional outcome			
Early	Good	Average	Good
Late	Good	Good	Good
Follow-up	Rectal endoscopy 1×/year	Pouch endoscopy 1×/3 years	Same as for sporadic CRC: pouch endoscopy 1×/3 years

AAPC = attenuated adenomatous polyposis coli; CRC = colorectal cancer; FAP = familial adenomatous polyposis; IPAA = restorative proctocolectomy with ileal pouch–anal anastomosis and mucosectomy; IRA = total colectomy with ileorectal anatosmosis; PC = proctocolectomy with permanent terminal ileostomy.

of the patient. The most common early postoperative complications include pouch leaks with or without pelvic sepsis (5 to 7%), and small bowel obstruction. In the literature, the overall complication rate ranges between 15 and 50%, whereas small bowel obstruction alone occurs in 20 to 25% of the cases. Less than half of these cases require reoperation. Unlike patients with ulcerative colitis, FAP patients rarely present with episodes of pouchitis (5% versus 20 to 25%).

In the short term, the functional outcome of IPAA is less favorable than that of IRA with regard to stool frequency, urgency, day- and nighttime continence, need for antidiarrheal medication, and diet. However, in the long term (more than 2 years), the IPAA functional results are similar to those of IRA. When necessary, conversion of IRA to IPAA seems to provide the same long-term favorable outcomes. Recent studies have reported that there is a decrease in fecundity (the ability to conceive) in women with FAP undergoing IPAA. This should be discussed with patients preoperatively. Finally, in patients with cancer of the upper or middle rectum, the oncologic resection can be included with the IPAA procedure by including total mesorectal excision.

Restorative proctocolectomy with IPAA and mucosectomy has become the operation of choice for most of our FAP patients. Our preference is also to do IPAA in cases with a familial history of desmoid tumors. In such families, we have experienced significant difficulties in trying to convert a previously performed IRA to an IPAA if a desmoid has developed. In fact, it may be difficult to perform a rectal excision and achieve enough length to exteriorize the ileum as an end-ileostomy in these individuals. A Kock pouch is contraindicated in view of the thickness of the mesentery.

The long-term fate of the mucosal lining of an ileal reservoir in patients with FAP is not completely known. Polyps develop in these pouches, and to date three cases of pouch cancer after IPAA in FAP patients have been reported. This underlines the need for endoscopic surveillance of the ileal reservoir. Options for treatment of ileal pouch adenomas include the use of photodynamic ablative laser therapy, and the long-term use of sulindac or other nonsteroidal anti-inflammatory drugs (NSAIDs).

Proctocolectomy and Permanent Terminal Ileostomy—Kock Pouch

This procedure is rarely indicated in FAP patients. In our experience, this operation is performed in patients with lower rectal cancer, when oncologic resection would be compromised by an IPAA procedure. Moreover, older patients with a previous IRA procedure and poor anal sphincter function may not be good candidates for an IPAA operation.

The construction of a continent ileal pouch (Kock pouch) may be an attractive option in these patients. Briefly, the Kock pouch is constructed using terminal ileum, with an intussuscepted ileal segment of the outlet known as the nipple valve created to achieve full continence. The valve is intubated when the pouch needs to be emptied. The most common complication is slippage of the nipple valve (10 to 20%). This complication usually requires reoperation. Small bowel obstruction occurs in approximately 6 to 15% of the cases. Overall satisfaction is high in patients with a Kock pouch, although morbidity and reoperation rates are high.

■ EXTRACOLONIC MANIFESTATIONS

Since the introduction of FAP registries and prophylactic colorectal surgery, a shift in mortality rate has occurred. Ampullary/duodenal cancer and desmoid tumors have become the most common causes of death in FAP patients.

The detailed management of desmoid tumors will be discussed in Chapter 61. However, it is worthwhile to mention that in our experience, it is better to avoid any attempt at surgical resection of large complex intra-abdominal desmoid tumors, as these tumors often encircle the major vasculature of the small bowel and cannot be excised for cure. The recurrence rate is exceptionally high (approximately 85%). For very complex and symptomatic cases, we have used cytotoxic drugs in combination: doxorubicin and dacarbazine followed by carboplatin and dacarbazine. In eight FAP patients with a mean follow-up of 42 months, two patients had complete tumor regression and four had partial, but significant, shrinkage. Symptoms, mainly of obstruction, have disappeared.

Epidemiologic studies have shown that FAP patients have a relative risk of ampullary and duodenal cancers 100 to 300 times that of a control population, respectively. Moreover, duodenal polyps develop in up to 90% of FAP patients, with polyps clustering around the ampulla. At our institution, upper gastrointestinal endoscopy is advised routinely in FAP patients by the age of 30 years. A side-viewing endoscope is used to visualize the ampulla of Vater. Multiple biopsies are taken from the gastric, duodenal, and ampullary mucosa, and from any visible lesions. We have developed a staging system and recommendations for surveillance and treatment (Table 60-2). Familial segregation has been demonstrated with respect to the severity of periampullary tumors in FAP kindreds. In our prospective study, 14 out of 74 patients (15%) developed advanced duodenal polyposis. For stage IV, we suggest either endoscopic or local surgical resection. Radical surgery (the Whipple procedure or pylorus-preserving duodenopancreatectomy) is performed in cases of large (>3 cm) ampullary adenomas, when rapid growth and severe dysplasia are observed, and in cases of cancer. As in other reports, endoscopic or surgical resection is associated with high recurrence rates. However, because recurrent polyps are small (<2–3 mm) and the natural history of duodenal polyposis is not completely understood at the genetic level (a possible role of carcinogens in the bile has also been suggested), it seems reasonable to suggest that many years may pass before these growths progress to large, severely dysplastic lesions. In our registry, follow-up remains too short to state whether death from duodenal/ampullary cancers is prevented by this strategy.

Table 60-2 Surveillance and Management of Duodenal Polyps in FAP Patients

STAGE	ENDOSCOPIC MORPHOLOGY	HISTOLOGY	SURVEILLANCE AND TREATMENT
I	Normal	Normal	EGD/each 5 years
II	Normal or polyp 1–2 mm	Adenoma	EGD/each 3 years
III	Polyp 2.1–10 mm	Adenoma	EGD/each 6 months
IV	Polyp >10 mm	Adenoma	Endoscopic/local surgical resection
V	Any polyp or mass	Adenocarcinoma	Radical surgery

EGD = esophagogastroduodenoscopy; FAP = familial adenomatous polyposis.

FAP patients are also at risk for developing other malignant tumors such thyroid, adrenocortical, hepatobiliary, pancreatic, and brain cancers. Because the occurrence of these tumors remains relatively low, we do not recommend any particular screening.

■ MEDICAL THERAPY

Polyp regression in FAP patients has been demonstrated with the use of sulindac, a NSAID that inhibits cyclo-oxygenase, a key enzyme in the conversion of arachidonic acid to eicosanoids. There are two cyclo-oxygenase enzymes: COX-1 and COX-2. Sulindac is active against both of them. Recent studies have shown that COX-2 plays a major role in the development of adenomas in colorectal carcinogenesis, and that COX-2 overexpression may result from an inability of the *APC* gene product to carry out its normal function. Celecoxib, a selective COX-2 inhibitor, was used in a double-blind, randomized, placebo-controlled study in 77 patients with FAP. After 6 months, patients receiving the higher dose of celecoxib (400 mg twice daily) showed a 28% reduction in mean number of polyps and a 30.7% reduction in the sum of polyp diameters. Further studies are planned.

Uncontrolled and randomized controlled trials of sulindac have demonstrated that this drug will also substantially reduce the number and size of adenomas in patients with FAP. However, polyp resolution is not generally complete, and recurrence is observed after cessation of therapy. Of concern are the anecdotal reports of rectal cancer development in FAP patients while on sulindac therapy. Finally, sulindac seems to be effective only on small polyps (<3 mm). Overall, these data suggest that medical therapy is not yet safe and effective to obtain consistent adenoma regression and prevent cancer in FAP. Therefore, these drugs, when indicated, should be given only to patients who have undergone prophylactic surgery.

■ SUMMARY

During the last decade, advances in the basic molecular genetic mechanisms have broadened our understanding of FAP as a global syndrome affecting different organs and systems. Predictive genetic testing and the knowledge of specific genotype-phenotype correlations have become important in the management of FAP patients and their relatives. In the near future, the awareness of specific germline mutations might guide the surgeon with regard to the choice of surgical therapy. For now, the IPAA procedure has gained more widespread acceptance as the operation of choice in these patients, whereas IRA and proctocolectomy with or without continent ileostomy still may be applicable in selected cases. Finally, further studies and treatments are necessary in patients with desmoid tumors and duodenal/ampullary adenomas in order to reduce the mortality rates from these extracolonic manifestations.

Suggested Readings

Church JM, Lowry A, Simmang C: Practice parameters for the identification and testing of patients at risk for dominantly inherited colorectal cancer—Supporting documentation. Dis Colon Rectum 2001;44:1404–1412.

Church JM, McGannon E, Burke C, Clark B: Teenagers with familial adenomatous polyposis: What is their risk for colorectal cancer? Dis Colon Rectum 2002;45:887–889.

Church JM, Simmang C: Practice parameters for the treatment of patient with dominantly inherited colorectal cancer (FAP on HNPCC). Dis Colon Rectum 2003;46:1001–1012.

deVos WH, Jarvinen HJ, Bjork J, et al: Worldwide survey among polyposis registries of surgical management of severe duodenal adenomatosis in familial adenomatous polyposis. Br J Surg 2003;90:705–710.

Fearnhead NS, Britton MP, Bodmer WF: The ABC of APC. Hum Molec Genet 2001;10:721–733.

Fodde R, Smits R: Disease model: Familial adenomatous polyposis. Trends Mol Med 2001;7:369–373.

Giardiello F: NSAID-induced polyp regression in familial adenomatous polyposis patients. Gastroenterology Clin North Am 1996;25:349–361.

Kartheuser AH, Parc R, Penna C, et al: Ileal pouch–anal anastomosis as the first choice operation in patients with familial adenomatous polyposis: A ten-year experience. Surgery 1996;119:615–623.

Nugent K, Phillips R: Rectal cancer risk in older patients with familial adenomatous polyposis and an ileorectal anastomosis: A cause for concern. Br J Surg 1992;79:1204–1206.

Poritz LS, Blackstein M, Berk T, et al: Extended follow-up of patients treated with cytotoxic chemotherapy for intra-abdominal desmoid tumors. Dis Colon Rectum 2001;44:1268–1273.

Soravia C, Berk T, Cohen Z: Molecular genetic testing and surgical decision making in hereditary colorectal cancer. Int J Colorect Dis 2000;15:21–28.

Soravia C, Berk T, Madlensky L, et al: Genotype-phenotype correlations in attenuated adnomatous polyposis coli. Am J Hum Genet 1998;62:1290–1301.

Steinbach G, Lynch PM, Phillips RK, et al: The effect of celecoxib, a cyclooxygenase-2 inhibitor, in familial adenomatous polyposis. N Engl J Med 2000;342:1946–1952.

Vasen HFA, van der Luijt RB, Slors JFM, et al: Molecular genetic tests as a guide to surgical management of familial adenomatous polyposis. Lancet 1996;348:433–435.

Wu J, Paul P, McGannon E, et al: APC genotype, polyp number, and surgical options in familial adenomatous polyposis coli. Ann Surg 1998;227:57–62.

61

DESMOID TUMORS

James M. Church, MBChB, M Med Sci, FRACS

Desmoid tumors are overgrowths of fibroaponeurotic tissue. They are rare in the general population but occur in 10 to 15% of patients with familial adenomatous polyposis (FAP). Although desmoid tumors are benign in that they don't metastasize, they can cause symptoms due to expansion and infiltration. Desmoid tumors cause major problems in the management of patients with FAP, owing to their effects on adjacent organs and the impact they have on surgical treatment of the large bowel. In this chapter the nature and incidence of desmoids will be discussed, along with current thoughts on their management.

■ DEFINITION, INCIDENCE, AND GENETICS

Clinically obvious desmoid tumors are relatively uncommon in patients with FAP, with the reported incidence ranging from 10 to 15%. They usually present as a mass lesion that causes symptoms by pressure effects on adjacent organs. Asymptomatic desmoids may be discovered incidentally during laparotomy or on computed tomographic (CT) scanning. The incidence of asymptomatic desmoid tumors is approximately 30%.

The term *desmoid tumor* implies a mass lesion (Fig. 61-1). *Desmoid reaction* has been used to describe the hard, white plaques that can be found on and within the small bowel mesentery of many patients with FAP (Fig. 61-2). Although asymptomatic, such plaques can have a major influence on clinical care by preventing ileal pouch–anal anastomosis.

Since the *APC* gene has been cloned, over 450 different mutations have been identified. Significant correlations exist between the site of the mutation and the severity of the polyposis, as well as the presence of CHRPE. A tendency for desmoids to occur more frequently in 3′ (downstream in exon 15) mutations is becoming apparent. A "desmoid tumor family," in which desmoids occurred in the absence of polyposis, has been described with an *APC* mutation at codon 1934. In other families with 3′ *APC* mutations extra-abdominal desmoids are found in infants, and relatively mild polyposis develops later. Such patients are at risk for postsurgical intra-abdominal desmoids and are a group in which surgery for polyposis should be delayed as long as possible. In general, the presence of a symptomatic desmoid in a family member increases the risk of desmoid formation in affected relatives.

■ PRESENTATION

FAP desmoids differ from sporadic desmoids in that most symptomatic tumors are intra-abdominal. Approximately 20% may be extra-abdominal or in the abdominal wall. Up to 80% develop after abdominal surgery, leading to a suspicion that trauma plays a role in their development. Evidence that desmoid tumors may be estrogen-dependent includes their predilection for women and their occasional response to estrogen-blocking drugs. Intra-abdominal desmoid tumors cause pain due to their mass effect or by obstruction of the bowel or ureter. Desmoid tumors may erode into blood vessels or bowel, causing necrosis, fistula, abscess, or hemorrhage. They may also liquefy. Submucosal desmoids can cause localized ischemia of the bowel leading to strictures and ulcers. Such patients may present with chronic anemia due to gastrointestinal bleeding. Desmoid reaction scleroses mesentery, causing kinking and puckering of the bowel and its mesentery, predisposing to subacute bowel obstruction with postprandial pain, nausea, and eventual weight loss.

■ NATURAL HISTORY

The natural history of desmoid tumors and desmoid reaction is hard to define. Many cases are incidental findings and may have been present without symptoms for a long time, yet in others the course is influenced by a variety of therapies. Some anecdotal reports describe rapid, relentless growth without response to any treatment, and others tell of spontaneous disappearance. Such extreme events are uncommon (about 7% each), although desmoid tumors are the second most common cause of death in patients with FAP. A recent review at the Cleveland Clinic suggests that most desmoid tumors are either inert or undergo cycles of growth and remission without ever threatening a patient's life.

A study from St Mark's Hospital has suggested that growing desmoid tumors can be distinguished from inert tumors by their appearance on abdominal magnetic resonance imaging (MRI). Growing tumors enhance in T2-weighted images but inert tumors do not.

■ PREVENTION

Nothing has been shown to effectively prevent desmoid tumors, although common sense suggests avoidance of circumstances thought to have a role in their stimulation: surgery, estrogens, or trauma.

Unnecessary surgery is avoided, and when surgery is inevitable it must be as gentle as possible. If surgery is to be done in a patient with a known desmoid tumor, premedication with sulindac may be beneficial. The use of oral contraceptives by any woman with FAP should be discouraged, and patients with known desmoid tumors should avoid pregnancy.

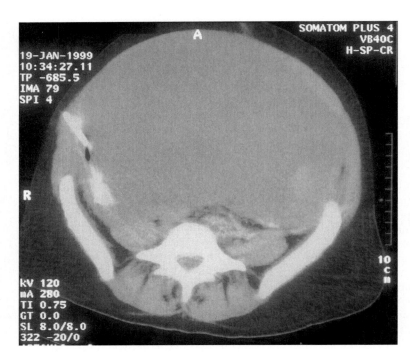

Figure 61-1
Abdominal computed tomographic scan showing a huge intra-abdominal desmoid tumor. This tumor was treated with cytotoxic chemotherapy but did not respond. The patient then underwent radiation, which killed the desmoid but produced enterocutaneous fistulas.

■ TREATMENT

Medical

Although many have been tried, no drug works reliably. The two most useful classes of medications are nonsteroidal anti-inflammatory drugs (NSAIDs) and estrogen blockers. One retrospective controlled study suggested that long-term sulindac treatment is better than nothing in inducing remission (150 mg twice daily for 2 years), and there are anecdotal reports of success with tamoxifen in doses up to 120 mg per day.

Chemotherapy

Antisarcoma-type chemotherapy using doxorubicin and dacarbazine has produced dramatic responses in some patients with life-threatening desmoid tumors. A recent report by Poritz and colleagues from Toronto describe two complete responses and four partial responses out of eight patients. A similar experience has been reported by other

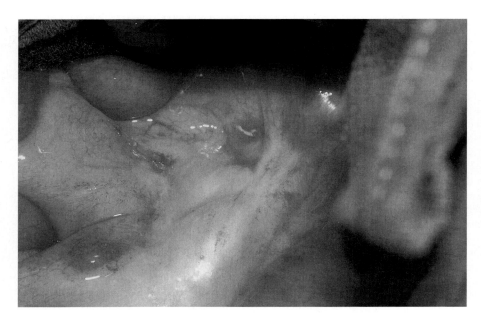

Figure 61-2
Desmoid reaction: a typical white plaque or sheet of tissue in the small bowel mesentery discovered during surgery to remove a patient's rectum and perform an ileal pouch–anal anastomosis. Despite this desmoid reaction, the surgery went ahead as planned.

institutions, establishing chemotherapy as an effective last resort.

RADIATION

Conflicting reports exist on the value of radiotherapy. Although external beam radiation does produce tumor shrinkage or tumor necrosis, the risk of radiation enteritis limits its use for intra-abdominal desmoid tumors.

Surgery

Excisional surgery for intra-abdominal desmoid tumors is associated with recurrence rates greater than 65%. This rate, along with the risks of short bowel syndrome, postoperative fistulas, and major hemorrhage and a need for permanent intravenous feeding, make attempts at removal of desmoid tumors very unattractive. Abdominal wall desmoid tumors, however, can sometimes be excised. Although the recurrence rate is still high, the morbidity is less serious. If abdominal wall tumors are growing despite sulindac, and if they are clearly apart from intra-abdominal structures, surgery is reasonable.

Desmoid Tumors and Surgery
Scenario 1. Surprise Desmoid at First Operation.
It is better to do a proctocolectomy and pouch, if possible, to avoid a later requirement for proctectomy. If a pouch will not reach the anal canal because of the desmoid, an ileorectal anastomosis (IRA) is reasonable for mild disease (<1000 polyps in the colon, <20 polyps in the rectum). If the patient has severe polyposis, do a proctocoletomy and ileostomy.

Scenario 2. Desmoid Found at Proctectomy after IRA.
In this case the rectum must be removed. Warn the patient preoperatively that if there is a desmoid, it may be impossible to do a restorative proctectomy and that a permanent ileostomy may be unavoidable. If there is a family history of desmoid disease, get a preoperative abdominal CT scan to exclude mass lesions and pretreat with sulindac, 150 mg two times daily for 3 months. (Note: There is no evidence to show that this works.)

Scenario 3. Prophylactic Surgery in a Patient with a Strong Family History of Desmoids.
These patients often have a mutation at the 3′ end of the *APC* gene and thus may have mild disease. It is tempting to do an IRA, which may be done laparoscopically under cover of sulindac. Alternatively, a proctocolectomy and pouch will minimize the need for future surgery. Surgery should be delayed as late as is safe. Yearly colonoscopy and treatment of polyps with an NSAID is a reasonable option for patients in their 20s.

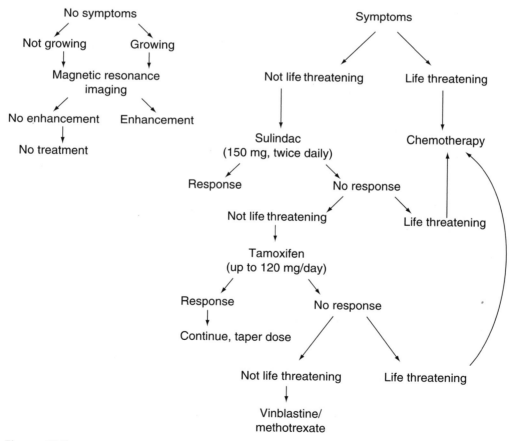

Figure 61-3
Algorithm for management of intra-abdominal desmoid tumor.

■ SUMMARY

Intra-abdominal desmoid tumors can cause major problems in patients with FAP. They cannot be removed surgically, do not respond predictably to anything, are rare enough to prevent a concerted trial of potential therapy, and horrific enough on occasion to cause fear in patients and physicians. The good news is that most desmoids are stable and follow a benign course regardless of what is done to them. The algorithm in Figure 61-3 provides some suggestions for their management.

Suggested Readings

Berk T, Cohen Z, McLeod RS, Stern HS: Management of mesenteric desmoid tumours in familial adenomatous polyposis. Can J Surg 1992;35:393–395.

Bertario L, Russo A, Sala P, et al: Genotype and phenotype factors as determinants of desmoid tumors in patients with familial adenomatous polyposis. Int J Cancer 2001;95:102–107.

Church JM: Desmoid tumors in familial adenomatous polyposis. Surg Oncol Clin North Am 1994;3:435–447.

Clark SK, Phillips RKS: Desmoids in familial adenomatous polyposis. Br J Surg 1996;83:1494–1504.

Farmer KCR, Hawley PR, Phillips RKS: Desmoid disease. In Phillips RKS, Spigelman AD, Thomson JPS (Eds.). Familial Adenomatous Polyposis and Other Polyposis Syndromes. London, Edward Arnold, 1994.

Gurbuz AK, Giardiello FM, Peterson GM, et al: Desmoid tumours in familial adenomatous polyposis. Gut 1994;35:377–381.

Hamilton L, Blackstein M, Berk T, et al: Chemotherapy for desmoid tumors in association with familial adenomatous polyposis: A report of three cases. Can J Surg 1996;39:247–252.

Healy JC, Reznek RH, Clark SK, et al: MR appearances of desmoid tumors in familial adenomatous polyposis. Am J Roentgenol 1997; 169:465–472.

Poritz LS, Blackstein M, Berk T, et al: Extended follow-up of patients treated with cytotoxic chemotherapy for intra-abdominal desmoid tumors. Dis Colon Rectum 2001;44:1268–1273.

62

HEREDITARY NONPOLYPOSIS COLORECTAL CANCER

Kevin M. Lin, MD
Alan G. Thorson, MD, FACS

Fifteen to 20% of the total colorectal cancer (CRC) burden in the United States is associated with a positive family history (cancer in one or more parents, siblings, or children). Hereditary nonpolyposis colorectal cancer (HNPCC) may account for 20 to 35% of such cancers or 4 to 7% of all cases of CRC. Approximately 150,000 new cases of CRC were diagnosed in the United States in 2002. Therefore, as many as 10,520 of those cancers could represent patients with HNPCC. Comparatively, familial adenomatous polyposis represents only about 1% of all cases of CRC. Inflammatory bowel disease, Peutz-Jeghers syndrome, and familial juvenile polyposis together contribute an additional 1% of all CRCs.

■ HISTORICAL PERSPECTIVE

For many years, familial adenomatous polyposis was the only entity known to represent hereditary CRC. However, hereditary CRC can arise in the absence of multiple colonic adenomas. This observation was first made by Aldred Warthin, MD, in 1913 in his study of Family G. His interest in this family was spurred by his seamstress, who remarked that she would die of gastric or uterine cancer because most of her family members had died from these cancers. Her prediction was accurate; she died of endometrial cancer at a young age.

Within Family G, Warthin originally observed an aggregation of gastric, colonic, and endometrial cancers. Gastric carcinoma was the predominant cancer in this first identified HNPCC family. Since then, gastric carcinoma has become less common in HNPCC, paralleling its decline in the general population. The mode of inheritance of these cancers was not appreciated until 1966 when Henry Lynch observed an autosomal dominant inheritance pattern of colorectal and extracolonic cancers in two extended midwestern kindreds.

■ MOLECULAR GENETICS

The fidelity of cellular DNA replication is enhanced by a system that identifies, excises, and corrects mismatched DNA pairings at the G_2/M phase of the cell cycle. Mismatches may occur during DNA replication by incorrect base pairings (A-C instead of G-C or G-T instead of A-T, where A = adenine, C = cytosine, G = guanine, and T = thymine) or by DNA polymerase slippage on the template strand, usually on long, repeating-nucleotide sequences. The repair of such mismatches requires the normal function of four protein subunits encoded by DNA mismatch repair (MMR) genes that are inherited in autosomal dominant fashion.

Tumors from HNPCC patients tend to exhibit genomic or microsatellite instability (MSI), which is the phenotypic marker, at the molecular level, of a defective MMR process. Microsatellites are mono-, di-, tri-, or tetra-dinucleotide repeats in the DNA genome that do not code for proteins and have no known function, although they are sometimes found within genes. A reference panel of five microsatellites (markers) has been proposed for testing colorectal neoplasms. In this system, tumors are characterized as high-frequency MSI (MSI-H) if two or more of the five markers show instability (insertion/deletion of base pairs in tumor DNA) when compared to normal tissue from the same patient. Low-frequency MSI (MSI-L) tumors are unstable in one of five markers, while microsatellite stable tumors (MSS) have no instability at all.

MSI is noted in 86% of HNPCC and 15% of sporadic colorectal tumors. MSI is also more frequently observed in HNPCC adenomas (57%) compared to sporadic colorectal adenomas (3%). Tumors with MSI (MSI-H) demonstrate significant clinicopathologic and prognostic differences when compared to tumors without MSI (MSI-L or MSS). A germline mutation in one allele of any of the six known DNA MMR genes (*MLH1*, *MSH2*, *MSH3*, *PMSI*, *PMS2*, or *MSH6*), followed by somatic loss or inactivation of the wild-type allele, results in a mismatch repair-deficient cell with resultant expression of MSI. Such cells accumulate mutations 1000-fold more frequently than normal cells, thus enhancing the potential for malignant transformation. MMR genes *MSH2* and *MLHI* account for 40% and 35%, respectively, of the germline mutations seen in HNPCC. As will be shown, there is marked variation in phenotypic expression between these HNPCC-causing mutations. Mutations of the recently discovered MMR gene *MSH6* (*GTBP*) account for a small subset of atypical HNPCC kindreds with a predominance of endometrial cancers that do not fulfill the Amsterdam criteria (see discussion under "Diagnosis").

In summary, an inherited germline mutation in one allele of a mismatch repair gene plus an acquired genetic change (somatic mutation or inactivation) at the same locus ("second hit") in the corresponding allele is responsible for MSI in HNPCC tumors.

MSI in sporadic tumors is caused inactivation of the MCH1 gene by a phenomenon known as *promotor methylation*. Gene expression is "switched off" by methylation of CpG islands in the promoter region of the gene. Early onset cancers in HNPCC can be explained by the fact that the first of the "two hits" occurs at birth, thus requiring only one additional sporadic event.

■ TUMOR BIOLOGY AND PROGNOSIS

Histopathologic features of HNPCC tumors include an excess of poorly differentiated (medullary, mucinous, and signet-ring) adenocarcinomas (Fig. 62-1*A* and *B*). We have noted poor differentiation in 44% of HNPCC tumors compared to 14% of sporadic tumors ($p = 0.002$). Ten percent of HNPCC tumors are signet-ring adenocarcinomas, which are rare in sporadic tumors. Balanced against these poor prognostic features is the tendency for HNPCC tumors to be more commonly diploid, less rapidly proliferating, and less vascularized than sporadic tumors.

Survival, both overall and stage for stage, has been compared between colorectal cancers associated with HNPCC and those of the general population. The Creighton experience with patients of *MLH1* and *MSH2* kindreds has shown a 10-year survival advantage for HNPCC (69% versus 48%). Likewise, Sankila and coworkers reported better 5-year overall survival for HNPCC patients (65% versus 44%). Some of this overall survival advantage could be accounted for by early diagnosis. In the Creighton registry, significantly more HNPCC cancers are diagnosed as TNM stage II and fewer as TNM stage IV (see "Presenting Tumor Stage"). Stage-for-stage comparisons in a second study found that TNM stage III HNPCC patients have improved 5-year survival ratesover their counterparts in the general population (60% versus 44%, $p = 0.012$).

We have also noted that full-thickness T3 colorectal cancers in HNPCC have fewer distant metastases than sporadic T3 CRCs in the general population (10% versus 22%, $p < 0.001$). Futhermore, for stage IV CRC, HNPCC patients present with fewer liver metastasis than patients in the general population (48% versus 71%, $p = 0.015$).

Several explanations have been proposed to explain these findings. The discrepancy between aggressive histologic features and more favorable prognosis in HNPCC could relate to host immune surveillance. A Crohn's-like lymphoid reaction (lymphoid aggregates, often with germinal centers, in peritumoral tissue) is more commonly seen in HNPCC tumors (49%) compared to sporadic tumors (27%) ($p < 0.05$) (Fig. 62-2). In addition, large

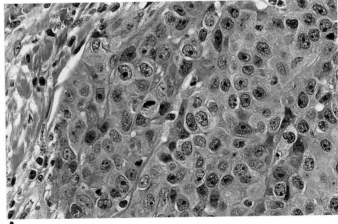

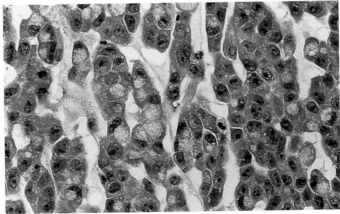

Figure 62-1
A, Poorly-differentiated (medullary) adenocarcinoma composed of irregular, solid sheets of large eosinophillic cells containing small glandlike spaces. *B*, Signet-ring adenocarcinoma.

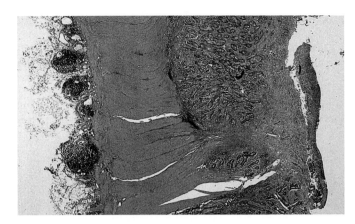

Figure 62-2
Crohn's-like lymphoid aggregation within a germinal center in the stroma inferior to the tumor.

numbers of tumor-infiltrating lymphocytes (TILs) are a feature of HNPCC and sporadic MSI-H tumors. As in malignant melanoma, sporadic colorectal cancers with dense TILs have been reported to have a survival advantage. TILs have been postulated to prevent tumor progression by expressing interleukin-4 (IL-4) and tumor necrosis factor-α (TNF-α) in response to human colon tumor antigen. In a recent preliminary study, we have found intraepithelial TILs in 53% of HNPCC tumors compared to 17% of sporadic CRC ($p < 0.002$). Histologically, TILs are recognized by a round nucleus surrounded by a clear halo (Fig. 62-3).

There are other theories for the favorable prognosis in HNPCC. As mentioned, 86% of colon cancers in HNPCC exhibit MSI-H compared to 15% of sporadic tumors. Sporadic colorectal cancers that are MSI-H demonstrate many features of HNPCC tumors, including right-sided predominance, exophytic growth pattern, peritumoral Crohn's lymphoid reaction, poor differentiation, extracellular mucin histology, and improved survival. The less aggressive behavior of MSI-H colon cancers may be a paradoxical effect of genomic instability. Under the assumption that malignant tumors in HNPCC retain the propensity to continually accumulate mutations, the malignant cells might eventually be burdened with such

an enormous mutational load that there is a loss of critical cell functions, including the ability to metastasize.

■ LIFETIME CANCER RISKS

The lifetime risk of cancer in HNPCC can be separated into extracolonic and colorectal manifestations. Each risk is considered separately.

Extracolonic Cancer

Benatti and coworkers reported on putative gene carriers ($n = 293$) from 40 families fulfilling HNPCC clinical criteria. They noted a 43% lifetime risk of endometrial cancers. They also reported the lifetime risk of other extracolonic cancers, such as stomach (19%), biliary tract (18%), urinary tract (10%), and ovaries (9%). Cancers of the breast, pancreas, liver, larynx, bronchus, lung, and esophagus as well as the central nervous system, hematologic system, and sarcomas have been observed in some HNPCC families but may represent coincidental associations.

Specific phenotypic variations between *MSH2* and *MLHI* genotypes have been reported by Vasen and coworkers. Although lifetime endometrial cancer risk was similar between *MSH2* and *MLHI* patients (61% versus 42%), only *MSH2* carriers had significantly increased rel-

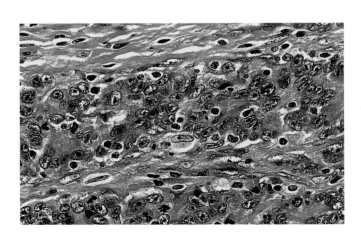

Figure 62-3
Tumor-infiltrating lymphocytes. (Courtesy of Tom C. Smyrk, MD, Associate Professor of Pathology, University of Nebraska College of Medicine.)

ative risk (RR) of cancer of the urinary tract (RR = 75.3), stomach (RR = 19.3) and ovaries (RR = 8.0) compared to the general population. Both *MSH2* and *MLHI* genotypes have shown a higher relative risk of small bowel cancer (RR > 100) compared to the general population, although the actual incidence remains quite low.

We have also noted significant phenotypic variations in cancer risks between *MSH2* and *MLH1* genotypes within the Creighton registry. Lifetime cancer risks were calculated for 49 *MSH2* germline mutation carriers (27 males) and 56 *MLH1* carriers (28 males). We found the lifetime risk of extracolonic cancer to be higher in *MSH2* than *MLH1* carriers (48% versus 11%).

Gender-specific differences in extracolonic cancer risk have been observed for *MSH2* but not *MLH1* carriers. *MSH2* females express a significant excess of extracolonic cancers over their male counterparts (69% versus 34%), not an unexpected finding considering the contribution from endometrial and ovarian cancers in females. The mean age of extracolonic cancer onset is older for *MSH2* males that *MSH2* females (55 years versus 39 years).

In addition to the lifetime extracolonic cancer risks in mutation carriers, we have studied the incidence of associated extracolonic cancers in CRC patients from known HNPCC kindreds (including family members who may not be gene carriers). A greater incidence of extracolonic cancers is noted in CRC patients from *MSH2* kindreds (33%) compared to *MLH1* kindreds (12%) or patients in the general population with CRC (7.3%) (Table 62-1). In fact, the extracolonic cancer incidence in CRC patients from *MLH1* kindreds is not statistically greater than CRC patients from the general population. This preponderance of extracolonic cancers in CRC patients from *MSH2* kindreds compared to the paucity in CRC patients from *MLH1* kindreds may explain the original observation of phenotypes that led to the categorization of HNPCC into Lynch I (site-specific CRC) and Lynch II (cancer family syndrome).

The marked excess of extracolonic cancers in *MSH2* mutation carriers provides evidence that germline mutations in different mismatch repair genes exhibit different phenotypic effects. This has recently been confirmed by Jager and coworkers who demonstrated that a specific founder mutation in the Danish population at *MLH1* intron 14 disrupts the splice donor site, thereby silencing the mutated allele, resulting in a milder phenotype with highly reduced frequency of extracolonic tumors.

Colorectal Cancer

In assessing overall lifetime colorectal cancer risk, we have observed no difference between *MSH2* and *MLH1* carriers (71% versus 84%). Vasen and coworkers also reported the lifetime CRC risk to be 80% for both groups. However, in *MSH2* carriers we have observed a higher CRC risk in males than females (96% versus 39%). This gender difference in CRC risk is not identified in *MLH1* carriers.

Using a population-based strategy, Dunlop and coworkers calculated the lifetime cancer risk associated with germline DNA MMR gene mutations from individuals not associated with known classic HNPCC families. They targeted genetic analysis to patients with early onset (mean age of 27) and MSI-H colorectal cancers to identify germline mutation carriers. They found the risk of CRC in these patients to be greater for males than females (74 versus 30%). Furthermore, they found that women had a higher risk for endometrial cancer (42%) than colorectal cancer.

■ CLINICAL FEATURES

Variations in clinical presentation have been observed between patients with the HNPCC genotypes, *MLH1* and *MSH2*, and the general population. We have compared 67 members of *MLH1* kindreds, 45 members of *MSH2* kindreds, and 1189 patients with "sporadic" CRC. Differences in age at cancer onset, presenting tumor stage, anatomic site distribution, and synchronous and metachronous CRC rates were noted.

Age at Cancer Onset

Although HNPCC patients form colonic adenomas at about the same rate as the general population, these adenomas may appear as early as age 35 or even younger. The mean ages of CRC onset are 44, 46, and 69 years for *MLH1*, *MSH2*, and the general population, respectively, so that the onset of CRC in HNPCC is about 20 years earlier than in the general population. The youngest HNPCC individual diagnosed with CRC was 13 years old.

Presenting Tumor Stage

When comparing the presenting TNM tumor stage of *MLH1* and *MSH2* patients to CRC patients in the general population, we have observed an overall lower stage of tumor presentation in HNPCC patients. Specifically, there are more stage II (43% versus 27%) and fewer stage IV (10% versus 22%) CRC in HNPCC. This observation may be due to either less aggressive nature of HNPCC tumors or increased screening and awareness in HNPCC families.

Table 62–1 Extracolonic Cancers in Colorectal Cancer Patients			
CANCER	**MSH2** (*n* = 45)	**MLH1** (*n* = 67)	**GENERAL POPULATION** (*n* = 1189)
Endometrium	5	3	6
Ovary	1	2	3
Breast	1	1	13
Kidney	3	0	7
Ureter	1	0	1
Bladder	1	1	10
Brain	0	1	1
Stomach	1	0	2
Esophagus	1	0	0
Thyroid	1	0	1
Other	0	0	43
Total	15 (33%)*	8 (12%)	87 (7.3%)

*$p < 0.001$ *MSH2* versus *MLH1* and the general population.
Source: Lin KM, Shashidharan M, Ternent CA, et al: Colorectal and extracolonic cancer variations in MLH1/MSH2 HNPCC kindreds and the general population. Dis Colon Rectum 1998; 41: 428–433.

Anatomic Site Distribution

There is a predominance of right colon cancer in *MLH1* (48%) and *MSH2* (41%) patients compared to the general population (25%) (Fig. 62-4). Accordingly, fewer sigmoid colon cancers are found in *MLH1* (16%) and *MSH2* (13%) patients compared to the general population (26%). With HNPCC genotype comparisons, the overall site distribution is significantly different between *MSH2* and *MLH1* patients. More rectal cancers are noted in *MSH2*-affected members (28%) than in *MLH1*-affected members (8%). In fact, in the Creighton registry, the incidence of rectal cancer in *MSH2* kindreds is comparable to that in the general population. Thus, the presence of rectal cancer in a patient should not preclude the possibility of HNPCC.

Synchronous and Metachronous Cancers

A greater number of synchronous colon cancers are noted in *MLH1* (7.4%) and *MSH2* (6.7%) patients compared to the general population (2.4%). Furthermore, the annual metachronous CRC rate is higher in both *MLH1* (2.1% per year) and *MSH2* (1.7% per year) patients than in general population (0.33% per year). These findings reinforce the importance of clearing or resecting the remaining colorectal mucosa when an index colorectal cancer is found.

■ DIAGNOSIS

Family History

Family history is the primary method of identifying patients with colorectal or endometrial cancer as possible members of an HNPCC family. The International Collaborative Group of HNPCC, comprising 30 leading experts from eight different countries, met in Amsterdam in August 1990 and proposed minimum clinical criteria to aid in the identification and study of colon and rectal cancer patients at risk for HNPCC.

These "Amsterdam criteria" required the following: (1) three or more relatives with histologically verified CRC, one of whom is a first-degree relative of the other two; (2) CRC involving at least two successive generations; (3) at least one relative diagnosed with CRC under the age of 50; and (4) the exclusion of familial adenomatous polyposis (FAP). About 70% of families who fulfill the Amsterdam criteria and undergo genetic testing will test positive for an HNPCC genotype. A negative test result does not necessarily exclude HNPCC, because all associated genotypes have not yet been identified.

With time, the Amsterdam criteria became misinterpreted as a clinical screening mechanism for HNPCC. However, by definition, the Amsterdam criteria are overly restrictive. By excluding patients with extracolonic cancers in the absence of CRC, the effectiveness of identifying HNPCC families is markedly diminished. This is especially true in *MSH2* kindreds with an excess of extracolonic cancers. In 1999 the Amsterdam II criteria for clinical diagnosis of HNPCC were published. They are similar to the original Amsterdam (I) criteria except that instead of three relatives with colorectal cancer, three with

any HNPCC-associated cancers are included. Thus, recognition and inclusion of the HNPCC tumor spectrum enhance the effectiveness of family history.

In 1996, a National Cancer Institute sponsor led to the development of the "Bethesda Guidelines" to assist in identifying at-risk patients. These guidelines broaden inclusion criteria and are meant to provide a rationale for testing of tumors for MSI as a screening for HNPCC. The criteria include:

1. Individuals with cancer in families that are Amsterdam positive
2. Individuals with two HNPCC-related cancers, including synchronous and metachronous CRC or associated extracolonic cancers
3. Individuals with CRC and a first-degree relative with CRC or HNPCC-related extracolonic cancer, at least one diagnosed under the age of 45 and a colorectal adenoma diagnosed under age 40
4. Individuals with CEC or endometrial cancer diagnosed under age 45
5. Individuals with right-sided CRC diagnosed under age 45 with poorly differentiated or undifferentiated histology (see Fig. 62-1*A*)
6. Individuals with signet-ring cell type CRC diagnosed under age 45 (composed of greater than 50% signet-ring cells) (see Fig. 62-1*B*)
7. Individuals with adenomas diagnosed under age 40

Genetic Testing and Counseling

Recent identification of some of the genes responsible for HNPCC has enhanced the ability to conclusively identify many affected patients by analyzing the DNA of peripheral blood leukocytes or the cancer specimen of an affected family member. Genetic testing might be considered in individuals with either of the following: (1) individuals with a family history fulfilling Amsterdam I or II criteria or (2) individuals who meet the "Bethesda Guidelines" and whose tumors exhibit MSI or fail to stain by immunohistochemistry or DNA mismatch repair proteins. Genetic testing is commercially available but should be undertaken in the context of a comprehensive hereditary cancer service to include both informed consent and genetic counseling. The current cost is about $2000 for the index member and $200 for each subsequent member, assuming that a mutation is found.

An informed consent should address the following issues:

1. Information regarding how the genetic test is performed
2. Implications of positive or negative test results
3. The possibility that the test may be inconclusive
4. The risk of insurance or employer discrimination
5. Confidentiality measures to protect the patient
6. The risk of psychological distress
7. The cost of genetic testing
8. The technical accuracy of the tests
9. The option for cancer risk estimation without genetic testing
10. The fact that further supportive counseling may be required to cope with emotions secondary to test results

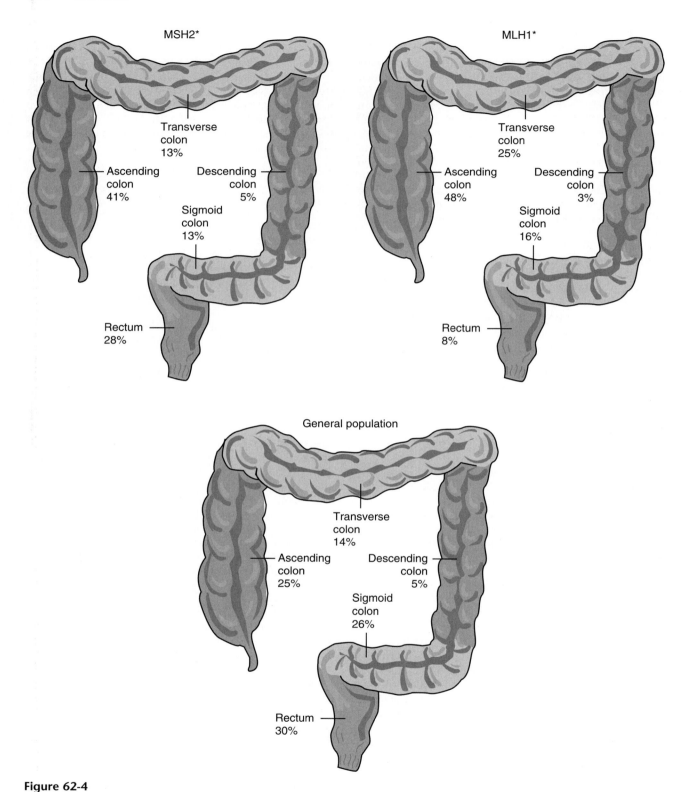

Figure 62-4

Variations in colorectal cancer site distribution are noted between *MSH2/MLH* kindreds versus the general population. In addition, the overall site distribution was different between *MSH* and *MLH*. *p = 0.036. (From Lin KM, Shashidharan M, Ternent CA, et al: Colorectal and exracolonic cancer variations in MLH1/MSH2 HNPCC kindreds and the general population. Dis Colon Rectum 1998;41:428–433.)

If genetic testing is the first major component of a hereditary cancer service, then genetic counseling is the second component. The physician or counselor must be prepared to perform counseling individually and collectively to family members. This process should start even before offering patients genetic testing and information regarding germline status. During counseling, the natural history and lifetime cancer risks in HNPCC must be carefully explained. Patients should be informed of the emotional and psychological stress of knowing one's DNA mutations. Anxiety, traumatic stress syndrome, and impairment of daily function are possible consequences after notifying patients of positive genetic mutation. A negative genetic result may also impose a psychological burden in the form of "survivor guilt." Ample time is needed to allow for patients' questions and concerns. The decision to accept genetic testing and pursue surveillance and management programs should be reached once all issues have been thoroughly explored.

In HNPCC, cancers do not occur with sufficient frequency in childhood or adolescence to justify genetic testing in children. There is no benefit to discovering the gene status of a child because recommendations for HNPCC cancer screening rarely start before age 20. Such a child could be unnecessarily burdened with fear, anxiety, and a sense of doom. Likewise, parents become overly protective, concerned, and guilty for passing on the hereditary gene. This is commonly known as the "fragile-child" syndrome. As the children of an HNPCC family reach adulthood (age 18 or older), appropriate counseling may then be offered so that they can participate in the decision regarding genetic testing, surveillance, and management.

■ MANAGEMENT

Colonoscopy Surveillance Studies

Surveillance studies have shown that HNPCC may be associated with an accelerated adenoma to carcinoma sequence which may be as short as 2 to 3 years. Lanspa and coworkers reported 55 asymptomatic individuals (ages 22 to 70) at risk for HNPCC that were screened for CRC. Eight individuals underwent polypectomies for adenomas and were followed with colonoscopy at 6-month intervals. The mean interval of finding new adenomas was 16 months. One adenocarcinoma was found arising in a tubulovillous adenoma. In the surveillance of 34 HNPCC patients, Mecklin and coworkers found nine adenomas and nine carcinomas arising within 3 years of a negative colonoscopy.

Mecklin and coworkers found high-grade dysplasia in 23% of adenomas in HNPCC compared to 13% in sporadic control subjects. Increased villous changes and high-grade dysplasia were also noted in HNPCC adenomas by Jass and coworkers. These findings suggest that HNPCC adenomas are more aggressive and thus more likely to undergo malignant transformation than sporadic adenomas.

Early and frequent screening with removal of adenomas in HNPCC has been shown to decrease cancer inci-

dence. Jarvinen and coworkers screened 133 patients from HNPCC kindreds (mean age 38.1 years) for CRC at 3-year intervals. Polypectomies were performed in 22 patients. A control group consisted of 118 HNPCC kindred members (mean age 38.6 years) who refused screening. Six colorectal cancers developed in the screened group compared to 14 cancers in the control subjects during 10 years of follow up. Thus, 3-year interval screenings more than halved the CRC rate (62% reduction) in at-risk members of HNPCC families. One cancer was prevented for every 2.8 polypectomies performed. In contrast, the National Polyp Study, which utilized data from the general population, found that 41 to 119 polypectomies were performed per cancer prevented.

Screening Recommendations

The International Collaborative Group on HNPCC recommends the following surveillance guidelines for members of gene-positive families and high-risk individuals based on clinical family history: (1) annual screening colonoscopy beginning at age 25 or 10 years earlier than the youngest family member diagnosed with CRC and (2) endometrial aspiration biopsy, transvaginal ovarian ultrasound, Papanicolaou smear, and bimanual pelvic examination every 2 years starting at age 30.

If there is a history of a specific HNPCC-associated extracolonic cancer within the family, the following additional measures should be taken: For stomach and biliary tract cancers, screen every 2 years with esophagogastroduodenoscopy, gastric brush cytology, transabdominal hepatobiliary ultrasound, and liver function test. For urinary tract cancer, begin at age 30 with yearly urinalysis and urine cytology, and 2 yearly cystoscopy and ultrasound.

Surgical Treatment

Colorectal Cancer

The accelerated adenoma to carcinoma sequence plus increased rates of synchronous and metachronous CRC support the recommendation to avoid segmental resection in favor of total colectomy with ileorectal anastomosis when an index colon cancer is diagnosed in HNPCC gene carriers (Fig. 62-5). This procedure is also recommended for patients presenting with CRC who are high-risk individuals based on family history but whose genetic status is unknown.

Lifetime proctoscopic surveillance following total colectomy is mandatory because of the risk of cancer in the residual rectum. Rodriguez-Bigas and coworkers showed that 8 of 71 patients (11%) had developed rectal cancer at a median of 158 months from their total colectomy for the index cancer. Thus, the risk of developing rectal cancer following abdominal colectomy is estimated to be 3%, every 3 years in the first 12 postoperative years.

Gynecologic cancers are the second most common manifestation of HNPCC. Therefore, gynecologic cancer screening and prophylactic surgery are the main extracolonic cancer prevention measures widely recommended in women with HNPCC. Prophylactic total abdominal hysterectomy with bilateral salpingo-oophorectomy should be offered to female HNPCC gene carriers and high-risk individuals who present with an index CRC, particularly if they are postmenopausal or have completed their families (see Fig. 62-5).

Without Colorectal Cancer

Some controversy exists to the best management for known HNPCC gene carriers without cancer. Prophylactic total colectomy with ileorectal anastomosis and lifetime proctoscopic surveillance appear to offer a reasonable alternative to lifetime annual colonoscopic surveillance. Such a recommendation is sound when the cancer risk is anticipated to be high (about 80% lifetime CRC risk for the overall HNPCC population). However, it may be that surgical recommendations in the future will be individualized based on genotype and gender. For example, in *MSH2* females, the lifetime CRC risk of 39% is less than the endometrial cancer risk of 61%. If these data are con-

firmed, such individuals might opt for endoscopic surveillance rather than colectomy.

Prophylactic total abdominal hysterectomy and bilateral salpingo-oophorectomy can be offered to female gene carriers without cancer who have completed their reproductive activity or who are postmenopausal. Although this procedure eliminates the risk of endometrial cancer, patients should be informed that there is a remote risk of extraovarian peritoneal serous papillary carcinoma, consonant with primary ovarian cancer.

■ SUMMARY

Current colorectal and extracolonic cancer surveillance and treatment recommendations are based on the overall respective lifetime cancer risks in HNPCC gene carriers. However, specific phenotypic variations are now being observed among identified genotypes. Ultimately,

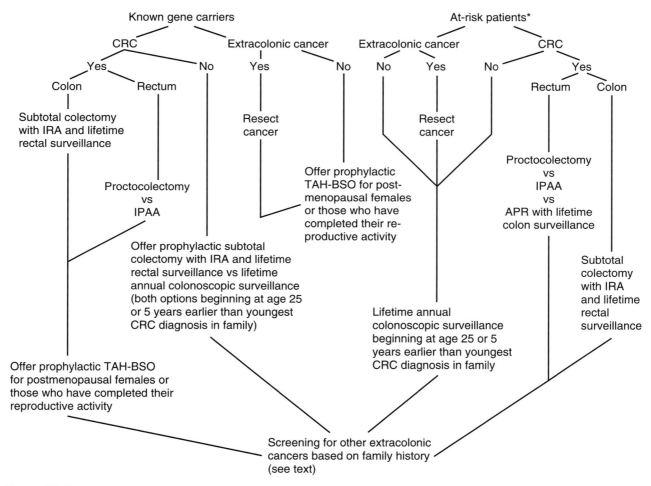

Figure 62-5
Recommendations for surgical treatment of HNPCC. *Based on clinical family history. APR, abdominal perineal resection; CRC, colorectal cancer; IPAA, ileal pouch–anal anastomosis; IRA, ileorectal anastomosis; TAH-BSO, total abdominal hysterectomy and bilateral salpingo-oophorectomy.

colorectal, endometrial, and other extracolonic cancer risk estimates for all five current HNPCC genotypes will be necessary for more precise planning of cancer prevention strategies in each genotypic subgroup. Additional surveillance in HNPCC families must be guided by the presence of specific extracolonic cancers within that family's history. In conclusion, as more HNPCC genotypes are discovered, knowledge of their specific phenotypic features will provide rationale for highly targeted screening, surveillance, and treatment recommendations for affected individuals.

Suggested Readings

Chung DC, Rustgi AK: DNA mismatch repair and cancer. Gastroentrology 1995;109:1685–1699.

Jager AC, Bisgaard ML, Myrhoj T, et al: Reduced frequency of extracolonic cancers in HNCPP families with monoallelic hMLH1 expression. Am J Hum Genet 1997;61:129–138.

Lin KM, Shashidharan M, Ternent CA, et al: Colorectal and extracolonic cancer variations in MLH1/MSH2 HNPCC kindreds and the general population. Dis Colon Rectum 1998;41:428–433.

Lin KM, Shashidharan M, Thorson AG, et al: Cumulative incidence of colorectal and extracolonic cancers in MLH1 and MSH2 mutation carriers of HNPCC. J Gastrointest Surg 1998;2:67–71.

Lynch HT, Shaw MW, Magnuson CW, et al: Hereditary factors in cancer: Study of two large midwestern kindred. Arch Intern Med 1966;117:206–212.

Ropponen KM, Eskelinen MJ, Lipponen PK, et al: Prognostic value of tumour-infiltrating lymphocytes (TILs) in colorectal cancer. J Pathol 1997;182:318–324.

Vasen H, Wijnen J, Menko F, et al: Cancer risk in families with HNPCC diagnosed by mutation analysis. Gastroenterology 1996;110:1020-1027.

Warthin AS: Heredity with reference to carcinoma. Arch Intern Med 1913;12:546–555.

63

CANCER OF THE APPENDIX AND PSEUDOMYXOMA PERITONEI SYNDROME

Paul H. Sugarbaker, MD, FACS, FRCS, FASAS

Malignant tumors of the appendix are rare gastrointestinal tumors. They constitute approximately 0.4% of all intestinal neoplasms. About 1% of all large bowel cancers arise from the appendix. Despite the diminutive size of this organ and the infrequent occurrence of such tumors, the histopathology of appendiceal malignancy has been confusing, and the approach to therapy is complex. Unfortunately, for adenocarcinoma of the appendix, a majority of the tumors have perforated at the time of definitive surgical treatment; consequently, the physician is required to manage the primary tumor and its peritoneal surface dissemination. Despite carcinomatosis, often present in large volume at the time of initial diagnosis, liver metastases and lymph node metastases are seldom present. To improve salvage of patients with perforated tumors and those with documented distant spread within the abdominal cavity, a new and curative approach to this previously uniformly lethal condition (the spread of tumor on peritoneal surfaces) is now widely accepted as a surgical responsibility.

■ PATHOLOGY OF APPENDICEAL MALIGNANT TUMORS

The two most commonly occurring malignant tumors of the appendix are carcinoid and adenocarcinoma. Approximately two thirds of all appendiceal malignancies are carcinoid. The other third are variations of adenocarcinoma (Table 63-1).

Carcinoid Tumors

By far the most common tumor within the appendix is the carcinoid. This lesion is usually found incidentally during the removal of an asymptomatic appendix. A small, hard tumor mass is found in the distal portion of the appendix. The appendix is the site of 45% of all gastrointesinal carcinoid tumors. Their incidence in females is higher than in males, probably because of the greater number of incidental appendectomies performed in women undergoing hysterectomy and cholecystectomy.

Although 90% of appendiceal carcinoids are incidental findings, approximately 10% result in acute appendicitis.

Rarely is the carcinoid syndrome the presenting feature. If the patient has the carcinoid syndrome, spread of tumor to the liver is inevitably present.

The selection of treatment options for carcinoid tumor depends on the size of the malignancy and, in large tumors, on the extent of local spread. It is extremely important to determine these clinical features at the time of exploration, because the histopathologic features of aggressive tumors are the same as those of tumors with no malignant potential.

Adenocarcinoid Tumors of the Appendix (Goblet Cell Carcinoid)

A small percentage of carcinoid tumors have malignant epithelial cells producing abundant mucus scattered among the carcinoid tumor cells. Usually these tumors have dissecting mucus diffusely infiltrating the wall of the appendix. In contrast non-mucinous carcinoid tumors present as an innocuous occurrence at the tip of the organ. Adenocarcinoid tumors present as acute appendicent more frequently than carcinoid tumors. The 5-year survival rate of such patients is greatly reduced compared to patients with carcinoid, because adenocarcinoid patients usually have peritoneal carcinomatosis at initial diagnosis. These patients have dissecting mucus produced in large quantity by the cancer. The wide distribution on peritoneal surfaces results in a grim prognosis unless they receive special treatments for peritoneal surface malignancy.

Adenocarcinoma of the Appendix

The most common varieties of epithelial malignancy within the appendix are mucinous adenomas or mucinous adenocarcinomas. The mucinous tumors are many times more common than the intestinal type of adenocarcinoma. In contrast, approximately 15% of colonic adenocarcinomas are of the mucinous variety. The preponderance of mucinous tumors in the appendix is probably related to the high proportion of goblet cells within its epithelium (Table 63-2).

On gross examination, it may be difficult or impossible to distinguish a mucinous tumor of the appendix from a benign mucocele. Both benign and malignant tumors of the appendix are likely to cause appendicitis, and there may be mucin collections within the right lower quadrant or throughout the abdominopelvic space. Two features should be sought that will histopathologically separate tumors as inconsequential with complete removal from those capable of causing death from progressive pseudomyxoma peritonei syndrome:

1. Invasion through the appendiceal wall by neoplastic glands
2. Atypical epithelial cells found within the extra-appendiceal mucin collection

If either one of these clinical features occurs, special follow-up and aggressive treatments are required.

The most common clinical entity arising from an appendiceal epithelial tumor is pseudomyxoma peritonei. This clinical entity has a perforated appendiceal adenoma

Table 63-1 Survey of Appendiceal Tumors*

FEATURE	CARCINOID	ADENOCARCI-NOID	PSEUDOMYXOMA PERITONEI	MUCINOUS ADENOCARCI-NOMA	ADENOCARCI-NOMA
Approximate incidence	66%	Rare	20%	Rare	10%
Location	Tip of appendix	Diffuse along appendix	Middle to tip of appendix	Diffuse along appendix	Base of appendix
Major symptom	Incidental finding	Expanding abdomen, ovarian mass	Expanding abdomen, ovarian mass, hernia, appendicitis	Appendicitis	Appendicitis
Prognosis	<1 cm, 100% cure >2 cm, 50% cure	Poor	Localized, 100% cure Adenomucinosis, 90% cure at 5 years	84% cure at 5 years if unperforated; 60% cure at 5 years if perforated	Follows Dukes' stages: A—80% cure B—50% cure C—20% cure
Histopathology of peritoneal surface implants	Carcinoid	Carcinoid plus mucinous adenocarci-noma	Adenomucinosis	Mucinous carcinomatosis	Intestinal type (nonmucinous) adenocarcinoma
Clinical syndromes	Carcinoid	Mucinous peritoneal carcinomatosis	Pseudomyxoma peritonei	Mucinous peritoneal carcinomatosis	Peritoneal carcinomatosis
Treatment	<1 cm, appendectomy only >2 cm, right colectomy + cytoreductive surgery	Appendectomy only or cytoreductive surgery + intraperitoneal chemotherapy	Appendectomy + cytoreductive surgery + intraperitoneal chemotherapy	Cytoreductive surgery + intraperitoneal chemotherapy	PAA Cytoreductive surgery + intraperitoneal chemotherapy if peritoneal implants

*In separating pseudomyxoma peritonei, adenocarcinoma, and mucinous adenocarcinoma, it must be remembered that these represent a spectrum of disease and are probably not distinct clinical entities. Benign mucocele is not included as an appendiceal tumor but is rather a cystic process. A perforated mucocele resulting from an appendiceal polyp usually develops into pseudomyxoma peritonei unless a chemotherapy wash is utilized. Tumors that histologically are between adenomucinosis and mucinous carcinomatosis are designated as hybrid type.

or villous adenoma as its primary site. Hyperplastic polyps, adenomatous polyps, and villous polyps within the appendix that have resulted in an appendiceal perforation are implicated in the pseudomyxoma peritonei syndrome (Higa et al, 1973; Ronnett et al, 1997). The mucus accumulations that are distributed in a characteristic fashion around the peritoneal cavity are referred to as adeno-mucinosis (Sugarbaker, 1994, 1996). Histologically, epithelial cells in single layers are surrounded by lakes of mucin. These epithelial cells show little atypia, absent mitosis, and result in mucinous tumor accumulations that follow the flow of peritoneal fluid within the abdomen and pelvis (Sugarbaker, 1994; Yan et al, 2001).

A second less common histologic type of appendiceal adenocarcinoma is the intestinal type of tumor, often referred to as the nonmucinous type. This cancer is usually located at the base of the appendix and resembles colonic adenocarcinoma in its histopathologic appearance. It is locally invasive and results in carcinomatosis proximal to the appendix, usually in the right paracolic sulcus and pelvis, especially in the cul-de-sac.

A third histologic type of appendiceal adenocarcinoma is the mucinous adenocarcinoma. This more invasive tumor type tends to involve the appendix diffusely. Yan and colleagues (2001) described three different variants as well-, moderately, and poorly differentiated. The poorly differentiated histologic type contains signet ring cells.

Ronnett and colleagues (1997) in their histologic description of the mucinous appendiceal tumors found a small proportion of patients with pseudomyxoma peritonei syndrome with small foci of mucinous adenocarci-

Table 63-2 Comparison of Colorectal and Appendiceal Malignant Tumors

FEATURE	COLON	APPENDIX
Adenocarcinoma incidence	85%	10%
Carcinoid incidence	<1%	70%
Mucinous adenocarcinoma	10–15%	20%
Signet ring adenocarcinoma	1/1000	1/10
Adenocarcinoid	Not reported	Rare
Differentiation of adenocarcinoma		
Well-differentiated	20%	60%
Moderately differentiated	60%	20%
Poorly differentiated	20%	20%
Associated malignancy	Unusual	Common

noma within the large volume of adenomucinosis. These tumors presented with the typical pseudomyxoma peritonei syndrome but had a poorer prognosis, similar to that of patients with mucinous carcinomatosis (Ronnett et al, 2001). Tumors with a predominant histologic type of adenomucinosis but foci (less than 5% of fields) of mucinous adenocarcinoma are referred to as hybrid histologic type.

■ DIAGNOSIS OF APPENDICEAL MALIGNANT TUMORS

Carcinoid

Ninety percent of carcinoid tumors are found as incidental findings upon removal of an otherwise normal appendix. Approximately 10% of patients with carcinoid have appendicitis, and only rarely does a patient present with the carcinoid syndrome. In patients with the malignant carcinoid syndrome, elevated urine levels of 5-hydroxyindoleacetic acid are routinely found. Also, elevated serum serotonin assays can be obtained. These patients almost invariably have liver metastasis.

Adenocarcinoma

The preoperative diagnosis in patients with adenocarcinoma of the appendix is usually appendicitis, a right lower quadrant abscess, or tumor mass (Table 63-3). Mucinous appendiceal cancer has usually perforated prior to diagnosis (Lyss, 1988). This perforation results in tumor spread to the ovaries, or the tumor may present as peritoneal carcinomatosis within a hernia sac. An aggressive mucinous adenocarcinoma may invade the retroperitoneum and appear as a mucus accumulation in the buttock or thigh. Also, abdominal wall invasion with an enterocutaneous fistula or bladder invasion with an enterovesical fistula may occur. Obstruction of the right ureter by a mucus-containing mass or invasion into the urinary bladder has also been described.

Pseudomyxoma Peritonei Syndrome

These minimally invasive appendiceal tumors have a high propensity for spread to peritoneal surfaces, but are unlikely to metastasize through lymphatic channels into lymph nodes, or through venules into the liver. Gonzalez-Morino and colleagues in a study of 501 patients reported lymph node metastasis in 2% and liver metastasis in 2%. After the appendiceal tumor ruptures the wall of the appendix, adenomucinosis may progress for months or even years within the abdomen and pelvis without causing other symptoms (Fig. 63-1). When this occurs, the resulting clinical syndrome is termed pseudomyxoma peritonei. The peritoneal cavity becomes filled in a characteristic way with mucinous tumor and mucinous ascites. The greater omentum is thickened (omental cake) and extensively infiltrated by tumor (Fig. 63-2). All dependent parts of the abdomen that tend to entrap malignant cells are also filled by tumor.

This process involves the undersurface of the right and left hemidiaphragms, the right subhepatic space, the splenic hilus, the right and left abdominal gutters, and especially the pelvis and cul-de-sac. An important clinical feature of pseudomyxoma peritonei is the relative sparing of the small bowel by this process (Fig. 63-3). Because the small bowel is spared of tumor involvement, removal of the involved parietal and visceral peritoneal surfaces by peritonectomy procedures combined with intraperitoneal chemotherapy may provide long-term disease-free survival in over 80% of patients.

Preoperative diagnosis of pseudomyxoma peritonei is quite different from appendiceal adenocarcinoma. The most common symptom in both men and women with pseudomyxoma peritonei syndrome is a gradually increasing

Table 63-3 Preoperative Diagnosis of Appendix Cancer at Time of Initial Laparotomy in 296 Case Reports

DIAGNOSIS	NO. OF PATIENTS	PERCENTAGE OF TOTAL
Acute appendicitis	139	47
Ruptured appendix with/without abscess	53	18
Intra-abdominal cancer or right lower quadrant mass	30	10
Inguinal hernia or chronic appendicitis	17	5
Incidental operations except for cholecystitis*	14	—
Cholecystitis (acute and chronic)†	10	—
Ovarian tumor or cyst	10	—
Small bowel obstruction	8	—
Right-sided groin mass or fistula	6	—
Acute abdomen	4	—
Appendiceal carcinoma	3	—
Hydronephrosis	2	—
Total	296	
Autopsy finding‡	10	

*Preoperative diagnosis includes gynecologic cases (eight) and one each of incisional hernia; gastric, esophageal, and sigmoid cancer; duodenal ulcer; and torsion of the small bowel.
†Not listed as incidental, because the present symptom complex may have been related to appendiceal disease in some cases.
‡Some patients died with postmortem diagnosis of metastatic malignancy.
Source: modified from Lyss AP: Appendiceal malignancies. Semin Oncol 1988;15:129–137.

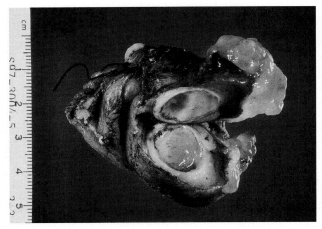

Figure 63-1
The distal appendix has ruptured from mucin within the mucocele. Adenomatous epithelial cells become widely distributed on peritoneal surfaces. The silk suture is on the base of the appendix.

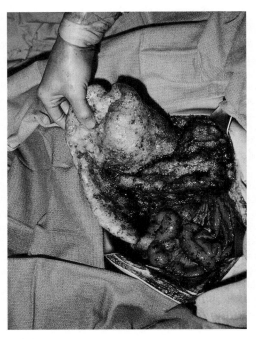

Figure 63-3
When the omentum is elevated, sparing of small bowel is common in pseudomyxoma peritonei.

abdominal girth (Esquivel and Sugarbaker, 2000). In women, the second most common symptom is an ovarian mass, usually on the right side and frequently diagnosed at the time of a routine gynecologic examination. In men, the second most common symptom is a new onset hernia. The hernia sac is found to be filled by mucinous tumor. In both males and females, the third most common presenting feature is appendicitis. This is the clinical manifestation of rupture of an appendiceal mucocele which

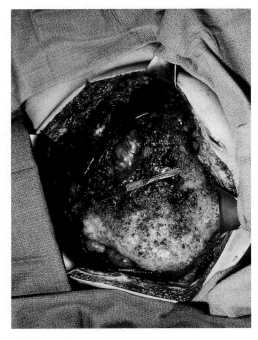

Figure 63-2
A thickened omentum (omental cake) is characteristically present in patients with pseudomyxoma peritonei.

contains intestinal bacteria. The symptoms and signs of pseudomyxoma peritonei syndrome are itemized in Table 63-4.

A caveat should be mentioned regarding the "benign mucocele" of the appendix. If a mucocele of the appendix is found at the time of a planned laparoscopic appendectomy, then open appendectomy should be performed (Jacquet et al, 1995). Laparoscopic resection of a mucocele is likely to cause rupture of that structure, and pseudomyxoma peritonei syndrome may then result within months or years. Resection of the appendiceal mass without traumatic rupture and without tumor spillage results in a complete eradication of the disease process.

When a patient presents with increasing abdominal girth as a result of presumed malignant ascites, a paracentesis or laparoscopy with biopsy is usually performed in order to establish a diagnosis. In many female patients, an ovarian neoplasm will be found. In others, a perforated adenocarcinoma from the colon, stomach, gallbladder, or appendix will be found. The remainder of these patients will have a peritoneal surface tumor such as peritoneal mesothelioma, papillary serous tumor, or peritoneal mucinous adenocarcinoma (of unknown primary site). In all instances, paracentesis or laparoscopy with biopsy should be performed directly within the midline and through the linea alba. These sites can be excised as part of a midline abdominal incision. No lateral puncture sites or port sites should be used, because incision in these areas will seed the abdominal wall with tumor and greatly interfere with disease eradication. Cytoreductive surgery and intraperitoneal chemotherapy are not effective for tumor within the abdominal wall.

Table 63-4 Symptoms and Signs of Patients Presenting with Pseudomyxoma Peritonei Syndrome

SYMPTOMS/SIGNS	NO. OF PATIENTS (%)	NO. OF MEN (%)	NO. OF WOMEN (%)
Appendicitis	58 (27)	36 (34)	22 (20)
Increased abdominal girth	49 (23)	28 (27)	21 (19)
Ovarian mass	44 (20)	—	44 (39)
Hernia	30 (14)	26 (25)	4 (4)
Ascites	9 (4)	5 (5)	4 (4)
Abdominal pain	8 (4)	5 (5)	3 (3)
Other	19 (9)	5 (5)	14 (12)
Total	217 (100)	105 (48)	112 (52)

Note: Values in parentheses are percentages.
Source: Esquivel J, Sugarbaker PH: Clinical presentation of the pseudomyxoma peritonei syndrome. Br J Surg 2000;87:1414–1418.

■ TREATMENT OF APPENDICEAL TUMORS

Carcinoid Tumors

With appendiceal cancer, as with almost all gastrointestinal cancers, the prognosis of the tumor depends on the stage at which it is diagnosed and the skill and experience of the surgeon. Fortunately for 90% of carcinoid tumors, the disease is in an asymptomatic state and cure is expected in nearly 100% of cases (Fig. 63-4). The prognosis depends on the size of the lesion and its capacity to invade locally. In patients with tumors 1 cm or smaller, simple appendectomy is all that is required. In this situation the prognosis is extremely good, with nearly all patients surviving free of disease. In patients with tumors 2 cm or larger, there is a greater likelihood for dissemination through lymph channels into lymph nodes or portal venules into the liver. If the tumor is over 2 cm in size, if there are involved lymph nodes, or if the tumor has invaded out of the appendix into the mesoappendix or nearby small bowel, an en bloc right hemicolectomy with peritonectomy of the periappendiceal surfaces is advised. Sometimes there is extensive spread of the tumor into the ileocolic mesentery. Even in this situation, a vigorous attempt is made to excise radically all tumor and involved adjacent organs en bloc.

In some patients a locally advanced carcinoid tumor will occur with hepatic metastases. Often these patients will have the carcinoid syndrome. If the local tumor can be excised even with minimal margins of resection, one should undertake its removal and also resection of hepatic metastases. Occasionally, several repeat hepatic resections may be required. A segmental approach or a metastasectomy procedure is preferred over a right or left hepatectomy. Whatever liver surgery is required to remove all visible deposits of tumor should be done to gain maximal long-term palliation.

Appendiceal Adenocarcinoma

In patients with adenocarcinoma of the appendix, a right hemicolectomy is suggested because it results in nearly twice the survival rate when compared to routine appendectomy (Hesketh, 1963). Therefore, all patients with invasive appendiceal adenocarcinoma, whether or not lymph nodes are involved, should receive a right hemicolectomy either during the same surgical procedure in which the appendectomy is performed or in a subsequent procedure. Certainly, when the surgeon performing an appendectomy finds that the appendix is infiltrated by an aggressive malignant process, emergency frozen sectioning should be performed. If there is adequate bowel preparation and if a diagnosis of adenocarcinoma can be made definitively, one should proceed without hesitation with a right hemicolectomy procedure. In some patients a cecectomy with preservation of the ileocecal valve has been utilized. This procedure is recommended if the appendiceal lymph nodes are negative by frozen sectioning.

Mucinous Tumors with Peritoneal Dissemination

A majority of patients with mucinous tumors of the appendix show perforation of the appendix at the time of exploration. In most of these patients, mucinous peritoneal carcinomatosis or pseudomyxoma peritonei is found at the time of appendectomy. In the past, this condition was always fatal. Recently, peritonectomy procedures combined with intraperitoneal chemotherapy have been employed for the treatment of pseudomyxoma peritonei and peritoneal carcinomatosis (Sugarbaker, 1999). The essential features of this approach are diagrammed in Figure 63-5. The surgeon is responsible for doing as much as possible to remove all tumor on peritoneal surfaces. This removal is accomplished by using a cytoreductive procedure in patients who have gross spread of tumor around the peritoneal cavity. This procedure involves a greater and lesser omentectomy and splenectomy, followed by peritonectomy procedures to strip tumor from the abdominal gutters, pelvis, right subhepatic space, and right and left subphrenic spaces (Sugarbaker, 1995). The primary appendicial tumor should be cleared by appendectomy unless the margins are positive or lymph nodes are positive (Gonzalez-Morino et al, 2004).

Perioperative Intraperitoneal Chemotherapy

After the resection, and with the abdomen open, the peritoneal space is extensively washed by the surgeon's hand using heated mitomycin C chemotherapy

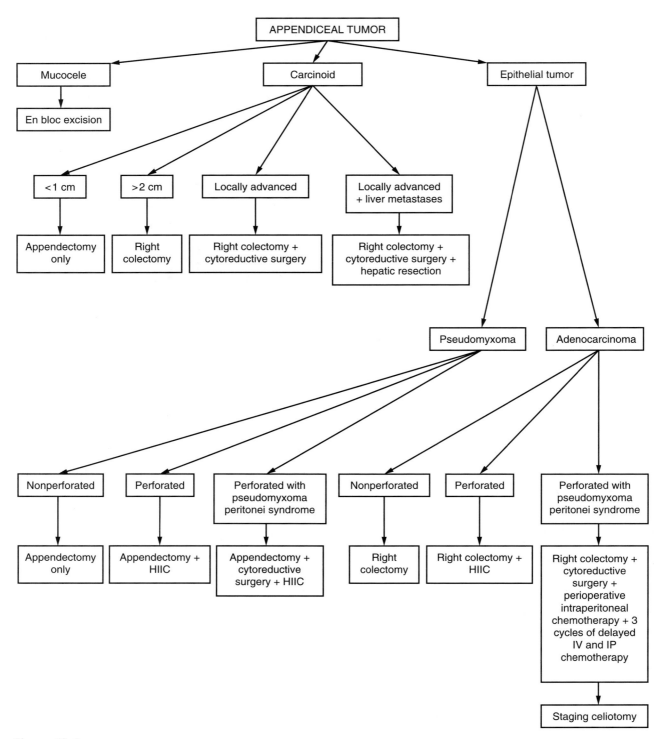

Figure 63-4
Algorithm for treatment of appendiceal malignancy. HIIC, heated intraoperative intraperitoneal chemotherapy; IP, intraperitoneal; IV, intravenous.

(Fig. 63-6). Also, a window of time exists in which all intraperitoneal surfaces are available for intraperitoneal chemotherapy utilizing 5-fluorouracil in the early postoperative period. Uniformity of treatment with intraperitoneal chemotherapy to all peritoneal surfaces, including those surfaces dissected by the surgeon, can be achieved if the intraperitoneal chemotherapy is used during the first postoperative week. As the chemotherapy is dwelling, distribution is facilitated by turning the patient alternately onto the right and left

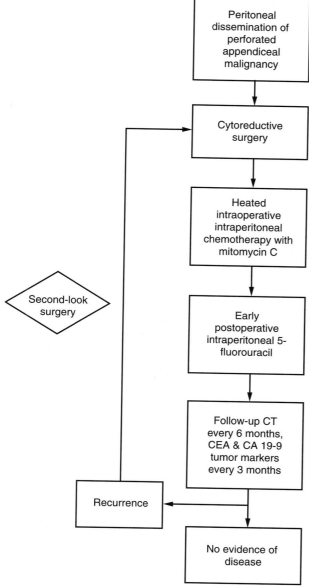

Figure 63-5
Approach to the treatment of peritoneal carcinomatosis from appendix cancer. CEA, carcinoembryonic antigen; CT, computed tomography.

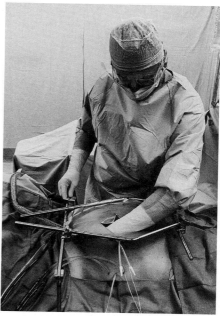

Figure 63-6
Coliseum technique for using intraperitoneal chemotherapy. The skin edges are suspended on a self-retaining retractor. Warm (41 to 42°C) chemotherapy solution is perfused while being manually distributed throughout the abdomen and pelvis.

sides as well as into the prone position (Sugarbaker, 1999).

This perioperative intraperitoneal chemotherapy (combination of heated intraoperative mitomycin C and early postoperative 5-fluorouracil) has been utilized in over 750 patients, and has not been associated with an increased incidence of anastomotic disruptions. In patients who have had extensive prior surgical procedures who require many hours of lysis of adhesions, there is an increased incidence of postoperative bowel perforation. This increased incidence is presumably a result of the combined effects of damage to small bowel from electro-surgical dissection of adhesions (seromuscular damage) and systemic effects of intraperitoneal chemotherapy on the intestine (mucosa and submucosa damage). In those patients who have high-grade appendiceal mucinous peritoneal carcinomatosis, intravenous chemotherapy is recommended. This chemotherapy is given once a month. Usually 5-fluorouracil, leucovorin, and irinotecan for 6 months is appropriate (Saltz et al, 2000).

In approximately one third of patients after the cytoreduction with perioperative chemotherapy a second-look surgery is required because of localized disease recurrence detected by follow up. If at the reoperative procedure small tumor foci are found in peritoneal fissures in the abdomen or pelvis, a final intraperitoneal chemotherapy treatment is performed.

Serial Debulking

It is important that definitive treatment of peritoneal carcinomatosis or pseudomyxoma peritonei be instituted in a timely fashion. Each nondefinitive (debulking) procedure jeopardizes subsequent surgical procedures, making potentially curative cytoreductive surgery more difficult. The relative sparing of the small bowel is seen only early in the natural history of peritoneal carcinomatosis and pseudomyxoma peritonei. After several surgical procedures have been performed, the fibrous adhesions that inevitably result become infiltrated by tumor, leading to extensive involvement of the small bowel by the malignant process. Eventually it becomes impossible to debulk the tumor safely, and the effects of the intraperitoneal chemotherapy by itself are not adequate to keep the patient disease-free.

Cytoreductive Surgery and Intraperitoneal Chemotherapy

The results of these treatments for peritoneal surface dissemination of appendiceal malignancies are unexpectedly good. The results of treatment of 385 patients with prolonged follow-up have been reported (Sugarbaker and Chang, 1999).

Survival by Completeness of Cytoreduction

The mean follow-up period of this group of 385 appendix malignancies was 37.6 months. After the completion of the cytoreductive surgery, all these patients had the abdomen inspected for the presence or absence of residual disease. A completeness of cytoreduction (CC) score was obtained for all patients. The completeness of cytoreduction score was based on the size of individual tumor nodules remaining unresected (Jacquet and Sugarbaker, 1996). A CC-0 score indicated no visible tumor remaining after surgery. A CC-1 score indicated tumor nodules less than 2.5 mm. A CC-2 score indicated tumor nodules between 2.5 mm and 2.5 cm. A CC-3 score indicated tumor nodules greater than 2.5 cm or a confluence of implants at any site. In Figure 63-7, the survival of patients who had a complete cytoreduction (CC-0 and CC-1) is compared with those with an incomplete cytoreduction (CC-2 and CC-3). Survival differences were significant ($p < 0.0001$); patients who left the operating room after cytoreductive surgery with tumor nodules less than 2.5 mm in diameter remaining were much more likely to sur-

vive long-term than were those with an incomplete cytoreduction. There were no significant differences in survival between patients with CC-2 and CC-3 cytoreductions (data not shown).

Survival by Histologic Assessment

At the time of cytoreductive surgery and whenever possible from a review of the primary appendiceal malignancy, a histologic assessment was made. The designations of adenomucinosis, hybrid, and mucinous adenocarcinoma have been described (Ronnett et al, 1997). Adenomucinosis included minimally aggressive peritoneal tumors that produced large volumes of mucous ascites. The primary appendiceal tumor was described as a cystadenoma. Hybrid malignancies showed adenomucinosis combined with isolated foci of mucinous adenocarcinomas (less than 5%). Mucinous adenocarcinoma showed an atypical histologic appearance. Often the signet ring morphology and poor differentiation was observed.

Figure 63-8 shows the survival distribution of these appendix malignancy patients by histologic type. The survival differences between patients with adenomucinosis and those with hybrid or mucinous adenocarcinoma were significant ($p < 0.0001$). A noninvasive histopathologic appearance is extremely important in selecting patients who are most likely to benefit from this treatment strategy. There were no significant differences between patients with hybrid and mucinous adenocarcinoma determined histologically.

Survival by Prior Surgical Score

When the previous operative notes on these patients were reviewed, a judgment was made regarding the anatomic sites of previous surgical dissections. The summation of

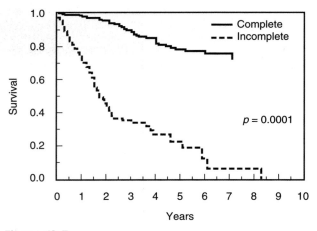

PERITONEAL SURFACE MALIGNANCY–APPENDIX
SURVIVAL BY CYTOREDUCTION

Figure 63-7
Survival rates by cytoreduction of appendiceal malignancy with peritoneal dissemination. (From Sugarbaker PH, Chang D: Results of treatment of 385 patients with peritoneal surface spread of appendiceal malignancy. Ann Surg Oncol 1999;6(8):727–731.)

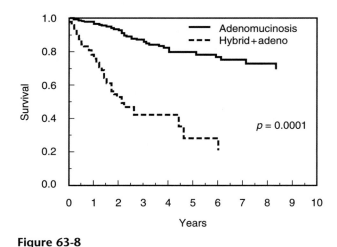

PERITONEAL SURFACE MALIGNANCY–APPENDIX
SURVIVAL BY HISTOLOGY

Figure 63-8
Survival rates by histologic type of appendiceal malignancy with peritoneal dissemination. (From Sugarbaker PH, Chang D: Results of treatment of 385 patients with peritoneal surface spread of appendiceal malignancy. Ann Surg Oncol 1999;6(8):727–731.)

these dissections was recorded on a diagram of the abdominopelvic regions (Esquivel and Sugarbaker, 1998). This review allowed an assessment of the anatomic locations in which previous surgery had been performed. In patients with a prior surgical score (PSS) of 0, diagnosis of peritoneal carcinomatosis was obtained through biopsy only, or by laparoscopy plus biopsy. PSS-1 indicated only a previous exploratory laparotomy. PSS-2 indicated exploratory laparotomy with some resections. Usually this procedure was a greater omentectomy or greater omentectomy plus a right colectomy. In PSS-3, patients had a prior attempt at a complete cytoreduction. This procedure was usually greater omentectomy, right colectomy, hysterectomy, and bilateral salpingo-oophorectomy, with the possibility of other resections from both abdominal organs or parietal peritoneal regions. The survival distribution by previous surgical score is shown in Figure 63-9. Patients with PSS scores of 0 through 2 had an improved survival compared with those with a PSS of 3 ($p = 0.001$).

Survival Analysis by Cox Semiparametric Model

All the significant clinical features were investigated to determine their status. The independent variables were determined to be complete versus incomplete cytoreduction. All the other clinical features investigated were found to have no independent predictive value. Complete versus incomplete cytoreduction had a risk ratio of 9.98. The 95% confidence limits were 4.23 to 23.09.

Treatment of Adenocarcinoid Appendiceal Malignancy

In the database at the Washington Cancer Institute 22 patients had a diagnosis of adenocarcinoid of the appendix. All patients had peritoneal seeding and most patients had high peritoneal carcinomatosis index. All patients were explored and cytoreduction attempted. If the cytoreduction was complete, intraoperative and early postoperative intraperitoneal chemotherapy was used. The survival distribution of all patients is shown in Figure 63-10. In selected patients an attempt at complete cancer resection is warranted, but the prognosis is guarded. If a debulking results in gross residual disease, only palliative surgical efforts associated with low morbidity and mortality rates are indicated because survival time is limited.

Morbidity and Mortality Rates

The extensive cytoreductive surgery combined with early postoperative intraperitoneal chemotherapy presents a major physiologic insult. Nevertheless, the mortality rate remains at 2% in this group of patients. Pancreatitis (7.1%) and fistula formation (4.7%) are the major complications. Anastomotic leaks were no more common in this group of patients than in a routine general surgical setting (2.4%). The overall grade III/IV morbidity rate was 27%. No morbidity or fatality was directly associated with the intraperitoneal chemotherapy administration. Rather, the incidence of complications depended on the extent of the surgery, number of peritonectomy procedures, and time required to complete the cytoreduction (Stephens et al, 1999).

■ SUMMARY OF NOVEL TREATMENT STRATEGIES FOR PERITONEAL SURFACE MALIGNANCY

Peritonectomy

In this treatment strategy for patients with peritoneal carcinomatosis from appendiceal malignancy, there were several distinct changes in the techniques used for surgery

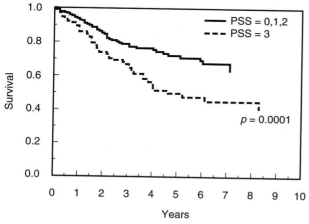

PERITONEAL SURFACE MALIGNANCY–APPENDIX SURVIVAL BY PRIOR SURGICAL SCORE

— PSS = 0,1,2
--- PSS = 3

$p = 0.0001$

Figure 63-9
Survival rates by prior surgical score (PSS) of appendiceal malignancy with peritoneal dissemination. (From Sugarbaker PH, Chang D: Results of treatment of 385 patients with peritoneal surface spread of appendiceal malignancy. Ann Surg Oncol 1999;6(8):727–731.)

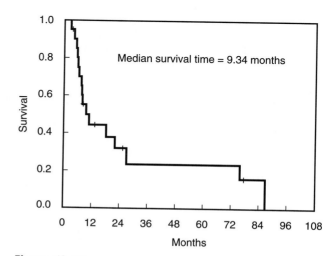

Median survival time = 9.34 months

Figure 63-10
Results of treament of 21 patients with carcinomatosis from adenocarcinoid of the appendix.

and methods of chemotherapy administration (Table 63-4). Surgery was more extensive and more meticulous than in other cytoreductive protocols. Because of the very limited penetration of tumor nodules by chemotherapy, the cytoreduction attempted to reduce the cancer within the abdomen and pelvis to its smallest volume (Sugarbaker, 1995). This required the use of peritoneal stripping procedures, now commonly referred to as peritonectomy procedures. These procedures often required many hours in the operating room. Frequently, they left the abdomen without peritoneal surfaces except that which was found on the small bowel. This approach represents a departure from the previous conservative surgical approach to peritoneal carcinomatosis.

Perioperative Intraperitoneal Chemotherapy

Several changes occurred in the use of chemotherapy in this patient population. First, the route of chemotherapy administration was changed from intravenous to intraperitoneal. Maximal doses of intraoperative intraperitoneal mitomycin C and early postoperative intraperitoneal 5-fluorouracil were used for the first 5 postoperative days. This chemotherapy was instilled perioperatively in order to contact all the abdominal and pelvic surfaces before the onset of wound healing. Once fibrinous deposits became organized, the chemotherapy would be unable to reach the residual tumors, and local recurrence would occur where the surfaces were adherent (Table 63-5).

The timing of chemotherapy administration was changed also. Chemotherapy was used in the perioperative period rather than 4 to 6 weeks after surgery in an adjuvant setting. Perhaps most important to the long-term favorable results, the selection of patients for treatment was changed. Patients with minimal peritoneal surface residual disease were treated more successfully. Patients with large volume residual disease in the abdomen after cytoreduction did not achieve a complete response. The target of these therapies was not metastases present at distant sites such as the liver, bone marrow, or lungs; rather, the target for these therapies was directed at macroscopic residual disease on both the parietal and visceral surfaces. Patients with metastases that could not be resected or gross residual peritoneal surface malignancy after completion of the cytoreductive surgery were excluded from these treatments.

Finally, it is hoped that with these changes in chemotherapy and changes in surgical approach, patients with peritoneal carcinomatosis can benefit from these aggressive treatment strategies. Perhaps the previous failures of palliative chemotherapy for peritoneal carcinomatosis and pseudomyxoma peritonei can be converted to success with this new combination of surgery plus regional chemotherapy.

Suggested Readings

Esquivel J, Sugarbaker PH: Elective surgery in recurrent colon cancer with peritoneal seeding: When to and when not to operate (editorial). Cancer Therapeut 1998;1:321–325.

Esquivel J, Sugarbaker PH: Clinical presentation of the pseudomyxoma peritonei syndrome. Br J Surg 2000;87:1414–1418.

Gonzalez-Moreno S, Sugarbaker PH: Right hemicolectomy does not confer a survival advantage in patients with mucinous carcinoma of the appendix and peritoneal seeding. Br J Surg 2004;91:304–311.

Hesketh KT: The management of primary adenocarcinoma of the vermiform appendix. Gut 1963;4:158–168.

Higa E, Rosai J, Pizzimbono CA, Wise L: Mucosal hyperplasia, mucinous cystadenoma and mucinous cystadenocarcinoma of the appendix. Cancer 1973;32:1525–1541.

Jacquet P, Averbach AM, Stephens AD, Sugarbaker PH: Cancer recurrence following laparoscopic colectomy: Report of two patients treated with heated intraoperative chemotherapy. Dis Colon Rectum 1995;38(10):1110–1114.

Jacquet P, Sugarbaker PH: Current methodologies for clinical assessment of patients with peritoneal carcinomatosis. J Exp Clin Cancer Res 1996;15(1):49–58.

Lyss AP: Appendiceal malignancies. Semin Oncol 1988;15:129–137.

Ronnett BM, Shmookler BM, Sugarbaker PH, Kurman RJ: Pseudomyxoma peritonei: New concepts in diagnosis, origin, nomenclature, and relationship to mucinous borderline (low malignant potential) tumors of the ovary. Anat Pathol 1997;2:197–226.

Ronnett BM, Yan H, Kurman RJ, et al: Pseudomyxoma peritonei associated with disseminated peritoneal adenomucinosis has a significantly more favorable prognosis than peritoneal mucinous carcinomatosis. Cancer 2001;92(1):85–91.

Saltz LB, Cox JV, Blanke C, et al, for the Irinotecan Study Group: Irinotecan plus fluorouracil and leucovorin for metastatic colorectal cancer. N Engl J Med 2000;343(13):905–914.

Stephens AD, Alderman R, Chang D, et al: Morbidity and mortality of 200 treatments with cytoreductive surgery and hyperthermic intraoperative intraperitoneal chemotherapy using the Coliseum technique. Ann Surg Oncol 1999;6(8):790–796.

Sugarbaker PH: Pseudomyxoma peritonei: A cancer whose biology is characterized by a redistribution phenomenon (editorial). Ann Surg 1994;219(2):109–111.

Sugarbaker PH: Peritonectomy procedures. Ann Surg 1995;221:29–42.

Sugarbaker PH: Observations concerning cancer spread within the peritoneal cavity and concepts supporting an ordered pathophysiology. In Sugarbaker PH (Ed.): Peritoneal Carcinomatosis: Principles of Management. Boston, Kluwer, 1996, pp 79–100.

Sugarbaker PH: Intraperitoneal Chemotherapy and Cytoreductive Surgery: A Manual for Physicians and Nurses, 3rd ed. Grand Rapids, MI, Ludann Co, 1999.

Sugarbaker PH, Chang D: Results of treatment of 385 patients with peritoneal surface spread of appendiceal malignancy. Ann Surg Oncol 1999;6(8):727–731.

Yan H, Pestieau SR, Shmookler BM, Sugarbaker PH: Histopathologic analysis in 46 patients with pseudomyxoma peritonei syndrome: Failure vs. success with a second-look operation. Mod Pathol 2001;14(3):164–171.

Table 63-5 Suggested Changes in the Use of Chemotherapy for Gastrointestinal Cancer

CHEMOTHERAPY APPLICATION	CHANGE
Route	Intraperitoneal vs. intravenous
Timing	Perioperative vs. systemic adjuvant
Patient selection	Minimal residual peritoneal surface disease vs. systemic disease
Target	Spread vs. metastases
Surgical approach	Peritonectomies vs. debulking
Results	Benefit vs. previous failure

64

MANAGEMENT OF CANCER OF THE COLON (INCLUDING ADJUVANT THERAPY)

Clifford L. Simmang, MD, MS
Philip J. Huber, Jr., MD

■ ETIOLOGY

The incidence of colon cancer varies, based on geographic location. In general, countries of the Western world have the highest incidence of colon and rectal carcinoma. Also, the risk of large bowel carcinoma is increased in urban populations when compared to rural populations. These variations correlate with socioeconomic status and culture, which may in turn be influenced by environmental impact and diet. Burkitt's observation of the low incidence of colorectal carcinoma in African natives prompted the idea that their high fiber intake was responsible for this finding. Western diets that are low in fiber are often high in animal fat and carbohydrates. Dietary fat enhances cholesterol and bile acid synthesis by the liver, resulting in increased levels of bile acids within the colon. When acted upon by anaerobic colonic bacteria, these compounds are converted to secondary bile acids that are promoters of carcinogenesis. Fermentable dietary fiber contains plant lignans, which may be protective against colorectal cancer, and resistant starch that by fermentation produces short-chain fatty acids. These short-chain fatty acids, in particular butyrate, have a stabilizing effect on colonocyte proliferation. Also possibly protective against colorectal cancer is ingestion of calcium, antioxidants, selenium, retinoids, plant steroids, sulfur compounds from onion and garlic, and aspirin. No convincing proof exists that any of these nutrients play a role in an individual's colorectal cancer predisposition, although some epidemiologic data are suggestive.

Colorectal cancer is a genetic disease in that its basic cause is genetic abnormalities in colonocytes leading to loss of control over DNA (deoxyribonucleic acid) repair, cell growth, differentiation, migration, senescence, and death. Although most of the genetic abnormalities are somatic and are probably acquired because of factors in the environment, some patients inherit a cancer-predisposing mutation. The classic examples of inherited colorectal cancer syndromes are familial adenomatous polyposis (FAP), which accounts for approximately 1% of colon cancer cases, and hereditary nonpolyposis colorectal carcinoma (HNPCC), commonly referred to as the Lynch syndrome, which is responsible for 2 to 3% of all colorec-

tal cancers. These inherited syndromes are fully discussed in Chapters 60 and 62.

Almost all colorectal cancers begin as an adenoma. However, only a tiny percentage of adenomas ever become malignant. The progression of adenoma to carcinoma from normal colon has been estimated to take about 10 years. It is accelerated in inherited syndromes of the disease. As the adenoma-carcinoma sequence progresses, adenomas tend to become larger and more dysplastic.

A subgroup of colorectal cancers may have their origin in hyperplastic polyps. These are likely to arise via a different genetic route than the common colorectal cancer. Serrated adenomas and mixed hyperplastic/adenomatous polyps are a likely intermediate step in this pathway.

■ RISK FACTORS

The average lifetime population risk for colorectal cancer in Western society has been estimated as about 6%. This population risk is age-related and increases with each passing decade. Several groups of patients are at particularly high risk for colorectal cancer, including patients who have already had an adenoma or cancer, those with a family history of colorectal neoplasia, and those with chronic ulcerative colitis or Crohn's colitis.

Certain features of adenomas are associated with a high risk of metachronous cancer. High-risk adenomas are tubular adenomas greater than 1 cm in diameter, adenomas with over 25% villous component, or adenomas with high-grade dysplasia. Multiple (>3) adenomas of any type confer increased risk. A past history of a colorectal cancer is associated with a 5 to 6% chance of a metachronous cancer.

An increased incidence of malignancy has been reported in first-degree relatives of patients with a colon and rectal cancer. As more relatives are involved and the age at diagnosis becomes younger, this association becomes stronger until it approaches the criteria required to make a diagnosis of HNPCC. Patients with ulcerative colitis, especially those who have had the condition for more than 10 years, have experienced onset in childhood, and have pancolonic (proximal to splenic flexure) involvement, have an increased cumulative risk of carcinoma that becomes greater than 30% after 25 years of disease. Crohn's disease has also been reported to increase the risk of colon cancer to 4 to 20 times greater than that for the general population.

A prior history of pelvic radiation has been associated with the diagnosis of rectal carcinoma following an interval of approximately 15 years. Ureterosigmoidostomy markedly increases the risk of sigmoid cancer up to 500 times that of the normal population. Currently, colon that remains in continuity with the fecal stream is seldom used for urinary diversion. Patients who have already had this operation should undergo endoscopic surveillance. Many studies have addressed the possible association between cholecystectomy and risk of colon cancer. The best evidence currently available does not support such an association.

Also, no increase in colorectal cancer in patients who have diverticulosis has been documented.

■ INCIDENCE

An estimated 147,500 new cases of colorectal cancer were expected in 2003, of which about 105,500 would be located within the colon. Over the past few decades there has been a gradual shift in distribution of large bowel cancers, from the left colon to the right. Certain geographic areas with a high incidence of colorectal cancer have a higher number of cancers located in the left colon compared to other geographic areas where there is a lower overall incidence of colorectal cancer but a right-sided predominance.

Synchronous colon cancers are found in about 5% of patients. Although metachronous cancer has previously been reported at about 5%, some centers with intensive surveillance programs have noted a lower incidence of metachronous cancer in the range of 1 to 2%.

■ EARLY DETECTION

Colon cancer is preventable. If adenomas are found and removed before malignant transformation, cancer is prevented. Because adenomas are usually asymptomatic, detection is dependent on screening. Screening guidelines for the early detection of colorectal cancer in an asymptomatic average-risk person have historically been an annual digital rectal examination and fecal occult blood test (FOBT) beginning at the age of 50, with flexible sigmoidoscopy every 5 years. A recent trend to recommending colonoscopy starting at age 50 years and repeated every 10 years has been driven by the relative lack of sensitivity of FOBT and sigmoidoscopy. A double-contrast barium enema, preferably combined with a flexible sigmoidoscopy, every 5 to 10 years is an alternative to colonoscopy, but is less sensitive and does not offer a therapeutic option. Guidelines produced by a consortium of five medical societies (American College of Gastroenterology, American Gastroenterological Association, American Society of Colon and Rectal Surgeons, American Society for Gastrointestinal Endoscopy, and Society of American Gastrointestinal Endoscopic Surgeons) were recently updated and revised. These guidelines are presented in detail and are evidence-based, and we would recommend that all physicians review these articles. New screening modalities that are under investigation include computed tomographic (CT) colography (virtual colonoscopy) and stool-based DNA testing. Therapy and surveillance of polyps is more fully discussed in Chapters 57 and 58.

■ PREOPERATIVE EVALUATION

The diagnosis of colon cancer is often made during colonoscopy. If colonoscopy is not the method of diagnosis, it should be done prior to performing a colectomy. If this approach is not possible, intraoperative colonoscopy can be performed to clear the proximal colon.

Preoperative laboratory studies include complete blood cell count, urinalysis, and a general chemistry screening panel. These tests assist in the assessment of the overall physiologic status for the patient, as well as the potential for liver metastases.

An electrocardiogram (ECG) is performed to evaluate the patient's cardiac status, and a chest x-ray serves not only to check for metastatic disease but also to evaluate the patient's pulmonary status. If there is a history of pulmonary dysfunction, such as chronic obstructive pulmonary disease, then pulmonary function tests should be obtained. More sophisticated evaluations need to be performed only if additional information is required to determine the significance of an abnormality detected during the above evaluation.

Measurement of carcinoembryonic antigen (CEA) completes the routine preoperative metastatic workup. Elevated levels of CEA have been reported in 70% of patients with colon cancer, but less than half of patients with localized disease have an elevated CEA. Therefore, CEA is not effective for screening. However, if the CEA were elevated preoperatively and returned to normal postoperatively, it is useful as a surveillance tool. Although the use and timing of CEA measurement for surveillance after resection for colon cancer remains controversial, a patient with a high preoperative CEA is usually followed by postoperative measurements. The interval ranges somewhere between 1 and 3 months for the first 2 years.

CT scans are not obtained routinely in patients with colon cancer. Situations in which CT scanning is more likely to provide information that might affect management decisions include patients who have abnormal liver function tests, patients with a palpable mass, and patients who have a near obstructing, annular, "apple core" cancer of the colon. In these situations, preoperative CT scanning may yield useful information. Demonstration of ureteral obstruction and hydronephrosis would change the preoperative plan to include urologic consultation, cystoscopy, placement of ureteral stents, and preparation for the possibility of having to perform an en bloc ureteral resection along with urinary tract reconstruction. Except for differentiating between a cyst or a solid hepatic mass that was detected by the CT scan, preoperative hepatic ultrasound is seldom used. On the other hand, intraoperative ultrasound of the liver is being used with more frequency. In a report by Rafaelsen and associates from Odense, Denmark, intraoperative ultrasonography was performed in 295 consecutive patients, taking an average time of 8 minutes. Synchronous liver metastases were detected in 64 (21.7%) of the 295 patients. Intraoperative ultrasonography detected liver metastases in 62 (96.9%) of the 64 patients with documented metastases. The sensitivities of serum levels of aspartate transaminase (AST), lactate dehydrogenase (LDH), and alkaline phosphatase in detecting these hepatic metastases from colon and rectal carcinoma were 9.4%, 46.9%, and 31.3%, respectively. Preoperative ultrasonography detected 45 of the 64 lesions, for a sensitivity of 70.3%. Fifty-four of the

64 lesions were detected by palpation of the liver during celiotomy, for a sensitivity of 84.4%. Intraoperative ultrasonography showed bilobar metastases in 9 patients who, by palpation at surgery, were thought to have metastases confined to only one lobe. Preoperative ultrasonography had identified bilobar metastases in only 1 of these 9 patients. This intraoperative finding obviates the need for a subsequent costly radiographic evaluation using studies such as hepatic CT portography.

■ PREOPERATIVE PREPARATION

A mechanical bowel preparation combined with both oral and intravenous antibiotic prophylaxis is routine. The most common form of mechanical bowel preparation is an oral lavage with polyethylene glycol–based electrolyte solution. Some patients have difficulty ingesting the large volume of solution, and for these individuals Fleet phosphosoda oral preparation is effective. The possible dehydration and electrolyte imbalance in patients taking Fleet phosphosoda almost never becomes clinically apparent, especially if the preparation is avoided in patients with renal or cardiac failure or who are taking diuretics. We use both oral and intravenous antibiotics. Patients receive 1 g neomycin and 1 g metronidazole by mouth at 2:00 PM and 7:00 PM 1 day prior to surgery. Approximately 30 minutes prior to the start of the operation, the patient receives cefotetan or Unasyn (Pfizer Inc., New York, NY) intravenously. Erythromycin, frequently used as one of the oral antibiotics, produces gastric side effects that are not seen with the combination of neomycin and metronidazole. Alternative bowel preparations are more fully discussed in Chapter 35.

Subcutaneous heparin or one of the low-molecular-weight heparin products is used for prophylaxis against deep venous thrombosis. Graded calf compression stockings are put on intraoperatively and continued postoperatively until the patient is walking.

Many patients prefer epidural anesthesia for postoperative pain relief. When this is requested, the epidural is placed prior to the induction of the general anesthetic. Once this has been performed, the patient is positioned. For lesions involving the right colon or the proximal transverse colon, the patient is positioned supine. If the lesion involves the distal transverse colon or the left colon, and anastomosis may be performed in the distal sigmoid or proximal rectum, then the patient is placed in low lithotomy position. We use Allen stirrups to provide the proper position. Attention to detail prevents the development of injury related to peroneal nerve, vascular, or muscular compression. When the lower extremities are properly positioned using Allen stirrups, all the weight will rest on the patient's heel and the portion underneath the leg will be angled below the calf, leaving a space and avoiding contact or compression.

In patients who have a cancer of the left colon, especially if it is in a distal location, rectal irrigation is performed using a 34 Fr mushroom or malecot catheter placed transanally. The bulbous portion is placed just above the levators, and the rectum is then irrigated with either saline or water until the return is clear. This is followed by irrigation with Betadine solution, which has the advantage of being tumoricidal as well as bactericidal. The catheter is then connected to a drainage bag to allow egress of residual colon contents.

A Foley catheter is inserted into the bladder. Although we do not routinely use a nasogastric tube postoperatively, either a nasogastric or orogastric tube is commonly inserted for the duration of the operation.

■ OPERATIVE PRINCIPLES

Exploration
A midline incision allows access to the pelvis and both flexures without the division of any muscles in the abdominal wall. Occasionally, we will select a low transverse incision. Although this incision has the disadvantage of transecting the lower rectus abdominis muscles, most patients report less postoperative discomfort and this incision may be cosmetically preferable for some patients.

Following entry into the peritoneal cavity, exploration should be performed. A wound protector may be placed to decrease wound contamination and possibly prevent tumor implantation. Mechanical retractors are used to provide exposure. The site of the primary lesion is identified to ensure that the incision is adequate to safely perform resection of that portion of the colon. Next, a methodical search throughout the abdomen should be performed to rule out the presence of metastatic disease and to identify incidental abnormalities. The pelvis is inspected to rule out "drop" metastases or Kruckenberg tumors. The entire bowel should be palpated from the ligament of Trietz to the rectum.

The liver must be evaluated using bimanual palpation, and any masses that are noted should be addressed. Increasing use of intraoperative ultrasound appears to improve the sensitivity of detecting hepatic metastases. If only a single lesion is encountered, this lesion may be excised if excision is easy and of low risk. This procedure usually means performing a wedge excision after the colectomy portion has been completed. Unresected lesions should be biopsied.

Principles of Resection
The goal of a curative procedure for colon cancer is the complete removal of all cancerous tissue. Carcinoma of the colon spreads in one of the following ways: direct continuity, transperitoneal spread, lymphatic spread, hematogenous spread, and implantation. It is unusual for microscopic intramural spread to occur more than 1 cm beyond the grossly visible tumor. Radial extension may occur through the bowel wall and result in adherence to other abdominal organs; 60% of such attached viscera will be invaded by cancer.

The operative techniques used to achieve complete excision of the cancer include removal of the primary lesion with an adequate margin, and the zone of lymphatic drainage. The size of the area removed is based on the arterial supply. Metastatic disease in the regional lymph nodes is found in about 50% of patients undergoing a curative colon resection. To achieve the appropriate mesenteric resection, the artery supplying the colonic segment in which the cancer is located is ligated and divided near its origin. If a cancer is located midway between two major arterial structures, then both arcades with the accompanying colon and mesentery in their distribution should be removed. Once this removal has been accomplished, proximal and distal margins are usually adequate. The one exception may be a cancer located in the distal sigmoid colon. In this case, the distal margin must include the proximal rectum to achieve adequate mesenteric margins. Division of the lymphovascular pedicle prior to mobilization of the primary tumor (the "no touch" technique) was advocated after the discovery that intraoperative manipulation of a colonic tumor was associated with shedding of tumor cells into the portal vein. Data from a randomized multicenter trial in the Netherlands showed a trend in reducing subsequent hepatic metastases using this technique, but the difference was not statistically significant.

Right Colon Cancer

Cancers that are located in the cecum or the ascending colon are removed by performing a right hemicolectomy, which encompasses the bowel served by the ileocolic, right colic, and, occasionally, the right branch of the middle colic vessels (Fig. 64-1). If the lesion is located in the area of the hepatic flexure, the right branch of the middle colic vessels is always included. Colonic mobilization is performed in the avascular embryonic fusion plane. Key steps when performing mobilization of the right colon include the following:

- Avoid injury to the duodenum as the mesentery is mobilized off the duodenum and the head of the pancreas.
- Avoid injury to the right ureter, which often remains behind a veil of retroperitoneal tissue. Additional dissection may be required if definitive visualization of the ureter on this side is required. At times the ureter can be identified where it crosses the iliac vessels and followed in the retroperitoneum by tenting the ureter.
- Avoid damage to the superior mesenteric artery and vein, especially when operating at the base of the transverse colon mesentery.

The anastomosis may be performed either with hand-sewn sutures or with staplers, depending upon the surgeon's preference.

Transverse Colon and Splenic Flexure Cancer

The appropriate boundaries of resection for carcinoma of the transverse colon have been controversial. Fulfilling the criteria for removal of the regional lymphatic drainage depends on the section of transverse colon that is involved. A lesion toward the right may require removal of the middle colic or right colic branches. Most surgeons favor performing an extended right colectomy with their

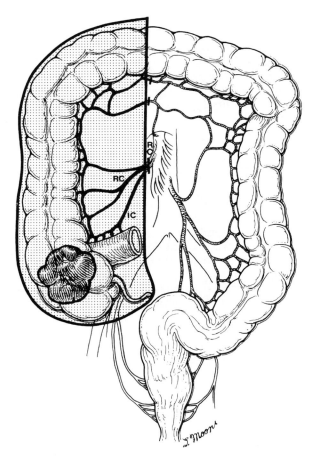

Figure 64-1
Areas resected for lesions of the cecum and proximal ascending colon. A 10- to 15-cm segment of terminal ileum is excised.

anastomosis placed in the left portion of the transverse colon (Fig. 64-2).

For a lesion located in the middle to distal transverse colon, several options may be appropriate. For a cancer in the middle of the transverse colon, a transverse colectomy is performed, although an extended right colectomy with an anastomosis to the proximal descending colon is another option. Similar options are advocated for cancers located near the splenic flexure. In this procedure, the left colic artery is divided after its takeoff from the inferior mesenteric artery (Fig. 64-3). Another alternative is to perform an extended left colectomy, with a transverse colon to rectal anastomosis. The transverse colon can be brought to the pelvis through a window in the ileal mesentery.

Water resorption occurs primarily in the right colon, and in some patients removal of this much colon will produce troublesome diarrhea. In order to improve the functional outcome, preservation of the proximal right colon has been suggested. In this procedure, the ileocolic vessels are preserved, maintaining blood flow to the cecum. The first sigmoid branch from the inferior mesenteric artery is divided with transection of the sigmoid colon in its midportion. A cecal-sigmoid anastomosis is then performed

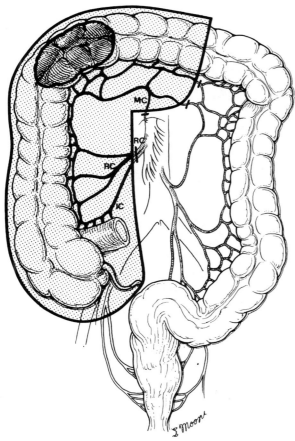

Figure 64-2
Extent of resection for a tumor of the distal ascending colon, hepatic flexure, and right transverse colon. A 5- to 10-cm segment of terminal ileum is removed.

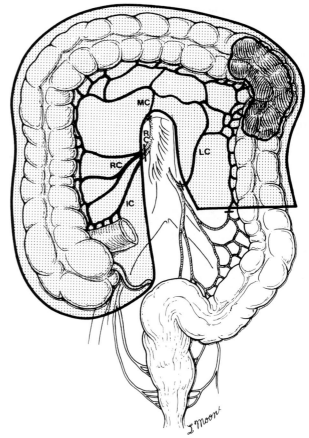

Figure 64-3
Enker's recommendations for resection for a tumor of the splenic flexure.

(Fig. 64-4). This procedure has the advantage of fulfilling oncologic criteria of an adequate resection and preserving the ileocecal valve, terminal ileum, and cecum for their resorptive and reservoir function. Its disadvantages are the likely disproportion between the diameter of the bowel ends and the lack of data showing its efficiency and safety. If the appendix is present, an appendectomy should be included. When performing resection for cancer of the transverse colon or splenic flexure, the adjacent omentum should be removed as well.

Mobilization of the splenic flexure is facilitated by incising the lateral peritoneal attachments along the descending colon and again mobilizing the colon along the avascular embryonic fusion plane. As the splenic flexure is approached, the splenocolic ligament can be defined by the passage of a finger along the colon wall under the veil of tissue, which can be elevated from the distal dissection. If the splenic flexure is high, the transverse colon should also be mobilized and the splenic flexure approached from both the proximal and distal directions. Excessive traction on the splenic flexure or the omentum may produce an avulsion of the inferior tip of the spleen. Should this occur, packing will most often result in hemo-

stasis. If packing fails to control bleeding, another approach is to place thrombostatic material, such as Avitene covered by thrombin-soaked Gelfoam, onto the injured area. When packing is removed, the Gelfoam remains in place and clots are not dislodged.

The appropriate surgical margin for sigmoid colon cancer remains controversial. No policy as to the exact length (left hemicolectomy versus sigmoid-colectomy), extent of lymph node excision, or level of ligation of the inferior mesenteric artery has shown a definite benefit. Rouffet and associates reported on a multicenter study from France involving 270 consecutive patients with left colon carcinomas. The patients were prospectively randomized to receive high ligation of the internal mesenteric artery (IMA) with formal left colon resection and anastomosis between the left third of the transverse colon and the supraperitoneal rectum (Fig. 64-5), or left distal segmental colectomy, also called sigmoidectomy. The sigmoid colon is removed along with lymph nodes accompanying the sigmoid artery, with the IMA being ligated immediately distal to the left ascending colic artery (Fig. 64-6). The lymph node at the origin of the IMA was examined in all cases. After 12 years of follow-up no difference in survival was found between the patients in

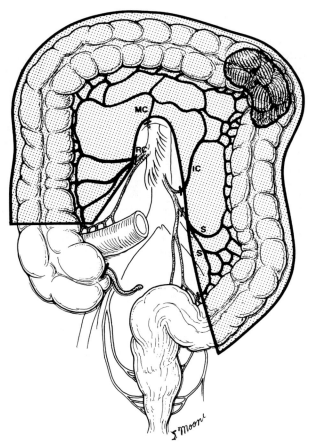

Figure 64-4
Alternative technique for resection of a splenic flexure tumor described by Rosi.

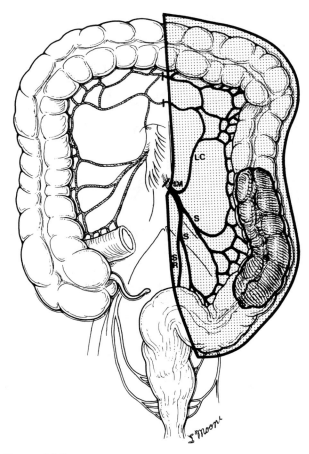

Figure 64-5
Areas of colon to be resected for tumors of the descending, proximal, and midsigmoid colons.

either treatment group, regardless of the Dukes' stage, showing that a similar outcome can be achieved from either procedure.

■ SPECIAL CONSIDERATIONS

Oophorectomy

Ovarian metastases have been reported in 2 to 8% of women with colorectal cancer. An additional 1 to 7% of women subsequently developed ovarian metastases. Prophylactic oophorectomy has not been shown to improve survival. Because of the poor prognosis associated with ovarian metastases, and the low morbidity of oophorectomy, this is considered for selected patients.

Metastases and Recurrence

Minor hepatic resections for isolated metastatic disease may be performed at the time of primary tumor resection, but major hepatic resection should be delayed for 3 to 6 weeks postoperatively. In the presence of unresectable hepatic metastases, a biopsy should be obtained if at all possible.

Patterns of failure after potentially curative resection indicate that the major risk is from disseminated cancer, with the liver being the chief site of metastases. In about one third of deaths due to colon cancer, the metastatic tumor is limited to the liver at autopsy, but in as many as two thirds, other sites also contain metastatic tumor. Autopsy series indicate locoregional recurrence in 25 to 50% of colon cancer deaths, but these recurrences are rarely clinically significant or isolated. One third to one half of recurrences involve peritoneal seeding.

Contiguous Involvement

Malignant invasion of contiguous organs has been reported in between 45 and 70% of the cases with adherence. Adhesions are inflammatory in the rest. Because malignant and inflammatory adhesions cannot be distinguished, the optimal operative treatment is en bloc resection of the carcinoma and all adherent structures without preliminary separation. From 66 to 89% of cases of carcinoma of the colon or rectum that invade adjacent organs arise in the rectum or sigmoid colon. Locally advanced carcinoma of the right colon and proximal transverse colon are adherent to adjacent organs in 11 to 28% of cases. Carcinomas of the right colon can invade the right kidney and ureter, liver, gallbladder, duodenum, and pancreatic head. Curley and associates from the

The distinction between malignant invasion and inflammatory adhesions cannot be determined by gross inspection and palpation. Biopsy of this area must not be performed as operative separation of a carcinoma of the colon and rectum and an adjacent structure involved by direct malignant extension produces local recurrence rates approaching 100% and markedly reduces the 5-year survival rate of these patients. Various reports have compared a 49 to 61% 5-year survival rate if there is no operative violation of the tumor reduced to a 0 to 23% 5-year survival rate if the tumor is entered during operation. Curley recommends that if a surgeon is not prepared to perform a radical extended resection that may include an en bloc pancreaticoduodenectomy, the incision should be closed and the patient referred immediately to a major oncologic center.

Another report from Landercasper retrospectively reviewed 54 patients during a 10-year period who underwent surgical treatment of colorectal carcinomas adherent to adjacent organs, the abdominal wall, or the retroperitoneum. Among the entire group of patients local recurrence developed in 16 (30%) and in 13 of these the recurrence was diagnosed within 18 months of surgery. Thirty-two (59%) of the 54 patients died during follow-up. Histologic evidence of tumor invasion into adherent structures was confirmed in 31 (57%) of their patients. The authors concluded that local failure and patient death almost invariably follow division of the malignant adhesion of colon cancer to adjacent structures. The poor outcome after such separation justifies radical en bloc resection whenever possible.

Obstruction and Perforation

About 15% of patients with colon cancer first present as surgical emergencies with intestinal obstruction, perforation at the site of tumor, or, rarely, a combination of both when perforation occurs in the distended colon proximal to the obstructing cancer. Emergency resection for cancer of the right colon is the generally accepted procedure, and primary ileocolic anastomosis is performed in almost all cases. Similarly, discontinuity resection of perforated tumors of the left colon has emerged as a standard surgical procedure. Improved long-term survival after primary resection of obstructing large bowel cancer has been reported. However, other studies have failed to show a significant difference. In a series of 77 patients who underwent emergency operation for colon cancer, Runkel and his colleagues reported that 57 of these operations were performed for obstruction, and 20 were performed for perforation (5 of this latter group had both obstruction and perforation). Perforation was at the site of the cancer in 75% of patients.

Complications were high after emergency surgery for colon obstruction. The overall mortality rate for all patients with obstructing carcinoma was 21%, and cardiac failure was the chief cause of death. For patients with perforated cancers, the overall mortality rate was 25%, and all deaths were related to sepsis. The infrequent combination of obstruction and perforation had the highest mortality rate at 40%.

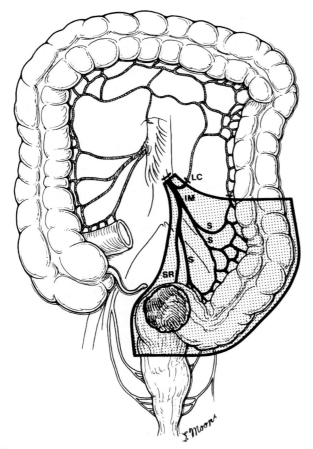

Figure 64-6
Areas of resection for distal sigmoid colon tumor.

M.D. Anderson Cancer Center reported on 12 patients who underwent extended resections of colon carcinomas involving the duodenum or pancreatic head. All 12 patients presented with symptoms related to locally advanced carcinoma of the colon. Seven of these patients underwent an extended right hemicolectomy with en bloc pancreaticoduodenectomy. No malignant invasion of the superior mesenteric vein was found, so the middle colic vein was divided at its junction. In five patients the locally advanced carcinoma involved the lateral aspect of the second or third portion of the duodenum, and an extended right hemicolectomy and en bloc lateral duodenectomy were performed. In one patient, the duodenum was closed primarily. The remaining four patients had large defects that were repaired with a Roux-en-Y limb of jejunum. No operative or postoperative deaths occurred, and mean postoperative stay was 12 days. Only 3 of the 12 patients had metastatic carcinoma in the lymph nodes. Malignant invasion of the wall of the duodenum or pancreatic head or both by carcinoma of the colon was confirmed in all 12 patients. Median follow-up of these 12 patients was 32 months, and at the time of the report, 8 patients were alive without evidence of recurrent or metastatic disease with a median survival time of 42 months.

Single-Stage Procedures for Obstructed Colon Cancer

Single-stage procedures using either segmental colectomy or subtotal colectomy are being performed with increasing frequency. In one prospective randomized study 91 patients were randomized to undergo subtotal colectomy ($n = 47$) or segmental colectomy following on-table colonic irrigation. The overall anastomotic leakage rate for both groups was 7% with no difference in overall complication rates. The postoperative (in hospital) mortality rate was 13% for the 47 subtotal colectomy patients (6 patients) and 11% for the 44 on-table lavage and segmental colectomy patients (5 patients).

A significantly greater number of patients have three or more bowel movements per day after subtotal colectomy (14 of 35) than after segmental resection (4 of 35). The authors note that their mortality rate is similar to unselected patients undergoing two-stage procedures, and although Hartmann's procedure avoids the risk of anastomotic leakage, it does so at the expense of the stoma, which is never closed in 32 to 62% of cases. Because of the functional disability from diarrhea and increased number of bowel movements in the patients that have undergone subtotal colectomy, segmental colectomy would be preferred in those patients in whom a primary anastomosis is considered.

Laparoscopic Colectomy

Laparoscopic colectomy is possible in many patients. Theoretical advantages include less postoperative pain, shorter hospital length of stay, improved cosmesis, and possibly a quicker and more complete recovery. Skilled surgeons have demonstrated that oncologic principles can be followed when performing laparoscopic surgery. They have demonstrated that the same resection margins can be obtained and the number of lymph nodes harvested from within the mesentery is comparable between both laparoscopic and open procedures. However, several reports of trocar site implantation of tumor have been disconcerting. This implantation has occurred in patients whose tumors were not transmural, and they occur at sites situated away from the area where the specimen was extracted. Several trials from both the United States as well as Europe have now been reported demonstrating no significant difference in tumor recurrence in an open incision or in a trocar site. It is felt that the trocar site recurrences were most likely from manipulation and were related to technique and not laparoscopy. The high incidence of tumor implantation in trocar sites occurred in a small series of surgeons who had not gained a large experience. Experienced surgeons may offer a laparoscopic colectomy depending on their own level of experience and the complexity of the procedure. Also, hand-assisted laparoscopic techniques may make the application for colorectal malignancy even more feasible.

■ PROGNOSIS AND FOLLOW-UP

The stage of disease is the most important determinant of survival after surgical resection. At present, the TNM system developed by the American Joint Committee for Cancer Staging has been adopted widely. Table 64-1 outlines the TNM classification for cancer of the colon and rectum. Table 64-2 outlines the stage grouping along with the corresponding Dukes' classification. In various series, survival rates differ considerably. Average crude 5-year survival rates for colon and rectal cancer using the stage group system are as follows: Stage 1, 75% (T1, 90%); Stage 2, 60%; Stage 3, 30%; Stage 4, 5%.

As previously discussed, the prognosis is adversely affected by complications, such as obstruction or perforation. Poorly differentiated tumors have a much worse prognosis than well-differentiated or moderately differentiated tumors. Other histologic features associated with the poor prognosis include mucinous and signet-ring cell adenocarcinomas, venous invasion, and perineural invasion. Probably the single most important prognostic variable in colon cancer is the presence or absence of lymph node metastases. The number of lymph nodes involved with metastases is also inversely correlated with the 5-year survival rate. When one node is affected, the 5-year survival rate is about 60%, compared to 35% when two to five nodes are involved and 20% when six or more nodes contain metastases. Newer prognostic markers are under investigation, including a number of genetic abnormalities. Microsatellite unstable tumors are felt to have a better prognosis than would be expected from their pathologic stage. Tumors with mutations or allelic loss of *p53* and *DCC* genes have worse prognoses than when these genes are functional. Certain mutations of the K-*ras* gene have

---

Table 64-1 TNM Staging for Colon Cancer

PRIMARY TUMOR (T)

TX	Primary tumor cannot be assessed
T0	No evidence of primary tumor
Tis	Carcinoma is situ
T1	Tumor invades submucosa
T2	Tumor invades muscularis propria
T3	Tumor invades through the muscularis propria into the subserosa or into nonperitoneal pericolic or perirectal tissues
T4	Tumor perforates the visceral peritoneum or directly invades other organs or structures

REGIONAL LYMPH NODES (N)

NX	Regional lymph nodes cannot be assessed
N0	No regional lymph node metastasis
N1	Metastasis in one to three pericolic or perirectal lymph nodes
N2	Metastasis in four or more pericolic or perirectal lymph nodes
N3	Metastasis in any lymph node along the course of a named vascular trunk

DISTANT METASTASIS (M)

MX	Presence of distant metastasis cannot be assessed
M0	No distant metastasis
M1	Distant metastasis

TABLE 64-2 Stage Grouping for Colorectal Cancer

STAGE	TUMOR	LYMPH NODES	METASTASES	DUKES' STAGE*	MAC*
0	Tis	N0	M0	—	—
I	T1	N0	M0	A	A
	T2	N0	M0	A	B1
IIA	T3	N0	M0	B	B2
IIB	T4	N0	M0	B	B3
IIIA	T1-T2	N1	M0	C	C1
IIIB	T3-T4	N1	M0	C	C2/C3
IIIC	Any T	N2	M0	C	C1/C2/C3
IV	Any T	Any N	M1	—	D

*Dukes' B is a composite of better (T3 N0 M0) and worse (T4 N0 M0) prognostic groups, as is Dukes' C (Any TN1 M0 and Any T N2 M0). MAC is the modified Astler-Coller classification.

also shown prognostic significance. None of these genetic prognostic markers are ready for routine clinical use.

The goals of follow-up and surveillance are the detection of recurrent, metastatic, or metachronous tumors while they are in a potentially curable stage. A vigorous debate continues between those who favor intensive follow-up and those who are more fatalistic in their approach. Results of several randomized studies and a meta-analysis favor aggressive follow-up as finding more curable recurrences. Patients can be triaged according to risk of recurrence. Those with stage I disease need little in the way of follow-up. For those with advanced disease, recommendations include routine physical examination with a complete blood cell count and liver function tests obtained every 3 months for 2 years, then every 6 months for 2 years, then annually. A chest x-ray is obtained every 6 months for 3 years, then annually. If CEA levels are to be monitored, they should be checked at an interval of between 6 and 12 weeks for 2 years, and every 3 to 4 months for 2 years, then annually.

If recurrent metastatic cancer is discovered, the patient is evaluated for potential resection of these lesions. Resection may be possible in some cases of hepatic or pulmonary metastases. Five-year survival rates of 37% for patients with solitary pulmonary metastases and 19% for those with two metastases have been reported.

If a single peripheral hepatic metastasis is encountered, this lesion can often be resected with a wedge resection at the same time as colectomy. Multiple lesions or central lesions should prompt a more thorough workup. Five-year survival rates approaching 30% have been reported following resection of hepatic metastases. Patients with a single metastasis have the best hope for cure; however, it is reasonable to perform a major hepatic resection if no more than four metastatic nodules are identified and they are all limited to one lobe. Patients with unresectable hepatic metastases have been treated with a number of modalities, including destruction by cryotherapy and radiofrequency ablation, and hepatic intra-arterial chemotherapy. Because of the significant toxicity and because a clear survival advantage has not been demonstrated, intra-arterial

chemotherapy remains investigational. Destruction of liver metastases and therapeutic chemotherapy are discussed in detail in other chapters.

■ ADJUVANT THERAPY

Both radiation therapy and chemotherapy have been used. The role of radiation therapy for colon cancer is limited. It may be considered for those patients in whom the tumor is unresectable, or following resection when a positive radial margin suggests residual tumor. Use of abdominal radiation is strictly limited by the potential for damage to the small intestine.

Adjuvant chemotherapy is administered using a combination of 5-fluorouracil and leucovorin. Randomized controlled trials have demonstrated that the addition of postoperative chemotherapy for patients with stage III disease significantly improves survival. Although the data are not as strong for stage II disease, most oncologists will offer adjuvant therapy for patients that have tumor that penetrates the serosa. Patients with stage I cancer are felt to be at low risk of recurrence and adjuvant chemotherapy is not recommended. New agents, irinotecan, oxaliplatin, and capecitabine show promise for more effective responses, especially for patients with metastatic disease.

Suggested Readings

Austgen TR, Souba WW, Bland KI: Reoperation for colorectal carcinoma. Surg Clin North Am 1991;71(1):175–192.

Bond JH: Colon polyps and cancer. Endoscopy 2001;33(1):46–54.

Busch ORC, Hop WCS, Hoynck van Papendrecht MAW, et al: Blood transfusions and prognosis in colorectal cancer. N Engl J Med 1993;328:1372–1376.

Cohen AM: Surgical considerations in patients with cancer of the colon and rectum. Semin Oncol 1991;18(4):381–387.

Colorectal cancer update. Prevention, screening, treatment, and surveillance for high-risk groups. Med Clin North Am 2000;84(5):1163–1182.

Curley SA, Evans DB, Ames FC: Resection for cure of carcinoma of the colon directly invading the duodenum or pancreatic head. J Am Coll Surg 1994;179:587–592.

Franklin ME, Ramos R, Rosenthal D, Schuessler W: Laparoscopic colonic procedures. West J Surg 1993; 17(1):51–56.

Krukowski ZH: SCOTIA Study Group. Single-stage treatment for malignant left-sided colonic obstruction: A prospective randomized clinical trial comparing subtotal colectomy with segmental resection following intraoperative irrigation. Br J Surg 1995; 82(12):1622–1627.

Kumar SK, Goldberg RM: Adjuvant chemotherapy for colon cancer. Curr Oncol Rep 2001;3(2):94–101.

Landercasper J, Stolee RT, Steenlage E, et al: Treatment and outcome of right colon cancer adherent to adjacent organs or the abdominal wall. Arch Surg 1992;127:841–846.

Lavery IC, Lopez-Kostner F, Pelley RJ, Fine RM: Treatment of colon and rectal cancer. Surg Clin North Am 2000;80(2):535–569.

Lumley SW, Fielding GA, Rhodes M, et al: Laparoscopic-assisted colorectal surgery: Lessons learned from 240 consecutive patients. Dis Colon Rectum 1996;39:155–159.

Macdonald JS, Astrow AB: Adjuvant therapy of colon cancer. Semin Oncol 2001;28(1):30–40.

Masaki T, Mori T, Matsuoka H, et al: Colonoscopic treatment of colon cancers. Surg Oncol Clin North Am 2001;10(3):693–708.

Michelassi F, Vannucci L, Ayala JJ, et al: Local recurrence after curative resection of colorectal adenocarcinoma. Surgery 1990; 108:787–793.

Moertel CG: Chemotherapy for colorectal cancer. N Engl J Med 1994;330:1136–1142.

Pikarsky AJ: Update on prospective randomized trials of laparoscopic surgery for colorectal cancer. Surg Oncol Clin North Am 2001;10(3):639–653.

Pitot HC, Goldberg RM: Future directions in adjuvant therapy for stage III colon carcinoma. Oncology 2001;15(3 suppl 5):31–36.

Rafaelsen SR, Kronborg O, Larsen C, Fenger C: Intraoperative ultrasonography in detection of hepatic metastases from colorectal cancer. Dis Colon Rectum 1995;38(4):355–360.

Rickard MJ, Bokey EL: Laparoscopy for colon cancer. Surg Oncol Clin North Am 2001;10(3):579–597.

Rouffet F, Hay JM, Vacher B, et al: Curative resection for left colon carcinoma: Hemicolectomy vs. segmental colectomy: A Prospective Controlled Multicenter Trial. Dis Colon Rectum 1994;37:651–659.

Runkel NS, Schlag P, Schwarz V: Outcome after emergency surgery for cancer of the large intestine. Br J Surg 1991;78:183–188.

Simmang CL, Provost D: Appendix and colon—Colon cancer. In McClellend RN (Ed.). Selected Readings in General Surgery. Dallas, University of Texas Southwestern Medical Center, 1996, p 23.

Winawer SJ, Fletcher RH, Miller L, et al: Colorectal cancer screening: Clinical guidelines and rationale. Gastroenterology 1997;112: 594–642.

Winawer SJ, Fletcher RH, Rex D, et al: Colorectal cancer screening and surveillance: clinical guidelines and rationale—Update based on new evidence. Gastroenterology 2003;124:544–560.

Wu JS, Fazio VW: Colon cancer. Dis Colon Rectum 2000;43(11): 1473–1486.

65

CHEMOTHERAPY FOR METASTATIC COLON CANCER

Neeraj Agrawal, MD
Robert J. Pelley, MD

In 2003, approximately 150,000 new cases of colorectal cancer were expected to be diagnosed in the United States, and more than one third of those patients are expected to eventually die of their disease. Early stage colorectal cancer has a high surgical cure rate but is essentially a disease without symptoms. Therefore, nearly one fifth of patients will present with metastatic disease and an equal number with regionally advanced disease with a high risk for recurrence (Cohen et al, 1997). Although a small fraction of patients with isolated liver metastases can be offered potentially curative surgery, the majority of patients with metastatic colorectal cancer (MCC) are candidates for palliative therapies only. This chapter will review the role of chemotherapy in the treatment of patients with unresectable MCC.

◼ 5-FLUOROURACIL

For over 40 years 5-fluorouracil (5-FU) has remained the mainstay of chemotherapy in patients with MCC. 5-FU was synthesized in 1957 based on the observation that fluorinated nucleosides were preferentially taken up by tumor cells (Heidelberger, 1963). 5-FU is a pro-drug and requires multiple enzymatic steps before being converted into the active phosphorylated forms. Although derivatives can be incorporated directly into both RNA and DNA, the most important metabolite is F-dUMP (5-fluorodeoxyuridylate monophosphate) which is a competitive inhibitor of thymidylate synthase (TS). TS is an obligatory step in the synthesis of thymidine, and its inhibition has a potent effect on DNA synthesis. The inhibition of TS by 5-FU is accentuated by reduced folates such as 5,10-methylene tetrahydrofolate (leucovorin), which stabilizes the ternary complex into a virtually irreversible complex (Bleyer, 1989). The process of leucovorin potentiating the activity of 5-FU is called biomodulation. A number of additional agents can modulate 5-FU activity through a number of biochemical interactions. These agents include cisplatin, interferon alpha, PALA (phosphonacetyl-L-aspartate), methotrexate, trimetrexate, thymidine, and uridine (Pinedo, 1988). Nonetheless, only leucovorin has found a continued role in the treatment of MCC.

As a single agent, bolus 5-FU has limited activity in colon cancer. When administered at its maximally tolerated dose, 5-FU produces partial responses in 10 to 15% of patients with MCC (Cohen et al, 1997). Toxicity commonly includes myelosuppression and gastrointestinal side effects such as diarrhea and mucositis. The severity of toxicity is dependent on the schedule of administration (Meta-Analysis Group in Cancer, 1998b). When combined with leucovorin (LV), cytotoxic activity increases in vitro and tumor response increases in vivo. This activity was demonstrated in numerous phase II trials utilizing diverse schedules of 5-FU and LV in patients with MCC (Machover, 1986). Over the years a series of phase III trials have compared 5-FU alone with 5-FU/LV. One meta-analysis of nine such randomized trials demonstrated a superior response rate (23% versus 11%) for the combination regimen (Advancer Colorectal Cancer Meta-Analysis Project, 1992). Similarly, additional randomized studies and meta-analyses have confirmed the increased tumor response rate for 5-FU/LV over 5-FU alone. Nonetheless, it is difficult to demonstrate a clinically significant improvement in survival for patients with MCC receiving 5-FU/LV over 5-FU alone (Lo Bello et al, 2000).

Schedules of 5-FU Administration

Since 1980, multiple schedules have been developed for the administration of 5-FU/LV utilizing bolus, short infusions and continuous infusion strategies. Many of the schedules developed in Europe have used infusion methods, whereas most North American schedules have used bolus administration. The two most commonly used regimens in the United States are the Mayo Clinic regimen (5-FU 425 mg/m^2 and LV 20 mg/m^2 days 1 through 5 every 4 to 5 weeks) and the Roswell Park regimen (5-FU 500 mg/m^2 and LV 500 mg/m^2 weekly for 6 weeks out of 8) (Poon et al, 1989; Petrelli et al, 1987). Multiple randomized clinical trials have compared these regimens, finding them equivalent for both tumor response rate and median survival (Buroker et al, 1994; Wang et al, 2000). Each schedule produces different toxicity profiles with weekly administration generating more diarrhea and the Mayo Clinic schedule producing more myelosuppression.

Continuous Infusion 5-FU

Because 5-FU is a cell cycle–specific agent and inhibits cells in S phase, it is more likely to be effective if prolonged drug levels are maintained within tumor tissue. This observation led to the design of a number of schedules for administering 5-FU as a continuous infusion. One of the most commonly used schedules for infusional 5-FU is the de Gramont regimen (LV 200 mg/m^2 IV over 2 hours followed by 5-FU 400 mg/m^2 IV bolus followed by an 22-hour infusion of 5-FU at 600 mg/m^2 repeated days 1 and 2 every 2 weeks). In a randomized trial comparing the Mayo Clinic regimen to the de Gramont schedule, patients receiving infusional 5-FU/LV had a superior tumor response rate and an improved median progression-free survival (de Gramont et al, 1997). A meta-analysis of six prospective randomized trials using different durations and doses of continuous infusion 5-FU confirmed a superior response rate in patients with MCC for regimens using infusional 5-FU versus bolus 5-FU (Meta-Analysis Group in Cancer, 1998a). However, significant differences in median survival are difficult to demonstrate. Although infusional 5-FU produces less myelosuppression and gastrointestinal (GI) toxicity, it is associated with a painful erythema of the hands and feet (palmar-plantar erythrodysesthesia) termed "hand-foot syndrome," which occurs in roughly 25% of patients. In addition, many infusional schedules are difficult to administer owing to expense, cumbersome equipment, and frequent office visits.

■ ORAL FLUOROPYRIMIDINES

Because the primary purpose of chemotherapy in patients with MCC is palliation, finding more convenient and less expensive methods for delivering 5-FU is a major objective for investigators. As with many chemotherapeutic agents, 5-FU has variable and unpredictable bioavailability when used orally. This effect is the result of the enzyme dihydropyrimidine dehydrogenase (DPD), which is the rate-limiting enzyme in the degradation of 5-FU. DPD is highly expressed in GI mucosa and liver and therefore degrades most 5-FU administered enterally. A number of agents and strategies have been devised to bypass or evade DPD by using either potent inhibitors of DPD or 5-FU analogs that are resistant to its activity. To accomplish this, either a pro-drug of 5-FU is administered or an inhibitor of DPD is coadministered with a source of 5-FU. These agents, known as oral fluoropyrimidines, are convenient to administer and achieve a sustained cytotoxic activity similar to that of infusional 5-FU.

Capecitabine

Capecitabine (Xeloda) is a fluoropyrimidine carbamate, a pro-drug of 5-FU rationally designed to be DPD-resistant. Following absorption, it undergoes a three-step activation into 5-FU. The first two steps of activation occur in the liver, and the final step is mediated by the enzyme thymidine phosphorylase, which is overexpressed intracellularly in colon and breast tumor cells (Miwa et al, 1998). Moreover, hypoxic cells have been shown to overexpress thymidine phosphorylase. This selective activation potentially reduces systemic exposure to 5-FU while maximizing the dose intensity within tumor cells.

Capecitabine has been compared to bolus 5-FU/LV (Mayo Clinic regimen) in a randomized study of chemotherapy naïve patients with MCC (Hoff et al, 2001). Capecitabine was equivalent to 5-FU/LV in terms of disease progression and median survival with a superior response rate (25% versus 16%; $p = .005$). Patients treated with capecitabine suffered less severe stomatitis, neutropenia, and neutropenic fever. As with patients receiving infusional 5-FU, patients receiving capecitabine had significantly more hand-foot syndrome and hyperbilirubinemia. Van Cutsem and associates (2001) also reported similar results with capecitabine as first-line therapy in MCC in a large randomized European trial. Based on the results of these two trials involving over 1200 patients, the FDA approved capecitabine for use as first-line treatment in patients with MCC.

Tegafur

Tegafur (FT) is another 5-FU pro-drug with excellent oral bioavailability. Surprisingly, in initial studies, it produced severe neurologic and GI toxicity. The addition of uracil to FT in a 4:1 molar ratio (UFT) improves its therapeutic index. Orzel is a commercially available combination of UFT with leucovorin. Two large phase III randomized trials have compared the combination of UFT/LV with intravenous 5-FU/LV (Mayo Clinic regimen) as first-line treatment of patients with MCC. The first trial randomized 816 patients and found the two arms to be statistically equivalent in response rate and median survival time (Pazdur et al, 1999). Similarly, in the second smaller trial involving 380 patients, the two treatment arms were equivalent in time to progression and median survival time (Carmichael et al, 1999). Despite UFT's favorable toxicity profile, this drug has not yet been licensed by the FDA for treatment of patients with MCC.

Eniluracil

Eniluracil (EU) is a potent irreversible inhibitor of DPD and increases the bioavailability of oral 5-FU to nearly 100% when coadministered. EU results in a prolongation of the plasma half-life of 5-FU from 10 minutes to approximately 5 hours. In addition, intratumoral DPD may be inactivated by EU. In phase I studies, the combination of 5-FU/EU mimics the pharmacokinetics of infusional 5-FU in a similar fashion to capecitabine. Two phase III multicenter randomized studies, one in North America and the other in Europe, have compared 5-FU/EU to 5-FU/LV (Mayo Clinic regimen) as first-line treatment for patients with MCC. In both studies, the overall survival of patients in the 5-FU/EU arms were inferior to the 5-FU/LV arms (Levin et al, 2001; Van Cutsem et al, 2001). In view of these findings, it is unlikely that EU will be clinically useful in the treatment of MCC.

The licensing of capecitabine and its availability in the United States is likely to inhibit the development of additional oral fluoropyrimidines in this country. This is especially true as emphasis turns to the development of new therapeutic agents and strategies, and away from further therapeutic refinement of fluoropyrimidine administration.

■ THYMIDYLATE SYNTHASE INHIBITORS

Because most of the cytotoxic activity of 5-FU is dependent on the target enzyme thymidylate synthase (TS), efforts have been made to develop specific inhibitors to TS. Raltitrexed (Tomudex) is a folate analog, synthesized with such an activity. As with other folates, this drug is dependent on active transport into tumor cells, but then can be polyglutamated and trapped, resulting in a long duration of activity. Thus, this drug requires a dosing schedule of only once every 3 weeks. In small phase II efficacy trials, raltitrexed showed promising response rates with reduced toxicity in patients with MCC. Therefore, three large randomized phase III trials were performed with over 1300 patients comparing raltitrexed monotherapy (3 mg/m² IV every 3 weeks) with 5-FU/LV (Mayo Clinic regimen) (Cocconi et al, 1998; Pazdur et al, 1997; Cunningham, 1998). Although response rates were comparable in all three trials, median survival time was superior in the 5-FU/LV arm in the study conducted in the United States (9.7 months versus 12.7 months, $p = .01$), while it was statistically equivalent in the other two multinational trials. An additional randomized trial comparing raltitrexed to infusional 5-FU demonstrated 5-FU to be superior in terms of time to progression, and quality of life (Maughen et al, 1999). This agent is currently approved for treatment of patients with MCC in Europe, Canada, Australia, and South America, but not in the United States. It is a logical choice for compassionate use in patients with DPD deficiency or for those with 5-FU-related cardiac toxicity.

Irinotecan

Irinotecan (CPT-11, Camptosar) is a semisynthetic derivative of the plant alkaloid camptothecin and represents almost 25 years of effort in drug development. Irinotecan is a pro-drug converted in vivo to the active metabolite SN-38, which is a potent inhibitor of the enzyme topoisomerase I. Topoisomerase I is necessary for unwinding DNA for self-replication and RNA transcription, and its inhibition produces DNA strand breaks and cytotoxicity (Vanhoefer et al). Irinotecan has a complex pharmacology with prolonged enterohepatic recirculation of SN-38 involving glucuronidation. The major toxicity of diarrhea may be linked to this complex metabolism. In phase II studies of patients with MCC, single-agent irinotecan demonstrated a 12 to 25% response rate. Initial trials also showed similar results in patients with 5-FU refractory MCC, indicating a lack of cross-resistance between the camptothecins and fluoropyrimidines.

Two randomized clinical trials have demonstrated the benefit of irinotecan given to patients with MCC refractory to 5-FU treatment. In the first trial, 279 patients with refractory MCC were randomized to supportive care alone versus irinotecan. Irinotecan produced an improved 1-year survival rate (36% versus 14%) and 3-month prolongation of median survival time (9 months versus 6 months) (Cunningham et al, 1998). In the second study, patients with refractory MCC received either irinotecan or infusional 5-FU as salvage therapy (Rougier et al, 1998). Survival was again prolonged in this trial for patients receiving irinotecan. Data from these trials led to the

FDA's approval of irinotecan for the salvage treatment of patients with 5-FU-refractory MCC in 1996.

The next logical step was to combine irinotecan with 5-FU/LV in an effort to increase efficacy in a disease that rarely responds to chemotherapy more than 30% of the time. Phase I trials were performed, and one schedule, which treated patients at weekly intervals, appeared to have tolerable toxicity and ease of administration (irinotecan 125 mg/m², leucovorin 20 mg/m² and 5-FU 500 mg/m², all given weekly for 4 of every 6 weeks). This schedule has become known as the Saltz regimen, or IFL (Saltz et al, 1996).

In March 2000, irinotecan combined with 5-FU/LV became the standard of care following completion of two landmark multinational randomized trials. Both studies randomized previously untreated patients with MCC to either standard 5-FU/LV regimens or triple drug therapy (Table 65-1). The first study was performed in Europe (Douillard et al, 2000) and added irinotecan to schedules of 5-FU/LV, which were the dominant infusional schedules at that time. Combination therapy with irinotecan/leucovorin/5-FU resulted in superior response rate (49% versus 31%) and improved median overall survival (17.4 months versus 14.1 months). Although both severe diarrhea and neutropenia were increased with combination therapy, toxicity seemed reversible and tolerable.

In a second study in North America by Saltz and associates (2000), patients were randomized to one of three treatments including either irinotecan alone (125 mg/m²/week for 4 weeks repeated every 6 weeks), 5-FU/LV (Mayo Clinic regimen) or combination therapy, IFL (Saltz regimen). Again, combination therapy produced an increased response rate (39%) and increased median overall survival (14.8 months versus 12.6 months). The single-agent irinotecan arm produced similar results to 5-FU/LV. Since March 2000, IFL has remained the standard combination regimen for patients with MCC and has served as the "control arm" therapy for any randomized trial in patients with MCC.

Toxicity from IFL, though tolerable, was not trivial. One year after approval by the FDA, an interim analysis of two trials showed an unexpectedly high rate of toxicity and mortality for patients receiving IFL (Sargent et al, 2001). A review panel identified two syndromes associated with irinotecan toxicity: one involving severe GI toxicity with diarrhea and neutropenia, and the second involving vascular events and thrombosis (Rothenberg et al, 2001).

Table 65–1 Combination FU/CPT-11 in MCC				
STUDY (NUMBER OF PATIENTS)	CHEMOTHERAPY	RESPONSE RATE (%)	MEDIAN PFS (MONTHS)	MEDIAN OS (MONTHS)
Saltz et al (683)	FU/LV/CPT-11	39 ($p < 0.001$)	7 ($p = 0.004$)	14.8 ($p = 0.04$)
	FU/LV	21	4.3	12.6
	CPT-11	18	4.2	12
Douillard et al (387)	FU/LV/CPT-11	41	6.7	16.8
	FU/LV	23 ($p < 0.001$)	4.4 ($p < 0.001$)	14 ($p = 0.03$)

CPT-11, irinotecan; FU, 5-fluorouracil; LV, leucovorin; PFS, progression-free survival; OS, overall survival.

The panel recommended that IFL should remain standard of care as front-line therapy but needed to be used cautiously by experienced physicians with early dose attenuation in appropriate patients.

Oxaliplatin

Oxaliplatin (L-OHP, Eloxatin) is a third-generation platinum analog that, unlike the related agents cisplatin and carboplatin, has unique activity in colorectal tumors. Like other platinum agents, oxaliplatin's cytotoxicity is mediated by the formation of covalent DNA adducts involving the complexed platinum atom. However, its large bulky diaminocyclohexane (DACH) ligand makes oxaliplatin adducts more difficult to repair presumably accounting for its unusual activity (Pelley, 2001).

As a single agent, oxaliplatin produces a response rate of 18 to 24% in previously untreated patients but only 10% in patients with MCC previously treated with 5-FU/LV (Armand et al, 2000). In preclinical testing, oxaliplatin had shown synergy with 5-FU both in vitro and in animal models, indicating some form of biomodulation between the drugs. This has been confirmed in phase II clinical trials in which response rates as high as 60% have been reported when oxaliplatin is combined with 5-FU/LV. Like other platinum agents, the toxicity of oxaliplatin includes myelosuppression, hypersensitivity reactions, and neurotoxicity. However, oxaliplatin produces not only a chronic reversible neuropathy, which is dose-dependent, but also a cold-induced hyperesthesia, which is rapidly reversible and without serious sequelae (Gamelin et al, 2002).

Multiple phase III trials have studied oxaliplatin in combination with 5-FU/LV in previously untreated patients with MCC. De Gramont and coworkers randomized 420 patients to infusional 5-FU/LV (de Gramont regimen) with or without oxaliplatin (85 mg/m^2 every 2 weeks), de Gramont 5-FU/LV versus FOLFOX4. The response rate of the combination therapy arm was superior to 5-FU/LV alone (51% versus 22%). However, patient survival was not statistically different possibly because of patient crossover to salvage therapy with irinotecan and oxaliplatin. These results were reproduced by a second large randomized trial in which patients were treated either with 5-FU/LV (Mayo Clinic regimen) or 5-FU/LV/oxaliplatin (oxaliplatin 50 mg/m^2 [LJ14]over 2 hours followed by 5-FU 2000 mg/m^2 over 24 hours and leucovorin 500 mg/m^2 on days 1, 8, 15, and 22, every 36 days) (Grothey et al, 2001).

In 1997, in an effort to establish the best chemotherapy for previously untreated patients with MCC, the North Central Cancer Treatment Group (NCCTG) designed a six-arm trial to be performed in the United States. They combined diverse chemotherapy combinations including 5-FU/LV (Mayo Clinic regiment), IFL (Saltz regimen), oxaliplatin/5-FU/LV (FOLFOX4), and three other combinations. In the year 2001, after the FDA redefined IFL as the standard of care for patients with MCC, the study was modified to only three arms by discontinuing the Mayo Clinic regimen arm and two regimens with excessive toxicity (Morton et al, 2001). Eventually, 795 patients with MCC were randomized to either IFL, FOLFOX4, or oxaliplatin/irinotecan. In May 2002, a preliminary report revealed that the patients treated with FOLFOX4 had significantly longer median survival times compared to patients first treated with IFL (18.5 months versus 14 months) (Goldberg et al, 2002). Time to progression and tumor response rate (38% versus 29%) were also superior in the FOLFOX4 arm. In addition, severe toxicity occurred less often with FOLFOX4. The oxaliplatin/Irinotecan arm produced results almost identical to IFL. The survival difference between the FOLFOX4 regimen and IFL was almost certainly the result of patients crossing over from FOLFOX4 to irinotecan for salvage therapy (52% of all patients). Because patients receiving IFL could not receive oxaliplatin as a salvage therapy, they in effect were limited to receiving only two drugs in contrast to the FOLFOX4 cohort who received three. In a complex decision, the FDA approved oxaliplatin (LOHP) for initial treatment of patients with MCC in August 2002. This approval has resulted in the acceptance of 5-FU/LV/oxaliplatin as front-line standard therapy of MCC with irinotecan as salvage therapy. The combination of all three drugs is currently undergoing testing but may prove to be too toxic as a standard therapy.

■ TARGETED THERAPY

Growth-regulating molecules and their receptors control a host of cellular processes within normal cells. Their aberrant or unregulated expression may result in, or contribute to, uncontrolled cell growth, tumor initiation, promotion, and metastases. Recent advances in understanding cancer biology and cancer genetics have made it possible to identify several such cellular pathways as potential targets for cancer therapy.

The epidermal growth factor receptor (EGFR) is a transmembrane tyrosine kinase protein that triggers cell signaling pathways important to the control of cell proliferation. EGFR is activated by binding growth factor ligands such as epidermal growth factor (EGF) or transforming growth factor alpha (TGF-α). This stage is followed by dimerization and activation of an intracellular tyrosine kinase domain that phosphorylates target proteins within the cell cytoplasm (Arteaga, 2001). EGFR overexpression has been noted in a number of solid tumors including lung, pancreas, and colorectal cancer. This receptor has served as a target for investigational agents that might inhibit its activity and thus malignant growth (Huang and Harari, 1999). Strategies for inhibition include the development of small molecules that act as competitive or irreversible specific inhibitors to the protein's tyrosine kinase activity [ZD 1839 (Iressa) or OSI-774 (Tarceva)]. An alternative approach has been the development and use of monoclonal antibodies that bind to the extracellular portion of the receptor blocking ligand binding and thus receptor activation.

IMC-C225 (cetuximab) is a chimeric monoclonal antibody that selectively binds EGFR and blocks its activation. In preliminary phase I trials, a number of remarkable tumor responses were seen in patients with MCC (Baselga, 2001). For this reason, a phase II study was performed (Saltz et al, 2001) with patients whose MCC tumors were resistant to 5-FU and irinotecan. Patients with tumors that were positive for EGFR protein, were treated with IMC-C225 while continuing irinotecan at the previous dose level. Approximately 72% of the screened tumors had positive staining for EGFR by immunohisto-chemistry. After 2 months of treatment, 27 of 120 patients (22%) had partial responses. An acne-like rash occurred in up to 60% of patients, and its intensity was associated with tumor responsiveness. Current clinical trials are exploring the use of cetuximab combined with 5-FU/LV, irinotecan, or oxaliplatin as salvage treatment in MCC.

A second important growth factor pathway involves the vascular endothelial growth factor receptor (VEGFR), which plays a critical role in tumor related angiogenesis (McMahon, 2000). Bevacizumab is a humanized monoclonal antibody directed against the growth factor ligand, VEGF. In preclinical testing, bevacizumab blockage of VEGF was able to inhibit growth of human tumor cells and xenografts in nude mice. A randomized phase II trial was performed with 104 patients with MCC who received either 5-FU/LV alone or 5-FU/LV in combination with either low or high doses of bevacizumab (Bergsland et al, 2000). The addition of low-dose antibody increased response rate (40% versus 17%), time to progression, and survival (21 months versus 14 months). Surprisingly, the cohort of patients receiving higher doses of bevacizumab did not achieve the same levels of apparent benefit. These data remain provocative and unexplained at the present time. A large nonrandomized phase II trial combining high-dose bevacizumab with IFL is ongoing and will determine if the apparent increase in response rate and survival is reproducible. Additional agents and antibodies are in various stages of testing to determine whether inhibition of tumor angiogenesis will benefit patients with MCC.

■ CONCLUSION

For 40 years, 5-FU has remained the mainstay of all chemotherapy options in colorectal cancer. Understanding of the metabolic pathways combined with methodical clinical trials has led to improvements in 5-FU's effectiveness through biomodulation and infusional schedules. The goal of finding new agents has been a frustrating one. However, the past decade has seen the emergence of two clinically useful drugs in oxaliplatin and irinotecan. These new agents have made conservative but steady progress in the treatment of metastatic colorectal cancer. Ongoing clinical trials will continue to refine the way we use these drugs in combination with radiation, surgery, and each other. In the coming decade, our growing understanding of tumor biology promises to generate new agents that will specifically inhibit signal transduction targets, providing less toxic therapies. It is hoped that this quiet revolution in pharmacogenetics will convert our current

palliative treatment of metastatic colorectal cancer into effective life-prolonging therapies.

Suggested Readings

Advanced Colorectal Cancer Meta-Analysis Project: Modulation of fluorouracil by leucovorin in patients with advanced colorectal cancer: Evidence in terms of response rate. J Clin Oncol 1992;10:896.

Armand JP, Boige V, Raymond E, et al: Oxaliplatin in colorectal cancer: An overview. Semin Oncol 2000;27:96.

Arteaga CL: The epidermal growth factor receptor: From mutant oncogene in nonhuman cancers to therapeutic target in human neoplasia. J Clin Oncol 2001;19:32s–40s.

Baselga J: The EGFR as a target for anticancer therapy: Focus on cetuximab. Eur J Cancer 2001;37(suppl 4):16–22.

Bergsland E, Hurwitz H, Fehrenbacher L, et al: A randomized phase II trial comparing rhuMAb VEGF (recombinant humanized monoclonal antibody to vascular endothelial cell growth factor) plus 5-fluorouracil/leucovorin (FU/LV to FU/LV alone in patients with metastatic colorectal cancer. Proc ASCO 2000;19:abstract 939.

Bleyer WA: New vistas for leucovorin in cancer chemotherapy. Cancer 1989;63(6 suppl):995–1007.

Buroker TR, O'Connell MJ, Wieand HS, et al: Randomized comparison of two schedules of fluorouracil and leucovorin in the treatment of advanced colorectal cancer. J Clin Oncol 1994;12:14.

Carmichael J, Popiela T, Radstone D, et al: Randomized comparative study of Orzel [oral uracil/tegafur (UFT) plus leucovorin (LV)] versus parenteral 5-fluorouracil (5-FU) plus LV in patients with metastatic colorectal cancer. Proc ASCO 1999;18:264a (abstract).

Cocconi G, Cunningham D, Van Cutsem E, et al: Open, randomized, multicenter trial of raltitrexed versus fluorouracil plus high-dose leucovorin in patients with advanced colorectal cancer. Tomudex Colorectal Cancer Study Group. J Clin Oncol 1998;16:2943–2952.

Cohen AM, Minsky BD, Schilsky RL: Cancer of the Colon. In DeVita VT Jr, Hellman S, Rosenberg SA (Eds.). Principles and Practice of Oncology. Philadelphia, Lippincott-Raven, 1997, p 1166.

Cunningham D: Mature results from three large controlled studies with raltitrexed ("tomudex"). Br J Cancer 1998;77(S2):15.

Cunningham D, Pyrhonen S, James RP, et al. Randomised trial of irinotecan plus supportive care versus supportive care alone after fluorouracil failure for patients with metastatic colorectal cancer. Lancet 1998;352:1413–1418.

de Gramont A, Bosset JF, Milan C, et al: Randomized trial comparing monthly low-dose leucovorin and fluorouracil bolus with bimonthly high-dose leucovorin and fluorouracil bolus plus continuous infusion for advanced colorectal cancer: A French intergroup study. J Clin Oncol 1997;15:808.

de Gramont A, Figer A, Seymour M, et al: Leucovorin and fluorouracil with or without oxaliplatin as first-line treatment in advanced colorectal cancer. J Clin Oncol 2000;18:2938.

Douillard JY, Cunningham D, Roth AD, et al: Irinotecan combined with fluorouracil compared with fluorouracil alone as first-line treatment for metastatic colorectal cancer: A multicentre randomised trial. Lancet 2000;355:1041.

Gamelin E, Gamelin R, Delva V, et al: Prevention of oxaliplatin peripheral sensory neuropathy by Ca^+ gluconate/Mg^+ chloride infusions: A retrospective study. Proc ASCO 2002;21:abstract 624.

Goldberg RM, Morton RF, Sargent DJ, et al: N9741: Oxaliplatin (Oxal) or CPT-11 + 5-fluorouracil (5FU)/leucovorin (LV) or oxal + CPT-11 in advanced colorectal cancer (CRC): Initial toxicity and response data from a GI Intergroup study. Proc ASCO 2002;21:abstract 511.

Grothey A, Deschler B, Kroening H, et al: Bolus 5-fluorouracil (5-FU)/folinic acid (FA) (Mayo) vs weekly high-dose 24 h 5-FU infusion/FA + oxaliplatin in advanced colorectal cancer. Results of a phase III study (abstract). Proc ASCO 2001;20:125a.

Heidelberger C, Ansfield FJ: Experimental and clinical use of fluorinated pyrimidines in cancer chemotherapy. Cancer Res 1963;23:1226–1243.

Hoff PM, Ansari R, Batist G, et al: Comparison of oral capecitabine versus intravenous fluorouracil plus leucovorin as first-line treatment in 605 patients with metastatic colorectal cancer: results of a randomized phase III study. J Clin Oncol 2001;19:2282.

Huang SM, Harari PM: Epidermal growth factor receptor inhibition in cancer therapy: Biology, rationale and preliminary clinical results. Invest New Drugs 1999;17:259–269.

Levin J, Schilsky R, Burris H, et al: North American phase III study of oral eniluracil (EU) plus oral 5-fluorouracil (5-FU) versus intravenous (IV) 5-FU plus leucovorin (LV) in the treatment of advanced colorectal cancer (ACC). Proc ASCO 2001;20:132a (abstract 523).

Lo Bello L, Pistone G, Restuccia S, et al: 5-Fluorouracil alone versus 5-fluorouracil plus folinic acid in the treatment of colorectal carcinoma: Meta-analysis. Int J Clin Pharmacol Ther 2000;38:553.

Machover D, Goldschmidt E, Chollet P, et al: Treatment of advanced colorectal and gastric adenocarcinomas with 5-fluorouracil and high-dose folinic acid. J Clin Oncol 1986;4:685–696.

Maughen TS, James RD, Kerr D, et al: Preliminary results of a multicentre randomized trial comparing 3 chemotherapy regimens (de Gramont, Lokich and raltitrexed) in metastatic colorectal cancer. Proc ASCO 1999;18:abstract 1007.

McMahon G: VEGF receptor signaling in tumor angiogenesis. Oncologist 2000;5(suppl 1):20–27.

Meta-Analysis Group in Cancer: Efficacy of intravenous continuous infusion of fluorouracil compared with bolus administration in advanced colorectal cancer. J Clin Oncol 1998a;16:301.

Meta-Analysis Group in Cancer: Toxicity of fluorouracil in patients with advanced colorectal cancer: Effect of administration schedule and prognostic factors. J Clin Oncol 1998b;16:3537.

Miwa M, Ura M, Nishida M, et al: Design of a novel oral fluoropyrimidine carbamate, capecitabine, which generates 5-fluorouracil selectively in tumours by enzymes concentrated in human liver and cancer tissue. Eur J Cancer 1998;34:1274–1281.

Morton RF, Goldberg RM, Sargent DJ, et al: Oxaliplatin (Oxal) or CPT-11 combined with 5FU/leucovorin (LV) in advanced colorectal cancer (CRC): An NCCTG/CALGB Study. Proc ASCO 2001;20: abstract 495.

Pazdur R, Douillard JY, Skillings J, et al: Multicenter phase III study of 5-fluorouracil (5-FU) or UFT in combination with leucovorin (LV) in patients with metastatic colorectal cancer. Proc ASCO 1999;18: 263a (abstract).

Pazdur R, Vincent M: Raltitrexed (Tomudex) versus 5-fluorouracil and leucovorin (5-FU + LV) in patients with advanced colorectal cancer (ACC): Results of a randomized, multicentre, North American trial. Proc ASCO 1997;16:abstract 801.

Pelley RJ: Oxaliplatin: A new agent for colorectal cancer. Curr Oncol Rep 2001;3:147–155.

Petrelli N, Herrera L, Rustum Y, et al: A prospective randomized trial of 5-fluorouracil versus 5-fluorouracil and high-dose leucovorin versus 5-fluorouracil and methotrexate in previously untreated patients with advanced colorectal carcinoma. J Clin Oncol 1987;5:1559.

Pinedo HM: Fluorouracil biochemistry and pharmacology. J Clin Oncol 1988;6:1653–1664.

Poon MA, O'Connell MJ, Moertel CG, et al: Biochemical modulation of fluorouracil: Evidence of significant improvement of survival and quality of life in patients with advanced colorectal carcinoma. J Clin Oncol 1989;7:1407.

Rothenberg ML, Meropol NJ, Poplin EA, et al: Mortality associated with irinotecan plus bolus fluorouracil/leucovorin: Summary of findings of an independent panel. J Clin Oncol 2001;19:3801–3807.

Rougier P, Van Cutsem E, Bajetta E, et al: Randomised trial of irinotecan versus fluorouracil by continuous infusion after fluorouracil failure in patients with metastatic colorectal cancer. Lancet 1998;352:1407.

Saltz LB, Cox JV, Blanke C: Irinotecan plus fluorouracil and leucovorin for metastatic colorectal cancer. Irinotecan Study Group. N Engl J Med 2000;343:905.

Saltz LB, Kanowitz J, Kemeny NE, et al: Phase I clinical and pharmacokinetic study of irinotecan, fluorouracil, and leucovorin in patients with advanced solid tumors. J Clin Oncol 1996;14:2959–2967.

Saltz L, Rubin M, Hochster H, et al: Cetuximab (IMC-C225) plus Irinotecan (CPT-11) is active in CPT-11-refractory colorectal cancer (CRC) that expresses epidermal growth factor receptor (EGFR). Proc ASCO 2001;20:abstract 7.

Sargent DJ, Niedzwiecki D, O'Connell MJ, Schilsky RL: Recommendation for caution in irinotecan, fluorouracil, and leucovorin for colorectal cancer. N Engl J Med 2001;345:144.

Van Cutsem E, Sorensen J, Cassidy J, et al: International phase III study of oral eniluracil (EU) plus 5-fluorouracil (5-FU) versus intravenous (IV) 5-FU plus leucovorin (LV) in the treatment of advanced colorectal cancer (ACC). Proc ASCO 2001;20:131a (abstract 522).

Van Cutsem E, Twelves C, Cassidy J, et al: Oral capecitabine compared with intravenous fluorouracil plus leucovorin in patients with metastatic colorectal cancer: Results of a large phase III study. J Clin Oncol 2001;19:4097–4106.

Vanhoefer U, Harstrick A, Achterrath, W et al: Irinotecan in the treatment of colorectal cancer: Clinical overview. J Clin Oncol 2001; 19:1501–1518.

Wang WS, Lin JK, Chiou TJ, et al: Randomized trial comparing weekly bolus 5-fluorouracil plus leucovorin versus monthly 5-day 5-fluorouracil plus leucovorin in metastatic colorectal cancer. Hepatogastroenterology 2000;47:1599.

66

MANAGEMENT OF COLORECTAL LIVER METASTASES

Eren Berber, MD
Allan E. Siperstein, MD

The liver is a frequent site of metastatic disease for tumors of colorectal origin. Colorectal cancer is responsible for up to 75% of liver metastases. It is the second leading cause of death from cancer in North America. There are over 150,000 new cases of colorectal cancer reported in the United States each year. As many as 25% of colorectal cancer patients will have liver metastases at presentation and another 50% will develop liver recurrence within the next 5 years. More than one third of patients presenting with liver metastases will have metastatic disease limited to the liver.

For untreated cases, median survival time is approximately 5 months, with a 20% 3-year survival rate and 1 to 2% 5-year survival rate. In the case of synchronous unresectable liver metastases, median survival time is 4 to 12 months with resection of the primary tumor, 2 to 8 months with stoma or bypass, and 2 to 3 months with biopsy only.

Liver metastases from colorectal cancer continue to be a therapeutic challenge for the surgeons and oncologists. Although surgical resection is the gold standard for treatment, only 10 to 20% of the patients will have resectable liver disease. The remaining patients would traditionally make a decision with their oncologist to either undergo systemic chemotherapy or do nothing. However, in recent years, a number of regional treatment methods have emerged to be options for these patients, including chemoembolization, intrahepatic arterial infusion pumps, cryotherapy, and radiofrequency thermal ablation.

■ DETECTION

Generally, patients with colorectal liver metastases do not develop symptoms in the early course of the disease. The diagnosis may be made during routine preoperative or intraoperative evaluation of the primary tumor. Follow-up computed tomographic (CT) scans, serial elevations of carcinoembryonic antigen (CEA), or liver function tests may identify metachronous hepatic lesions as well. Plasma CEA levels are elevated in 89 to 95% of the patients with colorectal liver metastases.

In about 60% of the patients with colorectal liver metastases, the presence of metastases is anticipated by preoperative studies. Computed tomography is the standard imaging modality to evaluate the liver for metastases. Improvements in CT imaging such as spiral studies, thin section scans, and arterial and portovenous imaging have largely replaced the need for invasive CT portography. Magnetic resonance imaging (MRI) is also used frequently to assess liver metastases. Both are sensitive for hepatic metastases that are at least 1 to 2 cm in diameter; nevertheless, longer scan times, higher cost, motion artifacts, and lower sensitivity for detecting extrahepatic disease in the abdomen are concerns for MRI.

Functional imaging using whole-body [^{18}F]-fluorodeoxyglucose positron emission tomography (FDG-PET) relies on the higher rate of glucose uptake and utilization in malignancies. Nevertheless, owing to the high background activity resulting from the hepatocytes, not all the tumors in the liver are able to be detected: Only about 21% of liver tumors smaller than 1 cm are visualized.

Intraoperative assessment involves bimanual palpation, which can feel tumors as small as 5 mm, though with less sensitivity for deep lesions and cirrhotic livers. Intraoperative ultrasonography is invaluable with its 98% sensitivity and ability to detect tumors as small as 4 mm. It allows for detection of additional liver tumors in up to 50% of patients compared to bimanual palpation. It can also be applied laparoscopically. Laparoscopic ultrasonography has been reported to demonstrate additional liver tumors not seen by preoperative triphasic CT scans in 20% of the patients undergoing laparoscopic radiofrequency ablation (RFA) (Fig. 66-1).

■ CHEMOTHERAPY

Most of the patients presenting with liver metastases from colorectal primary tumors are not candidates for surgical resection and even after curative liver resection, 60 to 70% of the patients experience recurrence that underscores the need for additional nonsurgical treatment modalities.

A widely used agent to treat metastatic colorectal cancer, the antimetabolite fluorouracil (5-FU) inhibits thymidylate synthase, an enzyme required for the synthesis of DNA (deoxyribonucleic acid). Leucovorin, a reduced folate (tetrahydrofolate), is commonly administered together to increase the affinity of fluorouracil for thymidylate synthase. In cases of unresectable liver metastases, 5-FU-based chemotherapy results in a 21 to 31% response rate with a median survival time between 6.4 and 13.7 months. With high-dose continuous intravenous infusions, response rate has been increased to 44% and mean survival time to 16.6 months.

Irinotecan (camptothecin, or CPT-11) is an inhibitor of topoisomerase I, a nuclear enzyme involved in the unwinding of DNA during replication. In a recent multicenter trial, 683 patients with metastatic colorectal cancer were randomized to receive either irinotecan, fluorouracil and leucovorin, or irinotecan alone. As compared with treatment with fluorouracil and leucovorin, treatment with irinotecan, fluorouracil, and leucovorin resulted in significantly longer progression-free survival time (median 7.0 vs. 4.3 months), a higher rate of confirmed response (39 vs. 21%), and slightly longer survival time (14.8 vs. 12.6 months). Results for irinotecan alone were similar to those for fluorouracil and leucovorin (Fig. 66-2).

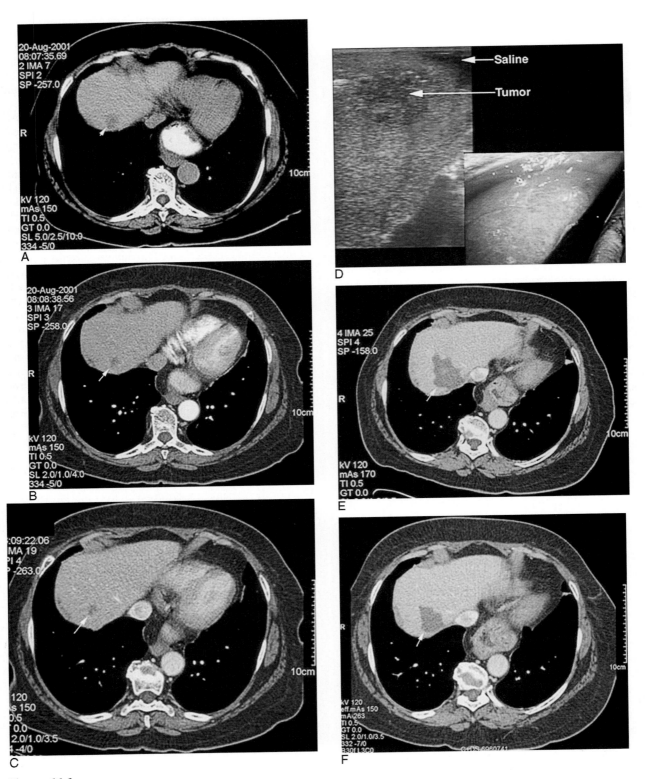

Figure 66-1

Computed tomographic (CT) and ultrasound images of a colorectal metastasis in a 72-year-old woman. Preoperative triphasic CT scan obtained in the noncontrast (*A*), arterial (*B*), and portovenous (*C*) phases demonstrated a lesion in the right lobe of the liver (arrow). Laparoscopic ultrasound in the operating room identified this 2-cm lesion in segment VIII (*D*), and the lesion was treated with radiofrequency ablation. Because the lesion was located superficially, the right upper quadrant was filled with saline to provide an acoustic medium for better visualization. The ablation zone was seen as a larger area in the postoperative 1-week CT scan (*E*), but the lesion gradually decreased in size in the 3-month (*F*) and 6-month (*G*) CT scans (arrow). Note that the lesion is seen as a hypodense subtle lesion on the CT scan, but laparoscopic ultrasound clearly demonstrates a 2-cm hypoechoic metastatic lesion with irregular borders.

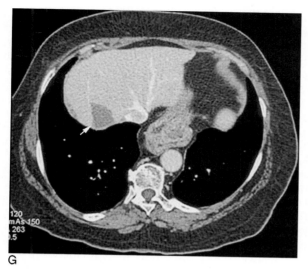

Figure 66-1 cont'd

In recent years, as the effectiveness of newer chemotherapy agents has been documented, there have been changes in initial and salvage chemotherapy regimens. In 2000, de Gramont and colleagues reported the results of a trial comparing 5-FU/leucovorin with 5-FU/leucovorin plus oxaliplatin, a new platinum-based agent. Response rates (22.3% vs. 50.7%) and median progression-free survival (6.2 months vs. 9 months) were significantly improved. A more recent study by Goldberg compared irinotecan/5-FU/leucovorin with oxaliplatin/5-FU/leucovorin (FOLFOX) and an irinotecan/oxaliplatin combination (IROX). Response rates were 31% for IFL, 45% for FOLFOX, and 35% for IROX. Median survival for FOLFOX was significantly better than that for IFL (19.5 months vs. 15 months) or IROX (17.4 months). Recently, the addition of monoclonal antibodies against EGFR (cetuximab, Erbitux) or VEGF (bevacizumab, Avastin) have improved response rates and survival. If the changes that have been occurring continue with the same trend, a persistent evolution in the chemotherapy regimens for initial and salvage therapy of colorectal liver metastases is expected.

Regional perfusion via hepatic artery infusion (HAI) delivers high concentration of drug with systematically tolerable drug levels. With this background, HAI has allowed for higher response rates, and downstaging of unresectable liver disease. More than 90% of fluorodeoxyuridine (FUDR) is taken up during a single pass via the hepatic artery compared to the 22 to 45% uptake for 5-FU. Randomized trials have shown increased intrahepatic response (41 vs. 14%) with HAI using FUDR compared to systemic chemotherapy. Nevertheless, randomized trials have failed to demonstrate a survival advantage. Moreover, a meta-analysis study failed to show a significant survival effect of HAI compared to intravenous administration of 5-FU or FUDR. The disadvantages of HAI using FUDR include ineffective systemic disease control and the complication of sclerosing cholangitis that eventually leads to liver failure. Several trials are under way to further evaluate which patients may benefit from this liver-directed therapy. Chemical hepatitis occurs in 26 to 79% of patients and biliary sclerosis in less than 10% of cases. Technically, hepatic artery placement entails cholecystectomy and devascularization of the distal lesser curve and superior aspect of the duodenum to prevent chemical cholecystitis and gastroduodenitis. The catheter is inserted via the gastroduodenal artery with the tip reaching the common hepatic artery.

Adjuvant Chemotherapy

Most patients surviving after liver resection die of recurrent disease, most commonly in the liver, so effective postoperative adjuvant therapy is needed. Nevertheless, no randomized trial has evaluated the role of adjuvant systemic therapy after complete resection of metastases in

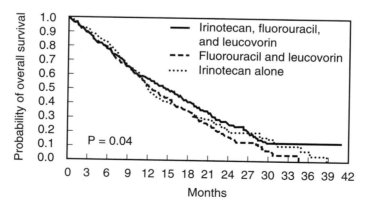

Figure 66-2

Kaplan-Meier curves showing overall survival of 683 patients who were randomized to receive irinotecan, fluorouracil, and leucovorin (231 patients), fluorouracil and leucovorin (226 patients), and irinotecan alone (226 patients). The median survival time of patients assigned to the first group was 14.8 months, as compared with 12.6 months for patients in the second group ($p = 0.04$). The median survival time of patients in the irinotecan group was similar to that for patients receiving fluorouracil and leucovorin (12.0 vs. 12.6 months). (From Saltz LB, Cox JV, Blanke C, et al: Irinotecan plus fluorouracil and leucovorin for metastatic colorectal cancer. N Engl J Med 2000;343:905–914.)

this patient population. HAI chemotherapy has been more extensively evaluated as an adjuvant therapy, but with a small number of patients reported in the studies. Lygidakis and coworkers, in a randomized study involving 40 patients, reported that adjuvant regional immunotherapy following resection increased the mean survival time from 11 months in the control group to 20 months. At present, it is best to conclude that the beneficial role of adjuvant therapy after resection of liver metastases from colorectal cancer is unproved.

Neoadjuvant Chemotherapy

A report by Bismuth and coworkers evaluated 330 patients with unresectable colorectal liver metastases who were treated with 5-FU, folinic acid, and oxaliplatin. After chemotherapy, 53 patients (16%) were found to have resectable disease with a 40% 5-year survival rate after liver resection. Although no current data support the use of neoadjuvant therapy for all patients with colorectal liver metastases, these results suggest that patients with unresectable colorectal liver metastases should be periodically assessed for possible resectability after chemotherapy.

■ SURGICAL RESECTION

In the past decades, appreciation of hepatic anatomy and physiology, the use of intraoperative ultrasonography, and improved surgical techniques have enabled liver surgery to evolve from imprecise resections with extensive hemorrhage to controlled anatomic procedures with acceptable risks. Indeed, hepatic resection is currently the only established treatment for patients with colorectal liver metastases that offers a possibility of cure with 20 to 40% 5-year survival rates after resection of all detectable disease. Median survival time after hepatectomy is 28 to 40 months. Ten-year survival rate is 23.6% and 20-year survival rate is 17.7% (Fig. 66-3).

Patient Selection and Prognostic Factors

The preoperative medical evaluation of patients is the same as for any other major surgical procedure. Age, gender, primary tumor grade, and location have not been shown to affect outcome after resection. Although some studies have shown an association between the number of metastases and survival when patients with less than three metastases are compared with patients with four or more metastases, others advocate that the number of metastases resected is no longer as important a predictor of survival as previously. The most consistent and important prognostic factors include the resection margin and coexisting extrahepatic disease at the time of liver resection. Complete excision of all tumor burden with 1 cm or greater clear resection margins has been shown to be critical. With margins less than 1 cm, long-term survival and cure are still possible, though somewhat reduced, if the margin is microscopically tumor-free. The presence of extrahepatic metastatic disease including hilar lymph node metastases should be regarded as a contraindication for curative liver resection. Two important exceptions are locally invasive disease that can be removed en bloc with the metastatic liver disease (most commonly diaphragmatic involvement) and resectable pulmonary metastatic disease. Prognostic criteria that worsen survival include the presence of symptomatic liver tumors, a brief (<12 months) interval between diagnosis of the primary cancer and metastatic liver disease, the presence of satellite lesions, high preoperative CEA level of greater than 200 ng/mL, and involvement of greater than 50% of the liver. Up to six anatomic segments or 75% of the liver volume can be resected without inducing postoperative liver failure. For patients undergoing such extensive liver resection, preoperative portal vein embolization of the affected segments, allowing for hypertrophy of the remaining liver, helps to preserve the hepatic function postoperatively.

Intraoperative Conduct

The detailed technical description of liver resection is beyond the scope of this chapter. Two important tools in the operating room include diagnostic laparoscopy and intraoperative ultrasonography. Laparoscopic evaluation of the liver and the abdominal cavity may identify unresectable metastatic disease, and cirrhosis or fatty infiltration in the non-tumor-bearing portion. Intraoperative ultrasonography defines the location of vascular structures, the extent of resection for adequate margins, and the presence of occult intra- or extrahepatic metastases. Laparoscopy allows the detection of unresectable disease in 25 to 50% of the patients. Laparoscopic ultrasonography identifies liver tumors not visible during laparos-

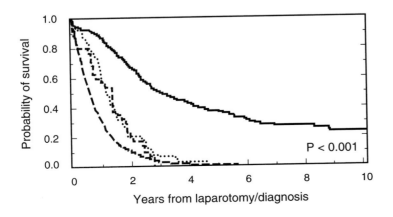

Figure 66-3
Survival times among 434 patients undergoing resection of liver metastases with curative intent (thick lines), divided into 366 potentially curative versus 68 nonradical procedures, including operative mortality rates. Thin lines indicate the two remaining patient groups undergoing deliberative debulking (solid thin line, n = 35) or no resection (broken thin line, n = 1249) of hepatic metastases. (From Scheele J, Stang R, Altendorf-Hofman A, Paul M: Resection of liver metastases. World J Surg 1995;19:59–71.)

copy in 33% of the patients and provides staging information in addition to that obtained by laparoscopy alone in 42% of patients with potentially resectable liver tumors.

Bleeding increases postoperative mortality and morbidity rates in liver resections. Operative strategies to minimize bleeding include temporary using of cell-savers, clamping of the gastrohepatic ligament (Pringle maneuver), total vascular exclusion, and keeping a low central venous pressure. The parenchyma then can be transected in many ways including the finger-fracture technique, using a Kelly clamp, ultrasound dissector (Cavitron ultrasonic aspirator, CUSA), and harmonic scalpel. Vessels and bile ducts are occluded by metal clips, ligatures, or staples. Hemostasis of the cut liver surface is obtained by suture ligations, fibrin sealant, or argon beam coagulation. The raw surface may also be covered with a pedicle of omentum.

The mortality rates of liver resection in recent series range between 2 and 4% and the complication rate exceeds 20%. Liver failure is the most common cause of death (1 to 5%). Pulmonary complications are the most frequent (10%), followed by biliary leak or fistula (3 to 4%), perihepatic abscess (1 to 9%), hemorrhage (1 to 3%), and myocardial infarction (1%). Median hospital stay is 9 days with 7% of the patients requiring intensive care (ICU) admissions.

Management of Synchronous Liver Metastases

The management of synchronous liver metastases at the time of primary surgery for colorectal cancer is controversial. The postoperative morbidity rate may be increased significantly when both resections are performed simultaneously. Synchronous open liver resection is not considered practical owing to difficulties with the incision, inadequate preoperative liver evaluation, absence of knowledge about the prognostic features of the primary cancer, and the medical status of the patient. Wedge resections of small, peripheral hepatic metastases are often performed at the time of colon resection, whereas major resections are usually performed in a staged manner.

Repeat Liver Resections for Recurrence

Recurrence is observed in about 60% of patients who undergo hepatic resection with a curative intent, and isolated liver recurrence develops in approximately 30% of these patients. Repeat liver resection may be performed with acceptable mortality, morbidity, and long-term survival rates in these cases. Postoperative mortality and morbidity rates do not differ from those reported after initial resections. Five-year survival rate ranges between 16 and 44%.

■ HEPATIC ARTERIAL LIGATION AND EMBOLIZATION

Liver tumors receive their blood supply from the hepatic artery in contrast to the parenchyma, which has dual blood supply also from the artery and portal vein. Hepatic arterial devascularization has therefore been tried as a treatment of liver tumors. However, metastatic colorectal tumors are relatively poorly vascularized, and emboliza-tion has produced poor results in the treatment of these tumors. Any benefit is temporary owing to the development of collaterals. Median survival rates have been no better than those obtained with chemotherapy.

Chemoembolization is performed by introducing a vascular occlusion agent combined with chemotherapeutics into the hepatic artery, causing both an ischemic and cytotoxic effect on the tumor. Most of the experience has been obtained in the treatment of hepatocellular carcinoma. Studies involving patients with colorectal liver metastases have reported tumor response between 29 and 63%, with a median survival time ranging between 8.6 and 14 months. Almost all patients experience the postembolization syndrome of liver pain and fever lasting for 3 to 6 days. Major morbidity rate ranges from 0 to 70%, including peritonitis, hemorrhage, liver abscess, gallbladder necrosis, myelosuppression, thrombosis, gastric ulcer, renal failure, and bile duct sclerosis, among others.

■ CRYOABLATION

Cryotherapy involves the use of a probe perfused with liquid nitrogen to produce an ice ball within the liver. Tissue destruction is caused by extensive formation of intracellular ice with disruption of cell membranes and cell death in the area adjacent to the probe, and cellular dehydration and microvascular thrombosis in the tissues at the rim of the process. Intracellular and extracellular formation of ice is responsible for cell death in the intermediate zone.

Intraoperative ultrasound has facilitated the efficacy of hepatic cryosurgery by overcoming the difficulties in detecting deep tumors and accurately monitoring the freezing of deeper hepatic tumors. Cryotherapy has been mostly performed using open techniques. The local recurrence after cryoablation of liver tumors has been reported to be 10 to 60% per lesion and 2.5 to 44% per patient.

In a study involving 136 patients with unresectable colorectal metastases treated by cyrotherapy, Weaver and asociates have reported a median survival time of 30 months with a 3.7% operative mortality rate. Complications included myoglobinuria (94%), hypothermia (6.3%), bleeding (3.7%), pleural effusion/atelectasis (3.7%), bile duct injury (3.2%), acute tubular necrosis (<1%), and hepatic abscess (<1%). Seifert and Morris have reported on 116 patients with colorectal hepatic metastases treated hepatic cryotherapy followed by hepatic arterial chemotherapy. Median survival time was 26 months with a 32.3% 3-year survival rate and 13.4% 5-year survival rate. Mortality rate was 0.9% and perioperative morbidity rate was 27.6%. In a study involving the adjunctive utilization of cryotherapy with surgical resection to treat all liver lesions in patients with colorectal liver metastases, median survival time in patients ($n = 52$) requiring cryoablation and liver resection to treat all evident liver disease was 20 months compared to 31 months for patients ($n = 34$) who required resection only. All patients develop a coagulopathy with elevated prothrombin times greater than 14 seconds as well as decreased platelet counts after hepatic cryotherapy.

■ RADIOFREQUENCY THERMAL ABLATION

Radiofrequency ablation (RFA) is a more recent method of locally destroying primary and secondary liver tumors. The basic principle of RFA includes generation of high-frequency alternating current (approximately 400 MHz), which causes ionic agitation that is converted to heat, which induces cellular death as a result of coagulation necrosis.

The procedure has been performed percutaneously and in open surgery with the first report of laparoscopic RFA in 1996. Although the percutaneous approach allows for rapid recovery, ultrasound guidance of the placement of the ablation catheter is difficult because of poorer percutaneous ultrasound resolution and respiratory movement of the liver, causing the procedure to yield higher recurrence rates than surgical approaches. Although the open approach overcomes these limitations and also allows for abdominal staging, it carries the morbidity of a laparatomy. The laparoscopic approach, on the other hand, is minimally invasive. Tumor targeting is facilitated by the upward movement of the diaphragm, eliminating liver respiratory movement, and laparoscopic ultrasonography allows for a highly sensitive staging of the liver. Percutaneously, lesions at the periphery of the liver may not be treated because of the risk of adjacent organ injury.

Patient Selection

In a significant number of patients with colorectal liver metastasis, the purpose is to debulk the liver in patients who are predicted to die of liver failure due to tumor progression. We currently use the following criteria to select the patients for RFA: (a) unresectable liver disease; (b) predominant liver disease, however, with minor additional extrahepatic disease; (c) enlarging liver lesions, worsening of symptoms, or failure to respond to other treatment modalities; (d) not more than eight liver lesions; (e) less than 20% of total liver volume replaced with tumor; (f) largest lesion smaller than 8 cm in diameter; and (g) normal biliary ductal diameters. Although we have generally performed RFA after the patients have failed chemotherapy, the optimal timing of RFA is controversial. An exception is synchronous ablation with resection in selective cases when liver metastases are detected at the time of surgery for primary disease, when concomitant liver resection may be too risky or not indicated.

Triphasic (noncontrast, arterial, and portovenous) CT scans and serum CEA levels are obtained 1 week before and after the thermal ablation procedure. The patients are then followed up with triphasic CT scans and tumor markers every 3 months.

Technique

The procedure is performed under general anesthesia. A diagnostic laparoscopy is first performed to obtain a biopsy of any suspicious extrahepatic disease. Laparoscopic ultrasonography of the liver is then performed, and the size and location of all suspected metastatic foci are determined. Color flow studies of the

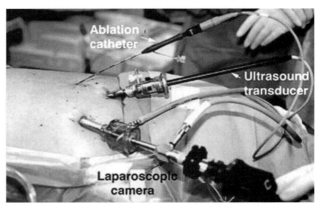

Figure 66-4
Placement of two subcostal 10-mm trocars for the laparoscope and laparoscopic sound transducer. The radiofrequency ablation catheter is placed through a separate percutaneous puncture.

metastatic lesions are done to assess their vascularity. Under ultrasound guidance, 18-gauge core biopsies are performed of the suspected metastatic foci for histologic confirmation. A minimum of two ports is required, one for the camera and one for the ultrasound transducer. An additional port may be required if extensive adhesions require dissection. The radiofrequency thermoablation catheter is then placed percutaneously into the lesion and the prongs are deployed. Laparoscopic ultrasound is used to guide needle placement to verify that the ablation zone is centered in all directions around the tumor. The radiofrequency ablation generator is run using various ablation algorithms depending on the technology used to ablate the tumor with a margin of normal tissue around it (Figs. 66-4 and 66-5).

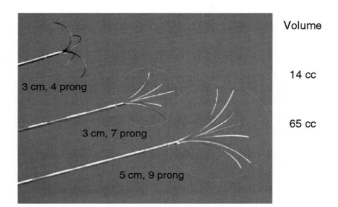

Figure 66-5
Radiofrequency thermal ablation catheters. The first-generation catheters could deploy out to 3 cm and had four or seven prongs. The second-generation catheters have nine prongs and can deploy out to 5 cm. An increase in the catheter deployment from 3 to 5 cm causes the ablation volume to increase significantly from 14 to 65 mL (4.6-fold).

The ablation process is assessed by (1) monitoring of thermocouple temperatures, (2) observation of outgassing of dissolved nitrogen into the heating tissues that creates a hypoechoic zone to encompass the area of ablation, and (3) observing the differences in tumor vascularity before and after ablation using color flow Doppler. In most cases, patients are monitored overnight and discharged home the morning following surgery.

Follow-up

Objective tumor response is assessed by measuring lesion size in follow-up CT scans. The lesion size is larger in the postablation CT scans owing to the ablation of a margin of normal tissue around the tumor, and gradually decreases or remains stable with successful ablation (Fig. 66-6).

Results

We treated 287 patients with 1003 primary and metastatic liver tumors using laparoscopic RFA between January 1996 and May 2002. Among these, 112 patients underwent 129 ablations for a total of 426 colorectal liver metastases. There were 72 men and 40 women with a mean ± SD age of 60 ± 13 years. The mean ± SD number of lesions treated per patient was 3.3 ± 2.5, with a range of 1 to 12. Mean tumor size was 3.9 ± 1.7 cm (range, 1 to 9 cm). With a mean follow-up of 9 months (range, 1 week to 25 months), local recurrence was detected in 65 lesions (15%). At the time of this analysis 88 (79%) patients were alive and 24 patients had died. Fifteen patients underwent repeat liver ablations to treat new or recurrent liver disease in follow-up.

In our total series of 287 patients, no perioperative deaths occurred. Complications were observed in

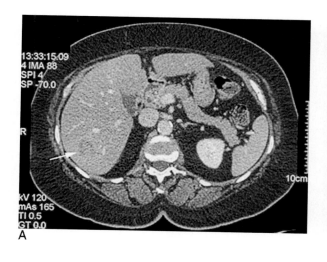
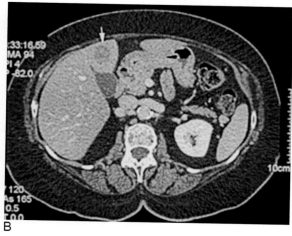
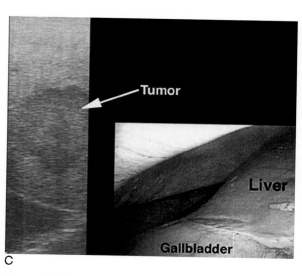
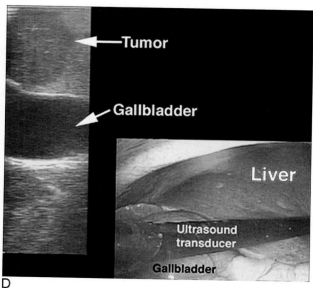

Figure 66-6

Preablation computed tomographic (CT) scan shows two metastases in the liver of a 71-year-old woman; they were discovered 4 months after her colon cancer diagnosis (*A* and *B*, arrow). Laparoscopic ultrasound in the operating room localized a 3.8-cm tumor in segment VI (*C*) and a 2.8-cm tumor in segment IV (*D*). Radiofrequency ablation was performed.

Continued

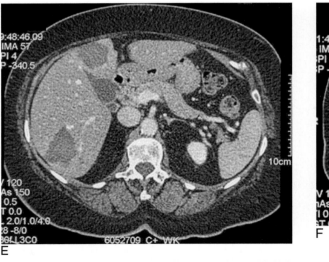

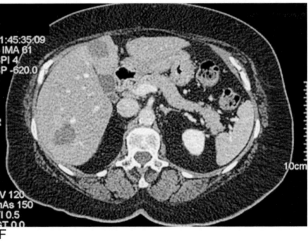

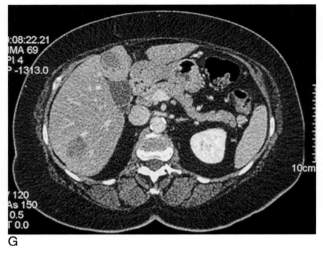

Figure 66-6 cont'd
In the CT scan obtained 1 week after ablation (*E*), the lesions appeared larger because of ablation of a rim of normal liver tissue around them. The ablated tumors gradually decreased in size in the postablation 3-month (*F*) and 6-month (*G*) CT scans. In this case, the lesion in segment IV was far enough from the gallbladder for the ablation to be performed without injuring the gallbladder. However, in cases in which the tumor is located too close to the gallbladder, cholecystectomy before ablation is warranted to prevent a thermal injury to the gallbladder.

7 patients (2.4 %), including liver abscess in 2 patients (treated with percutaneous drainage in one and antibiotics in the other), and transient atrial fibrillation, pulmonary embolism, postprocedure pain requiring admission, angioedema-urticaria, and recurrent ascites in 1 patient each.

In our whole series, 16% of the patients underwent RFA in combination with other procedures, including various colorectal operations in 14 patients. These procedures included laparoscopic-assisted colon resection in 5 patients, open colon resection in 2 patients, ileostomy closure in 5 patients, and colostomy formation and anal stricture dilatation in 1 patient each. Mean ± SD hospital stay was 2.8 ± 1.6 days. No patients died, and the only complication (2%) was the development of a right flank abscess after laparoscopic-assisted right hemicolectomy that was treated with percutaneous drainage. Although these patients undergoing laparoscopic RFA in combination with a clean-contaminated procedure could be at high risk for secondary infection of ablated foci, this complication was not observed. These data suggest that RFA may be used safely with colon resection in patients who may be resectable, but the morbidity of liver resection in a synchronous manner may be too risky.

■ CONCLUSIONS

Liver metastases from colorectal cancer continue to be a major health problem. Liver resection is the only treatment method that has been proved to provide long-term cure; nevertheless, the majority of the patients are not eligible for surgery. Chemotherapy has failed to provide more than a limited benefit for these patients. Hepatic artery ligation and embolization do not have a role in the management of these patients. Chemoembolization enables minimal survival advantage compared to chemotherapy, with a high rate of complications related to the therapy. Cryoablation is the classical method of local tumor destruction but carries a significant number of procedure-related complications. Radiofrequency ablation is a more recent technology providing an effective local tumor control in a minimally invasive manner with a significantly low morbidity rate. Nevertheless, no matter how well local tumor control is achieved with any therapy, two thirds of the patients experience recurrence, underscoring the need for systemic control to improve the current survival rates.

Suggested Readings

Berber E, Flesher NL, Siperstein AE: Initial clinical evaluation of the RITA 5-centimeter radiofrequency thermal ablation catheter in the treatment of liver tumors. Cancer J Sci Am 2000;6:S319–S329.

Bismuth H, Adam R, Levi F, et al: Resection of nonresectable liver metastases from colorectal cancer after neoadjuvant chemotherapy. Ann Surg 1996;224:509–522.

Cady B, Jenkins RL, Steele GD, et al: Surgical margin in hepatic resection for colorectal metastasis. A critical and improvable determinant of outcome. Ann Surg 1998;227:566–571.

de Gramont A, Figer A, Seymour M, et al: Leucovorin and fluorouracil with or without oxaliplatin as first-line treatment in advanced colorectal cancer. J Clin Oncol 2000;18:2938–2947.

Fong Y: Hepatic colorectal metastasis: Current surgical therapy, selection criteria for hepatectomy, and role for adjuvant therapy. Adv Surg 2000;34:351–381.

Foroutani A, Garland AM, Berber E, et al: Laparoscopic ultrasound vs triphasic computed tomography for detecting liver tumors. Arch Surg 2000;135:933–938.

Goldberg RM, Sargent DJ, Morton RF, et al: A randomized controlled trial of fluorouracil plus leucovorin, irinotecan and oxaliplatin combinations in patients with previously untreated metastatic colorectal cancer. J Clin Oncol 2004;22:22–30.

Link KH, Sunelaitis E, Kornmann M, et al: Regional chemotherapy of nonresectable colorectal liver metastases with mitoxantrone, 5-fluorouracil, folinic acid, and mitomycin C may prolong survival. Cancer 2001;92:2746–2753.

Lygidakis NJ, Ziras N, Parissis J: Resection versus resection combined with adjuvant pre- and post-operative chemotherapy-immunotherapy for metastatic colorectal liver cancer. A new look at an old problem. Hepatogastroenterology 1995;42:155–161.

Saltz LB, Cox JV, Blanke C, et al: Irinotecan plus fluorouracil and leucovorin for metastatic colorectal cancer. N Engl J Med 2000;343:905–914.

Sanz-Altamira P, Spence LD, Huberman MS, et al: Selective chemoembolization in the management of hepatic metastases in refractory colorectal carcinoma. A phase II trial. Dis Colon Rectum 1997;40:770–775.

Scheele J, Stang R, Altendorf-Hofman A, Paul M: Resection of liver metastases. World J Surg 1995;19:59–71.

Seifert JK, Morris DL: Prognostic factors after cryotherapy for hepatic metastases from colorectal cancer. Ann Surg 1998;228:201–208.

Siperstein A, Garland A, Engle K, et al: Local recurrence after laparoscopic radiofrequency thermal ablation of hepatic tumors. Ann Surg Oncol 2000;7:106–113.

Weaver ML, Ashton JG, Zemel R: Treatment of colorectal liver metastases by cryotherapy. Semin Surg Oncol 1998;14:163–170.

67

RESECTION OF COLORECTAL PULMONARY METASTASES

Thomas W. Rice, MD

Management of stage IV colorectal carcinoma is palliative in the majority of patients. Chemotherapy, the mainstay treatment of systemic disease, rarely results in long-term survival. Occasionally, in a patient with disease confined to the liver or lung, resection may be curative. Identification of patients who will benefit from an aggressive surgical approach is difficult, because the tumor and host factors that allow control of systemic disease with local therapy are unknown.

Pulmonary metastases are found in 20 to 50% of patients dying of colorectal carcinoma. In patients who undergo curative operation for colorectal carcinoma, pulmonary metastases will develop in 10 to 20%. Five percent of patients with metastatic colon cancer will have only pulmonary metastases; however, 80% of pulmonary metastases will be multiple. It is estimated that after curative resection of colorectal carcinoma, less than 10% of patients with pulmonary metastases will be candidates for pulmonary resection. Overall, less than 1% of all patients with colorectal pulmonary metastases will be candidates for pulmonary resection. Rectal cancers are four times more likely than colon cancers to metastasize to the lung.

■ PATHOLOGY

Colorectal pulmonary metastases are hematogenous and the majority originate from hepatic metastasis (cascade effect). Metastasizing cancer cells may bypass the liver via the systemic venous drainage of the rectum or by traveling through, but not arresting in, hepatic vessels. However, many metastases that are presumed to be isolated pulmonary metastases are the result of false negative clinical examinations of the liver. Although lymphangitic pulmonary metastases are theoretically possible, this pattern of metastasis is usually confined to the abdominal cavity.

■ DIAGNOSIS AND SCREENING

Because the majority of pulmonary metastases are peripheral, less than 10% of patients are symptomatic. Most colorectal pulmonary metastases are discovered on routine chest x-rays, the most cost-effective screening tool. Prior to the resection of a colorectal carcinoma, pos-teroanterior (PA) and lateral chest x-rays are mandatory. The follow-up of a patient with a resected colorectal carcinoma should include history, physical examination, carcinoembryonic antigen (CEA) test, colonoscopy, and chest x-rays. Following the resections of a colorectal carcinoma and a hepatic metastasis, part of the surveillance protocol should be computed tomographic (CT) scan of the abdomen. Frequency of follow-up varies, but the protocol should typically include a history and physical examination every 6 months; chest x-ray, CEA, and colonoscopy should be repeated annually for the first 5 years. It may be practical to intensify screening in the first 2 to 3 years by reducing examination periods from 6-month to 3-month intervals. An abnormal chest x-ray or rising CEA titer will raise the question of a pulmonary metastasis. CT scanning of the chest should be reserved for use at this time.

Screening with chest CT scan is problematic. CT examination is very sensitive but not positively predictive for pulmonary nodules. Depending upon nodule size, 25 to 50% of solitary pulmonary nodules in patients with colon carcinomas will be metastatic; others will be benign or an unrelated primary carcinoma.

■ PATIENT SELECTION

Surgery is the sole potentially curative therapy for patients with colorectal pulmonary metastases. It will be effective only if all metastatic disease is resected and the patient can survive the intended operation. Criteria for patient selection are as follows: (1) the primary colorectal carcinoma is controlled, (2) the lungs are the only site of metastases, (3) all pulmonary metastases are resectable, (4) the patient's pulmonary status is adequate for the planned resection, and (5) no major comorbidity is present.

Prognostic factors associated with long-term survival following resection of pulmonary metastases are the ability to completely resect all metastatic disease, the presence of a single metastatic focus, and a disease-free interval of 36 months or more. Considerable variation exists for factors retrospectively associated with a curative resection of a pulmonary metastasis of colorectal origin. Age, gender, and site of the colorectal primary cancer are not predictive of outcome. A favorable metastasis is asymptomatic, solitary, less than 3 cm in diameter, free of lymphatic metastases, slow growing (long tumor doubling time), well differentiated, diploid (by flow cytometry), and associated with a normal CEA level. Although absence of some factors does not preclude resection, lack of multiple factors should alert a surgeon that resection is unlikely to be curative.

The biologic behavior of a colon carcinoma and the host's defense mechanisms cannot be evaluated in the selection of patients for pulmonary resection. These factors are major determinants of the behavior of a pulmonary metastasis. Previously listed predictors can only approximate them. Until an understanding of tumor and host behavior is achieved, patient selection continues to be an educated guess.

PREOPERATIVE PREPARATION

After completion of a careful history, physical examination, and routine blood work, the local and metastatic status of the carcinoma is assessed and the health of the patient is evaluated. Colonoscopy is mandatory to assure local control. Metastatic survey should include a CT scan of the chest, abdomen, and pelvis. A brain scan should be considered because some nodules will be primary bronchogenic, and carcinomas that metastasize to brain are fatal. Positron emission tomographic (PET) scanning may prove the best single evaluation of local and distant extent of a colon carcinoma.

Spirometry and arterial blood gases are required for pulmonary assessment. Pulmonary assessment for patients who receive preoperative chemotherapy should include a diffusing capacity for the lung (DLCO). Quantitative perfusion scanning allows an estimation of the remaining pulmonary parenchyma following resection in patients with marginal lung function and in those requiring multiple or large resections. Exercise testing is indicated for patients with marginal pulmonary function. A cardiac stress test is prudent in patients over the age of 60 years and in those with a cardiac history. Other investigations are dependent upon comorbid conditions discovered at history or physical examination.

Tissue diagnosis is not mandatory prior to resection because a negative result for malignancy may reflect a false negative sampling error. If a diagnosis is required, the ascending order of sampling is sputum cytology, bronchoscopy with bronchial washings and brushings, transbronchial biopsy or percutaneous needle biopsy, and thoracoscopic biopsy. Sputum cytology is safe, easy, and well tolerated but more likely to provide a tissue diagnosis when the metastasis is central. Bronchoscopy is indicated for central lesions; cytologic examination of washings and brushings may be diagnostic in peripheral lesions. Transbronchial biopsy or percutaneous fine needle aspiration may yield a cytologic diagnosis. Thoracoscopic excision of a pulmonary nodule is performed for diagnosis only and should not be used with curative intent. The inability to palpate the lung at thoracoscopy results in a significant number of missed metastases and renders this approach diagnostic.

Preparation for pulmonary resection includes cessation of smoking and optimization of pulmonary function with bronchodilator therapy and cardiopulmonary rehabilitation. Patients with colostomies are instructed to do their routine care the night prior to surgery. The colostomy bag is emptied prior to the call to the operating room. It is draped out of the field and left alone.

OPERATIVE AND POSTOPERATIVE CARE

The surgical approach for unilateral metastases is via a muscle-sparing posterolateral thoracotomy. This provides excellent access to the ipsilateral lung and mediastinum. If lesions are bilateral, staged thoracotomies may be used.

The least involved lung is approached first, so that adequate pulmonary parenchyma is available for single lung ventilation when the major pulmonary resection is done approximately 6 weeks later. Bilateral metastases are generally approached via median sternotomy or a "clamshell" (bilateral anterior thoracotomies and transverse sternotomy) incision. Thoracoscopy has no role in patients selected for curative resection.

Possibilities of multiple or undetected metastases, contralateral surgery, or reoperation and re-resection mandates pulmonary sparing techniques. Because the metastatic process is hematogenous, many metastases are peripheral, and lymphatic spread is late. The standard resection is a nonanatomic wedge excision. For deeper lesions, a segmentectomy or lobectomy may be required. A pneumonectomy may be necessary for central metastases, but carries an increased operative mortality rate and is unlikely to be curative in patients with bilateral pulmonary disease. Pulmonary and mediastinal lymph node sampling (or lymphadenectomy) are mandatory because at least 15% of patients will have lymphatic metastases. A solitary adenocarcinoma in a patient at risk for primary bronchogenic carcinoma and who has had a colorectal carcinoma resected should be treated as if it were a lung cancer.

Pathologic evaluation of all resected nodules is essential for identification of benign and unrelated primary bronchogenic carcinomas. Typical histologic appearance of a colorectal metastasis is a rim of malignant glandular epithelium surrounding a necrotic center. The necrotic area is filled with nuclear and cytoplasmic debris (dirty necrosis), which is suggestive of colon metastasis. Special staining may further define the process but is unlikely to confirm the metastatic nature of the carcinoma. With many adenocarcinomas the diagnosis of a metastasis may be only presumptive.

Postoperative care of patients with colorectal metastases is similar to that of all patients undergoing pulmonary resection. Care must be taken to isolate a colostomy from the thoracotomy wound and chest tubes. The role of adjuvant postoperative chemotherapy following resection of colorectal pulmonary metastasis is unknown.

RESULTS

Operative mortality rate ranges from 0 to 1.4% in patients undergoing resections of colorectal pulmonary metastases. Operative mortality rate increases with advancing age and with pneumonectomy. In those patients, a 30-day postoperative mortality rate in the range of 1 to 2% can be expected. Reported 5-year survival rates vary from 13 to 60%. In carefully selected patients with all pulmonary metastatic disease resected, a 25 to 30% 5-year survival rate is anticipated.

History of a prior hepatic resection should not preclude the resection of metachronous pulmonary metastases if there is control of the primary and hepatic sites. Synchronous liver and lung metastases can sometimes be resected for cure. Again, careful patient selection, preparation, and complete resection are required to assure a reasonable chance of long-term survival. Isolated pulmonary recurrence following pulmonary metastasectomy is uncommon and is rarely amenable to repeat resection. Major cause of late death in most patients is recurrent carcinoma. This recurrence may be confined to the lung, but is usually disseminated.

Suggested Readings

Loehe F, Kobinger S, Hatz RA, et al: Value of systematic mediastinal lymph node dissection during pulmonary metastasectomy. Ann Thorac Surg 2001;72:225–229.

McAfee MK, Allen MS, Trastek VF, et al: Colorectal lung metastases: Results of surgical excision. Ann Thorac Surg 1992;53:780–786.

McCormack PM, Burt ME, Bains MS, et al: Lung resection for colorectal metastases. Arch Surg 1992;127:1403–1406.

McCormack PM, Bains MS, Begg CB, et al: Role of video-assisted thoracic surgery in the treatment of pulmonary metastases: Results of a prospective trial. Ann Thorac Surg 1996;62:213–217.

Okumara S, Kondo H, Tsuboi M, et al: Pulmonary resection for metastatic colorectal cancer: Experience with 159 patients. J Thorac Cardiovasc Surg 1996;112:867–874.

Robinson BJ, Rice TW, Strong SA, et al: Is resection of pulmonary and hepatic metastases warranted in colorectal carcinoma patients? J Thorac Cardiovasc Surg 1999;117:66–76.

The International Registry of Lung Metastases, Pastorino U, Buyse M, Friedel G, et al: Long-term results of lung metastasectomy: Prognostic analyses based on 5206 cases. J Thorac Cardiovasc Surg 1997;113:37–49.

68

NONEPITHELIAL COLORECTAL TUMORS

Guy R. Orangio, MD, FACS, FASCRS

Nonepithelial tumors of the colon and rectum are rare and represent less than 1% of all neoplasms of the colon and the rectum. They are categorized as benign or malignant lesions. This chapter will briefly discuss benign lymphoid hyperplasia, lipomas, and leiomyomas as well as leiomyosarcoma and the primary lymphomas of the colon and rectum. The majority of the chapter will deal with the cavernous hemangioma of the colon and rectum. Neurofibromas and rhabdomyosarcomas are extremely rare lesions; only nine cases of rhabdomyosarcoma have been recorded in the world literature. Endometriosis and the neuroendocrine tumors are discussed in other chapters in this text.

■ BENIGN NONADENOMATOUS LESIONS OF THE COLON AND RECTUM

Benign Lymphoid Hyperplasia

A benign lymphoid polyp is an aggregation of lymphoid tissue with a covering of normal rectal mucosa. These lesions are virtually all confined to the rectum and the distal sigmoid. They can be single or multiple, broad-based, or with a short pedicle. They are homogeneous, and can be reddish, purple, or gray. They vary in size from a few millimeters to several centimeters. These lesions are usually discovered incidentally, but they may be associated with hematochezia. They are not considered premalignant. If found during colonoscopy, they are removed, and their clinical appearance is nonspecific. Usually, the pathologist makes the diagnosis. Even if an endoscopist feels relatively sure that the lesion is a lymphoid aggregation, it should be removed.

Lipomas

Characteristic Features

Although lipomas are the second most common neoplasm of the colon after adenomas, they are uncommon. Their incidence is less than 1%, with a mean age of patients being 62.4 years, and an almost equal distribution between males and females. They are submucosal lesions ranging in size from 0.5 mm to 6.5 cm. They can be pedunculated (68.8%) or sessile (22.2%). The most common sites of occurrence are the cecum and ascending colon, followed in decreasing order of frequency by the transverse colon, sigmoid colon, and rectum. Most lipomas of the colon and rectum are asymptomatic and are usually found incidentally during routine barium enema or colonoscopy. The radiologic findings of a smooth polypoid lesion with sharp borders and a changing contour and configuration during manual application of external pressure (squeeze) should lead the radiologist to suspect that the lesion is a lipoma. The "squeeze" technique may be of historical note, however, and is not utilized currently. If a patient has an abnormal barium enema, a colonoscopy is indicated.

The typical endoscopic appearance of a submucosal lipoma is one of a yellowish, smooth, hemispheric polyp with a broad base or a short, thick stalk. The submucosal position of the lipoma causes stretching of the mucosa, allowing the endoscopist to visualize the normal blood vessels of the mucosa. Lipomas are rarely symptomatic but they can cause intermittent bowel obstruction (if the lipoma is near the ileocecal valve), colocolonic intussusception, or prolapse through the rectum. One patient passed a large lipoma per rectum. He had an acute onset of abdominal pain followed by hematochezia and passage of the lipoma. It was confirmed by histologic examination of the emergency room specimen. His follow-up colonoscopy showed a large ulceration of the rectosigmoid where the lipoma had resided. It was a large pedunculated lipoma, which had rotated on its stalk causing ischemia and autoamputation.

Therapeutic Alternatives

The therapeutic approach to lipomas of the colon and rectum is dictated by the clinical presentation. The approach to the asymptomatic patient depends on the size of the polyp and the findings at colonoscopy. The therapeutic approach to the symptomatic patient with a lipoma of the colon and rectum depends on the presentation and the position of the lipoma.

Several colonoscopic maneuvers can be used to make the endoscopist more secure in the diagnosis of a lipoma. Because the lipoma is soft, it can easily be indented with a closed biopsy forceps, and it will spring back to its previous shape after withdrawal of the forceps (cushion or pillow sign). When the "pillow" sign is present, most asymptomatic lipoma do not need to be treated. Their presence is noted for future reference. A pathognomic sign for a lipoma is the "naked fat sign." When diathermy snare is used to remove overlying mucosa, fat protrudes from this site. Once the diagnosis has been made, then the lipoma can be removed with a diathermy snare en toto or in a piecemeal fashion. An innovative technique for excision of larger lipomas of the colon and rectum has been described. The diathermy snare is placed around the lipoma, and the snare is gradually tightened. This ruptures the lipoma through the mucosa, thus allowing visualization and easier excision of the lesion. Only an experienced colonoscopist should attempt this technique and piecemeal excision of larger lipomas. As with any sessile lesion of the colon, the complication of perforation is always present, and prudence should be utilized. In fact, because of their high fat content, lipomas resist conduction of electricity more than adenomas. More current is required for snaring, and the risk of perforation is greater. Most lipomas should be left alone.

Symptomatic lipomas of the colon presenting with intussusception, obstruction, or bleeding require stabilization with intravenous hydration and antibiotics and appropriate surgical intervention.

When there is colonic obstruction or when a lipoma is ulcerated with inconclusive biopsies, then the lesion should be considered malignant and treated with surgical resection. Because the etiology of the colonic obstruction is very difficult to determine preoperatively, the lesion should be considered malignant. The surgical conduct of the operation should include minimal manipulation of the lesion, high vascular ligation, and wide margins with primary anastomosis.

Cavernous Hemangiomas

Characteristic Features

Relatively few histologically proved cavernous hemangiomas of the colon and rectum have been reported in the world literature. Most are found in the rectosigmoid. Hemangiomas of the gastrointestinal tract are classified as multiple phlebectasias, capillary hemangiomas, and cavernous hemangiomas. The majority are of the cavernous type, in which there are large, thin-walled vascular channels without true encapsulation, and typically with more smooth muscle fibers than capillary lesions. The pathogenesis of cavernous hemangiomas is a dynamic process of budding from ectopic mucosal implants of mesodermal tissue. This process of budding infiltration explains the transmural and mesenteric involvement of these lesions. There have been many reported cases of local infiltration into the uterus, urinary bladder and the sacrum. Figure 68-1 shows a rectal cavernous hemangioma invading the perirectal fat in a 3-year-old boy. Three years after resec-

tion he presented with a recurrence of the lesion not only involving the right buttock but the spinal canal near the cauda equina. He presented with a tender, right ischiorectal mass and associated anemia. Clinically, the mass measured 8 cm by 5 cm by 5 cm, was hard, and felt like a bag of "marbles." A computed tomographic (CT) scan revealed a recurrent cavernous hemangioma of the ischiorectal fossa, the pelvic wall, and the sacrum (Fig. 68-2). Selective angiography was performed and indicated internal iliac origin and spinal cord plexus origin. A magnetic resonance image (MRI) of the spinal cord indicated that the corda equina were involved with the hemangioma (Fig. 68-3). A multidisciplinary team including an interventional radiologist, pediatric neurosurgeon, and colorectal surgeon decided not to embolize or surgically approach this lesion because the child was minimally symptomatic. We also felt that arterial embolization was too dangerous because of the vessels of origin. Part of the lesion, involving the ischiorectal fossa, had spontaneously thrombosed, and he is still without abnormal neurologic findings.

The clinical triad of intermittent hematochezia, multiple ectopic phleboliths on x-ray, and cutaneous hemangiomas should alert the physician to the presence of an internal hemangioma as the cause of gastrointestinal hemorrhage. An important association between cutaneous and mucous membrane hemangiomas has been found on physical examination in this patient population. These lesions are usually seen on the skin, lips, mouth, tongue, pharynx, or perianal skin. There were cutaneous lesions in three of our six cases. Hematochezia was the presenting symptom in all of our cases and is found in 75% of the reported cases. This hemorrhage is usually intermittent, but it becomes progressively more severe with each successive bleeding episode. Bleeding usually begins at an early age and progresses through life. These patients can also present with multiple episodes of hematochezia, or with

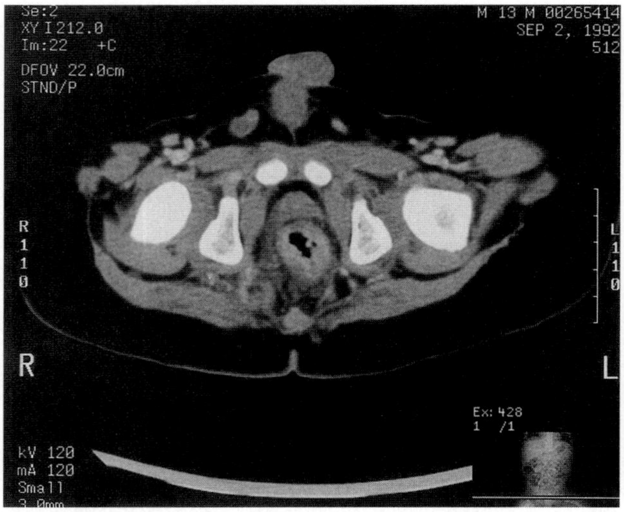

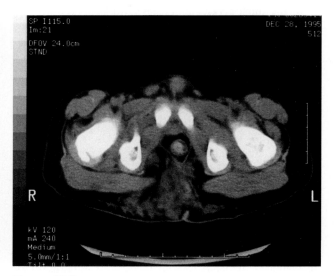

Figure 68-1
Computed tomographic scan illustrating thickening of the rectal wall and mesorectum and invasion into the pelvic wall.

Figure 68-2
Computed tomographic scan illustrating a recurrent cavernous hemangioma of the pelvic wall and ischiorectal fossa 3 years after resection of the primary lesion of the rectum.

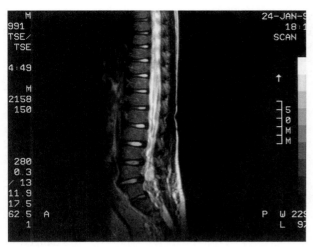

Figure 68-3
Magnetic resonance image of the spinal cord showing cavernous hemangioma of the corda equina area.

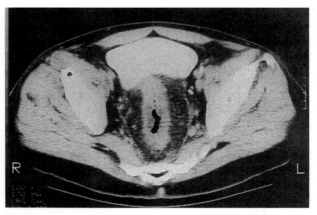

Figure 68-4
Computed tomographic scan illustrates transmural thickening of the rectal wall and mesorectum and the close adherence of the lesions to the posterior wall of the bladder and sacrum.

intestinal obstruction and tenesmus as the initial symptoms. In our series one patient was transferred to our care for massive lower gastrointestinal hemorrhage and an abnormal-appearing angiogram. The diagnosis of cavernous hemangioma of the rectum was made, and he underwent an emergency abdominoperineal resection with end–sigmoid colostomy. Unfortunately, the patient expired during the postoperative period because of multisystem organ failure. The most common error in diagnosis is bleeding internal hemorrhoids. Many patients have had multiple hemorrhoidectomies for local control of bleeding.

The pathognomonic endoscopic findings are dilated submucosal tumors that are typically soft and range in color from deep wine to plum. These tumors collapse upon insufflation, revealing the rectal mucosa in proximity to the dilated vascular channels to be congested and edematous. Biopsy is contraindicated because of the risk of hemorrhage. Laboratory abnormalities may include anemia, thrombocytopenia, defibrination, consumption coagulopathy, and depressed levels of factors V and VIII. Radiologic studies are helpful. Multiple ectopic phleboliths in clusters in the pelvis can be demonstrated roentgenographically in 50% of cases. A preoperative CT scan is important to define the extent of the lesion and possible local invasion into other pelvic structures (Fig. 68-4). Mesenteric angiography is essential for defining the arterial and venous origins of the lesions (Figs. 68-5 and 68-6). A colonoscopy is indicated preoperatively to define the anatomic extent of the lesion and find any synchronous lesions.

Therapeutic Options
Optimal therapy is surgery. The mortality rate is 50% in untreated patients. Attempts at mesenteric ligation or embolization, sclerosis, or local excision are suboptimal. Choice of surgical procedure for patients with rectosigmoid cavernous hemangiomas includes limited colon resection, low anterior proctosigmoidectomy with

colorectal anastomosis, modified Parks coloanal pull-through procedure, or abdominoperineal resection with end-colostomy. Sphincter-saving procedures should be the primary surgical option. Surgery is best done when the patient is not actively hemorrhaging. Intravenous vasopressin can help in decreasing the rate of hemorrhage in order to stabilize the patient for surgical intervention. In our experience sphincter salvage has been accomplished in five of the six patients (Table 68-1).

Surgical Technique
The patient is placed in the perineolithotomy position. The important technical considerations are early control of the inferior mesenteric artery and identification and protection of the autonomic nerve supply to the genitourinary system. The splenic flexure is mobilized, and the colon is divided at the anatomic division of the cavernous hemangioma and normal colon. This division is easily

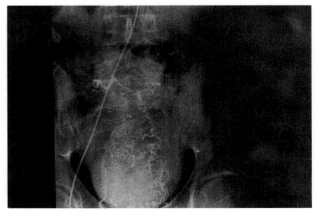

Figure 68-5
Angiogram of the inferior mesentery illustrates the abnormal vascular pattern of the rectosigmoid.

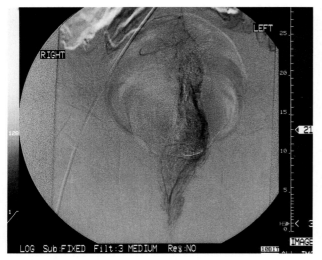

Figure 68-6
Angiogram of the inferior mesenteric artery in a 3-year-old boy with cavernous hemangioma of the rectum. Note the abnormal vasculature caused by these lesions.

determined because there are large subserosal serpentine vessels along the cavernous hemangioma. The involved colon is rigid and the mesentery is thickened. The pelvis is entered at the level of the sacral promontory anterior to the fascia of Waldeyer (presacral fascia). This thick fascia covers the presacral nerves of the hypogastric plexus. Posterior mobilization of the rectum is carried out sharply on the fascia propria of the rectum. Care is taken not to enter the rectal mesentery. Mobilization and division of the lateral ligaments are performed sharply down to the level of the levator muscles. The anterior dissection is done on the rectal side of Denonvilliers' fascia, thus preventing injury to the autonomic nerves. Dissecting in the correct plane ensures minimal blood loss and a low incidence of urinary and sexual dysfunction.

If a low anterior proctosigmoidectomy is done, a stapled colorectal anastomosis via the transanal approach is easiest. If the lesion involves the lower rectum, a modification of the Parks coloanal pull-through procedure can be done. The distal mucosal proctectomy is performed transanally. After submucosal infiltration of a local anesthetic with epinephrine solution, the mucosal stripping is begun 0.5 cm proximal to the dentate line. The remaining muscular cuff is approximately 2 to 3 cm in length. The descending colon or splenic flexure is brought down to the anus, and the coloanal anastamosis is hand-sewn. A proximal loop ileostomy is done in the right lower quadrant. The loop ileostomy is closed 8 to 12 weeks postoperatively.

Sphincter-saving procedures have been criticized because of recurrent bleeding. None of the five patients in our series have had recurrent bleeding. We could not have prevented the recurrence of the hemangioma in the young boy with an abdominoperineal resection. In the Saint Mark's Hospital experience, minor recurrent bleeding occurred in two patients, and no therapy was required. We therefore continue to advocate the sphincter-saving procedures over the abdominoperineal resection.

■ LEIOMYOMA AND LEIOMYOSARCOMA

Leiomyomas and leiomyosarcomas occur throughout the gastrointestinal tract. Approximately 50% of smooth muscle tumors of the colon and rectum are malignant. The overall incidence of leiomyosarcomas is 0.1% or less of all rectal malignancies. Smooth muscle tumors arise from the muscularis mucosa, the muscularis propria, or the smooth muscle of blood vessel walls. The median age of patients at presentation is 53 years old, with a higher incidence in women. These tumors range in size from a few millimeters to 15 cm. Presenting symptoms are bleeding, constipation, or a sense of fullness in the rectum. On palpation these lesions are smooth, firm submucosal tumors. They can be sessile or pedunculated. Approximately 86% of all smooth muscle tumors are within reach of the examiner's finger.

Characteristic Features
The diagnostic and therapeutic approaches to these lesions combine both clinical and pathologic findings. The gross specimen is firm, with yellow-white to reddish tan appearance on the cut surface. Size larger than 2.0 cm and ulceration of the mucosa suggest malignant lesions. The important microscopic feature is the number of mitoses per high-power field, and here the use of Broders' classification is helpful (Table 68-2). Sarcomas usually metastasize by blood-borne means, but local invasion and recurrence are common. Lymph node metastasis is rare. The cause of death is usually distant lung or liver metastasis. The preoperative evaluation of a patient with an established leiomyosarcoma includes CT scan, chest x-ray, and

Table 68-1 Cavernous Hemangiomas of the Colon and Rectum

PATIENT	SEX	AGE (YEARS)	LOCATION	OPERATION	FOLLOW-UP (YEARS)
	Female	49	Rectosigmoid	Coloanal*	10
	Male	46	Rectosigmoid	Proctosigmoidectomy	10
	Male	23	Rectosigmoid	Coloanal*	9.5
	Male	3	Rectosigmoid	Coloanal*	6
	Female	7	Sigmoid	Sigmoid resection	5
	Male	63	Rectosigmoid	Abdominoperineal resection	Postoperative mortality

*Low anterior resection, distal mucosectomy, hand-sewn coloanal pull-through anastomosis.

Table 68-2 Broder's Classification Applied to Leiomyosarcoma

Grade I	A greater abundance of cells is seen in leiomyosarcoma than in leiomyoma, and there is a slight increase in mitotic activity. Individual cells lack pleomorphism and anaplasia.
Grade II	Mitoses are found in one of five high-power fields. Nuclei maintain an elongated form, but the nuclear cytoplasmic ratio is greater than normal.
Grade III	Abundant mitotic figures, one to two per high-power field, are observed. Pleomorphic cells.
Grade IV	High degree of pleomorphism, cellularity, and mitoses.

bone scans. The 5-year mortality rate ranges from 15 to 40%. This variability is because there are so few reported cases.

Therapeutic Surgical Approaches

A lesion that is 3 cm or less from the dentate line is suitable for transanal excision. While the lesion is being removed, a small margin of normal tissue should be removed with it. For lesions that are inaccessible transanally, excision by the posterior trans-sphincteric approach (Mason) has been proposed as a surgical alternative. This operation requires familiarity with the anatomy of the area. There is disagreement in the literature as to the overall complication rate from this surgical technique, such as fistula, sepsis, and incontinence. The principles of the operation are to isolate and mark the muscle layers, as they are dissected, to maintain meticulous hemeostasis and to provide adequate local drainage. If a surgeon is not familiar with this technique, it may be better to refer the patient to a surgeon with experience or utilize a low anterior resection. Choice of the transanal or posterior trans-sphincteric approach to these lesions assumes that these lesions are benign. If the lesion is histologically malignant, a radical surgical excision is indicated.

A standard mechanical bowel preparation with oral or intravenous antibiotics should be utilized preoperatively. The surgical conduct of the operation is important to consider because malignant lesions recur both locally and via the blood. The use of high vascular ligation and wide pelvic dissection is essential. If an abdominoperineal resection is being performed, the perineal dissection is very wide, from the coccyx to the ischiorectal tuberosities. The use of adjuvant therapy with this patient population is beyond the scope of this chapter.

■ PRIMARY LYMPHOMA OF THE COLON AND RECTUM

Primary lymphoma of the gastrointestinal tract is a well-known entity. In a large review of primary lymphoma of the colon, the incidence was 0.65% of colonic neoplasms. The average age of onset is 50 years, with a 2:1 ratio of male to female. The cecum (70%) and rectum (11%) are the most common sites. The presenting symptoms are abdominal pain (100%), weight loss (100%), change in bowel habits (75%), painful palpable abdominal mass (80%), hematochezia or melena (10 to 30%), and obstruction (20 to 25%). By the most common pathologic classification (Rappaport), tumors are histocytic (43%), lymphocytic (29%), mixed cellular (14%), and Hodgkin's

disease (37%). Primary treatment is not surgical, although surgery may be necessary for making the diagnosis or for treating the complications. Chemotherapy and radiation therapy are beyond the scope of this chapter and will not be discussed.

The incidence of anorectal lymphoma is higher in association with acquired immune deficiency syndrome (AIDS). These lymphomas are undifferentiated or large-cell type with a B-cell phenotype, and tend to invade the perianal skin and ischiorectal areas. These patients have severe anal pain with associated hematochezia. The tissue is very hard and gritty to touch and appears as a severe infection of the perineum. However, it does not respond to antibiotics, and a biopsy of the area gives the diagnosis.

Recently, several cases of primary lymphoma of the colon presenting as ulcerative colitis or Crohn's colitis have been reported. No data support the theory of lymphoma associated with inflammatory bowel disease. These cases were probably atypical colitis that was unresponsive to standard therapy and in retrospect the biopsy interpretation may have been incorrect.

■ SUMMARY

Nonepithelial lesions of the colon and rectum are rare, but their signs and symptoms are similar to those for many common epithelial lesions. They form an important part of the differential diagnosis of atypical colorectal masses, and an understanding of their pathophysiology and surgical therapy is essential.

Suggested Readings

Borum ML: Cavernous colorectal hemangioma: A rare cause of lower gastrointestinal bleeding and a review of the literature. Dig Dis Sci 1997;42(12):2468–2470.

Byun JY, Kim AY, Cho KS, et al: Radiological features of leiomyomatous tumors of the colon and rectum. J Comp Assist Tomog 2000;24(3): 407–412.

DiSario JA, Burt RW, Kendrick ML, McWhorter WP: Colorectal cancers of rare histologic types compared with adenocarcinomas. Dis Colon Rectum 1994;37(12):1277–1280.

Djouhri H, Arrive L, Bouras T, et al: MR imaging of diffuse cavernous hemangioma of the rectosigmoid colon. AJR 1998;171(2):413–417.

Fan CW, Changchien CR, Wang JY, et al: Primary colorectal lymphoma. Dis Colon Rectum 2000;43(9):1277–1282.

Friesen R, Moyana TN, Murray RB, et al: Colorectal leiomyosarcomas: A pathobiologic study with long-term follow-up. Can J Surg 1992;35(5):505–508.

Hara AK, Johnson CD, Reed JE: Colorectal lesions: Evaluation with CT colography. Radiographics 1997;17(5):1157–1167.

Miettinen M, Sarlomo-Rikala M, Sobin LH: Mesenchymal tumors of muscularis mucosae of colon and rectum are benign leiomyomas that should be separated from gastrointestinal stromal tumors—A clinicopathologic and immunohistochemical study of eighty-eight cases. Mod Pathol 2001;14(10):950–956.

Romano G, Giordano P, Santangelo M, D'Alessandro V: Non-epithelial tumors of the colon-rectum. Our experience. Minerva Chirurg 1993;48(20):1161–1167.

Singland JD, Penna C, Parc R: Colorectal cavernous hemangiomatosis treated by total coloproctectomy and ileo-anal anastomosis. Ann Chirurg 1997;51(4):382–384.

Wang MH, Wong JM, Lien HC, et al: Colonoscopic manifestations of primary colorectal lymphoma. Endoscopy 2001;33(7):605–609.

69

COLONIC ISCHEMIA

Walter E. Longo, MD, MBA, FACS, FASCRS
Anthony M. Vernava III, MD, FACS, FASCRS

Intestinal ischemia produces a varied spectrum of diseases affecting the gastrointestinal tract. These syndromes can be acute or chronic and can affect the upper abdominal viscera as well as the small intestine and colon and rectum. They account for significant patient morbidity and mortality and continue to be the subject of clinical and laboratory investigation. The most common form of intestinal ischemia is ischemic colitis. Ischemic disease of the colon encompasses a diffuse spectrum of pathology. The pathophysiologic changes associated with this entity are related to numerous causative and aggravating factors. In certain circumstances, these factors are known and may be corrected; however, more often they remain unknown, and the treatment of colonic ischemia is symptomatic.

Cases of colonic gangrene were first described in the late 19th and early 20th centuries, but it was not until the 1960s that the pathophysiology of ischemic colitis was appreciated. In 1963, Boley described noniatrogenic, spontaneous colon ischemia in five patients. The term colonic ischemia, or ischemic colitis, was coined by Martson in 1966 when he described 16 cases of spontaneous colonic ischemia. Although occasionally occlusive in nature, as in left colon ischemia following aortic surgery, there is not usually a major vessel occlusion. The original insult precipitating the ischemic event often cannot be established. Many advances have been made in the diagnosis and treatment of patients with colonic ischemia since its original description by Boley and colleagues, and it is clear that the outcome depends on numerous factors, including the severity, extent, and rapidity of the ischemic insult as well as the therapy given. Increased awareness of this disease and knowledge regarding appropriate treatment are fundamental for its successful management.

■ ETIOLOGY AND PATHOGENESIS

Colonic ischemia has numerous causes (Table 69-1) which can be classified as either occlusive or nonocclusive. Occlusion of the blood supply to the colon may be related to trauma, thrombosis, or immobilization of the mesenteric arteries. Furthermore, obstruction or diffuse vasospasm involving the major arterial supply of the large intestine can result in severe ischemia to extensive regions of the colon or rectum. However, spontaneous episodes of ischemic colitis are by far more common and generally are viewed as localized forms of nonocclusive ischemia. Colonic blood flow is decreased by a variety of local and systemic physical and biochemical factors, through intensive vasoconstriction and arteriovenous shunting within the mesenteric circulation and bowel wall. Medications implicated in ischemic colitis include diuretics, beta-blockers, and cocaine. Colonic obstruction related to tumor, adhesions, diverticular disease, volvulus, or fecal impaction may contribute to colonic ischemia. In most cases, no cause or precipitating episode can be identified.

Several factors predispose the colon to ischemia. The colon has less blood flow per 100 g of tissue than does any other part of the gastrointestinal tract. The colon also frequently relies on a collateral arterial circulation. Another factor predisposing the colon to ischemic insult is the decrease in blood flow that accompanies functional motor activity of the colon. During hypotension, the colon does not autoregulate well compared with the rest of the gastrointestinal tract, and oxygen supply quickly reaches a critically low level, resulting in ischemia.

■ CLASSIFICATION

Clinically, the two principal forms of ischemic colitis are a nongangrenous type, subdivided into a transient reversible form and a chronic form, and a second form known as the gangrenous type (Fig. 69-1). The nongangrenous form of ischemic colitis accounts for 80 to 85% of cases. This nongangrenous transient form involves the mucosa or submucosa and is characterized by edema, submucosal hemorrhage, and partial mucosal necrosis. In general, transient ischemic colitis is followed by a complete structural and functional recovery within 1 or 2 weeks with no sequelae. The nongangrenous chronic form involves a more severe injury. Often, the damage penetrates beyond the submucosa into the muscularis propria. The damaged muscularis is replaced by fibrous tissue during a period of weeks to months and frequently results in a colonic stricture. These strictures may produce clinical sequelae. Chronic damage, in the form of persistent segmental colitis and strictures, occurs in 20 to 25% and 10 to 15%, respectively, of patients. Gangrenous ischemic colitis encompasses the remaining 15 to 20%. Gangrenous ischemic colitis involves a transmural necrotizing injury, which promotes sepsis and requires surgical resection of the involved colonic segment. Gangrenous ischemic colitis carries a mortality rate that approaches 50%.

Ischemic colitis may involve any portion of the colon and rectum although the splenic flexure, decending colon and sigmoid are most often affected. There is a variable degree of severity. Certain causes have a propensity to affect specific areas of the bowel. Ischemia secondary to systemic low flow states usually involves the right colon, most commonly its retroperitoneal surface. Localized, nonocclusive ischemia classically involves watershed areas of the colon such as the splenic flexure and the junction of the sigmoid and rectum. Ligation of the inferior mesenteric artery contributes to sigmoid colonic ischemia. The

Table 69–1 Causes of Colonic Ischemia

Idiopathic (spontaneous)	Hypolemia
Major vascular occlusion	Sepsis
Trauma	Neurogenic insult
Thrombosis, immobilization of mesenteric arteries	Anaphylaxis
Arterial embolus	Medications
Cholesterol embolus	Digitalis preparations
Aortography	Diuretics
Colectomy with inferior mesenteric artery ligation	Catecholamines
Midgut ischemia	Estrogens
Postabdominal aortic reconstruction	Danazol
Mesenteric venous trombosis	Gold
Hypercoaguable states	Nonsteroidal anti-inflammatory drugs
Portal hypertension	Neuroleptics
Pancreatitis	Colonic obstruction
Small vessel disease	Adhesions
Diabetes mellitus	Stricture
Rheumatoid arthritis	Diverticular disease
Amyloidosis	Rectal prolapse
Radiation injury	Fecal impaction
Systemic vasculitis disorders	Volvulus
Systemic lupus erythematosus	Strangulated hernia
Polyarteritis nodosa	Pseudo-obstruction
Allergic granulomatosis	Hematologic disorders
Scleroderma	Sickle cell disease
Behçet's syndrome	Protein C deficiency
Takayasu's arteritis	Protein S deficiency
Thromboangitis obliterans	Antithrombin III deficiency
Buerger's disease	Cocaine abuse
Shock	Long-distance running
Cardiac failure	

left colon and rectum remain the predominant location of colonic ischemia, being involved in approximately 75% of patients. The splenic flexure is involved in about one quarter of cases and the right colon in approximately 10%. Right colon ischemia may be a manifestation of midgut ischemia secondary to an embolus or thrombus in the superior mesenteric artery, because the midgut includes this part of the colon. Ischemic proctosigmoiditis is a rare event (see later discussion).

■ CLINICAL PRESENTATION

Ischemic colitis generally develops as an acute abdominal illness in patients older than 60 years of age who have had no previous colonic problems. However, this disease should not be discounted in the younger patient population. Signs and symptoms include abdominal pain, diarrhea, nausea, vomiting, and hematochezia. Blood loss in these patients is usually minimal, but "red currant jelly" stools may be present. The pain is sudden in onset, crampy, and often localized to the lower abdomen, frequently the left side. An acute urge to defecate frequently accompanies the pain. Anorexia, nausea, and vomiting, secondary to an associated ileus, may be present. The abdominal examination is often significant for mild distention and tenderness that usually corresponds to the site of the ischemia. A low-grade fever may be present. Rectal examination reveals heme-positive stool. A moderate leukocytosis with a left shift is often seen. In most cases, symptoms occur without sequelae. Patients with full-thickness gangrene involving variable amounts of colon

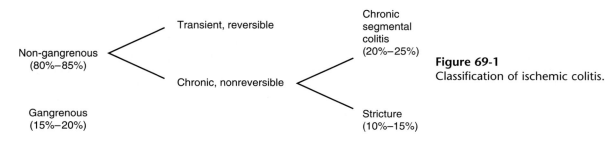

Figure 69-1
Classification of ischemic colitis.

present with signs and symptoms of a catastrophic abdominal event including sepsis and shock. Shock-associated ischemic colitis is a much more subtle process and will frequently be diagnosed only at the time of exploratory laparotomy in an intensive care unit patient being explored for sepsis and multiple organ failure.

Ischemic colitis is not limited to the elderly population. Colonic ischemia may affect younger people in whom identifiable etiologies include vasculitis, medication-induced reactions, coagulopathies, sickle cell disease, long distance running, and cocaine abuse. Because of few comorbidities, these patients usually tolerate both surgery and ischemia well.

■ DIAGNOSIS

A diagnosis of ischemic colitis is suggested by history and physical findings and supported by the presence of fever and leukocytosis. In a patient with suspected colonic ischemia, who has no signs of peritonitis and normal or nonspecific abdominal radiographs, colonoscopy should be performed. A plain radiograph that demonstrates free intra-abdominal air, air within the bowel wall, or portal venous gas signifies advanced ischemia or colon infarction and is an indication for immediate exploratory laparotomy. A plain radiograph may also demonstrate classical mucosal "thumbprinting" due to edema of the colonic mucosa. Computed tomography (CT) demonstrates only nonspecific findings, such as a thickened bowel wall. Barium enema should be avoided because of risk of perforation.

Colonoscopy is the preferred diagnostic study because it is more sensitive in diagnosing mucosal abnormalities, and biopsies may be obtained. Hemorrhagic nodules seen at colonoscopy represent bleeding into the submucosa and parallel the "thumbprints" or "pseudotumors" seen on barium studies. A segmental distribution of these findings, with or without ulceration, strongly suggests colonic ishemia. Colonoscopy is performed with special care. Distention of the bowel with room air to pressures greater than 30 mm Hg further diminishes colonic blood flow and actually may increase colonic ischemia. Chronically ischemic colon can be more fragile than normal and more prone to tear.

The precise endoscopic and histologic picture of ischemic colitis depends on the rate of the ischemic insult and the stage in the natural history of the disease at which the diagnostic studies are performed. Histologic evidence of mucosal infarction (ghost cells), although rare, is pathognomonic for ischemia. More common changes are vascular congestion and damage in the superficial half of the mucosa. There is loss of mucin and surface epithelial cells and a degeneration of normal crypt architecture, the extent of which depends on the overall degree of ischemic changes. Endoscopically, areas of gray-green or black mucosa and submucosa represent transmural infarction of the bowel wall. Mesenteric angiography is usually not indicated in the evaluation and management of colonic ischemia. Angiography is indicated when the diagnosis of acute mesenteric ischemia is being contemplated or when the initial colonoscopic examination is nonrevealing or demonstrates isolated right-sided colonic ischemia.

■ MANAGEMENT

The management of colonic ischemia depends on the etiology and severity of the disease process. Once the diagnosis has been made and if the clinical examination does not suggest intestinal gangrene or perforation, the patient is treated expectantly. Very mild cases can be managed on an outpatient basis. Generally, if the patient has abdominal pain, parenteral fluids are administered and empiric broad-spectrum antibiotics are given to cover aerobic and anaerobic bacteria. The bowel is placed at rest.

In most cases of colonic ischemia, signs and symptoms of the illness subside within 24 to 48 hours, and submucosal and intramural hemorrhages are resorbed. Clinical and radiologic resolution is virtually complete within 1 to 2 weeks. More severe ischemia with necrosis of the mucosa and submucosa produces ulceration, inflammation, and possibly chronic segmental ulcerating colitis or strictures. An initial attempt can be made to manage patients with chronic segmental colitis symptomatically.

Clinical deterioration, despite conservative therapy, is manifested as sepsis, peritoneal irritation, free intra-abdominal air, or extensive gangrene visualized endoscopically. This picture indicates colonic infarction and mandates immediate laparotomy and colon resection. Intraoperatively, assessment of colonic viability may be achieved by colonoscopy, evaluation of the antimesenteric serosal surface by hand-held, continuous-wave doppler, tonometric measurement of intramural pH, pulse oximetry of transcolonic oxygen saturation, or by using intravenous fluorescein. If the margins of the resected specimen are involved and performance of an anastomosis is contemplated, bleeding from the margins must appear grossly normal. Persistent concerns about remaining or ongoing ischemia mandate against an anastomosis and for a planned second-look laparotomy. It has been suggested that a primary anastomosis should not be attempted in patients with colonic gangrene, but a stoma and mucus fistula should be performed instead.

■ OUTCOME

Determining the outcome of spontaneous ischemic colitis is difficult because of the varying severity of the disorder. In a large series of 113 patients with spontaneous ischemic colitis reported in 1979, 66 patients had partial-thickness involvement and successfully recovered without an operation. An additional 26 patients underwent elective colon resections for strictures, with no mortality. Twenty-one patients underwent emergency surgery for gangrene, with a 53% mortality rate. Similar results were reported from our institution in 1986, with no deaths in patients with spontaneous ischemic colitis who did not require colon resection, whereas 60% of the patients undergoing colon resection for full-thickness necrosis and gangrene died.

Limited literature exists comparing patients with ischemic colitis who were treated surgically with those who did not undergo surgery. West and associates compared 13 patients managed conservatively with 12 patients who required intestinal resection. Although all 13 patients who were managed without surgery survived, no specific clinical patterns were identified to distinguish them from the operative group. Abel and Russell described the management of 18 patients with ischemic colitis, 9 of whom were treated conservatively and 9 of whom required operative therapy. The mortality rate was 55% in the operative group and 45% in the conservative group. All patients who died following conservative therapy had ischemic colitis confirmed at autopsy. Reeders and colleagues reported the results of treatment of 199 patients with ischemic colitis. Thirty-five patients underwent immediate surgery for peritonitis, and all died. The remaining 164 patients were initially managed nonoperatively. Of 98 patients who continued conservative treatment throughout their hospitalization, 57% died. Among the remaining 66 patients initially treated conservatively who ultimately required surgery for progression of disease, 51% died. Similar trends have been observed by others. In a recent study of 47 patients with ischemic colitis who were initially managed conservatively, it was demonstrated that duration of symptoms, coexisting medical diseases, initial hemodynamic instability, and prolonged ileus were significant predictors of outcome.

■ SPECIAL TOPICS

Ischemic Colitis After Aortic Surgery
Ischemic colitis following abdominal aortic reconstructive procedures remains a challenging problem. It usually involves the sigmoid colon and rarely involves the rectum. When postoperative colonoscopy is performed routinely on all patients, an incidence as high as 7% has been noted. When clinical criteria are used, the incidence is only 1 to 2%. It remains to be seen whether the new endoluminal grafting techniques for aortic surgery will have an impact on the incidence of ischemic colitis.

The incidence of ischemic colitis after repair of ruptured abdominal aortic aneurysms may be as high as 60%. Other risk factors include prior colectomy (because of collateral interruption), hypogastric or mesenteric arterial occlusive disase, advanced age, and preoperative hypotension. Patients with aneurysms may be at higher risk than those with occlusive disease because of better preformed collaterals in the latter group. On preoperative arteriography, retrograde filling of the superior mesenteric artery (SMA) and the inferior mesenteric artery (IMA) places the patient at a higher risk of postoperative ischemic colitis. IMA reimplantation is important in such cases, as it is for severe bilateral hypogastric artery stenosis. On the other hand, the presence of flow from the SMA to the IMA suggests adequate collateral colonic flow. If the IMA is found to be occluded or severely stenosed, ligation is believed to carry little risk of ischemic colitis. Ligation of the IMA should be carried out exactly at its origin to avoid disruption of collateral pathways. Finally, bypass to the femoral level may decrease pelvic circulation if retrograde flow to the internal iliac vessels is not assured.

Several criteria have been proposed in an effort to predict which patients might be at risk for postoperative ischemic colitis. Such efforts are based on the assumption that direct colonic or pelvic revascularization at the time of aortic reconstruction might lessen the risk of postoperative ischemic colitis. Indeed, in one study, in which such aggressive revascularization was undertaken, the incidence of endoscopically proved ischemic colitis was reduced to 3% with all cases being mild and nonfatal. Intraoperatively, the presence of IMA back-bleeding does not guarantee protection from ischemic colitis. However, the presence of an IMA stump pressure/systemic pressure ratio greater than 0.4 has been reported to be associated with a low likelihood of postoperative colonic ischemic after IMA ligation.

Prevention of ischemic colitis after aortic surgery is important because its development is associated with a very high mortality rate. In a recent report of U.S. veterans who developed such a complication, the overall mortality rate was 54%. Colectomy was required in two thirds of patients, and in that subgroup, the mortality rate was 89%. Mean hospitalization time was greater than 1 month after the diagnosis of ischemic colitis was made. None of the patients developed evidence of aortic graft infection in the immediate postoperative period.

Early recognition of postoperative ischemic colitis is equally important to allow the institution of supportive measures. Warning symptoms include bloody or Hemoccult-positive diarrhea, especially early after surgery; increased fluid requirements; fever of uncertain causes; unexplained leukocytosis or thrombocytopenia; abdominal distention; and acidosis. Treatment is similar to that for ischemic colitis in other patients, although the threshold for colectomy should be lower to avoid possible perforation. Patients treated nonoperatively should undergo flexible sigmoidoscopy every other day to assess the status of the disease. Those who come to surgery require colectomy, vigorous abdominal irrigation, omental patch covering of the retroperitoneum, and long-term antibiotic coverage.

Colonic Ischemia Following Cardiopulmonary Bypass
Colonic ischemia after cardiopulmonary bypass, although uncommon, is a lethal complication, often associated with sepsis and multiple organ failure. The incidence of bowel ischemia in this circumstance ranges between 0.06% and 0.2%. Mortality rate averages 76%.

Evaluation of critically ill postoperative cardiac patients is difficult because they are often ventilated and sedated. The presence of blood in the stools, hemodynamic instability, or cardiac parameters suggesting sepsis mean that colonoscopy should be strongly considered. This can be done with a bowel preparation or after proctoscopy and gentle enemas. Physicians are often reluctant to submit these patients to major abdominal surgery in the period immediately following cardiac surgery. However, surgical intervention, per se, is not associated with a significant increase in mortality rate.

Gastrointestinal mucosal ischemia after cardiopulmonary bypass is likely to be related to the low flow state of bypass and is maintained by splanchnic vasoconstriction. Contributing factors include systemic hypovolemia, hypotension, and hypothermia. Cardiopulmonary bypass exposes the blood to abnormal surfaces, resulting in blood coagulation abnormalities, alterations in cells and proteins, liberation of biologically active substances, and activation of the complement cascade. This sequence of events results in a reduction of blood flow throughout the intestinal microcirculation. However, long bypass times, postoperative use of inotropes, which may induce splanchnic vasoconstriction, and the intra-aortic balloon pump act as cumulative insults.

Ischemic Colitis Associated with Colon Carcinoma and Obstructing Colon Lesions

Patients may have symptoms of colonic ischemic or symptoms related to primary cancer. Acute ischemic colitis may also masquerade as colonic carcinoma. A biopsy should prove definitive. Repeat interval endoscopy will add further assurance.

Obstructing lesions, including diverticulitis, volvulus, fecal impaction, and strictures from prior ischemic insults, operations, or radiation therapy may cause diminished colonic blood flow by the profound effects of sustained increased intraluminal pressure. Because the tension in the bowel wall is greatest in the cecum, it is this part of the colon that is usually ischemic.

Total Colonic Ischemia

A rare fulminating form of colonic ischemia, involving all or most of the colon and rectum has been identified in a few patients. These patients present with a sudden onset of bleeding, fever, severe diarrhea, abdominal pain, and tenderness, often with signs of peritonitis. They have sustained systemic insults that render the entire colon susceptible to ischemia. The clinical course typically accelerates rapidly. Management of the condition, similar to that for other forms of fulminating colitis, requires with total abdominal colectomy and ileostomy. Further clinical deterioration mandates proctoscopy to evaluate any ischemia that may involve the rectum.

At our institution, we sought to determine the outcome of patients with ischemic colitis, comparing those with segmental disease to those with total colonic ischemia. Forty-three consecutive patients with ischemic colitis were identified and were grouped into those with segmental ischemic colitis and total colonic ischemia. The mean age was 68.8 years; 28 of the 43 (65%) were males. The diagnosis was established by colonoscopy in 31 of 43 (40%) of the patients during admission for an unrelated illness. In 6 (14%) of these 43 patients, ischemic colitis developed following surgery. Segmental colitis was present in 31 of 43 (72%), and 12 (35%) of

these 31 patients were successfully managed nonoperatively. In the patients with segmental colitis who required surgery, the 30-day mortality rate was 22%. Among 12 of 17 (71%) with segmental ischemia treated by resection and stoma, 9 (75%) underwent eventual stoma closure. All 12 patients with total colonic ischemia required surgery, and 9 of the 12 (75%) died. Total colonic ischemia carries a worse prognosis than segmental colonic ischemia.

Ischemic Proctosigmoiditis

Rectal ischemia is rare because the blood supply derives from three arteries with independent origins. Although rectosigmoid ischemia is usually accompanied by more proximal colonic involvement, it may occur alone. A retrospective review of all patients diagnosed as having colonic ischemia at the Mayo Clinic from 1976 to 1991 revealed 10 of 328 patients with ischemia of the rectosigmoid extending to no more than 30 cm above the dentate line. Among these 10 patients, 6 were chronic and 4 were acute. These patients were predominantly elderly with atherosclerosis. An identifiable precipitating factor such as a major illness or hemodynamic disturbance was identified in a number of these patients. CT often revealed rectal wall thickening, and angiography demonstrated atherosclerosis of the aortoiliac vessels. The authors concluded that, in contrast to generalized colonic ischemia, patients with acute rectal ischemia often have a clearly identifiable cause. Conservative management fairs well for acute disease, but patients with chronic disease may develop complications such as stricture or perforation.

■ CONCLUSIONS

Ischemic colitis usually occurs in patients hospitalized for other reasons, and the diagnosis requires an informed, astute, and attentive clinician. Management depends on the presence or absence of peritonitis and the severity of the comorbid illness. Most patients can be successfully managed nonoperatively with attention paid to hemodynamic and respiratory support. Operation is indicated for those who deteriorate despite appropriate medical intervention. Unfortunately, the mortality rate for this disorder remains high because of the associated comorbidities. Further investigation may concentrate on methods of preserving colonic blood flow during aortic and cardiovascular surgery and cytoprotective measures for ischemia and reperfusion.

Suggested Readings

Abel ME, Russell TR: Ischemic colitis: Comparison of surgical and non-operative management. Dis Colon Rectum 1983;26:113–115.

Bharucha AE, Tremaine WJ, Johnson CD, Batts KP: Ischemic proctosigmoiditis. Am J Gastroenterol 1996;91:2305–2309.

Boley SJ, Schwartz S, Lash J, Sternhill V: Reversible vascular occlusion of the colon. Surg Gynecol Obstet 1963;116:53–60.

Ghandi SK, Hanson MM, Vernava AM, et al: Ischemic colitis. Dis Colon Rectum 1996;39:88–100.

Longo WE, Ballantyne GH, Gusberg RJ: Ischemic colitis: Patterns and prognosis. Dis Colon Rectum 1992;35:726–730.

Longo WE, Lee TC, Barnett MG, et al: Ischemic colitis complicating abdominal aortic aneurysm in the U.S. veteran. J Surg Res 1996;60:351–354.

Longo WE, Ward D, Vernava AM, Kaminski DI: Outcome of patients with total colonic ischemia. Dis Colon Rectum 1997; 40:1448–1454.

Reeders JWAJ, Tytgat GNJ, Rosenbusch G: Ischemic Colitis. The Netherlands, Martinus Nijhoff, 1984.

Toursarkissian B, Thompson RW: Ischemic colitis. Surg Clin North Am 1997;77:461–470.

Vernava AM, Moore BA, Long WE, Johnson FE: Lower gastrointestinal bleeding. Dis Colon Rectum 1997;40:846–858.

West BR, Ray JE, Gathright JB: Comparison of transient ischemic colitis with that requiring surgical treatment. Surg Gynecol Obstet 1980;151:366–368.

70

MANAGEMENT AND TREATMENT OF COLON AND RECTAL TRAUMA

Andreas Platz, MD
Susan Galandiuk, MD

■ ETIOLOGY

Many different types of trauma cause injury to the colon and rectum. The frequency of these injuries will vary according to practice location and patient demographics.

Colonic Trauma

Stab wounds and low-velocity gunshot wounds represent 85 to 95% of colon injuries in the civilian environment. The colon is injured in 30% of all abdominal gunshot wounds and in 5% of stab wounds. Iatrogenic injuries are infrequent, but occur most commonly with colonoscopy and barium enema. Blunt trauma accounts for less than 15% of colonic injuries and is usually caused by motor vehicle accidents, pedestrian trauma, and falls. Delayed colonic wall disruption, which may occur with blunt trauma such as seat belt contusions, is associated with high rates of morbidity, usually because of delayed diagnosis.

Rectal Trauma

Rectal injury can be caused by trauma to the perineum. Rectal injuries can also occur in association with compound pelvic fractures, but may be overlooked as a result of severe associated injuries. Among male homosexuals, foreign bodies are frequently reported as a cause of rectal perforation.

■ PREOPERATIVE ASSESSMENT

Physical Examination

As with all trauma, evaluation of the patient's injuries begins with the ABCs, ensuring that the patient has a patent airway (A), is breathing adequately (B), and can maintain satisfactory circulation (C) as measured by systolic blood pressure.

The patient's abdomen, both flanks, back, and perineum are examined for signs of external injury such as penetrating wounds or ecchymosis. Abdominal distention may indicate major hemoperitoneum. Fifteen to 25% of alert patients with colorectal trauma do not exhibit peritoneal signs. A digital examination is performed both to examine for blood within the rectum and, in male patients, to ascertain the position of the prostate. The presence of blood in the rectum or a high-riding prostate can indicate severe pelvic injury. Pelvic fractures, especially those with disruption of the symphysis, are frequently associated with rectal injury.

Diagnostic Peritoneal Lavage

Diagnostic peritoneal lavage (DPL) has in the past been widely used to evaluate abdominal trauma, but is not always diagnostic in patients with colonic injury. A small incision is made below the umbilicus in cases of abdominal trauma without associated pelvic injury, and above the umbilicus in cases of suspected pelvic hematoma or pregnancy. One liter of normal saline is infused into the peritoneal cavity via a small catheter and then allowed to flow out of the abdomen by gravity through the same catheter. The results of DPL are considered positive for intra-abdominal injury if there are over 100,000 red blood cells/mL fluid, bacteria, or vegetable matter. The presence of either of the latter indicates probable colonic injury. Hemodynamically unstable patients require emergent laparotomy without prior DPL.

Abdominal Sonography

Sonography is very effective in detecting both free intraperitoneal fluid and solid organ injury. In the hemodynamically stable patient, sonography has virtually replaced DPL in the evaluation of the trauma patient. The Focused Assessment with Sonography for Trauma (FAST) includes evaluation of the pericardium, right and left upper quadrants, and pelvis. Although the quality of sonography is dependent on the person performing the examination, it is relatively inexpensive, not invasive, and a rapid bedside procedure that can be repeated frequently (Fig. 70-1).

Computed Tomography

Computed tomography (CT) is sensitive and specific in detecting intra-abdominal injuries, but it has no place in the evaluation of the hemodynamically unstable patient. Both the presence of free fluid within the abdominal cavity and extent of solid organ injuries can be determined by CT. As with ultrasound, hollow organ injuries are not detected as well as injuries to solid organs. CT is especially useful in evaluating the retroperitoneum, including retroperitoneal areas of the ascending and descending colon as well as retroperitoneal hematomas. CT is used extensively in the evaluation of the pediatric patient and in the evaluation of the stable patient with a flank injury. Triple-contrast CT, with contrast per os, per rectum, and intravenously, is helpful in such cases to evaluate the presence of intraperitoneal injury.

Assessment of Injury

Numerous trauma scores have been devised to assess the severity of the injury. These scores enable one to predict the likelihood of septic complications independent of the chosen operative treatment. The Injury Severity Score and

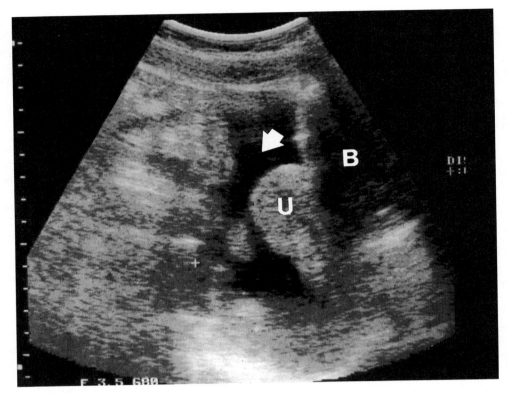

Figure 70-1
Sagittal view of lower abdominal ultrasound using 7-mHz transducer reveals free intraperitoneal fluid (arrow). B = bladder, U = uterus.

APACHE are two of the more common scoring systems in use.

■ TREATMENT OF COLONIC INJURY

A midline incision is preferred for exploratory laparotomy, because it permits rapid evaluation of all intra-abdominal organs. The first priority during initial surgical exploration is the control of hemorrhage and life-threatening injury. During the operation, fecal soilage can be minimized by clamping the colon distal and proximal to the site of injury. Colon injuries can be treated by the following methods:

- Debridement with primary repair
- Resection with anastomosis
- Exteriorization with or without resection
- Resection and diversion
- Resection and packing

True prophylactic antibiotic coverage of a trauma patient is not applicable because, by definition, contamination occurs after the trauma. With penetrating injuries, broad-spectrum antibiotics should be started in the emergency room and are usually continued for 24 hours. Meticulous irrigation of the abdominal cavity to remove particulate matter should be performed prior to closure.

Primary Repair

Many trials have shown primary repair to be safe, with equivalent or fewer complications than treatment by resection and diversion. Many trauma surgeons feel that primary repair can be used for both blunt and penetrating injuries, provided that no significant fecal contamination has occurred and if the surgery is performed within 8 hours after injury. Colon injuries due to low-velocity gunshot or stab wounds may also be suitable for primary repair.

To achieve best results and acceptable morbidity risk with primary closure, apply the following guidelines:

- The patient should be hemodynamically stable with few other injuries.
- The injury should not encompass more than 50% of the circumference of the colon.
- The blood supply of the injured segment should be intact.

After careful débridement and assessment of the severity of the colon injury, many injuries can be repaired by primary suture using either a one- or two-layer technique with absorbable suture. With primary repair, tension must be avoided. Longitudinal ruptures should be treated by longitudinal closure.

Stone and Fabian demonstrated in a randomized study that low-risk patients undergoing primary repair had lower colon-related morbidity rates than patients undergoing colostomy. Recent prospective studies from Sasaki and coworkers and from Gonzales and coworkers have also demonstrated that primary repair is a safe procedure compared to diversion and has a lower overall complication rate. In another series George and associates reported primary repair of penetrating colon injuries in 93% of patients.

Resection with Anastomosis

If more than 50% of the circumference of the colon wall has been injured or the blood supply to the bowel is compromised, resection and primary anastomosis should be considered. This procedure is most often performed for ascending colon injuries. Because ileostomies are associated with a significant morbidity rate, primary ileocolic anastomosis is preferable in patients without shock and in the absence of generalized peritonitis and other injuries. The treatment of left colon injuries is more controversial, however, as surgeons increasingly favor either primary repair or resection and anastomosis in hemodynamically stable patients.

Exteriorization with or without Resection

If there is any doubt about bowel viability after primary repair or resection and anastomosis or about the repair, this segment of bowel can be exteriorized to safeguard against leakage. Many surgeons feel that this type of procedure offers no advantage. If there are any doubts about bowel viability, a planned "second look" operation can be performed within 24 hours and, if necessary, a colostomy can be created at that time.

Resection and Diversion

Over the past years, the indications for colostomy have become more narrow. Colostomy is performed in patients in shock, in those with significant fecal contamination, or in those with other significant injuries. Mucous fistulas are generally not constructed for left-sided injuries.

Resection and Packing

Patients in unstable condition must be recognized as such and treated differently from patients without other associated injuries. Hypothermia (core temperature 34°C or less), acidosis (pH <7.2), and coagulopathy must be avoided. The only goal of surgery is to assess the injury and stabilize the patient. The injured colon should be resected by using a stapler, and the stapled ends are left in the abdomen. The abdomen can be packed or closed with mesh. A planned "second look" operation is performed 24 to 48 hours later, or when the patient has been stabilized. This plan may be necessary with significant hepatic or pelvic injury.

Laparoscopy

The role of laparoscopy in the trauma patient is limited, but has been shown to be of value in determining which penetrating abdominal injuries traverse the peritoneal cavity, especially in patients in whom the wound trajectory is unclear.

Treatment of Anorectal Injury

If a rectal injury is suggested either by digital rectal examination or by the mechanism of the trauma, sigmoidoscopy is mandatory. Depending on the severity of the injury, two types of treatment are possible. Minor injuries to the rectal wall without full-thickness perforation require no further treatment. Full-thickness perforations into the abdominal cavity or extraperitoneal space mandate intravenous antibiotics, débridement, proximal diversion, and drainage. A divided sigmoid colostomy with mucous fistula usually is performed in such cases. The site of the rectal injury should be surgically closed whenever possible, either transanally or transabdominally, at the time of the diversion. The benefit of a rectal "washout" with povidone-iodine has not been documented in a prospective clinical trial. If washout is performed, the anal sphincter should be dilated and irrigation performed using low pressure. If this procedure is not done, the risk of further contamination is increased. All rectal injuries require drainage. In some cases, a drain is placed through a separate incision posterior to the anus. Large setons or drains should not be passed through intact rectal wall (Fig. 70-2).

Anal injuries are, for the most part, caused by mechanisms similar to rectal injuries. In cases of sphincter disruption, anatomic reconstruction should be performed as soon as the patient is stable. Most surgeons agree that a temporary sigmoid colostomy is part of the management of severe anal injuries. Complications of anal trauma include sphincter dysfunction or anal stenosis due to scarring. In the stable patient, endoanal ultrasound can be used to evaluate sphincter integrity (see Fig. 70-2).

■ MANAGEMENT OF COLORECTAL INJURY IN SPECIAL SITUATIONS

Pregnancy

In addition to examination of the abdomen of the mother, the fetus must be monitored. Ultrasound is the diagnostic modality of choice. If free intra-abdominal fluid is detected by ultrasound without signs of injury to solid organs, laparotomy should be performed to exclude or confirm colonic injury.

Iatrogenic Rectal Injuries

Many iatrogenic injuries of the colon and rectum, like colonoscopic perforation, can be treated nonoperatively with systemic antibiotics and close observation. In cases of bowel perforation during barium enema examination, immediate laparotomy with fecal diversion is required owing to the high morbidity and mortality rates associated with barium peritonitis.

Pelvic Fracture and Rectal Trauma

The first step in management is control of hemorrhage by stabilization of the pelvis using external fixation or by MAST (medical antishock trousers) devices. In the case of pelvic hemorrhage, angiographic embolization is a preferred option, if available. Fecal diversion usually is

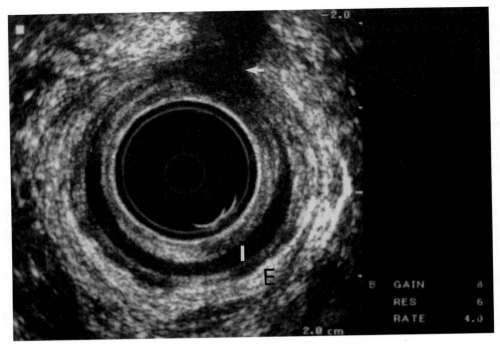

Figure 70-2
Endoanal ultrasound using 10 mHz transducer shows severe sphincter injury secondary to incorrect placement of drain through lower rectum and anal sphincter in a patient with rectal wall disruption following an impalement injury (arrow). E = external anal sphincter, I = internal anal sphincter.

performed after hemodynamic stabilization. Patients with this combination of injuries are at especially high risk of developing septic complications.

■ POSTOPERATIVE COMPLICATIONS

Several risk factors are associated with an increased rate of postoperative complications after colon trauma (Table 70-1). Intra-abdominal abscess is the most frequent severe postoperative complication of colorectal trauma, occurring in up to 20% of all patients.

CT- or ultrasound-guided percutaneous drainage is the preferred treatment for most intra-abdominal abscesses. Chapuis and coworkers prospectively randomized their trauma patients, regardless of risk factors, and demonstrated that outcome was dependent on injury severity, but not on the method of treatment. The incidence of intra-abdominal abscess or infection in the diversion group and primary repair group were 14 and 11%, respectively.

■ COLOSTOMY

Colostomy was formerly the treatment of choice to reduce the complication rate following colorectal trauma. If a colostomy is created, the two options are end-colostomy and Hartmann procedure, or end-colostomy and mucous fistula. Specific complications of a diverting stoma include parastomal hernia, stomal necrosis, peristomal abscess, and obstruction. These complications occur in approximately 5% of patients. There is no optimal time for stoma closure. This depends on the patient's condition and associated injuries. After trauma, the mean time of closure is usually between 6 weeks and 3 months postoperatively. In patients with rectal injury, the sphincter should be carefully examined prior to stoma closure. Barium enemas or proctosigmoidoscopy can be performed to ensure no fistulas are present; however, these studies are of low yield.

Fecal fistulas are rare in colostomy patients, but occur in 1 to 2% of patients following primary repair. Wound infec-

Table 70-1 Risk Factors for Postoperative Complications after Colorectal Trauma
Shock, systolic blood pressure <80 mm Hg
Intraoperative blood loss >1000 mL
Injury of more than 2 intra-abdominal organs
Delay in operation >8 hr
Excessive fecal contamination
Colon injury requiring resection
Major abdominal wall loss

tion is, however, more common in patients with diversion. In patients with limited contamination, the skin and the subcutaneous tissue can be closed primarily. In patients with significant contamination, wound infection can be avoided by leaving the skin and subcutaneous tissue open to close by secondary or delayed primary intention.

■ CONCLUSION

Systematic, careful evaluation and individualization of treatment are necessary in the management of the trauma patient with colorectal injury. Complication rates are related to the degree of injury but can be minimized by choosing the safest treatment based on thorough evaluation of associated injuries, reducing or eliminating contamination, and the time of surgery.

Suggested Readings

Ahmad W, Polk HC Jr: Blunt abdominal trauma: A prospective study with selective peritoneal lavage. Arch Surg 1976;111:489–492.

Carrillo EH, Somberg LB, Ceballos CE, et al: Blunt traumatic injuries to the colon and rectum. J Am Coll Surg 1996;183:548–542.

Chapuis CW, Frey DJ, Dietzen CD, et al: Management of penetrating colon injuries. Ann Surg 1991;213:492–498.

Dawes LG, Aprahamian C, Condon RE, Malangoni MA: The risk of infection after colon injury. Surgery 1986;100:796–803.

Flint LM, Vitale GC, Richardson, JD, Polk HC Jr: The injured colon. Relationships of management of complications. Ann Surg 1981;193:619–623.

Galandiuk S: Colorectal trauma. In Keighley MRB, Pemberton JH, Fazio VW, Parc R (Eds.). Atlas of Colorectal Surgery. New York, Churchill Livingstone, 1996, pp 345–356.

George SM, Fabian TC, Voeller GR, et al: Primary repair of colon wounds. Ann Surg 1989;209:728–734.

Gonzales RP, Merlotti GJ, Holevar MR: Colostomy in penetrating colon injury: Is it necessary? J Trauma 1996;41:271–275.

Rozycki GS, Ballard RB, Feliciano DV, et al: Surgeon-performed ultrasound for the assessment of truncal injuries: Lessons learned from 1540 patients. Ann Surg 1998;228:557–567.

Sasaki LS, Allaben RD, Golwala R, Mittal VK: Primary repair of colon injuries: A prospective randomized study. J Trauma 1995;39: 895–901.

Stone HH, Fabian TC: Management of perforating colon trauma: Randomization between primary closure and exteriorization. Ann Surg 1979;190:430–436.

Vitale GC, Richardson JD, Flint LM: Successful management of injuries to the extraperitoneal rectum. Am Surg 1983;49:159–162.

71

ENDOMETRIOSIS OF THE COLON AND RECTUM

H. Randolph Bailey, MD

Endometriosis, defined as functioning endometrial tissue outside the uterus, occurs in 4 to 17% of women in the reproductive age group, of whom only 5 to 10% have colorectal involvement. The most widely accepted theory of pathogenesis is the retrograde passage of endometrial cells through the fallopian tubes at the time of menstruation. These cells implant on the peritoneum and other locations. The most common sites of involvement are in the cul-de-sac of Douglas and the ovaries, and the most frequent locations of large bowel involvement are the rectum, rectosigmoid colon, and the appendix.

Significant symptoms of colorectal endometriosis include severe pelvic pain, dyspareunia, cyclic rectal bleeding, and bowel irregularity associated with menses. Only rarely do patients have overt obstructive symptoms of the large bowel. These complaints usually begin after age 20 and become progressively more severe. The differential diagnosis of intestinal endometriosis includes primary carcinoma, metastatic carcinoma (Blummer's shelf), diverticulitis, inflammatory bowel disease, pelvic inflammatory disease, radiation colitis, and ischemic stricture. Although cyclic rectal bleeding may be seen in up to a third of women with rectosigmoid involvement, the mucosa is rarely invaded by the endometriosis.

Most patients with endometriosis are initially evaluated and diagnosed by their gynecologist. Others may be found to have an intestinal lesion at the time of laparotomy without benefit of workup or bowel preparation. These patients present a particular management challenge. Most women with endometriosis are young and many desire to become pregnant. The choice of treatment modality depends on the age, parity, endocrine status, extent of disease, and attitude of the patient toward childbearing.

■ MEDICAL TREATMENT

The medical treatment of endometriosis involves hormonal manipulation, including the induction of pseudopregnancy with combination estrogen-progesterone (oral contraceptive agents), and induction of pseudomenopause with agents such as danazol and gonadotropin-releasing hormone (Gn-RH) agonists. Danazol functions as an antiestrogen, shutting down its production by the ovaries. The significant androgenic side effects of danazol have made its administration intolerable for many patients. Gn-RH agonists such as leuprolide acetate (Lupron) and nafarelin acetate (Synarel) have demonstrated equivalent antiestrogen activity with much lower androgenic side effects. These agents are quite effective in the treatment of small endometrial implants of the peritoneal surfaces, but do not have a major impact on the large endometrial deposits seen in ovarian endometriomas or colorectal nodules. They may be of value in the preoperative preparation of patients for infertility surgery because they decrease the vascularity of implants. The medical therapy of endometriosis is largely administered by the treating gynecologist and usually requires 3 to 6 months of treatment to produce significant benefit.

■ TIMING AND APPROACH TO SURGERY

Most decisions for operative intervention are again made by the gynecologist based on the severity of symptoms and response to medical treatment. Pain and infertility are the two most common symptoms that lead to surgical intervention. Colorectal endometriosis may also be encountered unexpectedly at the time of abdominal exploration. Its appearance may be difficult to distinguish from that of malignant neoplasia, and the true diagnosis may not be discovered until after radical surgery has been carried out. Endometrial implants on the bowel may appear as small pigmented nodules on the peritoneum or as larger lesions with puckering of the serosa that is indistinguishable from carcinoma. The submucosa may be involved, but extension of the lesions into the mucosa is quite rare. In the patient found to have a lesion of the bowel at laparotomy, treatment depends on making the proper diagnosis and on whether a significant obstructive component is present. Biopsy and frozen section may make the diagnosis, but intraoperative endoscopic evaluation of the bowel mucosa will assist in ruling out the possibility of primary bowel neoplasia. Obstructing or near-obstructing endometriomas should be resected and, if the bowel has not been adequately prepared, traditionally require a Hartmann procedure. If the diagnosis of endometriosis can be confirmed and there is no significant obstruction, the wisest course is often to close the abdomen and consider definitive treatment of the patient after bowel preparation and possible medical therapy. Nevertheless, some authors have suggested that primary anastomosis is safe in unprepared bowel. This approach may be particularly important for the cohort of patients who undergo unexpected resection for nonobstructing lesions.

■ INVESTIGATION

The patient suspected of bowel involvement with endometriosis, either because of laparoscopic findings or signs and symptoms, should be further evaluated and colorectal surgical consultation obtained prior to definitive surgery. Because of the uncertainty of preoperative diagnosis, patients are frequently inadequately prepared for resection of the colon and rectum when endometriosis is encountered. The most striking physical findings are nodularity and tenderness of the cul-de-sac and uterosacral ligaments, as well as adherence of the rectal wall to the cul-de-sac. With experience, the invasive nature of the cul-de-sac endometriosis can be appreciated on bidigital rectovaginal examination. Rigid sigmoidoscopy rarely reveals masses that extend completely through the mucosa but will often demonstrate flattening and puckering of the mucosa secondary to infiltration of the submucosa. These findings are subtle and may be overlooked by a less experienced examiner. The rigid proctoscope, as opposed to the flexible sigmoidoscope or colonoscope, may serve as an extension of the examiner's finger in "palpating" firm masses on the rectal wall, which are also tender when manipulated with the scope. Endometriosis is seldom positively diagnosed on endoscopic biopsy.

Diagnostic laparoscopy has been valuable in confirming the diagnosis of pelvic endometriosis. Many patients can be treated definitively through the laparoscope for their gynecologic disease. A frequent laparoscopic finding is that of cul-de-sac obliteration by rectosigmoid endometriosis. Although there are a few reports by highly skilled laparoscopists performing bowel resections for endometriosis, the difficulty of the pelvic dissection in most patients with colorectal endometriosis may render these patients unsuitable for laparoscopic colectomy.

Solid column barium enema has been more helpful than air contrast studies in evaluating the extrinsic involvement of the bowel by endometriosis. The presence of intact mucosa over the lesion helps rule out malignancy. Excretory urography (intravenous pyelogram) may be performed to assess possible ureteral involvement by the endometriosis (seen in approximately 15% of patients), and to look for congenital abnormalities such as duplication of the ureter or absence of the kidney.

Pelvic ultrasonography is utilized widely by gynecologists in making the diagnosis of endometriosis. Intrarectal ultrasound has not been as useful owing to tenderness of the rectal wall nodules and angulation and narrowing of the bowel, which make inserting the probe difficult.

■ SURGICAL TREATMENT

The issue of surgical management of colorectal endometriosis is controversial. For lesions producing partial obstruction, most authors advocate resection. Recommended options in dealing with less extensive lesions include oophorectomy or induction of hormonal menopause, excision without entering the mucosa, and segmental resection.

The traditional management of colorectal endometriosis has been ovarian ablation; most surgeons are reluctant to resect the colon or rectum. Although oophorectomy may cause regression of the endometrial nodule, large implants on the bowel may scar and ultimately lead to obstruction. This observation has been particularly true with castration by radiotherapy. Several authors have reported an incidence as high as 7% of bowel endometriosis in postmenopausal women. If women with colorectal endometriosis are treated by oophorectomy without hormonal replacement, they develop severe menopausal symptoms, accelerated atherosclerosis, osteoporosis, and atrophic vaginitis. If they are given hormonal replacement, the endometrial implants in the bowel may reactivate and grow. Although rare, endometrial implants may also undergo malignant transformation.

Recently, a number of reports have advocated bowel resection for severe endometriosis. Although bowel involvement with endometriosis is relatively common, involvement severe enough to require bowel resection occurs infrequently enough that few surgeons have an opportunity to see enough cases to develop an organized approach to the management of this disease.

We favor an aggressive approach to the evaluation and management of colorectal endometriosis, attempting to resect all visible and detectable endometriosis, whenever technically possible, and preserving fertility whenever feasible and desired by the patient. A large majority of patients with bowel involvement with endometriosis will have failed to respond to hormonal therapy prior to surgery. Some patients will develop the disease even after bilateral salpingo-oophorectomy due to residual ovarian tissue left on the pelvic side wall.

We obviously prefer to have an opportunity to evaluate and prepare the patients prior to their gynecologic procedure. A discussion of the risks of resection may be of more importance in patients with endometriosis than those with neoplasms or inflammatory problems of the large bowel, because the management of those diseases is less controversial. A full mechanical and antibiotic bowel preparation should be carried out preoperatively in anticipation of a possible bowel resection.

During the surgery, the gynecologist performs whatever procedure is necessary to remove the endometriosis from the genital organs. This approach can range from hysterectomy and bilateral salpingo-oophorectomy to a conservative, fertility-preserving procedure (leaving the uterus and at least one tube and ovary).

At the time of laparotomy, the gynecologist can assess the situation, and if superficial involvement of the bowel with endometriosis is encountered, it can often be resected or vaporized with the CO_2 laser. If deeply infiltrating nodules are encountered, however, the colorectal surgeon should be called to evaluate the situation and carry out the appropriate resection. The large majority of involvement will be encountered in the cul-de-sac, with complete obliteration of the cul-de-sac and dense adherence of the rectum to the posterior uterus and vagina. The ovaries and ureters may also be pulled into this mass as well. Dissection of larger lesions off the intact large bowel mucosa may be difficult because the submucosal dissection is quite bloody and the planes become indistinct. Recurrences may also be encountered when endometriomas are managed in this fashion. Full-thickness excision of the involved bowel, either by disk excision of smaller isolated lesions or segmental resection for larger lesions, may be technically more satisfactory, yielding a lower incidence of recurrence.

The most difficult portion of the resection may involve the anterior dissection. This area is best approached after first mobilizing the rectum posteriorly and laterally. The plane between the rectum and vagina can be dissected bluntly below the area of involvement and then the uterosacral ligaments and/or vaginal muscularis can be resected with the rectum, removing all the disease. A margin of 1 cm of soft, uninvolved bowel is sufficient. If the patient is not in a lithotomy position to allow access to the anus with a stapler, it may be preferable to perform a hand-sutured anastomosis in lieu of changing the position of the patient.

Among the arguments offered against colorectal resection for endometriosis have been the potential morbidity of the resection and anastomosis, as well as increased incidence of adhesions and consequent decrease in fertility. It is essential, therefore, if one is going to undertake an aggressive approach for benign, non-life-threatening disease, that it be done with low morbidity. In experienced hands, an aggressive approach, as outlined here, can provide excellent relief of symptoms in the vast majority of patients. The operations can be performed with minimal morbidity and maintenance of fertility in those women who desire to become pregnant.

Suggested Readings

Bailey HR: Colorectal endometriosis. Perspect Colon Rectal Surg 1992;5:251–259.

Bailey HR, Hoff SD: The handsewn colorectal anastomosis. Probl Gen Surg 1992;9:765–770.

Brooks JJ, Wheeler JE: Malignancy arising in extragonadal endometriosis: A case report and summary of the literature. Cancer 1977;40:3065–3073.

Burke P, Mealy K, Gillen P, et al: Requirement for bowel preparation in colorectal surgery. Br J Surg 1994;81:907–910.

Duepree HJ, Senagore AJ, Delaney CP, et al: Laparoscopic resection of deep pelvic endometriosis with rectosigmoid involvement. J Am Coll Surg 2002;195:754–758.

Howard FM: An evidence based medicine approach to the treatment of endometriosis-associated chronic pelvic pain: Placebo-controlled studies. J Am Assoc Gynecol Laparosc 2000;7:477–488.

Prystowsky JB, Stryker SJ, Ujiki GT, Poticha SM: Gastrointestinal endometriosis. Incidence and indications for resection. Arch Surg 1988;123:855–858.

Sievert W, Sellin JH, Stringer CA: Pelvic endometriosis simulating colonic malignant neoplasm. Arch Intern Med 1989;149:935–938.

Urbach DR, Reedijk M, Richard CS, et al: Bowel resection for intestinal endometriosis. Dis Colon Rectum 1998;41:1158–1164.

72

PNEUMATOSIS CYSTOIDES INTESTINALIS

Susan Galandiuk, MD

Pneumatosis cystoides intestinalis refers to the occurrence of multiple gas-filled cysts of the gastrointestinal tract that are subserosal, submucosal, or both. It is a fairly uncommon finding; only 410 cases had been described as of 1974. The entity of pneumatosis cystoides intestinalis was first described by Du Vernoi in 1730 in his description of a cadaver dissection, and it has long been noted in animals. Two types of pneumatosis cystoides intestinalis can occur: the fulminant form, which usually requires immediate surgical intervention, and the benign form, which is usually seen as an incidental finding at laparotomy for other reasons.

■ ETIOLOGY

Several different etiologic factors have been implicated in pneumatosis cystoides intestinalis. The most notable of these are mechanical and bacterial mechanisms. The mechanical theory suggests that gas is forced into the bowel wall by one or more mechanisms: (1) pulmonary action, (2) trauma, (3) mucosal breaks, (4) anastomoses, (5) obstruction, (6) increased pressure, or (7) increased peristalsis. Chronic obstructive pulmonary disease can be associated with pneumatosis cystoides intestinalis. Because coughing, artificial insufflation of the lungs, straining, and alveolar ectasia lead to alveolar rupture, air is thought to dissect into the mediastinum, along the great vessels to the retroperitoneum, and along the perivascular space, through the mesentery, to the bowel serosa. Experiments done in the early 1960s showed that injection of air into a catheter inserted into the mediastinum of animals resulted in subserosal pneumatosis cystoides intestinalis of the colon and sigmoid. The distribution of pneumatosis cystoides intestinalis is related to the bowel vascular pattern and has been reported following traumatic procedures such as sigmoidoscopy, colonoscopy, and mucosal biopsy. Breaks in mucosal integrity, such as ulcerations, may permit entry of intraluminal gas into the bowel wall. Pneumatosis cystoides intestinalis has been reported after end-to-end anastomoses, and with increased frequency in patients who have undergone jejunoileal bypass. In these patients, this condition affects the bypassed small bowel, usually the midjejunum. Some investigators believe that the ileosigmoid anastomosis permits large bowel flora to enter the ileum, with subsequent increased gas production and cyst formation. Others feel that the absence of bile may increase bacterial growth, leading to increased hydrogen production and cyst formation.

A bacterial etiology of pneumatosis cystoides intestinalis is supported by several analyses of cyst gas, which have demonstrated a hydrogen content of up to 50%. Because normal intestinal gas contains only 14% hydrogen and hydrogen is produced by bacteria, it has been suggested that bacteria may be responsible for pneumatosis cystoides intestinalis. Several investigators have injected organisms such as *Escherichia coli, Enterobacter aerogenes,* and *Clostridium perfringens* into intestinal submucosa in experimental animals and were able to induce pneumatosis cystoides intestinalis. It is thought that a functional break in the mucosa, with penetration of bacteria into the submucosa or subserosa or both, may be involved in the formation of intestinal gas cysts. Decreased intestinal mucosal resistance to infection or ulceration may lead to severe fulminant pneumatosis cystoides intestinalis, which is occasionally seen in adults. The bacterial etiology of pneumatosis cystoides intestinalis is also supported by breath-hydrogen analyses of affected patients. Many of these patients have increased breath hydrogen levels, leading some investigators to postulate that the high amount of hydrogen produced by bacteria may be responsible for the persistence of cysts.

■ CLASSIFICATION

Pneumatosis cystoides intestinalis is a relatively rare finding. It can be classified as either adult or infantile and may demonstrate benign and fulminant forms. Infantile pneumatosis cystoides intestinalis is usually submucosal and runs a fulminant course, with acute necrotizing enterocolitis, edema of the bowel wall, and dilatation of lymphatics. In adults, pneumatosis cystoides intestinalis is usually benign, although fulminant forms can occur, resulting in a high mortality rate despite surgery. The benign form can be divided into primary idiopathic and secondary. The cysts are submucosal, subserosal, or both, and are usually an incidental finding at laparotomy. Secondary pneumatosis cystoides intestinalis can be associated with a proximal gastrointestinal lesion such as pyloric stenosis or with chronic obstructive pulmonary disease. Pneumatosis cystoides intestinalis affecting the small bowel and ascending colon is thought to be secondary, whereas that affecting the descending colon is thought to be idiopathic or primary. The secondary form of the disease accounts for approximately 85% of cases. Table 72-1 illustrates some conditions associated with secondary pneumatosis cystoides intestinalis. One of the largest reviews of patients with pneumatosis cystoides intestinalis was reported by Koss; 58% of the patients in his series had a pyloric lesion, usually peptic ulcer with pyloric stenosis. The patient's age is usually between 30 and 50 years.

Table 72-1 Conditions Associated with Secondary Pneumatosis Cystoides Intestinalis

GASTROINTESTINAL

Necrotizing enterocolitis
Pseudomembranous colitis
Ulcerative colitis
Crohn's disease
Diverticulitis
Appendicitis
Cholelithiasis
Volvulus
Intestinal obstruction or strangulation
Intestinal anastomosis
Tuberculous enteritis
Refractory sprue
Mucosal trauma
Idiopathic megacolon
Neurogenic bowel dysfunction
Esophageal stricture
Peptic ulcer disease, including pyloric channel lesion
Pyloric stenosis

NONGASTROINTESTINAL

Chronic obstructive pulmonary disease, including
  emphysema and asthma
Cystic fibrosis
Collagen vascular diseases
Systemic sclerosis
Dermatomyositis
Exposure to alkyl halides, including chloral hydrate and
  trichloroethylene
Steroid therapy
Cancer chemotherapy
Transplantation immunosuppression
Kidney transplantation
Heart transplantation
Hepatic transplantation
Graft-versus-host disease, as in bone marrow
  transplantation
Lactulose treatment
Cytomegalovirus infection
Acquired immune deficiency syndrome
Leukemia
Lymphoma

Source: Wong SL, Galandiuk S: Pneumatosis cystoides intestinalis. In Zuidema GD, Yeo CJ (Eds.). Surgery of the Alimentary Tract, Vol. V, 5th ed. Philadelphia, WB Saunders, 2002, pp 461–466.

■ HISTOLOGY AND GROSS PATHOLOGY

The histologic changes observed in pneumatosis cystoides intestinalis can be replicated by injecting air into subcutaneous tissue. After several days there is a foreign body reaction with inflammation, development of a histiocytic lining, and pericyst fibrosis. The intestinal gas cysts of pneumatosis cystoides are also surrounded by foreign body giant cells and macrophages (Fig. 72-1). Serosal cysts usually occur near the mesenteric border, with a few cysts occurring on the antimesenteric margin. Cysts are fre-

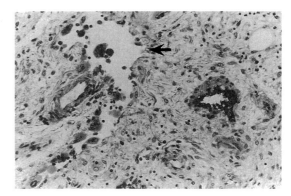

Figure 72-1
High magnification photomicrograph of pneumatosis cystoides intestinalis illustrating a gas cyst (arrow), lined in part by multinucleated giant cells. (From Galandiuk S, Fazio VW, Petras RE: Pneumatosis cystoides intestinalis in Crohn's disease: Report of two cases. Dis Colon Rectum 1985;28:951–956.)

quently located on loops of dilated bowel and range in size from a few millimeters to several centimeters. They can occur singly or in clusters, occasionally appearing like soap bubbles on the serosa (Fig. 72-2). Submucosal cysts, although not visible, give the bowel a spongy consistency. Cyst gas is under pressure and causes a hissing sound when the cysts are punctured.

■ SYMPTOMS

Symptoms of pneumatosis cystoides intestinalis are generally nonspecific and may include diarrhea and distention.

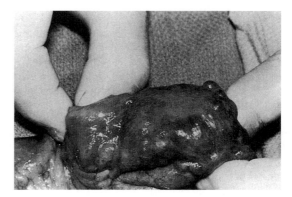

Figure 72-2
Benign pneumatosis cystoides intestinalis with subserosal cysts on the mesenteric margin of the ileum distal to a small bowel stenosis. (From Galandiuk S, Fazio VW, Petras RE: Pneumatosis cystoides intestinalis in Crohn's disease: Report of two cases. Dis Colon Rectum 1985;28: 951–956.)

If the lesion is located in the terminal ileum or colon, constipation, rectal bleeding, passage of mucus per rectum, abdominal pain, vague abdominal discomfort, weight loss, malabsorption, and excessive flatus may occur. Hemorrhage associated with pneumatosis cystoides intestinalis is probably due to congested mucosa overlying the cysts. If partial bowel obstruction secondary to cysts develops, vomiting and abdominal distention may occur. Diarrhea and abdominal distention are the most frequent presenting symptoms in patients with jejunoileal bypass and pneumatosis cystoides intestinalis. Increased or abnormal peristalsis due to the presence of cysts may lead to volvulus. Spontaneous pneumoperitoneum is seen more frequently with small bowel pneumatosis cystoides intestinalis. Complications of this condition are volvulus, pneumoperitoneum, intussusception, intestinal obstruction, tension pneumoperitoneum, intestinal perforation, and hemorrhage. Cysts can also lead to extrinsic compression of the bowel and may cause obstructing adhesions to form. The lack of symptoms is common, however, although only for the benign form of pneumatosis cystoides intestinalis. Fulminant pneumatosis cystoides intestinalis, as in necrotizing enterocolitis, may cause pneumoperitoneum, diarrhea, abdominal pain, bleeding per rectum, and ultimately an elevated white blood cell count with signs of peritonitis and sepsis.

■ DIAGNOSIS

In fulminant cases, a flat film of the abdomen may show gas in the bowel wall and pneumoperitoneum (Fig. 72-3). Rectal examination may reveal crepitance. There is often ischemic or hemorrhagic necrosis of the bowel with vascular thrombosis. In infantile pneumatosis cystoides intestinalis, one form of fulminant pneumatosis, concentric rings of gas in the small bowel are pathognomonic. Gas-filled cysts may protrude into the lumen, and streaks of air may separate loops of bowel. Gas may also be seen in the portal and mesenteric veins.

The benign forms of pneumatosis cystoides intestinalis may present with free air under the diaphragm or retroperitoneal gas outlining the kidneys, indicating spontaneous perforation with pneumoperitoneum or pneumoretroperitoneum. Pneumatosis cystoides intestinalis can result in prolonged recurring idiopathic and asymptomatic pneumoperitoneum without peritonitis. The small bowel is usually involved in these cases. Persistent pneumoperitoneum implies that gas enters the peritoneum at a rate equal to its absorption. Some investigators have suggested that subserosal cysts rupture, followed by repair of rupture sites and refilling of cysts. Repeated rupture occurs, with fibrosis and obliteration of older cysts. In the absence of pneumoperitoneum, pneumatosis cystoides intestinalis of the small bowel cannot be diagnosed on abdominal plain films. Cysts are difficult to differentiate from the small bowel gas pattern. Pneumatosis cystoides intestinalis of the colon may mimic the appearance of polyps on barium enema. Cysts can be differentiated from polyps and intramural hematomas, because the entire cyst

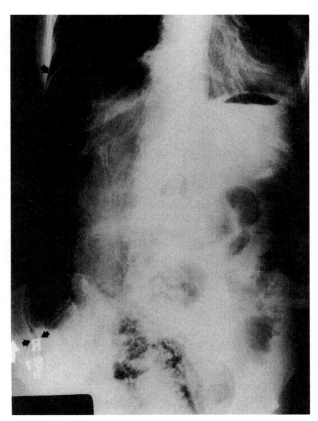

Figure 72-3
Flat film of the abdomen, revealing pneumoperitoneum and air in the bowel wall (dark arrow in right lower quadrant). (From Galandiuk S, Fazio VW, Petras RE: Pneumatosis cystoides intestinalis in Crohn's disease: Report of two cases. Dis Colon Rectum 1985;28:951–956.)

outline is visible. Unlike polyps, cyst size changes on distention of the colon, with flattening of the base. In addition, the radiolucency extends into the bowel wall. In some cases, pneumatosis cystoides intestinalis can be diagnosed by sigmoidoscopy or rectal examination. Differential diagnosis is rarely a problem; the condition is usually an incidental finding at laparotomy. On barium enema, cysts may mimic the appearance of polyposis. Enterogenous intestinal cysts may be confused with pneumatosis cystoides intestinalis, but these cysts are usually single and intramural, and they are most frequently seen in the terminal ileum. They are lined by intestinal mucosa and occur in young adults and children. Diffuse emphysema is usually secondary to a gas-producing infection and different from pneumatosis cystoides intestinalis, because gas is distributed in all tissue spaces. In emphysematous gastritis, gas is present in the stomach wall, but unlike pneumatosis cystoides intestinalis, this condition is characterized by hematemesis, pain, and leukocytosis. Lymphangioma of the peritoneum is a very rare entity that may resemble pneumatosis cystoides intestinalis. In lymphangioma of the peritoneum, however, cysts contain lymph rather than gas and are not lined by giant cells. In sclerosing lipogranulomatosis, which usually occurs in fat tissue, cystic spaces are lined by macrophages and giant cells, but these spaces are filled with fat rather than gas. Lymph nodes involved by Whipple's disease appear similar to those in pneumatosis but are associated with intestinal lipodystrophy, whereas those in pneumatosis are not.

■ THERAPY

The therapy of pneumatosis cystoides intestinalis is usually benign neglect, because it is frequently an incidental finding at laparotomy. If a segment of bowel affected with subserosal cysts is found during the course of a laparotomy, an effort should be made to ensure that no obstruction is present and that there is no loss of integrity of the bowel wall itself. If an obstruction is found, it should be relieved by resection or, in certain cases, strictureplasty. Selected patients with Crohn's disease with isolated short fibrotic strictures may be suitable for strictureplasty. If nonviable areas of bowel are found, the affected segments must be resected. The most important goal prior to therapy is to recognize the entity. As a result of carelessness, colectomies have been performed for pneumatosis cystoides intestinalis that appeared to be multiple polyps on barium enema study. In addition, abdominoperineal resections have been performed for lesions that were thought to be malignant but were actually cysts of pneumatosis intestinalis. If there is no obstruction and the affected bowel shows no vascular compromise, no therapy is indicated.

In the rare cases of symptomatic benign pneumatosis cystoides intestinalis, several treatment options are available. The recurrence rate after treatment is very high. Pneumatosis cystoides intestinalis has been successfully treated with high-flow oxygen breathing or hyperbaric oxygen therapy. This is based on the fact that gas cysts are filled mostly with gases other than oxygen at a pressure above atmospheric. Increasing the concentration of inhaled oxygen results in a higher partial pressure of oxygen and a lower partial pressure of nitrogen. Most of the oxygen is metabolized as it passes through tissue and the end capillary gas pressure decreases, resulting in a pressure gradient with diffusion of cyst gas into the blood. Several investigators have used inhalation of 70% oxygen via non-rebreather mask or head tent, resulting in a partial oxygen pressure of approximately 250 mm Hg for 4 to 10 days. This results in partial or complete radiologic and colonoscopic resolution of pneumatosis cystoides intestinalis and associated symptoms. Only hyperemic and edematous mucosa are visible on follow-up colonoscopy. In order to avoid pulmonary and central nervous system toxicity, hyperbaric oxygen treatment at 2.5 atm for 2.5 hours for 2 to 3 consecutive days has also been used. Recurrence after such treatment has been reported as early as 1 year after treatment and may occasionally occur immediately. The other type of therapy for patients with symptomatic benign pneumatosis cystoides intestinalis is an elemental diet for a 2-week period. High fasting hydrogen breath levels decrease after this diet, and gas production is decreased, because the elemental diet does not reach the colon and less hydrogen is formed by bacteria. Recurrence rates after this form of treatment are also high, and cysts have been reported to occur as early as 4 months after resuming a regular diet. Another alternative treatment is chronic oral antibiotic therapy with agents such as neomycin or Flagyl. The recurrence rate is likewise high after cessation of treatment.

In patients with fulminant pneumatosis cystoides intestinalis, the treatment is determined by the patient's clinical condition. The presence of pneumoperitoneum or air in the bowel wall on abdominal plain film in a patient with an increasing white blood cell count, pyrexia, and a deteriorating clinical course should alert the physician to the possibility of fulminant pneumatosis cystoides intestinalis with hemorrhagic or ischemic necrosis of the bowel. In these cases, the patient's condition is usually poor, and resection of the involved segment with exteriorization of the ends of the bowel is usually safest. Failure to operate may lead to excessive bowel necrosis, sepsis, and death. Even with surgery, the mortality rate is high.

Suggested Readings

Galandiuk S, Fazio VW: Pneumatosis cystoides intestinalis: A review of the literature. Dis Colon Rectum 1986;29:358–363.

Koss LK: Abdominal gas cysts (pneumatosis cystoides intestinalis hominis): An analysis with report of a case and critical review of the literature. Arch Pathol 1952;53:89–94.

Masterson JS, Fratkin LB, Osler TR, Trapp WG: Treatment of pneumatosis cystoides intestinalis with hyperbaric oxygen. Ann Surg 1978;187:245–247.

van der Linden W, Marsell R: Pneumatosis cystoides coli associated with high H_2 excretion: Treatment with an elemental diet. Scand J Gastroenterol 1979;14:173–174.

73

CONSTIPATION

Tonia M. Young-Fadok, MD, MS, FACS, FASCRS
John H. Pemberton, MD

Constipation is the reason for 2.5 million physician visit each year—a prevalence of 1.2% in the general population. Among the general population not seeking medical care, however, the prevalence varies from 2 to 28%. Most patients are seen by general and family practitioners (31%), internists (20%), and pediatricians (15%), and only 4% are seen by gastroenterologists. The magnitude of the problem is further illustrated by the $400 million spent on laxatives annually. Constipation itself is not a disease and, thus, has no single etiology or mechanism of pathogenesis; rather, constipation is a symptom or more often a constellation of symptoms. Depending on the individual patient, "constipation" may mean infrequent bowel movements, small hard pellet-like stools, straining to evacuate, incomplete evacuation or painful evacuation, and, in some patients, even the absence of a daily stool. Because the definition of constipation varies so markedly among individuals, it is important that the physician clarify the patient's intended meaning. A recent international conference attempted to delineate more clearly the parameters by which to diagnose constipation. The definitions presented required two or more of the following features to be present for 12 months when not taking laxatives:

Fewer than three bowel movements per week
Straining more than 25% of the time
Incomplete evacuation more than 25% of the time
Hard pellet-like stools more than 25% of the time
Fewer than two bowel movements per week, present for 12 months

Making the diagnosis of constipation is merely labeling a symptom; establishing the underlying etiology is frequently more complex, but is of vital importance in determining the appropriate therapy. The focus of this chapter is primarily on those forms of severe lifestyle-altering constipation considered to be the result of abnormalities in the motility or function of the colon or the pelvic floor muscle. The rarity of such severe constipation is illustrated by the fact that, of patients referred to gastroenterologists in a tertiary care setting for severe chronic constipation considered not amenable to further aggressive management, only 7% are surgical candidates. The checkered history of surgical intervention for constipation is almost entirely due to lack of understanding of underlying pathophysiology. This has only relatively recently been elucidated, allowing identification of appropriate surgical

candidates. Surgical intervention is appropriate only for patients in whom a diagnosis of colonic slow transit constipation (STC) has been made. Such patients comprise a very small fraction of all patients presenting with a complaint of constipation, but may be dramatically helped by surgery. This is not the case for patients with other causes of constipation. The availability of new tests and improved analysis of colonic motility and pelvic floor function have allowed identification of those patients with colonic STC who can be improved by surgical intervention.

As patient selection is by far the most critical aspect determining success of the surgical approach, an orderly workup is extremely important. This evaluation may be considered in three stages, each of which will be discussed in detail. First, it is necessary to differentiate between colonic and extracolonic causes of constipation. Second, if a colonic cause is suspected (by excluding or correcting extracolonic causes), it is important to differentiate between functional and structural causes. Third, once a functional cause has been established (by excluding a structural etiology), further investigations allow classification into one of four groups: slow transit constipation (STC), pelvic floor dysfunction (PFD), combined STC and PFD, and irritable bowel syndrome (IBS).

■ COLONIC VERSUS EXTRACOLONIC CAUSES

The establishment of a colonic cause of constipation relies on exclusion of extracolonic causes. Although numerous extracolonic causes can precipitate constipation (Table 73-1), the majority of them are usually relatively simply ruled out by a careful history and physical examination. This evaluation may often reveal the cause of constipation, such as medications, coexistent medical problems such as hypothyroidism, or symptoms and signs of cancer. The severity of the patient's symptoms should be clarified, as this will indicate the patient's level of distress associated with the complaint. The number of stools per week may be formally evaluated with a daily diary. Treatments already tried are important in assessment of severity. The exact nature of the symptoms should be elicited, as this may help to suggest the underlying mechanism; for example, infrequent bowel movements suggest STC, but daily, difficult evacuation suggests PFD. The report of hard stools or excessive straining may be more objectively assessed by inquiring about the need for enemas or digital disimpaction.

The vast majority of patients are helped by conservative measures, which include addition of fiber to diet, an exercise regimen, and possibly bulk-forming laxatives. Obviously, recent changes in bowel function, or factors such as the patient's age or family history, would prompt colonic screening prior to a trial of conservative therapy.

■ FUNCTIONAL VERSUS STRUCTURAL CAUSES

Determining that a functional cause of constipation exists requires exclusion of structural abnormalities. The history

Table 73-1 Extracolonic Causes of Constipation

Endocrine and Metabolic Disorders

Carcinomatosis
Diabetes mellitus
Glucagonoma
Hypercalcemia
Hyperparathyroidism
Hypokalemia
Hypopituitarism
Hypothyroidism
Milk-alkali syndrome
Pheochromocytoma
Porphyria
Pregnancy
Uremia

Neurologic Disorders

Peripheral
    Autonomic neuropathy
    Chagas' disease
    Hirschsprung's disease
    Hypoganglionosis
    Intestinal pseudo-obstruction (myopathy, neuropathy)
    Multiple endocrine neoplasia, type IIB
    von Recklinghausen's disease
Central
    Cauda equina syndrome
    Cerebrovascular accident
    Ischemia
    Meningocele
    Multiple sclerosis
    Paraplegia
    Parkinson's disease
    Shy-Drager syndrome
    Tabes dorsalis
    Trauma to nervi erigentes
    Tumors

Collagen Vascular and Muscle Disorders

Amyloidosis
Dermatomyositis
Myotonic dystrophy
Scleroderma

Table 73-2 Drugs Associated with Constipation

Analgesics
Anticholinergics
Antispasmodics
Antidepressants
Antipsychotics
Antiparkinsonian drugs

Cation-Containing Drugs

Aluminum (antacids, sucralfate)
Barium sulfate
Calcium (antacids, supplements)
Iron supplements
Metallic intoxication (arsenic, lead, mercury)

Others

Anticonvulsants
Antihypertensives
Calcium channel blockers
Ganglionic blockers
Monoamine oxidase inhibitors
Opiates
Vinca alkaloids

may be suggestive of some of the causes listed in Table 73-2. For example, a prior history of diverticulitis may suggest a sigmoid stricture. The physical examination includes palpation of the abdomen, observation of the perineum, and a digital rectal examination. Observation of the patient while straining is an important aspect of the physical examination. Straining in the left lateral position allows observation of descent and elevation of the perineum during simulated evacuation and retention squeeze; while straining on the toilet may help identify constipation due to rectal prolapse. The digital anal examination should evaluate sphincter tone at rest and during efforts to squeeze. The external sphincter will be recruited during squeeze efforts; the internal sphincter will not tighten. The puborectalis muscle should be palpated and compressed to determine if this elicits pain along the border of the muscle, suggestive of puborectalis spasm syn-

drome. The patient may also be instructed to attempt to expel the examiner's finger. Vaginal examination may reveal the presence of a rectocele.

More invasive investigations start with a colonoscopy or barium enema (combined with a rigid or flexible sigmoidoscopy). Either approach can help to establish or rule out a structural abnormality, but the two together frequently provide complementary information. Information regarding functional abnormalities may also be obtained from the endoscopic examination, by asking the patient to strain during inspection of the rectum and observing for "occult" rectal prolapse; such information is not always wholly accurate, however. Solitary rectal ulcer, although a structural abnormality (with characteristic histology), is indicative of a functional abnormality of the pelvic floor. Further contrast studies, in the form of a defecating proctogram, are helpful in diagnosing pelvic floor dysfunction and the presence of rectoceles and enteroceles (again, structural abnormalities resulting from a functional problem). Structural causes of constipation may be considered in two categories: either isolated anatomic abnormalities or abnormal anatomic presentation of an underlying defect in pelvic floor function. The former (Table 73-3) can usually be approached surgically. The latter (Table 73-3) may be best treated either by pelvic floor retraining or by a combination of surgery and retraining; surgery alone is not often helpful. These disorders are covered in other chapters.

■ DETERMINING THE CAUSE OF FUNCTIONAL CONSTIPATION

When an anatomic abnormality of the colon has been excluded as a cause for constipation, then functional

Table 73-3 Structural Causes of Constipation

Isolated Anatomic Defect
Carcinoma
Crohn's stricture
Diverticular stricture
Hirschsprung's disease
Large polyp
Volvulus
Anatomic Defect and Pelvic Floor Dysfunction
Descending perineum syndrome
Occult rectal prolapse
Rectal prolapse
Rectocele
Solitary rectal ulcer syndrome

constipation is likely. Further workup includes both an assessment of colonic activity and an assessment of pelvic floor function.

Colonic motility, measured by transit study, is assessed to determine if movement of fecal material through the colon is excessively prolonged. The two types of transit studies are marker and scintigraphic studies. Marker studies involve the ingestion of 20 marker tablets taken at the same time on 3 consecutive days. Plain abdominal radiographs are then taken on days 4 and 7, and transit time through different segments of the colon (right, left, and rectosigmoid) can then be calculated. Mean transit time in normal control subjects is 36 ± 4 hours. Patients who have a transit time of greater than 72 hours are considered to have slow transit constipation. This study has the advantage of being inexpensive and widely available, but requires 7 days to complete.

Scintigraphic transit studies require the ingestion, with a mixed meal, of technetium and indium particles in a delayed-release capsule coated with the pH-sensitive polymer methacrylate. Each capsule contains technetium (^{99m}Tc)-radiolabeled Amberlite resin particles to assess gastric and small bowel transit; and indium-111 particles in a coated capsule that disperse in the ileocecal region to assess regional colonic transit. Scanning at 24 and 48 hours allows determination of the geometric mean. Median values for healthy control subjects are 3.53 ± 0.57 and 4.18 ± 0.4.

An evaluation of pelvic floor function is extremely important in determining whether surgical intervention is appropriate in patients with severe constipation. Possibly the most useful single test is anal manometry, with inclusion of a balloon expulsion test. Different versions of anal manometry are in use, but one common version uses an 8-channel perfused catheter, which is inserted in the anal canal, allowing pressures to be measured at predetermined points in the canal as the catheter is withdrawn. Resting and squeeze pressures are measured, in addition to rectal compliance and determination of the presence or absence of the rectoanal inhibitory reflex. The balloon expulsion test is an excellent assessment of overall pelvic floor function. It does not measure a specific physiologic abnormal-

ity, but it indicates the ability of the individual to coordinate pelvic floor function in such a manner that defecation is possible. This study involves inserting a balloon containing 50 mL of warm water into the rectum and having the patient attempt to expel the balloon. If this is not possible, gradually increasing weights are added to assist in expulsion. Of healthy patients who could not pass the balloon spontaneously, a mean weight of 126 ± 41 g is required; patients with PFD require a mean weight of 590 ± 114 g. An abnormal result is considered to be a requirement of more than 200 g in weight to assist expulsion. The presence of an anorectal inhibitory response can also be determined during manometry testing; it is useful for excluding the rarely seen adult presentation of Hirschsprung's disease.

Additional tests of pelvic floor function are performed if necessary. These tests include studies of the mechanism of defecation, such as a defecating proctogram or scintigraphic defecography. The defecating proctogram visualizes the anatomy of the rectum and anal canal during straining, and hence is useful for demonstrating occult prolapse and physiologically significant rectoceles (those that obstruct defecation or require digitation or manipulation for emptying). Scintigraphic balloon topography can demonstrate abnormalities in the anorectal angle (which opens 17 ± 3 degrees in healthy control subjects but only 4 ± 4 degrees in patients with PFD. It can also assess descent of the perineum, which is 2.3 ± 0.2 cm in normal control subjectss, but only 0.5 ± 0.1 cm in patients with PFD, demonstrating a relatively immobile perineum.

If all the foregoing tests are normal, both slow transit constipation and pelvic floor dysfunction are excluded. Such patients frequently have constipation due to IBS. Surgery will not produce resolution of symptoms in such patients, who are best managed by a gastroenterologist with an interest in IBS.

■ MEDICAL THERAPY FOR CONSTIPATION

Given the prevalence of the complaint of constipation, careful consideration must be given to the potential for excessive health care expenditure. The majority of patients with simple constipation can be identified with a careful history and physical examination, and can be appropriately treated with increased dietary fiber (up to 20 g per day), increased fluid intake, and an exercise regimen. Others may require adjustment of medication or treatment of underlying comorbidities. The majority (85%) of physician visits for constipation, however, result in a prescription for laxatives or cathartics.

Even the 4% of patient visits to a gastroenterologist have the potential for significant impact on health costs. In one study of 51 patients seen in a tertiary referral center, the average expenditure for the diagnostic evaluation was $2752. Still, 61% had constipation of no clear etiology despite a rigorous evaluation. This statistic underscores the need for an orderly approach to all patients with constipation and particularly for those with severe symptoms.

■ MEDICAL THERAPY FOR FUNCTIONAL CONSTIPATION

Slow Transit Constipation

Slow transit constipation (STC) is identified in 7 to 24% of patients presenting to tertiary referral centers with severe constipation. In such patients dietary fiber is often unhelpful and may exacerbate symptoms of pain and bloating. Lesser grades of STC may be helped by a bowel training regimen: evacuating with an enema or glycerine suppository as needed, taking an osmotic diuretic if necessary (lactulose, Milk of Magnesia, magnesium citrate), and at a consistent time of day, providing a distraction-free 15 to 20 minutes on the toilet. Mineral oil, agents that provoke intestinal secretion (e.g., docusaste), or stimulant laxatives (senna, bisacodyl) are often not recommended because of the chronicity of the problem and the risk of side effects, but may be reserved for failure of the preceding regimen, prior to consideration of polyethylene glycol (PEG) solution or even surgery. Cisapride, which is a 5-HT4 agonist, has been found to be effective only in mild constipation. Newer 5-HT uptake inhibitors hold promise of acting in a more specific manner to increase stool frequency in constipation. With more severe forms, even PEG solution may eventually become ineffective. Such patients have severe, lifestyle-altering constipation, many of them having hospital admissions for disimpaction before they consider surgery as a reasonable alternative to improve their quality of life.

Pelvic Floor Dysfunction

An intensive course of pelvic floor retraining may help some patients with pelvic floor dysfunction. This approach involves treatment by a multidisciplinary team, including a surgeon or gastroenterologist, specialist in rehabilitation medicine, psychiatrist, and physical therapist trained in techniques of biofeedback. These courses require a strong commitment on the part of the patient.

Pelvic floor retraining comprises biofeedback and relaxation training. As an intervention, such a therapy is free of morbidity, although it is demanding of the patient. Biofeedback enhances a process of relearning and trains patients to gradually suppress the nonrelaxing activity of the pelvic floor and to coordinate relaxation with pushing in order to achieve defecation.

Biofeedback has been shown to reduce obstructive symptoms with an increase in the frequency of bowel movements, a more obtuse anorectal angle during defecation, and more dynamic pelvic floor movements when the anal sphincter is contracted. One series of 69 patients with documented pelvic floor discoordination (determined by measurements of anorectal angle, perineal descent, scintigraphy, and balloon expulsion) underwent a 10-day inpatient retraining program consisting of dietary manipulation, relaxation, and coordination retraining and biofeedback. The median weight required to expel a balloon from the rectum before retraining was 284 g, but after training it was 0 g. At 2 months 80% had improved defecation function, the mean number of stools per week was 7, 94% did not use finger disimpaction, 69% did not need enemas, and 67% passed stool spontaneously. At 3 years, 65% were still passing stools spontaneously, and 88% did not require enemas. Hence, these patients with pelvic floor dysfunction recovered defecation function and experienced long-term relief after a retraining program.

■ SURGICAL THERAPY FOR FUNCTIONAL CONSTIPATION

Surgical intervention is appropriate only for documented severe STC. This point cannot be overemphasized, as the results that are obtained from surgical intervention are directly related to the thoroughness of the preoperative assessment and exclusion of inappropriate candidates. Many small series of colectomy performed for constipation exist in surgical literature with unacceptable results, such as persistent constipation, or dissatisfaction with the procedure in up to 50% of cases. Closer inspection of the evaluation protocols employed in such series will often reveal doubt regarding the presence of colonic STC, failure to rule out pure pelvic floor dysfunction, or failure to identify and treat PFD when it coexists with STC.

A rigorous preoperative evaluation will identify a highly select group of patients with STC, who have been shown to benefit from surgical intervention. In one series, 1009 patients with severe chronic constipation considered not amenable to further aggressive management by the referring physicians were assessed in a large tertiary referral center. All patients underwent a full history and physical examination to exclude extracolonic causes of constipation, followed by colonoscopy or barium enema to rule out structural abnormalities. Excluded from this series were patients with megacolon, megarectum, volvulus, prolapse, colonic pseudo-obstruction, tumors, and polyps. Patients were then evaluated with marker or scintigraphic colonic transit studies, pelvic floor function studies including anorectal manometry, balloon expulsion, scintigraphic measurements of anorectal angle and pelvic floor descent, scintigraphic evacuation, and a defecating proctogram. (In our routine practice, only the first two of these studies are routinely employed.) Seventy-four patients (68 women) with STC were identified: 52 with STC alone and 22 with STC and PFD. The patients with combined STC and PFD underwent pelvic floor retraining prior to surgery. Postoperatively, all patients were able to pass a stool spontaneously, 97% of patients were satisfied with the results of surgery, and 90% had a good or improved quality of life. There were no operative deaths and the morbidity rate was 9% with small bowel obstruction and 12% with a prolonged ileus. There was no difference in outcome of surgery in patients with STC alone compared with those having both STC and PFD.

No evidence suggests that any form of surgical procedure provides benefit to patients with pure PFD or with IBS. As noted previously, those patients in whom there is a combined presentation of STC and PFD should undergo pelvic floor retraining prior to consideration of an operation for the slow transit component of their constipation.

Even patients with pure STC and no evidence of PFD may benefit from evaluation by a physical therapist familiar with pelvic floor retraining, as patients with normal pelvic floor function tests may still have acquired abnormal patterns of straining.

The timing of surgery is frequently best decided by the patient, often when all conservative measures have failed to result in an acceptable quality of life. Preoperative counseling includes discussion of standard operative risks such as bleeding, wound infection, and anastomotic leakage, and an admonition that symptoms such as cramping and bloating may or may not be improved by the procedure.

Preparation for the procedure is more involved than with most other operations on the colon. These patients are frequently employing electrolyte solutions merely to have a bowel movement once a week, and hence a single application often will not be sufficient to produce an adequate bowel preparation. Multiple enemas and laxatives, in addition to 48 hours of a liquid diet, may be necessary. Perioperative intravenous antibiotics with or without oral antibiotics (as part of one's standard bowel preparation) are also given.

The procedure of choice is subtotal colectomy (total abdominal colectomy) and requires removal of the colon from the terminal ileum to the rectosigmoid junction and creation of an ileorectal anastomosis. Performance of a less extensive procedure, for example, ileosigmoid anastomosis or a segmental colectomy alone, produces poor results and has been one of the factors responsible for the notoriety of surgical intervention for constipation. Less extensive operations are frequently followed by the need to complete the operation eventually and perform an ileorectostomy. Transit studies, marker or scintigraphic, do not demonstrate segmental differences in the colon of patients with STC, probably explaining the poor results from segmental resections. The anastomosis may be constructed in a side-to-end fashion, if there are discrepancies in caliber between the rectum and the terminal ileum, or in an end-to-end fashion if the two lumens are closely matched.

Patients are counseled that in the early postoperative period stools may be not only frequent but loose, with a risk of incontinence. Surprisingly few, however, do in fact experience loss of control and most soon settle into a more regular habit, with a median of two to four bowel movements per day. Approximately 10% use some form of antidiarrheal (e.g., diphenoxylate and atropine) to control frequency of bowel movements immediately after surgery; this use is not necessary by 1 year postoperatively. More than 90% of patients have either solid or semisolid stools by 6 months, and in series with longer-term follow-up, these stools tended to become more solid up to 3 years later.

In summary, patients with severe lifestyle-altering constipation are relatively rare despite the high prevalence of the complaint of constipation. These patients need a carefully planned investigation to determine the most appropriate course of therapy. Only patients with colonic STC are candidates for surgery. When STC coexists with pelvic floor dysfunction, it should be identified and treated prior to proceeding with operative therapy. In carefully selected patients, the results of surgical therapy are excellent, with improved quality of life in the vast majority of patients.

Suggested Readings

Bartolo DCC, Kamm MA, Kuijpers H, et al: Working Party Report: Defecation disorders. Am J Gastroenterol 1994;89:S154-S159.

Juhasz ES, Pemberton JH, Rath DM: Early and late results of pelvic floor retraining for pelvic floor discoordination. Gastroenterology 1993;1104:A530.

Nyam DCNK, Pemberton JH, Ilstrup DM, Rath DM: Long-term results of surgery for chronic constipation. Dis Colon Rectum 1997;40:273-279.

Piccirillo MF, Reissman P, Wexner SD: Colectomy as treatment for constipation in selected patients. Br J Surg 1995;82:898-901.

Whitehead WE, Chaussade S, Corazziari E, Kumar D: Report of an International Workshop on Management of Constipation. Gastroenterol Int 1991;4:99-113.

74

SMALL BOWEL OBSTRUCTION

David W. Dietz, MD

Small bowel obstruction is one of the most common conditions encountered by colorectal surgeons. A recent analysis of Health Care Financing Administration data found that 14% of patients undergoing abdominal surgery will require hospitalization for small bowel obstruction within 2 years and that 2.4% will require adhesiolysis; colorectal procedures, in particular, seem to carry the highest risk. Approximately 300,000 operations are performed each year in the United States for this disorder at a cost of over $1 billion.

Postoperative adhesions are the most common cause of small bowel obstruction, accounting for 50 to 75% of cases in recent series. Hernias and malignancy account for most of the remainder (20 to 40%), and volvulus, Crohn's disease (Chapter 77), chronic radiation enteritis (Chapter 82), intussusception, and gallstone ileus make up only a fraction.

Perhaps the most critical components in the management of patients with bowel obstruction are the recognition and prevention of significant bowel ischemia. Timely surgical intervention, prior to the development of transmural necrosis, will limit complications and improve outcome. In one recently published series of over 1000 patients undergoing surgery for small bowel obstruction, nonviable strangulated bowel was present at laparotomy in only 16% of cases but the risk of death in this group was increased fourfold.

■ PRESENTATION AND DIAGNOSIS

Nausea and vomiting, crampy pain, abdominal bloating, and obstipation are the hallmark signs of small bowel obstruction. The degree to which each of these contributes to the clinical picture will depend on the location, degree, and duration of the obstruction. A thorough history and physical examination should be performed. The patient is questioned regarding previous surgical procedures, known hernias, prior abdominal or pelvic radiation therapy, history of malignancy, signs or symptoms of undiagnosed cancer, or personal or family history of Crohn's disease. Significant comorbidities should also be sought. A general assessment of the patient's toxicity is made and vital signs obtained. The presence or absence of distention, surgical scars, or ventral and groin hernias is noted, and the abdomen is palpated to assess for peritonitis, masses, or incarcerated hernias not obvious on inspection. Percussion may reveal tympany from gas-filled bowel loops, and on auscultation characteristic high-pitched, tinkling bowel sounds may be heard. A digital rectal examination should always be done in order to exclude an obstructing rectal cancer.

Laboratory tests include white blood cell count, hematocrit, electrolytes, serum bicarbonate, blood urea nitrogen, and creatinine. Amylase and lipase are usually requested to rule out pancreatitis with associated ileus. Serum lactate levels may be obtained, but they should not be relied upon as a sole indicator of ischemia.

Commonly accepted signs of strangulated bowel are fever, tachycardia, leukocytosis, sepsis, peritonism, and the presence of continuous as opposed to intermittent pain. If any of these signs are found, the suspicion of ischemia should be high; however, these signs may also be found in many patients without strangulation and are, therefore, nonspecific. In general, the diagnosis of strangulated bowel should be made based on a combination of clinical experience and the foregoing indicators. In many cases, however, this determination is not made until laparotomy. Timely surgical intervention, therefore, may be the best means of avoiding the progression to bowel ischemia. This fact is underscored by a report from Sarr and colleagues, who found that the traditional clinical parameters usually employed to predict strangulation were neither sensitive nor specific. Nearly one third of patients with strangulation were not diagnosed until the time of surgery.

■ RADIOGRAPHIC STUDIES

Plain Radiographs

An acute abdominal series is the initial imaging study performed in most patients suspected of having small bowel obstruction and consists of both upright and supine abdominal films and an upright chest x-ray. Typical findings include dilated, air-filled loops of small bowel; air-fluid levels; and an absence or paucity of colonic air. These findings may be absent, however, when the obstruction is proximal or the dilated bowel loops are mostly fluid-filled. The sensitivity of plain radiographs in detecting small bowel obstruction is approximately 60%. The finding of pneumatosis intestinalis or portal vein gas is worrisome for advanced bowel ischemia.

Computed Tomography

Abdominopelvic computed tomographic (CT) scanning is being used increasingly as a primary imaging modality in patients with small bowel obstruction. In addition to establishing the diagnosis, CT scan may also be able to precisely define a transition point and reveal secondary causes of obstruction such as tumors, hernias, intussusception, volvulus, or inflammatory conditions such as Crohn's disease and radiation enteritis. CT scan may also reveal closed loop obstruction or signs of progressive ischemia, such as bowel wall thickening, pneumatosis, or portal vein gas. Several studies have shown that the sensitivity of CT in diagnosing small bowel obstruction approaches 90 to 100%.

Contrast Studies

Contrast studies employing water-soluble agents are frequently used in patients with acute small bowel obstruction. In patients with distal small bowel obstruction, a contrast enema is an efficient means by which colonic obstruction can be excluded. Antegrade studies of the small bowel can help to differentiate partial from complete obstruction, and may therefore predict the need for surgical intervention. In fact, some authors have used small bowel contrast studies as a "screening test" for patients presenting with adhesive obstructions. Failure of contrast material to reach the colon by 24 hours is used as an indication for surgical exploration. Several studies have also shown that the antegrade administration of contrast agents may speed the resolution of partial small bowel obstruction, presumably through an osmotic effect. However, conflicting data exist, and the therapeutic effects of the small bowel contrast study remain to be defined.

Barium studies have no role in the evaluation of patients with acute obstruction, but they can be valuable in those with chronic or relapsing symptoms. Perhaps the most sensitive test in these cases is enteroclysis, for which barium is administered beyond the pylorus via a nasoenteric catheter. This method minimizes the dilution of the barium as it passes distally and can reveal mucosal lesions not evident on routine small bowel studies. Another diagnosis that should be kept in mind in patients with chronic obstructive symptoms is intestinal malrotation. The typical finding of the duodenum not crossing to the left of the spinal column on plain films or contrast studies may be overlooked by even experienced clinicians.

■ INITIAL THERAPY AND NONOPERATIVE MANAGEMENT

Once the diagnosis of small bowel obstruction is made, the patient is admitted to the hospital. Those with peritonitis, perforation, signs of ischemic bowel, or irreducible incarcerated hernias are immediately prepared for laparotomy with prompt fluid resuscitation. A urinary catheter is inserted to guide resuscitation, with the end points being resolution of tachycardia and hypotension or achieving a urine output of at least 0.5 mL/kg/hr. Broad-spectrum antibiotic coverage is begun, and a nasogastric tube is inserted to decompress the stomach, as these patients are at risk for aspiration on induction of general anesthesia. Patients with no prior surgical history and no obvious hernias on examination may be taken for laparotomy after resuscitation, or further imaging studies such as CT scanning may be obtained. Patients with suspected large bowel obstruction should undergo a contrast enema.

If signs of perforation or ischemia are not present, a trial of observation may be undertaken. Patients with partial small bowel obstructions secondary to adhesions will resolve with nonoperative therapy in 80% of cases. The success rate for patients initially presenting with complete obstruction is significantly lower. The nonoperative management of small bowel obstruction consists of fluid and electrolyte replacement, bowel rest, and tube decompression. The debate between standard nasogastric tube versus long nasoenteric tube decompression has mostly settled in favor of the nasogastric tube. This preference is in part due to the fact that long tubes with mercury-weighted tips are no longer available for use. Long tubes are also more difficult to place, requiring special expertise, serial radiographic studies, or fluoroscopy to guide insertion. Recently, interest in the use of nasoenteric tubes has resurfaced, mostly among radiologists.

Narcotic analgesics may be administered to comfort the patient, but not to the point of diminishing mental status. The practice of withholding pain medication for the purpose of obtaining a baseline examination is probably unnecessary. Serial abdominal examinations should be performed to assess for increasing tenderness or the presence of peritoneal signs. Any change in the patient's condition that suggests developing bowel ischemia (constant pain, peritonitis, signs of sepsis, etc.) mandates exploratory laparotomy. In general, a nonoperative course may be followed for 24 to 48 hours. If the obstruction has not resolved within that time period, it is unlikely to do so and laparotomy is advised.

■ INDICATIONS FOR SURGERY

A number of studies have attempted to define certain criteria that would reliably predict the presence or absence of strangulated bowel. Common signs used are fever, tachycardia, hypotension, leukocytosis, metabolic acidosis, and elevated lactate levels. Unfortunately, none of these indications have been shown to be particularly accurate. The best predictor remains sound clinical judgment. Certainly, patients with fever, peritonitis, pneumoperitoneum, or overt sepsis should undergo emergent laparotomy, for these signs are hard evidence of transmural bowel necrosis. The presence of early ischemia, however, is much more difficult to discern. It is not uncommon for patients with small bowel obstruction to present with tachycardia, relative hypotension, mild acidosis, and leukocytosis, all of which may be secondary to dehydration. These patients should be aggressively rehydrated with isotonic intravenous fluids, and the same parameters should be reassessed. Persistence of any of these signs after adequate rehydration should prompt immediate laparotomy. Adherence to this simple algorithm should minimize the progression to strangulation while limiting the number of unnecessary laparotomies.

Distinguishing between partial and complete obstruction is also a key element in deciding which patients should be taken for early operation. As already stated, the likelihood of resolution of a complete obstruction with expectant management is low (20%) and carries the risk of delaying operative therapy until after a nonviable strangulation or perforation has occurred, complications which substantially increase the mortality rate. Although this distinction may be difficult clinically, some useful caveats can be applied. The passage of stool or flatus cannot be relied upon as an accurate predictor because patients with complete obstruction may continue to pass stool and flatus until the bowel distal to the site of obstruction is evacuated. However, if this continues for more than 12 hours after the onset of obstructive symptoms, the likelihood of complete obstruction is diminished. The passage of large volumes of watery stool in the face of vomiting and distention is pathognomonic for partial small bowel obstruction. The onset of flatus, however, usually signals the beginning of resolution of the obstruction.

Radiographic studies can also aid in making the distinction between complete and partial obstruction. Serial plain films of the abdomen that show persistent colonic air are good indicators of the presence of a partial as opposed to complete obstruction. Small bowel contrast studies may suggest complete obstruction when the contrast agent fails to reach the cecum, usually within 24 hours. Finally, CT scan can also differentiate complete obstruction from ileus or partial obstruction, and may reveal the underlying cause. CT scan is especially useful in cases in which a cause of obstruction other than adhesions is suspected.

■ SURGICAL TECHNIQUE

Adhesive Obstruction

Once the decision has been made to operate, the adequacy of resuscitation is confirmed and broad-spectrum antibiotics active against enteric pathogens are administered. The peritoneal cavity is entered through the previous incision (usually midline). At this point in the operation the risk of inadvertent enterotomy is very high because bowel loops are distended and usually adhesed to the undersur-

face of the abdominal wall. Once the fascia is encountered, the application of gentle pressure with the bevel of the scalpel blade, rather than a cutting stroke, is used to breach the peritoneal cavity. Using this technique, the surgeon is usually able to recognize an adherent bowel loop before enterotomy occurs.

In the best scenario, a single constricting band will be encountered which can be sharply divided to relieve the obstruction. In the worst cases, the peritoneal cavity will be totally obliterated by scar tissue. An orderly and systematic approach to adhesiolysis is advised in these instances. First, the underside of the midline scar is cleared so that the entire length of the incision can be opened, if necessary. Next, adhesions to the abdominal wall are dissected laterally in both directions until the paracolic gutters are reached. This stage will allow the placement of a self-retaining retractor to facilitate exposure. If bowel distention is severe, needle decompression may be used to gain additional working space. Attention is then turned to the pelvis, where the most difficult adhesions are often encountered. Rather than separating individual bowel loops at this stage, the small bowel residing in the pelvis should be mobilized "en masse" by lysing adhesions to the pelvic structures in an anterior-to-posterior fashion in order to "roll" the mass of intestine up and out of the pelvis. The final portion of this stage of the operation involves mobilizing the plane between the small bowel mesentery and the retroperitoneum until the duodenum is encountered. Only at this point are all adhesions between individual bowel loops lysed in order to free the entire length of the small intestine. The bowel is then inspected for any coexisting disease and for enterotomies or serosal tears created in the course of mobilization.

Assessment of bowel viability is usually possible by using the triad of color, peristalsis, and mesenteric pulsations. If these signs are questionable, the ischemic segment should be wrapped in warm, wet packs and viability reassessed after 15 minutes. If still in doubt, use of the Doppler flow probe or systemic injection of fluorescein dye followed by inspection of the bowel under a Wood's lamp may aid in decision making. If the area in question is a short segment, it may be best to proceed with resection. If an extensive segment is of questionable viability, then a second-look operation 24 hours later should be planned before committing the patient to a massive small bowel resection.

Some debate exists as to the need for complete adhesiolysis when the point of obstruction is encountered early in the operation. It is our policy to divide the majority of adhesions if this can be done safely. This practice will facilitate inspection of the entire length of the small bowel and allows for the placement of antiadhesion barriers if desired (see Prevention of Adhesions).

Hernias

Incarcerated hernias account for 10 to 20% of cases of small bowel obstruction. These patients usually require urgent operation as they are at significant risk for strangulation and are not likely to resolve their obstruction spontaneously. This situation is especially true for femoral hernias, which, due to the narrow defect, are especially prone to ischemic complications. Both incarcerated inguinal and femoral hernias are usually readily identified on physical examination. Obturator hernias, on the other hand, are easily overlooked. The complaint of pain along the inner aspect of the thigh in a patient with bowel obstruction should alert the clinician to this entity. Ventral hernias in morbidly obese patients may also be difficult to appreciate on examination and in these cases a CT scan will help make the diagnosis.

Findings of erythema and edema of the skin overlying the incarcerated hernia along with tenderness are signs of strangulation. In these cases, immediate surgery should be performed. If these signs are not present, then a gentle attempt at reduction is appropriate. If successful, elective repair may be performed in the near future. A waiting period of at least 24 hours is advised to allow edema within the tissues to resolve.

Incarcerated inguinal hernias are approached through a standard inguinal incision. Once the hernia sac is opened, the bowel can be inspected for viability. If viable, the bowel is returned to the peritoneal cavity, the sac excised, and standard hernia repair performed. Necrotic bowel can usually be resected via the inguinal approach, and after healthy small bowel is delivered through the defect, an anastomosis is performed. If this is not possible or bowel of questionable viability escapes back into the peritoneal cavity, a midline incision should be made for thorough exploration. Repair of an inguinal hernia that contains strangulated bowel is best performed using a layered repair with permanent monofilament suture. Mesh should not be employed owing to the risk of infection. Incarcerated femoral hernias can be approached via a low inguinal incision, preperitoneal approach, or low midline incision. In these cases, it is usually necessary to convert to a lower midline incision if necrotic bowel is present.

Malignancy

Small bowel obstruction secondary to malignant disease usually results from metastases or involvement of the small intestine by advanced cancer in a nearby organ. Primary small bowel cancers, usually adenocarcinomas or gastrointestinal stromal cell tumors, are less common causes. The surgical mortality rate in this group of patients ranges from 10 to 40%, with median survival time after the perioperative period measured only in months. Although the prognosis in these patients is grim, a limited palliative procedure in cases of obstruction secondary to advanced systemic malignancy can improve quality of life. Resection may offer better palliation than bypass, but the findings at the time of operation should dictate the procedure performed. In cases of a frozen abdomen from carcinomatosis, creation of a loop stoma in the bowel proximal to the obstruction is adequate palliation. If no amount of small bowel can be mobilized, then a gastrostomy tube is placed for decompression. If this situation is recognized preoperatively, then placement of a percutaneous gastrostomy tube and institution of hyperalimentation may allow the patient to return to home for the remainder of their life. Involvement of a palliative care specialist in these cases is important, as the administration of narcotic pain medication, antiemetics, anticholinergics, and somatostatin analogs will be the mainstay of treatment.

■ SPECIAL SITUATIONS

Early Postoperative Bowel Obstruction

Early postoperative bowel obstruction is generally defined as mechanical obstruction occurring within 1 month of abdominal or pelvic surgery. This condition is special in that attempts at relaparotomy in the early postoperative period frequently result in disastrous complications. The mantra of "never let the sun rise or set on a patient with bowel obstruction" should not be broadly applied in this group. An intense inflammatory response usually begins within the abdomen at 7 to 10 days postoperatively and persists for at least 6 weeks. If forced to operate during this period, the surgeon is likely to encounter dense hypervascular adhesions that may obliterate the peritoneal cavity. The risk of enterotomy and subsequent fistulization is extremely high. In addition, vascular injury or extensive deserosalization of the bowel may lead to massive resections. Therefore, immediate reoperation for early postoperative bowel obstruction is not advised, especially considering the fact that the development of strangulation in this setting is extremely rare. These patients should be managed conservatively with nasogastric suction and intravenous fluids. If resolution does not occur within the first 5 to 7 days, a percutaneous gastrostomy tube is placed for longer-term decompression and the patient is started on hyperalimentation. We will frequently discharge patients from hospital on this regimen and then perform laparotomy in 3 to 6 months if the obstruction has not resolved. However, if peritonitis or signs of sepsis are present initially or develop during the course of nonoperative therapy, surgery must be performed immediately. There is a place for very early exploration within the first 5 to 7 days postoperatively if obstruction is recognized promptly. The adhesions encountered during this time period have not usually become severe and can be dealt with safely.

Intussusception

Although common in the pediatric population, intussusception accounts for only 1% of cases of small bowel obstruction in adults. In 90% of adult cases, the intussusception is caused by an intraluminal neoplasm being pulled into the more distal bowel by peristalsis. As the proximal segment (the intussusceptum) is drawn further into the distal bowel (the intussuscipiens), the mesentery is compressed and ischemia of the intussusceptum may result. These patients may describe intermittent episodes of obstruction that are frequently accompanied by the passage of bloody stool mixed with mucus ("red currant jelly"). The diagnosis may be made by contrast studies, CT scan, or occasionally colonoscopy, but in many cases it is an unexpected finding at laparotomy. Attempts at reduction of the intussusception, either hydrostatic or at surgery, are not advised. Because most cases are secondary to neoplasm, formal resection of the involved segment is the treatment of choice.

Gallstone Ileus

Gallstone ileus is another rare cause of small bowel obstruction, accounting for 3% of cases with intestinal obstruction. Patients are usually elderly, and a strong female predominance is seen. The pathologic picture is that of a large gallstone eroding from the gallbladder directly into an adjacent segment of bowel (duodenum, jejunum, or hepatic flexure colon), the two structures being adherent due to chronic cholecystitis. This stone then passes distally in the intestinal tract until it becomes impacted, usually in the terminal ileum. The classic radiographic features of gallstone ileus are small bowel obstruction, a radiopaque gallstone outside the right upper quadrant, and pneumobilia. Termed *Rigler's triad*, this combination of findings is present in less than 10% of cases, mostly because the majority of gallstones are radiolucent.

Surgery is necessary in all cases. At the time of laparotomy, the entire small bowel should be carefully palpated to identify multiple stones if present (5% of cases). The obstructing gallstone can usually be "milked" proximally to healthy bowel, where an enterotomy is made for stone extraction. If the stone is so tightly impacted that it cannot be moved, then resection of the segment is indicated. Some controversy exists as to whether the biliary tract disease should be addressed at the same operation. This approach is usually discouraged owing to the dense inflammation often present within the right upper quadrant in patients with biliary enteric fistulas. Additionally, these patients are typically elderly, have extensive comorbidities, and come to operation late in the course of the obstruction. Cholecystectomy can be performed electively at a later date, if necessary. The risk of recurrent obstruction secondary to passage of a new stone in the interim is less than 10%.

■ PREVENTION OF ADHESIONS

Over 90% of patients undergoing abdominal surgery will develop adhesions. Adhesion formation can occur wherever the visceral or parietal peritoneum has been disturbed. Once an area of injury is established, fibrin is deposited and then organizes to form a matrix for collagen deposition. Bowel motility and endogenous lubricants attempt to counteract this process, but in most cases, adhesions will eventually result as the deposited collagen matures. As discussed earlier, the progression from early to mature adhesions usually takes approximately 6 weeks.

A number of strategies have been developed to minimize, prevent, or influence adhesion formation. Gentle handling of tissues, avoiding the deposition of talc by wearing powder-free gloves, and copious lavage of the peritoneal cavity at the conclusion of the operative procedure are simple means that should be employed in all cases. When particularly severe adhesion formation can be anticipated, for instance, in patients with multiple recurrences of small bowel obstruction, the use of long intestinal tubes placed at the conclusion of surgery to "splint" the bowel open during adhesion formation has been advocated. Recently, several chemoprophylactic agents have been developed in an attempt to reduce or eliminate adhesions through a barrier mechanism. The best studied of these is a bioresorbable membrane of modified sodium hyaluronate and carboxymethylcellulose. A large multicenter study by Becker and associates has shown that this material substantially reduces the incidence, severity, and amount of adhesion formation. Its efficacy in reducing the incidence of adhesive bowel obstruction, however, has not yet been reported.

Suggested Readings

Beck DE, Opelka FG, Bailey HR, et al: Incidence of small-bowel obstruction and adhesiolysis after open colorectal and general surgery. Dis Colon Rectum 1999;42:241–248.

Becker JM, Dayton MT, Fazio VW, et al: Prevention of postoperative abdominal adhesions by a sodium hyaluronate-based bioresorbable membrane: A prospective, randomized, double-blind multicenter study. J Am Coll Surg 1996;183(4):297–306.

Fevang BT, Fevang J, Stangeland L, et al: Complications and death after surgical treatment of small bowel obstruction. A 35-year institutional experience. Ann Surg 2000;231(4):529–537.

Jenkins JT, Taylor AJ, Behrns KE: Secondary causes of intestinal obstruction: Rigorous preoperative evaluation is required. Am Surg 2000;66:662–666.

Legendre H, Vanhuyse F, Caroli-Bosc FX, et al: Survival and quality of life after palliative surgery for neoplastic gastrointestinal obstruction. Eur J Surg Oncol 2001;27:364–367.

Macari M, Megibow A. Imaging of suspected acute small bowel obstruction. Semin Roentgenol 2001;36:108–117.

Sarr MG, Buckley GB, Zuidema GD: Preoperative recognition of intestinal strangulation obstruction: Prospective evaluation of diagnostic capability. Am J Surg 1983;145:176–182.

75

SHORT BOWEL SYNDROME

Marc Brand, MD
Douglas Seidner, MD
Ezra Steiger, MD

Short bowel syndrome (SBS) occurs as a result of an extensive loss of functional intestinal surface area. Usually, SBS is the consequence of extensive small bowel resection due to mesenteric ischemia, intestinal volvulus, trauma, malignancy, inflammatory bowel disease, or congenital abnormalities. Intestinal obstruction due to intra-abdominal adhesions and primary and secondary forms of pseudo-obstruction are less common causes of this syndrome. The clinical features include chronic diarrhea, dehydration, electrolyte abnormalities, and malnutrition, which are caused by the malabsorption of fluid, electrolytes, and nutrients. This chapter will review how extensive intestinal resection affects gastrointestinal physiology so that a rational approach can be taken toward the nutritional care of patients with this devastating condition.

■ GASTROINTESTINAL PATHOPHYSIOLOGY FOLLOWING INTESTINAL RESECTION

Surgical resection or bypass of up to 50% of the small intestine can be tolerated quite well so long as a portion of this does not include the distal ileum. Resection of 50 to 75% of the small intestine often can be managed through dietary manipulation, oral supplementation, and the use of medications aimed at enhancing intestinal absorption. Prolonged parenteral support is almost certainly required when more than 75% of the small intestine is resected. In terms of small bowel length, 150 cm ending in a stoma or 60 to 90 cm anastomosed to a moderate length of colon can be used as a point of reference to help determine who will and who will not require long-term parenteral nutrition. However, it is the overall function and not just the length of remaining bowel that will determine the intensity of support a patient will require. Some of these factors are outlined in Table 75-1.

The region of bowel resection clearly has a bearing on the consequences of SBS. For nutrient absorption, proximal resection involving the jejunum is better tolerated than resection of an equivalent length of ileum because the ileum can easily adapt to the absorption of amino acids, sugars, and water-soluble vitamins while retaining its unique role in the absorption of vitamin B_{12} and bile

salts. Resection or bypass of the duodenum is also well tolerated in this regard; however, supplementation with calcium, iron, and folate may be needed because the duodenum, along with the proximal jejunum, is the primary site for the absorption of these nutrients. Fluid absorption can be maintained with proximal small bowel resection because the colon is capable of increasing its absorptive capacity from 2 to 6 L per day. Although nutrient absorption can often be maintained with distal intestinal resection, dehydration may develop if the colon is also resected because of the inability of the remnant bowel to absorb the proximal gastrointestinal secretions. This problem can sometimes be compensated for by using oral rehydration solutions, which take advantage of the active cotransport of sodium and glucose. Finally, gastric acid hypersecretion is a common phenomenon that can occur after extensive small bowel resection. This excess acid can cause peptic ulceration of the proximal gastrointestinal tract and can aggravate malabsorption by inactivating pancreatic enzymes and bile salts, which work best at a neutral pH. This hypersecretion usually lasts no more than a few months to a year and is best managed with a histamine (H_2)-blocking agent or a proton pump inhibitor.

The terminal ileum plays a unique role in the absorption of vitamin B_{12} and bile salts. Vitamin B_{12} injections should be started after surgical resection of more than 100 cm of the terminal ileum to avoid the development of the hematologic and neurologic consequences that occur with the deficiency of this vitamin. When a lesser resection is undertaken, one should keep in mind that other conditions may contribute to the development of vitamin B_{12} deficiency, including atrophic gastritis, gastric resection, bacterial overgrowth, and pancreatic insufficiency, so vitamin B_{12} injections may be required in these patients, too. As far as bile salts are concerned, the bile salt pool can be maintained when only a portion of the distal 100 cm of terminal ileum is resected or involved with mucosal disease because fecal losses are low and hepatic synthesis can compensate to make up for these losses. A secretory diarrhea, which has been termed *choleraic diarrhea,* can develop if a sufficient quantity of bile salts come in contact with the mucosa of the colon. With a slight decrease in the bile salt pool, steatorrhea is usually mild, with less than 20 g of fat being lost in the stool each day. Cholestyramine is often helpful in controlling diarrhea in this setting. When

---

Table 75-1 Factors Favoring Intestinal Absorption after Extensive Bowel Resection

Length of remaining bowel
   >60–90 cm of small bowel with colon
   >150 cm of small bowel alone
Jejunum versus ileum resected
Ileocecal valve present
Absence of mucosal disease
Presence of colon
Normal hepatic and pancreatic function
Adequate intestinal adaptation

more than 100 cm of distal ileum is removed or diseased, a normal bile salt pool cannot be maintained because intestinal losses exceed the synthetic capacity of the liver. Under these circumstances, steatorrhea can be modest to severe, with more than 20 g of fat being lost in the stool each day. A low-fat diet can be helpful in these patients because a component of the diarrhea results from the secretory effect that unabsorbed long-chain fatty acids has on the mucosa of the colon. Because it is often difficult to determine the extent of intestinal resection based on surgical or pathologic reports, it may be necessary to determine the severity of fecal fat losses by performing a Sudan stain of a stool sample or providing the patient with a therapeutic trial of cholestyramine or a low-fat diet.

Small bowel motility is also altered following extensive intestinal resection. More distal portions of the intestine tend to increase the transit time of chyme through the previous segments of bowel. In the small bowel, this effect is most prominent for the ileum and has been termed the *ileal brake*. Hence, resection of the jejunum will have a less detrimental effect on intestinal motility when compared to an equivalent length of ileal resection. Furthermore, the presence of the ileocecal valve and colon will increase intestinal transit time when compared to transit time when these segments are absent.

The number of bacterial species, especially anaerobic ones, and the density of their growth can be increased following resection of the ileocecal valve. Bacterial overgrowth can lead to the deconjugation of bile salts, which are then less able to emulsify dietary fats; will interfere with the absorption of vitamin B_{12}; and can result in direct mucosal injury. Oral antibiotics may help improve the malabsorption associated with bacterial overgrowth. In addition, D-lactic acidosis should be considered in patients with SBS who develop a metabolic encephalopathy and an anion gap positive metabolic acidosis. These patients are colonized with bacteria that produce D-lactic acid, which cannot be metabolized by humans. Management requires restriction of dietary carbohydrates and an oral nonabsorbable antibiotic.

Nephrolithiasis and cholelithiasis can also complicate extensive intestinal resection. Nephrolithiasis usually results from hyperoxaluria, which is common following small bowel resection when all or a portion of the colon remains. Dietary oxalate normally passes harmlessly through the gut as an insoluble calcium salt; however, with steatorrhea, the calcium has a higher affinity for the fatty acids than the oxalate, and the oxalate remains in a soluble form, which is absorbed by the colon and is finally excreted by the kidney. Management of this problem, described in more detail later, includes restriction of dietary fat and oxalate and supplementation with oral calcium. In cases refractory to this approach, cholestyramine, which works by binding intraluminal oxalate, can be given. Cholelithiasis is the result of a diminution in the size and concentration of the bile salt pool. Because the management of complications associated with cholelithiasis may be more difficult in patients with SBS, it has been argued that a prophylactic cholecystectomy is in order for patients who undergo massive small bowel resection.

■ INTESTINAL ADAPTATION

Intestinal adaptation is a process that takes place following extensive small bowel resection whereby the remnant bowel improves its ability to absorb nutrients. This process has been shown to begin immediately after intestinal resection and to progress for the next 1 to 2 years or more. Clinical improvement may be observed over time and includes a decrease in diarrhea and malabsorption and improved tolerance toward enteral feeding. Structurally, the remnant bowel is seen to both elongate and dilate and have an increase in villus height, crypt depth, cell proliferation, and mucosal enzyme activity. Although the exact mechanisms that lead to intestinal adaptation are not known, similar changes have been shown to occur on an experimental basis with various nutrients and neurohumoral factors. An understanding of these factors may help to optimize the care of patients with SBS.

Dietary nutrients play a pivotal role in the adaptive response of the intestinal tract, with a whole diet leading to a greater degree of adaptation than an elemental diet. The effect of nutrients on intestinal morphology is due to the direct effect of these metabolic substrates, the simulation of the enteric nervous system and local hormones in the gut, and to a lesser degree direct mechanical stimulation. Secretin and cholecystokinin are released by the duodenum and proximal jejunum in response to a meal and in turn lead to the secretion of pancreatic enzymes and bile salts, respectively, into the intestinal lumen. These gastrointestinal hormones and digestive secretions have been shown to directly stimulate mucosal proliferation. Enteroglucagon, epidermal growth factor (EGF), growth hormone (GH), and insulin-like growth factor-1 (IGF-1) are other hormones that have been shown to have potent trophic effects on the intestine. Enteroglucagon and EGF originate from the gastrointestinal tract, and GH and IGF-1 are systemically derived. Of these hormones, GH has been the most extensively studied. GH enhances mucosal hyperplasia in the small bowel and colonic mass following extensive intestinal resection in animals. GH can also increase the transport of sodium and water in the small and large bowel and amino acid transport in the jejunum.

Glutamine is the preferred oxidative fuel for the mucosa of the small intestine and is an important substrate for cells with a rapid turnover, including enterocytes and lymphocytes. Glutamine-enriched parenteral nutrition has been shown to prevent mucosal atrophy and intestinal permeability in critically ill patients and has been shown to enhance postresection hyperplasia following massive small bowel resection in animals. Enteral glutamine enhances glucose and sodium absorption.

These observations have led to two clinical trials that have studied the effect of GH and glutamine on bowel adaptation and nutrient absorption. In a study of 47 patients with TPN-dependent SBS, Byrne and coworkers were able to significantly reduce the need for TPN through the provision of GH, glutamine, and a modified diet. After the 1-month study period, 40% of the patients were weaned from TPN while an equal number were able to significantly reduce their reliance on this therapy. The relative importance of the hormonal therapy versus the diet modification in this study has been questioned, as the GH was provided for only 21 days. More recently, Scolapio and associates performed a randomized, double-blind, placebo-controlled, crossover study with a similar treatment aim in eight patients with SBS and was able to show only a modest improvement in electrolyte transport and delayed gastric emptying. Small bowel morphology, stool volume, and macronutrient absorption did not improve, raising a question about the efficacy of this approach. Currently, the individual components of this program are being investigated.

■ MANAGEMENT AFTER SMALL BOWEL RESECTION

Optimal patient care requires a thorough assessment to determine the integrity of the remaining small bowel and the nutritional deficits that might be present. Each patient's treatment plan must be individualized and should include appropriate dietary instructions, vitamin and mineral supplementation, and medications to promote digestion and minimize nutrient, fluid, and electrolyte losses. An overview of one approach can be seen in Figure 75-1. Careful monitoring is an integral part of this program and ensures that the nutritional and metabolic needs of each SBS patient are met. Many of the adverse consequences of SBS can be avoided through proper and timely intervention.

Parenteral Nutrition

Parenteral nutrition (PN) should be started soon after intestinal resection in patients who will likely suffer from SBS. PN assures that protein and energy needs are met so that wound healing and recovery following surgery are successful. Typical requirements range from 1.5 to 2.0 g/kg/day for protein and 35 to 40 kcal/kg/day for energy and are usually maintained at this stage and after hospital discharge to promote weight gain in individuals who have lost weight prior to surgery.

Maintenance of a patient's fluid status can be challenging, especially in those with proximally diverted small bowel. Our approach is to initially provide 35 mL/kg/day

TREATMENT OF THE SHORT BOWEL SYNDROME

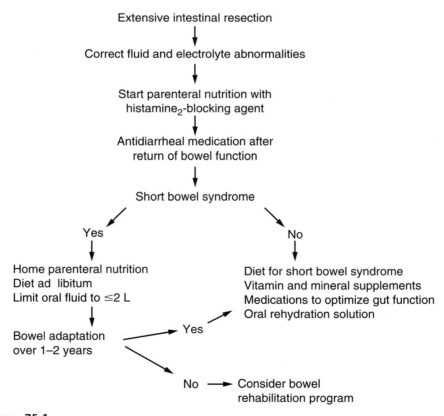

Figure 75-1
A typical approach for the management of a patient following extensive intestinal resection. Short bowel syndrome initially occurs if there is less than 60 to 90 cm of small bowel anastomosed to the colon or 150 cm of small bowel ending at an enterostomy. See text for discussion of other factors that may affect the absorptive function of the remaining bowel.

of fluid in adult patients as a standard maintenance requirement and to run a second intravenous line to meet gastrointestinal losses. Once the average volume of intestinal losses is known, this volume can be added to the PN solution. When oral intake is resumed, it may become necessary to restrict the volume and type of oral fluid intake because intestinal secretions can overwhelm the absorptive capacity of the gut, as was previously discussed. This need can be determined by closely monitoring the intake and output of enteral fluids. Patients who are found to be secretory are advised to take in no more than 2 L of oral fluid, and if they have excessive thirst due to dehydration, extra intravenous fluids and not oral fluids will be needed. If fluid requirements are in excess of the 4 L that can be provided in most PN containers, it may be necessary to provide octreotide subcutaneously to control intestinal secretions. The major drawback to this approach is that octreotide is a potent suppressor of intestinal hormone secretion and thus may impair the ability of the remaining bowel to undergo adequate adaptation.

The PN solution can also serve as a vehicle for the delivery of an H_2-blocking agent, which, as previously discussed, is required for several months following extensive intestinal resection. Finally, a sufficient amount of micronutrients must be added to the PN to meet a patient's requirements. A typical PN formula for an adult with SBS is illustrated in Table 75-2.

Dietary Management

The goal of dietary management in patients with SBS is to minimize the symptoms associated with severe malabsorption while optimizing nutrient absorption so that reliance on specialized nutritional support can be diminished. By adhering to the principles discussed regarding the pathophysiologic consequences of intestinal resection, a logical approach can be followed to reach this end point.

Food should be consumed in small quantities and divided into five or more meals each day. Protein should be of high biologic value, and carbohydrates should be of the complex type. The intake of concentrated sweets, especially in the form of fruit juices, should be minimized, as they tend to exaggerate the underlying osmotic diarrhea. Further dietary recommendations depend on whether the colon is present or absent and are outlined in Figure 75-2.

Fat, lactose, and oxalate restrictions are not necessary when the colon is absent or out of continuity with the small bowel. The percentage of fat absorbed is constant over a broad range, and so the calories derived from fat increase as the amount of fat consumed is increased. Stoma losses of fluid and electrolytes do not increase significantly with a high-fat diet in patients with small bowel enterostomy. On the other hand, patients with an intact colon develop a secretory diarrhea secondary to the effect that unabsorbed fatty acids have on the colonic mucosa, and so these patients require fat restriction. Lactose malabsorption is common in SBS because of lost intestinal mucosal surface area; however, symptoms generally occur as a result of fermentation of the unabsorbed disaccharide in the colon. Therefore, dairy products, which are a rich source of calcium, vitamin D, riboflavin, and protein, can

Table 75-2 Parenteral Nutrition for Short Bowel Syndrome

NUTRITIONAL COMPONENT	AMOUNT
Standard amino acids[1]	105 g
Total calories[1]	2450 kcal
Nonprotein calorie distribution[2]	Dextrose 70%
	Fat 30%
Total volume[3]	3500 mL
Infusion rate[4]	146 mL/h
Sodium chloride[5]	120 mEq
Sodium acetate	100 mEq
Potassium chloride	80 mEq
Calcium gluconate	15 mEq
Magnesium sulfate	15 mEq
Phosphate (as sodium)	30 mEq
Adult multiple vitamin-12	10 mL
Multiple trace elements (Zn, Cu, Cr, Mn)	1 mL
Selenium[6]	120 µg
Heparin[7]	3500 U
Additives[8]	3500 U

[1]Based on a weight of 70 kg providing protein 1.5 g/kg/24 h, calorie 35 kcal/kg/24 h.
[2]Nonprotein calorie distribution equals 100%. Total calorie distribution is protein 420 kcal (17%), dextrose 1421 kcal (58%), and fat 609 kcal (25%).
[3]Maintenance fluid requirements, 35 mL/kg/24 h plus 1000 mL for stool losses.
[4]Rate for infusion over 24 h. Infuse over 12 h if patient sent home on parenteral nutrition.
[5]Infused electrolytes account for typical urinary excretion plus stool losses.
[6]Extra zinc, selenium, and chromium may be needed for stool losses.
[7]Low-dose heparin decreases the risk of catheter-associated venous thrombosis.
[8]H_2 blockers and insulin may be added as needed.

be given to patients with small bowel enterostomies, but some restriction may be necessary for patients who still have their colons. Last, although oxalate restriction may be necessary in patients with their colons, if they adhere to a low-fat diet and take a calcium supplement, the absorption of oxalate in the colon may be low and so an additional restriction can sometimes be avoided. Our approach is to first initiate a diet with 60 to 70 g fat (approximately 20% of total calories) and 1500 mg of calcium carbonate and to then measure oxalate in a 24-hour urine sample. If the quantity of oxalate is above normal or if a patient develops calcium oxalate kidney stones with a normal value, then oxalate should be restricted in the diet.

Enteral fluids may be advanced beyond the previously stated 2-L restriction once the enteral intake and output balance is positive. Patients with small bowel enterostomies may require oral rehydration solutions, which take advantage of the active cotransport of sodium and glucose to maintain hydration. Sodium concentrations range from 45 to 90 mmol/L in these solutions, and glucose is provided at a concentration of 20 g/L. Higher concentrations of sodium, even up to 120 mmol/L, may be needed for patients with very short guts. Cereal- or rice-based oral rehydration solutions have been recommended by some

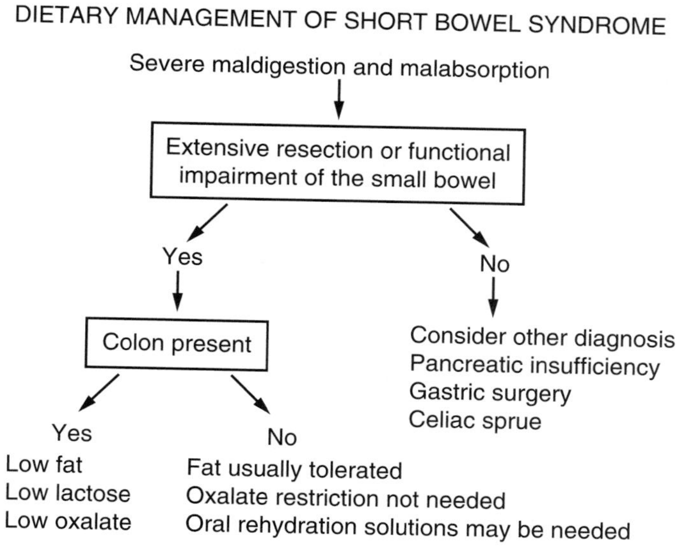

DIETARY MANAGEMENT OF SHORT BOWEL SYNDROME

Figure 75-2

Factors to consider when prescribing a diet for short bowel syndrome. Small, frequent meals with limited fluid intake during meals and sips of fluid between meals will maximize absorption. Multiple vitamins and calcium supplement are needed for all patients, with other micronutrients being prescribed as needed. Measure 24-hour urinary oxalate on low-fat calcium supplement to determine need for restriction.

Severe maldigestion and malabsorption

Extensive resection or functional impairment of the small bowel

Yes → Colon present

No → Consider other diagnosis
Pancreatic insufficiency
Gastric surgery
Celiac sprue

Colon present:

Yes
Low fat
Low lactose
Low oxalate

No
Fat usually tolerated
Oxalate restriction not needed
Oral rehydration solutions may be needed

because of the lower osmolarity, which may lessen the severity of diarrhea. Patients may also benefit from taking their meals with a minimal amount of fluid and to take fluids between meals, as do patients with postgastrectomy syndrome, to slow the emptying of nutrients from the stomach. In contrast, patients with at least one half of their colons often have adequate sodium absorption so long as there is an adequate amount in the diet and oral rehydration solutions are not necessary.

In the past, a low-fiber diet has been recommended for SBS because of the observation that dietary fiber leads to an increase in intestinal transit time and fecal weight. There has also been some concern that insoluble fiber, such as wheat bran, may decrease the availability of certain divalent cations such as calcium, magnesium, and zinc. Pectin, a soluble fiber, has been shown to delay gastric emptying and increase intestinal transit, two factors that are desirable in SBS. In addition, the fermentation of soluble fiber in the colon results in the production of short-chain fatty acids, which are the preferred substrate of the colonocyte and have been shown to promote mucosal proliferation in the colon. Our current practice is to encourage patients with an intact colon to try a variety of dietary fibers to most optimally manage the consistency of their bowel habit. We are not concerned with the development of vitamin and mineral deficiency because supplements are provided.

Medium-chain triglycerides (MCTs) are occasionally used in patients with SBS. These dietary fats are easily hydrolyzed by pancreatic lipase and do not require emulsification with bile salts for intestinal absorption. Once they gain entry into the enterocyte, medium-chain fatty acids are re-esterified into MCTs, which pass directly to the liver via the portal circulation, whereas long-chain triglycerides pass via the intestinal lymphatics into the systemic circulation. Unfortunately, MCTs have an unpleasant taste, can cause diarrhea when given in large doses, and may impair intestinal adaptation. It must also be kept in mind that MCTs do not provide essential fatty acids,

and so patients with severe fat malabsorption may require parenteral lipid emulsions to meet this dietary requirement. We currently advise no more than 30 g per day of this dietary supplement when it is used.

Medications and Dietary Supplements

A variety of medications often may be necessary to manage patients with SBS. The type and indication for these medications are outlined in Table 75-3. Many of these medications have already been discussed in the context of preventing complications of SBS. The antidiarrheal medications are essential to control the loss of fluid and electrolytes from stool and to maximize the absorptive function of the remnant bowel. Despite the potential for abuse of these medications, we find that most patients take them to control their diarrhea and not for their euphoric effect.

Commonly used fat-soluble vitamins and mineral supplements are presented in Table 75-4. These supplements are required only in patients being transitioned from parenteral to enteral nutrition or for those who are maintained on enteral nutrition alone. A multiple vitamin with minerals should be taken two or three times daily. Most patients require calcium for reasons already discussed and to avoid metabolic bone disease. Magnesium salts, which solubilize readily, should be used to foster maximal absorption exacerbation of diarrhea. Zinc supplements are sometimes needed, especially when moderately severe diarrhea is present. Mineral and trace element supplementation should be based on monitoring of blood levels and urinary losses.

■ SURGICAL MANAGEMENT OF SHORT BOWEL SYNDROME

Although SBS is the result of intestinal resection, a number of important surgical issues must be considered in

Table 75-3 Oral Medications Used in Short Bowel Syndrome

MEDICATION	FORM*	STRENGTH AVAILABLE	TYPICAL REGIMEN
H₂ BLOCKERS			
Cimetidine	tab	200 mg, 300 mg, 400 mg, 800 mg	400–800 mg bid or qid
	liq	300 mg/5 mL	
Ranitidine	tab	150 mg	150 mg bid
	liq	150 mg/10 mL	
Famotidine	tab	20 mg, 40 mg	20 mg bid
	susp	40 mg/5 mL	
PROTON PUMP INHIBITORS			
Omeprazole	cap	20 mg, 40 mg	20–40 mg bid
Lansoprazole	cap	15 mg, 30 mg	15–30 mg bid
PANCREATIC ENZYMES			
Pancrelipase	tab or cap	lipase = 8000 U protease = 30,000 U amylase = 30,000 U	1–8 tabs with meals and snacks
ANTIDIARRHEALS			
Diphenoxylate	tab	2.5 mg (with 25 µg atropine)	2 tabs or 10 mL ac qid (maximum)
	liq	2.5 mg (with 25 µg atropine)/5 mL	
Loperamide	cap	2 mg	2 tabs or 10 mL ac qid (maximum)
	liq	1 mg/5 mL	
Opium tincture	tinc	1% morphine anhydrous	10–20 drops qid
Paregoric	tinc	0.04% morphine anhydrous	5–10 mL qid
ANTIMICROBIALS FOR BACTERIAL OVERGROWTH			
Metronidazole	tab	250 mg	250–750 mg tid
Tetracycline	cap	100 mg, 250 mg, 500 mg	1–2 g in 2–4 divided doses
	susp	125 mg/5 mL	
Cephalexin	cap	250 mg, 500 mg	1–2 g in 2–4 divided doses
	susp	125 mg/5 mL, 250 mg/5 mL	
BILE ACID–BINDING RESINS			
Cholestyramine	powd	4 g/packet (tsp)	1–6 packets in water or other beverage; 1–4 divided doses
Colestipol	powd	5 g/packet (tsp)	1–6 packets in water or other beverage; 1–4 divided doses
Colestipol	tab	1 g	5–30 g in 1–2 divided doses

*cap, capsule; liq, liquid; powd, powder; susp, suspension; tab, tablet; tinc, tincture.

order to prevent or minimize the sequelae of extensive intestinal resection. In addition, a few patients with established SBS might benefit from surgical techniques that have been developed to optimize intestinal absorption and hence diminish the reliance on specialized nutritional support. Finally, advances in immunosuppressive medications have led to the ability to perform small bowel transplantation in a select group of patients with intestinal failure. This section will briefly explore these issues.

Early Surgical Treatment

Early surgical treatment of the patient with intestinal ischemia is directed toward limiting the loss of viable bowel and controlling sepsis. Control of sepsis implies resection of nonviable intestine and drainage of associated abscesses. Timely operative intervention is necessary to reduce the extent of irreversible intestinal ischemia, so the implication is that one must have a high index of suspicion in the diagnosis of this condition. Methods of restoring blood flow to ischemic tissues, such as reduction of intestinal volvulus or strangulated hernia and arterial embolectomy, should be undertaken prior to resection of ischemic bowel. After allowing the revascularized bowel to recover, only obviously nonviable bowel should be resected. Any bowel of questionable viability should be reinspected in 24 to 36 hours at a so-called "second look" laparotomy. Margins of resection should be kept to a minimum, and the ileocecal valve and colon should be preserved if at all possible.

Table 75-4 Oral Vitamin and Mineral Supplements for Adults with Malabsorption

NAME	FORM*	STRENGTH AVAILABLE	TYPICAL REGIMEN
VITAMINS			
Vitamin A	cap	5000–50,000 IU	5000–10,000 IU/day
	liq	50,000/mL	
Vitamin D$_2$ (ergocalciferol)	cap	25,000, 50,000 IU	50,000 IU 2–3 times/week
	liq	8000 IU/mL, 200 IU/drop	
Vitamin D$_3$ (calcitriol)	cap	0.25, 0.50 µg	0.25–1 µg/day
Vitamin E	tab	200, 400 IU	100–400 IU/day
(D-α-tocopherol)	liq	50 mg/mL (1.49 IU = 1 mg)	
Vitamin K	tab	5 mg	5–10 mg/day
(phytonadione)			
MINERALS†			
Calcium carbonate‡	tab	1.25 g (500 mg)	1000–3000 mg/day
	ch tab	750 mg (300 mg)	
	susp	1.25 g/5 mL	
Calcium citrate	tab	950 mg (200 mg)	
Calcium glubionate	syr	5.4 g/15 mL (345 mg)	
Calcium gluconate	ch tab	500 mg (45 mg), 1 g	
Calcium lactate	tab	325 mg (42 mg), 650 mg	
Magnesium gluconate‡	tab	450 mg (27 mg)	50–500 mg/day
Magnesium lactate	tab	840 mg (84 mg)	
Potassium chloride	tab	10 mEq, 20 mEq	As needed
	liq	10% solution = 20 mEq/15 mL	As needed
Phosphate as sodium and potassium	cap	250 mg (8 mM) PO$_4$ (7.125 mEq each of Na and K)	
Sodium bicarbonate	tab	650 mg	1300–5200 mg/day
Bicitra	liq	1 mL = 1 mEq Na, HCO$_3$	As needed
Polycitra	liq	1 mL = 1 mEq Na, K, 2 mEq HCO$_3$	
Zinc sulfate‡	cap	220 mg (50 mg)	50–150 mg/day

*cap, capsule; ch, chewable; liq, liquid; susp, suspension; syr, syrup; tab, tablet.
†Minerals should be taken in divided doses two to four times each day.
‡Amounts of calcium, magnesium, and zinc are listed as total dose of salt, and dose of parent mineral is given in parentheses.

The temptation to restore intestinal continuity at the time of initial resection should be resisted in the majority of cases of acute intestinal ischemia. A risky anastomosis can compromise potentially viable bowel and thus may be more detrimental than creation of a temporary jejunostomy. Restoration of continuity should be reserved for those few patients who are hemodynamically stable and in whom viability of the remaining bowel is certain, remaining small bowel length is at least 90 cm, and anastomosis to the colon is not needed.

Laparotomy following massive small bowel resection is to be avoided between the seventh day and third month after the primary surgical procedure, because adhesion formation is maximal at this time and places viable bowel at risk for iatrogenic injury and thus additional loss of functional intestine. Abdominal and pelvic abscesses should be managed by placement of radiographically directed percutaneous drains whenever feasible, and as often as necessary. Postoperative bowel obstruction may best be managed by long-term gastric decompression and parenteral nutrition so long as the patient does not demonstrate any signs of peritonitis. Only those patients with uncontrolled intra-abdominal hemorrhage, recurrent ischemic bowel, and abscesses that cannot be ade-

quately drained by radiographic techniques should be considered for reoperation during this critical period.

Surgical Procedures to Enhance Remnant Bowel Function

Surgical techniques to enhance the function of the remaining bowel are directed toward prolonging the transit time and increasing the absorptive surface of the intestine. The most obvious and reliable means to this end is to replace diverted intestine into the fecal stream. Although this approach seems simple, surgeons and patients are sometimes reluctant to accept "elective" surgery following what most likely was a catastrophic event leading to extensive intestinal resection. The best time to restore intestinal continuity is usually 3 to 6 months after the last abdominal operation. In many instances, patients can be weaned from nutritional support following the restoration of intestinal continuity. However, for patients who continue to rely heavily on nutritional support, an observation period of 12 to 24 months must occur to allow the bowel to fully adapt before considering other procedures to improve intestinal function.

Distended loops of bowel may be the result of chronic partial small bowel obstruction. If adhesive obstruction is clearly documented, relief of the obstruction can significantly improve bowel function. Stricturoplasty has become quite popular in managing strictures in Crohn's disease when maintaining as much small bowel as possible may delay or prevent a patient's reliance on specialized nutritional support. On the other hand, short segment bypass is preferred in the case of radiation enteritis with segmental obstruction when healing might be suboptimal.

Diffuse bowel dilatation without a transition point or clinical evidence of obstruction may result in stasis and bacterial overgrowth. Short segments of stagnant loops of small bowel can be resected and may lead to improved absorptive function. Alternatively, tapering enteroplasty can achieve the same goal. However, both interventions can waste viable mucosal absorptive surfaces. Intestinal plication techniques have been designed to retain the absorptive surface of the bowel but may result in mechanical obstruction. Finally, long, stagnant segments of small bowel can be divided along both the antimesenteric and mesenteric side of the bowel in a technique described by Bianchi. This procedure, which doubles the length of involved small bowel, initially improves intestinal motility and with time leads to dilation and hence an increase in the mucosal surface of the bowel. Intestinal leaks and obstruction are formidable complications of this procedure and thus have limited its use.

The management of patients with rapid intestinal transit with an adequate absorptive surface area has included bowel interposition of antiperistaltic segments of small bowel or isoperistaltic segments of colon and the creation of a nipple valve in an attempt to normalize motility. These techniques have met with variable success. However, experience with these techniques is limited, and these procedures are advised infrequently because of potential complications, such as bowel obstruction, bleeding from colitis of the interposed colon, or concern that a critical amount of bowel length may be compromised in creating a nipple valve.

Small Bowel Transplantation

Improved surgical techniques and the introduction of the antirejection drug FK 506 (tacrolimus, Prograf) have led to the recent advancement of small bowel transplantation. Isolated small bowel, liver–small bowel, and multivisceral transplantation have been offered to patients with intestinal failure on an experimental basis. Although early results suggest that overall survival is best for recipients of isolated small bowel transplants, time has shown that graft survival is the worst in this group. In addition, survival is optimal if both the donor and host are cytomegalovirus negative. Epstein-Barr virus–associated B-cell lymphoma is a serious complication of transplantation and is related to the high levels of immunosuppressive medications necessary to prevent graft rejection. Because of these factors and a graft survival of only 50% at 3 years, small bowel transplantation can be advised only for patients with TPN-dependent SBS who develop life-threatening complications from TPN.

Suggested Readings

Bianchi A: Intestinal loop lengthening: A technique for increasing small intestinal length. J Pediatr Surg 1980;15:145–151.

Byrne TA, Persinger RL, Young LS, et al: A new treatment for patients with short-bowel syndrome: Growth hormone, glutamine, and a modified diet. Ann Surg 1995;222:243–255.

Lennard-Jones JE: Oral rehydration solutions in short bowel syndrome. Clin Ther 1990;12:101–110.

O'Keefe SJD, Peterson ME, Fleming CR: Octreotide as an adjunct to home parenteral nutrition in the management of permanent end-jejunostomy syndrome. JPEN 1994;18:26–36.

Scolapio JS, Camilleri M, Fleming CR, et al: Effect of growth hormone, glutamine, and diet on adaptation in short-bowel syndrome: A randomized, controlled study. Gastroenterology 1997;113:1074–1081.

Todo S, Reyes J, Furukawa H, et al: Outcome analysis of 71 clinical intestinal transplantations. Ann Surg 1995;222:270–282.

Wilmore DW, Byrne TA, Persinger RL: Short bowel syndrome: New therapeutic approaches. Curr Probl Surg 1997;34:398–444.

76

CROHN'S DISEASE OF THE DUODENUM, STOMACH, AND ESOPHAGUS

David J. Schoetz, Jr., MD

Crohn's disease, a granulomatous inflammatory disease of unknown etiology, may affect the entire gastrointestinal tract from the mouth to the anus. Despite the propensity to involve the terminal ileum and colon more often than other parts of the digestive system, Crohn's disease of the esophagus, stomach, and duodenum are well-described conditions that present challenges in diagnosis and management, in part because of their relative rarity.

Isolated clinically significant esophageal Crohn's disease is unusual, representing less than 2% of complaints in patients suffering from Crohn's disease. The most common symptom is the rapid development of painful dysphagia with subsequent substantial weight loss resulting from restriction of oral intake. Absence of heartburn and regurgitation is an important differentiating point from the more common reflux esophagitis. Approximately half of patients affected by Crohn's esophagitis will have a history of involvement of other portions of the gastrointestinal tract. Active treatment with immunosuppressive agents for the intestinal disease raises the possibility that the esophageal symptoms are caused by superinfection of the esophagus with Candida or viral agents.

Gastroduodenal Crohn's disease affects between 0.5 and 4% of people in most large series of patients with Crohn's disease. As with esophageal involvement, more than half of affected patients will be known to have pre-existing Crohn's disease elsewhere; furthermore, with long-term follow-up, the majority of patients without known Crohn's disease will subsequently prove to have other sites of granulomatous intestinal disease. Early symptoms of gastroduodenal involvement are nonspecific and indistinguishable from acid-peptic disease. As the disease progresses, fibrosis of the duodenum results in duodenal obstruction with postprandial vomiting of undigested food and weight loss. Anemia from chronic blood loss is common, whereas brisk upper gastrointestinal tract hemorrhage is distinctly unusual (Fig. 76-1).

Once the possibility of esophageal, gastric, or duodenal Crohn's disease is entertained, the diagnosis is established by the performance of upper gastrointestinal endoscopy or barium contrast radiography. Radiologic study should be performed with detailed fluoroscopy. Continuation of the study as a small bowel series should be routinely ordered so that the remainder of the small bowel can be examined for associated and perhaps previously unsuspected Crohn's disease.

Esophageal Crohn's disease tends to be confined to the distal half of the esophagus, where early radiographic findings include thickened mucosal folds, asymmetric irregularity of the esophageal wall, and aphthous ulcers. Similar mucosal abnormalities are observed in early gastroduodenal Crohn's disease; the distribution of disease is most often contiguous involvement of the distal stomach and proximal duodenum, followed by isolated proximal duodenal Crohn's disease. For unknown reasons, isolated distal duodenal and proximal gastric Crohn's disease is extremely unusual (Fig. 76-2).

Progression of the inflammatory process results in fibrosis with resultant obstruction. Tubular stenosis of the esophagus is the end result of fissuring ulcers deepening into the submucosa and muscularis propria. Similar findings are observed in the duodenum, with cobblestoning and fissuring ulcers leading to stenosis and obstruction.

Endoscopy with biopsy should be performed in all patients with suspected upper gastrointestinal tract Crohn's disease. Visual findings are generally nonspecific and include hyperemia, friability, granularity, and nodular mucosal thickening. Aphthous ulcers and serpiginous ulcerations are more common in gastroduodenal disease than with esophageal involvement. Multiple biopsies should be obtained from affected mucosa. Histologic findings are generally nonspecific acute and chronic inflammation, with granulomas in about 10% of patients. However, multiple biopsies will exclude the presence of cancer and fungal or viral infection. Regarding gastroduodenal Crohn's disease, the relatively recent demonstration of the importance of Helicobacter pylori infection in the pathophysiology of gastritis and ulcer disease must be considered and appropriate biopsies obtained to exclude this specific diagnosis.

■ MEDICAL THERAPY

Treatment of patients with Crohn's disease, by either pharmacology or surgery, is indicated only for symptoms resulting from complications of the disease; therapy for asymptomatic patients with incidental radiographic or endoscopic findings is not justified. Medical management of patients with Crohn's disease continues to be nonspecific. Anti-inflammatory drugs are the cornerstone of therapy, combined with other medications that relieve symptoms. Corticosteroids are the treatment of choice in both esophageal and gastroduodenal Crohn's disease. Steroid therapy regimens should be designed such that the dosage is tapered rapidly enough to minimize the risk of permanent steroid side effects, including osteoporosis, cataracts, and aseptic necrosis of joints. Alternate-day dosing may be associated with fewer side effects.

Aminosalicylates (5-ASA drugs) are activated in the distal small bowel or colon and thus have not been proved to be beneficial in the treatment of patients with Crohn's disease in the upper gastrointestinal tract. Acid reduction in esophageal Crohn's disease is indicated only when

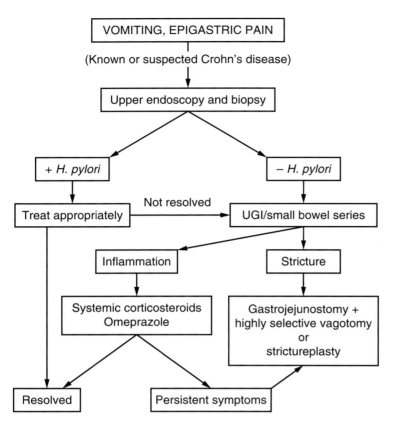

Figure 76-1
Evaluation of suspected gastroduodenal Crohn's disease.

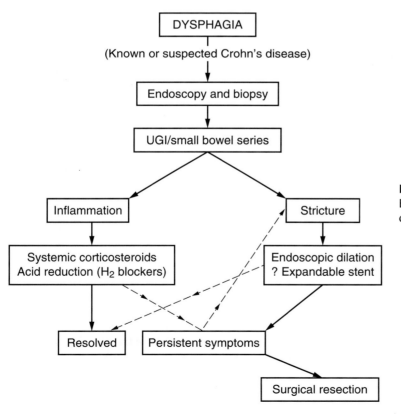

Figure 76-2
Evaluation of suspected esophageal Crohn's disease.

associated reflux symptoms are present, although gastro-duodenal mucosal protection is usually advised in patients prescribed systemic steroids. Regarding gastroduodenal Crohn's disease, the addition of the proton pump inhibitor omeprazole has been recommended to prevent progression to pyloric or duodenal stenosis. Associated *Helicobacter pylori* infection should be treated with any of the accepted double or triple antibiotic combinations before initiating steroid therapy.

Other drugs used to treat more distal intestinal Crohn's disease, such as metronidazole, 6-mercaptopurine, aza-thioprine, and newer biologic modifiers, have not been employed frequently enough in proximal disease to show proof of efficacy, although many patients may require them for their distal disease.

■ SURGICAL THERAPY

The end point of drug therapy is symptomatic relief with control of the inflammatory process, which, left unchecked, results in permanent luminal narrowing requiring more aggressive therapeutic intervention to relieve obstruction. Approximately one third of patients with gastroduodenal Crohn's disease will require operation, whereas esophageal Crohn's disease mandates surgery in 10 to 20% of patients. Pain without obstruction has been the indication for surgical intervention in 15 to 20% of earlier series of gastroduodenal Crohn's disease, but this will nearly vanish with more accurate early diagnosis and more effective nonoperative treatment of the acid-peptic components of the symptom complex.

Because obstruction usually results in an inability to ingest solid food and subsequent weight loss, patients being considered for operation should undergo a period of nutritional repletion before elective surgery. If liquids can be tolerated, appropriate protein/calorie enteral preparations are preferable to total parenteral nutrition. Complications from the use of the gastrointestinal tract are significantly less, as are costs. Although it is not necessary to restore ideal body weight, reversal of the catabolic state and restoration of a normal immune status should be the goals of nutritional therapy.

In considering operative intervention for patients with upper gastrointestinal tract Crohn's disease, assessment of the need for surgical treatment of other portions of the gastrointestinal tract must be undertaken. Combined treatment of proximal disease and distal disease may be necessary to restore health. Conversely, the performance of a laparotomy to treat esophageal or gastroduodenal disease should not push the surgeon to remove portions of the intestine that would not otherwise be considered for excision.

Before open abdominal surgery, the possibility that endoscopic techniques might relieve the obstruction should be entertained. Dilation of esophageal strictures with simple bougienage or pneumatic dilation may obviate the need for thoracotomy or laparotomy. Expandable metal stents may also play a role in esophageal strictures if the stent can be placed completely above the lower esophageal sphincter. It is only a matter of time until application of these techniques will extend to strictures involving the pylorus and duodenum. In the near future, creative endoscopic and advanced laparoscopic techniques may obviate the need for open surgery in the majority of patients.

If medical treatment and esophageal dilation fail to relieve esophageal obstruction, surgery is required. With fewer than 200 cases of esophageal Crohn's disease reported and with surgery required in only about 20%, little can be dogmatically stated regarding the preferred operation. Resection of the strictured segment is required; reconstruction of the intestine's continuity will be accomplished by whatever means the remainder of the anatomy permits. Anastomosis of the esophagus to the stomach will be feasible in the majority of patients. Interposition of either small or large bowel will rarely be considered, particularly in light of the high incidence of Crohn's disease elsewhere that had previously been diagnosed or even treated surgically.

Regarding gastroduodenal Crohn's disease, the preferred operation is bypass by means of a gastrojejunostomy. Resection of the stomach or duodenum should not be performed unless there is a realistic concern over the presence of cancer, which has yet to be reported as a complication of gastroduodenal Crohn's disease. Resection, compared with bypass, is associated with significantly higher morbidity and mortality rates. More recently, strictureplasty has been safely employed in many of the patients with nonperforated duodenal Crohn's disease, and is constructed in a Finney or Heineke-Mickulicz manner, depending on the length and position of the strictured segment. Strictureplasty should be reserved for patients with fibrotic strictures without active inflammation; performance of strictureplasty in inflamed bowel is associated with a sizable incidence of anastomotic leak. Surgeons have long realized that truncal vagotomy at the time of gastrojejunostomy or gastroduodenostomy may aggravate pre-existing diarrhea, but marginal ulceration may result from failure to decrease gastric acid production by fundal denervation. However, prior controversy regarding the need for truncal vagotomy has been rendered moot because highly selective vagotomy has supplanted truncal vagotomy. At present, the preferred operation for patients with obstructing gastroduodenal Crohn's disease is gastrojejunostomy with highly selective vagotomy. Strictureplasty is favored for isolated duodenal disease, and is combined with vagotomy only when the pylorus is disrupted. Laparoscopic techniques have been described for accomplishing these operations in other settings and may be useful in appropriately selected patients with gastroduodenal Crohn's disease.

■ SUMMARY

In summary, upper gastrointestinal tract Crohn's disease is unusual, esophageal involvement being less common than gastroduodenal disease. Both present with early nonspecific symptoms, requiring endoscopy and radiography to establish a diagnosis. Early treatment is medical, with an emphasis on acid reduction and systemic corticosteroids in an attempt to control symptoms while preventing progression of the inflammatory process to fibrotic obstruction. Involvement of the distal gastrointestinal tract must be excluded in most instances, either concomitant with or subsequent to establishing the initial diagnosis. Failure of medical management requires resection of esophageal strictures, bypass of gastroduodenal disease, and strictureplasty for duodenal strictures; coincident surgical removal of distal Crohn's disease is warranted only when the distal disease is sufficient to require operation on its own merits. Finally, endoscopic dilation and stenting may replace open surgery in the majority of patients in the future.

Suggested Readings

Geboes K, Janssens J, Rutgeerts P, Vantrappen G: Crohn's disease of the esophagus. J Clin Gastroenterol 1986;8:31–37.

Lamers C: Crohn's disease of the upper gastrointestinal tract. In Allan RN, Rhodes JM, Hanauer SB, et al (Eds.). Inflammatory Bowel Diseases. London, Churchill Livingstone, 1997, pp 583–588.

Maffei VJ, Zaatari GS, McGarity WC, Mansour KA: Crohn's disease of the esophagus. J Thorac Cardiovasc Surg 1987;94:302–311.

Murray JJ, Schoetz DJ Jr, Nugent FW, et al: Surgical management of Crohn's disease involving the duodenum. Am J Surg 1984;147:58–65.

Nugent FW, Roy MA: Duodenal Crohn's disease: An analysis of 89 cases. Am J Gastroenterol 1989;84:249–254.

Roberts PL, Schoetz DJ Jr: Gastroduodenal Crohn's disease. Semin Colon Rectal Surg 1994;5:199–203.

Schoetz DJ Jr: Gastroduodenal Crohn's disease. Perspect Colon Rectal Surg 1992;5:145–154.

Worsey MJ, Hull TL, Ryland L, Fazio VW: Strictureplasty is an effective option in the operative management of duodenal Crohn's disease. Dis Colon Rectum 1999;42:596–600.

77

CROHN'S DISEASE OF THE SMALL BOWEL

Scott A. Strong, MD

Crohn's disease is a chronic remitting inflammatory disorder of the intestinal tract that presents with varied symptoms and signs depending upon the distribution and nature of the disease. Although the etiology and pathogenesis of the disorder are poorly understood, Crohn's disease tends to affect genetically predisposed persons exposed to initiating or triggering events that likely include environmental and microbial factors. For many years, the resultant condition has been classified by its anatomic site of involvement, but more recently it has been described by its clinical behavior (Table 77-1). The ileocecal region is the most common site for initial presentation, observed in 40% of individuals, although small bowel disease is witnessed in nearly 30% of these patients. In patients with ileocecal or small bowel disease, the probability of surgery within 5 years of onset is 75% and 50%, respectively, and these numbers increase to 90% and 70%, respectively, after 10 years of symptoms. The operative management of these individuals is based upon multiple variables, including prior therapy, clinical disease behavior, and associated complications, and primarily consists of resection and strictureplasty performed by conventional or laparoscopic approaches.

■ CLINICAL PRESENTATION

Ileocecal disease typically causes symptoms of cramping abdominal pain, borborygmi, diarrhea, and low-grade fever with physical examination commonly revealing a tender mass in the right lower abdomen. Extension of the inflammatory process can irritate surrounding structures and instigate renal colic or dysuria. Transmural disease can penetrate into adjacent mesentery, bowel, bladder, abdominal wall, or vagina, and can produce an abscess or fistulous communication between the affected bowel and the target organ. Less commonly, free perforation occurs and causes peritonitis with systemic signs of sepsis.

The symptoms and signs of small bowel Crohn's disease are partially determined by the extent and behavior of the disease. Some findings are a direct result of the disease, similar to those witnessed with ileocecal involvement, and others are indirect manifestations representing the systemic effects of the condition. As the length of involved intestine increases, the amount of effective digestive and absorptive surface diminishes, precipitating problems with malabsorption and enteric loss of nutrients. The malabsorption of minerals (e.g., niacin), electrolytes (e.g., calcium, magnesium), and vitamins (e.g., folate, vitamin B_{12}, vitamin D) leads to various maladies, including pellagra, neuromuscular dysfunction, coagulopathy, anemia, and osteopenia. An alteration in bile salt absorption causes steatorrhea, whereas enteric loss of protein results in hypoalbuminemia. In the pediatric patient with small bowel Crohn's disease, growth retardation is occasionally encountered and primarily originates from malnutrition linked to poor nutritional intake and severe disease involvement.

■ EVALUATION

Any patient presenting with ileocecal or small bowel Crohn's disease should undergo an interview about his or her illness and past medical history, followed by a thorough physical examination. The results of this effort enable the clinician to decide how to further evaluate the patient utilizing a variety of potential methods, including hematologic testing, endoscopy, and radiographic imaging.

Hematologic testing is used to determine abnormalities in blood cell counts and aberrations in electrolytes, proteins, liver enzymes, and coagulation pathways. These values can help the surgeon identify and appropriately treat anemia, electrolyte abnormality, malnutrition, and coagulopathies. Furthermore, blood levels of leukocytes, acute phase reactants such as C-reactive protein, and prothrombotic clotting factors can help discriminate between the inflammatory and fibrostenotic patterns of Crohn's disease. They are typically elevated in cases of inflammatory disease but relatively normal in patients with a fibrostenotic disease pattern.

Endoscopy permits evaluation of the upper and lower intestinal tracts. Upper endoscopy is only occasionally employed in persons requiring operative management of their ileocecal or small bowel disease and is reserved for individuals whose symptoms suggest gastroduodenal disease. Conversely, colonoscopy is utilized in most patients to exclude primary or secondary large bowel involvement. Concomitant colonic resection may be necessary if colonic disease or an enterocolic fistula is identified. Moreover, permanent fecal diversion might be warranted if severe rectal disease is encountered. Thus, the endoscopic appearance of the large bowel assists the surgeon in planning the operation and counseling the patient.

Radiographic imaging includes contrast studies, ultrasonography, and nuclear medicine studies. Contrast studies have long been considered the best radiologic method for diagnosing Crohn's disease and demonstrating the mucosal extent of the inflammatory process. Small bowel series and enteroclysis can be used to examine the small intestine, and the overall accuracy of the two techniques is similar, assuming they are performed by an experienced radiologist with careful attention to detail. Computed tomography (CT) has recently become a valuable diagnostic tool and complements, rather than replaces, the traditional contrast studies. Thus, barium

Table 77-1 Clinical Presentation of Crohn's Disease Based on Clinical Behavior

FEATURE	INFLAMMATORY DISEASE	FIBROSTENOTIC DISEASE
Preoperative disease duration	Short	Long
Operative indication	Inflammatory mass, fistula, perforation	Refractory disease, obstruction, stricture
Postoperative recurrence rate	High	Low
Postoperative duration of remission	Short	Long

studies demonstrate mucosal disease, and CT imaging accurately identifies extension of the disease into the bowel wall and adjacent structures. Used in combination, these imaging modalities are useful for demonstrating strictures, fistulas, sinus tracts, and ulcerations that might indicate the need for an operation, but sometimes fail to recognize more subtle abnormalities identified at the time of surgery. Therefore, these imaging tests can be used to justify operative intervention, but the surgical procedure should not be directed at correcting only those findings seen during the radiologic testing. The roles of magnetic resonance imaging and ultrasonography continue to evolve, but promising results are coming from European centers where these modalities are more commonly utilized. Nuclear scintigraphy is also emerging as a useful technique for identifying actively inflamed bowel, which allows differentiation of inflammatory disease that might respond to medical therapy from fibrostenotic disease that is best treated by operative management.

■ OPERATIVE MANAGEMENT

Goals

The primary goal of Crohn's disease management should be to safely minimize disease-associated symptoms and preserve small bowel function using appropriate medical and operative approaches. This notion is based upon an understanding that the disease is an incurable disorder that often afflicts young persons who will be faced with multiple disease-associated events during their lifetime. The patient's long-term care should always be considered, and procedures that jeopardize small bowel function should be avoided. Accordingly, if a diseased small bowel segment does not appear to be linked to hemorrhage, perforation, obstruction, or malignancy, the segment should be left undisturbed.

Indications

In general, the operative indications for ileocecal or small bowel Crohn's disease are categorized as failed medical therapy or acute and chronic disease complications.

Failed Medical Therapy

Medical therapy is initiated for most patients suffering from disease symptoms unless the presentation mandates emergent operative treatment. Antibiotics, 5-aminosalicylates, steroids, immunomodulating agents, or biologic modifiers are prescribed and delivered topically, enterally, or parenterally. Many individuals with Crohn's disease eventually fail their medical therapy, and this failure is classified as one of the following:

- Lack of response
- Incomplete response
- Intolerant of medication
- Noncompliant with medication

Patients started on medication for disease treatment should be informed about potential side effects and adverse reactions. Additionally, the objectives of therapy should be explained from the outset while clearly defining the goals for symptom management and treatment duration. If the therapy fails to adequately reduce the specified symptoms within the dictated time interval, the medication should be supplanted or supplemented. If significant disease symptoms persist after employing reasonable medical alternatives, surgery is warranted. Alternatively, some patients will not tolerate or will become noncompliant with the prescribed medications. In either instance, operative intervention should be contemplated.

Acute Disease Complications

Acute disease complications include the following:

- Massive hemorrhage
- Perforation

Hemorrhage is a rare complication of ileocecal or small bowel Crohn's disease, but more commonly results from other unrelated causes such as peptic ulcer disease or gastritis. Consequently, gastric aspiration and upper endoscopy are often required to exclude sources of hemorrhage indirectly associated with the primary disease.

Perforation can present as a free or contained perforation, with the latter group including abscesses and fistulas. Free perforation of the bowel is seen infrequently and typically occurs during an acute exacerbation of chronic disease in a region just proximal to a strictured intestinal segment.

Chronic Disease Complications

Chronic disease complications include the following:

- Obstruction
- Malignancy
- Growth retardation
- Extraintestinal manifestations

Obstruction is a common complication of ileocecal or small bowel Crohn's disease. Acute obstruction is due to stenotic disease, and usually resolves with rehydration, bowel rest, and nasogastric decompression. Conversely, chronic obstruction is typified by recurring episodes that do not respond to long-term medical therapy, and require elective operative treatment.

The association between malignancies of the alimentary tract and Crohn's disease is well recognized, and a variety of cancers occur with greater frequency in Crohn's disease compared to the general population. Small bowel adenocarcinoma complicating Crohn's disease is acknowledged and thoroughly described. Less reported associations include carcinoid tumors, lymphoma, and malignant melanoma. Overall, small bowel malignancy is an extremely rare complication of Crohn's disease, but tends to be seen more commonly in bypassed bowel segments.

Growth retardation occurs in nearly one quarter of children affected by Crohn's disease. If retarded growth persists despite adequate medical and nutritional therapy, operative intervention is recommended before the onset of puberty. Otherwise, the loss in stature will not be recovered because longitudinal growth is halted after epiphyseal closure.

Extraintestinal manifestations affect more than one quarter of Crohn's disease patients. Some of the manifestations are associated with the intestinal disease, but others are discordant. Typically, the cutaneous, ocular, and peripheral joint manifestations are linked to gut inflammation, and ankylosing spondylitis and primary sclerosing cholangitis behave independently. Occasionally, operative treatment of asymptomatic intestinal disease is required to control symptomatic manifestations affecting selected extraintestinal sites.

Options

Several types of operations are used in the surgery of ileocecal or small bowel Crohn's disease:

- Bypass
- Resection
- Strictureplasty

The role of laparoscopy in treatment of persons with Crohn's disease continues to evolve, and initial criticism has been largely dispelled. After the approach's feasibility and safety were established, studies have focused on other outcome measures, including physiologic function, length of stay, quality of life, disease recurrence, and cost. In many instances, the results obtained with laparoscopic surgery have surpassed those seen with a conventional surgical approach.

For ileocecal disease, laparoscopic mobilization of the terminal ileum and right colon can be readily performed in most instances through either a lateral or medial approach. Early division of the ileocolic pedicle will release the specimen from the retroperitoneum except at the areas of intense inflammation, which are addressed later. Following adequate mobilization, a small (4 to 8 cm) midline incision allows exteriorization of the specimen, control of remaining mesenteric vessels, bowel division, and extracorporeal anastomosis. Any areas of proximal bowel inadequately visualized at the outset of the laparoscopic procedure must be delivered through the midline incision and inspected for occult strictures.

The safety and benefits of this approach have been examined in many prospective as well as retrospective stud-

ies. The laparoscopic procedure offers a faster recovery of pulmonary function with fewer minor complications and a shorter length of stay compared to conventional surgery. Also, several retrospective studies have reported less narcotic use, quicker return of intestinal function, and reduced cost of hospital admission. At some other centers, conversion rates are high (17 to 40%), suggesting patient selection, time constraints, and surgeon experience might influence successful completion of the laparoscopic approach. However, many experienced surgeons report that intraabdominal abscesses and fistulas do not increase their rates of conversion or perioperative morbidity.

Bypass

Although bypass operations have been largely abandoned because of risk for continued disease activity and malignant degeneration, they are still considered as options in specific circumstances. Exclusion bypass is very reasonable for a complicated ileocolic phlegmon associated with dense attachments to the iliac vessels or retroperitoneum, with plans for definitive resection in later months. In such cases the proximal end of the excluded ileal segment should be exteriorized as a mucous fistula to vent the mucosal secretions that could instigate dehiscence of the ileal stump.

Resection

Resection is the procedure of choice for most persons undergoing operation for Crohn's disease of the ileocecal region. Even with scattered proximal skip lesions that may be amenable to strictureplasty, the distal ileal segment is typically the most severely affected area and warrants resection. In persons with isolated small bowel disease, resection is less commonly employed but is still used more frequently than strictureplasty alone.

The configuration of an ileocolostomy has been evaluated in a randomized controlled trial that compared side-to-end anastomosis to end-to-end configuration and another study that contrasted side-to-end anastomosis with side-to-side configuration. In neither reports did the side-to-end anastomosis improve safety or delay recurrence. However, some recent retrospective reviews report that early anastomotic recurrence is less common after side-to-side anastomosis compared to conventional end-to-end anastomosis, and proponents hypothesize that a larger anastomotic cross-sectional area is associated with a lower risk for recurrence.

The anastomosis can be constructed with suture or stapling devices depending upon the surgeon's preference without affecting safety or recurrence. However, in persons undergoing surgery for chronic obstruction, the bowel wall of the proximal limb can be quite thickened, whereas the distal limb is normal. In these instances, a hand-sewn anastomosis is recommended because the wall thickness may exceed the specifications of the stapling device, which risks anastomotic bleeding and leakage.

Strictureplasty

The surgical therapy for Crohn's disease has shifted toward conservative approaches over the past 2 decades. For patients with multiple strictures of the small bowel, intestinal conservation may be maximally achieved by surgically widening each stricture. The strictureplasty procedure has proved effective in relieving obstructive symptoms with weight gain that accompanies improved food tolerance. In addition, despite diseased segments being left unresected, steroid medication can often be withdrawn or reduced in dosage. Initial concerns about suture line healing and the occurrence of intra-abdominal abscesses or fistulas have been calmed by appropriate patient selection.

As experience with the procedure has grown, strictureplasty is considered in the following situations:

- Diffuse involvement of the small bowel with multiple strictures
- Stricture(s) in a patient who has undergone previous major resection(s) of small bowel (>100 cm)
- Rapid recurrence of Crohn's disease manifested as obstruction
- Stricture in a patient with short-bowel syndrome
- Nonphlegmonous fibrotic stricture

The contraindications to strictureplasty are as follows:

- Free or contained perforation of the small bowel
- Phlegmonous inflammation, internal fistula, or external fistula involving the affected site
- Multiple strictures within a short segment
- Stricture in close proximity to a site chosen for resection
- Colonic strictures
- Hypoalbuminemia (<2.0 g/dL)

A Weinburg strictureplasty technique is used for short (<10 cm) strictures, a Finney method is recommended for medium-length (10 to 20 cm) strictures, and a side-to-side isoperistaltic strictureplasty can be safely performed for longer (>20 cm) strictures. In this latter instance, the strictured segment's middle third is sometimes resected to facilitate a tension-free anastomosis.

Strategy

Certain guidelines should be evoked when operating for ileocecal or small bowel Crohn's disease, regardless of the presentation and clinical behavior pattern. These principles include the following:

- Multiple perioperative factors and intraoperative findings influence the surgeon's decision making; the planned operative procedure must be often altered and occasionally aborted.
- Nondiseased bowel can be affected. Inflammatory disease can frequently affect nondiseased bowel segments as well as adjacent organs. In most instances, this target organ is bluntly teased from the diseased bowel, débrided, and primarily closed.
- Mesenteric division can be difficult. The mesentery of diseased segments is typically thickened and friable; division of the mesentery requires overlapping placement of suture ligatures to maximize hemostasis and minimize the likelihood of hematoma.
- Resection margins should be conservative. Bowel length is conserved with limited (2 cm), macroscopically normal resection margins that are associated with

recurrence rates comparable to extensive, macroscopically or microscopically normal resection margins. Similarly, the configuration and construction of the anastomosis seem not to impact future recurrence.

- Septic foci require long-term drainage. Extensive, long-term drainage and omentum interposition will minimize the risk for recurrent sepsis and secondary involvement of a newly created anastomosis.

Hemorrhage

If the bleeding originates from a diseased segment within the small bowel, mesenteric angiography aids in localization of the bleeding site. Moreover, this diagnostic tool can become therapeutic with selective infusion of vasopressin, which often controls the hemorrhage. If the bleeding cannot be arrested, the mesenteric arterial catheter is left in place and used intraoperatively to accurately identify the bleeding site and facilitate limited bowel resection. Overall, one third of patients with Crohn's disease will experience recurrent hemorrhage typically within 3 years of their initial episode. Given the potential efficacy of radiographic and medical treatment, a nonoperative approach is suggested as first-line therapy in most patients.

Perforation

In cases of free perforation, resection is preferred over simple suture closure because the associated mortality rate is reduced 10-fold to approximately 4%.

Abscess

Most abdominal abscesses in ileocecal or small bowel Crohn's disease arise from penetrating fissures or ulcers. Although some surgeons advocate primary management by laparotomy, an enteroparietal abscess is usually best treated by preliminary CT-guided external drainage if the cavity is accessible or surgical drainage if the abscess is unapproachable despite imaging guidance. Subsequent resection of the diseased intestinal source is carried out when the abscess has resolved. Recent reports have challenged the notion that an abscess ultimately mandates laparotomy with resection. In one series, more than half of persons undergoing a CT-guided drainage procedure avoided subsequent operative intervention, and most of these patients had evaded surgery and remained asymptomatic after 3 years of follow-up.

Intramesenteric abscesses arise when a mesenteric ulcer penetrates the bowel wall, and the abscess spreads between the leaves of the mesentery, extending toward the mesenteric root. Resection of the bowel with a mesenteric cuff risks secondary peritoneal contamination and difficulty with vascular pedicle ligation. These pedicles are particularly fragile and slippage or premature erosion of the ligature can instigate major secondary hemorrhage. Instead, the abscess should be identified by intraoperative needle localization, and emptied by needle aspiration as well as manual compression of the mesenteric leaves. The bowel associated with the affected mesentery is then excluded by dividing the intestine on either side, creating proximal and distal mucous fistulas, and constructing an enteroenterostomy to restore bowel continuity. The excluded segment is resected 6 months later.

Posterior or retroperitoneal perforation of the ileocecal area may be well circumscribed or poorly localized because of deep extension behind the psoas fascia. A small simple abscess is managed by CT-guided drainage followed by elective resection of the diseased segment. A larger multiloculated abscess is best treated by surgical drainage. An incision is created over the site, the oblique muscles are separated, the abscess is localized with a large-bore needle, the pyogenic membrane is incised, and loculations are disrupted. Then, a catheter is inserted and remains until the cavity has collapsed as evidenced by sinography. If an unsuspected psoas abscess is identified at laparotomy, the ileocecal segment is mobilized, the bowel is resected, an anastomosis is completed, the abscess is unroofed and drained extraperitoneally, and omentum is interposed between the bowel and the residual cavity.

Fistula

Fistulas complicating ileocecal or small bowel Crohn's disease typically originate from a diseased intestinal segment and involve nondiseased adjacent organs such as bowel, bladder, abdominal wall, or vagina. Many of these fistulas can be ignored if they are relatively asymptomatic or successfully treated with immunomodulators and biologic modifiers. If this approach is unjustified or unsuccessful, the principles of operative management focus on resection of the primary offending bowel, suture closure of the secondary target site, excision or drainage of sepsis, and interposition of tissue between the involved organs. A primary anastomosis can be constructed and left nondiverted in most instances unless the patient suffers from poor nutrition, excessive intraoperative blood loss, or unresolved sepsis. When another segment of intestine is the target site, the mucosa of this bowel must be carefully inspected to exclude concomitant disease involvement because this will lead to breakdown of the repair and postoperative sepsis. When a loop of small bowel is nondiseased and secondarily affected, a wedge excision is typically performed and the enterotomy is closed. For an ileal-sigmoid colon fistula, the fistula tract commonly enters the nondiseased large bowel at its mesenteric margin, making débridement with primary closure difficult in some instances. Instead, a sleeve resection of the sigmoid colon with end-to-end coloproctostomy is often preferred to assure a safe anastomosis. For nonintestinal secondary sites, simple débridement with or without primary closure is recommended.

Outcome

The outcome of surgery for Crohn's disease may be considered under several headings: mortality, morbidity, recurrence, and quality of life. In long-term studies, the overall frequency of surgery averages 2.5 operations per patient, with the typical patient undergoing an operation every 10 years.

Mortality

Long-term studies report an approximate twofold excess mortality rate for Crohn's disease patients, although this appears to be lessening in modern times. The mortality rate is highest in the first 3 years following diagnosis, death being due to the disease and its intestinal complications. The relative and cumulative effect of aging appears independent of disease duration. In fact, except for emergencies, patients developing Crohn's disease after 40 years of age are at no particular increased risk of death.

Morbidity

Major postoperative complications occur in 10 to 20% of patients with a 4 to 8% reoperative rate and are most commonly intra-abdominal abscess, wound infection, enteric fistula, or bowel obstruction. Serious complications are more common in cases of pre-existing intra-abdominal abscess and preoperative steroid use, ranging in one study from a 0.6% complication rate (no steroids and abscess) to 16% (both steroids and abscess).

Recurrence

Recurrence of Crohn's disease is generally listed as a complication, despite the probable panenteric nature of the condition and the limitations of medical or surgical therapy in providing a cure. Several factors have been purported to be linked with recurrence, including age of disease onset, gender, tobacco use, anatomic pattern of disease, clinical pattern of disease, extraintestinal manifestations, duration of preoperative symptoms, previous resection, operative indication, blood transfusion, extent of resection, and pathologic features of resected bowel. The only variables that consistently predict an increased risk for recurrence are tobacco use and absence of fecal diversion.

With regard to ileocecal and small bowel disease specifically, a number of studies have looked at the association between the amount of affected bowel and recurrence. Although some clinicians contend that patients with more than 50 cm of disease are more likely to experience clinical recurrence, the association is likely due to the fact that multiple-site versus single-site involvement is associated with an increased recurrence rate, rather than the notion that absolute length of affected bowel predicts recurrence.

Clinicians have recently attempted to decrease the incidence of postoperative recurrence with prophylactic medications such as antibiotics, 5-aminosalicylates, and immunomodulating agents. Although 3 months of metronidazole therapy reduced the likelihood of clinical relapse at 1 year, this benefit was not seen after 2 years of follow-up. The aminosalicylates appear to provide a sustained protective effect in persons with ileal disease, but 6-mercaptopurine remains the most effective therapy at reducing relapse after resection for Crohn's disease.

Quality of Life

The physical and mental limitations imparted on life quality experienced by both nonoperated and postoperative patients with Crohn's disease are difficult to quantify. No one denies that limitations exist and sometimes can be serious. Late complications and side effects associated with medical or operative therapy affect the quality of life enjoyed by most patients. Also, mental disturbance, particularly depression, has been reported in 33 to 100% of patients with Crohn's disease. However, patients are most concerned about the uncertain nature of the disease and feel this uncertainty affects their quality of life more than other factors. This worry can be best alleviated through physician counseling of patients about what to expect from their disease. Accordingly, the overall outcome is still promising. More than two thirds of patients will report that they are in good or excellent health at the time of follow-up, encouraging many clinicians to maintain an optimistic attitude about the affected patient's eventual outcome.

■ SUMMARY

Operative management of Crohn's disease involving the ileocecum or small bowel is warranted in persons whose disease is refractory to appropriate medical therapy as well as those individuals with acute or chronic disease complications. After thorough patient evaluation, the surgical procedure may employ a combination of operative options dictated by multiple perioperative factors and intraoperative findings that influence the surgeon's decision. The patient's postoperative life quality will likely return to a relatively normal level, which can be enhanced if the person is counseled about his or her condition and medical prophylaxis is employed to delay disease recurrence.

Suggested Readings

Ayuk P, Williams N, Scott N, et al: Management of intra-abdominal abscesses in Crohn's disease. Ann R Coll Surg Engl 1996;78:5–10.

Fazio VW, Marchetti F, Church J, et al: Effect of resection margins on the recurrence of Crohn's disease in the small bowel: A randomized controlled trial. Ann Surg 1996;224:563–573.

Lochs H, Mayer M, Fleig WE, et al: Prophylaxis of postoperative relapse in Crohn's disease with mesalamine: European Cooperative Crohn's Disease Study VI. Gastroenterology 2000;118:264–273.

Milsom JW, Hammerhofer KA, Bohm B, et al: A prospective, randomized trial comparing laparoscopic versus conventional surgery for refractory ileocolic Crohn's disease. Dis Colon Rectum 2000;44:1–9.

Rubesin SE, Scotiniotis I, Birnbaum BA, Ginsberg GG: Radiologic and endoscopic diagnosis of Crohn's disease. Surg Clin North Am 2001;81:39–70.

Strong SA: Crohn's disease: Quality of life and cost. Clin Colon Rectal Surg 2001;14:175–180.

Tichansky D, Cagir B, Yoo E, et al: Strictureplasty for Crohn's disease: Meta-analysis. Dis Colon Rectum 2000;43:911–919.

Williams JG, Wong WD, Rothenberger DA, Goldberg SM: Recurrence of Crohn's disease after resection. Br J Surg 1991;78:10–19.

78

SMALL BOWEL NEOPLASMS

Howard S. Kaufman, MD
John L. Cameron, MD

Tumors of the small bowel are uncommon, insidious in presentation, and frequently represent a diagnostic challenge. The small intestine contributes greater than 90% of the mucosal surface area of the alimentary tract and 75% of its entire length. However, small bowel tumors are much less common than neoplasms of the stomach and colon and account for only 2% of all gastrointestinal malignancies. Approximately 3000 cases of small bowel cancer are reported annually. The majority of neoplasms of the small intestine are found within the duodenum, proximal jejunum, and terminal ileum, with relative sparing of the intervening distal jejunum and proximal ileum. Benign tumors of the small bowel are more common than malignant tumors and are encountered in 0.5% of autopsy cases.

Certain groups of patients have a higher incidence of neoplasms of the small intestine than the general population. Patients with Crohn's disease have an increased incidence of adenocarcinoma of the terminal ileum. Adenocarcinoma and T-cell lymphoma occur with increased frequency in patients with celiac disease. Immunosuppressed patients have an increased incidence of Kaposi's sarcoma and lymphoma. Adenomatous polyps and adenocarcinoma of the small bowel commonly occur in patients with familial adenomatous polyposis and other syndromes of inherited colorectal cancer.

■ CLINICAL PRESENTATION

Nonspecific abdominal symptoms are common in patients with small bowel neoplasms. Benign tumors of the small bowel are usually asymptomatic and are detected at autopsy or at laparotomy for other intra-abdominal disease. Symptomatic benign neoplasms of the small intestine may produce pain (25%), obstruction (20%), and bleeding (10 to 20%). Pain may be vague and nonspecific or crampy secondary to intermittent intussusception, causing episodes of partial obstruction. The tumor often serves as a lead point for an intussuscepting segment of small intestine. Bleeding may be overt or occult and may lead to chronic iron deficiency anemia.

Malignant small bowel tumors usually present at a late stage with signs and symptoms of advanced cancer. Nearly all patients have lost weight and may be moderately to severely malnourished. Over 50% of patients with small bowel malignancies present emergently with complications of bleeding or obstruction. Unlike the chronic intermittent intestinal obstruction seen with benign small bowel neoplasms, malignant tumors usually present with progressive narrowing of the intestinal lumen by circumferential tumor growth. The resulting obstruction is therefore usually high grade, partial or complete. Obstruction may also occur from volvulus of a loop of small bowel around the fixed site of tumor invasion. Ulceration of malignant tumors usually leads to more pronounced anemia than is seen with benign tumors. Rarely, small bowel tumors may perforate and present with localized abscess formation, if walled off, or with generalized peritonitis. Finally, periampullary duodenal tumors may present with obstructive jaundice.

■ DIAGNOSIS

In the case of complete small bowel obstruction, the diagnosis of a small bowel tumor may not be made until laparotomy is performed. Plain abdominal radiographs are usually nonspecific for tumors of the small intestine. In patients with intermittent or partial small bowel obstruction, barium contrast examination of the small bowel is the procedure of choice. Enteroclysis or small bowel enema is preferable to an upper gastrointestinal series with "small bowel follow-through" because air contrast techniques, fluoroscopic manipulation, and compression techniques will increase the sensitivity of detecting mucosal or extraluminal abnormalities. Extrinsic compression of the intestinal lumen is also nicely demonstrated by computed tomography (CT) with oral contrast examination, which may also allow detection of nodal or hepatic metastases for more complete preoperative staging.

Capsule Endoscopy

Recently, wireless capsule endoscopy has become available for evaluation of the small bowel. The endoscopic capsule (11 × 26 cm) contains a lens, 4 LEDs (as a light source), a color camera, batteries, a radiofrequency transmitter, and an antenna. The capsule is advanced by peristalsis, and the patient may be ambulatory and perform normal activities. Images are captured via an ultra-high-frequency bowel radiotelemetry belt worn by the patient. Stored images are viewed subsequently on a video monitor. In small series, capsule endoscopy has been useful in identifying a bleeding source in 55 to 70% of patients with obscure or uncontrolled GI bleeding. Future studies will be necessary to determine the role of this technology in the diagnosis of small bowel tumors.

The clinically stable patient with evidence of iron deficiency anemia has had an unremarkable endoscopic evaluation of the upper and lower gastrointestinal tract. In this setting, an enteroclysis study should be obtained. The clinician should not fall into the trap of attributing microcytic hypochromic anemia to iron deficiency without appropriate radiologic evaluation of the small intestine. Endoscopy can be helpful in diagnosing duodenal and terminal ileal neoplasms. Esophagogastroduodenoscopy (EGD) with biopsy of suspicious lesions may provide a tissue diagnosis of duodenal and ampullary adenomas or adenocarcinomas. Colonoscopy with direct visualization of the terminal ileum can provide tissue diagnosis of neoplasms of the terminal ileum. Small series have been published describing experience with enteroscopy; however, this technique has not been widely applied to evaluation of the small bowel.

■ MANAGEMENT

Small bowel tumors usually produce mechanical problems. The management of these neoplasms is therefore surgical and is designed to relieve obstruction, stop bleeding, or treat rare cases of perforation. Patients who present with acute intestinal obstruction without previous abdominal surgery or obvious hernias should be decompressed with a nasogastric tube and volume-resuscitated in preparation for laparotomy. Patients who have acute small intestinal bleeding should be resuscitated in preparation for laparotomy. Large-bore intravenous access should be obtained, and a Foley catheter should be placed to guide the adequacy of resuscitation. If endoscopic evaluation of the esophagus, stomach, and duodenum is negative, a technetium-labeled red blood cell scan or selective angiography should be obtained to localize the source of bleeding. In addition, selective embolization of bleeding small bowel neoplasms may arrest ongoing bleeding until laparotomy can be performed.

■ BENIGN TUMORS

Benign tumors of the small intestine are usually incidental findings at laparotomy or are detected in autopsy series. The incidence of various types of benign tumors of the small intestine is shown in Table 78-1. Adenomatous polyps, leiomyomas, and lipomas are the most common neoplasms of the small intestine.

Adenomas
Small bowel adenomas occur most commonly in the duodenum. These lesions may be classified as tubular adenomas, villous adenomas, and Brunner's gland adenomas. Tubular adenomas of the small intestine behave in a similar fashion to their counterparts in the colon. Small tubu-

lar adenomas have a low malignant potential but have more propensity for malignant change as they enlarge. Small intestinal adenomas may be found in up to 50% of patients with familial adenomatous polyposis. Tubular adenomas of the duodenum are best managed by endoscopic resection but on occasion may require surgical resection. Larger tubular adenomas of the jejunum or ileum, which have been identified radiographically, are managed by laparotomy or laparoscopic-assisted surgery. Once the involved segment of small intestine is identified, polyps may be removed through an enterotomy with local polyp excision or with segmental small bowel resection and primary anastomosis. Because palpation of the small intestine is usually necessary to localize a polyp, laparoscopic-assisted techniques may be helpful in delivering a suspicious segment of bowel up to a smaller abdominal wound for resection by an enterotomy or segmental enterectomy. Villous adenomas are also most common in the duodenum. Approximately one third of these lesions contain an area of invasive carcinoma. Duodenal villous adenomas may be excised via snare polypectomy techniques with or without submucosal saline injection. Periampullary duodenal villous adenomas are best managed by duodenectomy with wide excision of the lesion. The tumor should be pathologically examined by frozen section, and if malignant transformation has occurred, a more extensive resection by pancreaticoduodenectomy is the procedure of choice. Pancreas-sparing duodenectomy should be performed for villous adenomas of the third and fourth portion of the duodenum that have undergone malignant transformation.

Yearly follow-up endoscopy should be performed in patients who have had endoscopic or local resections of tubular or villous adenomas of the duodenum. Brunner's gland adenomas are benign lesions that represent hyperplasia of the submucosal exocrine glands of the first portion of the duodenum. These lesions are most often incidental findings at endoscopy but may bleed. Treatment of ongoing bleeding requires endoscopic or operative resection.

Leiomyomas
Leiomyomas of the small bowel usually occur in the jejunum and ileum. These tumors tend to be solitary and occur with equal distribution in males and females. They are most commonly found in the sixth decade and have an autopsy incidence of 1 to 2 per 10,000. Leiomyomas arise from the smooth muscle of the intestinal wall and produce an eccentric narrowing of the intestinal lumen. On contrast examination, the intestinal mucosa is usually intact in the setting of an extrinsic filling defect (Fig. 78-1). Small bowel leiomyomas may serve as a lead point for intussusception. Larger leiomyomas are likely to outgrow their blood supply, resulting in central necrosis and luminal ulceration. Rarely, extraluminal hemorrhage may occur if the ulceration is present on the serosal aspect of the intestinal wall. Tumors larger than 5 cm are considered malignant, although the biologic behavior of this type of tumor is often difficult to predict (see later discussion of gastrointestinal stromal tumors). The management of

Table 78-1 Incidence of Benign Tumors of the Small Bowel	
TYPE OF TUMOR	**PERCENTAGE**
Leiomyoma	30–40
Adenomatous polyp	20–30
Lipoma	15–20
Hemangioma	<10
Lymphangioma	<5
Fibroma	<5

found in the ileum and have an equal distribution in the duodenum and jejunum. As with leiomyomas, these tumors present with eccentric filling defects on small bowel contrast studies. A CT scan may be helpful in distinguishing a lipoma from a leiomyoma based on the presence of fat density within the suspicious lesion (Fig. 78-2). If a lipoma of the small bowel is diagnosed by CT scan and remains asymptomatic, it can be followed. Occasionally, these tumors will increase in size and cause obstruction or bleeding. Segmental resection may be performed via laparotomy or laparoscopy.

Hamartomas

The polyps in the Peutz-Jeghers syndrome are hamartomas and are found frequently in the jejunum and ileum and less commonly in the stomach and large bowel. The syndrome is characterized by autosomal dominant transmission, and affected patients have characteristic abnormal epithelial pigmentation, which is usually found on the perioral area as well as on fingers and toes. The intestinal polyps tend to be slow growing and are not pigmented. These hamartomas have no malignant potential and range in size from several millimeters to several centimeters in diameter. Larger lesions may present with bleeding or obstruction due to intussusception. Only symptomatic polyps warrant resection, which may be carried out endoscopically or surgically.

Hemangiomas

Hemangiomas of the small intestine represent less than 10% of benign small bowel neoplasms. They can arise from the mucosa, submucosa, or muscle of the small intestine. They may be solitary or multiple and can involve the entire gastrointestinal tract. Small intestine hemangiomas may be associated with similar lesions in the skin and buccal mucosa, as found in the Osler-Weber-Rendu syndrome. When symptomatic, hemangiomas usually present with acute intermittent blood loss. Diagnosis is

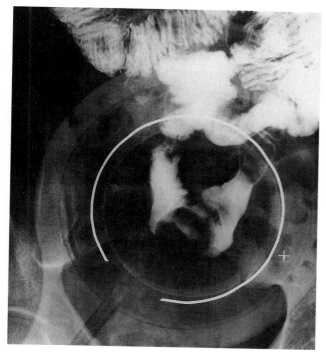

Figure 78-1
Enteroclysis study from a patient with a leiomyoma (gastrointestinal stromal tumor) of the small bowel. The tumor creates an eccentric filling defect with surrounding normal small bowel mucosa.

small intestine leiomyomas is surgical resection, even if they are asymptomatic. Resection can be performed via laparotomy or laparoscopic-assisted techniques.

Lipomas

Lipomas represent the third most common type of benign small intestine neoplasms. They are most likely to be

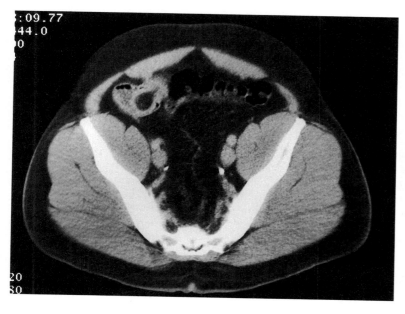

Figure 78-2
Computed tomographic scan revealing an ileal lipoma. The intestinal lumen is compressed by this mass with fat density.

made by endoscopy or angiography. If accessible to the endoscope, lesions may be obliterated by electrocautery or laser. Lesions identified angiographically may be treated with superselective embolization.

■ MALIGNANT TUMORS

The four major types of malignant neoplasms of the small intestine are adenocarcinomas (40 to 50%), carcinoid tumors (30 to 40%), lymphomas (20 to 25%), and leiomyosarcomas or gastrointestinal stromal tumors (10 to 15%). Adenocarcinomas are more commonly found in the duodenum than the ileum. Small intestine gastrointestinal stromal tumors (GISTs) are nearly evenly distributed within the jejunum and ileum but are rarely found in the duodenum.

Adenocarcinoma

Adenocarcinoma is the most common malignant tumor of the small intestine. These cancers are found with decreasing frequency as one progresses distally through the small intestine. Adenocarcinoma of the small intestine has been reported in association with Crohn's disease, villous adenomas, hereditary nonpolyposis colorectal cancer, and familial adenomatous polyposis. The surgical management of adenocarcinoma of the small intestine is determined by the location of the tumor. Tumors should be excised widely with a 6-inch margin of small bowel on either side of the primary tumor. An adequate lymphadenectomy by resection of the mesentery draining the involved segment of small intestine should also be performed. Unfortunately, there is usually more proximal and unresectable lymphadenopathy than can be excised safely. Following resection, a primary end-to-end anastomosis is performed. If a tumor involves the terminal ileum, a right hemicolectomy with ileotransverse colostomy should be performed. Patients with advanced disease manifested by extensive lymph node involvement or hepatic metastases should be treated by palliative segmental small bowel resection with primary anastomosis to prevent further symptoms of bleeding or obstruction. Prognosis for jejunal and ileal adenocarcinoma is usually poor, with 5-year survival rates of 20 to 25%. Owing to the rarity of this tumor, no prospective randomized studies of adjuvant therapy have been done in this setting. However, most patients will be offered 5-fluorouracil-based chemotherapy for advanced-stage disease.

Adenocarcinoma of the duodenum is usually diagnosed preoperatively by endoscopy with biopsy. Pancreaticoduodenectomy is the procedure of choice for adenocarcinoma of the first or second portion of the duodenum. Tumors of the third and fourth portion of the duodenum are treated by segmental resection of the third and fourth portion of the duodenum with end-to-end or end-to-side reconstruction to the second portion of the duodenum. A recent series of 55 patients treated at Johns Hopkins with duodenal tumors has demonstrated that survival is better for patients who have periampullary adenocarcinoma of the duodenum than adenocarcinoma of the third and fourth portions of the duodenum. Patients with resectable node-negative adenocarcinoma of the duodenum have a survival rate greater than 50%. Long-term survival rate is less than 15% for patients with node-positive disease.

Gastrointestinal Stromal Tumors

Leiomyosarcomas are a subtype of this group of tumors, which were initially thought to originate from gastrointestinal smooth muscle. As more specific cellular markers have become available and have been applied by immunohistochemical staining and electron microscopy techniques, these tumors have been further differentiated according to their mesodermal origin. GISTs may occur from the esophagus to the rectum. When benign GISTs are included, this group of tumors represents the second most common form of small bowel neoplasm. Tumors less than 5 cm in diameter are often benign and are usually grouped with leiomyomas. Tumors larger than 5 cm in diameter often behave in a malignant fashion and are further subtyped according to cell of origin. In a recent review and classification of these tumors collected over 20 years at the Memorial Sloan-Kettering Cancer Center, gastrointestinal autonomic nerve tumors (GANTs) were the most common subtype of GIST and occurred in over 50% of patients. Other cell types occurring with decreasing frequency included mixed leiomyosarcoma/neural tumors, spindle cell leiomyosarcomas, and epithelioid leiomyosarcomas.

Gastrointestinal stromal tumors are usually diagnosed by CT scan or by barium contrast study. Extrinsic compression of the intestinal mucosa may be seen endoscopically. Biopsy of these lesions is often unreliable due to their submucosal location. As tumors enlarge, patients may present with a palpable abdominal mass. Because these tumors may become large and outgrow their blood supply, central necrosis may occur, leading to intraluminal or free intraperitoneal bleeding.

Management of small intestine GISTs is surgical resection. Segmental enterectomy with primary anastomosis is the procedure of choice for distal duodenal, jejunal, and ileal GISTs. Tumors in the periampullary region should be treated with pancreaticoduodenectomy. Because these tumors metastasize through hematogenous spread and direct peritoneal implantation, wide lymphadenopathy is of no added benefit to the procedure. If distant disease is present, palliative resection should be performed to control or prevent bleeding or obstruction.

Although subclassification of these tumors has made histologic delineation more accurate, there is controversy regarding predictive factors for biologic behavior of these tumors. Factors that suggest a poor prognosis include large size (>8 cm), high mitotic index, high tumor grade, and the presence of positive margins. In general, survival after resection of low-grade lesions can be greater than 60%, yet it is less than 20% after resection of high-grade tumors. However, long-term survivors have been reported despite the presence of poor prognostic factors.

Until recently, adjuvant chemotherapy had no proven benefit in the treatment of GISTs. Gleevec, a tyrosine kinase inhibitor initially approved for use in chronic myelogenous leukemia, was found to have potent activity against GISTs that contained a *C-kit* proto-oncogene mutation that resulted in tyrosine kinase activity. Two multicenter trials have been conducted in the United States and Europe investigating the role of Gleevec in unresectable or metastatic GISTs. Radiographic response rates have been reported in 53 to 70% of patients. Gleevec received FDA approval for use in unresectable or metastatic GISTs in May 2002. Ongoing trials are investigating the role of Gleevec in the adjuvant and neoadjuvant setting for GISTs.

Carcinoid

Carcinoid tumors account for 30 to 40% of small bowel tumors and are the second most common malignancy of the small intestine. After the appendix, which accounts for 85% of all carcinoids, the terminal ileum is the next most common site. Thirty percent of patients have more than one primary tumor. Although most carcinoid tumors of the appendix are benign, 90% of carcinoid tumors of the terminal ileum are associated with metastases. Carcinoid tumors arise from enterochromaffin cells within the intestinal crypts of Lieberkühn and are capable of producing serotonin and other vasoactive substances. Approximately 50% of patients will have increased plasma serotonin levels, and 5-HIAA (5-hydroxyindoleacetic acid), a serotonin metabolite, may be found in increased quantities in the urine of patients with carcinoid tumors. Carcinoid tumors may occur at any age; however, the most common age of patients at the time of diagnosis is in their sixth and seventh decades. Males are more commonly affected than females by a ratio of 2:1.

Patients with carcinoid tumors may present with intestinal obstruction or with the carcinoid syndrome when hepatic or other extraintestinal metastases are present. Primary tumors are usually over 2 cm in diameter but may cause an intense desmoplastic reaction within the adjacent mesentery (Fig. 78-3). This fibrous reaction may be so intense that it results in occlusion of mesenteric blood vessels and segmental bowel ischemia or infarction. This desmoplastic reaction is thought to be due to a local release of serotonin.

The surgical management of carcinoid tumors is dependent on their location and size. Segmental resection of small bowel with wide mesenteric resection should be performed for tumors of the jejunum or ileum. Terminal ileal lesions should be treated by ileocecectomy. The remaining small bowel should be carefully examined for synchronous lesions. Small carcinoid tumors of the duodenum may be enucleated or included in a segmental resection. Larger tumors or those near the ampulla may require pancreaticoduodenectomy. Because these tumors tend to be slow growing even in the face of advanced local disease or hepatic metastases, resection of involved small bowel and mesentery is advocated to prevent further symptoms from obstruction, bleeding, or the intense desmoplastic response of the mesentery. Resection or debulking of hepatic metastases is advocated to prevent or decrease symptoms of the carcinoid syndrome and may actually prolong survival.

The carcinoid syndrome is an uncommon clinical entity that occurs when serotonin and other vasoactive substances secreted by carcinoid tumors reach the systemic circulation. The majority of malignant carcinoids secrete these substances into the portal circulation, where they are then inactivated by the liver. When metastases are present in the liver or in other sites that drain into the systemic circulation, such as ovaries, testes, lungs, or the abdominal wall, these vasoactive substances cause a cluster of symptoms known as the carcinoid syndrome. Flushing occurs in 25 to 75% of patients and may be interspersed with attacks of cyanosis. Diarrhea may be present in up to 85% of patients. Other less common symptoms include bronchospasm and congestive heart failure

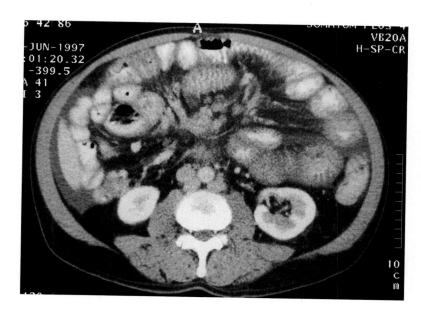

Figure 78-3
Computed tomographic scan from a patient with ileal carcinoid. The mesentery shows a characteristic desmoplastic response with resulting foreshortening.

secondary to right-sided fibrotic valvular heart disease. Physical examination may reveal flushing during an episode. Abdominal examination frequently reveals borborygmi. Signs of right-sided heart failure usually occur in the disease process.

Systemic chemotherapy is of little benefit for patients with metastatic carcinoid. Doxorubicin, 5-fluorouracil, and streptozocin have been used with response rates of 20 to 30% and no effect on long-term survival. Symptomatic patients with the carcinoid syndrome who are not completely resectable may be successfully palliated with octreotide. This synthetic somatostatin analog decreases circulatory serotonin levels and has been shown to decrease flushing and diarrhea in up to 85% of patients. Successful palliation of symptoms by octreotide persists for over 2 years in one third of patients.

Lymphoma

Lymphomas account for approximately 15% of small bowel malignancies. The average age of presentation is in the fifth to sixth decades, and males are twice as likely to be affected as females. Patients with celiac disease or Crohn's disease and immunosuppressed patients are at higher risk for developing small intestinal lymphomas. Most of these tumors arise in the terminal ileum owing to presence of increased lymphoid tissue in this area. Primary small bowel lymphomas can be differentiated from intestinal involvement of systemic lymphoma by the absence of leukocytosis and peripheral and mediastinal lymphadenopathy. Most small bowel lymphomas are of B-cell lineage, although lymphomas arising in the setting of celiac sprue arise from T cells.

Patients with primary lymphoma of the small intestine have nonspecific symptoms including fatigue, weight loss, malaise, and abdominal pain. One third of patients will have a palpable abdominal mass. Perforation is more common from lymphoma than from other small bowel neoplasms. Patients may also present with obstruction or bleeding. Diagnosis may be

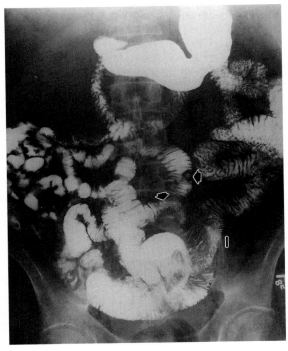

Figure 78-4
Barium contrast image from a patient with multifocal small bowel lymphoma. Several primary submucosal tumors (arrows) are seen narrowing the intestinal lumen. In addition, a segment of bowel is intussuscepted and displays a characteristic coiled spring appearance.

made preoperatively on an enteroclysis study with the appearance of submucosal nodules (Fig. 78-4). CT findings include bowel thickening and lymphadenopathy (Fig. 78-5). The Ann Arbor system (Table 78-2) is the most widely used classification for staging of gastrointestinal lymphoma.

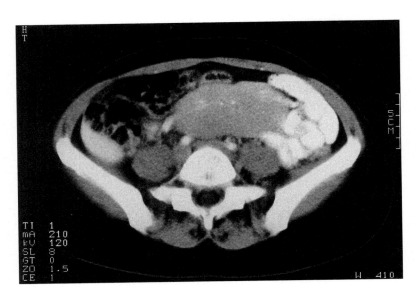

Figure 78-5
Computed tomographic scan from a patient with multifocal small intestine lymphoma demonstrating extensive mesenteric adenopathy.

Table 78-2 Modified Ann Arbor Classification of Primary Non-Hodgkins Gastrointestinal Lymphoma

STAGE	DESCRIPTION
I_E	Tumor confined to small intestine without nodal involvement
II_E	Tumor involving a localized segment of bowel with regional lymph node involvement
III_E	Bowel involvement with lymph nodes beyond the regional basin
IV_E	Spread to other nonlymphatic organs

Patients with localized small intestinal lymphoma (stages I_E and II_E) should be treated by resection of the involved bowel with its adjacent mesentery. A thorough exploration of the abdomen is necessary and liver biopsy as well as sampling of periaortic and mesenteric nodes outside the field should be performed for staging purposes. Splenectomy is not indicated. Patients with diffuse disease should be debulked to avoid later complications of bleeding, obstruction, or perforation provided that sufficient bowel can be left to allow for adequate enteral nutrition. The role of adjuvant therapy for stages I_E and II_E disease remains controversial, while patients with residual abdominal disease are usually offered chemotherapy. Overall 5-year survival rate is 20 to 40% with prognosis dependent upon stage. Patients with localized disease have a 5-year survival rate of 60%. Most patients with stages III_E and IV_E die within a year of prognosis.

Metastatic Tumors

Metastases to the small bowel are less common than primary small bowel malignancies. The most common tumors that metastasize to the small intestine are malignant melanoma, hypernephroma, Kaposi's sarcoma, and adenocarcinoma of the breast and lung. Patients may present with intestinal bleeding or obstruction from these tumors. Palliative resection should be undertaken unless metastatic disease is widespread and life expectancy is short.

Suggested Readings

Davila RE, Faigel DO: GI stromal tumors. Gastrointest Endosc 2003;58(1).

DiSario JA, Burt RA, Vargas H, McWhorter WP: Small bowel cancer: Epidemiological and clinical characteristics from a population-based registry. Am J Gastroenterol 1994;89:699–701.

Erlandson RA, Klimstra DS, Woodruff JM: Subclassification of gastrointestinal stromal tumors based on evaluation by electron microscopy and immunohistochemistry. Ultrastruct Pathol 1996;20: 373–393.

Frost DB, Mercado PD, Tyrell JS: Small bowel cancer: A 30-year review. Ann Surg Oncol 1994;1:290–295.

Lewis BS, Swain P: Capsule endoscopy in the evaluation of patients with suspected small intestinal bleeding: Results of a pilot study. Gastrointest Endosc 2002;56(3).

Moertel CG: An odyssey in the land of small tumors. J Clin Oncol 1987;5:1503–1522.

Sohn TA, Lillemor KD, Cameron JL, et al: Adenocarcinoma of the duodenum: The influence of site on survival. J Gastrointest Surg (in press).

79

CARCINOID TUMORS OF THE LARGE AND SMALL BOWEL

Dieter Hahnloser, MD
Heidi Nelson, MD, FACS

Carcinoids are rare indolent neuroendocrine tumors, mainly located in the gastrointestinal tract (74%). The term *karzinoid* was first used by Oberndorfer in 1907 to describe the typical pathologic features of the tumor, characterized by positive reaction to silver stains and to markers of neuroendocrine tissue. Intestinal carcinoids usually present as diagnostic dilemmas owing to nonspecific symptoms. When symptoms do occur, they are due to either local tumor effects or the bioactive products of the neoplasm. The release of serotonin and other hormonal products into the systemic circulation is thought to cause the carcinoid syndrome. The syndrome is uncommonly seen in intestinal carcinoids, but is typically associated with extensive hepatic metastases and portends a poor prognosis. The treatment protocols for each site are remarkably similar, and determined largely by site, extent of disease, functioning status of the tumor, and the ability to surgically excise the lesion with microscopic clear margins. Although surgery is frequently curative in early lesions, prolongation of life and palliative care often can be achieved in advanced metastatic cases by a combination of aggressive surgical and medical therapy.

The exact etiology of carcinoid tumorigenesis is unknown, although experimental studies indicate that the nuclear oncogenes N-myc and c-jun are involved. Another common event in intestinal carcinoids is allelic deletions on chromosome 18. Detected in 88% of tumors, these deletions are thought to indicate an important event in tumorigenesis.

■ DIAGNOSIS

Diagnosis of intestinal carcinoids may be difficult, and the indolent nature of their growth dictates that they are often asymptomatic until locally advanced or widespread. Up to 53% of carcinoid tumors are found incidentally at autopsy, endoscopy, or surgery for other causes. Two scenarios in diagnosing intestinal carcinoids can be distinguished: (1) those tumors suspected as carcinoids before surgery and (2) tumors diagnosed after surgery or biopsy.

Carcinoid Tumor Suspected before Surgery

Rarely is a carcinoid tumor suspected before surgery. The classical carcinoid syndrome occurs in fewer than 10% of patients with intestinal carcinoids. It is usually attributed to high serotonin production and release into the systemic circulation from the primary site or, more commonly, from metastatic sites. Increased levels of plasma substance P, serotonin, or increased 24-hour urinary 5-hydroxyindolacetic acid (5-HIAA) can be measured. If results are equivocal, the test should be repeated and other markers of neuroendocrine tumors, such as chromogranin A, should be measured. It is particularly helpful in rectal carcinoids with normal urinary 5-HIAA excretion and, in addition, is useful in the early detection of recurrences and follow-up of patients after intervention treatment. If chromogranin A is elevated and the urinary 5-HIAA and plasma amines are equivocal, the use of a provocative study such as the pentagastrin test may be of value. Pentagastrin can be administered in a provocative test to induce facial flushing and gastrointestinal symptoms in patients with liver metastases but not in healthy patients.

If biochemical tests are abnormal, the precise localization of the primary tumor and its metastases should be undertaken. Somatostatin receptor scintigraphy (SRS), is the initial imaging procedure of choice to localize the primary. Approximately 80 to 90% of carcinoid tumors demonstrate receptors that have moderate to high affinity for somatostatin and its analogs. SRS has an accuracy of 83% and a positive predictive value of 100%. Because of the ability to obtain whole body images with SRS, it is also useful for visualizing extrahepatic and extra-abdominal tumor spread. Furthermore, it is a predictive test for sensitivity to somatostatin analog treatment. The sensitivity of the study can be further enhanced by the simultaneous use of single positron emission computed tomography (SPECT) imaging. Positron emission tomography (PET scan) with ^{11}C-labeled serotonin precursor 5-hydroxytryptophan ($[^{11}C]5$-HTP) may prove to be a superior method to visualize carcinoids, as it has been shown to detect more liver and lymph node metastases than CT scan or SRS in some recent studies, but its use is not widespread. CT scan, ultrasonography, and magnetic resonance imaging (MRI) often fail to localize small primary tumors. Selective angiography has been used to localize small tumors, but this procedure is invasive and often yields false positive results. Endoscopic ultrasound is a new technique, which is relatively sensitive but not available in all centers. Ultrasonography performed intraoperatively has shown the greatest sensitivity.

The site of the primary carcinoid has implications for the diagnostic workup. The majority of *appendiceal* lesions are found incidentally at operation. They are rarely anticipated prior to operation, and hence, no approach to preoperative diagnosis need be formalized. *Colonic* carcinoids are usually diagnosed late, when complications of the disease or metastases become clinically apparent. If suspected, colonic carcinoids can usually be diagnosed by endoscopic biopsy. Early *rectal* carcinoid may be diagnosed incidentally at screening endoscopy; however, more established lesions may cause a variety of clinical manifestations, often mimicking adenocarcinoma. Endorectal ultrasonography may yield valuable information regarding the size and depth of penetration, useful for therapeutic decision making. Diagnosis of early *small bowel* carcinoids remains a challenge. Enteroclysis is frequently recommended, but yields a diagnostic return of approximately 40%. Regional lymph node involvement is found in 45% of tumors that are less than 1 cm in size. This pattern of spread produces the classic kinking, angulation, and separation of small bowel loops that can be seen radiologically and on CT scan. The lesions may also be visualized at laparoscopy.

Carcinoid Tumor Diagnosed after Surgery or Biopsy

Because the diagnosis of carcinoid tumor so often is made after surgical intervention or biopsy, all pathologic findings and operative notes should be reviewed first. Biochemical testing of platelet 5-hydroxytryptamine (5-HT) urinary 5-HIAA and serum chromogranin A should be performed next. Patients who are asymptomatic with normal biochemical test results and with no residual disease are followed up by biochemical and radiologic investigations on a yearly basis. Patients who are asymptomatic but have known residual disease should undergo SRS scanning, CT scans, and other investigations to assess surgical resectability. CT scanning has remained the mainstay of detection of advanced lesions, and will detect the majority of liver metastases. On MRI, the primary carcinoid tumor presents either as a nodular, well-defined soft tissue mass or as regional, relatively uniform bowel wall thickening. The majority of carcinoid liver metastases are hypervascular and can show several patterns of gadolinium enhancement on MRI. Ultrasonography may be of value in guiding percutaneous biopsy. If the residual dis-

ease is judged unresectable, systemic treatment with interferon-α, iodine-131-labeled metaiodobenzylguanidine ($[^{131}I]$MIGB), or chemotherapy is instituted. Furthermore, echocardiography should be done regularly to recognize carcinoid heart disease. The three most common cardiac lesions include pulmonary stenosis (90%), tricuspid insufficiency (47%), and tricuspid stenosis (42%). Enlargement of the right heart and paradoxic septal contraction patterns are less frequent.

Common to all carcinoid tumors is the high percentage of coexisting noncarcinoid tumors and multicentricity, warranting a meticulous evaluation during diagnosis and treatment. Gastrointestinal carcinoid tumors are at least twice as likely to be associated with second primary malignancies than are other tumors. Adenocarcinomas of the large bowel are the most common second primary malignancies, and the majority of them are found synchronously with the carcinoid tumor. It is prudent to search for these primary tumors, either at endoscopy or intraoperatively, as the overall prognosis depends primarily on the more aggressive second primary malignancy. The etiology of the increased risk of other primaries is not clearly defined, but it may be the result of accumulated growth stimulation by the neuroendocrine factors elaborated by the carcinoid.

■ TREATMENT OF LOCALIZED INTESTINAL CARCINOIDS

Localized carcinoids can be defined as macroscopically resectable neoplasms with histologically clear margins. Cure rates with long-term survival of 90% can be achieved. Despite marked variations in the frequency and presentation of carcinoids at various sites in the small and large bowel (Table 79-1), the recommended treatment algorithm remains similar. Lesions smaller than 1 cm

Table 79-1 Clinical Characteristics of Small and Large Bowel Carcinoids

CHARACTERISTIC	APPENDIX	SMALL BOWEL	COLON	RECTUM
Percentage of all carcinoid tumors	8–19%	20–29%	4–11%	10–13%
Usual site	75% at tip of appendix	Ileum > jejunum	Cecum > transverse > sigmoid	4–13 cm above dentate line
Age at onset (decade)	Fourth to fifth	Sixth or seventh	Seventh	Sixth
Presentation	Incidental, 75% <1 cm in size	Nonspecific gastrointestinal symptoms	Abdominal mass, mean size = 5 cm	50% incidental, 80% <1 cm in size
Local complication	Appendicitis	Obstruction, hemorrhage, infarction	Obstruction	Rectal bleeding
Carcinoid syndrome	<10%	Common with liver metastases	<5%	Very rare
Incidence of multiple tumors	4%	30–40%	Infrequent	1–4%
Incidence of second primary malignancy	13–32%	29–52%	20–35%	5–32%
Overall 5-year survival rate	>90%	55%	33–42%	70–80%

require less aggressive surgery to achieve clear margins. For lesions larger than 2 cm, segmental bowel resection, including generous resection of draining lymph node fields, is indicated. For those lesions between 1 and 2 cm, consideration needs to be given to the general state of the patient, the anatomic site of the lesion, histologic features, the consequences of definitive resection (e.g., sphincter loss), and the feasibility of postresection surveillance.

Small Bowel Carcinoids

Small bowel carcinoids are most frequently located in the distal ileum and are often multicentric. Long-term survival correlates closely with the stage of the disease at presentation, and the majority of patients present with metastases to the lymph node or to the liver. Tumor size is an unreliable predictor of metastatic disease, and metastases have been reported even from tumors measuring less than 0.5 cm in diameter. The diagnosis of a small, isolated carcinoid tumor in the small bowel is rare, and usually is made as an incidental finding at laparotomy for some other indication. The presentation of established lesions may be one of obstruction or of intestinal ischemia. Occlusion of the mesenteric vessels results from a number of factors characteristic of these lesions, including a profound desmoplastic reaction, vascular elastosis, and tumor secretion products.

For isolated small bowel carcinoid, "segmental" resection of small bowel is indicated, with wide local margins. Generally, a margin of around 10 cm on either side of the lesion is appropriate, and may be tailored to the size of the primary tumor and its location. Because small bowel carcinoids have the highest rates of second primary malignancies (29 to 52% of all carcinoid tumors) and because of the high frequency of metachronous lesions in small bowel carcinoids (30 to 40%), a thorough exploratory laparotomy is mandatory, concentrating particularly on the rest of the small bowel and the large bowel. Aggressive reoperative procedures are justified, because debulking can enhance the palliative success rate of subsequent treatments. An algorithm for the evaluation of small bowel carcinoids is presented in Figure 79-1.

Appendiceal Carcinoids

Although appendiceal carcinoids were previously recognized as the most frequently occurring carcinoid, their relative frequency appears to have decreased over time. One possible explanation may be the decreased surgical commitment to incidental appendectomy in the past 2 decades. Less than 10% of appendiceal carcinoids cause symptoms, because 75% are located in the tip of the appendix, where they are unlikely to cause obstruction (Fig. 79-2).

The overall risk of metastases is between 2 and 8%. Those lesions smaller than 1 cm are almost universally associated with an excellent outcome, and should be treated with appendectomy alone. The only exception to this rule is in the setting of local invasion of the cecum, in which case right hemicolectomy is indicated. Invasion of the mesoappendix per se does not mandate hemicolectomy. Lesions between 1 and 2 cm in size are associated with a 0 to 11% rate of metastases, and hence, the management of these lesions should be tailored to the individual patient, giving consideration to such factors as age, general health, the presence of angiolymphatic invasion, and the presence of clinically involved nodes. Lesions larger than 2 cm metastasize in 30 to 60% of cases and should be treated with right hemicolectomy. When right hemicolectomy is performed, lymph nodes adjacent to the superior mesenteric artery should be removed with care. Multicentricity occurs in approximately 4% of cases, and hence, thorough examination of the small bowel should be performed concurrent with the appendectomy. Overall, the 5-year survival rate for appendiceal carcinoid is over 90%.

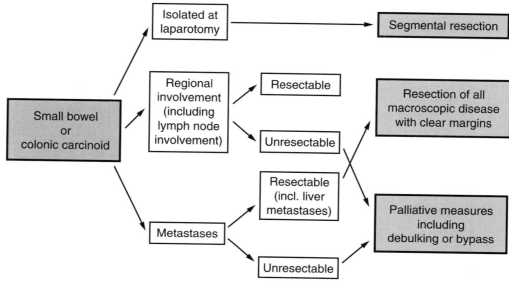

Figure 79-1

Treatment algorithm for small bowel and colonic carcinoid.

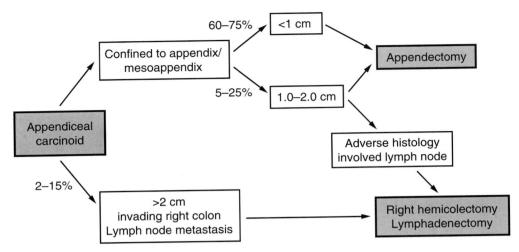

Figure 79-2
Treatment algorithm for isolated appendiceal carcinoid.

Colonic Carcinoids

Colonic carcinoids are most commonly found in the cecum: The incidence diminishes further along the distal colon. The average tumor diameter at presentation is 5 cm, and over two thirds of patients have either nodal or distant disease at the time of presentation. The finding of an early, resectable colonic carcinoid is a rare event. The 5-year survival rates are 70% for patients with local disease, 44% for those with regional metastases, and 20% for those with distant metastases. Carcinoid syndrome is rare with colonic carcinoids. Colonic lesions should be treated by standard segmental resection, including a wedge of mesentery and draining lymph nodes: the same surgical approach as for adenocarcinoma. Unresectable tumors should be debulked provided that the projected surgical morbidity of such a procedure is reasonable.

Rectal Carcinoids

These lesions are often diagnosed incidentally at the time of screening endoscopy and fortunately are associated with a good prognosis (Fig. 79-3). Predicted survival in rectal carcinoid is dependent on stage of disease. In the absence of metastases, the 5-year survival rate is 92%. If nodes are involved, the rate is 44%, falling to 7% if distant and unresectable metastases are present. The carcinoid syndrome is virtually unknown with rectal carcinoid. The majority are found in patients greater than 50 years of age. Most neoplasms are found between 4 and 13 cm above the dentate line, and hence are often palpable on digital rectal examination.

Tumor size and microinvasiveness are probably the two most important prognostic factors. Approximately 80% of the lesions are less than 1 cm in size, submucosal, and show

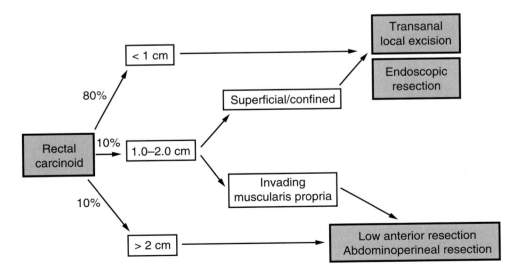

Figure 79-3
Treatment algorithm for rectal carcinoid.

no metastatic spread, and a minor procedure can be advocated. Lesions in the lower half of the rectum are usually best managed by transanal resection. Higher rectal lesions may be removed through an endoscope, typically using snare cautery. Cure rates of 100% can be anticipated.

If the neoplasm is 2 cm or greater (10% of cases) or a muscular invasion or lymph node metastases are present, radical surgery (low anterior resection or abdominoperineal resection) should be performed. The value of these procedures in the treatment of rectal carcinoids has recently been questioned, because they do not appear to extend survival beyond that observed with local excision in retrospective series. An individualized approach taking into account the patient's age and coexisting conditions may therefore also be appropriate in deciding on a surgical approach to large rectal carcinoids.

The management of lesions of intermediate size, from 1 to 2 cm, needs to be tailored to the individual patient. The frequency of metastases is this setting is approximately 11%. Usually, local excision is adequate, but unfavorable factors, particularly invasion of the muscularis propria, may suggest the need for more extensive resection. Endorectal ultrasonography may be of value in determining the depth of invasion. Decision making should be tailored to the general condition of the patient and the risk of sphincter loss.

A difficult scenario is the referral of a patient with incomplete removal of a rectal carcinoid, particularly after attempted endoscopic resection. Initial assessment should include accurate assessment of the size of the original lesion (if this is possible) followed by repeat endoscopy to macroscopically assess the site. Repeat biopsy of the base of site of excision may demonstrate residual tumor. In this case, ultrasonography, although difficult to interpret in this setting, may define the relationship of the lesion to the muscularis propria. If the lesion is reliably determined to be smaller than 1 cm, cautery ablation of the base of the resection site may be all that is required. If the lesion is larger or repeat biopsy is positive, then formal resection of the bed will be required. If the lesion is small and confined to the superficial tissues, then transanal local excision will suffice. If the lesion is larger than 2 cm or has invaded the muscularis propria, then formal resection is preferable.

■ TREATMENT OF INTESTINAL CARCINOIDS WITH REGIONAL INVOLVEMENT

Lesions that extend from the bowel to include local structures, or in whom lymph node metastases are present, are still curable using aggressive surgical management. The aim of operation should be the resection of all macroscopic disease, including nodal and peritoneal disease with clear histopathologic margins. If this goal can be achieved, then excellent cure rates are again attainable, with a 5-year survival rate in the region of 70%. The risk of local recurrence is increased in this setting.

■ TREATMENT OF METASTATIC INTESTINAL CARCINOIDS

The clinical course of patients with metastatic carcinoid disease is highly variable, and some patients remain free of symptoms for years. Survival up to 2 years even in the presence of liver metastases is common. If the patient is asymptomatic at the time of presentation, observation may be the most appropriate course of action (Fig. 79-4). The major aim of therapy in the presence of metastatic disease is palliation of symptoms, although enrollment of

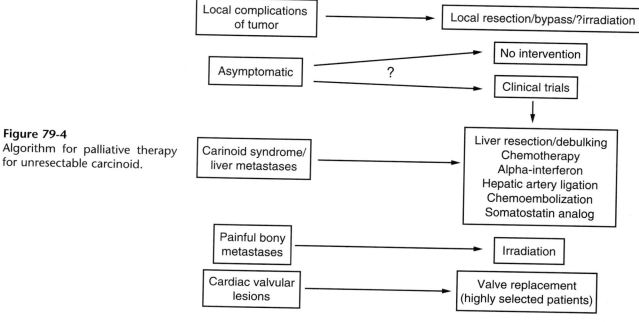

Figure 79-4
Algorithm for palliative therapy for unresectable carcinoid.

patients into clinical trials of nonsurgical modalities, with a view to producing prolongation of survival, is entirely appropriate. Randomized controlled data pertaining to these techniques are difficult to produce given the rarity of these lesions.

The options for active management of metastatic disease are discussed in the following sections.

Surgical Management

Specific complications of disease within the peritoneal cavity that may be palliated by surgical resection include obstruction of small bowel, regional ischemia, and infarction. In patients with unresectable disease, bypass, debulking, and stoma formation may all be appropriate.

Metastatic involvement of the liver tends to be diffuse, and can rarely be resected with curative intent. There is a clear role for palliative hepatectomy or enucleation of liver metastases in the presence of the carcinoid syndrome. Both cryosurgery and radiofrequency ablation have been used with mixed results. Liver transplantation has also been used to treat otherwise unresectable disease. Survival rates of 60% at 5 years have been achieved in one study.

Chemotherapy

There is no clear standard chemotherapy for carcinoid tumors. Most oncologists use a combination of 5-fluorouracil (5-FU) and streptozocin for advanced, progressive, and nonresectable carcinoid tumors; the results are mostly poor and the benefit seldom counterbalances the toxicity. The best criteria for initiating chemotherapy seem to be young age, good pathologic stage, unresectable tumor, and failure of chemoembolization or tumor extension preventing local-regional treatments. In case of tumor regression it is important to evaluate an eventual secondary resection of the main metastases. Interferon alfa preparations have been demonstrated to produce transient control of symptoms in carcinoid syndrome, and to produce short-lived slowing of tumor growth. Survival of patients with unresectable intestinal carcinoids has increased substantially as a result of interferon-α administration. Unfortunately, 20% of patients do not respond to treatment and their disease progresses. The combination of interferon-α and 5-FU has been demonstrated to produce antitumor activity, and may provide useful palliation. Symptomatic patients should be considered for chemotherapy combinations in a trial setting.

Embolization and Chemoembolization

In patients with liver disease too diffuse for surgical management, embolization and chemoembolization in combination with chemotherapy has been used to selectively target tumor tissue growth. However, the duration of its positive effect is usually transitory, lasting less than 1 year. There does not appear to be a significant difference in reported series between the two methods.

Radiation Therapy

The use of radiation in the treatment of carcinoid disease is restricted to symptomatic palliation, particularly of painful bony metastases. Somatostatin receptor–targeted radiotherapy reaches and destroys tumor DNA exclusively, but the therapy is still investigational. [131I]-MIBG has been demonstrated to reduce symptoms in preliminary studies.

■ MANAGEMENT OF CARCINOID SYNDROME

The most common cause of carcinoid syndrome is metastatic liver disease arising from small bowel carcinoid tumor. The release of serotonin and other vasoactive substances into the systemic circulation is thought to cause carcinoid syndrome, the manifestations of which are episodic flushing, wheezing, diarrhea, and eventual right-sided valvular disease.

Treatment of carcinoid syndrome should be directed at resection of the primary tumor or debulking of hepatic metastases and at blocking of the systemic effects of serotonin. For those patients in whom invasive techniques fail to control symptoms, the somatostatin analog *octreotide* is highly effective. Symptomatic improvement is reported in 70 to 90% of patients, biochemical response (reflected as >50% reduction in urinary 5-HIAA levels) in 30 to 70%, and temporary stabilization of tumor growth in as many as 85% of patients. While treated with somatostatin analogs, patients benefit from substitution with pancreatic enzyme supplements to avoid steatorrhea. The administration of general anesthesia is prone to produce *carcinoid crisis* in predisposed individuals, including attacks of life-threatening hypotension or bronchospasm. The usual recommended dose of somatostatin analog is 50 μg subcutaneously either before induction of anesthesia or before tumor manipulation. Further, preoperative proper hydration, correction of hypoproteinemia, hyperglycemia, and electrolyte abnormalities, as well as premedication with blocking agents such as antihistaminics, antiserotonin agents, and glucocorticoids are recommended. Regional anesthesia and specific pharmacologic agents such as morphine, suxamethonium, beta-adrenergic receptor agonists, tubocurarine, halothane, and atracurium should be avoided.

In summary, although patients with advanced carcinoid disease and carcinoid syndrome have benefited from recent therapeutic advances, there is no uniform agreement regarding ideal treatment strategies. Management options for patients with advanced disease or syndrome should be individualized according to the disease process and patient's condition. When possible, these patients should be entered into therapeutic trials.

Suggested Readings

Ganim RB, Norton JA: Recent advances in carcinoid pathogenesis, diagnosis and management. Surg Oncol 2000;9:173–179.

Habal N, Sims C, Bilchik AJ: Gastrointestinal carcinoid tumors and second primary malignancies. J Surg Oncol 2000;75:310–316.

Kulke MH, Mayer RJ: Carcinoid tumors. N Engl J Med 1999;340:858–868.

Memon MA, Nelson H: Gastrointestinal carcinoid tumors: Current management strategies. Dis Colon Rectum 1997;40:1101–1118.

Skogseid B: Nonsurgical treatment of advanced malignant neuroendocrine pancreatic tumors and midgut carcinoids. World J Surg 2001;25:700–703.

80

ENTEROCUTANEOUS FISTULA

Scott W. Gibson, MD
Josef E. Fischer, MD

Management of the enterocutaneous fistula is still one of the most daunting problems that a surgeon will face. An enterocutaneous fistula is defined as an abnormal communication between bowel and skin, which may be lined with epithelium. Once the epithelium reaches the skin, the fistula will not close spontaneously. Seventy-five to 85% of enterocutaneous fistulas are iatrogenic in origin, and arise most often as a complication of operation for intestinal obstruction. Occasionally, neoplastic disease or inflammatory bowel disease (Crohn's disease) will present with spontaneous fistulas. Less frequently, fistulas originate from sites of bowel anastomosis, in cases of diverticulitis, or as a late complication of abdominal radiation. The underlying cause of the fistula can have a profound influence on the chance that the fistula will close without surgical intervention. For instance, fistulas resulting from radiation or carcinoma are unlikely to resolve spontaneously, whereas those arising from inflammatory bowel disease sometimes close with bowel rest and reopen when enteral feeding resumes. Fistula output is also prognostic, as low-output postoperative fistulas often close with conservative management, so long as there is no distal obstruction.

Enterocutaneous fistulas always result in the external loss of fluid, electrolytes, trace minerals, and protein. They are divided into three categories based on the volume of this output: (1) high-output fistulas (greater than 500 mL/24 hours), (2) moderate-output fistulas (200 to 500 mL/24 hours), and (3) low-output fistulas (less than 200 mL/24 hours). High-output fistulas usually originate from the small bowel, and low-output fistulas tend to arise from the colon. Fistulas may be further defined by describing their anatomic course (e.g., gastrocutaneous), which helps to determine the likelihood of spontaneous closure, and is useful for planning medical management and any necessary operative approach. The three major complications seen in these patients are sepsis, electrolyte imbalance, and malnutrition. These complications are directly tied to fistula output, with higher output corresponding to higher morbidity and mortality. Indeed, the mortality rate of this disease has been reported to be up to 20%, largely due to sepsis and malnutrition. In addition, malignancy accounts for 30 to 40% of deaths associated with fistulas.

■ MANAGEMENT

The majority of enterocutaneous fistulas appear postoperatively. The likely presentation is that of a patient 5 to 6 days after a reoperative abdominal procedure who has a persistent ileus and is febrile. The patient will have electrolyte imbalances and evidence of fluid loss. A wound infection will appear, and drainage, usually of pus in the initial stages, will result in defervescence. In the next 24 to 72 hours, enteric contents will be seen coming from the wound, signaling the presence of a fistula.

The goals of treatment in the patient with an enterocutaneous fistula are closure of the defect and reestablishment of intestinal continuity through operative or nonoperative means. In order to deal with the complicated course of these patients, we have divided the management into a sequence of six phases: (1) prevention, (2) recognition and stabilization, (3) investigation, (4) decision, (5) definitive therapy, and (6) healing (see Table 80-1).

Prevention

Because most enterocutaneous fistulas are iatrogenic, it is logical to consider steps aimed at their prevention. Commonly, fistulas occur in patients who have undergone an emergency procedure for intestinal obstruction with inadequate preoperative preparation. Poor preoperative nutritional status can play a significant role in anastomotic breakdown, and may result in a diminished response to infection. Strict attention to detail and the application of sound surgical principles in all intestinal operations will help minimize the occurrence of enterocutaneous fistulas.

In the case of emergency procedures, the patient should be fully resuscitated prior to operation, perioperative antibiotics should be given, and ongoing efforts should be aimed at maintaining tissue perfusion. In the elective case, preoperative nutritional status must be assessed. Patients with more than a 10 to 15% loss of body weight over 3 to 4 months, a serum albumin level less than 3.0 g/dL, a serum transferrin concentration less than 220 mg/dL, or an inability to perform usual activities due to weakness are at an increased risk for anastomotic breakdown and will likely need preoperative nutritional support. Mechanical bowel preparation, especially in operations in which colonic anastomoses are anticipated, is generally used in the elective setting, although prospective studies report no benefit. No clear evidence indicates that intraluminal antibiotics greatly decrease rates of anastomotic breakdown or wound infection in intestinal surgery when adequate perioperative systemic antibiotics are given. However, it is our practice to use a neomycin and erythromycin base for bowel preparation. Perioperative systemic antibiotics (1 g cefoxitin is suggested) should be given prior to the induction of anesthesia.

During any bowel procedure, anastomotic technique should be meticulous, using well-prepared bowel with a good blood supply. The anastomoses should be tension-free. In instances of unfavorable conditions, we prefer to use a

Table 80-1 Management Phases for Enterocutaneous Fistula

PHASES	GOALS	TIME COURSE
Prevention	Adequate patient preparation for abdominal operation Meticulous surgical technique	Prior to development of disease
Recognition/stabilization	Rehydration Correction of anemia Drainage of sepsis Electrolyte repletion Oncotic pressure restoration Nutrition support institution Control of fistula drainage Institution of local skin care	Within 24–48 hours
Investigation	Fistulogram to define anatomic and pathophysiologic conditions CT to localize collections and to stage cancer, when present EGD or colonoscopy as indicated	After 7–10 days
Decision	Assess likelihood of spontaneous closure Plan therapeutic course Decide surgical timing	From 7–10 days to 4–6 weeks
Definitive therapy	Plan operative approach Bowel resection with end-to-end anastomosis Ensure secure abdominal closure Gastrostomy Jejunostomy	When closure is unlikely or after 4–6 weeks; with difficult fistulas operation will be easier after 4 months
Healing	Continue nutritional support Transition feedings	From 5–10 days after closure

CT, computed tomography; EGD, esophagogastroduodenoscopy.
Source: Adapted from Berry SM, Fischer JE: Enterocutaneous fistulas. Curr Prob Surg 1994;31:469.

two-layer, interrupted 4-0 silk anastomosis. The need for meticulous hemostasis cannot be understated. All bowel wall serosal tears and mesenteric traps should be closed. Drains need to be kept away from the anastomosis.

Recognition and Stabilization

The initial management of the patient with a new fistula should be geared toward timely resuscitation. Priority should be given to ventilation, circulation, and tissue oxygenation. The patient is likely to display signs of significant intravascular fluid deficits due to sequestration in the bowel and bowel wall. Crystalloid should be given to offset these losses, depending on estimates of intravascular volume depletion. Electrolyte imbalances should be corrected as they arise, and commonly involve potassium, sodium, magnesium, phosphate, and zinc.

Concurrent with resuscitation, any obvious abscess should be drained promptly. This must be completed 24 hours prior to placement of central venous catheters intended for parenteral nutrition to avoid bacterial seeding of the line. Because sepsis can lead to death in these patients, they are likely to receive multiple antibiotics during their hospital stay. This practice selects for resistant organisms over time. Antibiotics should be reserved for

the patient with obvious sepsis who displays evidence of mental status changes, hemodynamic instability, high fevers, or signs of impaired organ function. The most common organisms causing sepsis in these patients originate from the bowel. Staphylococcus is also frequently present because the fistula communicates with the skin surface. In most instances, systemic organ dysfunction is due to an undrained septic focus. Thus, prompt investigation and drainage should follow, generally by computed tomographic (CT)-guided drainage.

The fistula wound requires special care, because surgical procedures for permanent closure should not be performed through a septic, indurated, infected, or denuded abdominal wall. Drainage from the fistula is best controlled with a sump, preferably a soft latex catheter. This sump will improve local skin care and will allow for the measurement of fistula output. Output records are necessary for adequate fluid and electrolyte replacement, and to track fistula progress. The skin around the wound needs to be protected from maceration and breakdown once drainage is under control. Several preparations are useful, such as karaya powder or seal, ileostomy cement, glycerine, or ion exchange resins that keep the skin acidic and prevent activation of pancreatic enzymes by a basic environment. Protective dressings (stomadhesive) are also effective in promoting local skin healing. Recently, adhesive suction dressings have been designed which can be applied to complex, large open wounds with fistulas in the base. These lesions are otherwise difficult to control. The suction dressings also help to promote fibrosis and shrinkage of the wound over a relatively short period of time.

Over time, the external drainage of a fistula can become demoralizing and humiliating for the patient. The services of a trained ostomy nurse are invaluable. Continued reassurance from the physician will help in this situation. If necessary, psychotropic medications or treatment by the psychiatric service may prove valuable.

In conjunction with proper resuscitation and control of the external component of the fistula, the clinician should begin treatments aimed at reducing enteric volume and subsequent fistula output. Even though fistula output does not correlate with spontaneous closure rates, this can make the metabolic and electrolyte changes easier to manage. Unless the fistula is high in the intestinal tract, or the intestine is obstructed, the use of a nasogastric tube should be avoided. These tubes are uncomfortable and can result in impaired cough, serous otitis media, pharyngitis, alar necrosis, mucosal erosion, and esophageal reflux with late esophageal stricture. The fistula patient should be started on therapeutic doses of an H_2 antagonist or an H^+-K^+ ATPase inhibitor if there are no contraindications. Stress and prolonged periods of taking nothing by mouth predispose patients to peptic ulceration. These drugs directly affect the gastric mucosa by decreasing gastric acid secretions and intraluminal volume. Furthermore, this decrease in gastric acid secretion may lead to an indirect decline in pancreaticobiliary secretions.

Once sepsis has been controlled, prompt initiation of nutritional support is necessary. It is important to accurately calculate the patient's nutritional need to avoid both underfeeding and overfeeding. Because these patients are in a hypercatabolic state, we recommend feeding at a rate 1.3 to 1.5 times higher than the basal energy expenditure. This rate can be adjusted downward for fistulas with a relatively low output or in patients without sepsis. Weight gain should not be the goal of nutritional therapy because it tends to reflect fluid retention rather than nutritional repletion. The goal of nutrition in this setting should be achieving nitrogen equilibrium while maintaining or improving structural and functional protein synthesis. The protein requirement of the patient with an enterocutaneous fistula is 1.5 to 2.5 g of protein/kg/day, which is greater than that given to other patients receiving parenteral nutrition because of external losses and metabolic stress. The combination of increased protein and calorie intake should maintain protein synthesis in the hypermetabolic patient. Fluid requirements for maintenance can be estimated from either body weight or body surface area and adjusted for existing deficits and ongoing fistula losses. Electrolytes, vitamins, and trace elements should be supplemented as necessary. Fistula patients frequently lose significant amounts of copper, zinc, and magnesium in addition to the commonly monitored electrolytes. It is useful to check magnesium levels biweekly and supplement if a deficiency is noted. Copper is usually supplemented adequately if two ampules of commercially prepared vitamins and trace elements are given daily. For high-output fistulas, 10 to 20 mg per day of elemental zinc should be added to the nutrition regimen.

In patients with low-output fistulas that are not expected to close spontaneously, diet or enteral feeding may be considered. Not only does the patient have the psychological support of oral ingestion, but enteral nutrition may improve systemic immunity and the response to infection. In addition, enteral nutrition stimulates hepatic protein synthesis, which may improve fistula outcome. Feeding a portion of the daily nutritional requirement (20 to 30% of calories) enterally may afford these benefits. When used, duodenal or jejunal feeding is usually tolerated better and carries a lower risk of aspiration than gastric feeding. The practice at our institution is to use formulations that minimize the enteral glucose or carbohydrate load by increasing lipids and medium-chain triglycerides. Glucose- or oligosaccharide-based formulations tend to be poorly tolerated in patients with diseased bowel due to high osmolarity. Physiologic and metabolic parameters should be determined at regular intervals in the patient receiving enteral feeds. Weekly assessment of the short turnover proteins transferrin, prealbumin, and retinol-binding protein is helpful, as these protein levels indicate the nutritional state of the patient. Fistula output may increase for a few days after enteral feeding is started but should resolve. If output continues to increase, the feedings will need to be decreased or stopped.

Patients who cannot tolerate enteral feeding, or are not candidates for enteral nutrition due to intestinal obstruction, should begin parenteral nutrition. A 15% dextrose formula with 5% amino acids and 250 mL of 20% lipids should be given daily. This will provide a calorie-to-nitrogen ratio of 100:1 while supplying 25 to 40% of calories as lipid. If this solution fails to improve serum protein concentrations after 1 week, then the amino acid content can be increased to 6 to 8%, as long as the patient does not have an elevated blood urea nitrogen (BUN) concentration. As with enteral nutrition, the clinician should monitor electrolytes and metabolic indicators in patients receiving parenteral nutrition, adjusting the formulation to meet day-to-day needs. Parenteral nutrition should be administered through a single-lumen central venous catheter dedicated solely to this purpose. Multiple-lumen catheters carry a significantly higher rate of infection and should be replaced at 72-hour intervals. Central venous catheters used for parenteral nutrition should be placed in the upper body whenever possible.

The use of somatostatin in the fistula patient has received much attention in recent years. In the case of pancreatic fistulas, it clearly decreases output volume, but has not been demonstrated to increase closure rates in prospective studies. Its role in treatment of other forms of fistulas is even less clear. Somatostatin is known to accelerate gastric emptying while inhibiting motility in the rest of the intestinal tract. Long-acting somatostatin preparations are currently available, with a dosing schedule ranging from 100 to 600 µg per day given in two to four divided doses. In some studies, conservative treatment with parenteral nutrition alone leads to fistula closure rates of 60 to 75%, while treatment with parenteral nutrition and somatostatin leads to similar closure rates of 60 to 92%. In contrast, the average time to closure of 50 days seen in patients treated with parenteral nutrition alone is decreased to 5 to 10 days in *selected* patients when somatostatin is added to the regimen. The clinician should note that even though somatostatin treatment is promising in some patients, it has little use in fistulas that are unlikely to undergo spontaneous closure, such as those caused by radiation or neoplasia.

Investigation

The fistula may be investigated radiographically 7 to 10 days after onset, when the tract has matured and the patient is resuscitated, although this is necessary only if there are plans to take the patient to surgery early in the course of development of the fistula. Whenever performed, the examination should involve injection of the fistula tract with contrast medium under fluoroscopy. This procedure should be performed in the presence of the senior surgeon in charge of the patient and an experienced radiologist in order to obtain the maximum information. In our practice, water-soluble contrast fluid is injected through a No. 5 or No. 8 Fr pediatric feeding tube, and early films obtained before loss of contrast. The fistulogram obtained in this fashion usually yields accurate and detailed information regarding bowel continuity, the location of the fistula, the presence of an abscess, the presence of intestinal obstruction, the length of the fistula tract, the size of the bowel wall defect, and the cause of the fistula. Other studies, such as an upper gastrointestinal series, small bowel follow-through, and barium enema, are usually redundant and unnecessary. The use of CT scan or magnetic resonance imaging (MRI) is usually limited in the evaluation of the fistula patient without sepsis. However, CT scan is a valuable tool in the search for abdominal abscesses in the septic fistula patient, and can be used to place percutaneous catheters for abscess drainage.

Therapeutic Decisions

The management of the patient with a gastrointestinal-cutaneous fistula will ultimately lead to decisions geared toward resolution of the fistula and, if possible, restoring the bowel to normal function. Many fistulas will close spontaneously with the medical management described previously. The average rate of spontaneous closure varies considerably, depending on location of the fistula in the gastrointestinal tract. The clinician can plan a time course for nonoperative management based on this knowledge. For instance, esophageal and lateral duodenal fistulas can close in 15 to 25 days, colonic fistulas in 30 to 40 days, and small bowel fistulas (especially ileal) may take 40 to 60 days, if they close at all. Only one third of complicated cases will resolve spontaneously. Moreover, a mere 10 to 20% of fistulas close without surgery if they are still open after 4 to 5 weeks of sepsis-free nutritional therapy. The fistula is likely to become lined with epithelium from both ends by this time and become a mature tract. In any case, the ability to accurately predict which fistulas will close on their own is imprecise. Several favorable and unfavorable factors have been discussed in the literature and can help the clinician make management choices (Table 80-2).

Once the surgeon has determined that the fistula warrants operative closure, the patient should start a period of definitive nutritional therapy. Usually, parenteral nutrition is administered in this setting, and should last for at least 7 to 10 days and usually much longer. This will allow time for the patient's abdominal skin to heal, for nutritional repletion, and for possible spontaneous closure.

Fistulas that result from malignancy are indicative of advanced transmural disease and have a poor prognosis. However, malignancy does not contraindicate aggressive fistula management, because many patients with malignancy can be treated and have a reasonable life expectancy. Each case should be tailored according to the kind of tumor involved. The surgeon should keep in mind that fistulas arising from malignancy are not prone to close spontaneously, and will likely require adjunctive therapy to achieve disease-free intervals or survival.

Table 80-2 Predictive Factors for Spontaneous Closure of Enterocutaneous Fistula

FACTOR	FAVORABLE	UNFAVORABLE
Anatomic location	Oropharyngeal, esophageal duodenal stump, pancreaticobiliary, and jejunal	Gastric, lateral duodenal, ligament of Treitz, and ileal
Nutritional status	Well nourished	Malnourished
Sepsis	Absent	Present
Cause	Appendicitis, diverticulitis postoperative	Crohn's disease, cancer, foreign body, radiation
Condition of bowel	Healthy adjacent tissue, small leak, quiescent disease, no abscess	Total disruption, abscess, distal obstruction, active disease (Crohn's disease, tumor)
Miscellaneous	Tract >2 cm long Defect size <1 cm²	Epithelialization, foreign body
Transferrin	>200 mg/dL	<200 mg/dL

Source: Berry SM, Fischer JE: Enterocutaneous fistulas. Curr Prob Surg 1994;31:469.

■ DEFINITIVE THERAPY

Surgical correction is indicated in patients with an anatomically unfavorable fistula that is unlikely to spontaneously close. It is also indicated in patients with a more anatomically favorable fistula that fails to show signs of closing after 4 or 5 weeks of sepsis-free nonoperative management. Of course, the development of sepsis should prompt urgent investigation with drainage of any abscess found. Correction of the fistula at this time is appropriate if the surgeon feels that the patient can withstand the stress of a prolonged procedure. In fragile patients, surgical drainage of the abscess should be performed, along with proximal diversion of the gastrointestinal tract to control continued soiling. Definitive repair of the fistula is saved for a later time, when the patient is stable and initial dense adhesions have settled, allowing a safer surgical approach.

Indeed, the timing of surgery is an important issue. Many of these complex patients develop obliterative adhesions that are so dense that adhesiolysis is fraught with the risk of further enterotomy and fistula formation. This period lasts from 3 weeks to 3 months after the index event. Thus, it is often advisable to wait 4 months or more before contemplating relaparotomy, by which time the adhesions have frequently become more manageable. In rare cases re-laparotomy is impossible because of the severity of adhesions. In these patients it is sometimes possible to bring out a proximal loop of small bowel, often in the left upper quadrant, to divert stool from a difficult enterocutaneous fistula into a stoma appliance. A definitive laparotomy can then be performed several months later.

As previously indicated, operations to correct a fistula need to be conducted under optimal conditions whenever possible. The well-prepared patient will be nutritionally replete as evidenced by adequate short turnover protein levels. Meticulous skin care and control of fistula drainage will allow the surgeon to enter the abdomen through a healthy abdominal wall, which enhances the chance of a secure abdominal closure. The fistula drainage needs to be cultured to guide intravenous antibiotic therapy. Prophylactic antibiotics should be given. Enteral nutrition should be stopped several days before surgery to decrease related abdominal distention that may hinder abdominal closure. Parenteral nutrition should be given before and after the procedure.

To begin the operation, some surgeons prefer to enter the abdomen through a new incision, to help keep the major operative field relatively clean. The authors prefer a transverse incision. Other surgeons prefer to reuse the midline incision, keeping as much as possible of the abdominal wall available for future stoma sites, particularly in the patient with inflammatory bowel disease. The entire length of the bowel, from the ligament of Treitz to the rectum, should be freed of adhesions. With this completed, the surgeon should proceed to definitive resection of the fistula tract and involved bowel. An end-to-end anastomosis of the bowel should be performed with two layers of 4-0 silk in a clean field, away from any abscess cavities or the fistula site. This approach is consistently associated with the highest rates of permanent fistula closure and the lowest incidence of complications. Other methods of closure, such as exteriorization and bypass, offer inferior results and should be performed only if resection and anastomosis are not feasible (Fig. 80-1). In cases with complex repairs of multiple fistula sites, it may be prudent to consider temporary fecal diversion using a proximal loop stoma for a period of 8 to 12 weeks.

After the anastomosis is complete, the omentum should be placed in its anatomic position. The omentum is used to separate the anastomotic site from the abdominal incision. Meticulous technique and hemostasis is essential to prevent further fistula formation. The abdominal wall must be closed securely. A plastic surgery consultation may be helpful in the event of a complicated closure. The surgeon should avoid using prosthetic materials for abdominal closure because they can lead to recurrent fistulization, and may need to use techniques such as a lateral release of the external oblique aponeurosis to

OPERATION

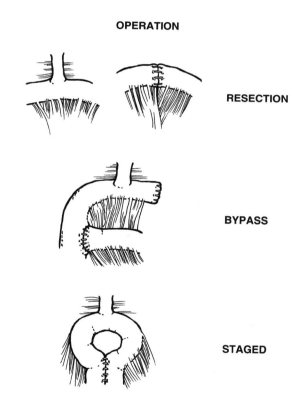

RESECTION

BYPASS

STAGED

Figure 80-1

Options for operative fistula management. *Top,* Resection with end-to-end anastomosis is the preferred method for surgical fistula management. *Middle,* Permanent bypass, although no longer recommended, may be necessary in certain palliative circumstances, such as in patients with an unresectable tumor and a short life expectancy. *Bottom,* Staged bypass with delayed resection may be considered in patients whose medical condition will not permit extensive operative procedures. (From Berry SM, Fischer JE: Enterocutaneous fistulas. Curr Prob Surg 1994;31:469.)

allow closure. Ventral hernias can always be repaired later with synthetic mesh. Prior to closure, a gastrostomy and feeding jejunostomy can be considered for postoperative gastric drainage and nutritional access.

■ HEALING

Nutritional support in the postoperative period is essential to ensure proper wound healing and resistance to infection. Parenteral nutrition should be given until ileus resolves, and then continued as a supplement until at least 1500 kcal per day of enteral nutrition is tolerated. Regardless of whether the fistula is closed operatively or heals spontaneously, the surgeon must be aware that fistulas can recur in many instances, especially when the fistula is caused by a persistent problem such as inflammatory bowel disease, malignancy, or irradiated bowel.

Patients who have undergone multiple resections for recurrent fistulas are at risk for short bowel syndrome. In these cases, parenteral nutrition will be necessary indefinitely. At least a portion of calories should be provided enterally to stimulate the remaining bowel. The surgeon should also watch for other late complications such as anastomotic stricture and adhesive small bowel obstruction. Overall, most patients with an appropriately treated enterocutaneous fistula can expect a good prognosis.

Suggested Readings

Berry SM, Fischer JE: Enterocutaneous fistulas. Curr Probl Surg 1994;31(6):469–576.

Fischer JE: Gastrointestinal-cutaneous fistulas. In Nyhus LM, Baker RJ, Fischer JE (Eds.): Mastery of Surgery, 3rd ed. Boston, Little, Brown, 1997, pp 1378–1383.

Surgical management of gastrointestinal fistulas. Surg Clin North Am 1996;76(5):1009–1203.

81

ACUTE AND CHRONIC MESENTERIC ISCHEMIA

Susan Galandiuk, MD
Todd Waltrip, MD

Mesenteric ischemia can be either acute or chronic. Acute mesenteric ischemia is a life-threatening disease of sudden onset and has several distinctly different causes. The majority of patients who are diagnosed with acute visceral ischemia have progressed to the point of bowel necrosis. Early recognition of acute ischemia is essential to permit timely intervention prior to bowel necrosis, irreversible multisystem organ failure, and death.

Chronic visceral ischemia, on the other hand, is a manifestation of systemic atherosclerosis and is rarely life-threatening. The quality of life for patients with chronic ischemia can be significantly improved by surgical revascularization of one or more visceral arteries.

■ ACUTE MESENTERIC ISCHEMIA

Acute mesenteric ischemia is being encountered with increasing frequency. The consequences of unrecognized ischemia and infarction of the viscera are devastating, with multisystem organ failure and death nearly unavoidable in many cases. The causes of acute mesenteric ischemia are listed in Table 81-1. The most frequent causes are embolization to the superior mesenteric artery (SMA) and thrombosis of the SMA, accounting for 50 and 25% of cases, respectively. Arterial emboli, which occur most commonly in the SMA, usually lodge 3 to 10 cm distal to the vessel origin, particularly where the vessel begins to narrow at the origin of the middle colic artery. SMA thrombosis, on the other hand, generally occurs at its origin. Patients who present with thrombosis often have

chronic mesenteric ischemia, which predisposes them to sudden occlusion of an already stenotic vessel.

Nonocclusive mesenteric ischemia (NOMI) accounts for 25% of cases of intestinal ischemia and results from hypovolemia, cardiac failure, sepsis, digitalis therapy, and alpha-adrenergic agents. Digitalis may cause abnormal mesenteric vasospasm and is at least partially involved with the majority of cases of NOMI. Mortality rates from NOMI are as high as 70% because of the difficulty of early diagnosis. Hemodialysis patients who develop periods of hypotension during dialysis are at risk for NOMI. These patients classically present with an occluded dialysis shunt that is an indicator of the hypotensive episode. NOMI typically involves the watershed areas of the splenic flexure and left colon, except in rare instances of hypotension related to trauma, which leads to right colon ischemia.

Acute mesenteric venous thrombosis is caused by hypercoagulable states and results in massive influxes of fluid into the bowel wall and lumen. Conditions associated with visceral venous thrombosis include any of the inherited hypercoagulable states (Table 81-2), cirrhosis, inflammatory bowel disease, trauma, pancreatitis, and cancer. The mortality rate with mesenteric venous thrombosis is greater than 80%.

Other, more unusual causes of acute mesenteric ischemia include aortic dissection, cardiopulmonary bypass, and median arcuate ligament compression. Some patients with aortic dissection will develop visceral artery occlusion, which is an indication for repair of the dissection. Mesenteric ischemia has been described in patients after cardiopulmonary bypass and appears to be a type of NOMI. Patients who develop NOMI after cardiopulmonary bypass are often, but not always, those with intraaortic balloon pumps or vasopressor support for cardiac dysfunction. Median arcuate ligament compression of the SMA or celiac axis is another unusual cause of mesenteric ischemia that may require surgery to release the ligament and revascularize the involved vessels.

Presentation

Patients with acute mesenteric ischemia have sudden onset of abdominal pain that is often "out of proportion" to the findings on physical examination. Patients may have nausea, vomiting, and gastrointestinal bleeding, either frank or occult. Obtaining a thorough patient history is crucial in the early differentiation of the various forms of mesenteric ischemia. Specific history taking should include prior cardiac arrhythmias, pain with weight loss, malignancy, and hematologic abnormalities. Presentation may follow an episode of hypotension or recent institution of digitalis therapy (both suggestive of NOMI).

Acute ischemia has three phases of presentation:

1. The initial phase is extremely painful and may consist of abdominal pain, vomiting, diarrhea, and gastrointestinal hemorrhage.
2. The intermediate phase is more vague and nonspecific.
3. The final phase is when bowel necrosis has occurred.

Table 81-1 Causes of Acute Mesenteric Ischemia		
CAUSE	**SOURCE**	**INCIDENCE (%)**
SMA embolus	Cardiac	50
SMA thrombosis	Underlying atherosclerosis	25
NOMI	Low-flow states, medication	20
Mesenteric venous thrombosis	Hypercoagulable states	5

SMA, superior mesenteric artery; NOMI, nonocclusive mesenteric ischemia.

Table 81-2 Hypercoagulable States

Protein C and S deficiency
Antithrombin III deficiency
Dysfibrinogenemia
Abnormal plasminogen
Polycythemia vera
Factor V Leiden mutation
Thrombocytosis
Sickle cell disease

Evaluation

Patients with acute mesenteric ischemia may have leuko-cytosis, fever, metabolic acidosis, and peritonitis, but these are usually late signs, when bowel necrosis has already occurred. Serum amylase and lactate will often be elevated. Lactate may be the most useful laboratory test, because it is often elevated in the early stages of ischemia, when other tests are uninformative. New diagnostic assays including D-lactate, intestinal fatty acid binding protein, and the isoenzyme of glutathione S-transferase have been reported, but none have reached clinical practice at the current time. Diagnostic peritoneal lavage has been used, but may only demonstrate white blood cells in the presence of frank bowel necrosis or perforation.

Plain radiographs are generally nonspecific but are useful to exclude other intra-abdominal processes. Radiographic signs that suggest visceral ischemia include bowel wall thickening, intestinal pneumatosis, and portal vein gas, the latter being a sign of advanced disease. Intraluminal contrast medium administration is contraindicated, because it can interfere with later arteriography.

Ultrasonography, to demonstrate flow in the SMA or celiac axis, is frequently obscured by dilated, gas-filled bowel loops. A computed tomographic (CT) scan of the abdomen and pelvis can show bowel wall thickening, pneumatosis in bowel wall, or portal vein gas. The CT scan is the diagnostic study of choice in mesenteric venous thrombosis and can demonstrate thrombus in the portal or superior mesenteric vein.

The gold standard for diagnosis of acute mesenteric ischemia continues to be biplanar mesenteric arteriography. Both anteroposterior and lateral views of the visceral vessels are necessary to fully visualize all three visceral vessels. Angiography can usually differentiate emboli from thrombosis, and the vasospasm of NOMI is readily apparent in smaller, branching arterioles (Fig. 81-1).

Treatment

Initial treatment of acute mesenteric ischemia, which begins during patient evaluation, includes fluid resuscitation, correction of acidosis, and broad-spectrum antibiotics. Systemic anticoagulation with heparin is necessary to prevent further clot propagation. Patients with peritoneal signs should be operated on without delay, for they will uniformly have some degree of bowel necrosis. In patients without peritonitis or other evidence of bowel necrosis, some authors have advocated angioplasty, if possible, with selective utilization of thrombolytic therapy or intravascular stenting as appropriate.

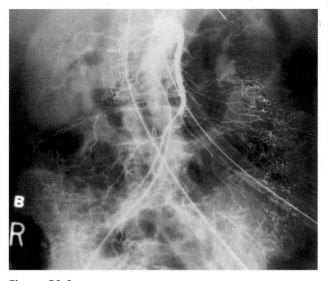

Figure 81-1
Superior mesenteric arteriogram in a patient with nonocclusive mesenteric ischemia, typified by tapering of distal arterial branches. (From Allen KB, Salam AA; Lundsen AB: Acute mesenteric ischemia after cardiopulmonary bypass. J Vasc Surg 1992;16:393, with permission from Vascular Surgery and The American Association for Vascular Surgery.)

SMA embolization is treated operatively with embolectomy. A transverse arteriotomy is made in the SMA to avoid the narrowing vessel when it is closed. Embolectomy catheters are then passed proximally and distally. SMA thrombosis is treated operatively with either transaortic mesenteric endarterectomy or bypass.

Treatment of mesenteric venous thrombosis is primarily systemic anticoagulation and resection of any necrotic bowel. Venous thrombectomy has been shown to be of little benefit, because the thrombus typically extends into small vein branches.

The treatment of NOMI is resection of necrotic bowel, continuous infusion of papaverine through a catheter in the SMA (both intra- and postoperatively), and discontinuation of digitalis and other vasoconstrictors. Papaverine is a vasodilator that reverses mesenteric vasoconstriction. Heparin should never be administered through the same line as papaverine because precipitation results when the two agents are combined. Papaverine infusion should continue until the patient is asymptomatic and when repeat arteriography no longer shows vasospasm. Figure 81-2 presents an algorithm for evaluation and treatment of patients with acute mesenteric ischemia.

Long-term anticoagulation following acute mesenteric ischemia is controversial. Some advocate anticoagulation with warfarin for venous thrombosis or arterial embolism and use of platelet inhibitors for arterial thrombosis or NOMI.

Bowel Viability

Determining bowel viability in the early ischemic period can be difficult. The best criteria for determining viability

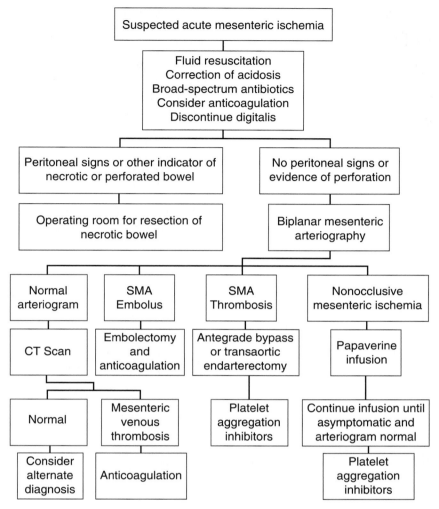

Figure 81-2
Algorithm for the treatment of acute mesenteric ischemia.

include color, palpable mesenteric pulses, and visible peristalsis. These combined criteria are better indicators of bowel viability than intraoperative Doppler, though Doppler can also be useful. Active bleeding from adjacent mesenteric fat can also be an indicator of adequate perfusion. Merely cutting a small segment of the adjacent fat will allow visualization of adequate or inadequate bleeding. Another technique for determining viability is fluorescein administration. Viable bowel will absorb fluorescein dye, which will fluoresce when viewed under a Wood's lamp. Fluorescein diffuses into all fat-containing tissues with time and is useless as a viability marker if not assessed early after administration.

The stability of the patient and pattern of ischemic involvement of the intestine determine whether or not primary reanastomosis is performed after resection of necrotic bowel. If the margins of the ischemia are not clearly defined, as may occur in NOMI, then reanastomosis should not be performed, and a proximal enterostomy should be fashioned, often with a mucous fistula. A sec-ond-look laparotomy is performed at 24 to 48 hours. If clearly viable margins are found, anastomosis may be performed in the stable patient. There should be a low threshold for second-look laparotomy at 24 to 48 hours. If a second-look laparotomy is planned at the time of surgery, then this plan should not be changed simply because the patient appears to be doing well in the postoperative period. Most surgeons do not perform any resection if the entire small bowel is necrotic, because it would relegate the patient to parenteral nutrition for the remainder of his or her life. In younger patients, however, more heroic efforts will be attempted; certainly the ethical dilemmas involved in such decision making are significant.

Laparoscopy

Laparoscopy has been applied to selected patients with acute mesenteric ischemia in selected cases. Some medically unfit patients with acute occlusion of the SMA have successfully undergone intra-arterial fibrinolytic therapy followed by laparoscopy. Diagnostic laparoscopy has been used to verify that all bowel is viable. Fluorescein coupled with laparoscopy has been used to assess bowel viability and is as accurate as open laparotomy for detecting nonviable bowel. Using the laparoscope, however, an argon beam laser must be used instead of a Wood's lamp.

■ CHRONIC MESENTERIC ISCHEMIA

Chronic mesenteric ischemia is caused by atherosclerotic disease that involves two or more visceral vessels. The large number of collateral vessels in the mesenteric circulation explains the rarity of symptomatic ischemia with only single-vessel disease. The percentage of patients with chronic mesenteric ischemia who will progress to bowel infarction is not known, but the symptoms of chronic ischemia are so debilitating that operative treatment is desirable in many cases.

Presentation
Symptoms typically include postprandial abdominal pain and weight loss. Weight loss occurs because the postprandial pain causes the patient to develop "food phobia." An abdominal bruit can occasionally be detected on physical examination. The majority of patients with chronic mesenteric ischemia are women, and, as with other forms of atherosclerotic disease, smoking and hypertension are common factors in these patients.

Evaluation
The diagnostic study of choice for mesenteric ischemia is biplanar arteriography. Mesenteric arteriography may cause visceral infarction and therefore should be performed only in centers capable of addressing this. Figures 81-3 and 81-4 demonstrate some typical arteriographic findings in patients with stenosis or occlusion of one or more visceral arteries.

Operative Treatment
No single surgical technique is best for all cases of chronic mesenteric ischemia. The two most favored techniques are antegrade bypass with one or more vessels and retrograde bypass. Antegrade bypass originates from the supraceliac aorta and, whenever possible, should revascularize multiple visceral arteries. The supraceliac aorta can be difficult to expose, but is less often diseased than other areas of the

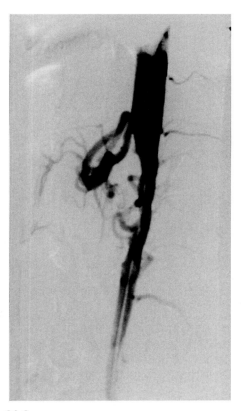

Figure 81-3
Aortogram in a patient with severe infrarenal atherosclerotic disease and occlusion of the superior mesenteric artery (SMA). (Courtesy of Tom Bergamini, MD, Department of Surgery, University of Louisville, KY.)

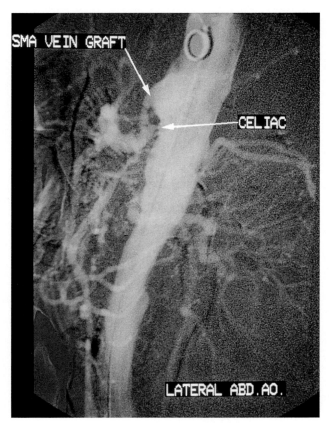

Figure 81-4
Aortogram in a patient with a previous patent antegrade bypass to the superior mesenteric artery (SMA). Very tight celiac stenosis can be seen just below the origin of the saphenous vein bypass. (abd. ao. = abdominal aorta.) (Courtesy of Seyhan Senler, MD, Department of Radiology, University of Louisville, KY.)

aorta. The benefits of antegrade bypass include reduction in kinking and turbulent flow, along with greater ease of multivessel revascularization. Antegrade bypass requires cross-clamping of the aorta above the renal vessels and therefore has a risk of renal ischemia.

Retrograde bypass originates from either the infrarenal aorta or the iliac arteries and usually revascularizes only the SMA. It is technically easier to expose the infrarenal aorta, and cross-clamping above the renal arteries is not required. Either type of bypass may be performed with autogenous vein or prosthetic graft.

Three-year survival rates are between 75 and 86% following bypass, and symptomatic graft failures occur in about 15% of patients. Primary patency does not appear to differ between antegrade and retrograde bypasses, with both having greater than 85% patency 6 years after operation. Primary patency may be overestimated, however, because many studies evaluate only symptomatic patients, and many asymptomatic patients may have undetected failed bypasses.

Angioplasty

Percutaneous angioplasty with stent placement in visceral arteries (which is still under investigation) is technically more difficult than in iliac or other lower extremity arteries. Success has been reported with angioplasty of the celiac artery, SMA, and inferior mesenteric artery, but limited follow-up periods have yielded restenosis rates as high as 50%.

■ CONCLUSION

Acute mesenteric ischemia is a cause of significant morbidity and carries a tremendous mortality rate, most likely because of the difficulty in early diagnosis. Because the consequences of missed or delayed diagnosis are so devastating, clinicians who encounter patients with typical, or even suggestive, symptoms should suspect acute visceral ischemia until the diagnosis can be firmly excluded.

Chronic mesenteric ischemia, although not a life-threatening condition, is often difficult to diagnose. Patients without significant weight loss either do not have chronic visceral ischemia, or do not have ischemia severe enough to warrant an attempt at revascularization. Those patients with uncertain diagnoses but no weight loss, however, should receive close follow-up to assess for other intra-abdominal disorders, along with the possibility of chronic ischemia that will worsen and require revascularization.

Suggested Readings

Klempnauer J, Grothues F, Bektas H, Pichlmayr R: Long-term results after surgery for acute mesenteric ischemia. Surgery 1996;121: 239–243.

McKinsey JF, Gewertz BL: Acute mesenteric ischemia. Surg Clin North Am 1997;77:307–317.

Moawad J, Gewertz BL: Chronic mesenteric ischemia. Surg Clin North Am 1997;77:357–367.

Stoney RJ, Cunningham CG: Acute mesenteric ischemia. Surgery 1993;114:489–490.

82

RADIATION ENTERITIS AND PROCTOCOLITIS

John Dvorak, MD
David W. Dietz, MD

Radiation therapy has become an important adjunctive treatment for the local and regional control of gastrointestinal, genitourinary, and gynecologic malignancies. Although this modality contributes greatly to our oncologic armamentarium, collateral damage to adjacent organs is unavoidable in many cases. Radiation injury to these normal tissues is a significant source of morbidity and death, especially considering that approximately 50% of all cancer patients receive radiation therapy during the course of their treatment.

The small and large intestine are two of the organs most commonly injured. The spectrum of radiation enteritis ranges from relatively mild acute inflammation, which is mostly self-limited, to severe chronic cases in which the bowel strictures or even perforates. Early management of radiation enteritis focuses on its underlying inflammatory pathology. Many of the same medications commonly used in the treatment of inflammatory bowel disease are also used in managing acute radiation enteritis. In fact, these agents have become the standards by which new therapies are compared. When the disease reaches a chronic stage, however, medical treatments have little to offer. The operative management of patients with chronic radiation enteritis is one of the most difficult problems in surgery. However, by combining attention to detail, adherence to basic principles, and careful patient selection, the palliation of symptoms can be achieved with acceptable morbidity and mortality rates.

This chapter will focus on radiation injury to the small and large intestine. Data regarding the pathophysiology and natural history of the disease will be presented, and a practical approach to managing this challenging problem will be outlined.

■ EPIDEMIOLOGY

Fifty to 75% of patients undergoing abdominopelvic radiation therapy will suffer acute symptoms such as diarrhea, abdominal cramping, tenesmus, and hematochezia. These symptoms are often self-limited and subside when the course of treatment is terminated. The occurrence of these acute symptoms does not necessarily predict future development of chronic radiation injury.

The true incidence of those who progress to chronic radiation enteritis is unknown, but is widely reported to be 5 to 15%. These unfortunate patients may experience gastrointestinal bleeding, obstruction, pelvic sepsis, fistulization, or the development of cancer. Nearly 50% of patients presenting with chronic symptoms will eventually need surgery.

Most radiation treatments are directed against gynecologic and urologic pelvic malignancies. Therefore, 75% of patients with radiation enteritis will have involvement of the rectum. Although the rectum is relatively radioresistant, its proximity to the target organs and its fixed position in the pelvis place it at risk. Fifty percent of patients with radiation enteritis will have involvement of those portions of the small and large intestine that either are fixed within the pelvis or are mobile enough to move into the radiation field. The cecum and sigmoid colon are often affected because of their fixed position at the pelvic brim. The ileum easily slides into the pelvis, particularly in women who have a wider pelvic inlet. Occasionally, an adhesion holding the transverse colon in the pelvis will lead to damage. On the other hand, the hepatic and splenic flexures are almost never involved, as they are fixed outside the radiated field.

■ RADIATION THERAPY TECHNIQUES

Radiation therapy can be delivered by several different techniques, which are often combined as part of a comprehensive treatment plan. All treatments are designed to conform the radiation field to the shape of the tumor in order to maximize the oncologic effect while minimizing damage to normal tissues. Enhancements to each of these delivery methods have improved treatment. External beam radiation therapy (EBRT) uses multiple ports, which direct the beam through three or more planes focusing on the tumor. EBRT limits the exposure of harmful radiation to normal tissues. Brachytherapy is the ultimate form of conformal therapy. In this method, selective placement and exposure of radioactive beads within the tumor bed allows for maximal radiation to be delivered to the tumor, while limiting damage outside the field of radiation. Intracavitary radiation therapy is administered at the time of operation. Radiosensitive normal tissues are easily retracted and shielded.

In spite of recent advances in delivery mechanisms, therapeutic doses remain limited by the tolerance of the most sensitive normal tissues in the radiated field. There is a narrow line between effective therapy and toxicity. For this reason, minimal and maximal tolerance doses are described. TD5/50 is the dose at which 50% of patients will experience side effects of radiation at 5 years. Table 82-1 shows the different dose tolerance levels for various intra-abdominal organs. Generally, the goal of the radiation oncologist is to choose a delivery path and dose that will yield the highest local control of the tumor yet not exceed a 5% risk of developing late complications.

Table 82-1 Tolerance Dose Levels

ORGAN	MINIMAL DOSE (TD5/5) (CGY)	MAXIMAL DOSE (TD50/5) (CGY)
Liver	3500	4500
Stomach	4500	5000
Small bowel	4500	6500
Colon	4500	6500
Rectum	5000	8000
Esophagus	6000	7500

Radiation therapy is usually given in doses of 3000 to 7000 cGy in divided fractions of 150 to 200 cGy over 4 to 8 weeks. Complications from radiation therapy are directly related to total dose given, volume of tissue irradiated, and fraction size. In general, higher doses over shorter time intervals increase toxicity.

■ PREDISPOSING FACTORS

A number of predisposing factors are thought to influence the development of radiation enteritis. Although the relative importance of the factors has been debated, it is estimated that two thirds of patients with chronic radiation enteritis had some factor placing them at increased risk of developing the injury. Patients with mesenteric vascular disease may be at increased risk as fixed luminal stenoses secondary to atherosclerotic plaque can compromise the ability to maintain adequate perfusion after the development of the obliterative endarteritis caused by radiation therapy. Patients with a history of previous abdominal or pelvic surgery are also more likely to develop radiation injury. This injury may occur from interruption of collateral blood flow by a previous bowel resection or from adhesions that entrap bowel near or adjacent to an irradiated field. Body habitus may also be an important risk factor for radiation enteritis. Thin elderly female patients are more likely to have small bowel within the pelvis leading to greater absorption of radiation than in a robust individual with a narrow pelvis.

Chemotheraputic agents that are known radiation sensitizers or cytotoxic agents have been reported to augment the effects of radiation on both malignant and normal tissues. Drugs commonly used for these purposes include adriamycin, 5-fluorouracil, methotrexate, and actinomycin. The degree to which these drugs influence the development of chronic radiation injury is unclear, but their effect seems to be equivalent to raising the total dose of radiation given. It is also known that the total dose of radiation given has a direct effect on the development of long-term symptoms. Individuals receiving excessive doses have a much higher incidence of chronic radiation enteritis.

Pre-existing inflammatory conditions such as diverticulitis or inflammatory bowel disease may be exacerbated by radiotherapy. Technical factors also contribute, with higher complication rates seen with the use of less than three treatment fields or the administration of fractions greater than 200 cGy per day. Finally, the addition of chemotherapy not only increases radiation toxicity but may also cause significant leukopenia.

■ PATHOPHYSIOLOGY OF RADIATION INJURY

How Radiation Kills Cells

Radiation therapy has its highest kill effect on rapidly dividing cells such as those found in tumors and mucosal linings. Electrons from the generating apparatus execute their lethal effect in two ways: direct ionization of DNA and production of toxic oxygen-free radicals.

During cellular division, helical DNA is sensitive to mutation, deletion, or abnormal reconstitution of the genetic code. This loss of genetic integrity leads to cell death. Because radiation injury is greatest in rapidly dividing cells, effects first appear in the mucosa, and then progress to involve the submucosa, muscularis, and serosa. Ionizing radiation also results in the production of oxygen-free radicals. These molecules interact with nuclear DNA, disrupting its integrity and leading to programmed cell death (apoptosis).

Therapeutic radiation therapy to the abdomen and pelvis affects the intestines in two distinct ways. Acutely, the rapid division and turnover of mucosal cells is halted. Subsequent alterations in the supportive vasculature (vaso recta) then impair blood supply.

Acute Injury

Acute injury occurs during radiation therapy and may last up to 6 months. It is directly related to fraction size, frequency of treatment, and total volume of tissue irradiated. Generally, higher doses over shorter time intervals induce greater toxicity. Cells at the crypt base normally divide, travel upward along the villus, and are then exfoliated. Complete cellular turnover normally takes 5 to 6 days. Depletion of actively dividing crypt cells results in a lag time between replacement and regeneration, resulting in shortened villi. Consequent loss of absorptive capacity results in malabsorption of carbohydrates, proteins, and bile salts. The primary symptoms experienced are diarrhea, tenesmus, and mucous discharge (50 to 75% of patients). Continued damage results in complete loss of the mucosal lining in areas. This disruption has the endoscopic appearance of an ulcer and can produce hematochezia. Should intestinal ulceration continue, bacterial translocation and systemic infection can result. Once therapy is halted, however, regeneration of the crypts ensues and the patient's symptoms usually resolve in a matter of days to weeks. Histologic recovery is usually complete by 6 months.

Chronic Injury

Late effects of radiation therapy generally appear at 6 to 12 months. In late injury a progressive change in the supportive microvasculature results from an irregular proliferation of endothelial cells. Fibrotic capillaries result in stasis and inefficient oxygen delivery to tissues. This process has been called an "obliterative vasculitis" and leads to further changes in the extracellular milieu. A fibrous proliferation ensues and progresses until a steady state is reached and surviving parenchymal cells are able to be sustained by the microvasculature.

This process of obliterative vasculitis results in architectural changes within the bowel that can be identified clinically. Endoscopic examination may reveal mucosal telangiectasias, which can be a source of gastrointestinal bleeding. Abdominal pain, distention, and diarrhea may also be seen and are early signs of ischemia or obstruction. In this instance, contrast studies will demonstrate bowel wall thickening or strictures. Patients may also develop painful ulcers, draining fistulous tracts, pelvic sepsis, or carcinoma. As previously stated, these complications are not correlated with early acute symptoms, but are directly related to the total dose of radiation received and the volume of tissue irradiated.

■ RADIATION INJURY OF THE SMALL BOWEL

Acute Radiation Enteritis

Acute radiation injury to the small bowel develops in up to 75% of patients receiving radiation therapy for pelvic malignancies. Symptoms are the result of damage to the mucosa and include nausea, vomiting, abdominal pain, and diarrhea, typically beginning during the second or third week of therapy. In the majority of cases, the illness is self-limited and can be managed with a combination of antiemetics, a low-residue diet, antispasmodics, and anticholinergics. A number of studies have evaluated the ability of 5-ASA compounds to prevent or treat acute radiation enteritis, but the results have been conflicting. When acute radiation injury is not responsive to these conservative measures, the dose of radiation may need to be reduced. Rarely, therapy must be discontinued secondary to severe toxicity. The acute symptoms will usually resolve within 6 weeks of stopping treatments.

Chronic Radiation Enteritis

Complications

Chronic radiation enteritis is the end result of a progressive and unrelenting obliterative endarteritis that affects the small nutrient blood vessels of the bowel wall. This leads to ischemic injury manifested by ulceration, hemorrhage, perforation, fistulization, and fibrosis with stricture formation. Clinically, the most common presentation is that of intestinal obstruction, which may occur 2 months to 30 years after radiation treatments. Although this obstruction is usually secondary to fibrotic stricturing, the possibility of recurrent cancer should always be entertained. A smaller number of patients will develop gastrointestinal bleeding or septic complications such as abscess or fistula. Free perforation is unusual.

Diagnostic Studies

In most cases, the diagnosis of chronic radiation enteritis can be confirmed by a contrast study of the small intes-

tine. This study will typically show a long strictured segment within the terminal ileum with proximal bowel dilatation. Multiple strictures may also be seen within a long segment of disease. Computed tomographic (CT) scans may be helpful when an abscess or perforation is expected. Colonoscopy is obtained when large bowel involvement is suspected. If signs of urinary obstruction are present, then an intravenous pyelogram should be performed to rule out ureteral strictures.

When surgical treatment is indicated, a thorough evaluation of the small and large bowel using the preceding imaging tests should be obtained preoperatively. This evaluation will help define the location, extent, and clinical significance of multiple lesions and serve as a guide for planning the operation. Failure to obtain these studies can lead to uncertainty at the time of laparotomy, predisposing to poor decisions and poor outcomes.

Medical Management

Although many patients with chronic radiation enteritis will require surgery, those with mild obstructive symptoms may be managed medically with a low-residue diet. In patients in whom oral intake is limited secondary to obstruction or malabsorption, total parenteral nutrition (TPN) may be needed, either as a permanent measure or temporarily in preparation for surgery. Survival rates for patients maintained on home TPN for chronic radiation enteritis range from 65% at 3 years to 54% at 5 years, with the majority of deaths due to further complications of radiation enteritis or recurrent cancer. However, in patients in whom surgery is not an option, TPN can provide some degree of palliation. Currently, no effective medical treatment exists for reversing the changes of chronic radiation enteritis.

Surgical Management

Indications for Surgery. Up to 50% of patients with chronic radiation enteritis will eventually need surgery. In broader terms, this amounts to between 1 and 4% of all patients treated with abdominopelvic radiation therapy. The most common indication for surgery is obstruction secondary to small bowel stricturing. Fistula, perforation, bleeding, and cancer are less frequent complications. Most patients can achieve good palliation of symptoms with surgery. Adhering to the principles outlined here should keep mortality and morbidity rates below 10 and 30%, respectively, making the risk-benefit ratio favorable for most patients. In those patients who are judged to be extremely high risk for complications after surgical intervention, obstruction can be palliated with a percutaneous gastrostomy tube and hyperalimentation. Fistulas, once controlled, can also be managed in this way. It should always be remembered, however, that radiation enteritis is progressive over time. Recurrent symptoms will develop in over 50% of patients following surgery, and a large number will be due to new lesions remote from the original. Patients and physicians should understand that the goal of surgery for chronic radiation enteritis is not to cure the disease, but rather to deal with complications as they arise.

Preparation for Surgery. Once the decision to operate has been reached, every effort should be made to optimize the patient's condition prior to surgery. Malnutrition is frequently present, usually from anorexia related to obstruction with or without functional short bowel syndrome. If malnutrition is severe (weight loss >15% ideal body weight or serum albumin <2.5 g/dL), a period of preoperative hyperalimentation may be beneficial. Although data support this practice in patients with upper abdominal malignancy, similar studies have not been reported in patients with chronic radiation enteritis. The end points of preoperative hyperalimentation are not clear, but a reasonable approach consists of 7 to 10 days of administration followed immediately by surgery. Hyperalimentation is continued in the postoperative period until adequate oral caloric intake is achieved. If malnutrition is not severe, the patient may be taken to surgery as soon as anemia and fluid and electrolyte deficits are corrected.

Immediately prior to surgery, broad-spectrum antibiotics as well as subcutaneous heparin are administered. Informed consent is obtained from the patient and the possibility of stoma creation is discussed. Potential sites for stoma apertures are marked in all four quadrants of the abdomen to provide the surgeon with multiple options. Marking should be done with the patient in an upright sitting position and should involve an enterostomal therapy nurse if available. Bowel preparation using a polyethylene glycol solution is given if obstructive symptoms are minimal. If bowel preparation is not possible, the patient is restricted to clear liquids for several days prior to surgery.

Operative Strategy. Laparotomy is typically performed in the modified lithotomy position using Lloyd-Davies or Allen stirrups. This position allows ready access to the perineum if needed. Bilateral ureteral stents are often placed, as the surgeon can anticipate a difficult pelvic dissection in all cases of chronic radiation enteritis. Stents will not necessarily prevent ureteric injury, but they do facilitate its recognition and repair at the time of surgery. If ureterolysis is anticipated due to hydronephrosis on preoperative imaging studies, then these stents are mandatory.

The peritoneal cavity is entered through a midline incision. As many of these patients have had prior abdominal or pelvic surgery, adhesions should be anticipated. One point of controversy in the intraoperative management of chronic radiation enteritis is the degree of adhesiolysis to be performed. Some authors advocate limiting dissection to only that which is necessary to define and correct the problem at hand. They cite a high incidence of postoperative enterocutaneous fistulas with extensive adhesiolysis. Certainly, these patients are at higher risk for developing such postoperative complications, as radiated bowel is extremely fragile, relatively ischemic, and very unforgiving. Others, however, advocate just the opposite. These authors feel that complications can be minimized by careful attention to detail during adhesiolysis and that complete abdominal exploration should be done so that the full scope of the radiation damage to bowel and other organ systems can be assessed and synchronous lesions

dealt with. Ultimately, however, each operation is tailored to each patient's individual situation.

Most patients will be benefited by a full exploration, at which time all the small bowel is inspected from the ileocecal valve to the ligament of Treitz. The appearance of bowel affected by chronic radiation varies, but the serosal surface is typically pale gray or mottled in color. The bowel wall and its mesentery are thickened and fibrotic, resulting in decreased pliability. Areas of stricturing can be seen within these affected segments and, if clinically significant, will usually be preceded by upstream dilatation. Fistulas may be uncovered during separation of adherent loops of bowel, and chronic abscess cavities found during adhesiolysis. Radiation damage is most commonly seen in the terminal ileum and decreases as one moves proximal, although any segment of bowel fixed within the pelvis is assumed to be affected. The cecum, sigmoid colon, and rectum are also frequently involved. The liberal use of preoperative diagnostic studies should define significant segments of disease and guide this exploration. If possible, all strictures encountered should be treated in order to minimize the risk of recurrence.

In some cases, however, extremely dense "hostile" adhesions are encountered. The most difficult of these usually involve the pelvis, where a significant portion of the small bowel may be entrapped. In these situations, a decision must be made as to whether or not to attempt mobilization of the small bowel up and out of the pelvis with the risk of extensive serosal tears, enterotomies, or vascular injury, which could result in the loss of large amounts of small intestine or uncontrolled pelvic bleeding. In such cases, it may be wise to abandon pelvic dissection and bypass the diseased segment instead.

Another point of controversy in the management of chronic radiation enteritis is whether resection or bypass is the surgical procedure of choice. Proponents of bypass emphasize the relatively high anastomotic leak rates seen after resection. A seminal paper on this topic by Swan and associates reported a 36% leak rate and 21% mortality rate in patients undergoing resection, compared with a 6% leak rate and 10% mortality rate in those treated with bypass. However, this difference has not been the experience of more recent authors. A retrospective, multi-institutional study by Regimbeau and colleagues found no significant differences in leak rates or mortality rates in patients managed by resection versus bypass (9 and 5% vs. 12 and 0%). The only factor found to be predictive of operative death was emergency surgery. This improvement in results may be due to a better understanding of the subtleties of radiation enteritis. Through experience, surgeons have learned that despite a fairly normal appearance, the terminal ileum, cecum, and ascending colon are usually affected by some degree of radiation damage and should be avoided when constructing anastomoses. With the implementation of this policy, Galland and Spencer reported a decrease in leak rate after resection from 52 to 7% and a dramatic fall in mortality rate from 42 to 0%.

Supporters of resection cite the persistence of symptoms, further complications, or early recurrence of disease in patients whose diseased segment remains in situ after bypass or diversion. These events have been reported in 30 to 50% of patients. In addition, at least one study has found decreased long-term survival in patients managed by bypass rather than resection, mostly due to gastrointestinal hemorrhage. Leaving radiated bowel behind also places the patient at a small but definite risk of developing cancer within that segment.

Based on the foregoing data, we favor resection over bypass for the management of chronic radiation enteritis. Adhering to the principle of constructing anastomoses from nonirradiated bowel should minimize leak rates and risk of operative death while providing the patient with the benefits of a definitive operation. Good judgment and flexibility by the surgeon are critical to optimizing outcomes, however. In patients in whom mobilization of diseased bowel may lead to major complications, bypass or simple diversion remains the best option.

One situation involves special mention. Occasionally, the surgeon will encounter several "dominant" strictures occurring in a background of extensive radiation enteritis. In such cases, performing a resection to encompass the *entire* diseased bowel will inevitably result in short gut syndrome. Bypass is equally unattractive, as it will also lead to functional short bowel with the added risk of bacterial overgrowth in isolated segments between the strictures. In these very unusual cases, we have performed strictureplasty to address these dominant lesions and have reported a satisfactory outcome in five patients (Dietz and coworkers). There were no anastomotic leaks and all patients avoided permanent hyperalimentation. It should be stressed, however, that these were desperate situations in which the risk of complications from the strictureplasty suture line were felt to be less than the risk of the morbidity of a major resection.

Surgical Technique. Several technical points must be emphasized in dealing with chronic radiation enteritis. First, all anastomoses should be constructed from nonirradiated bowel, if at all possible. This approach avoids segments with the typical gross changes of radiation enteritis as well as those which appear relatively normal but are known to have been included in the pelvic radiation field (terminal ileum, cecum, rectum, and ascending and sigmoid colons). In the typical case of terminal ileal radiation enteritis, this choice will result in a proximal ileum to transverse colon anastomosis. Our preference is for hand-sewn anastomoses in almost all instances, as stapling devices may not be reliable in the setting of chronically obstructed bowel. If omentum is available, it is placed over the anastomosis in order to provide a covering of well-vascularized tissue. Omentum can also be interposed between the anastomosis and any chronic abscess cavity. If conditions are not suitable for anastomosis, an end-stoma is created. Such conditions include diffuse fecal peritonitis and questionable viability of the bowel ends.

The mesentery adjacent to segments of radiation-damaged intestine may also be affected, showing the same fibrosis, thickening, and decreased pliability as the bowel wall. Conventional division using Kelly clamps can be com-plicated by retraction of the vessels when ties are applied, leading to mesenteric hematomas or intraperitoneal bleeding. To avoid this complication, we have adopted a technique whereby the mesentery is divided sequentially between Kocher clamps and then the vessels are suture ligated with heavy (No. 1) chromic sutures. If minor bleeding persists, the cut edge of the mesentery can also be oversewn with a locking suture of the same material.

■ PREVENTING RADIATION ENTERITIS

Perhaps the best approach to the problem of radiation enteritis is prevention. A number of methods have been advanced in hopes of reducing the frequency and severity of the disease. Refinements in the technique of radiation delivery are meant to limit the volume of surrounding normal tissues being radiated. The use of pretreatment imaging studies (CT scan, small bowel series) will show the location and mobility of the small bowel. Maneuvers such as prone positioning, bladder distention, and abdominal wall compression may then be used to move the small bowel out of the treatment field. One published study has demonstrated a 50% reduction in the number of chronic bowel complications by utilizing this approach.

Certain drugs may lessen the potential for radiation toxicity. *Radiosensitizers* such as 5-fluourouracil increase the sensitivity of the tumor to radiation but not the surrounding normal tissues. *Radioproctectants* work by augmenting the ability of normal cells to withstand the effects of radiation. The most widely studied radioprotectant is amifostine, an agent that acts by scavenging oxygen free radicals and stabilizing the DNA. It has been shown to decrease the incidence of moderate or severe late radiation toxicity in patients undergoing treatment for rectal cancer.

When pelvic radiation therapy is anticipated after surgery, mechanical measures to exclude the small bowel from the pelvis are warranted. It is well established that prior pelvic surgery is a risk factor for developing radiation enteritis, as the small bowel can become trapped within the pelvic radiation field by adhesions. A number of methods have been described to isolate the small bowel from the pelvis at the time of surgery. Most commonly, a sling using omentum or absorbable mesh acts as a barrier to hold the small bowel out of the pelvis. Alternatively, the omentum may be mobilized as a "pedicle graft" and used to fill the pelvis, thereby excluding the small bowel. A number of reports have supported the efficacy of these techniques, but they may be of diminishing importance in view of the recent shift to preoperative adjuvant radiation therapy for patients with rectal cancer.

■ RADIATION INJURY TO THE RECTUM

Natural History

Only retrospective studies looking at the natural history of radiation proctosigmoiditis exist. By far the most common side effect of radiation is rectal bleeding, occurring in more than 95% of patients. The peak incidence of bleeding occurs approximately 1 year from treatment but is usually resolved by 18 months in the majority of patients. Failure of resolution leads to further problems, such as persistent or severe bleeding, change in bowel habits, and rectal pain. The need for surgery secondary to complications of radiation proctocolitis is estimated at 5 to 10%, although considerably higher rates have been reported in some series. Older surgical series were plagued by morbidity and mortality rates as great as 80% and 50%, respectively. More recent reports, however, have shown better results with mortality rates as low as 3% and morbidity rates at 9%, presumably due to improved patient selection. Fistulas are the most frequent postoperative complication, but wound dehiscence, bowel obstruction, and sepsis are also common.

Treatment

Radiation injury to the large bowel occurring during treatment is initially managed conservatively, using the same measures outlined earlier for acute radiation enteritis. Hydrophilic stool softeners, local anesthetics, steroid enemas, and 5-aminosalicylic acid (5-ASA) suppositories may be especially useful, and most symptoms will resolve over 1 to 2 weeks as the crypts regenerate. Diarrhea can lead to electrolyte disturbances, with both potassium and magnesium being depleted. At least one study as supported the use of a long-acting magnesium chloride preparation to help prevent early symptoms of acute radiation-induced proctosigmoiditis. However, some feel that magnesium may also provide protection to tumor cells.

Many different treatments have been proposed for chronic radiation-induced proctocolitis, but none have proved ideal. Original strategies described using steroids in combination with 5-ASA compounds, or sucralfate enemas to reduce mucosal inflammation. More significant or recalcitrant bleeding can be addressed by coagulating the mucosa, with topical formalin solutions or lasers. Hyperbaric oxygen has been described, but its expense and limited availability make it impractical. Resective surgery remains the option of last resort.

In most cases, steroid enemas, either alone or combined with oral sulfasalazine, are considered as the first line treatment of radiation proctitis. One study compared 2 mg sucralfate enemas every 12 hours to a 20 mg prednisolone retention enema every 12 hours along with 1 g of oral sulfasalazine three times a day and found a statistically significant improvement in the sucralfate group by clinical assessment, but no difference in endocsopic appearance. Further studies have shown that sucralfate enemas can produce a lasting result in over 90% of patients if used on a regular basis. No long-term data are available on whether these topical treatments effect a histologic change.

Nonoperative Management

The use of topical formalin for the treatment of radiation proctitis was first described in the mid-1980s, having been adapted from its use in radiation cystitis. The procedure is typically performed in the operating room under either a regional or general anesthetic. After the rectum is evacuated, a 4% formalin solution is applied directly to the areas of bleeding with a sponge or cotton-tip applicator directed through the rigid proctoscope. Contact is maintained for several minutes or until bleeding ceases. At the conclusion of treatment, the rectum should be copiously irrigated with saline. Studies show topical formalin therapy to be effective in 80% of patients after one or two applications. However, about 30% of those treated will eventually develop recurrent bleeding. Acute proctocolitis, anococcygeal pain, and stricture formation are all reported complications of topical formalin therapy.

Laser coagulation of the rectal musosa has become a popular modality for the management of bleeding radiation proctitis. Lasers can be used in the awake or sedated patient through a rigid proctoscope or flexible endoscope and often require several sessions for adequate response. The neodymium:yttrium-aluminum-garnet (Nd:YAG) laser has been able to achieve deep penetration to provide more homogeneous coagulation of vessels. However, reports of stricture, ileus, and postcoagulation abdominal pain syndrome have been described. Because of these risks, its use should be limited to those with experience. A recent study of the Nd:YAG laser in radiation proctitis reported cessation of bleeding in 25% of patients failing local drug therapy and a significant decrease in bleeding in an additional 15%. An average of three treatments is generally necessary and there is a high rate of recurrent bleeding (70%), requiring further sessions. The argon plasma coagulator (APC) has recently sparked interest and has a number of potential advantages. It is able to treat larger areas by "painting" the surface of the bowel. It provides a uniform 2- to 3-mm burn penetration, which limits transmural necrosis, stricturing, perforation, and fistula formation. Further, blood is "blown" off the tissue surface by argon gas flow, resulting in a direct effect of electrocoagulation current on the bleeding lesion. Side effects of bloating and anal pain have been described. Care must be taken to withdraw excess air from the colon. The treatment of lesions close to the dentate line requires sedation of the patient.

Surgical Management

With the success of nonoperative measures in the treatment of radiation proctitis, surgical management can be delayed and many times avoided altogether. Patients considered for surgery are those with severe complications such as pelvic sepsis from perforation, fistulas, rectal strictures, recalcitrant bleeding, pain, or carcinoma. All these problems are challenging for the surgeon and are made more so because these patients often are not good surgical candidates. When contemplating surgery, one should consider the overall health and nutrition of the patient, anatomy of their rectal disease, the type of radiation therapy received, and life expectancy. Preoperative preparation consists of optimizing nutritional status, correcting anemia, and administering broad-spectrum antibiotics. In most cases, ureteric stents are placed prior to commencing surgery.

A diverting ostomy is a simple approach for the acutely symptomatic patient. It can help alleviate pain from a deep anal ulcer, can help control sepsis when combined with local drainage, can bypass a rectal stricture, and has low morbidity and mortality rates. It is not indicated for hemorrhage because bleeding tends to continue after diversion. Several important principles should be adhered to when creating an ostomy for complications of radiation proctitis. First, the stoma should not be formed with diseased bowel. Up to one third of stomas created from irradiated bowel develop necrosis, stricture, prolapse, or bleeding. Second, serious consideration should be given to performing a diverting ileostomy, as this is perhaps the most expeditious way to achieve diversion. Third, if a diverting colostomy is to be undertaken, then care should be taken not to sacrifice its blood supply. The right transverse colon is perhaps the best place to form a colostomy because it is rarely affected by radiation enteritis and preserves the middle colic artery and splenic flexure. Preserving these vessels assures good blood supply and easier mobilization for any future reconstruction. Much of this, however, is dictated by the distribution of radiation damage.

Resection and primary anastomosis can be considered for localized disease. Occasionally, the transverse colon will have been trapped in the field of radiation and will develop a stricture. Under these circumstances simple resection and colon-colon anastomosis can usually be performed. A bypass of the affected area may seem attractive, but would not address the ongoing bleeding that often plagues these patients. When the cecum is affected, an ileocolic resection can be safely carried out using nonirradiated proximal ileum and ascending or transverse colon. In all cases, the surgeon should follow the standard principles of bowel anastomosis—no tension and adequate blood supply. Consideration should be given to a diverting stoma based on nutritional status, overall health of the patient, and the quality of anastomosis.

The vast majority of radiation injury of the colon is limited to the rectosigmoid. After proctosigmoidectomy, a low rectal or coloanal anastomosis is feasible if the very distal rectum is relatively healthy and the anal sphincters are intact. It is always preferable to join two nonirradiated ends of bowel together, but acceptable leak rates of 7 to 10% have been achieved when only one end of the bowel was not affected. Whenever possible, an omental pedical graft based on the left gastroepiploic vessel should be placed around the anastomosis. Introducing well-vascularized tissue into an irradiated field will help prevent fistulization and help contain a localized anastomotic leak. Although some retrospective studies have reported good results without a covering stoma for low colorectal or coloanal anastomoses, we consider fecal diversion mandatory.

Fistulas often develop after radiation to the pelvis. The most commonly seen types are rectovaginal, but ileorectal, ileovaginal, and vesicovaginal fistulas are also encountered. Prior to any definitive surgical intervention, it is important to delineate the anatomy of such fistulas. These studies include the liberal use of fistulograms, small bowel studies, contrast enemas, and examinations under anesthesia. This foreknowledge helps with planning surgery and determining the extent of resection. The principles of management are complete resection of diseased bowel, anastomosis if safe, and interposition of healthy, well-vascularized tissue. As stated earlier, fecal diversion is mandatory.

Rectovaginal fistulas are common and pose substantial challenges. Local repair by mucosal advancement flap will invariably fail and should be avoided. The approach most often required is laparotomy with dissection of the rectum to a level well below that of the fistula. Excision of the fistula is not necessary, but interposition of an omental pedicle flap, or other nonirradiated tissue (rectus abdominis or gracilis muscle) is necessary to prevent recurrent fistula. Alternatively, a coloanal pull-through procedure could achieve the same effect by bringing nonirradiated bowel adjacent to the fistula. A delayed coloanal anastomosis as described by Turnbull and Cutait may be indicated in this situation. A diverting stoma is always created.

Occasionally, the surgeon is faced with extremely severe pelvic radiation damage manifested by multiple fistulas, perforations, and chronic sepsis—the aptly named *frozen pelvis*. Under these circumstances, proctectomy is extremely difficult, as dense fibrosis surrounds the rectum and tissue planes are nonexistent. If proctectomy can be achieved, the surgeon is frequently "rewarded" with a rigid pelvic cavity and perineum, which either cannot be closed or will invariably break down in the postoperative period. In this instance, omentum may be used to fill the pelvis. This tissue will serve as a barrier to exclude the small bowel and provides a vascularized tissue bed for granulation of the perineal wound. If omentum is not available, a rectus muscle flap is an alternative. If the rectum cannot be safely resected, a diverting colostomy or ileostomy is created. This procedure should be done in a loop configuration or with an associated mucous fistula, as stricturing may progress to the point of rectal obstruction in the future. In some cases, the urinary system will also be involved. If so, ureterolysis, cystectomy, or placement of nephrostomy tubes may be necessary.

■ CONCLUSION

With the widespread use of radiation for pelvic malignancies, surgeons will continue to be called upon to treat patients with radiation proctitis and enteritis. Further refinements in the delivery of radiation therapy using multiple ports, conformal therapy, and radioprotectors will help reduce damage to the bowel, but will not eliminate it. The natural history of the disease is a tendency toward improvement over time. Generally, aggressive medical therapy should be the first line of treatment, with surgery reserved for complicated and recalcitrant disease.

Suggested Readings

Baker DG: The response of the microvascular system to radiation: A review. Cancer Invest 1989;7(3):287–294.

Dietz DW, Remzi F, Fazio VW: Strictureplasty for obstructing small bowel lesions in diffuse radiation enteritis—Successful outcome in 5 patients. Dis Colon Rectum 2002;44(12):1772–1777.

Galland RB, Spencer J: Surgical management of radiation enteritis. Surgery 1986;99(2):133–139.

Kochhar R: Natural history of late radiation proctosigmoiditis treated with topical sucralfate suspension. Dig Dis Sci 1999;44(5):973–978.

Nussbaum ML: Radiation-induced intestinal injury. Clin Plast Surg 1993;20(3):573–580.

Regimbeau JM, Panis Y, Gouzi JL, et al: Operative and long term results after surgery for chronic radiation enteritis. Am J Surg 2001;182:237–242.

TagKilidis PP: Chronic radiation proctitis. Aust N Z J Surg 2001;71:230–237.

Waddell BE, Rodriguez-Bigas MA, Lee RJ, et al: Prevention of chronic radiation enteritis. J Am Coll Surg 1999;189(6):611–624.

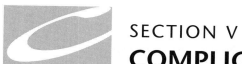

COMPLICATIONS (AND OTHER MISCELLANEOUS TOPICS)

83

COLORECTAL SURGERY IN THE HIGH-RISK PATIENT

Walter A. Koltun, MD

Increased life expectancy coupled with the high prevalence of colorectal (especially malignant) disease has resulted in the increasing need for surgeons to be able to operate on patients with comorbid medical conditions. Generally, patients with disease in one or more organ systems in addition to their primary colorectal ailment will have a higher probability of complication or death from colorectal surgery. Identifying the high-risk patient is the first step in minimizing operative morbidity and mortality.

■ IDENTIFICATION OF THE HIGH-RISK PATIENT

The increasing interest in surgical outcomes research has led to studies establishing specific and statistically validated criteria that relate morbidity after colorectal surgery to preoperative risk factors. Ondrula and workers reviewed 972 colorectal procedures using multivariate discriminant function analysis and found 11 factors that predicted operative outcome, each of which could be assigned a value that could then be used to generate a "risk score" (Table 83-1). Mortality rate in four patient groups was directly proportional to the risk score (0 to 4 points, 1%; 5 to 8 points, 10%; 9 to 13 points, 19%, and greater than 13 points, 33%). Two risk factors, cirrhosis and renal insufficiency, could not be accurately assigned risk values because they were associated with such high mortality rates and because relatively few of these patients were in the study, causing a disproportionate statistical effect. The 11 identified factors having a negative impact on outcome affirmed the clinical intuition of most colorectal surgeons.

Their identification and management should be the surgeon's preoperative focus in order to improve a patient's readiness for surgery.

Other scoring systems, such as POSSUM (Physiological and Operative Severity Score for enUmeration of Mortality and morbidity), have also been developed to allow comparison among different institutions by applying validated formulas that allow comparison of predicted and observed morbidity and mortality rates. Despite some concerns about overprediction of complications with these systems, alterations such as the Portsmouth modification have been applied with greater accuracy, allowing standardization among institutions and direct comparison of outcomes in specific groups of patients such as those undergoing colorectal or laparoscopic surgery or the elderly.

■ MINIMIZING THE RISK ASSOCIATED WITH EMERGENCY SURGERY

Emergency surgery is conventionally associated with a two- to threefold increase in operative mortality and morbidity rates, and in the Ondrula study, it received the highest index value. Why emergency surgery has such a negative impact on surgical outcome is unclear but is probably multifactorial, relating in part to advanced presentation of disease, an unprepared colon, and secondary organ effects of sepsis, stress, or dehydration.

Clearly, the patient with an acute abdomen or signs and symptoms of an intra-abdominal catastrophe cannot avoid the operating room for long. Through the use of increasingly sophisticated radiologic or endolaparoscopic modalities, however, the initial nonoperative management of the emergency colorectal patient may allow a subsequent definitive operation to take place under semielective or even fully elective circumstances, so decreasing operative risk.

Emergency colorectal procedures can be largely grouped under those associated with sepsis (acute diverticulitis, pelvic abscess), obstruction (large bowel cancer, volvulus), or bleeding (diverticular, diffuse colitis). In each of these instances, patients will first require the usual fluid resuscitation (with blood products, if necessary) and diagnostic maneuvers including plain x-rays, proctosigmoidoscopy, and possibly computed tomographic (CT) scan or angiography. In the case of

Table 83-1 Risk Factors and Relative Values Predicting Morbidity and Mortality in Colon and Rectal Surgery

RISK FACTOR	RELATIVE VALUE
Emergent surgery	6
Age ≥75 years	4
Congestive heart failure	4
Prior radiation	3
Albumin <2.7 g/dL	2
Prior myocardial infarction	2
Chronic obstructive pulmonary disease	1
Diabetes	1
Steroid therapy	1

Source: Ondrula DP, Nelson RL, Prasad ML, et al: Multifactorial index of preoperative risk factors in colon resection. Dis Colon Rectum 1992; 35:117–122.

abdominal sepsis from diverticulitis, CT-guided percutaneous drainage of an identified abscess can be done. This drainage will allow the subsequent performance of a single-stage colectomy with minimal morbidity after interval drainage and intravenous antibiotic treatment (usually 5 to 7 days) and oral bowel preparation. Acute colonic obstruction mandates either colonoscopy or Gastrografin enema, either of which can be therapeutic in the case of volvulus, obviating the emergency and allowing elective correction. With a malignancy causing obstruction, a so-called "trephine" stoma can be made proximal to the obstruction directly through the stoma site without laparotomy, usually in less than 1 hour and under light general or spinal anesthesia. This procedure will then allow further semielective workup and time to treat the usually encountered malnutrition and fluid and electrolyte disturbances. In addition, in the case of low-lying malignancies, definitive resection can then take place some weeks later after completion of adjuvant chemoradiation therapy. For persistent lower gastrointestinal bleeding, the site of hemorrhage must be accurately determined, and this may require angiography. Such localization results in improved operative morbidity rate because the subsequent resection can then be more limited. The acute presentation of the patient with obstruction from known Crohn's disease can nearly always be treated with high-dose intravenous steroids and hyperalimentation after ruling out an abscess by CT scanning. Operation can be done several days later when the acute inflammation in the adjacent bowel loops uninvolved with Crohn's disease has calmed, so minimizing the extent of resection.

■ MINIMIZING THE RISK ASSOCIATED WITH CARDIAC DISEASE

Numerous studies have been done looking at factors predictive of cardiac complications in patients undergoing major noncardiac general surgery. Most of these (such as those by Goldman and Eagle, see Table 83-2) have been done in patients largely undergoing surgery for peripheral vascular disease (PVD) and therefore do not directly apply to the colorectal patient. It is interesting to note, however, those factors predictive of morbidity in Ondrula's work that are also found in these other studies. Specifically, history or presence of congestive heart failure (CHF), previous myocardial infarction (MI), old age, diabetes mellitus, and emergency surgery are recurring features in these investigations. It should be pointed out that as many as 60% of patients who have PVD will also have significant, silent coronary vascular disease. The presence of PVD should alert the colorectal surgeon to possible cardiac disease even in the asymptomatic individual. Asymptomatic carotid stenoses may also be present, but general opinion is that they are of low risk to the individual prior to abdominal surgery and do not mandate endarterectomy.

If significant cardiac disease is suspected or identified, further testing may be necessary to assess preoperative risk. Typically, this assessment involves some form of stress test (exercise, the administration of dipyridamole or dobutamine) and then some form of imaging (electrocardiogram, thallium redistribution, echocardiography). The dobutamine stress echocardiogram is more commonly done than the dipyridamole thallium scan, because of its presumed physiologic similarity to the release of catecholamines during the surgical experience. Both these studies, however, have a very high negative predictive value, usually greater than 90%, and a positive predictive value of 10 to 50%. Patients who have significant coronary artery disease and a positive stress test will be at very high risk for noncardiac

Table 83-2 Factors Predisposing to Cardiac Morbidity in Noncardiac Surgery

GOLDMAN'S SERIES*	EAGLE'S SERIES*
1. Congestive heart failure, S₃ heart sound	1. Q waves on ECG
2. Myocardial infarction within 6 months	2. History of ventricular arrhythmia/congestive heart failure
3. >5 premature ventricular contractions/min	3. Diabetes
4. Rhythm other than sinus or premature atrial contractions	4. >70 years old
5. >70 years old	5. History of angina
6. Abdominal/chest or aortic surgery	
7. Emergency surgery	
8. Aortic stenosis	
9. Poor metabolic condition	

*See references under Suggested Readings.

surgery without first undergoing optimization of cardiac status, including possible coronary revascularization. A proposed algorithm for identification and management of the potential cardiac patient is shown in Figure 83-1.

Perioperatively, cardiac medications should be continued, especially any beta blockade, both to avoid rebound tachycardia and to prevent the myocardial ischemic effects of catecholamines released during surgery. Effective pain control is similarly very important. Pulmonary artery catheter monitoring is usually reserved for those patients of at least moderate risk. If used, it should be maintained through the postoperative period of fluid mobilization, usually 48 to 72 hours after surgery.

■ MINIMIZING RISK ASSOCIATED WITH PREVIOUS RADIATION

Acute radiation injury usually causes bowel wall edema and can precipitate obstruction. Radiation injury usually resolves with cessation of radiation, bowel rest, and nasogastric decompression. Chronically, strictures and bleeding can occur. Preoperative preparation involves decompression and oral antibiotics, even in the case of small bowel strictures, because bacterial overgrowth can occur. It is important to recognize that the pathophysiology of radiation enteritis relates to small vessel obliteration with result-

ant tissue ischemia, so surgery involves meticulous technique. Strictureplasty is not advised, but rather resection and anastomoses created in healthy, nonirradiated tissue. The use of the omentum to wrap or separate one or more anastomoses from adjacent organs to avoid fistula, and the creation of temporary, protecting stomas is wise. Parenteral alimentation in patients with malnutrition should be considered during the perioperative period.

■ MINIMIZING RISK ASSOCIATED WITH MALNUTRITION

It is clear that significant nutritional compromise can worsen operative morbidity. Factors used to assess nutritional state include albumin, prealbumin, weight loss, triceps skinfold thickness (as a measure of fat stores), and serum transferrin. Generally, an albumin level below 3.0 g/dL and serum transferrin less than 170 mg/dL bespeaks moderately severe malnutrition that will worsen surgical morbidity. It is more difficult to document, however, that preoperative intervention, specifically with total parenteral nutrition (TPN), will improve surgical outcome. Certainly, any form of nutritional intervention requires more than a few days' administration to invoke a significant benefit.

The colorectal surgeon should keep in mind certain principles in managing perioperative malnutrition. These can be

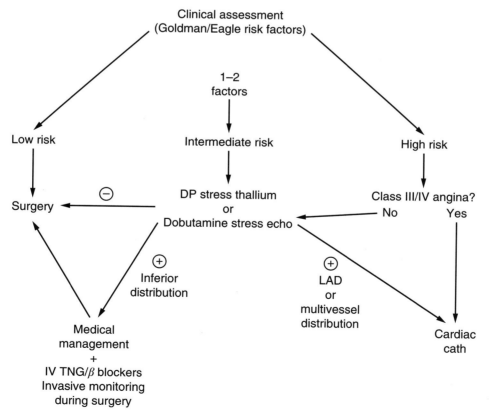

Figure 83-1
Algorithm for cardiac workup of the colorectal surgical patient.

classified by recognizing the cause for malnutrition (lack of intake, lack of absorption, increased losses/catabolism). If the patient is not eating but has an intact and patent gastrointestinal tract, then placement of a feeding tube for enteric feeding is best. This option should be kept in mind especially during the operative procedure itself, because the surgical placement of a gastric or gastrojejunal feeding tube can improve and simplify postoperative management immeasurably, especially in the critically ill patient. Similarly, malnutrition secondary to an obstructing cancer may best be handled by a diverting stoma prior to definitive resection, allowing the patient to resume an oral diet.

Short gut or other intrinsic intestinal disease provides a better rationale for the use of TPN. When preoperative patients will be without a regular oral diet for more than a few days, such as those with acute diverticulitis or flaring Crohn's disease, the combination of TPN for the majority of caloric requirements, with a restricted amount of low-residue oral supplements, helps to maintain nutrition and the integrity and defensive barrier function of the intestinal epithelium.

Finally, patients with excessive nutritional requirements, as exemplified by the medically unresponsive ulcerative colitis, should be managed by definitive surgical resection. TPN cannot hope to replace the excessive loss of albumin, blood, and other critical serum proteins from a severely diseased colon. Delaying surgery will simply result in further nutritional deterioration if medical management of the colitis has clearly failed.

■ MINIMIZING RISK ASSOCIATED WITH PULMONARY DISEASE

Patients who cannot climb two flights of stairs at a steady pace without dyspnea, those who have a smoking or other pulmonary history, or those who on pulmonary testing have less than 70% of predicted values for timed forced expiration (correlates with coughing ability), tidal volume, and maximum voluntary ventilation should be considered at increased risk. Preoperative preparation should include the culture of sputum, if present, and appropriate antibiotic treatment; institution of bronchodilators, if necessary; abstinence from smoking; and patient education in the use of incentive spirometry. Carbon dioxide retention or an oxygen tension of less than 50 mm Hg on room air blood gas predicts ventilator dependency postoperatively. In such higher-risk patients, awake epidural anesthesia can be used for the operative procedure, because the avoidance of intubation and general anesthesia, coupled with excellent postoperative pain control, facilitates pulmonary function and may even minimize some of the other adverse effects associated with the stress of surgery.

■ MISCELLANEOUS RISK FACTORS

The risk associated with diabetes relates largely to the chronic secondary organ effects of the illness, so the col-

orectal surgeon should evaluate such patients keeping in mind the possibility of silent myocardial disease, PVD, and chronic renal failure.

Patients on chronic steroids will require perioperative stress dosages that are tapered postoperatively to their baseline levels within 3 to 5 days. The rapidity with which steroids can be totally discontinued in the chronic user can be estimated by evaluating intrinsic adrenal function using a cosyntropin test. This test is especially worthwhile in septic patients who cannot tolerate the immunosuppressive effects of steroids given for another illness, for example, the chronic obstructive pulmonary disease patient with diverticulitis.

Hepatic failure is a significant risk factor for colorectal surgery. Risk of fatality is commonly assessed using the relatively well-known Child's classification based on nutritional status, serum bilirubin and albumin levels, and the presence or absence of ascites and encephalopathy. Mortality rates of approximately 50% for Child's C patients (bilirubin >3, albumin <3, poorly controlled ascites, and encephalopathy) come from early reports of patients undergoing surgery for portal decompression but are probably better when less major surgery is planned, especially with newer methods of critical care management. Nonetheless, the perioperative care of the patient with cirrhosis is a significant undertaking requiring careful management of volume, coagulation, and nutritional status. Colectomy with anastomosis in such patients can result in peritoneal sepsis secondary to contaminated ascites, whereas the creation of a stoma can also lead to problematic ascitic leaks or peristomal varices. Colorectal surgery in severely cirrhotic patients should be limited to treating critical life-threatening or malignant disease.

Suggested Readings

Eagle KA, Coley CM, Newell JB, et al: Combining clinical and thallium data optimized preoperative assessment of cardiac risk before major vascular surgery. Ann Intern Med 1989;110:859–866.

Evans BA, Wijdicks EF: High-grade carotid stenosis detected before general surgery: Is endarterectomy indicated? Neurology 2001;57:1328–1330.

Fischer JE, Tiao GM: Cirrhosis and jaundice. In Wilmore DW, Brennan MF, Harken AH, et al (Eds.). Care of the Surgical Patient. New York, Scientific American, 1995.

Goldman L, Caldera DL, Nussbaum SR, et al. Multifactorial index of cardiac risk in noncardiac surgical procedures. N Engl J Med 1977;197:845–850.

Koltun WA, McKenna KJ, Rung G: Awake epidural anesthesia is effective and safe in the high-risk colectomy patient. Dis Colon Rectum 1994;37:1236–1241.

Ondrula DP, Nelson RL, Prasad ML, et al: Multifactorial index of preoperative risk factors in colon resections. Dis Colon Rectum 1992;35:117–122.

Stephenson ER, Ilahi O, Koltun WA: Stoma site creation through the stoma site: A rapid, safe technique. Dis Colon Rectum 1997;40:112–115.

Tekkis PP, Kocher HM, Bentley AJ, et al: Operative mortality rates among surgeons: Comparison of POSSUM and p-POSSUM scoring systems in gastrointestinal surgery. Dis Colon Rectum 2000;43:1528–1532.

Wong CB, Porter TR: Cardiac management of patients undergoing major noncardiac surgery. Nebraska Med J 1995;80:350–353.

84

REOPERATIVE PELVIC SURGERY

M. Jonathan Worsey, MA, MBBS, FRCS, FACS
Dana P. Launer, MD, FACS

Reoperative pelvic surgery presents one of the most difficult challenges a colon and rectal surgeon must face. A combination of anatomic, postsurgical, and disease-specific factors conspire to test the skills of even the most experienced pelvic surgeon. An ordered and logical pre- and perioperative approach is essential to minimize morbidity and maximize the chance of a successful outcome.

■ FACTORS COMPLICATING REOPERATIVE PELVIC SURGERY

Anatomic Factors

The pelvis is a bony cavity lined with muscle and fascia containing gastrointestinal, urologic, and gynecologic organs. In the anatomic position it resembles a forward-tilting basin, and this position, combined with the unyielding margins and the relative lack of free space (particularly in the male "android"-type pelvis), limits visualization and access.

Important urologic, vascular, and nervous structures run within the pelvis and are susceptible to injury during pelvic reoperation. The distal half of the ureter lies within the pelvis, crossing the pelvic brim at the bifurcation of the iliac artery and then coursing downward along the lateral pelvic sidewall before turning upward and medially to enter the base of the bladder at the pelvic floor. The many branches of the internal iliac artery provide a rich blood supply to the pelvic viscera, which are drained by corresponding pelvic veins. Beneath the presacral fascia is an extensive venous plexus connecting directly with the sacral basivertebral veins. The pelvic sympathetic nerves follow the inferior mesenteric artery to enter the pelvis and lie on the presacral fascia. Once these nerves have joined the parasympathetic nerves in the pelvic plexuses on the pelvic sidewalls, nerves to the anus, rectum, bladder, urinary sphincter, and penis are formed and pass caudally and medially to their respective end organs. Of particular note is that the nerves to the urinary sphincter and penis pass behind the prostate but in front of the fascia of Denonvillier, and if the rectum is dissected behind this fascial layer, they will not be damaged.

Postoperative Factors

Small Intestinal Adhesions

Following operation in the pelvis the loops of small intestine become fixed in the pelvis to varying degrees. Dense adhesions are especially likely if there has been sepsis, significant bleeding, a large raw area, or irradiation.

Loss of Normal Tissue and Fascial Planes

Identification of and dissection within the correct tissue planes is the key to avoiding injury. In reoperative cases these planes may be difficult to define or completely obliterated.

Ectopic Position of Important Structures

Following pelvic surgery, especially where there has been prior mobilization of the rectum, the ureters may be in unusual locations. At the pelvic brim the ureters may assume a more medial position, sometimes even being fused to the mesorectum or a rectal stump after proximal rectal resection. Likewise, following previous resection of the colon, the abdominal portions of the ureters can be encountered surprisingly quickly during lateral abdominal dissection. They may be closely related to the small bowel as it fuses to the retroperitoneum and remnant of the mesocolon

Disease-Specific Factors

Some common reasons for pelvic reoperation are sepsis, recurrent cancer, and obstruction due to adhesions or irradiation. In each of these situations the operative field is significantly distorted, adding further to the difficulty of safe dissection.

■ APPROACH TO REOPERATIVE PELVIC SURGERY

Preoperative Planning

Timing of Reoperation

To reduce the difficulty and potential morbidity attributable to adhesions, 3 to 6 months should be allowed in nonurgent cases before attempting reoperative pelvic surgery. In cases with significant sepsis or irradiation at least 6 months and perhaps a year or longer should be allowed. If early reoperative pelvic surgery is unavoidable, during a "window" of 10 to 14 days adhesions can be lysed with relative ease and safety. After 2 weeks adhesions become denser and are associated with an inflammatory reaction, predisposing to bowel injury. In these circumstances if the patient does not have to be urgently explored, alternative approaches such as percutaneous abscess drainage, proximal fecal diversion, or parenteral nutrition should be utilized to "buy time."

Preparation of the Patient

Pelvic reoperation often involves prolonged operative and anesthetic times, and, therefore, careful preoperative patient preparation may help reduce postoperative complications.

The nutritional status of the patient should be optimized, preferably by the enteral route, but parenterally if needed. In older patients particular attention to cardiopulmonary status is important because bleeding may cause intraoperative blood pressure fluctuations, and prolonged anesthetic times and large incisions may predispose to pulmonary problems. Epidural analgesia may allow earlier postoperative mobilization and should be considered. In view of the high risk of pelvic and lower extremity venous thrombosis, compression stockings and subcutaneous heparin are routine. In those at highest risk or in whom heparin may be contraindicated for fear of bleeding, vena caval filter placement is occasionally needed. Mechanical bowel preparation and appropriate preoperative antibiotics (oral, intravenous, or both) should be administered.

Defining Anatomy

A preoperative "plan of attack" is important, especially in cases of recurrent tumors or planned bowel reanastomosis or when the conduct of previous operations is unclear. Computed tomographic (CT) scanning usually provides the most helpful information; however, under certain circumstances magnetic resonance image (MRI) scanning, may give better three-dimensional anatomy by virtue of its ability to scan in different planes. Antegrade and retrograde contrast studies of the intestine can help define the anatomy of enteric fistulas or the suitability of "out of circuit intestine" for reanastomosis. Positron emission tomographic (PET) scanning can be very useful in the face of malignant disease, as unappreciated, unresectable, or distant disease may change the aggressiveness of the approach. It may also differentiate postoperative changes from recurrent cancer.

Anticipating Problems and Complications

Sudden, significant blood loss is a risk of reoperative pelvic surgery, and blood should be available. If clinically indicated, coagulation parameters are checked. A cell saver may be useful in certain circumstances when fecal contamination is not anticipated. Easy access to platelets, fresh frozen plasma, and cryoprecipitate is also advisable in case massive transfusion is required.

Plan for a long difficult case and the potential need for other specialists' help, such as urologic or gynecologic surgeons, should the disease be more extensive than anticipated or inadvertent injury to other organs occur. Schedule the case to start early in the day and enlist the most senior help available as assistants. Provide the anesthetist with advance notice of potential for blood loss and a long difficult procedure and allow time to place appropriate lines, monitoring devices, and warming blankets.

Intraoperative Conduct

Patient Positioning and Preparation

Placing the patient on a beanbag that can be molded to fit may be useful in stopping the patient from slipping down the table when in the steep Trendelenburg position. Tuck both arms securely at the patient's side, even if the patient is obese, to avoid jeopardizing access to the pelvis. The legs are placed in carefully positioned and padded Lloyd-Davies stirrups or Allen stirrups, the latter having the advantage of being more easily maneuvered to allow access to the perineum. Skin is prepared from nipples to perineum and draped so that access to the perineum can be obtained without contaminating the abdominal field. The vagina should also be prepared, especially when operating low in the pelvis when there is a risk of inadvertent entry.

Optimizing Visibility and Exposure

Long midline incisions are safest with the distal end carried down to the pubis, including the overlying skin. The proximal extent of the incision should be high enough to gain safe entry to the abdomen away from the worst adhesions or fistulas. Enterocutaneous fistulas are left in place until the bowel around them is fully mobilized to avoid injury to noninvolved bowel. A self-retaining retractor is used and either a "C-arm" is attached to it or a malleable retractor is folded into a U shape to retain the viscera in the upper abdomen. A bladder blade is attached to the self-retaining retractor and fixed snugly against the pubic bone. A large chromic suture is often placed in the dome of the uterus and then tied around the bladder blade to pull the uterus up and out of the pelvis. Once the small bowel has been delivered from the pelvis, placing the patient in the Trendelenburg position will help keep the pelvic field clear, although excessive head-down positioning will make visualization deep in the pelvis, especially anteriorly, more difficult.

Good lighting is essential, and an operating room with several easily maneuverable and well-functioning lights is important. Newer lightweight headlights are brighter and less likely to cause neck and back ache than older models and are often helpful. In addition, we use lighted retractors and occasionally the free light cord in particularly awkward situations. The lighted Deaver retractor has a relatively shallow curve and is a short instrument, being ideal for the early part of the posterior rectal dissection. As the rectal dissection progresses deeper into the pelvis, longer instruments are used, including two further types of retractor. The Bright-Track retractor is a 15-inch-long and 1.5-inch-wide lighted instrument. Its narrow profile is ideal for anterolateral retraction of the seminal vesicles and prostate in men and the vagina in women as well as the most inferior part of the posterior rectal dissection. In our experience the most useful retractors are the curved deep pelvic retractors, which have wide or narrow blades. These retractors are especially useful in lifting the rectum forward with some degree of force to accentuate the correct plane of dissection behind the rectum. Also, it can be used to retract the bladder and prostate or vagina forward to assist with the anterior dissection.

Gaining Access to the Pelvis

Adhesions are taken down carefully, the preferred technique being to mobilize matted loops of bowel into the wound and then separate the individual loops. This procedure is particularly difficult when one or more loops of small bowel descend into the pelvis and are fused to the vagina, levators, or sacrum. In this instance it is best to try to identify the afferent and efferent loop descending into the pelvis and gently retract the apex of the loop with a sponge in the nondominant hand. Sharp dissection is performed close to the bowel wall, and the loop is separated from the dense fibrous adhesions. Enterotomies or myotomies may be unavoidable, but are preferable to injuring blood vessels, nerves, or ureters. The bowel should then be repaired or resected as appropriate. Once the loops of bowel are delivered into the wound, their separation is not usually too difficult. Grade IV adhesions fusing the bowel together or to the abdominal wall or the presence of an enterocutaneous fistula may pose problems. With enterocutaneous fistulas the uninvolved bowel should be mobilized first, leaving the fistulous connection to last and then detaching it sharply. Dissection of the densest adhesions may be facilitated by infiltrating the fused area with saline using a small-gauge needle (hydrodissection). The saline will preferentially expand the correct plane for dissection and reduce the likelihood of bowel injury. Sometimes this procedure does not help, and if a relatively small area is fused to the abdominal wall, it may be mobilized by leaving a small disk of dissected abdominal wall attached to the bowel. Hydrodissection may also be of value in finding a plane between the vagina and the previously mobilized rectum.

Identification of Specific Pelvic Structures

A scarred obliterated pelvis may become reperitonealized, and it may appear at first glance that the entire rectum, bladder, and uterus have been removed because of the deceptive smooth concavity of the pelvis. Therefore, identification and avoidance of injury to specific structures are of utmost importance.

Ureters. A thorough understanding of ureteral anatomy and the potential effects of pelvic surgery upon this area are the most important factors in identifying and avoiding injury to the ureters in the postoperative pelvis. Identification of the ureters may be facilitated by ureteric stent placement at the beginning of the operation. Unfortunately, in the most difficult cases, when the stents may be of special value, the ureter may be kinked or angulated because of adhesions or inflammation, and stent placement may not be safely undertaken. In addition, the use of stents may give a false sense of security, and because dense adhesions may make palpation of even stented ureters difficult, the first sign of a stent may be when the ureter is transected. Early identification, with or without stenting, is the key to avoiding ureteric injury, and the ureters are found proximally and traced to the pelvis. They may be marked by loosely placed encircling ligatures and then are constantly referred to during the dissection. Stenting may increase cost and time, and stents have not been proven to reduce rates of ureteric injury. However, one of the great disasters of pelvic surgery is the missed ureteric injury, and this problem is much more obvious with a stent in place.

Bladder. The bladder is usually relatively easy to identify; however, if the previous abdominal incision was extended to the pubis for maximal exposure and the bladder likewise mobilized to allow its anterior retraction, the bladder may be densely adherent beneath the midline fascia in the lower part of the wound. Care is necessary in re-entering the abdomen to avoid inadvertent injury to the bladder at this point. After radiation there may be a tight, restrictive, crescent-shaped band in the deep pelvis corresponding to a fibrous bladder base, which will limit exposure of the lower rectum. This restriction can be eased by placing superficial cautery incisions in the bladder base, being careful to take into account the entrance of the ureters, and then stretching this narrow entrance.

Rectal Stump. The ease of identification of the rectal stump is often determined by the prior surgery. If the rectum was divided at or just below the sacral promontory, the stump may be adherent to the presacral fascia, the great vessels, or the ureters, with all being at risk of injury. Under these circumstances the dissection should start lateral to the midrectum in "virgin tissue" developing the plane of the mesorectum. Once the peritoneum has been incised the dissection is facilitated by retracting the rectum medially using the lighted Deaver retractor and then using electrocautery to follow the mesorectum posteriorly to the presacral space. The proximal part of the rectal stump is then mobilized by sharp dissection or electrocautery exactly in the midline over a 1- to 2-cm area to allow development of the plane between the posterior mesorectum and the presacral fascia. The dissection is then kept on the posterior wall of the mesorectum and attached ureters or vessels are dissected free. With appropriate narrow retractors the plane is developed to meet the presacral dissection commenced from laterally and this dissection carried distally as far as needed. The remainder of the lateral attachments and lateral stalks can then be divided if required.

When the rectum has been divided below the peritoneal reflection it can be very difficult to find and to mobilize. The initial identification and subsequent mobilization can be facilitated by placing a large bougie or proctoscope transanally, which can be palpated or seen from above. This placement should be done with some care because a stricture may develop in a defunctionalized rectum. With a very low rectal stump bimanual palpation is a useful technique to identify the rectum and to accurately assess the level of the dissection in relation to the sphincters. Here an additional sleeve and glove are donned to allow placement of the surgeon's finger through the anus into the distal rectum. The other hand palpates the rectum from above. Once the apex of the rectum is identified, mobilization can be facilitated by grasping it with an Allis or Babcock clamp.

Vagina. As in rectal dissection, an obturator or bougie may be extremely helpful in identification of the vagina and prevention of injury here. The use of hydrodissection to expand an obliterated rectovaginal plane is also useful. Occasionally, bimanual palpation with one finger in the rectum and one in the vagina will facilitate the separation of the most distal aspects of rectum and vagina.

Control of Bleeding

Bleeding is a major concern in any reoperative pelvic operation and will be discussed in more detail in a separate section. However, it is worth making a few brief points. Anticipation of significant bleeding and appropriate preoperative crossmatching of blood are essential. Bleeding is usually encountered in a few key areas:

1. Bleeding from presacral and lateral sacral veins caused by inadvertent breaching of the presacral/Waldeyer's fascia above the S3-S4 level.
2. Internal iliac vein bleeding by tearing or shearing of branches from the main trunk.
3. Anterolateral bleeding from rectovaginal, retroprostatic, and paravesical veins, which is difficult to expose and control under direct vision.

General measures for control of bleeding include good lighting, more than one suction, and good exposure to identifying the source of the bleeding. Specific measures include suture placement or thumbtack placement in small breaches of the presacral fascia, use of Surgicel or rectus muscle for tamponade, and packing either for a few minutes or, if the bleeding cannot be adequately controlled, for 24 to 48 hours. The key to the management of massive uncontrollable bleeding is initial control with a finger or a pack while additional suction and retraction are obtained and sutures are readied. If control of bleeding cannot be obtained quickly, it may be wise to make the decision to place packs before a huge amount of blood is lost, leading to hypothermia, coagulopathy, and acidosis, which will compound the problem. The patient is then taken to intensive care for resuscitation and stabilization. Removal of packs at 24 to 48 hours usually reveals a dry field.

Drainage

We use drains routinely if there is a significant amount of dissection and raw surface, especially if continued oozing of blood is expected postoperatively. A single Jackson-Pratt or Atraum suction drain may suffice, but if there has been significant blood loss or fecal contamination, then sump drains are used and brought out through a separate stab incision. These drains are continuously irrigated for 24 to 48 hours postoperatively (at a rate of 0.5 to 1 L every 8 hours) and then usually are removed on postoperative day 3 when the effluent diminishes and clears.

An omental pedicle graft, usually mobilized to the left and outside the epiploic arcade, is useful for filling dead space or quarantining abscess cavities, which would otherwise fill with small bowel. Perineal drains are rarely used.

■ COMMON CLINICAL SITUATIONS

Small Bowel Obstruction

Along with staged procedures small bowel obstruction is probably the most common scenario encountered during reexploration of the pelvis. Small bowel obstruction is more likely if either the uterus or rectum has been removed, creating a large empty space where the mobile loops of small intestine will find their way by gravity. Pelvic node dissections creating a large raw surface, sepsis, and irradiation often cause the worst adhesions. Under most circumstances the above-described techniques will be successful. However, if the small bowel is fused deep in the pelvis as a result of irradiation or recurrent pelvic cancer, sometimes a bypass between the afferent and efferent loops is safest.

Reversal of Hartmann's Procedure

The problem of finding the rectal stump for anastomosis has been discussed. Performing the anastomosis to the out-of-circuit rectum, as in the second stage of a Hartmann's procedure, may also pose problems. There may be a midrectal stricture that may or may not have been appreciated preoperatively, which makes passage of the stapler impossible. Usually, the serial passage of dilators per rectum will remedy this, but occasionally further rectal resection to distal healthy rectum is needed. If more than half the rectum is removed, consideration should then be given to a colonic J-pouch or coloplasty to improve early function. When considering an end-to-end anastomosis it may be tempting to pass the cartridge of the stapler without the anvil per rectum and drive the trocar through the presumed end of the rectum. However, the end of rectum typically has a lot of scar around it, and this results in the distal donut being excessively thick, preventing adequate staple closure and causing tearing of the anastomosis upon withdrawal. Similarly, if the trocar is brought through the rectum, close to but not at the end, ischemia may develop between the anastomosis and the oversewn end of rectum, with the risk of subsequent perforation. Under these circumstances a number of techniques may be used, including resecting and opening the distal rectum for either a double purse-string technique or even a hand-sewn anastomosis or an end-to-side anastomosis well below the stapled end.

Leak at a Low Rectal Anastomosis

If there is generalized peritonitis, early re-exploration with disconnection of the anastomosis and an end-colostomy is necessary. If adhesions and inflammation do not allow safe access to the pelvis, proximal diversion with either a loop ileostomy or colostomy and drain placement can be done. A localized abscess may be amenable to percutaneous or transanastomotic drainage.

An early leak with perianastomotic sepsis frequently causes both stricturing and angulation so that, even if the leak heals, function is significantly impaired. Under these circumstances revision will often be necessary, and it is usually better to wait 6 to 12 months before attempting this.

If the leak and abscess from a very low anastomosis manifest as a perineal fistula that fails to close with local measures, then a further low or coloanal anastomosis will run the significant risk of a similar fistula. Under these circumstances a delayed coloanal anastomosis such as a Turnbull-Cutait procedure may be helpful.

Repeat Ileal-Pelvic Pouch Procedure

For ileal-pelvic pouch procedure, the original procedure required extensive pelvic dissection with removal of the entire rectum and creation of a neorectum placed into the pelvis in which the blood supply is dependent upon a single posterior blood vessel. Not surprisingly, this operation may be one of the most challenging of all pelvic reoperations. Ureteric stents are routinely placed to reduce the chance of inadvertent injury. The pelvic dissection requires sharp and precise mobilization of the pouch, which is usually fused to the presacral fascia, to prevent breaching the presacral fascia posteriorly or damaging the superior mesenteric artery anteriorly. Adhesion of the pouch deep within the pelvis requires careful use of retractors and lighting to allow safe mobilization under direct vision. Bleeding is sometimes a problem, requiring the maneuvers described earlier. Care should also be taken anteriorly in the male pelvis, where damage to the seminal vesicles and autonomic nerves may easily occur. Drainage with either sump or passive drains is combined with mobilization and placement of the omentum deep within the pelvis around the pouch.

The overall results of a series of repeat pelvic pouches at the Cleveland Clinic highlights the success that can be achieved with experience and a well-organized approach to the reoperative pelvis. Of 35 patients undergoing "redo" pelvic pouches, over 80% had a functioning pouch 6 months later. In the subset of ulcerative colitis patients (22 of 35), all but one (95%) had a functioning pouch at 6 months.

Recurrent Malignancy

In these circumstances the chances of cure or palliation must be clearly defined preoperatively, and features such as sciatic pain, lower limb lymphedema, bilateral ureteric obstruction, retroperitoneal para-aortic node involvement, and fixation to the side walls of the pelvis are usually ominous signs. Preoperative imaging studies are thus very important, and recently PET scanning has been useful not only in differentiating cancer from postoperative changes in the pelvis but also in determining the presence or absence of distant disease. Radical resections including exenterations and sacral resections may sometimes be indicated for cure or palliation in experienced hands if acceptable complication rates can be achieved. Trial dissection of the presacral space may be performed until fusion of recurrence disease to the sacrum is encountered. Under these circumstances the risks and benefits of dissection posterior to the presacral fascia must be weighed.

In summary, a very selective approach with a strong emphasis on preoperative staging may yield rewarding palliation and cure rates in experienced hands.

■ TECHNIQUES TO EASE SUBSEQUENT PELVIC SURGERY

Whether or not reoperation is planned, a few techniques can be used at the original surgery to make a subsequent operation easier and safer:

1. When performing a Hartmann's procedure leave a long rectal stump or even divide the bowel at the distal sigmoid colon, assuming that it is not involved by the disease process. The divided sigmoid can be brought through the distal portion of the abdominal wound and sutured in place to lay subcutaneously, minimizing the effect of a "stump blowout" and making subsequent identification straightforward. The presacral space is rarely violated in this procedure.
2. Minimize unnecessary pelvic dissection, mobilizing the rectum only as far as is needed for a good margin and a safe anastomosis.
3. Routinely use the mobilized omentum to fill "dead space" in the pelvis where the small bowel will become adherent. This measure is especially important if postoperative radiation is planned.
4. Use antiadhesion preparations beneath the abdominal wall.
5. Consider adequate drainage of the pelvis because blood and persistent sepsis are potent stimulators of dense adhesions.

■ CONCLUSION

Reoperative pelvic surgery may challenge even the most experienced colon and rectal surgeon. However, careful preoperative preparation and well-planned and methodical intraoperative conduct may lead to successful and gratifying outcomes.

Suggested Readings

Delaney CP, Fazio VW, Senagore AJ, et al: "Fast track" postoperative management protocol for patients with high co-morbidity undergoing complex abdominal and pelvic colorectal surgery. Br J Surg 2000;88:553–558.

Fazio V, Wu J, Lavery I: Repeat pelvic pouch-anal anastomosis to salvage septic complications of pelvic pouches. Clinical outcome and quality of life assessment. Ann Surg 1998;228:588.

Mantyh CR, Hull TL, Fazio VW: Coloplasty in low colorectal anastomosis: Manometric and functional comparison with straight and colonic J-pouch anastomosis. Dis Colon Rectum 2001;44(1):37–42.

Remzi FH, Oncel M, Strong SA, et al: The Turnbull-Cutait adominoanal pull-through excision (in preparation).

Wanebo HJ, Antoniuk P, Koness RJ, et al: Pelvic resection of recurrent rectal cancer: Technical considerations and outcomes. Dis Colon Rectum 1999;42:1438–1448.

85

NUTRITIONAL SUPPORT

Thomas E. Hamilton, MD, FACS, FAAP
John L. Rombeau, MD

Nutritional support, consisting of parenteral and enteral nutrition, is a mandatory component of the perioperative care of severely malnourished patients requiring colorectal surgery. Parenteral and enteral nutrition provide optimal metabolic subtrates as well as minerals and micronutrients to assist in wound healing and restoration of positive nitrogen balance. This chapter reviews nutritional assessment, nutrient requirements, indications for, and delivery of perioperative nutritional support for patients in need of colorectal surgery.

Colon and rectal cancer and inflammatory bowel disease are among the most common indications for elective colorectal surgery. Patients with these diseases, who are also severely malnourished, need perioperative nutritional support. Severe malnutrition is associated with increased postoperative morbidity and mortality rates. Examples of morbidity include wound and anastomotic dehiscences, immunodeficiency and ensuing infection, atelectasis, pneumonia, and respiratory failure. At the time of evaluation for surgery it is imperative to identify the colorectal surgery patient who is severely malnourished or at risk for becoming malnourished. Expeditious, cost-effective assessment is especially important in the current health care setting in which home bowel preparation and short hospital stays are the norm. When high-risk patients are identified, the provision of appropriate enteral and parenteral nutritional support becomes an integral component of patient care. Total nutritional supportive care is best delivered under the aegis of a multidisciplinary nutritional support team.

■ NUTRITIONAL ASSESSMENT

Nutritional assessment is the process of diagnosing malnutrition and determining nutrient requirements. It should be performed soon after hospital admission to provide baseline information prior to possible effects from iatrogenic factors such as blood transfusions, chemotherapy, radiotherapy, administration of drugs, or emergency operations. The subjective global assessment (SGA) in conjunction with serum albumin level has been used and validated in hospitalized patients, and is based on body weight loss, anticipated duration of illness, and status of gastrointestinal function. The SGA classifies the patient's nutritional status into three categories based on the medical history and physical examination: (1) well nourished,

(2) moderately malnourished, and (3) severely malnourished (Table 85-1). It should be emphasized that only severely malnourished patients appear to benefit from nutritional support. This SGA is indeed subjective, and consequently it has no absolute values in its measurement. Consideration of the complete clinical picture and the physician's common sense and judgment determine the value of the SGA. This SGA combined with measurement of the serum albumin level is superior or equal to single objective parameters in predicting the development of nutritionally related complications in patients undergoing major operations, including colorectal surgery.

Body Weight Loss
Patients with a minimum of 15% nonvolitional loss (10% is severely stressed) of usual body weight are arbitrarily defined as moderately to severely malnourished and should receive some form of nutritional support. Body weight loss has the greatest clinical outcome importance when it has occurred within the 6 months prior to admission.

Serum Albumin Level
Serum albumin is the most important biochemical index of malnutrition. Significant decreases in levels of serum albumin reflect chronic protein depletion; however, they are poor measures of early protein malnutrition because of the long half-life of serum albumin (20 days) and large total body pool of albumin. Falsely altered levels occur during volume overload, dehydration, or loss of capillary integrity. In general, serum albumin levels lower than 3 g/dL correlate with increased morbidity and mortality rates of postoperative patients. Various degrees of chronic protein depletion are reflected by the following serum albumin levels: mild depletion as 2.8 to 3.5 g/dL, moderate depletion with 2 to 2.7 g/dL, and severe depletion being less than 2.1 g/dL.

Dietary Intake
Reduced dietary intake or malabsorption is the primary cause of malnutrition in colorectal surgical patients. The reduced intake can be identified easily by asking the patient to list the foods consumed during a recent 24-hour period. A clinical dietitian is often helpful with this analysis. Symptoms that decrease dietary intake such as anorexia, nausea, vomiting, and diarrhea are common in the colorectal surgical population. The nutritional impact of such symptoms varies with severity, duration, and frequency of the primary disease.

Disease Type and Catabolic Effects
Weight loss has been reported in 19 to 80% of patients with inflammatory bowel disease. The causes of weight loss in these patients include inadequate dietary intake, excessive nutrient losses, increased nutrient requirements, and corticosteroid administration. Malnutrition may be associated with colonic obstruction or metastatic tumor.

Physical Examination
The important physical features of malnutrition include evidence of weight loss, decreased fat stores, impaired

Table 85-1   Classification of Nutritional Status: Subjective Global Assessment

CRITERIA	WELL NOURISHED	MODERATELY MALNOURISHED	SEVERELY MALNOURISHED
Medical History			
Body weight change in the last 6 months	Loss <5%	Loss 5–10%	Loss >10%
Dietary intake	Balanced diet that meets requirements	70–90% of required intake	<70% of required intake
Gastrointestinal symptoms (vomiting, diarrhea)	No	Intermittent	Daily for >2 weeks
Functional capacity	Full capacity	Reduced	Bedridden
Physical Examination			
Subcutaneous fat	Normal	↓	↓↓
Muscle mass (quadriceps, deltoids)	Normal	↓	↓↓
Edema (ankle, sacral)	No	+	++
Ascites	No	+	++
Serum albumin	>4.0 g/dL	3.0–4.0 g/dL	<3.0 g/dL

↓ = minimally decreased; + = minimally increased; ↓ ↓ = moderately decreased; ++ = moderately increased

muscle mass, and presence of edema. Visible areas of moderate weight loss are noted in the patient's face and hands. The loss of subcutaneous fat in the skinfolds in the triceps region and in the midaxillary line at the level of the lower ribs is easily measured. Measurements of skinfolds are imprecise but provide an impression of the degree of subcutaneous tissue loss. Depleted muscle mass is noted in wasting of the quadriceps and deltoid muscles as determined by loss of bulk and tone. Finally, ankle and presacral edema and the presence of ascites may be due to major nutritional deficits such as hypoproteinemia.

Energy Requirements

Determination of energy requirements is an integral component of nutritional support. It must first be clearly established whether the objective for nutritional support is to replete or maintain lean body mass (fat-free energy-consuming tissue of the body). Patients who are critically ill have increased circulating levels of catabolic hormones including cortisol, catecholamines, glucagon, and proinflammatory cytokines such as tumor necrosis factor-α (TNF-α) and interleukin-6 (IL-6). This hormonal milieu impairs nitrogen retention and inhibits anabolism; therefore, the caloric goal in these severely stressed patients is to maintain and not replete lean body mass. Nutritional repletion is possible only in a hormonal environment that supports an anabolic phase of recovery. Delivery of excess nutrients will not convert a catabolic patient into an anabolic state. In fact, excess delivery of nutrients in the catabolic phase of illness, especially in the presence of stress or sepsis, results in increased lipogenesis, leading to hepatic fat and glycogen deposition and a potentiation of the stress response. Thus, the caloric goal for the catabolic patient is maintenance of nutritional status. Primary treatment must be directed at the underlying cause of the catabolic state. When the catabolic state resolves, the hormonal milieu supports anabolism, and the goal for nutritional support is to replete existing deficits.

Energy determination is based on age, gender, body build, activity level, and disease state. No single test measures the energy needs for all patients. Estimates for energy requirements are calculated by standard formulas or measured by indirect calorimetry.

The formula most commonly used to predict resting metabolic expenditure (RME) is the Harris-Benedict equation:

$$RME\ male = 66 + 13W + 5H - 6.8A$$
$$RME\ female = 655 + 9.6W + 1.8H - 4.7A$$

where RME is measured in kcal/day, W is weight in kilograms, H is height in centimeters, and A is age in years.

After determination of the RME, energy requirements are adjusted for physical activity and illness (Table 85-2).

Protein Requirements

Protein utilization is influenced by energy intake, and depends in part on the nonprotein calorie/nitrogen ratio, which varies considerably in different clinical conditions.

Table 85-2   Correction Factors for Predicting Energy Requirements for Hospitalized Patients

CLINICAL CONDITION	CORRECTION FACTOR (× RME)
Physical activity	
Confined to bed	1.2
Out of bed	1.3
Starvation	0.7
Fever	1.0 + 0.13 per degree Celsius
Elective surgery	1.0–1.2
Peritonitis	1.2–1.5
Soft tissue trauma	1.14–1.37
Major sepsis	1.4–1.8

RME = resting metabolic expenditure (see text for calculation).
Source: Adapted from Bernard MA, Jacobs DO, Rombeau JL: Nutritional and Metabolic Support of Hospitalized Patients. Philadelphia, WB Saunders, 1986, p 13.

In the nonstressed patient, the optimal ratio of nonprotein calorie/nitrogen is 150:1. In critically ill patients this ratio decreases to 100:1 owing to requirements for synthesis of acute phase proteins and tissue repair. Precise amounts of protein required for different levels of caloric intake have not been defined; however, practical guidelines have been created for initial protein and calorie prescriptions. Adjustments of protein and calories should be made according to measurements of nitrogen balance and changes in clinical course.

Electrolytes and Micronutrients Requirements

Requirements for sodium, potassium, bicarbonate, chloride, magnesium, calcium, and phosphate are determined by baseline levels, calculated losses, and maintenance needs (Rombeau and Caldwell).

Vitamins should be administered daily in quantities recommended by the Nutritional Advisory Group of the American Medical Association. Standard amounts of trace elements are included in most commercially available enteral formulas.

■ MONITORING

Patients who receive nutritional support require careful monitoring, which is best performed by a multidisciplinary nutrition support team. A monitoring protocol may be helpful in institutions where physicians of variable levels of experience are responsible for writing orders for nutritional support. Daily physical examination is essential for critically ill patients when dysfunction of the gastrointestinal tract may produce intolerance to enteral formulas. Intolerance is manifest as abdominal distention, diarrhea, nausea, and excessive gastric residuals. Nitrogen balance (nitrogen loss measured by 24-hour urea nitrogen + estimate of 4 g for fecal losses), body weight, and serum protein levels are monitored at least weekly and these values are used in calculating nutrient requirements as discussed previously. Complementary use of total parenteral nutrition (TPN) with enteral feeding is sometimes necessary to reach nutritional goals during the early postoperative period when there can be intolerance to large amounts of enteral nutrients. Detailed attention to metabolic status and fluid balance are also essential when treating critically ill patients. When standardized monitoring is followed, potential complications can be averted pre-emptively often by simple maneuvers, such as changing the dietary infusion rate, caloric density, or formulation.

■ INDICATIONS

Preoperative Nutritional Support

Only severely malnourished colorectal surgical patients benefit from or justify the risk and cost of preoperative nutritional support. Severe malnutrition usually includes a body weight loss minimum of 15% of usual body weight, marked decrease in dietary intake (as identified by dietary history), significant gastrointestinal symptoms (anorexia, nausea, vomiting, and diarrhea) of greater than 2 weeks' duration, functional status (cancer, severe inflammatory bowel disease), and abnormal physical findings such as loss of subcutaneous fat, muscle wasting, and the presence of ankle and presacral edema. The time needed to preoperatively replete the malnourished patient should be realistic (7 to 10 days) and should not unduly delay surgery. A home regimen can be arranged if a prolonged period of preoperative nutritional support will be needed prior to an elective operation.

The urgency of the operation is another important determinant in preoperative nutritional decisions. For patients in need of emergency surgery (e.g., megacolon), preoperative nutritional support cannot be given. However, nutritional assessment should be performed briefly even before emergency operations to identify those patients in need of intraoperative access, such as gastrostomy, jejunostomy, or special central venous catheters to provide long-term postoperative nutritional support.

Prior to elective colorectal surgery the anticipated duration of nutritional support should be estimated. Preoperative nutritional regimens of less than 4 days have no benefit in reducing the rates of postoperative morbidity and mortality, and continuing the nutritional regimen for more than 14 days preoperatively cannot be justified in today's health care economy. When the aforementioned criteria of severe malnutrition are present, we recommend in-hospital preoperative nutritional support for 7 days.

Postoperative Nutritional Support

Postoperative nutritional support is indicated for conditions in which inordinate delays (7 to 10 days) in postoperative oral intake either has occurred or is anticipated. Examples include severe preoperative malnutrition, metastatic colorectal cancer, peritonitis, severe sepsis, and prolonged ileus. Parenteral nutrition is preferred in the early postoperative period of many colorectal surgical patients because of the potential risks associated with enteral feeding proximal to new enteric anastomoses. In conditions such as Crohn's disease, radiation enteritis, prolonged obstruction, ischemia, peritonitis (diffuse or localized), multiple bowel anastomoses, urinary and biliary diversion, immunosuppression, shock, or sepsis, it is prudent to wait for clinical evidence of return of bowel function prior to initiating enteral nutrition. Patients who receive TPN for severe malnutrition are usually continued on this regimen until normal bowel function returns. Patients who are normally nourished and in whom no delay in oral intake is anticipated do not need postoperative nutritional support. However, these patients should be monitored to identify possible ensuing severe malnutrition during their hospital stay.

■ PROVISION OF NUTRITIONAL SUPPORT

Oral Intake

If the patient is able to eat 75% of his or her calculated requirements, it is usually possible to meet the remaining nutrient needs with oral supplements. However, in patients with complicated inflammatory bowel disease or colorectal cancer in whom anorexia is a common manifestation, it is often difficult to give sufficient nutrients solely via the oral route. Wexner and associates recently reported a prospective randomized trial of oral feeding after elective colorectal surgery versus the "traditional" way of feeding only after resolution of postoperative ileus. There were no significant differences in the rate of vomiting, nasogastric tube reinsertion, length of hospital stay, or overall complications in the two groups. However, the patients in the early feeding group tolerated a regular diet earlier than did the patients in the regular feeding group (2.6 ± 0.1 days versus 5 ± 0.1 days; $p < 0.001$). This study demonstrated the safety and efficacy of early oral feeding in the majority of patients after elective colorectal surgery (Table 85-3).

Enteral Nutrition

Enteral nutrition is defined as the direct administration of liquid formula diets into the gut. This method of nutritional support is preferred in most postoperative patients because of the beneficial effects on bowel structure and function, safety, and low cost when compared to TPN. Enteral nutrition preserves normal nutrient metabolism and utilization and maintains intestinal integrity and hormonal balance. It has fewer metabolic complications than TPN, especially abnormalities of liver function often present in patients with chronic inflammatory bowel disease. Enteral nutrition is recommended if the gut is functioning and can be used safely and effectively. Contraindications to enteral feeding include vomiting, intestinal obstruction, severe ileus, abdominal distention, and significant gastrointestinal hemorrhage.

Enteral nutrition is administered by several routes, depending on the anticipated duration of feeding and potential risk for aspiration. The oral route is preferred. However, it requires an alert patient with an intact gag reflex, who requires only supplementation with meals. Other methods for delivery of enteral nutrients include nasogastric tubes, nasoenteric tubes, gastrostomy, jejunostomy, and combined gastrojejunal tubes.

Access: Nasogastric and Nasoenteric Tubes

Nasogastric and nasoenteric tubes are best used for patients who have intact gag reflexes and a competent lower esophageal sphincter and who require short-term enteral feeding. Ideal candidates include patients with poor oral intake such as that secondary to cancer-induced anorexia. The stomach is the most preferred and physiologic site of delivery; however, if gastroparesis exists or if the patient is at increased risk for aspiration, a nasoenteric tube should be advanced into the jejunum. The interventional radiologist or endoscopist is often helpful with tube placement into the jejunum.

Percutaneous Endoscopic Gastrostomy/Operative Gastrostomy

The percutaneous endoscopic gastrostomy (PEG) is the safest and most cost-effective method of tube placement in the stomach for long-term enteral feeding. PEG is contraindicated in patients with strictures or obstructing lesions of the esophagus. An operative gastrostomy can be performed on patients undergoing ensuing abdominal surgery. Indications for operative gastrostomy include the inability to insert a PEG or in association with a concomitant laparotomy.

Operative Jejunostomy

Operative jejunostomy is indicated for those patients at high-risk for aspiration, or in whom the stomach cannot be used for feeding. Jejunostomies are also indicated as an adjunctive procedure when a prolonged postoperative delay in oral intake is anticipated. Adjunctive jejunostomy is recommended for operative patients with colorectal cancer and in need of either chemotherapy or radiation therapy.

Gastrostomy-Jejunostomy Tubes

Combined gastrostomy-jejunostomy (G-J) tubes have been devised for simultaneous jejunal feeding and gastric decompression. They are placed surgically and are indicated in the malnourished patient at increased risk for aspiration and in need of postoperative enteral feeding.

Total Parenteral Nutrition

TPN is indicated when enteral nutrition cannot or should not be used. Patients with high-output intestinal fistulas, intestinal obstruction, severe ileus, or upper gastrointestinal bleeding and conditions in which bowel rest is desired, such as preoperative bowel preparations, are all indications for TPN.

Therapeutic Decision Making

Figure 85-1 summarizes the decision-making approach to nutritional management of colorectal surgical patients. Appropriate use of nutritional support is based not only

Table 85-3 Comparison of Results of Early and Regular Postoperative Feeding			
FACTOR	EARLY FEEDING	REGULAR FEEDING	*p* VALUE
Tolerating early feeding	79%	—	—
Vomiting	21%	14%	>0.05
Nasogastric tube insertion	11%	10%	>0.05
Resolution of ileus (days, range)	3.8 ± 0.1 (1–8)	4.1 ± 0.1 (1–9)	>0.05
First meal ingestion (days, range)	2.6 ± 0.1 (2–8)	5.0 ± 0.1 (2–10)	>0.001
Length of hospital stay (days, range)	6.2 ± 0.2 (2–12)	6.8 ± 0.2 (3–12)	>0.05

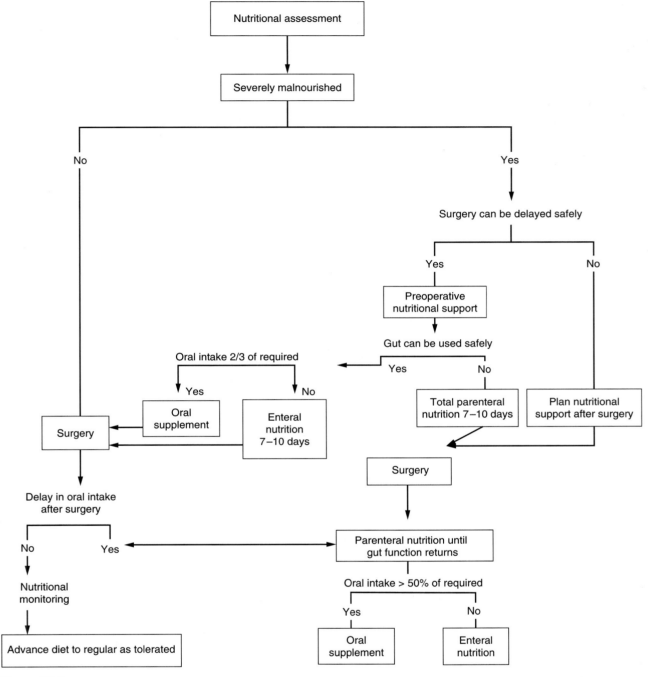

Figure 85-1
Algorithm for decision-making approach for nutritional management in colorectal surgical patients.

on recognizing malnourished patients at increased risk of developing nutritionally related complications but also on anticipating conditions that may interfere with the maintenance of a normal nutritional status.

Complications

Similar to any medical treatment, nutritional support is associated with complications. The most common complications of parenteral and enteral nutrition are listed in

Table 85-4. A detailed discussion of these complications can be found in the suggested readings.

■ SUMMARY

Nutritional assessment is a mandatory component of the perioperative care of patients requiring colorectal surgery. Preoperative nutritional support is reserved for severely

Table 85-4 Common Complications of Nutritional Support

MECHANICAL		METABOLIC		SEPTIC		GASTROINTESTINAL	
ENTERAL	PARENTERAL	ENTERAL	PARENTERAL	ENTERAL	PARENTERAL	ENTERAL	PARENTERAL
Nasopharyngeal irritation	Pneumothorax	Overhydration	Hyperglycemia	Aspiration pneumonia	Bacteremia	Diarrhea	Acalculous cholecystitis
Tube obstruction and displacement	Arterial laceration	Hyperglycemia	Hypoglycemia	Otitis media	Septic embolism	Vomiting	Mucosal atrophy
	Hemothorax	Electrolyte and mineral imbalance	Electrolyte and mineral imbalance	Sinusitis	Candidiasis	Distention	
	Venous thrombosis		Fatty liver				

malnourished patients as identified by the subjective global assessment. Placement of enteral feeding tubes or central venous access should be considered intraoperatively if postoperative nutrition support is anticipated. When appropriate principles are followed, early postoperative enteral feeding is safe in the majority of patients undergoing elective colorectal surgery. Currently, many colorectal surgeons prescribe a more rapid progression of postoperative dietary intake when compared to traditional teachings of waiting for the resolution of postoperative ileus and for return of normal bowel function.

Suggested Readings

Barot LR, Rombeau JL, Feurer ID, Mullen JL: Caloric requirements in patients with inflammatory bowel disease. Ann Surg 1982;145:214–218.

Detsky AS, McLaughlin JR, Baker JP, et al: What is subjective global assessment of nutritional status? JPEN 1987;11:8–13.

Detsky AS, Baker JP, O'Rourke K, et al: Predicting nutrition-associated complications for patients undergoing gastrointestinal surgery. JPEN 1987;11:440–446.

Grant JP: Percutaneous endoscopic gastrostomy. Initial placement by single endoscopic technique and long-term follow up. Ann Surg 1993;217(2):168–174.

Hamilton TE, Rombeau JL: Enteral nutrition. In Nyhus LM, Baker RJ, Fischer JE (Eds.). Mastery of Surgery, 3rd ed. Boston, Little, Brown, 1996.

Hickman DM, Miller RA, Rombeau JL, et al: Serum albumin and body weight as predictors of postoperative course in colorectal cancer. JPEN 1980;4:314–316.

Reissman P, Teoh TA, Cohen SM, et al: Is early oral feeding safe after elective colorectal surgery? A prospective randomized trial. Ann Surg 1995;222(1):73–77.

Rombeau JL, Rolandelli RH (Eds.). Clinical Nutrition: Parenteral Nutrition, 3rd ed. Philadelphia, WB Saunders, 2001.

Rombeau JL, Rolandelli RH (Eds.). Clinical Nutrition: Enteral and Tube Feeding, 3rd ed. Philadelphia, WB Saunders, 1996.

86

PREVENTION AND MANAGEMENT OF SEPSIS

Robert B. Noone, Jr., MD

Over the last century, advancements in surgical technique, antisepsis, and antibiotic therapy have resulted in a drastic decrease in the rate of surgical infections. Infectious complications still occur as a result of a complex interaction among the virulence and dose of infectious agents, patient factors, technical issues, and the wound environment. Prevention of infection is one of the primary goals in intestinal surgery. It is important to understand the risk factors for development of infection in order to decrease the chance of complications. Prompt recognition and appropriate treatment of infection that does occur is critical to successful outcome.

■ BASIC PRINCIPLES

Bacterial Factors

The type and number of bacteria that are introduced to a wound from external or endogenous sources determine the risk of infection. Bacteria have specific mechanisms to avoid host clearance, such as encapsulation to avoid phagocytosis (e.g., *Klebsiella* and *Streptococcus pneumoniae*). Gram-negative organisms (e.g., *Escherichia coli*, *Enterobacter*) have surface toxins (endotoxin or lipopolysaccharide) that enhance infectious ability. Other organisms secrete exotoxins (certain *Staphylococcus* and *Clostridium* species) that cause local wound necrosis and dramatically enhance infection with a small inoculum. Decreasing the load of the infectious organisms in a wound is critical to avoiding infection.

The most important organisms that are encountered in community-acquired abdominal infection or in elective bowel surgery are *Escherichia coli* and *Bacteroides fragilis*, and antibacterial therapy should be directed routinely against these organisms. Infections that occur within the hospital often include organisms such as *Pseudomonas* species, *Enterococcus* species, fungi, and *Staphylococcus epidermidis*.

Local Wound Factors

Good surgical technique is important to prevent a conducive environment for bacterial growth. Dissection in proper surgical planes, avoidance of excessive cautery, and maintenance of hemostasis are important. "Prophylactic" drains in the abdominal cavity have, in general, been shown to increase the chance of infection. Drains, partic-

ularly closed suction drains, are useful when a potential space that will collect fluid or blood, or a cavity such as a localized abscess exists. Skin bacteria will "wick" along the drain, and so its removal in a timely fashion is recommended.

Preoperative shower with an antibacterial soap such as chlorhexidine has been shown to decrease wound infections. The patient can do this at home the evening before surgery. Preoperative shaving the night before has been shown to increase the chance of wound infection, presumably from bacterial growth in small cuts in the skin. Thus, shaving should be avoided, if possible. Skin trauma may be minimized by the use of clippers immediately before skin preparation. Depilatory cream also can be used.

The length of preoperative hospitalization has been shown to correlate with risk of infection, particularly with resistant organisms. Special care with skin decontamination is important for patients who have been in the hospital for more than a few days prior to surgery.

■ RISK FACTORS

Patient Factors

Several underlying patient factors increase the chance of complications from infection (Table 86-1). Diabetics have been shown to have higher risks of wound infection. Elevated HbA_{1c} levels have been associated with infection, and evidence suggests that carefully monitored perioperative blood glucose levels can decrease infection risk. Elderly and very young patients are at increased risk. High doses of corticosteroids inhibit wound healing and can predispose to surgical site infection. Avoidance of intraoperative hypothermia and use of supplemental postoperative oxygen helps decrease the infective risk. Remote infection at the time of surgery doubles the risk of wound infection.

Procedure Factors

Table 86-2 summarizes the National Research Council (NRC) classification of surgical wounds and expected infection rates for closed wounds. These rates are affected by comorbid factors and are higher with underlying illness. The Study of the Efficacy of Nosocomial Infection

---

Table 86-1 Patient Risk Factors for Infection

Duration of preoperative hospitalization
Poor nutrition
Hypothermia
Diabetes mellitus
Presence of distant infection
Smoking
High-dose corticosteroid use
Extremes of age
Hypoperfusion
    Hypovolemic shock
    Vasopressors

Table 86-2 Classification of Surgical Wounds

CLASS	DEFINITION	EXAMPLE	RISK OF WOUND INFECTION
Clean	Atraumatic; no entry of respiratory, urinary, gastrointestinal, or biliary tracts; no inflammation; no break in sterile technique	Breast biopsy	1 to 3%
Clean-Contaminated	Controlled entry into gastrointestinal, genitourinary, respiratory, or biliary tracts; minor break in technique	Elective bowel resection	5 to 10%
Contaminated	Traumatic wound, gross spillage from gastrointestinal tract, acute nonpurulent infection, major break in technique	Appendectomy for acute appendicitis	15%
Dirty	Existing purulent infection, perforated viscus	Hartmann's procedure for perforated diverticulitis	40%

Control (SENIC) defined four independent risk factors for surgical site infection: operations on the abdomen, surgery lasting longer than 2 hours, three or more associated medical diagnoses (at time of discharge), and NRC classification as dirty or contaminated. The number of these risk factors accurately predicts risk of infection and is used to stratify cases for hospital infection control programs.

Specific techniques are used to prevent wound infection in dirty and contaminated wounds. In wounds that have a high risk of infection, delayed primary closure (DPC) or leaving the wound open to heal by second intention is effective. DPC is done by packing the wound and covering with a sterile dressing for 3 days. The wound is then examined. If it is clean with no necrotic tissue or exudates, the wound is redressed sterilely and is closed on postoperative day 4 with Steri-strips or sutures placed at the time of surgery.

The goal in emergency surgery in dirty cases is to remove the source of contamination to prevent further sepsis. For example, perforated diverticulitis is best managed by removal of the involved colon and not with diversion alone. Hartmann's procedure is performed to prevent anastomotic breakdown. In select cases a primary anastomosis may be performed, with or without a proximal stoma. This procedure is done only in an otherwise healthy patient, who is not in extremis, when adequate bowel preparation is possible (or intraoperative lavage can be done) and substantial (particularly fecal) peritoneal contamination is absent.

■ PREVENTION

Bowel Preparation

Prior to elective colon surgery, removal of stool by mechanical bowel preparation decreases the total amount of bacteria present and allows for technical ease at surgery. Any remaining stool after preparation has the same bacterial load per unit weight. Mechanical preparations can lead to complications such as preoperative dehydration and electrolyte abnormalities, and it has been suggested that avoiding preparation may be beneficial. Although several reports have demonstrated that the avoidance of a mechanical bowel preparation is not associated with adverse consequences, a mechanical bowel preparation remains the standard of care for elective colon surgery.

Bowel preparation is usually done on an outpatient basis the day prior to surgery in otherwise healthy, nonobstructed patients. A clear liquid diet is consumed. Effective bowel preparation is done with a polyethylene glycol (PEG) and electrolyte lavage (CoLyte, GoLYTELY), 1 gallon the day prior to surgery. Better tolerated by many patients and as effective is preparation with oral sodium phosphate (Fleet Phospho-Soda), 1.5 oz in 8 oz of liquid, given as two doses the night before surgery. This laxative may cause significant electrolyte abnormalities and volume depletion and is avoided in patients with renal insufficiency and significant cardiac disease. Oral hydration solutions (e.g., Gatorade) help to avoid these problems in healthy patients. Table 86-3 offers an example of patient instructions for preparation at home.

In the case of emergency surgery, intraoperative lavage may be used to empty the colon of stool in the absence of preoperative mechanical preparation. Lavage is particularly useful in surgery for acute diverticulitis or colonic obstruction in the patient who is otherwise a candidate for primary anastomosis. A urinary balloon catheter is placed through the appendix or through a purse-string suture in the terminal ileum. Both flexures are mobilized for best results. Large-bore tubing such as plastic respiratory ventilator tubing is placed in the distal colon and secured with a hernia tape. The tubing is directed off the surgical field into a disposal bucket. Warm saline solution is then run through the colon from the balloon catheter until the bowel is clean (Fig. 86-1).

Antibiotic Prophylaxis

Antibiotics are directed against the predominant bacterial species in the bowel: the coliform gram-negative rods

Table 86-3 Outpatient Preoperative Bowel Preparation Instruction Sheet

Outpatient Cleaning of the Large Intestine Before Surgery	*Schedule for Preoperative Bowel Preparation*
NAME: _____ Date of Surgery: _____	Your surgery is scheduled for _____
The large intestine stores stool that is mostly made of germs. Infection after surgery is one of the most serious problems (complications) that occurs when operating on the large intestine (your colon and rectum). By cleaning out the large intestine and giving antibiotics by mouth before surgery, the rate of postoperative infection is reduced from 40% (40 patients out of every 100 having surgery) to less than 5% (5 patients out of every 100).	Begin your clear liquid diet at ___ AM/PM on _____
It is important to prepare your large intestine before having surgery on it. You must follow a clear liquid diet, drink your medicine that cleans out the colon, and take your antibiotics by mouth as your doctor and nurse have explained to you. This will make your operation safer by lowering your risk of having an infection after surgery on the large intestine.	Start drinking your Colyte or GoLYTELY at ___ AM/PM on _____. You must drink 4 liters of this over 3–4 hours. This is easy to do if you drink 8–10 oz. of this medicine every 15 minutes. If necessary, mix Colyte solution as directed by the pharmacist in 4 liters of water at ___ AM/PM on and refrigerate. *Do not add ice to Colyte solution once mixed;* this would make it too watery.
Begin the clear liquid diet as below on _____	In the afternoon of _____ begin taking your antibiotics by mouth. Swallow 1 gram of erythromycin (2 tablets) and 1 gram of neomycin (2 tablets) together at 1 PM, 2 PM, and 11 PM on _____. You might have some nausea. Call your doctor if vomiting continues or if you have abdominal swelling or pain.
Coffee, decaffeinated coffee (no milk or cream) Tea, herbal tea Carbonated beverages (soft drinks), regular and sugar-free Gelatin dessert, plain or fruit flavored Apple juice, grape juice, cranberry juice Gatorade, Kool-Aid, lemonade, limeade Hawaiian Punch, Delaware Punch Clear fat-free beef or chicken broth Bouillon, clear consomme Snowball (water-ice, flavored), popsicles Hard candy, sugar, salt	Drink 1 quart of 10-K or Gatorade on the evening of _____.
Note: Avoid any liquids not specifically listed above. Alcohol is not permitted unless you check with your physician or nurse.	This will replace the salts and water lost during the cleansing of your large intestine. Eat or drink nothing after midnight, the night before your surgery. Stop all aspirin or aspirin-containing medicine before surgery, 2 weeks before if possible. Be sure to ask your doctor or nurse any questions that you may have about cleaning the intestine before surgery or about the operation itself. If a problem develops, call _____

Source: Holmes JW, Nichols RL: Sepsis following colorectal surgery. In Fazio VW (Ed.). *Current Therapy in Colorectal Surgery*. Philadelphia, WB Saunders, 1990.

and anaerobes. Nichols and coworkers introduced an oral regimen in 1972 that was very effective in decreasing the rate of infection after elective colon surgery from 40% to less than 10% compared to mechanical preparation alone. Erythromycin (anaerobic coverage) and neomycin (aminoglycoside directed against gram-negative bacteria) are administered orally in three doses the night before surgery. Metronidazole is often substituted for erythromycin and is the author's preference, as it is better tolerated.

An equivalent reduction in infectious risk can be achieved with the perioperative use of parenteral antibiotics with gram-negative and anaerobic coverage. This regimen has the advantage of achieving much higher systemic antibiotic levels at the time of potential contamination. Most often, a second-generation cephalosporin is used. This agent gives good gram-negative and anaerobic coverage. Cefotetan has a longer half-life than cefoxitin and is preferred. Acceptable substitutes are metronidazole with a third-generation cephalosporin (e.g., cefotaxime) or quinolone (e.g., ciprofloxacin) or a broad-spectrum combination antibiotic such as amoxicillin-clavulanic acid. Timing of administration is important—it should be given at time of anesthetic induction and not "on call to OR." Antibiotics must be administered no later than 30 minutes after the start of the procedure.

The majority of colon and rectal surgeons surveyed use both oral and parenteral antibiotics. Some studies show a marginal improvement in infection rates over the use of one alone. Several randomized studies have shown no advantage to adding oral antibiotics to perioperative parenteral antibiotics. No study or meta-analysis has demonstrated any benefit from using more than a single dose of parenteral antibiotics, as long as the dose is repeated if the surgery lasts more than 4 hours.

■ INFECTIOUS COMPLICATIONS

Nonsurgical Infections
The most common source of infection in the surgical patient is in the urinary tract. Many patients require an indwelling catheter, which increases the risk. Although urinary tract infection (UTI) is readily recognized and usually is easily treated, it can be a significant cause of morbidity. Bladder catheters should be inserted under sterile conditions, should be kept to sterile closed

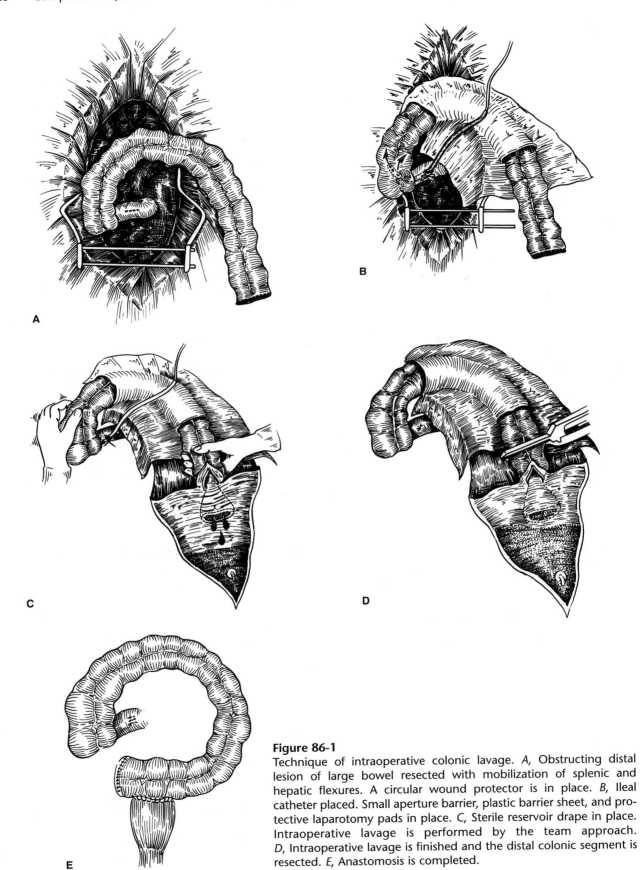

Figure 86-1
Technique of intraoperative colonic lavage. *A,* Obstructing distal lesion of large bowel resected with mobilization of splenic and hepatic flexures. A circular wound protector is in place. *B,* Ileal catheter placed. Small aperture barrier, plastic barrier sheet, and protective laparotomy pads in place. *C,* Sterile reservoir drape in place. Intraoperative lavage is performed by the team approach. *D,* Intraoperative lavage is finished and the distal colonic segment is resected. *E,* Anastomosis is completed.

drainage, and should be removed as quickly as possible to minimize infectious risk.

Pneumonia is the third leading cause of postoperative infection after UTI and surgical site infection (SSI), and the most common cause of death from hospital-acquired infection. Pneumonia may be difficult to diagnose, especially in the postoperative patient with significant atelectasis. The most common cause of pulmonary effusion and atelectasis after surgery is an abdominal inflammatory process.

Antibiotic-associated diarrhea represents a postoperative infection that requires increasing attention. This infection is usually caused by overgrowth of *Clostridium difficile* and may be severe and occasionally fatal. Stool from patients with postoperative diarrhea should be checked for *C. difficile* toxin. Repeated samples for the assay should be sent if suspicion is high. Similarly, empiric treatment should be started in the ill patient while awaiting the assay results. *C difficile* infections can be present in patients with ileal pouches (whether continent ileostomy or ileoanal pouch) and rarely in patients with an end-ileostomy. Initial treatment is with metronidazole, but aggressive treatment for severe cases may require intravenous metronidazole, oral vancomycin, and even vancomycin enemas.

■ SURGICAL SITE INFECTION

Wound Infection

Superficial wound infections are recognized by erythema, swelling, drainage, and warmth at the wound site. Fever may be present. Exploring a small section of the wound by removing one or two sutures or staples may release occult fluid when infection is suspected. Gram stain of fluid sampled from the wound will differentiate infection from benign drainage such as fat necrosis or edema fluid. When the wound is opened to treat infection, the fascia is examined for deep wound involvement and dehiscence. Superficial wound infections should be opened to drain the entire cavity, and the wound should be packed with gauze. Any devitalized tissue should be débrided. Wound dressing changes are then started, and the wound is allowed to close by secondary intention. The patient can irrigate the wound in the shower daily if possible. Antibiotics are unnecessary unless cellulitis is present.

Deep infection of the muscle and fascia may result in wound dehiscence. Although small areas of dehiscence may be managed expectantly, larger areas or complete wound dehiscence require operative debridement and reclosure of the wound with retention sutures to prevent evisceration.

The special case of the early postoperative wound infection should be noted. Invasive soft tissue infection with beta-hemolytic streptococcus or clostridial species (usually *C. perfringens*) may present within the first 36 hours after surgery, at a time when wound infection often is not suspected as a source of postoperative fever. The wound must be examined, and fluid from the wound examined by Gram stain to make the diagnosis. The fluid is thin and often not obviously purulent. Both organisms tend to cause severe wound pain, sometimes in the setting of a normal-appearing wound (especially clostridial myonecrosis.) Invasive streptococcal infection will usually present with marked wound inflammatory changes. Both types of infection require aggressive débridement and antibiotic coverage with high-dose penicillin.

Intra-abdominal Infection or Abscess

Early recognition of intra-abdominal infection can be difficult in the postoperative period. Rarely, early infection in the first 36 hours after surgery may be due to bowel injury with intraperitoneal leak of contents. This infection is recognized by signs of systemic toxicity: fever, tachycardia, tachypnea, diffuse abdominal pain (nonincisional), and abdominal tenderness. Hemodynamic changes may progress to hypotension and oliguria, and volume requirements are large. The abdominal pain can be most prominent after laparoscopic surgery as incisional tenderness is often minimal and inadvertent bowel injury may be unrecognized. In this setting, early examination by repeat laparoscopy is recommended.

Unexplained fever or new onset of undue abdominal pain in the postoperative period should start the search for infectious complications. Other signs include leukocytosis, ileus, focal tenderness, or palpable abdominal mass. Sometimes respiratory distress is the only indicator of a subtle abdominal problem such as a small anastomotic leak. After left colon, colorectal, coloanal, or ileoanal anastomoses, a water-soluble contrast study of the anastomosis is recommended in the patient who is not following the expected postoperative course and develops septic manifestations or pain suspicious of leak. Early recognition and management of anastomotic complications improve ultimate outcome.

Computed tomography (CT) is the procedure of choice to evaluate suspected intra-abdominal infection. Oral and intravenous contrast material is used, and localized fluid collections or extravasation of contrast medium may be seen. Unfortunately, the local inflammatory process associated with surgery is difficult to separate from infectious processes. It is uncommon to have a true positive CT scan for intra-abdominal infection within the first postoperative week, and the author waits at least 5 days after surgery to get a CT if indicated. Early fluid collections should undergo diagnostic aspiration to differentiate benign postoperative fluid from infection. Localized abscess may often be drained percutaneously under CT or ultrasound guidance. The advantage of CT is that surrounding structures are well visualized and a tract can often be found even to deeper collections without violating vascular or visceral organs. Pelvic collections may be accessed successfully through the sciatic foramen, although these catheters may be quite uncomfortable for the patient. If a pelvic collection relates to an anastomotic leak, it should generally be drained transanally through the anastomosis.

If an abscess is successfully accessed, a pigtail catheter is placed and put to a suction apparatus or to a drainage bag. Catheters draining thick fluid often require intermittent flushes with saline solution to keep the lumen patent. The patient is then monitored closely for clinical improvement. The cavity may be restudied 24 to 48 hours later by repeat CT or by fluoroscopic contrast injection to confirm decrease in abscess size, particularly for those with unexpectedly slow clinical improvement. Connections to the bowel can be demonstrated by contrast studies. If the catheter does not drain freely and the abscess does not collapse, occasionally exchange of the catheter for a larger size may help. If the patient does not clinically improve and the cavity does not resolve, open operative drainage is necessary. CT drainage of simple abscess cavities is ultimately successful in 60 to 90% of cases. Multiple abscess cavities, complex multiloculated collections, abscess with enteric connection, and infection associated with necrotic tissue or tumor are more likely to require operative drainage. Other situations in which percutaneous drainage is not as successful are fungal abscess, infected hematoma, and inter-loop abscesses.

Broad-spectrum antibiotics are started when intra-abdominal infection is diagnosed. These drugs can be tailored to specific organisms when culture data are available after drainage or débridement of the infection. The Surgical Infection Society published a consensus statement in 1992 on the antibiotic therapy of abdominal infection. This list has been updated by several authors based on more recent controlled trials and is summarized in Table 86-4.

Source Control

Any patient with signs and symptoms of intra-abdominal infection after intestinal anastomosis should have an evaluation to exclude anastomotic leak. Colorectal and low pelvic anastomoses can be well evaluated by water-soluble contrast study. More proximal anastomoses are not as easily seen in this fashion secondary to dilution of the contrast material and should be examined using CT with intravenous, oral, and rectal contrast media ("triple contrast"). Clinical features of anastomotic dehiscence may range from asymptomatic to frank peritonitis. Completely asymptomatic leaks may be demonstrated incidentally on contrast studies at a rate that is approximately four times higher than the rate of symptomatic leaks. These leaks do not require specific treatment besides clinical observation.

The acutely ill patient with gross peritonitis requires laparotomy, disconnection of the anastomosis with a stoma, mucous fistula, or Hartmann's procedure. Diversion without resection of the anastomosis may be used selectively; however, candidates must be chosen with great care because the septic source is not removed and patients who fail this approach have poorer outcomes. Suitable patients are those with a small defect in an otherwise well-perfused, intact anastomosis, who have a nonfecal peritonitis, and who are otherwise healthy. The defect can be sutured, the anastomosis is wrapped in omentum, the bowel is defunctioned proximally with a loop ileostomy, and soft rubber drains are placed close to the anastomosis.

In the ill patient with a leak that has been demonstrated, but no gross peritonitis, and has no demonstrable

Table 86-4 Recommendations of Empiric Antibiotic Therapy for Intra-abdominal Infection

Community-acquired infection, mild to moderate severity
  Cefoxitin*
  Cefotetan*
  Ticarcillin/clavulanate
  Ampicillin/sulbactam
Severe sepsis or hospital-acquired infection, particularly with recent antibiotic use
  Imipenem
  Meropenem
  Piperacillin/tazobactam
Or

Gram-Negative ± Gram-Positive Coverage	and	Antianerobe
Aminoglycoside		clindamycin*
Third-generation cephalosporin*		metronidazole
Cefotaxime		
Ceftizoxime		
Ceftriaxone		
Ceftazidime		
Cefepime		
Aztreonam		
Quinolone		
Ciprofloxacin		
Ofloxacin		
Levofloxacin		

*Note: Although any antibiotic use may lead to *Clostridium difficile*–associated diarrhea, clindamycin and cephalosporin use (especially oral and third-generation intravenous cephalosporins) have higher incidences of *C. difficile* infections. For this reason, the author avoids the use of these drugs when possible in the hospital setting.

abscess, conservative therapy with bowel rest and antibiotics may be attempted for up to a week. These patients often need parenteral nutrition. Failure to improve necessitates surgery. If there is no peritoneal soilage and the anastomosis is grossly intact, diversion with proximal colostomy or ileostomy and placement of soft rubber drains close to the anastomosis may be attempted.

If an abscess is found, drainage is indicated. Pelvic anastomoses may have dehiscence visible by proctoscopy and be treated by opening the site and placing a transanal drain that may be irrigated. Other abscesses are drained by percutaneous methods as outlined previously, if possible. Percutaneous drainage of anastomotic abscess may result in enterocutaneous fistula. In the absence of distal obstruction, foreign body, malignancy, persistent abscess, or sepsis, most fistulas will close spontaneously. Oral nutrition should be continued unless fistula output is too high to manage, in which case bowel rest, total parenteral nutrition (TPN), and octreotide (somatostatin analog) are used.

Tertiary Peritonitis

Tertiary peritonitis is defined as recurrence of intra-abdominal infection after apparent initial control of abdominal sepsis. The organisms involved are often less intrinsically virulent but drug-resistant and include *E. coli*,

Enterococcus species, *Staphylococcus epidermidis*, *Candida* species, *Pseudomonas aeruginosa*, and *Enterobacter*. The mortality rate is high in this situation. It is felt that the cause is inadequate treatment of the original infection, although it may as well be an acquired nosocomial infection in an otherwise ill patient. Management includes physiologic support, antibiotic therapy, and intervention to control the source of infection. These patients require careful search for drainable collections and culture-directed antibiotic therapy. Localized collections should be drained percutaneously or surgically as necessary. Scheduled repeat laparotomy without demonstrated drainable collection has not been shown to improve outcome.

Suggested Readings

Bohnen JMA: Antibiotic therapy for abdominal infection. World J Surg 1998;22:152–157.

Church JM: Surgical management of anastomotic leaks and intra-abdominal sepsis. Probl Gen Surg 1992;9:634–640.

Dellinger EP: Surgical infections and choice of antibiotics. In Townsend CM, Beauchamp RD, Evers BM, Mattox KL (Eds.). Sabiston Textbook of Surgery, 16th ed. Philadelphia, WB Saunders, 2001.

Harford FJ: Sepsis. In Hicks TC, Beck DE, Opelka FG, Timmcke AE (Eds.). Complications of Colon and Rectal Surgery. Baltimore, Williams & Wilkins, 1996.

Lewis RT: Oral versus systemic antibiotic prophylaxis in elective colon surgery: A randomized study and meta-analysis send a message from the 1990s. Can J Surg 2002;45(3):173–180.

Malangoni MA: Evaluation and management of tertiary peritonitis. Am Surg 2000;66(2):157–161.

Nichols RL, Smith JW, Garcia RY, et al: Current practices of preoperative bowel preparation among North American colorectal surgeons. Clin Infect Dis 1997;24(4):609–619.

Song F, Glenny AM: Antimicrobial prophylaxis in colorectal surgery: A systematic review of randomized controlled trials. Br J Surg 1998;85:1232–1241.

87

ANASTOMOTIC LEAK AFTER COLON AND RECTAL RESECTIONS

Theodore R. Schrock, MD

■ INCIDENCE

Anastomotic leakage is an uncommon complication after elective colonic resection. It is more likely to occur after emergency resection, particularly if the colon has not been prepared or if there was peritonitis or an abscess at the time of operation. Extraperitoneal rectal anastomoses leak more often than intraperitoneal rectal or colonic anastomoses.

The incidence varies with the method of detection. Leaks are apparent clinically in 1 to 2% of patients following elective anastomosis of the colon and in 3 to 7% of patients following elective anastomosis in unprepped colon or in the presence of peritoneal infection. Subclinical leaks may be detected in an additional 5% of patients who are studied prospectively with sigmoidoscopy or contrast enema radiographs.

■ GENERAL PRINCIPLES

Management of anastomotic leak depends on its cause, size, location, effects on the patient, and the patient's general condition.

Cause

Anastomotic leaks can be the result of technical, local, or systemic factors singly or in combination. When an anastomosis leaks, the surgeon should attempt to analyze the cause. An anastomosis can dehisce because of a single major adverse factor, such as overextensive clearing of mesocolic vessels or hypoxemia from chronic pulmonary disease. In other instances, two or more lesser factors may combine to cause dehiscence; for example, diabetes and postoperative hypovolemia together may result in leakage. Recognition of underlying problems helps determine the optimal method of treating the complication. However, often the surgeon cannot be certain about the cause of the leak, particularly when the problem is technical.

Size

The size of a leak and the cleanliness of the bowel determine the extent of paracolic or pararectal fecal contamination. In general, small leaks are minor and large leaks have major consequences, although even small areas of dehiscence can have devastating effects on debilitated patients.

Location

Leakage of stool into the peritoneal cavity may be walled off by omentum, small bowel, parietal peritoneum, or other viscera. Leaks into the presacral space from the extraperitoneal rectum are not controlled by abdominal viscera because omentum and small bowel may not be in the vicinity. Also, the normal circulation of fluids in the peritoneal cavity that clears bacteria through the diaphragm may not reach the postoperative pelvis, and small leaks can be serious. Bacterial clearance also is impaired when fibrinous adhesions obstruct fluid circulation in the abdomen.

Effects on the Patient

Minor leaks may be subclinical and escape detection altogether. Some subclinical leaks are found on radiologic studies as part of a research protocol or prior to further procedures, such as taking down of diverting colostomy or ileostomy. These leaks, of course, have no ill effects on the patient.

Larger leaks cause pain, fever, and leukocytosis. If host defenses fail to control leakage into the abdominal cavity, spreading peritonitis and eventually generalized peritonitis result. Large abscesses and peritonitis may cause septic shock. The clinical consequences of leakage are major factors in determining the method of management.

The Patient's General Condition

The general condition of the patient, associated diseases, disease for which colonic resection was done initially, and postoperative complications other than anastomotic leak have an important bearing on management decisions when an anastomosis dehisces. Competence of the patient's immune system is critically important; acquired immune deficiency syndrome and chemotherapy for malignancy are commonly encountered reasons for impaired immunity in urban health centers today. The ability of a patient's defenses to cope with the infection has obvious implications. Age of the patient, although it should be considered in the equation, is much less important than physical and mental condition.

■ MANAGEMENT OF MINOR LEAKS

A minor leak by definition contributes little to morbidity and is not life-threatening. Short-term fecal drainage or incidental radiologic detection of sinus tracts and abscesses is characteristic of this group. About one half of leaks from rectal anastomoses are minor, and one third of colonic anastomotic dehiscenses fit into this category.

Subclinical leaks detected by radiologic studies require no treatment. One might delay taking down a diverting stoma if a preoperative contrast study shows a small leak, but if a tiny cavity drains freely into the lumen of the bowel, usually it is obliterated in 2 to 3 weeks.

Minor leaks become apparent clinically by causing low-grade fever, pain, and leukocytosis. Minor colonic anastomotic leakage does not cause peritonitis, and the systemic response is minimal. Most leaks cause symptoms 5 to 10 days postoperatively. A search for the problem usually begins with a CT scan of the abdomen or pelvis. Water-soluble contrast material communicating with the lumen is the rule. In rare cases, a fistula travels along a drain tract or leads directly to the abdominal wound.

Symptomatic minor anastomotic leaks should be treated with antibiotics and supportive care. Sinus tracts and fecal fistulas generally close without reoperation or fecal diversion. Small abscess cavities undergo progressive obliteration over a period of 4 to 6 weeks.

Leaks from extraperitoneal rectal anastomoses usually arise in the posterior midline. Drainage of an infected collection of fluid from the presacral space through the anastomosis into the lumen is commonly blamed for this complication, although proof of this sequence is seldom found. Minor leaks from low rectal anastomoses can be treated by transanal passage of a catheter through the anastomosis into the abscess cavity or sinus tract to improve drainage and to allow irrigation of the cavity. This procedure should be done under anesthesia to fully evaluate the situation. A transanal catheter is inconvenient and uncomfortable, however, particularly if the patient is passing stools per rectum. Another option is percutaneous drainage through the buttock or perineum under computed tomographic (CT) guidance. This method carries the risk, although small, of resulting in an extrasphincteric fistula. Fortunately, most minor leaks do well without intervention.

■ MANAGEMENT OF MAJOR LEAKS

Major leaks lead to large abscesses, persistent fecal fistulas, spreading peritonitis, septic shock, and sometimes death. There is a wide spectrum of these consequences, and details of management vary according to severity. These patients have large defects in the anastomosis due to extensive necrosis, technical errors, or other unfavorable local or systemic factors. Most of the morbidity and all deaths due to anastomotic leakage occur in this group.

A major anastomotic leak produces fever, abdominal pain, leukocytosis, peritonism, abdominal mass, fecal fistula, and septic shock, or some combination of these problems. Systemic response to infection is prominent, except in patients who are too debilitated to mount a defense. Spreading peritonitis occurs if stool leaks freely into the peritoneal cavity. A mass develops if a large abscess forms. Septic shock ensues in patients with major leaks if they are not treated promptly. Pneumoscrotum is an early sign of anastomotic leak after low rectal resection, with gas presumably entering the scrotum through the raw pelvic surface. If the pelvic floor peritoneum is left open, which is the practice of most surgeons, this complication does not occur.

Anastomotic leakage in the presence of drains may not result in emergence of feces or pus through the drain tract.

It is well known that drains become walled off by fibrin that prevents communication with abdominal spaces.

Sometimes cardiovascular collapse is an early manifestation of extensive anastomosic leakage. Clearly some catastrophe has occurred, but it may not be immediately apparent whether the problem is abdominal, cardiac, or pulmonary. Prompt operation in such situations, even without proof of a leak, may be lifesaving. Less harm is inflicted by a policy of immediate reoperation than by waiting for proof of a complication that rapidly becomes difficult to control. If the patient's condition permits and there is doubt regarding the diagnosis of anastomotic leak, CT scans may be obtained.

Intravenous antibiotics and supportive care are begun immediately. Further management depends on the presence of spreading peritonitis and cardiovascular instability.

No Peritonitis, Patient Stable

Patients with major anastomotic leaks and good defense mechanisms may localize the contamination to form a large abscess with or without an external fistula. If there is no spreading peritonitis and the patient is stable, management by percutaneous drainage may be appropriate. A large abscess visible on CT scan can be drained percutaneously by the interventional radiologist under CT guidance, presuming there is a window that avoids risk of injury to other viscera. If an abscess is drained externally, a fecal fistula may be established; it can be dealt with later if it does not close.

A major anastomotic leak that spontaneously results in an external fistula invariably has an associated abscess that may not be drained adequately as the fistula forms. Interventional radiology techniques are used to explore the tract, detect and drain associated abscesses, and provide drainage close to the site of the intestinal leak (Fig. 87-1). Attentive radiologic management involves repeated fistulograms and repositioning of catheters as needed; when good systemic management is added, most patients recover.

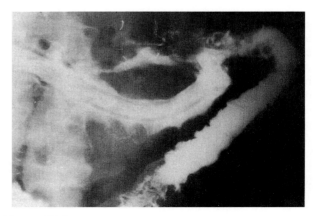

Figure 87-1
Large catheter passed through fistula tract and positioned near leaking ileocolic anastomosis following resection for Crohn's disease in 41-year-old man.

Peritonitis or Patient Unstable

With rare exceptions, the presence of spreading or generalized peritonitis, with or without septic shock, requires prompt laparotomy. Laparoscopic approaches may be used by surgeons who have the necessary skills, especially if the initial colonic resection was performed laparoscopically. Systemic antibiotics and intravenous fluid resuscitation are essential.

The goal of surgical treatment of major leaks with peritonitis or sepsis is removal of the sources of infection from the abdominal cavity. Theoretical surgical options are listed in Table 87-1. Despite the length of this list, resection of the anastomosis with an end stoma and a distal mucous fistula or Hartmann procedure is the safest option for removing the source of sepsis from the abdomen or pelvis. Persistent leakage through the anastomotic defect and continuing contamination of the peritoneal cavity despite the presence of drains contribute to ongoing morbidity and even death.

Suture of small anastomotic defects, perhaps with proximal diversion, is tempting at times, but may not be the best alternative. Proteolytic enzymes in the colonic wall soften the tissues so that new sutures will not hold. Attempts to close a defect may only enlarge it as the sutures cut through.

Proximal diversion alone should be discouraged. A transverse colostomy, cecostomy, or ileostomy leaves a column of stool from that point to the site of leakage, and stool can continue to leak into the peritoneal cavity. If a leak is large enough to cause septic shock or spreading peritonitis, it must be excluded from the abdomen. A leaking colorectal anastomosis should not be treated by division of the remaining left colon to form a left-sided colostomy because that risks interruption of the blood supply to the colon distally from the colostomy down to the anastomosis.

Another undesirable option is exteriorization of the leaking segment, a tempting alternative if the bowel is sufficiently mobile to reach the abdominal wall. Exteriorization leaves the patient with a bulky colostomy that is difficult to manage. Further, if the leak is not precisely on the antimesocolic border, stool can leak into the subcutaneous tissues and cause devastating infection. It is better to resect a leaking anastomosis than to exteriorize it as a loop.

Resection of the anastomosis, or simply taking it apart in the case of a low rectal anastomosis, is the most widely applicable method of management. Attempts to reanastomose the bowel in these circumstances face a high chance of failure. The proximal end is used to form an end-ileostomy or colostomy, and the distal end is oversewn or exteriorized as a mucous fistula, depending on location. Occasionally, it is impossible to close the distal rectal stump in a very low anastomosis; transanal drains through the open end of rectum may lead to stricture and closure of the rectal stump.

■ SUBSEQUENT MANAGEMENT

Patients who recover and have a stoma or develop a tight anastomotic stricture need definitive surgical reconstruction after a minimum of 3 months. These operations can be difficult. In patients with a rectal stump, the intraluminal stapling device or the dilators that accompany this device can be passed transanally to help identify the distal bowel. It is usually unnecessary to dissect out the rectal stump fully in order to do an end-to-end anastomosis. Fistulas associated with persistent abscesses deep in the pelvis can be very difficult problems. Some can be managed by endoanal anastomosis, and a few are impossible to reconstruct with the hope of good anorectal function. The

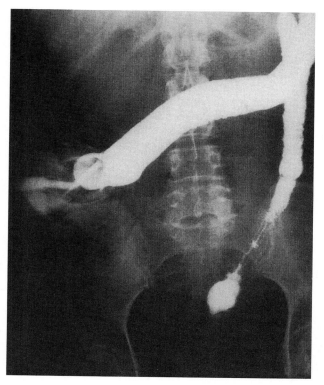

Figure 87-2
Barium x-ray study via transverse colostomy in 50-year-old woman showing complete obstruction at strictured colorectal anastomosis. Anastomotic leakage after anterior resection for rectal carcinoma led to fecal fistula, which healed.

Table 87-1 Operative Management of Major Anastomotic Leaks
External drainage
Suture defect
Suture defect with proximal diversion
Proximal diversion
Proximal diversion with drainage
Exteriorize leaking segment
Resect anastomosis with reanastomosis
Resect anastomosis with end stoma and mucous fistula or Hartmann's pouch

patient in this situation can be left with a Hartmann operation, or the rectal stump can be excised, depending on the original problem, the patient's condition, and other factors. Restoration of continuity after diversion and construction of a mucous fistula is fairly straightforward.

Anastomotic stricture can develop if a major leak is not managed by resection (Fig. 87-2). Strictures result from fibrosis as the associated abscess cavity heals. Minor strictures, particularly in the rectum, can be dilated transanally. Resection may be needed for tight strictures. In some cases with a very distal stricture, the rectum cannot be salvaged.

■ OUTCOME

Anastomotic leakage prolongs hospital stay and causes much morbidity. Approximately 10% of colonic anastomotic leaks are fatal, a lower mortality rate than 2 decades ago, probably because of improved perioperative management.

Suggested Readings

Ambrosetti P, Robert J, Mathey P, et al: Left-sided colon and colorectal anastomoses: Doppler ultrasound evaluation of 200 consecutive elective cases. Int J Colorectal Dis 1994;9:211–214.

Averbach AM, Chang D, Koslowe P, et al: Anastomotic leak after double-stapled low colorectal resection. Dis Colon Rectum 1996;39:780–787.

Bruce J, Krukowski ZH, Al-Khairy G, et al: Systematic review of the definition and measurement of anastomotic leak after gastrointestinal surgery. Br J Surg 2001;88:1157–1168.

Dehni N, Schlegel RD, Cunningham C, et al: Influence of a defunctioning stoma on leakage rates after low colorectal anastomosis and colonic J pouch–anal anastomosis. Br J Surg 1998;85:1114–1117.

Golub R, Golub RW, Cantu RJ, et al: A multivariate analysis of factors contributing to leakage of intestinal anastomoses. J Am Coll Surg 1997;184:364.

Hirsch CJ, Gingold BS, Wallack MK: Avoidance of anastomotic complications in low anterior resection of the rectum. Dis Colon Rectum 1997;40:42–46.

Jex RK, Van Heerden JA, Wolff BG, et al: Gastrointestinal anastomoses. Factors affecting early complications. Ann Surg 1987;206:138–141.

Karanja ND, Corder AP, Bearn P, et al: Leakage from stapled low anastomosis after total mesorectal excision for carcinoma of the rectum. Br J Surg 1994;81:1224–1226.

Moore JW, Chapius PH, Bokey EL: Morbidity and mortality after single- and double-stapled colorectal anstomoses in patients with carcinoma of the rectum. Aust NZ J Surg 1996;66:820–823.

Sagar PM, Hartley MN, Macfie J, et al: Randomized trial of pelvic drainage after rectal resection. Dis Colon Rectum 1995;38:254–258.

Schrock TR, Deveney CW, Dunphy JE: Factors contributing to leakage of colonic anastomoses. Ann Surg 1973;177:513–518.

Vignali A, Fazio VW, Lavery IC, et al: Factors associated with the occurrence of leaks in stapled rectal anastomoses: A review of 1,014 patients. J Am Coll Surg 1997;185:105–113.

88

COMPLICATIONS OF COLONOSCOPY

Graham L. Newstead, MBBS, FRACS, FRCS
(Eng), FACS, FASCRS, FACP (Hon) (GBI),
FRSM (Hon)

The most common serious complications of colonoscopy are perforation and hemorrhage. Death is extremely rare. Most complications can be prevented by careful technique, dependent upon supervised training; acquisition of cognitive skills; and maintenance of those skills by continuing experience.

■ RANGE

A variety of complications other than those of a more technical nature may be encountered (Table 88-1).

Preparation
Imperfect bowel preparation due to failure by the patient to complete the preparation, vomiting during the preparation, severe constipation, or incomplete obstruction may make it impossible to complete the examination. Dehydration and electrolyte imbalance, particularly in the elderly with compromised cardiac status, may occur. Use of an oral osmotic agent without adequate oral fluid supplementation may reduce intracellular potassium and cause significant fluid depletion, resulting in arrhythmia on induction of sedation or general anesthetic. Diabetics will need special attention, anticoagulants may need reversal, and aspirin (and related products) should normally be ceased well in advance of planned therapeutic colonoscopy. Glutaraldehyde may cause colitis if the instrument is not properly rinsed.

Procedure
The incidence of bacteremia is reported as low as 1% and as high as 20%. Antibacterial prophylaxis should be considered in patients with cardiac valvular disease or implanted prostheses, those with immune depression, cirrhosis, or ascites, and patients with known intra-abdominal infection. Septicemia is rare but may occur, with endotoxemia being reported in 10% of patients. Insufflation of air, increased abdominal pressure during the procedure, and the presence of a hiatal hernia all contribute to the risk of regurgitation and potential aspiration, particularly if the cough reflex is suppressed under sedation. The use of mannitol as an osmotic agent producing hydrogen by bacterial action on the disaccha-

ride causes a significant risk of explosion during therapeutic endoscopy. Use of inert osmotic agents has significantly reduced this risk. Mechanical failure of the instrument, light source, or accessories poses potential hazards, which can mostly be avoided by the provision of stand-by equipment. Missed polyp rates vary, depending on the subspecialty and experience of the endoscopist. This may include even a small percentage of missed cancer. This risk may also be worthwhile to emphasize at the time of consent.

Sedation
The use of pulse oximetry will allow early recognition of hypoxia due to oversedation. Appropriate equipment must be available to deal with an arrhythmia or respiratory or cardiac arrest. Supportive equipment should include an electrocardiograph machine, a defibrillator, endotracheal intubation equipment, oxygen supply, and suction apparatus with appropriate pharmacologic agents to reverse narcotics and treat cardiac arrest. The presence of a pacemaker should be noted when considering the use of diathermy equipment. It may merit turning the pacemakers off during the procedure and turning them on right after the procedure. Conversely, the presence of significant circular muscle hypertrophy, creating a tortuous lumen or colonic redundancy, will often require a greater level of intravenous sedation to diminish pain.

Postprocedure Complications
Vasovagal episodes will usually be avoided if a proper period of observation and gradual mobilization are observed. Oral replacement of fluids following recovery from sedation will assist, and an escort should accompany the patient on discharge. Gas trapping and abdominal bloating resulting in abdominal discomfort occur regularly, particularly in the presence of significant irritable bowel spasm or in patients with a narrow tortuous sigmoid colon associated with muscle thickening. Limited but adequate air insufflation during the procedure and careful aspiration of insufflated air on gradual withdrawal of the colonoscope will help avoid this problem. The recolonization of colonic flora is a process that will normally take a few days but can, on occasion, extend to a week or two. Spicy and irritating foods should be avoided, and colonized yogurt may be of benefit.

■ TECHNICAL PROBLEMS

Inability to Complete the Procedure
A fine balance between the ability to complete assessment to the cecum with surety and ensuring safety while doing so is required. Supervision during training is therefore essential, as is certainty in the recognition of cecal intubation. As experience increases, the safe completion rate should rise. The need for mucosal slide should diminish in favor of luminal view. Failure to complete the procedure will always be a factor, some of the causes being extreme redundancy, intense sigmoid circular muscle hypertrophy,

Table 88-1 Nontechnical Complications of Colonoscopy

Preparation
    Incomplete
    Dehydration
    Electrolyte imbalance
    Mechanical obstruction
    Medical: diabetes
    Colitis: glutaraldehyde
Procedure
    Bacteremia and septicemia
    Aspiration
    Explosion
    Mechanical failure
    Missed polyp rates
Sedation
    Oversedation and undersedation
    Arrhythmia; respiratory and cardiac arrest
Postprocedure
    Vasovagal
    Gas trapping
    Diarrhea

fixed angulation points, and problems of sedation or of a medical nature.

Colonoscope Entrapment

Failure to be able to progress or withdraw the colonoscope may occur when a volvulus is created by instrumental looping in the unfixed cecum, the redundant sigmoid, and in the small intestine. Gentle instrumental manipulation should be carried out using derotation techniques under radiologic control. Forcible extraction of the instrument should not be attempted. It may be necessary to transfer the patient with the colonoscope in situ to a facility with the availability of screening. Reported cases of entrapment of the colonoscope in both inguinal and incisional hernias should also be dealt with in a like manner but will include the application of gentle pushing.

Stomal Intubation

Before passage of a colonoscope through a colostomy (or ileostomy), clinical assessment, including careful digital examination, should be carried out to exclude the presence of a parastomal hernia. Forcible introduction of the instrument into a stoma that is redundant within the subcutaneous layer may fail to identify the lumen as the stoma passes through the abdominal muscular wall, creating the potential for mural damage. Usage of a pediatric colonoscope may help in these circumstances.

■ MAJOR INJURIES

Perforation and thermal injury (and occasionally a combination of both) are the significant potential injuries about which patients undergoing colonoscopy should be made aware by informed consent for the procedure. Some common mechanisms are demonstrated in Figure 88-1.

Most series report a perforation rate of around 0.1%. A greater incidence occurred during the early days of diagnostic colonoscopy when those who are now teaching colonoscopy were learning themselves. The original instruments were stiff and unforgiving, of wide diameter, and with a relatively poor view through an eyepiece delivering a poor image. The advents of flexible instruments, video imaging, and training programs have greatly diminished the risk of perforation during diagnostic colonoscopy.

The improvement reported in published series should not diminish the care required at all times and particularly during difficult colonoscopies. However, perforation and transmural burns are more likely to be encountered occasionally, owing to the nature of the procedure and the potential for thermal injury. This problem is not confined to large or difficult polyps. Once again, experience is particularly important.

Despite large published series, the majority of perforations probably remain unreported. Figures provided by the Federal Department of Health in Australia indicate that only 2% of colonoscopy practitioners perform more than 500 procedures each year. Of significance, 50% perform less than 20 colonoscopies per year. This lack of

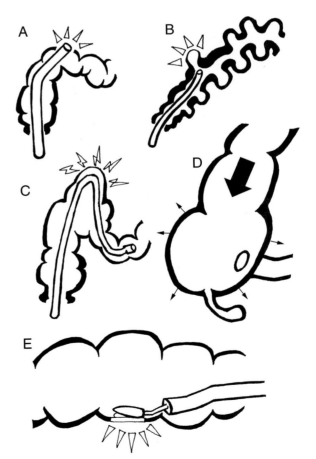

Figure 88-1
Common mechanisms of perforation are mechanical (*A, B, C*), barotrauma (*D*), and thermal (*E*).

experience might be presumed to be relevant in the risk of complications. The overall incidence of hemorrhage following polypectomy is likewise unknown but, again, in published series is around 2%. Death is rare and may be related to underlying medical conditions rather than the colonoscopy itself but should certainly be included when compiling audit. The management of perforations is summarized in Figure 88-2.

Mechanical Perforation

Mechanical perforation most frequently occurs in the segment between the distal descending colon and the proximal rectum. Continuing to apply significant pressure to the colonoscope while experiencing difficulty negotiating the junction of the descending and sigmoid colons may result in overstretching of the sigmoid wall. This stretching will usually result in a longitudinal split. As the tip of the instrument is already more proximal than the damaged segment, the colonoscopy will frequently be completed and the defect not recognized until the withdrawal phase of the examination (see Fig. 88-1C). Direct pressure with the tip of the instrument may occur anywhere in the colon, made more hazardous by a persistence of attempted mucosal slide without luminal vision (see Fig. 88-1A). Visualization of intraperitoneal fat and intestine should result in careful but immediate withdrawal of the instrument and concomitant aspiration of insufflated air. Difficult sigmoid intubation due to intense circular muscle hypertrophy with consequent luminal tortuosity may cause the inadvertent passage of the tip of the colonoscope into a diverticulum and, with excessive pressure, through the tip of the diverticulum, composed only of mucosa and serosa. The diverticular orifices are often larger than the residual slitlike colonic lumen.

If there is no doubt about the colonic wall having been breached, there is little to be gained by abdominal radiologic examination. Cessation of the procedure, commencement of intravenous fluids and antibiotic cover, preparation for transfer to the operating room, and notification of the patient's relatives should occur immediately. It is inappropriate to manage such patients conservatively. The defect is often longer than expected, peritoneal soiling is minimal or absent, and laparotomy with lavage of the abdominal cavity and simple repair of the defect should provide a very good outcome. If the tear is longitudinal, transverse closure in the manner of a pyloroplasty should be considered in order to prevent stricture.

If the defect is not recognized during the procedure, then severe abdominal pain with rebound tenderness should become evident in the recovery period. Chest and abdominal radiographs should then be obtained to confirm pneumoperitoneum prior to laparotomy.

Barotrauma

Modern colonoscopic equipment is capable of delivering pressures of more than 300 mm Hg. Serosal tears, pneumatosis, and transmural rupture occur at less than 225 mm Hg. Sigmoid rupture occurs at approximately 170 mm Hg, but the cecum can tear at only 80 mm Hg owing to the law of LaPlace, with the wide cecal diameter allowing generation of a greater tension in the cecal wall (see Fig. 88-1D). A process of repeated insufflation/aspiration should be maintained as passage through each colonic segment is achieved. If aspiration is inadequate, then petechial hemorrhages may occur in the cecal mucosa. Rarely, significant pressure may cause mural damage. It is very important to recognize that the pathophysiologic

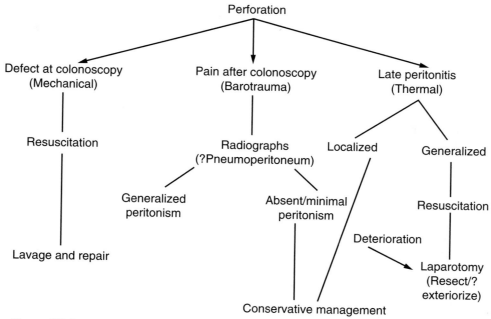

Figure 88-2
Algorithm for the management of colonic perforation.

sequence is that the serosa splits first, followed by splaying of the muscle, and then herniation of the mucosa with ultimate rupture.

Barotrauma, direct instrumental mechanical damage, and thermal injury can all produce leakage of air, which might not be associated with a major mural defect and may not require surgical intervention. Pneumoretroperitoneum, pneumomediastinum, pneumoscrotum, or asymptomatic pneumoperitoneum may all occur and cause minimal (or absent) peritonism. These patients should be managed with intravenous fluids and antibiotics, bowel rest, and observation.

Thermal Injury

Mural burns following the application of diathermy current to the base of a polyp are probably more common than currently recognized. Laparotomy for elective colectomy following recent colonoscopy with polypectomy will sometimes demonstrate the presence of an appendix epiploica or perhaps omentum sealed against the site of polypectomy. This finding does not necessarily indicate a full-thickness burn, but relates to the transmission of thermal current from within the colonic wall. The application of diathermy current is three-dimensional, and a judicious balance of coagulation and cutting currents should be determined according to the morphology of the polyp and its site (see Fig. 88-1*E*). Short bursts of current are obviously preferable to long applications. The wall of the cecum is thin and that of the sigmoid is often quite thick. Multiple tiny metaplastic polyps may be as hazardous as a large polyp with a thick stalk. It is not necessary to destroy all of a tiny polyp when using hot biopsy. A fine white collar at the base of the polyp is sufficient. A sessile polyp may need to be "tested" by trial snaring to determine whether it can be pedunculated sufficiently to remove it safely. If the head of the polyp is particularly large, then careful piecemeal removal may be appropriate. Lipomas can generally be recognized and should not be removed. The fat within the polyp is liquid at body temperature and the heat generated by diathermy may boil the oil, adding to the thermal injury.

Complete perforation due to polypectomy may occur and be recognized at the time of colonoscopy, in which case it should be treated as for mechanical injury. A ring of necrosis will be present at the site of injury, and the edges may need to be trimmed. Again, it should be possible to carry out primary repair.

Significant thermal injury will, however, usually present several days following the procedure. The pain may be localized and persistent. If there is no pneumoperitoneum and no significant sepsis, conservative management with intravenous fluids, bowel rest, and antibiotics will usually be sufficient. If the pain is of more sudden onset, producing a generalized symptomatic and objective peritonitis, then resuscitation and preparation for laparotomy are appropriate. Turbid, often purulent fluid will usually be encountered, extensive lavage is required, and if the defect is large, local resection with possible exteriorization will be necessary.

Air-Trap Injury

Perforation of the small intestine has been reported. This complication will usually occur in patients who have undergone colonic resection and who have extensive intra-abdominal adhesions. It is presumed that a closed valve effect occurs and the mechanism is therefore barotrauma.

Damage to Other Organs

Excessive stretch applied to the colonic wall, particularly the sigmoid, may result in an omental hematoma. This damage is more likely if there are adhesions or a point of fixity present. Such injuries may be asymptomatic or may result in abdominal pain without signs of peritonitis and without evidence of pneumoperitoneum. Particular care must be taken in patients on anticoagulants (which have not been reversed) and immunosuppressive agents. Hemorrhage from spleen and liver are both reported, the latter being much less common. These injuries result from excessive traction at the flexures. The phrenicocolic ligament will frequently have attachments to the lower pole of the spleen. Severe left upper quadrant pain, absence of radiologic pneumoperitoneum, local tenderness, and, of course, tachycardia with hypotension may necessitate a computed tomographic (CT) scan and possible laparotomy.

■ HEMORRHAGE

Bleeding following polypectomy (Fig. 88-3), usually by snare, may be immediate and may be seen while the

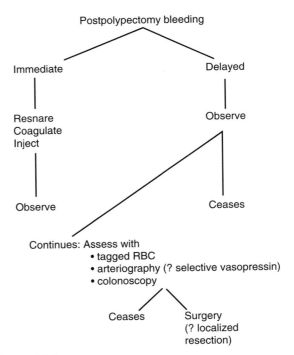

Figure 88-3
Algorithm for the management of postpolypectomy hemorrhage.

instrument is still at the site. If there is sufficient mucosal stalk, then it may be resnared and further coagulation current can be applied. When there is a large polyp with a thick stalk, it is not uncommon to encounter a large primary arterial vessel. The use of hot biopsy forceps to further coagulate the base may be possible but should be carried out with great care given the risk of transmural burn. Chasing a vessel into the submucosa is hazardous. Injection of saline containing a vasoconstricting agent may assist. Observation with the instrument in situ will usually result in cessation of the bleeding.

Delayed hemorrhage will usually present at 5 to 10 days following polypectomy. Knowledge of the site of bleeding will, of course, depend on whether one polyp or many were removed. Ninety percent of secondary hemorrhage presentations settle spontaneously with conservative management and observation. If the bleeding continues, then use of radiolabeled red blood cells may indicate the site of bleeding. Should surgery become necessary because of persistence of bleeding, then localized surgery may be carried out. If localization fails, then arteriography may be employed with consideration of vasopressin instillation by selective catheterization. Reports of the efficacy of repeat colonoscopy vary widely and probably depend upon the experience of the operator and the amount of bleeding. It may be possible to identify a site and carry out repeat local therapy, thus avoiding laparotomy.

■ PREVENTION

A prospective training program carried out under supervision which includes both diagnostic and therapeutic procedural skills and a detailed understanding of colonic anatomy, pathology, and pathophysiology are undoubtedly the major factors in diminishing the risks from colonoscopy. Maintenance of skills by sufficient experience and continuing audit are equally important. Colonoscopy should be carried out with appropriate support in a well-equipped facility that offers high standards of patient care.

Suggested Readings

Church JM: Risks and complications: Prevention and treatment. In Church JM (Ed.). Endoscopy of the Colon, Rectum, and Anus. New York, Igaku-Shoin, 1995, pp 197–213.

McRae FA, Tan KG, Williams CB: Towards safer colonoscopy: A report on the complications of 5000 diagnostic or therapeutic colonoscopies. Gut 1983;24:376–385.

Opelka F: Colonoscopic perforations. In Wexner SD, Vernava AM (Eds.). Clinical Decision Making in Colorectal Surgery. New York, Igaku-Shoin, 1995, pp 477–480.

Standards of Training Committee, ASGE: Principles of training in gastrointestinal endoscopy. Gastrointest Endosc 1992;38:743–746.

U.S. Multi-Society Task Force on Colorectal Cancer: Quality in the technical performance of colonoscopy and the continuous quality improvement process for colonoscopy: Recommendations of the U.S. Multi-Society Task Force on Colorectal Cancer. Am J Gastroenterol 2002;97:1296–1308.

89

THE MANAGEMENT OF HEMORRHAGE DURING PELVIC SURGERY

Clifford Y. Ko, MD, MS, MSHS
Marvin L. Corman, MD

The most common cause of hemorrhage during pelvic surgery is bleeding originating from the presacral venous plexus. The prevalence of this intraoperative complication is difficult to determine, but has been variously reported to be from 3 to 7%. As one would expect, the consequences are minimal if the bleeding is controlled; if not, it can be fatal. In the latter situation, the bleeding cannot be stopped by the usual techniques of hemostasis, such as electrocautery, suture ligation, or packing. To meet a presumed need, a number of other methods for establishing hemostasis have been developed.

Presacral bleeding is not specific to colon and rectal surgery, but is a potential occurrence in any pelvic operation, including spine (e.g., presacral neurectomy) and gynecologic procedures (e.g., abdominal sacral colpopexy). Familiarity with the techniques for controlling presacral hemorrhage is mandatory for any surgeon operating in the pelvis. The objective of this chapter is to review the techniques used to control presacral bleeding.

■ ANATOMY

Qinyao and colleagues advanced our understanding of presacral bleeding by performing anatomic studies on the sacrum and its related venous plexus system. They found that the sacrum may have one or more large foramina through which the sacral basivertebral veins penetrate. The veins emerge from the inner surface of the sacrum and serve to connect the internal and external vertebral venous systems, the latter of which includes the presacral venous plexus. Pertinent for the surgeon to understand is the fact that the adventitia of the basivertebral veins blend with the sacral periosteum at the opening of the foramina. Thus, dissection in the presacral space may result in the fascia being lifted off the sacrum. One can readily understand how the presacral or basivertebral veins can tear and even retract into the foramina, making hemostasis extremely difficult. This observation is not uncommon, as one of the most common causes of severe presacral hemorrhage is blunt, nonvisualized separation of the posterior rectal fascia propria from the presacral concavity.

■ TECHNIQUES FOR HEMOSTASIS

Once presacral bleeding is encountered, the surgeon should attempt to pack the area, remove the specimen (if possible), and obtain an adequate exposure as quickly and safely as possible. Once this is accomplished, not only should the point of bleeding be identified, but it is important to determine which veins are bleeding (e.g., the presacral venous plexus versus the basivertebral veins). This identification is necessary because the hemostatic techniques may differ, depending on which vessel is responsible.

To determine which veins are bleeding, the surgeon should perform the following maneuver. Maintain sufficient pressure with gauze or with fingers on the presacral area in order to effect hemostasis. Then the gauze is slowly rolled back or the surgeon's fingers are withdrawn until the area of bleeding is visualized. If the bleeding can be controlled by compressing the veins *adjacent* to the bleeding point, the source of hemorrhage is most likely from the presacral venous plexus. In this situation, a suture ligature or application of direct pressure to the area with gauze will usually stop the bleeding, especially if held for 10 to 15 minutes. Conversely, if the bleeding can be controlled only by pressing directly onto the bleeding point, then the source is likely to be a basivertebral vein, possibly retracted into one of the foramina. In this case, suture ligature or direct pressure is unlikely to be effective. In this circumstance special techniques are usually required to control the hemorrhage.

One well-described approach involves occluding the bleeding vessel with a thumbtack inserted into the bone. This method is probably the most efficient method for controlling presacral bleeding from a basivertebral vein. While some reports simply use stainless steel upholstery tacks that have been sterilized, a more recent study by Stolfi and coworkers demonstrates the efficacy of using a titanium occluder pin. This pin looks like a thumbtack but has monodirectional beveled grooves that reduce the possibility of the pin being dislodged. Whichever pin or tack is chosen, its application involves placing the thumbtack directly over the area of bleeding, and seating it into the bone so that the head is flush with the bony cortex. If bleeding continues, one must consider the possibility of additional sites for tack placement. Care should be taken when multiple tacks are used to avoid overlapping the heads.

Another method described for presacral hemostasis involves applying pressure over the bleeding area with a muscle fragment while indirect coagulation is delivered through the muscle. This technique involves taking a piece of muscle about 2×2 cm in size, usually from the rectus abdominis near the incision. The muscle fragment is used to maintain hemostasis instead of the surgeon's finger. After any accumulated blood is suctioned off, electrocautery is delivered to the muscle fragment until it and the underlying presacral tissue begin "boiling." Pressure on the muscle fragment is gradually decreased to ascertain if bleeding recurs. If so, the electrocoagulation is repeated. After hemostasis is achieved, the muscle is usually left in place because it tends to adhere to the presacral tissue.

The use of staples has also been suggested to control presacral bleeding. With an endoscopic stapling device designed for mesh hernia repair, titanium staples can be delivered into the sacral bone to compress the vein against the bone. This technique is probably most appropriate for bleeding from the presacral venous plexus and not from the basivertebral veins.

Two additional methods appropriate for presacral venous plexus bleeding employ the principle of pressure tamponade to the bleeding area. This method involves the application of pressure to the bleeding area through the use of either a tissue expander or a plastic bowel isolation bag filled with vaginal packing or roller gauze. Both methods have advantages over simple gauze packing of the bleeding area. First, the implant can be inflated or deflated, depending on the amount of pressure required. In addition, the expander is designed to remain in the body for an extended period. The risk of infection is, therefore, not as worrisome as when gauze is used. The bowel bag also can be filled with a varying amount of gauze as determined by the circumstances. If the procedure is an abdominal perineal resection, the bag is placed in the presacral space, and the perineal wound can be closed with the neck and strings of the bag exposed. When bleeding ceases, the gauze can be unraveled and removed through the perineum. When all the gauze is removed, the bag can then be easily extracted. Conversely, if the procedure is a low anterior resection, the bag is similarly placed in the presacral space; however, a second procedure will be required for its removal. As is the case with the implant, the plastic bag is advantageous in that it doesn't absorb blood, a concern which may give the surgeon a false sense of security. Also, the bag does not stick to the adjacent tissue and cause exacerbation of hemorrhage during its removal.

For the purposes of completeness of the discussion, the use of bone wax has been offered as another way to stop presacral bleeding. The technique involves breaking the foramen containing the bleeding vessel with a blunt instrument and then packing with bone wax. This approach is generally felt to be marginally effective.

It is important to note that ligation or embolization of the internal iliac arteries is not recommended because the bleeding is generally venous. Furthermore, ligation of bilateral internal iliac veins also will not control presacral bleeding because this maneuver will cause more blood from the obturator and gluteal veins to be directed to the injury through lateral sacral veins. In addition, the blood flow from the vertebral venous system will continue to drain into the presacral venous plexus even when the iliac veins are ligated. The surgeon should not waste precious time in attempting to perform these ineffective or even harmful exercises.

■ PREVENTION

Prevention of presacral bleeding is the key. Direct visualization of the presacral space by sharp dissection is less likely to tear the fascia and cause presacral bleeding. Using the sigmoid colon to retract the distal part of the bowel forward and dissecting laterally between the rectum and lateral walls of the pelvis should initially be undertaken to obtain a wider operative field before mobilizing the distal part of the posterior rectal wall in the deep posterior pelvic hollow. By following these steps, the surgeon should be able to identify exactly what can be divided safely, thereby minimizing the risk of producing presacral bleeding.

Suggested Readings

Cosman B, Lackides G, Fisher D, Eskenazi L: Use of tissue expander for tamponade of presacral hemorrhage. Dis Colon Rectum 1994; 37:723–726.

Hill A, Menzies-Gox N, Darzi A: Methods of controlling presacral bleeding. J Am Coll Surg 1994;178:183–184.

Khan F, Fang D, Nivatvongs S: Management of presacral bleeding during rectal resection. Surg Gynecol Obstet 1987;165:275–276.

Metzger P: Modified packing technique for control of presacral pelvic bleeding. Dis Colon Rectum 1988;31:981–982.

Nivatvongs S, Fang D: The use of thumbtacks to stop massive presacral hemorrhage. Dis Colon Rectum 1986;29:589–590.

Qinyao W, Weijin S, Youren Z, et al: New concepts in severe presacral hemorrhage during proctectomy. Arch Surg 1985;120:1013–1020.

Remzi FH, Oncel M, Fazio VW: Muscle tamponade to control presacral venous bleeding: Report of two cases. Dis Colon Rectum 2002;45(8):1109–1111.

Stolfi V, Milsom J, Lavery I, et al: Newly designed occluder pin for presacral hemorrhage. Dis Colon Rectum 1992;35:166–169.

Xu J, Lin J: Control of presacral hemorrhage with electrocautery through a muscle fragment pressed on the bleeding vein. J Am Coll Surg 1994;179:351–352.

90

UROLOGIC COMPLICATIONS OF COLORECTAL SURGERY

George K. Chow, MD
Drogo K. Montague, MD

Because of the intimate anatomic relationship of the genitourinary and enteric organs within the pelvis, urologic complications are the most common extraintestinal complications of colorectal surgery. These complications can be classified as injury to the ureter, bladder, urethra, and autonomic nervous system.

■ URETERAL INJURIES

The ureter is vulnerable to injury during colorectal surgery. Inflammation, neoplasm, previous surgery, or radiation can be the cause of marked deviation of the ureter from its normal anatomic position. The most common perioperative urology consultation requested by the colorectal service at our institution is for the placement of ureteral catheters. Ureteral catheterization aids the surgeon in both intraoperative identification of the ureter to prevent injury, and recognition of ureteral injury once it occurs.

If the ureter is inadvertently cut, the proximal and distal ends should be mobilized sufficiently to permit a tension-free anastomosis. Care should be taken not to completely strip the ureter of its investing tissue, as its blood supply is contained therein. One ureteral end is spatulated along its anterior surface, and the other end is spatulated on its posterior surface. The ends are then approximated by interrupted, full-thickness sutures of 5-0 chromic (Fig. 90-1). Before the last sutures are placed, a double J ureteral stent is positioned within the lumen. This stent permits urinary drainage from the renal pelvis to the bladder to allow anastomotic healing. The stent can be removed cystoscopically in 6 weeks. Intravenous urogram can then be performed to confirm that the injury has healed.

When the ureter is cut distally, close to the bladder, reimplantation of the ureter into the bladder is performed. The distal ureter is mobilized so that it will form a tension-free anastomosis with the bladder. The bladder is opened anteriorly, and a stab incision wide enough to admit the ureter is made through the posterolateral wall (Fig. 90-2A). The ureter is brought through the stab incision, and a submucosal tunnel is created down through

the trigone (Fig. 90-2B). The length of this tunnel, which prevents vesicoureteral reflux, should be two to three times the width of the ureter. The ureter is drawn down into the submucosal tunnel, spatulated, and sutured to the bladder with interrupted 5-0 chromic. The mucosa at the upper end of the tunnel is closed with 5-0 chromic (Fig. 90-2C and D). The anterior cystotomy incision is then in two layers, a running, full-thickness layer of 4-0 chromic followed by a second layer of interrupted 3-0 chromic.

If there is inadequate length of distal ureter to reach the bladder, a *Boari flap* may be fashioned. This anterior bladder flap is fashioned into a tube to which the ureter can be anastomosed (Fig. 90-3). Another option, the *psoas hitch*, involves suturing the bladder to the psoas muscle to try to stretch the bladder superiorly to reach the distal ureter. Additionally, a *transureteroureterostomy* can be performed. This procedure starts with a retroperitoneal tunnel being created in front of the aorta from the side of the severed ureter to the contralateral ureter (Fig. 90-4A). The injured ureter is brought through this tunnel across the midline. It is then spatulated and an end-to-side anastomosis is made with the normal ureter (Fig. 90-4B). If the ureter is

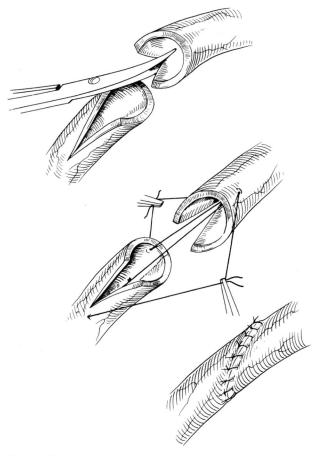

Figure 90-1
Ureteroureterostomy is performed after spatulating ureteral ends on opposing surfaces to create a wide anastomosis.

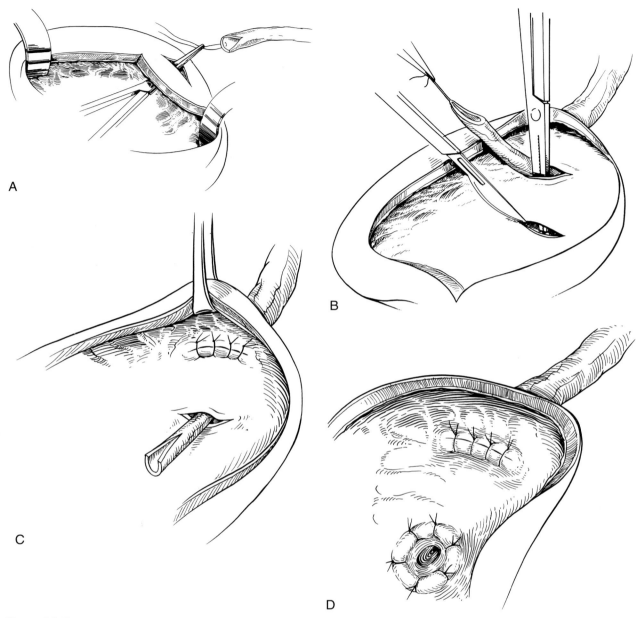

Figure 90-2

A, Ureteroneocystostomy is begun by opening the bladder anteriorly and making a stab incision for the ureter. *B,* A submucosal tunnel is created to prevent vesicoureteral reflux. *C,* The ureter is brought through the tunnel, and the mucosa at the upper end is closed. *D,* Ureteroneocystostomy is completed by anchoring the end of the ureter to the bladder wall.

severely foreshortened, an *ileal interposition* or *ileal ureter* interposition can be performed. A segment of the ileum of adequate reach is mobilized, and passed retroperitoneally through the mesocolon. The ileal segment is then anastomosed proximally to the renal pelvis and distally to the bladder. Finally, if all else fails, an *autotransplantation* of the kidney into the *iliac fossa* can be performed.

When the ureteral injury is not identified intraoperatively, the patient may develop postoperative urinary obstruction, fistula, or extravasation. Urinary obstruction,

or hydronephrosis, may be associated with flank pain or urosepsis. Diagnosis is by imaging studies such as ultrasound, computed tomographic (CT) scan, or urogram. Initial management consists of placement of a percutaneous nephrostomy tube to provide proximal drainage. Definitive repair with one of the previously discussed procedures could be performed 6 weeks later.

Ureterocutaneous fistula and urinary extravasation may present as copious drainage from the incision site. The drainage fluid can be sent for laboratory evaluation.

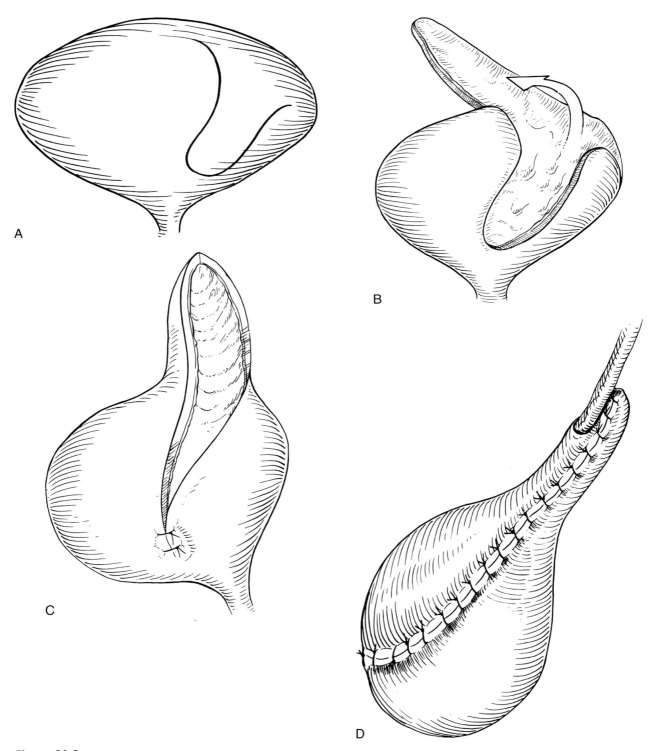

Figure 90-3
A, The creation of a Boari flap is begun by outlining an anterior bladder flap. *B*, The bladder flap is raised. *C*, Closure of the bladder is begun. *D*, The ureter is anastomosed to the upper end of the Boari flap.

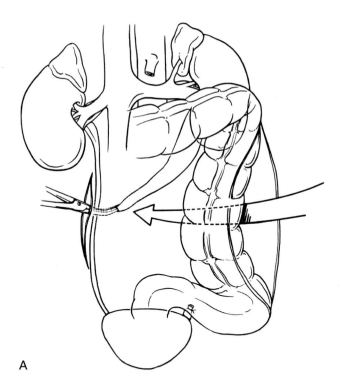

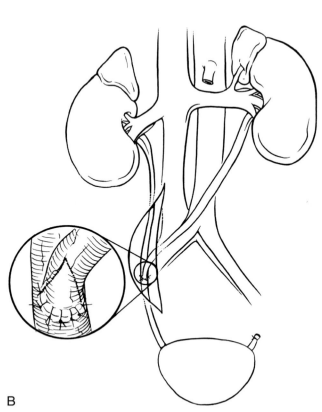

If the creatinine level is equal to that of serum creatinine, the fluid is peritoneal fluid; if the level is higher than the serum creatinine level, it is urine. To identify the fistula tract or ureteral defect, imaging studies such as retrograde pyelography or intravenous urography can be helpful. Once again, management is based on diversion of urine, either via percutaneous nephrostomy tube or indwelling ureteral stent. Definitive repair should be delayed for about 6 weeks because some fistulas spontaneously resolve with diversion of urinary flow (Fig. 90-5).

■ BLADDER INJURY

Though uncommon, the bladder can be perforated due to resection of an invasive colonic lesion or by inadvertent injury. If injury is suspected intraoperatively, the instillation of methylene blue in the bladder via Foley catheter can help localize the defect. Postoperatively, bladder perforation usually presents as extravasation or as urinary fistula. Any fluid drainage from the abdomen can be identified as urine if its creatinine level exceeds the serum

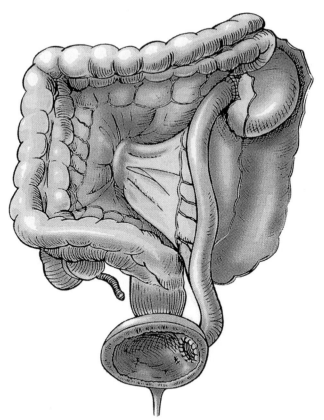

Figure 90-4
A, In transureteroureterostomy, the short ureter is brought retroperitoneally in front of the aorta to the contralateral ureter. *B*, Transureteroureterostomy is completed by making an end-to-side anastomosis with the recipient ureter.

Figure 90-5
Ileal ureter. Left colon is reflected medially to reveal transposed ileum, which is retroperitoneal and anastomosed to renal pelvis and bladder. Note the window in mesocolon for ileal mesentery.

creatinine level. In the postoperative period, diagnosis of bladder perforation can be made by cystography. Small perforations can be managed conservatively by several days of Foley catheter drainage. Larger defects require surgical repair. These repairs can be managed successfully by performing an anterior cystotomy and closing the defect from inside the bladder with a full-thickness running 4-0 chromic suture. The first layer is reinforced by a second layer of interrupted 3-0 chromic suture placed from the outside of the bladder. A Penrose drain is left in the perivesical space, and a Foley catheter is left in the bladder. Unless it is draining urine, the Penrose drain is removed on the third or fourth postoperative day, and the Foley catheter removed about 10 days after surgery.

Colovesical fistulas can result from iatrogenic injury as well as a number of colonic disease entities such as diverticulitis, inflammatory bowel disease, or neoplasm. Presenting symptoms include pneumaturia, fecaluria, and persistent urinary tract infection with enteric pathogens. Diagnosis can be made by cystogram, barium enema, and in some instances, CT scan. Another useful diagnostic technique is to have a patient drink an activated charcoal slurry, such as that used to treat drug overdoses. The appearance of charcoal in the urine indicates the presence of a colovesical fistula. Postoperative cystoscopy should be performed to identify the location of the fistula and its proximity to the ureteral orifices. Surgical management consists of resection or repair of the colonic disease and closure of the bladder as described earlier. Omentum can be mobilized to cover the repair if deemed necessary. Drainage of the perivesical space and bladder is performed as described earlier. Because of the reduction in the bladder capacity, increased urinary frequency may be noted in the early postoperative period; however, the bladder rapidly increases in size and normal voiding intervals soon reappear.

■ URETHRAL INJURY

Injuries in the urethra are not common, but when they occur, they most frequently involve the membranous urethra. The prostatic urethra is the second most commonly involved segment. Clinical manifestations of these injuries include periurethral abcess, urethroperineal fistula, and urethral stricture.

Periurethral abcesses are managed by incision and drainage. Urethroperineal fistulas, if small, can be managed by suprapubic cystostomy tube drainage. If this is inadequate, surgical repair is required. Both abdominal and perineal approaches have been described. The fistula tract is excised and a layered closure is performed with interposition of omentum or gracilis muscle flap to promote healing. Urethral stricture often results after traumatic instrumentation of the urethra or after periurethral abscesses at the membranous urethra. Dilatation of the urethral strictures almost always provides only temporary relief. The initial treatment of the urethral strictures is usually internal urethrotomy, a procedure in which an endoscopically guided knife is used to incise the stricture. If internal urethrotomy fails, urethroplasty can be performed.

■ NEURAL INJURY

Injury to the pelvic autonomic nervous system during colorectal surgery can result in chronic urinary retention, erectile dysfunction, or ejaculatory failure.

Urinary Retention

Temporary urinary retention is common following abdominal and pelvic surgery, and its etiology is often multifactorial. Prolonged bed rest, narcotic analgesia, alpha-adrenergic medication, and anticholinergic medication can contribute to postoperative urinary retention. Management consists of Foley catheter drainage for several days followed by further trials of voiding. If the patient fails repeated trials to void in the absence of any etiologic factors, the urinary retention is considered chronic, and it then presents a problem with regard to long-term management.

Chronic urinary retention in colorectal patients is usually a result of damage to the pelvic nerves. The neurologic damage can usually be documented by urodynamic evaluation or cystometry. The most common urodynamic finding in this setting is that of detrusor areflexia. This condition is characterized by atony or hypocontractility of the bladder muscle.

Chronic urinary retention is best managed initially by clean intermittent self-catheterization (CIC). In spite of their initial aversion to the idea of catheterizing themselves, most patients adapt readily to CIC. Once patients see how easily CIC is performed, they usually welcome it, because it frees them from the discomfort of an indwelling catheter. Sterile catheterization is unnecessary; clean catheterization is safe, economical, and convenient in the outpatient setting. The procedure is usually performed with a well-lubricated 12 to 14 Fr straight catheter inserted every 4 to 6 hours. Most patients develop bacteriuria whether the technique is sterile or not. Bacteriuria in CIC patients is usually asymptomatic and is not treated. If the patient develops a symptomatic urinary tract infection on CIC, short-term antibiotic therapy is given.

Neurologic impairment of bladder function in these patients is often transient and is presumably due to postoperative inflammation and edema. If bladder function is going to return, it usually does so within 6 months: if bladder function has not returned within a year, dysfunction is usually permanent. Because the patient on CIC does not have an indwelling catheter, he or she is the first to note when voiding resumes. When voiding resumes, the patient is instructed to start keeping a record of the time and amount of each voiding. In addition, the patient performs self-catheterization after each void, and records the amount of residual volume. When the patient is voiding in reasonable amounts at normal intervals and the residual volume is consistently less than 50 to 100 mL; we obtain a urine culture, and then instruct the patient to discontinue CIC.

In males over the age of 40, neural damage from colorectal surgery may complicate any pre-existing bladder outlet obstruction from benign prostatic hypertrophy. If bladder function in these men does not return to normal in a timely fashion, we recommend treatment of the prostate, either by transurethral resection or laser ablation. Medical treatment with alpha agonists, which relax the bladder neck, such as terazosin, doxazosin, or tamsulosin, may also be considered.

Erectile Dysfunction

Injury to the pelvic autonomic nerves in a male can also result in erectile dysfunction (ED), the inability to obtain and maintain an erection that is satisfactory for coitus. Because the stress of a major illness and surgery can result in psychogenic disturbance in erectile function, it is important to be able to differentiate erectile dysfunction due to psychogenic reasons from that due to pelvic nerve injury. This determination can usually be done by obtaining a detailed patient sexual history and by performing nocturnal penile tumescence studies. These studies are useful in this regard because normal men and men with psychogenic ED have normal sleep erections, whereas most men with organic ED have measurable impairment in sleep erections.

Men with psychogenic ED following colorectal surgery should be offered a trial of sex therapy. Sex therapy, a form of behavioral modification treatment for the male patient and his sexual partner, is designed to reduce performance anxiety and other stresses that promote continued dysfunction.

Male patients with organic ED following colorectal surgery also frequently have neurogenic bladder dysfunction. Once again, the neural injuries associated with these disorders are often temporary, and these patients should be given 6 months to allow their erectile function to return. If function is not returned within a year, the erectile dysfunction is likely to be permanent.

Treatment of patients with organic ED consists of oral therapy (sildenafil or vardenafil), vasoactive intracavernous pharmacotherapy, vacuum erection device (VED), or implantation of a penile prosthesis. The direct injection of vasoactive drugs into the penile corpora cavernosa bypasses the nervous system, and produces usable erections in patients with reasonable normal penile circulation. Papaverine hydrochloride, a potent vasodilator and smooth muscle relaxant, is often combined with phentolamine, an alpha-adrenergic blocking agent, for vasoactive intracavernous pharmacotherapy. Prostaglandins with smooth muscle relaxing properties are often used as well. Male patients are taught how to inject these medications through the 27-gauge needle to produce an erection each time they want to have coitus. Surprisingly, there is little discomfort from the injection, and the dose of medication is adjusted to produce an erection that lasts about an hour. Complications of intracavernous pharmacotherapy, which are infrequent, include priapism, fibrosis, hematoma, infection, and hepatic dysfunction.

An alternative to vasoactive intracavernous pharmacotherapy is the usage of a vacuum erection device (VED). The VED consists of a cylinder, a pump mechanism, and a constricting elastic band. The cylinder is placed over the flaccid penis, and the pump is used to evacuate air from the cylinder. The negative pressure resulting from the vacuum created draws blood into the penis. Sliding the elastic band off the base of the cylinder onto the base of the penis prevents blood from leaving the penis, and thus maintains penile tumescence.

A more invasive option for managing organic ED is the implantation of a penile prosthesis. Men with organic ED following pelvic surgery often maintain normal libido and penile sensation. The only sexual disability these patients have is the inability to develop enough penile rigidity for coitus. The prosthesis supplies this needed rigidity by replacing the erectile tissue in the corpora cavernosa with either an inflatable cylinder or malleable rod. Because of the permanent loss of erectile tissue in the corpora after prosthesis placement, a penile prosthesis should not be placed until it is likely that normal erectile function is not going to return. These prostheses are implanted under general or spinal anesthesia. Complications include mechanical failure, infection, and erosion.

Ejaculatory Failure

Occasionally after colorectal surgery male patients may experience ejaculatory failure instead of erectile dysfunction. These patients can obtain normal erections and experience orgasm; however, no semen is ejaculated from the penis. This dysfunction results from damage to either the lumbar sympathetic chain or to the sympathetic hypogastric plexus. In some instances, the bladder neck fails to close during ejaculation, and the semen is propelled backward into the bladder (retrograde ejaculation). In others, seminal emission is absent, and no semen is deposited into the prostatic urethra. In most instances, these abnormalities do not interfere with the ability to enjoy coitus, and a simple explanation is all the patient requires.

In young men, these abnormalities may cause problems with infertility. To differentiate between retrograde ejaculation and absence of seminal emission, a postmasturbatory urine sample is collected and checked for the presence of fructose or sperm. If sperm are found in bladder urine after orgasm, they can be recovered and used for artificial insemination of the partner. Additionally, the administration of sympathomimetic agents such as phenylpropamine, 50 mg, or ephedrine, 25 mg, 1 hour before coitus may result in the return of antegrade ejaculation in some of these patients.

91

PREVENTION AND TREATMENT OF COMPLICATIONS OF LAPAROSCOPIC INTESTINAL SURGERY

Thomas E. Read, MD, FACS, FASCRS
James W. Fleshman, MD

Laparoscopic intestinal surgery is more complex and technically demanding than other common laparoscopic procedures performed by general surgeons (e.g., cholecystectomy, appendectomy, herniorrhaphy, fundoplication). The need to accurately identify the site of intraluminal lesions, mobilize long segments of bowel, control and divide mesenteric vessels, extract a large specimen, and create an anastomosis requires advanced laparoscopic skills. The laparoscopic intestinal surgeon must be able to operate from multiple viewpoints, recognize anatomy from unfamiliar aspects, and be proficient with complex laparoscopic instruments. Several studies have demonstrated a learning curve for laparoscopic intestinal surgery. Surgeons who perform higher volumes of such cases have lower complication rates.

Complications of laparoscopic intestinal surgery can be divided into two broad categories: complications related to laparoscopy in general; and those specifically related to intestinal operations. Laparoscopic complications include those related to needle or trocar placement, peritoneal insufflation, hypercarbia, deep venous thrombosis, the use of electrocautery in an enclosed spaced, and trocar site hernias. Complications of intestinal operations include those related to obtaining exposure, patient positioning, identifying intraluminal lesions, bowel manipulation and mobilization, dissection of the mesentery, removal of the specimen, reestablishing bowel continuity, and avoiding dissemination of tumor cells in the peritoneal cavity. A summary of key points that may help avoid intraoperative complications is provided in Table 91-1.

■ COMPLICATIONS OF LAPAROSCOPY

Absolute contraindications to laparoscopic surgery today are very few. The inability to tolerate general anesthesia or laparotomy is the only absolute contraindication. In addition, laparoscopic techniques severely limit the ability to explore, irrigate, adequately drain, and débride the peritoneal cavity in the setting of diffuse fecal or purulent peritonitis. Prior laparotomy, obesity, pregnancy, and pulmonary disease are now considered relative contraindications. The addition of a hand-assisted approach may further limit the relative contraindications to laparoscopic colorectal surgery. Severe inflammation, adhesions, difficult mobilization, and localization of diseases may be overcome using a hand-assisted laparoscopic surgery (HALS) approach.

Peritoneal Access and Pneumoperitoneum

Veress needle insertion can be complicated by puncture of intra-abdominal or retroperitoneal viscera and by misplaced insufflation of nonperitoneal spaces. The bladder and stomach should be decompressed prior to attempting needle insertion to reduce the risk of perforating these organs. Aspiration of blood or enteric contents through the needle indicates a puncture injury of a vessel or hollow viscus. Exploration to search for the site of injury is mandatory. If the patient is stable, this exploration can be performed initially using laparoscopy. However, cases in which the extent of injury cannot be assessed accurately and cases involving injury to large retroperitoneal vessels are probably best managed by open laparotomy. Selection of Veress needle for establishment of pneumoperitoneum should be limited to patients who have had no previous abdominal operations and minimal inflammation in the area of the umbilius. Movement to an unaffected quadrant for insertion may allow Veress needle insertion, but usually an open insertion of a trocar is more appropriate.

Improper placement of the Veress needle can cause subcutaneous emphysema, or more rarely, pneumomediastinum, pneumothorax, and pneumopericardium. Subcutaneous emphysema will usually resolve over several hours postoperatively with minimal patient discomfort. However, large amounts of carbon dioxide sequestered in the subcutaneous tissues can sometimes overwhelm endogenous clearance mechanisms, resulting in hypercarbia and acidosis. Treatment requires immediate evacuation of intraperitoneal carbon dioxide and prolonged mechanical hyperventilation of the patient. If subcutaneous emphysema cannot be limited during the laparoscopic procedure by using a lower pressure pneumoperitoneum (<15 mm Hg), or a life-threatening complication of gas migration occurs, the procedure should be converted to open laparotomy or abandoned.

Carbon dioxide gas embolism is a rare but potentially fatal complication of misdirected insufflation. If large amounts of carbon dioxide are introduced into the venous circulation, a "gas lock" may form in the right atrium, leading to sudden cardiovascular collapse. Treatment involves placing the patient in the head-down, left lateral decubitus position, ventilating with 100% oxygen, and attempting to aspirate gas from the right ventricle through a central venous catheter.

The safest access procedure is the open technique using a Hasson trocar. The open technique is recommended for patients with prior laparotomies, small bowel obstruction,

---

Table 91-1 Avoiding Laparoscopic Complications: Top Ten Surgical Tips

1. For splenic flexure dissection, avoid applying excessive downward traction on the transverse and descending colon so that vessels are not torn from the splenic capsule.
2. Identify the ureters early in the procedure, during the initial phases of dissection.
3. Pick up the peritoneum with grasping instruments and pull vigorously away from the ureters before using electrocautery.
4. The mesocolic and gonadal vessels sometimes look just like the ureter, but the *ureter never branches*.
5. If the ureter cannot be located, convert the laparoscopic procedure to a conventional open procedure or a hand-assisted laparoscopic surgical (HALS) approach.
6. Extensively irrigate the abdomen with heparinized saline solution (3000 to 5000 U/L). During the operation; use a laparatomy sponge via the HALS approach or insert a 4×4 gauze pad through a 10-mm trocar to soak up the blood. Once clots are formed in the abdomen, the hemoglobin absorbs light, and the quality of the image deteriorates.
7. Always keep the full view of the exposed surface of the cutting or dissecting instrument in the center of the camera field of view.
8. In a right colectomy, the antimesenteric border of the terminal ileum is followed proximally to ensure that a volvulus of the small bowel was not caused during construction of the anastomosis.
9. The teniae on the antimesenteric surface of the transverse colon and left colon are examined for signs of torsion after a left-sided anastomosis.
10. Difficult-to-identify mesenteric vessels can be identified by transillumination, use of a HALS approach, or a Doppler device.

---

or ascites, where air-filled loops of bowel are anterior in the peritoneal cavity. Some surgeons advocate the use of direct trocar insertion without first establishing pneumoperitoneum. Although the reported complication rate is comparable to Veress needle insertion, the risks of this technique far overweigh its few benefits.

Intraperitoneal insufflation with carbon dioxide can lead to major alterations in acid-base balance and cardiopulmonary physiology. Patients with preexisting cardiopulmonary disease are particularly at risk. Hypercarbia and acidemia can lead to bradycardia and asystole. Pneumoperitoneum in excess of 20 mm Hg can impair venous return, decrease renal perfusion, and decrease cardiac output. Continuous monitoring with end-tidal capnography, low-pressure (10 to 12 mm Hg) pneumoperitoneum, and awareness of both the surgeon and anesthesiologist will minimize these risks. Because prolonged hypercarbia risks the development of cardiac arrhythmias, end-tidal carbon dioxide level greater than 60 mm Hg warrants deflation of the abdomen, hyperventilation, and monitoring until end-tidal carbon dioxide returns to less than 40 mm Hg.

Venous stasis in the lower extremities is potentially increased by the effects of intraperitoneal insufflation pressure and the reverse Trendelenburg position often utilized during laparoscopic procedures. Routine use of intermittent pneumatic compression stockings actually increases blood return to the heart above that of open procedures. Low-dose subcutaneous heparin pre- and postoperatively improves further the prophylaxis against venous thrombosis.

Electrosurgical Complications

Use of electrocautery during laparoscopic procedures can result in unrecognized injury to organs outside the field of vision of the laparoscope. This risk is magnified somewhat during laparoscopic intestinal surgery because dissection often involves a large area in the abdomen, requiring changes in port position of various instruments. Both electrocautery and ultrasonic dissection instruments can generate considerable amounts of heat, which may cause an unrecognized bowel burn that can progress to transmural perforation. Such an injury may manifest within hours or days, and usually produces ileus, peritoneal irritation, fever, and leukocytosis. Obvious intestinal perforation with peritonitis postoperatively is best managed by laparotomy. A small burn on the bowel recognized intraoperatively can be managed by suture imbrication; larger burns are best managed by segmental resection. Serious consideration should be given to open laparotomy at the time such injures are recognized.

Unrecognized energy-related bowel injuries can be minimized by keeping the entire metal surface of the instrument in the visual field when cutting or cauterizing. The best method to avoid damage to structures beyond the point of interest is to compensate for the two-dimensional vision of laparoscopy by using an angled or flexible laparoscope. These scopes are especially valuable in laparoscopic intestinal surgery, which requires multiple fields of view to allow careful dissection of vessels, segments of bowel, or pelvic structures. Reusable instruments, especially scissors, should be checked regularly for insulation defects along the instrument shaft away from the usual cutting surface. Unanticipated current release may result in intestinal damage, which will remain undetected until manifested as intraperitoneal sepsis.

■ COMPLICATIONS OF LAPAROSCOPIC INTESTINAL SURGERY

Localization of Intraluminal Lesions

Laparoscopy precludes manual palpation of a mass lesion in the bowel or liver. To avoid missing a targeted colonic lesion in the resected specimen, the optimal approach is to verify its position with a contrast enema examination preoperatively. Alternatively, a simple abdominal radiograph may be obtained at the time of colonoscopy with the tip of the scope positioned at the site of the lesion. India ink injection at the time of colonoscopy may be helpful, although the site may be missed intraoperatively if the ink is placed on the mesenteric border of the bowel or if the needle penetrates the bowel, and ink is dispersed throughout the peritoneal cavity. If a colonic lesion cannot be located at the time of laparoscopic exploration, either hand-assisted laparoscopy or intraoperative colonoscopy should be employed. Specimens should always be opened in the operating room to confirm removal of the target lesion. Preoperative computed tomographic (CT) scans are used to assess the liver in cases of malignancy. Laparoscopic ultrasound can now be used to accurately stage hepatic lesions at the time of resection of a colon primary lesion.

Positioning

Because laparoscopic intestinal surgery often requires frequent changes in position, an electric table is preferred. The patient is often placed in extremes of position to allow small bowel to fall away from the area of dissection, and thus patient slippage is a concern. A bean bag mattress can help support and fix the patient; the bean bag is attached to the table with large Velcro strips. After all exposed or bony prominences are carefully padded, arms tucked to the sides, and the bean bag wrapped around the patient's shoulders, sides, and buttocks, the bag is deflated and hardens. The table is then rotated into all the extremes of position to ensure that the patient does not slip during the operative procedure. Virtually all laparoscopic intestinal operations are performed in modified lithotomy position to allow access to the rectum, and to allow the surgeon or assistant to stand between the patient's legs.

Port Sites

A modified anchor configuration of port sites is adequate for almost all laparoscopic colon resections (Fig. 91-1). An additional right upper quadrant trocar is helpful in performing a left colectomy. This configuration allows access to all sides of the abdomen without interference. If a stoma is anticipated, one of the port sites will be placed at the preselected stoma position. Trocars are placed under direct vision, and care is taken to avoid puncturing the epigastric vessels. Although the complication of port site hernia is rare, we close all fascial wounds where trocars 10 mm or larger have been used. The simple technique of closing the inner aspect of all 10-mm trocar sites has been adequate to prevent trocar site hernia in our patients. Long-term follow-up shows that rate of hernia formation at the specimen extraction site is the same as for open incision but that trocar hernias are minimal.

Bleeding

Bleeding is one of the most common complications of laparoscopic intestinal resection. Other than the aforementioned injuries to large vessels at the time of Veress needle insertion, the major source of intra-abdominal hemorrhage associated with laparoscopic intestinal surgery is the mesenteric vessels. Various methods have been employed to approach and control mesenteric vessels. After skeletonizing the major feeder vessels at their origin, clips can be applied, and harmonic scalpel or bipolar cautery can be used as to control and divide the vessels. A pretied surgical ligature may be placed on the mesenteric stump for additional security. An alternative or more time-efficient method is to divide the mesentery using a laparoscopic linear stapler with short staple height. Although the stapler may be a more rapid method, it is also more expensive. If the surgeon loses control of a vessel, an attempt should be made to isolate the vessel and reclamp it prior to applying a clip or pretied ligature. Blind clipping or blind application of a stapler risks injury to other structures. If the vessel cannot be promptly regrasped and the area becomes obscured by blood, pressure can be applied to the area with a clamp while an

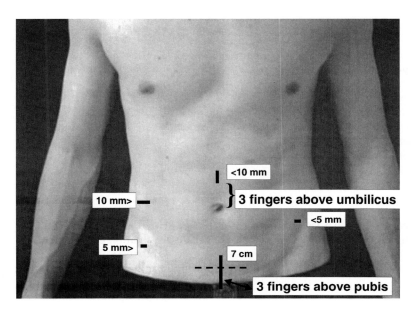

Figure 91-1
A modified configuration of port sites for almost all laparoscopic colon resections.

assistant irrigates and dries the field. If all these measures are unsuccessful, the bleeding is vigorous, or the vessel retracts into the mesentery and a hematoma forms, the patient may be best served by prompt laparotomy. A suction device with a 1-cm aspirator tip is needed to clear an area of clot and fluid during the laparoscopic intestinal resection. Hand-assisted laparoscopic techniques have the advantage that vessel control may be much easier and less adventuresome than with pure laparoscopic techniques.

During mobilization of the splenic flexure, excessive traction on the transverse and descending colon or the omentum can lacerate the splenic capsule. Care must be taken during this portion of the procedure because the lack of tactile sensation afforded by long endoscopic instruments can make it difficult to judge how much tension is being applied to tissue. Positioning the patient in steep reverse Trendelenburg position can reduce the need for traction during splenic flexure mobilization. Proceeding from lateral to medial allows the surgeon to use the avascular plane anterior to the left kidney as a guide and avoids dissection on the spleen. A medial to lateral left mesentric dissection prevents all traction on the spleen and leaves only the flimsy peritoneal attachments in the left upper quadrant after completion.

Postoperative bleeding may occur as a result of improperly secured large mesenteric vessels or bleeding from small veins. The pressure of the pneumoperitoneum may prevent small venous injuries from becoming apparent intraoperatively. Careful cautery or ultrasonic control of hepatic flexure and splenic flexure attachments will limit venous ooze postoperatively. After the pneumoperitoneum is released, the decrease in pressure may allow hemorrhage. Spontaneous cessation of bleeding from these small vessels depends on thrombus formation. For this reason, care should be taken in the postoperative period with the use of antiplatelet agents such as aspirin and ketorolac. If a patient requires reexploration for hemorrhage and is hemodynamically stable, it is reasonable to make an initial attempt at laparoscopic exploration, because it is rare to find often a definitive bleeding site.

Contamination

Contamination of the peritoneal cavity and trocar sites with enteric bacteria and tumor cells should be avoided. Mechanical and antibiotic bowel preparation should be performed in patients without evidence of bowel obstruction. The rectal lumen should be irrigated clean after induction of anesthesia if a rectal anastomosis is contemplated. Bowel should be grasped with atraumatic forceps and great care taken not to create traction injury or twist the grasper and tear the intestine. The use of steep Trendelenburg or Fowler's positions with rotation of the table to the left or right is extremely helpful to allow the small bowel to fall away from the area of dissection. This technique obviates the need for extensive and repeated grasping of the bowel. It is safest to use closed grasping clamps as retracting probes when loops of bowel being retracted are out of the field of vision during the procedure. The bowel which is to be included in the resected specimen is grasped for retraction. A plastic wound drape

at the site of specimen extraction further protects the wound from contamination.

Controversy exists over the merits of totally intracorporeal laparoscopic intestinal resection versus a laparoscopically assisted technique in which a portion of the operation (usually the resection and reanastomosis) is performed extracorporeally through a minilaparotomy or a hand-assisted approach. Despite the advances in laparoscopic instrumentation and technique which make intracorporeal anastomosis feasible, specimen removal still mandates that a small abdominal wall incision be made in most cases of intestinal resection (abdominoperineal resection being the most notable exception). When the hand-assisted technique is used, this wound is made at the beginning of the procedure so that it can be used to accommodate the surgeon's hand. Given that bowel division and reanastomosis is faster and potentially safer when performed under direct vision, we perform the vast majority of intestinal resections using a laparoscopically assisted technique. The bowel is mobilized and the mesentery is divided intracorporeally. A small incision is then made to bring the mobilized bowel out of the abdomen, where it is divided and anastomosis performed. The incision is usually placed in the midline at the umbilicus for right colectomies, and in the midline just above the pubis for left colectomies. We feel that this technique has less risk of contamination than the technique of totally intracorporeal anastomosis, with little added morbidity because a small incision is needed in either case.

The issue of trocar site implantation with malignant cells at the time of laparoscopic colectomy for carcinoma has been put to rest. Numerous anecdoctal reports exist of wound implantation in patients with both early- and late-stage carcinomas. This development most likely represents violation of surgical technique during resection with dissemination of cells by the pneumoperitoneum. A multi-institutional randomized trial of laparoscopic versus open colectomy for malignancy has been completed and shows no increase in tumor recurrences in laparoscopic cases. Every effort should be made to avoid manipulation of tumors during the course of dissection. Use plastic wound isolation drapes or laparoscopic specimen bags during specimen removal, and evacuate intraperitoneal gas and liquid via trocars rather than through open wounds. It is also presently advisable to perform laparoscopic colectomy for malignancy only after the extensive learning curve for laparoscopic colectomy has been accomplished. Surgeons must be able to perform a true cancer operation with "no touch" mobilization of the tumor-bearing segment, high vascular ligation, adequate bowel margins, adequate mesenteric resection, and complete containment of the tumor during extraction and anastomosis.

Anastomotic Torsion

A well-known complication of intestinal resection, especially right colectomy, is malrotation or torsion of one of the bowel limbs, leading to early postoperative bowel obstruction. This complication can be best prevented after a right colectomy or ileocolic resection by conscientiously closing the mesenteric defect prior to returning the bowel to the abdomen after completion of the anastomosis. It is difficult to close the mesenteric defect on the left, but it is possible to follow the teniae on the antimesenteric surface from the transverse colon to the level of transection to ensure that no twisting has occurred prior to performing the anastomosis. Returning the small intestine to its anatomic position, either overlying the left colon after a left-sided colectomy or falling into the pelvis after a right colectomy, will prevent internal herniation or volvulus around the anastomosis.

Urologic Complications

Ureteral injury is the most common urologic complication of laparoscopic colon surgery. As the indications for laparoscopic bowel resection broaden to include inflammatory conditions such as Crohn's disease and diverticulitis, great care must be taken to avoid ureteral injury. Knowledge of pelvic and retroperitoneal anatomy is essential. An avascular, areolar tissue plane separates the left and right colon from the retroperitoneal structures and should be used to guide the dissection anterior to the ureter and gonadal vessels. Identifying the ureters early in the course of the dissection, and pulling the peritoneum away from the ureter before using electrocautery will help prevent injury. In cases in which inflammation is anticipated, ureteral stents can be helpful. The stent can even be felt using laparoscopic instruments. We have found that fiberoptic stents are not as useful because the laparoscope lamp must be dimmed to appreciate them. It is possible, though difficult, to safely dissect inflamed bowel away from ureter and bladder because magnification facilitates the procedure. However, if any concern for injury exists, it is important to document that the ureter is intact by giving intravenous indigo carmine or methylene blue after the dissection is complete. The HALS approach has made this portion of the procedure much easier and much safer.

If a ureteral injury is recognized intraoperatively, it should be repaired. Urologic consultation is strongly advised. Although repair can be performed laparoscopically, given the time and expertise required, we would recommend open laparotomy. Trocar injuries to the bladder can usually be repaired primarily with prolonged catheter drainage postoperatively. The management of urine leaks discovered postoperatively is identical to that after open procedures.

■ CONCLUSION

Laparoscopic intestinal surgery can be performed safely. Complications, when they occur, should be managed using standard techniques and principles. The decision to convert the procedure to an open operation, when an intraoperative complication occurs, should depend on the severity of the complication and the skill of the surgeon. Good judgment is the surgeon's best tool.

Suggested Readings

Bennett C, Stryker S, Ferreira R, et al: The learning curve for laparoscopic colorectal surgery. Arch Surg 1997;132:41–44.

Callery M, Strasberg S, Soper N: Complications of laparoscopic general surgery. Gastro Endosc Clin North Am 1996;6(2):423–444.

Fleshman J, Nelson H, Peters W, et al: Early results of laparoscopic surgery for colorectal cancer. Retrospective analysis of 372 patients treated by Clinical Outcomes of Surgical Therapy (COST) Study Group. Dis Colon Rectum 1996;39:S53–S58.

Jager R, Wexner S (eds): Laparoscopic colorectal surgery. New York, Churchill Livingston, 1996.

Jones DB, Guo LW, Reinhard MK, et al: The impact of pneumoperitoneum on trocar site implantation of a colon cancer in a hamster model. Dis Colon Rectum 1995;38:1182–1188.

Lacy A, Garcia-Valdecasas J, Delgado S, et al: Postoperative complications of laparoscopic-assisted colectomy. Surg Endosc 1996;11:119–122.

Milsom J, Bohm B: Laparoscopic colorectal surgery. New York, Springer, 1996.

Monson J, Darzi A: Laparoscopic colorectal surgery. Oxford, Isis Medical Media, 1995.

Ramos R: Complications in laparoscopic colon surgery: Prevention and management. Semin Colon Rectal Surg 1994;5(4):239–243.

Regadas FS, Rodrigues LV, Nicodemo AM, et al: Complications in laparoscopic colorectal resection: Main types and prevention. Surg Laparosc Endosc 1998; 8(3):189–192

Schlachta CM, Mamazza J, Seshadri PA, et al: Determinants of outcomes in laparoscopic colorectal surgery: A multiple regression analysis of 416 resections. Surg Endosc 2002;14(3):258–263.

Schmidt CM, Talamini MA, Kaufman HS, et al: Laparoscopic surgery for Crohn's disease: Reasons for conversion. Ann Surg 2001;233(6):733–739 [erratum appears in Ann Surg 2001;234(2): following table of contents].

Senagore AJ, Madbouly KM, Fazio VW, et al: Advantages of laparoscopic colectomy in older patients. Arch Surg 2003;138(3):252–256.

Weeks JC, Nelson H, Gelber S, Sargent D, Schroeder C, Clinical Outcomes of Surgical Therapy (COST) Study Group: Short-term quality-of-life outcomes following laparoscopic-assisted colectomy vs. open colectomy for colon cancer: A randomized trial. JAMA 2002;287:321–328.

Winslow ER, Fleshman JW, Birnbaum EH, Brunt LM: Wound complications of laparoscopic vs open colectomy. Surg Endosc 2002;16(10):1420–1425.

Wu J, Fleshman J: Colorectal surgery. In Jones D, Wu J, Soper N (Eds.). Laparoscopic Surgery. Principles and Procedures. St. Louis, Quality Medical Publishing, 1997, pp 258–287.

92

PREVENTION AND MANAGEMENT OF STOMA COMPLICATIONS

James W. Fleshman, MD

■ PREOPERATIVE STOMA SITING

The majority of stoma complications can be prevented by preoperative stoma site marking. Preoperative stoma marking is important to avert skin and appliance problems. Selection of a stoma site is best accomplished before surgery with the patient sitting, standing, and supine while wearing clothes typical of his or her lifestyle (Fig. 92-1). This allows selection of potential sites which are visible to the patient; do not interfere with clothes, belts, bony prominences, or scars; and coincide with the apex of any fat fold. Visibility of the stoma for appliance placement should be the primary concern. A scar can be used to site the stoma if it is flat and narrow or can be flattened with reconstructive surgery. Positioning the site above the umbilicus is an option if visualization of the stoma is poor when placed below the umbilicus. If possible, the stoma should be placed within the rectus abdominis muscle sheath. This tends to give a better base for the ostomy appliance and brings the stoma more to the midline for two-handed management. Several authors have suggested, however, that the incidence of complications of hernia or prolapse may not be affected by transrectus placement of the stoma.

A properly placed stoma can improve the patient's quality of life even though the patient does not suffer recognized "surgical complications." The time spent marking a stoma preoperatively, even in an emergency, is time well spent. The patient avoids annoying inconveniences when clothing dislodges the appliance, loss of independence when poor visibility interferes with pouch changes, and occasionally disabling skin irritation when body folds prevent proper skin barrier function. Proper stoma placement also saves money because the economic cost is very high when an appliance must be changed more frequently than the expected every 4 to 7 days for a well-sited stoma.

■ CONVENTIONAL ILEOSTOMY

Altered Physiology

Output greater than 1000 mL from a mature ileostomy may result in sodium and water depletion that may eventually produce clinically significant dehydration requiring parenteral replacement of fluid and electrolytes. High ileostomy output occurs in the setting of ileus, bacterial overgrowth, gastroenteritis, radiation enteritis, partial small bowel obstruction, short bowel syndrome, Crohn's disease, and intra-abdominal abscess. The risk of dehydration in a proximal ileostomy, such as a diverting loop ileostomy for a pelvic pouch procedure, may be as high as 20%. The chronic dehydration and acid urine may lead to formation of uric acid renal calculi, which are the most common stones associated with an ileostomy. The simple addition of 4 g of $NaHCO_3$ to the diet and adequate fluid intake may prevent uric acid stone formation. The patient should become adept at tracking ostomy output and adjusting oral intake accordingly. Athletic electrolyte solutions may be used to replace losses and avoid intravenous replacement. A significant deficit in vitamin B_{12} absorption is unusual if less than 10 cm of ileum is resected. In fact, vitamin B_{12} levels have been shown to be normal even in patients with 30 to 40 cm of terminal ileum used to create a reservoir. Vitamin B_{12} levels should be checked in the first month after ileostomy construction and a replacement schedule formulated accordingly.

Peristomal skin irritation has been reported in a significant number of patients with an ileostomy (15 to 79%), and bacterial or fungal infection of the skin occurs commonly (11%). The most common stoma-related infection in the immediate postoperative period is *Candida albicans* (*Monilia*). Mycostatin powder can be sprinkled over the skin before applying a well-fitted faceplate to restore the affected skin. Coliform bacteria, bile acids, and proteolytic enzymes that attack the keratin layer of the epidermis cause odor and skin irritation if the effluent comes in contact with the skin.

Conditions which predispose to skin irritation include a flush or retracted stoma, an improperly placed stoma (near a bony promontory, through a dimpling scar, in a fold, under a belt), inadequate care of a well-made stoma (improper fitting of an appliance, infrequent appliance change), and an allergy to adhesive materials on the bag. Skin irritation is usually preventable. Proper stoma siting and construction, in conjunction with appliance maintenance, can eliminate the majority of significant skin problems in patients with an ileostomy.

Pyoderma gangrenosum (or necrotizing granulomatous ulceration of the skin) may occur around the ileostomy in patients with Crohn's disease or ulcerative colitis. It most commonly occurs in patients after colectomy who have active disease elsewhere. In the majority of these patients, pyoderma will respond to steroids with 5-aminosalicylic acid (5-ASA) or cyclosporine; however, it is sometimes necessary to remove the active disease or relocate the stoma. Intensive efforts to protect the diseased skin are also effective. Calcium alginate crystals, steroid creams, and antifungal powder applied beneath a telfa cutout all under the adhesive wafer of an appliance may allow healing. Pressure from ostomy belts should be avoided.

Ileostomy Necrosis

Ischemic necrosis of the stoma has been reported in 2.3 to 17% of patients undergoing ileostomy construction.

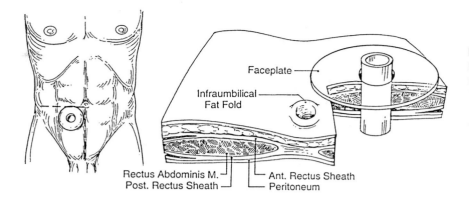

Figure 92-1
Location for ileostomy. (From Fleshman JW: Ostomies. In Hicks TC, Beck DE, Opelka FG, et al (Eds.). Complications of Colon and Rectal Surgery. Baltimore, Williams & Wilkins, 1996, pp 357–381.)

Skeletonization of the terminal ileum may be the most frequent cause of an acute problem. Ileostomy necrosis may also result when the abdominal wall is thickened by subcutaneous fat and the panniculus is very mobile, the mesentery is thickened by inflammation or fat, and the abdominal opening is inadequate.

Ileostomy necrosis should be evaluated to determine the level of necrosis. The physician can insert a small, clear test tube into the stoma and, with flashlight illumination, look for pink mucosa. A pediatric (10 mm) proctoscope gives better visualization of the stoma. If viable tissue is present above the fascial level, conservative therapy is usually possible. Good pouching techniques, dietary manipulation, and even bowel rest and total parenteral nutrition (TPN) may allow the surgeon to temporize in the unstable or immediately postoperative patient until the stoma can be revised by local exploration.

Necrosis below the level of the fascia requires immediate exploratory laparotomy. In patients with thickened mesentery due to obesity or inflammation, a loop ileostomy should be considered. This prevents skeletonization of the distal ileum and maintains adequate vasculature to the body of the stoma. A loop end-ileostomy can be constructed to provide an adequate spigot and a minimal blind pouch (Fig. 92-2). The stapled end of the ileostomy may be left below the fascia if necessary as long as the mucous fistula opening is maintained at skin level in the nonfunctional (distal) limb.

Flush Stoma

Stoma retraction occurs in as many as 15% of patients. Obesity, improper construction or siting, or tension may cause stoma retraction, while ischemic necrosis may result in a skin level stoma due to loss of bowel above the skin. If an inadequate scar forms in the everted stoma, the stoma may flatten. Recurrent Crohn's disease may also cause retraction of the ileostomy. Severe skin excoriation is the result of poor appliance adherence to a flush stoma.

Local revision to reconstruct a protruding 2.5-cm spigot is usually possible. Bidirectional seromyotomies placed 1 cm apart on the surface of the bowel from skin level upward may induce adequate scarring to prevent unfolding and retraction of the spigot (Fig. 92-3). Suspension of the cut edge of the mesentery of the ileum from the anterior abdominal wall peritoneum may prevent tension of the stoma. Use of four tripartite sutures (bowel edge, serosa at skin level, and dermal layer) or separate sutures from serosa to Scarpa's fascia around the stoma may also maintain eversion of the stoma until the normal fibrosis of healing can occur to prevent retraction. Recurrent retraction may require more drastic measures such as placing a serosal strip within the stoma or stapling the stoma in its everted position with a bladeless linear cutting stapling instrument.

Obstruction

Ileostomy obstruction within the first 6 months after construction is usually caused by a food bolus lodging behind the stoma. Small bowel obstruction occurs frequently (11%) after loop ileostomy construction for temporary diversion after pelvic pouch construction. Food bolus obstruction proximal to a new ileostomy usually responds to nasogastric decompression and a diagnostic/therapeutic water-soluble contrast stoma injection. Patients should be rehydrated intravenously and started slowly on liquid oral intake.

Late obstruction of an ileostomy is most likely caused by an adhesive band or stenosis at the stoma, food bolus obstruction, or recurrent inflammatory bowel disease. A stoma injection study using a water-soluble contrast medium is again helpful in diagnosis and may provide relief of the blockage without surgery or excessive manipulation. Stenosis due to previous ischemia or serositis at the stoma is best treated with local revision or relocation of the stoma.

Recurrent stenosis, due to scar formation after revision or resiting, may require revision of the stoma site using a square or modified elliptical opening to prevent recurrence of the stenosis. A double Z-plasty of the peristomal skin also provides excellent long-term results (Fig. 92-4).

Ileostomy Prolapse

Ileostomy prolapse is an unusual complication (6%) of a Brooke ileostomy. Prolapse is usually associated with a parastomal hernia, obesity, a stoma site outside the rectus sheath, or stoma placement in an area of previous incisions. Prolapse may be prevented by suspending the mesentery of the ileum from the abdominal wall along the cut edge of the mesentery; this is not always successful, however. A prolaps-

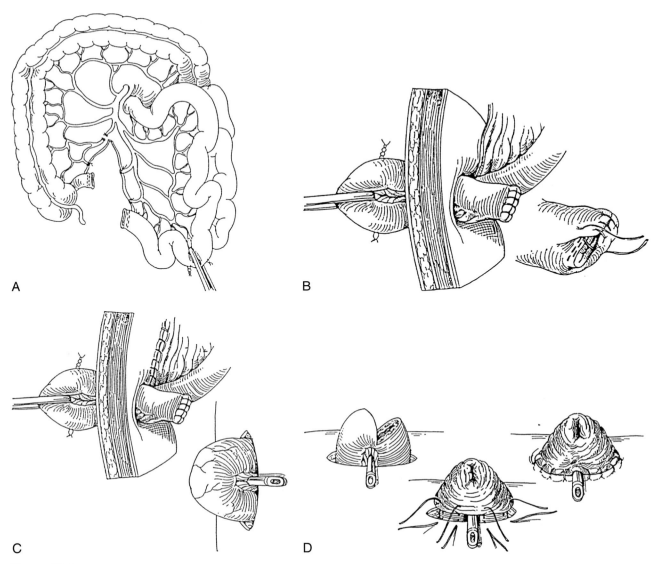

Figure 92-2
Construction of a loop end-ileostomy. *A,* A tracheostomy tape is placed around the loop of intestine, with the mesentery mobilized but completely preserved. *B,* The end of the ileum is closed. *C,* The intestine is pulled through the abdominal wall so that the functional limb will be in the inferior position, and the closed end is allowed to reside just within the abdominal cavity. *D,* The mesentery of the ileum is fixed to the abdominal wall because this is meant to be the permanent stoma.

ing ileostomy should be repaired to prevent ileostomy obstruction or ischemia and to avoid cosmetic problems.

Repair of a prolapsed ileostomy usually requires repair of the associated parastomal hernia. Local revision is rarely successful over long-term follow-up but is a reasonable first effort when trying to avoid a full exploratory laparotomy and stoma relocation. The prolapsing ileum should not be excised because the terminal ileum is extremely important physiologically. Reduction of the prolapse, repair of the abdominal wall hernia with per-

manent suture, and revision of the ostomy site to its original 1¼ inch are the major components of the local approach to this problem. The use of bidirectional seromyotomies and tripartite sutures around the ileostomy may provide adequate scarring to prevent future prolapse. Occasionally, a piece of synthetic mesh is needed to either bolster the hernia repair or induce scarring between the serosal layers of the ostomy spigot. Infection and fistula formation are the obvious major concerns with this approach.

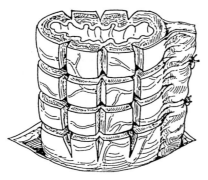

Figure 92-3
Two-directional myotomy. Incisions are made through the muscular layers, but not the mucosa, of the exteriorized ileum. The ileostomy is then fashioned as described to prevent retraction of the stoma. (From Fry RD: End ileostomy: Techniques for construction and management of complications. Semin Colon Rectal Surg 1991;2:86–92.)

The ultimate method of repair involves relocation of the stoma, suspension of the ileal mesentery from the abdominal wall, wrapping the inner aspect of the ileostomy with a strip of fascia, and primary maturation as usual.

Parastomal Hernia

Parastomal hernia is not as common after ileostomy (3%) as it is after colostomy (up to 58%). Patients with obesity, chronic obstructive pulmonary disease, and a previous repair are at risk for parastomal herniation. These patients are also at risk for abdominal hernia at sites other than at the stoma. Placement of the stoma outside the rectus muscle may increase the development of parastomal hernias, although this is controversial. Patients may complain of local pain, visceral pain, or obstruction. The hernia may prevent adequate maintenance of an appliance and result in skin irritation as the primary complaint. The symptomatic patient without physical findings is best evaluated with a computed tomographic (CT) scan of the abdominal wall.

As with prolapse, local fascial repair of the hernia to restore the abdominal wall opening to two fingerbreadths is rarely successful. Relocation of the stoma is usually needed to achieve success. Resiting to the opposite side rectus muscle can sometimes be done through the existing stoma site if adhesions are not prohibitive. However, when relocation is not possible due to body habitus or previous incisions, a permanent synthetic mesh overlay repair of the fascia closure at the existing site may be successful in nearly two thirds of patients. The cut edge of the mesh placed over the fascial repair (usually in a donut configuration) should not come in contact with the stoma. Special

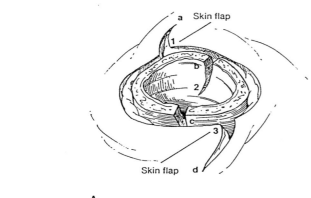

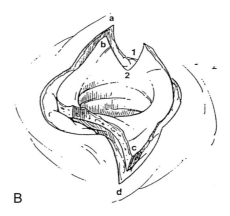

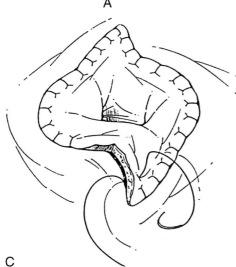

Figure 92-4
A, Skin incisions are made on opposing sides of the stoma. Corresponding incisions are made in the ileum. Skin between *a* and *1* and *d* and *3* is mobilized to create two flaps. B, Skin flaps are rotated into the grooves cut in the ileum; *b* is brought to *a*, and *1* is brought to *2*; similarly, *c* is brought to *d*. C, New mucocutaneous junction is sewn with interrupted 3-0 absorbable sutures. (From Gorfine SR, Bauer JJ, Gelent IM: Continent stomas. In MacKeigan JM, Cataldo PA (Eds.). Intestinal Stomas. Principles, Techniques and Management. St. Louis, Quality Medical Publishing, 1993, pp 154–187.)

care to avoid gross fecal contamination of the mesh is also prudent.

Inadequate Diversion

Fecal diversion after a coloanal or ileoanal anastomosis is now most commonly achieved with a loop ileostomy. However, a loop ileostomy is associated with a significant risk for complications, and surgeons who perform large numbers of pouch operations now attempt the procedure without a diverting ileostomy in selected patients. The complications associated with a loop ileostomy include obstruction, parastomal herniation, skin irritation, and retraction. Complications also occur after loop ileostomy

closure and include anastomotic leak and small bowel obstruction. These procedures carry a higher complication rate than that associated with a Brooke ileostomy. The most significant problem is inadequate diversion, which occurs in 6% of cases. This problem can be reduced by ensuring a 2.5-cm spigot and completely recessed distal limb opening of the loop ileostomy. Even so, occasionally a loop ileostomy will not accomplish the goal of completely diverting the fecal stream. In those circumstances, a divided end-loop ileostomy should provide adequate diversion (Fig. 92-5). A staple line is placed across the defunctioned end, and the antimesenteric corner of the staple line is tacked to the dermis at the inferior aspect of

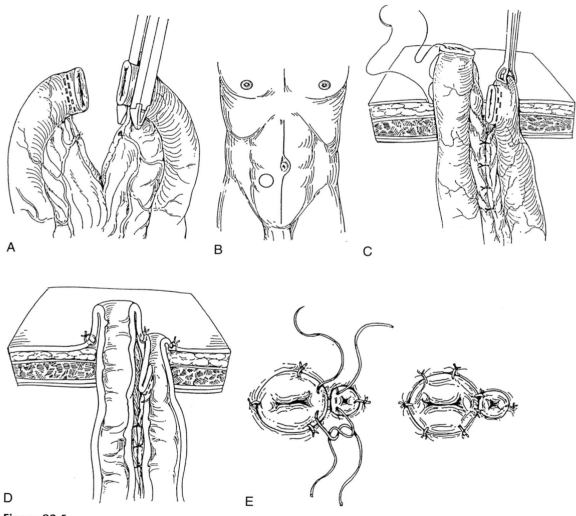

Figure 92-5
End-loop ileostomy. *A,* The ileum is divided with the linear-cutting stapler at a point where the proximal and distal limbs can be drawn through the abdominal wall without tension. *B,* The ileostomy incision is placed in the right lower quadrant overlying the rectus muscle. *C,* The divided end of the proximal ileum and the antimesenteric corner of the distal ileum are gently drawn through the opening in the rectus muscle. The mesenteric defect is closed. *D,* Sagittal view of the completed end-loop ileostomy. *E,* Two transition sutures are placed to help mature the distal "mini-stoma." (From Hicks TC, Beck DC, et al: Complications of Colon and Rectal Surgery, Baltimore, Williams & Wilkins; 1996.)

the stoma. The proximal functioning limb is matured as a Brooke ileostomy. Rotating the ileostomy to place the defunctionalized distal opening superiorly in the stoma site has not improved the diverting properties of the stoma and has caused an increase in obstruction at the stoma.

■ COLOSTOMY

Altered Physiology

A colostomy usually functions with the bowel pattern the patient experienced before the operation. A left-sided colostomy will produce solid stool. Only a right-sided colostomy produces liquid stool and a risk for dehydration. The indications for a right colostomy are extremely rare, because a well-constructed ileostomy is a much better stoma. Only in the case of impending short bowel syndrome should a right colostomy be considered.

Skin Problems

Parastomal skin irritation is less common around a colostomy (6 to 14%) than it is around an ileostomy. A colostomy producing solid stool is usually constructed as a flush stoma. A left-sided stoma which is irrigated on a daily basis will rarely have skin irritation since a degree of continence is achieved. However, liquid stool from a right-sided or transverse colostomy will cause local skin irritation because the appliance cannot achieve a water-tight seal around the flat stoma. Malpositioning of the stoma on a scar, within a crease, or near a bony prominence will also contribute to skin irritation, for a left colostomy as well as a right. The irritation of the skin is mostly minor excoriation and redness and rarely will be due to fungal or bacterial skin infection. The majority of skin problems can be managed by aggressive hygiene, enterostomal therapy consultation, and use of stoma adhesive bolstering and local antimicrobial application. A malpositioned stoma may require relocation.

Colostomy Ischemia and Gangrene

Colostomy necrosis is influenced by the same factors which predispose a patient to ileostomy necrosis: obesity, tension on the bowel, inadequate opening in the fascia, and skeletonization of the terminal portion of the bowel. Necrosis of the colostomy above the fascial level may be due to an inadequate abdominal wall opening or skeletonization of the terminal portion of the bowel. When colostomy necrosis is suspected, the level of necrosis or viability should be documented. The same techniques used to evaluate a compromised ileostomy apply to the ischemic colostomy. If the necrosis is above the fascia, a conservative approach is possible. Incision of the mucosa may confirm a submucosal/muscle blood supply. The long-term result of superficial necrosis of a colostomy is stenosis, which can be revised locally in most cases by simply excising the scarred skin and drawing the soft, pliable colon wall to the level of the skin to create a flush stoma. This procedure should not be attempted until the tissue around the stoma has become soft and nonindurated.

Ostomy necrosis which extends below the level of the fascia and is therefore intraperitoneal, should be managed by immediate re-exploration and revision of the colostomy. If the blood supply is difficult to maintain because of tension or body wall thickness, a divided loop end-colostomy may be helpful. The divided loop end-colostomy is constructed similarly to the divided loop end-ileostomy (Fig. 92-5) but without a spigot. The anti-mesenteric corner of the distal stapled end is tacked to the dermis of the stoma site at its most inferior portion and covered by the sutured mucocutaneous junction of the proximal functioning end of the colon.

Retraction

Colostomy retraction is not as clinically significant as retraction of an ileostomy. If the stoma separates from the skin and releases into the peritoneum, urgent operative intervention is required. Retraction (not complete separation) occurs in up to 10% of cases in most series. Lateral space closure does not prevent retraction of the colostomy. Revision of the stoma with fascial-level sutures as well as mucocutaneous sutures may help prevent recurrence. Complete freedom from the tension on the colon is essential and probably the most significant factor in preventing recurrence. A tension-free colostomy may require mobilization of the splenic flexure of the colon or even division of the inferior mesenteric artery and vein at their origin in the extremely obese patient.

Obstruction

Obstruction at the colostomy is most commonly due to the late formation of a paracolostomy hernia or a stenosis at the skin level. Fecal impaction behind an otherwise normal colostomy is easily treated with injection of water-soluble contrast into the stoma during fluoroscopy to control the distention of the colon. The water-soluble contrast acts as a laxative and stool softener. The patient should then be advised to take fiber and increased liquid on a daily basis. Stool softeners are sometimes useful for patients on diuretics. Cathartics and irritative laxatives on a regular basis should be avoided to preserve overall colonic function on a long-term basis.

Colostomy Prolapse

Colostomy prolapse occurs in up to 5% of cases in most reported series. Immediate postoperative colostomy prolapse may be due to improper construction. However, colostomy prolapse usually occurs in conjunction with parastomal hernia. As a result, prolapse has been shown to occur more frequently in stomas placed in the exploratory laparotomy incision. Colostomy prolapse is a frequent problem in the paraplegic population who have had a colostomy placed for decubitus ulcers, constipation, rectal prolapse, or incontinence. The best initial colostomy in paraplegic patients is an end-sigmoid colostomy. This provides a muscular portion of colon at the stoma and allows the patient to irrigate for bowel control. A high percentage of right-sided or transverse colostomies have been found to prolapse after long-term follow-up. Loop transverse colostomies typically prolapse the distal end of the colostomy, not the functioning proximal limb.

The treatment of colostomy prolapse is not urgent. Loss of blood supply to the prolapsed segment is unusual. However, colostomy prolapse causes discomfort, anxiety, and a concern for appearance. An elective procedure to excise the redundant segment and fix the colon laterally should be the initial effort. This procedure is successful in approximately one third of cases. If the prolapse recurs, resiting the stoma should be considered; eventually, colectomy with ileostomy may be necessary to achieve control of the recurring prolapse.

Stenosis

Colostomy stenosis or stricture occurs in up to 9% of patients. The scar which results from early ischemia or separation of the mucocutaneous junction is the cause of the stricture. Fortunately, it is rarely significant. The majority of patients will respond to a local excision of the scar (96%) and resiting is only rarely required. Multiple operations to revise the scarred stoma may be required (and should be attempted if necessary) before the problem resolves.

Hernia

The most common complication experienced by patients with a colostomy is a paracolostomy hernia. The risk of a colostomy hernia over the patient's lifetime can be as high as 58%. A parastomal hernia is clinically significant when the patient is unable to maintain an ostomy appliance, experiences pain in the parastomal area, or intestinal incarceration and obstruction occur. Paracolostomy hernias usually occur within the first 2 years after construction. Herniation increases with age, length of follow-up, morbid obesity, chronic pulmonary disease, and development of other abdominal wall hernias. Herniation probably does not occur more frequently when the stoma is placed outside the rectus muscle or in the incision itself. The determining factor for placement of the stoma should, therefore, be the best site for patient accessibility, visibility, and comfort when marked preoperatively.

Fortunately, only a minority of patients with a paracolostomy hernia require repair. These patients are usually operated on for psychological stress, pain, or difficulty irrigating. A relatively small group of patients require operation for incarceration or obstruction. Local repair of the paracolostomy hernia can be very successful (53%). Permanent sutures placed in the fascia to approximate the edges of the herniated fascia with or without mesh reinforcement on the anterior surface of the fascia is the simplest method. The mesh should be kept well away from the serosal surface to avoid erosion. A drain is placed in the subcutaneous space and brought out through a lateral site. It prevents a seroma collection and may reduce the risk of infection. If the local repair fails and the hernia recurs, the stoma should be resited. The lower quadrants, either the right or left, and midline at the umbilicus seem to be the best choices. However, an upper quadrant stoma should function well if it is properly constructed. The risk of recurrent hernia is affected more by the previously mentioned factors than the upper quadrant site.

Other Complications

Daily irrigation of the colostomy for bowel control is usually quite safe. Irrigation is safe in 90% of elderly patients, and continence can be achieved in 97.8% of patients. Stenosis, prolapse, bleeding, hernia, and displacement of the colostomy loop occurred in 10% of a large Italian series. Perforation of the colostomy can be avoided by using an irrigating cone rather than a red rubber catheter. Irrigant should be introduced gently and with a pressure no greater than a 3-foot column of water. Overdistention of the colon by excessive volume should be avoided. Only lukewarm water should be used because the stoma may be burned if irrigating fluid is too hot.

Perforation of the colostomy has been caused by a bone caught behind the relative stenosis of the colostomy with a subcutaneous paracolostomy abscess.

Fistula formation due to suture placement occurs occasionally. Eliminating the tacking of the serosa to the fascia can prevent the perioperative subcutaneous infection and fistula formation. A colostomy can be flush with the skin; thus, there is no advantage to placing serosal sutures to cause eversion in the majority of patients.

Suggested Readings

Brooke BN: The management of an ileostomy including its complications. Dis Colon Rectum 1993;36:512–516.

Fazio VW, Tjandra JJ: Prevention and management of ileostomy complications. J ET Nurs 1992;19:48–53.

Fleshman JW: Ostomies. In Hicks TC, Beck DE, Opelka FG, Timmcke AE (Eds.): Complications of Colon and Rectal Surgery. Baltimore, Williams & Wilkins, 1996;39:15–22.

Fleshman JW, Lewis MG: Complications and quality of life after stoma surgery: A review of 16,470 patients in the UOA data registry. Seminars in Colon and Rectal Surgery 1991;2:66–72.

Kodner IJ, Fry RD, Fleshman JW, Birnbaum EH: Colon, rectum and anus. In Schwartz SI (Ed.): Principles of Surgery, 6th ed. New York, McGraw-Hill, 1993, Chap. 26, pp 1191–1306.

Londono-Schimmer EE, Leong APK, Phillips RKS: Life table analysis of stomal complications following colostomy. Dis Colon Rectum 1994;37:916–920.

Pearl RK: Parastomal hernias. World J Surg 1989;13:569–572, 1989.

Pemberton JH: Management of conventional ileostomies. World J Sug 1988;12:203–210.

Oritz H, Sara MJ, Armendariz P, et al: Does the frequency of paracolostomy hernias depend on the position of the colostomy in the abdominal wall? Int J Colorectal Dis 1994;9:65–67.

Rubin MS, Schoetz DJ Jr, Matthews JB: Parastomal hernia: Is stoma relocation superior to fascial repair? Arch Surg 1994;129:413–419.

Tjandra JJ, Hughes LE: Parastomal pyoderma gangrenosum in inflammatory bowel disease. Dis Colon Rectum 1994;37:938–942.

Venturini M, Bertelli G, Forno G, et al: Colostomy irrigation in the elderly: Effective regardless of age. Dis Colon Rectum 1980;33:1031–1033.

93

STOMA AND WOUND CONSIDERATIONS: NURSING MANAGEMENT

Paula Erwin-Toth, MSN, RN, ET, CWOCN, CNS
Barbara J. Hocevar, BSN, RN, ET, CWOCN

Rehabilitation of the patient with a stoma or wound is the responsibility of the entire health care team. Understanding the principles and techniques of ostomy and wound management are essential for successful patient rehabilitation. As Dr. Rupert B. Turnbull, Jr. discovered in the 1950s, collaboration with an enterostomal therapy (ET) nurse can facilitate this goal.

■ PREOPERATIVE PREPARATION

Successful rehabilitation begins with initial patient interactions. The patient and family must have a thorough understanding of the surgical procedure and resultant changes. The alterations in anatomy, bowel and bladder function, pouching, and activities of daily living with a stoma should be discussed.

An essential component of preoperative preparation is the selection of the stoma site(s). Whether the stoma is to be temporary or permanent is irrelevant. A poorly sited and constructed stoma can be a nightmare for the patient with a temporary ostomy even over a relatively short time. Skin problems, pouching difficulties, and social isolation are a few of the consequences.

The best sites are usually found in the right or left lower quadrants. Patients should be evaluated while supine, sitting, and standing because the abdominal contours can significantly change with repositioning. Scars, creases, and bony prominences should be avoided. Patients with multiply scarred abdomens will particularly benefit from preoperative stoma site selection. Some patients with pendulous abdomens or those who require constant use of a wheelchair may require an upper quadrant site. The procedure for selecting and marking the stomal site is provided in Table 93-1.

Occasionally, preoperative stoma site selection for the patient undergoing a pelvic pouch procedure may be problematic. If the ideal site is located in the upper quadrant, it may be technically inadvisable to construct the stoma in this location because of the need to use a very proximal bowel loop for the stoma. A less-than-ideal lower quadrant site may have to be used with the knowledge that successful pouching may be difficult. Stomal marking for patients undergoing a continent diversion generally follow the same guidelines as for conventional stomas. However, the clinician may elect a site slightly lower on the abdomen.

■ POSTOPERATIVE MANAGEMENT

From a fitting standpoint, the ideal stoma is matured primarily and is budded. A flush, retracted, or excessively elongated stoma can pose pouching difficulties. A clear pouch with a skin barrier should be applied in the operating room. The aperture in the pouch should be approximately ⅛-inch larger than the base of the stoma. The skin should be cleansed with a nonlotion soap and dried prior to pouch application. The procedure for the application of a one-piece pouch is included in Table 93-2. If a rod is present, a flexible skin barrier should be fitted over, not under, the rod, and the pouch labeled "rod underneath" to prevent accidental dislodgement and mucosal trauma.

The pouch should be changed on the first postoperative day. The stoma, mucocutaneous junction, and peristomal skin are assessed at this time. Early and late postoperative stoma and peristomal skin complications and their management are described in Tables 93-3 and 93-4. Stomas that are retracted or flush as well as patients with a soft abdomen may benefit from a convex pouching system. Principles of fitting are highlighted in Table 93-5.

The need to minimize lengths of hospital stay provides the impetus to begin patient/family education as soon as possible. Learner readiness, considered essential for effective patient education, is not always feasible. All patients should be able to empty and manage pouch closure prior to discharge. If the patient is unable to independently change the pouch, a "significant other" is taught or home care or subacute care services are arranged. Although the pouch change procedure is generally not complex, learning can be complicated by the effects of pain medications, anesthesia, and the emotional adjustment to the stoma.

■ SPECIAL CONSIDERATIONS

Continent Ileostomy

To maintain patency of the catheter, gentle irrigation with 30 mL of normal saline every 2 hours is advisable in the immediate postoperative period. This interval can be modified based on individual patient needs. Patients with continent diversions will be discharged wearing a catheter and leg bag with a bedside drainage bag available at night. One convenient way to stabilize the catheter can be to use a stoma plate and baby bottle nipple.

Intubation instructions are conducted approximately 3 to 4 weeks after operation in the ambulatory care setting. Patients are asked to perform and repeat the demonstration and are given written instructions to reinforce the information regarding technique and frequency of intubation. The frequency of intubation is generally every 2 hours the first week and the interval is increased an hour

Table 93-1 Criterion Checklist for Stoma Site Marking

1. Explain procedure to patient.
2. Wash hands.
3. Assemble equipment at bedside.
4. Apply nonsterile gloves.
5. With patient in supine position, locate the border of the rectus muscle.
   a. Ask the patient to lift head from bed, cough, or laugh.
   b. Palpate the abdomen to identify border of rectus muscle.
6. With patient in supine position, locate possible stoma site in the following manner:
   a. Place marking disk on the abdomen within the anatomically appropriate quadrant for type of stoma.
   b. Position marking disk on area of smooth surface within quadrant, avoiding umbilicus, bony prominences (e.g., iliac crest, symphysis pubis), creases/folds, wrinkles, scars, belt line, areas of previous radiation treatment.
   c. Using water-soluble pen, mark possible stoma site with an x or circle in center opening of the marking disk.
7. Use marking disk as needed to assess initial stoma site with patient sitting, standing, and bending; relocate site if necessary to avoid creases, wrinkles, and irregular contours that become apparent with change of patient's position; mark relocated site with water-soluble pen.
8. With patient sitting and standing, determine that site is located on summit of the infraumbilical fat mound.
9. Assess patient's ability to see and reach the stoma site by asking the patient to touch the stoma site while in sitting and standing position.
10. With the patient in supine position, tattoo or indelibly mark the selected stoma site.
    a. Tattoo method (preferred method).
       (1) (Optional) Cleanse site with alcohol and allow to dry.
       (2) Drop a small amount of India ink on site.
       (3) Using sterile 25-gauge needle, puncture skin three times through drop of ink.
       (4) Spread skin.
       (5) Cleanse residual ink from skin with dry gauze followed by alcohol wipe.
       (6) If necessary, circle tattoo with indelible ink with contrasting color.
       (7) Apply a small adhesive bandage as needed.
    b. Indelible marker method.
       (1) Using indelible pen, mark preferred stoma site with an x or circle.
       (2) Cover mark with transparent film dressing.
11. Remove gloves.
12. Wipe pen and marking disk with alcohol wipes.
13. Discard waste in appropriate container.
14. Wash hands.
15. Document in progress notes.

per week up to every 4 to 5 hours. Patients may elect to maintain constant drainage at night or set an alarm to awaken them. It is important for patients to prevent overdistention of the pouch. All patients with stomas, but especially those with continent diversions, should be urged to wear a medical identification tag to alert emergency care personnel to their medical status.

Detailed written information regarding pouch and wound care procedures, frequency of change, specific ordering information for supplies (including names and stock numbers), and source of supply should be provided. Dietary guidelines and other information relating to activities of daily living are also included (Table 93-6). Patients need to order their pouching supplies prior to or immediately upon discharge because minimal equipment will be sent home with them. A listing of patient resources should be made available.

■ WOUND MANAGEMENT

A patient who experiences a fistula, mucocutaneous separation, parastomal ulcer, or complex abdominal/perineal wounds will benefit from the advances in wound management made in recent years.

The goals in managing most types of wounds are the same: removal of necrotic tissue; prevention and elimination or control of infection; absorption of exudate; maintenance of a moist wound environment; protection of the wound from trauma; and protection of the skin around the wound. When a draining wound or fistula is present, creative combinations of pouching and wound care products can result in cost-effective, comfortable systems. Patients with these complex conditions will benefit from the expertise of an ET nurse.

Wound care dressings can be categorized as transparent adhesive films, hydrocolloids, hydrogels, exudate absorbers, foams, antimicrobials, lubricating sprays or emollients, and nonadherent and gauze dressings. Appropriate use of these products can promote healing and enhance patient comfort (Table 93-7). Adjunctive technology, such as negative-pressure wound closure, may prove useful in promoting healing of wounds and improve control of drainage in selected patients.

■ POSTDISCHARGE FOLLOW-UP

Patients returning for postdischarge care should have a thorough examination and evaluation of stoma, wound, skin, and management methods. Remeasurement and refitting of the pouching system, modification of wound care regimen, and treatment of stoma/peristomal skin problems should be done (see Tables 93-3, 93-4, and 93-5). Recommendations for basic ostomy and wound care supplies, which the surgeon should have available in the office, are given (Table 93-8).

■ COLOSTOMY STIMULATION AND IRRIGATION

A patient with a sluggish bowel may benefit from colostomy stimulation. Although this procedure will not relieve a persistent ileus, it can facilitate release of flatus and stool in patients with some peristalsis. The procedure is usually performed with descending or sigmoid

Table 93-2 Procedures for Changing Pouches

HOW TO CHANGE YOUR DISPOSABLE, ONE-PIECE, CUT-TO-FIT POUCH WITH ATTACHED SKIN BARRIER	HOW TO CHANGE YOUR DISPOSABLE, TWO-PIECE POUCH WITH CUT-TO-FIT SKIN BARRIER FLANGE

1. Gather the following supplies:
   Washcloths or paper towels
   Nonoily soap (Ivory and Dial are recommended brands)
   Scissors
   Plastic bag or newspaper
   New pouch
   Accessory products
2. Prepare the new pouch.
   Trace the pattern (sized to fit within ⅛ inch of stoma) onto the cover paper of the skin barrier.
   Cut out the skin barrier; be careful not to cut through the front of the pouch.
   Remove the cover papers from the skin barrier and the adhesive surface of the pouch.
   Set the pouch aside, sticky side up.
3. Remove the worn pouch.
   Holding the pouch upright, remove the clip from the end of the pouch.
   Empty the waste from the pouch into the toilet.
   Remove the worn pouch by:
   —Applying light pressure on the skin with one hand.
   —Gently pulling the pouch from the skin with the other hand.
   Wrap the worn pouch in newspaper, or place in a plastic bag and discard.
4. Cleanse the skin around the stoma.
   Wash the area around the stoma with nonoily soap and warm water.
   Rinse the area thoroughly with warm water.
   Pat the skin dry with a washcloth or paper towel.
5. Apply the new pouch.
   Center the pouch opening over the stoma and press into place.
   Smooth the sticky surface of the pouch onto the skin.
   Hold the pouch firmly in place for a few moments.
6. Close pouch end securely.
   Fasten the pouch end securely with the clip.
	1. Gather the following supplies:
	   Washcloths or paper towels
	   Nonoily soap (Ivory and Dial are recommended brands)
	   Scissors
	   Plastic bag or newspaper
	   New pouch
	   Accessory products
	2. Prepare the new pouch.
	   Trace the pattern (sized to fit within ⅛ inch of stoma) onto the cover paper of the skin barrier flange.
	   Cut out the skin barrier flange.
	   Remove the cover papers from the skin barrier and the adhesive surface of the flange.
	   Set the skin barrier flange aside, sticky side up.
	3. Remove the worn pouch.
	   Holding the pouch upright, remove the clip from the end of the pouch.
	   Empty the waste from the pouch into the toilet.
	   Remove the worn pouch by:
	   —Applying light pressure on the skin with one hand.
	   —Gently pulling the pouch from the skin with the other hand.
	   Wrap the worn pouch in newspaper, or place in a plastic bag and discard.
	4. Cleanse the skin around the stoma.
	   Wash the area around the stoma with nonoily soap and warm water.
	   Rinse the area thoroughly with warm water.
	   Pat the skin dry with a washcloth or paper towel.
	5. Apply the prepared pouch.
	   Center the skin barrier flange opening over the stoma and press into place.
	   Smooth the sticky surface of the skin barrier flange onto the skin.
	   Snap the pouch securely onto the skin barrier flange.
	   Hold the pouch firmly in place for a few moments.
	6. Close pouch end securely.
	   Fasten the pouch end securely with the clip.

colostomies on the sixth or seventh postoperative day (Table 93-9).

A colostomy irrigation may be appropriate for patients with established descending or sigmoid colostomies. Irrigation is done to regulate bowel function, cleanse the bowel prior to procedures, or administer medications. A cone or soft catheter and baby bottle nipple should always be used when instilling solutions into the colostomy to avoid bowel perforation (Table 93-10).

■ ILEOSTOMY LAVAGE

An ileostomy (ileal) lavage may be performed as a diagnostic or therapeutic intervention for patients with sus-

pected food bolus obstruction. To facilitate the passage of the catheter and patient tolerance of the procedure, premedication with a narcotic analgesic or muscle relaxant is advisable (Table 93-11).

■ CONCLUSION

Provision of comprehensive pre- and postoperative care can maximize the probability for cost-effective and successful rehabilitation of patients with stomas or wounds. The collaboration between surgeon and ET nurse facilitates this process.

Table 93-3 Selected Stomal Complications

PROBLEM	CHARACTERISTICS	INTERVENTIONS
Early Complications		
Mucocutaneous separation	Separation of suture line at the junction of stomal mucosa and skin. Erythema around area of separation; may have pain, drainage at site. Can be partial or circumferential; shallow or deep.	Assess depth of separation: if peritoneal contamination is a concern, resuture stoma to skin. Shallow separation: use skin barrier powder to fill defect, pouch. Deep separation: gentle packing with gauze may be necessary; cover with transparent film or other dressing, pouch. If large volume of fluid is draining from separation, include area in pouch opening.

Necrosis	Mucosal color dark red to purple, or cyanotic hue; also seen as brown-black color. Stoma is dry, flaccid.	Utilize clear pouch in postoperative period to allow for ongoing mucosal assessment.
		 Assess depth of necrosis:
		    If below fascial level, reoperation with reconstruction of stoma.
		    Superficial necrosis, conservative management with tissue allowed to slough.

Parastomal abscess or fistula	Abscess area adjacent to stoma. Fistula may be present.	Systemic antibiotics. Incision and drainage of abscess site; best done with mushroom-tipped catheter. Contrast studies to define extent of fistula. Surgical intervention as needed. Modification of pouching system based upon location and extent of fistula or abscess.
Late Complications		
Food bolus obstruction	Severe, crampy abdominal pain with nausea, vomiting. Output may cease or become watery and odorous. Stomal edema common. Patient relates recent history of ingesting high-fiber foods such as peanuts, popcorn, string vegetables.	Conservative management: warm bath, peristomal massage, liquids. Supportive measures: intravenous fluid replacement, pain medications, massages, nasogastric tube. Ileal lavage (see Table 93-11)
Hernia	Hernia around stoma presents as a bulge that can interfere with pouch seal, causing mechanical or irritant dermatitis.	Use of support belt. Pouch modification to accommodate change in contour. Consider discontinuing routine colostomy irrigation. Surgical repair plus or minus relocation.
Melanosis coli	Viable stoma appears dark brown or black secondary to fecal stasis or overuse of anthracine-containing cathartics.	Recognition of condition.
Prolapse	Telescoping of the bowel through the stoma, length and diameter of mucosa increases with potential for laceration.	Conservative: reduce prolapse; apply binder with prolapse overbelt; reassess pouching system for proper aperture size. Surgical management.
Retraction	Stoma recedes below skin level, causing a variety of pouching and peristomal skin difficulties.	Refitting of pouching system usually by increasing degree of convexity. Assess for recurrent disease such as Crohn's disease. Surgical revision if pouching modifications are not successful.
Stenosis	Narrowing of the lumen of the stoma can lead to partial stomal obstruction.	Preventive measures such as an appropriate pouching system, prompt treatment of pseudoverrucous lesions, avoidance of routine dilatation of stoma. Surgical revision.
Trauma	Laceration or bruising of mucosa. Lacerations are seen as yellow to white linear marking in the mucosa.	Identify and eliminate causative factor for the trauma, e.g., correct aperture, clothing alterations.

Table 93-4 Selected Peristomal Skin Conditions

CONDITION	CHARACTERISTICS	INTERVENTIONS
Allergic contact dermatitis	Allergic response caused by patient sensitivity to a particular product. Area of response generally conforms to exposed area. Skin appears erythematous, edematous, eroded, weepy, or bleeding.	Remove offending product, avoid other irritants, protect skin. Modify pouching system as needed, possible use of nonadherent system. Patch test with other products as needed. Use of corticosteroid agents as needed.
Candidiasis	Generally diffuse erythematous papules. Often papules coalese to form a plaque with characteristic advancing border with satellite lesion. Proliferation of *Candida albicans* is fostered by warm, dark, moist environment. Severe pruritus is common.	Eliminate moisture; use pouch covers; dry tapes with blow dryer on cool setting. Assess pouching system for leakage. Apply topical antifungal preparations.
Caput medusa or peristomal varices	In patients with portal hypertension, the pressure at the portal systemic shunt in the mucocutaneous junction increases, creating venous engorgement, seen as area of bluish purple discoloration of skin around the stoma. The area blanches when pressed, displaying irregular, small blood vessels. Profuse bleeding can occur at the mucocutaneous junction. If stoma is relocated, varices eventually recur around the new stoma.	If bleeding occurs, direct pressure or use of hemostatic agents, e.g., silver nitrate, cautery, or suture ligation. Careful pouch removal. Avoid aggressive skin barriers.
Folliculitis	Inflammation of hair follicle due to traumatic removal of hair with resultant bacterial infection. Lesions arise from hair follicle and are erythematous pinpoint pustules.	Use proper pouch removal techniques. Use adhesive removers and skin sealants. Shave peristomal skin. Apply topical antibacterial powders as needed.
Irritant dermatitis	Chemical destruction of the skin is caused by pouch leakage or topical products. Skin appears red, moist, shallow with erosion and is painful.	Cover large weepy lesions with nonadherent gauze. Dust denuded area with skin barrier powder. Refit pouching system based on stoma size and abdominal contours. The abdomen is assessed in the supine and sitting positions. Review product usage and techniques. Revise as needed.
Mechanical trauma	External item or force causes damage to skin from pressure, laceration, friction, or shear. Seen as pressure ulcer, red or denuded lesions with irregular borders. Painful.	Assess equipment and pouching technique. Modify equipment and accessories to prevent reinjury. Treat denuded tissue with skin barrier powder or other topical dressing as dictated by wound characteristics.
Parastomal ulcer	Area of ulceration adjacent to stoma; varies in size, contour, level of pain. Not uncommon in patients with Crohn's disease.	Unroof ulcer as needed. Give intralesional steroid injection. Topical management depends on size: options include skin barrier powder, nonadherent gauze, hydrogel, astringent solution, hydrocolloid wafer, and foam. A nonadherent pouching system can be fashioned with a one-piece pouch with belt tabs and extra gasket. Treatment of systemic disease.
Pseudoverrucous lesions or hydration (formerly called PEH)	Overgrowth of tissue caused by overexposure to moisture. Appears as raised, moist lesions with wart-like appearance. Begin at base of stoma and extend outward. Painful. Difficulty with pouch adhesion.	Properly size aperture and convexity of pouching system. In severe cases, sharp débridement of skin or relocation of stoma may be required.
Radiation injury	Red, thinned skin. Ulceration possible. Tissue easily traumatized by removal of skin adhesives.	Gently cleanse skin with cool water. Select pouching system with easy-to-remove barrier. Cautious use of solvents or skin sealants due to frequent sensitivities.

Table 93-5 Principles of Fitting: Pouches, Stomas, and Accessories

Pouching Systems

TYPE	FEATURES AND VARIETIES
One-piece drainable, closed-end, urostomy	Flexible, semiflexible, firm, with or without skin barrier attached
	Flat and with convexity ranging from shallow to very deep; precut and cut-to-fit types
	Clear or opaque pouches, adult or pediatric sizes
	Drainable, generally odor-proof pouches
	Urostomy odor-resistant pouches
	Belt hooks or optional gasket if use of belt is desired
	Built-in gas/deodorizing filters
Two-piece system	With or without adhesive tape collar
	Precut and cut-to-fit varieties
	Flat or built-in convexity or option of convex insert
	Adult and pediatric sizes
	Pouch removable without disturbing flange
	Clear and opaque pouches
	Variety of sizes and shapes of pouches, irrigation sleeves, and stoma caps
	Belt hooks for optional belt use

Abdomen/Stoma Considerations

ABDOMINAL TYPE	STOMA TYPE	APPROPRIATE POUCH
Firm	Flush	Flat/flexible
	Retracted	
	Budded	
Soft	Flush	Semiflexible; shallow to medium convexity
	Retracted	
	Budded	Flat or semiflexible; shallow convexity
Very soft	Flush	Firm; deep to very deep convexity*
	Retracted	
	Budded	Firm; deep convexity*

Accessory Products

PRODUCT	USE
Paste	Enhances seal by filling the space between the stomal and pouch barrier edge. To apply paste, use one of the following methods (but not both): Put the paste around the edges of the skin barrier opening, and let dry for at least 1 minute before applying to the skin. Put the paste on the skin around the stoma, and let dry for at least 1 minute before applying the pouching system.
Powder	Provides an absorbent, protective layer for sore or moist skin. When using powder, be sure to dust off the excess powder so that the pouch will stick securely to the skin.
Sealant	Provides protective film surface to help prevent tearing of the skin when the sticky pouch adhesive is removed. The sealant is placed under the tape collar of the pouch.
Barrier	Protects the skin around the stoma from bowel drainage and creates a level pouching surface. Barriers are also used to treat peristomal skin loss due to injury. Barriers are available in regular and extended wear.
Pouch deodorant	Assists in controlling odor. When using pouch deodorant, it is best to place it in the lower half of an empty pouch. Oral, aerosol, and charcoal filter products are used to assist with odor management.
Belt	Provides support to the pouch at the 9 o'clock and 3 o'clock positions. They are available in several adult and pediatric sizes. Some belt brands can be used with any pouch, and other brands must be used with the pouch system of the same manufacturer.
Binders	Help hold the pouch in place. They have Velcro closures and come in widths from 3 to 9 inches. They also can be ordered with a prolapse overbelt. The binder opening that accommodates the pouch can be custom-ordered to match the location of the pouch.
Convex inserts	Provide curvature and additional support for certain two-piece pouching systems. These inserts force the pouch to have more curve to fit the abdominal contour better. The insert must be carefully sized to clear the stoma by ¼ inch (internal diameter) and to fit the skin barrier flange (external diameter). These inserts must be used with the pouch system of the same manufacturer.
Pouch covers	Control moisture between the pouch and skin. They help make the pouch less noticeable, which can enhance body image. They are available in several adult and pediatric sizes to fit various pouches.

Table 93-5 Principles of Fitting: Pouches, Stomas, and Accessories

PRODUCT	USE
Bedside drainage systems for urinary stomas	Help reduce or eliminate trips to the bathroom to empty the pouch during the night. These systems use plastic bags or bottles and have attached drainage tubing. An adapter is required to attach the urinary pouch to the drainage tubing. These drainage systems can be secured to the bed frame or placed in a plastic wastebasket on the floor.
Underwear and swimwear	Support the pouch while making it less noticeable, which can enhance body image. They are available in several sizes and styles.
Stoma guide strips	Assist patient in centering the pouch. Guide strips are inserted into the pouch opening. Because they are made of rice paper, guide strips dissolve when they come in contact with moisture.
Tapes	Secure the pouch in place. They are available from a variety of manufacturers in many sizes and types. Waterproof tapes are available for patients who participate in water sports or activities.
Solvents	Help remove the pouch and adhesive that is left on the skin between pouch changes. Most solvents are petroleum-based and are available in liquid and "wipe" forms. After using solvents, be sure to wash and rinse the skin thoroughly to prevent sore skin.

*Inappropriate use of firm convexity can result in peristomal skin necrosis.

Table 93-6 Frequently Asked Questions for Ostomy Care

When Should I Change the Pouch?

- Schedule routine pouch changes during periods of reduced stomal activity, such as before breakfast or in the evening before going to bed.
- Plan regular pouch changes every 3 to 5 days.
- Date the tape on the pouch or mark your calendar to remind you when the pouch was last changed.
- Change the pouch promptly if you experience an itching or burning sensation on the skin around the stoma; these sensations may indicate a potential leakage.

How Should I Empty the Pouch?

- "Cuff" the bottom of the pouch before emptying it so you can keep your fingers clean.
- Empty the pouch when it is ⅓ to ½ full so that the pouch won't overfill or lose its adhesive seal. The pouch will be much easier to empty. Also, a ⅓ to ½ full pouch won't be as noticeable under your clothes.
- Float toilet tissue in the toilet bowel or flush the toilet as you empty the pouch to minimize splashing.
- Clean and dry the bottom of the pouch with toilet paper before applying the closure clip.
- To rinse the pouch without removing it, use a baster, cup, or squeeze bottle to pour cool water into the drain end.
- Use wet wipes or tissues in public rest room facilities to make it easier to clean the pouch.

How Should I Care for the Stomal Area?

- The stoma and surrounding skin require the same cleanliness as the rest of the body. It is not necessary to use sterile materials to cleanse this area.
- Trim body hair around the stomal area with blunt-end scissors or an electric razor.
- Avoid using oils or ointments on the skin around your stoma. They may prevent the pouch from adhering to your skin.

Are There Any Special Bathing Recommendations?

- You may shower or bathe with the pouch on or off, although the ostomy may keep working while you're showering or bathing.
- You can replace, air dry or blow dry (with a hair dryer on a low setting) the pouch tape after showering or bathing.

How Should I Care for the Pouch During Exercise?

- Stretch underwear can be worn by both men and women to support the pouch during physical activity. Wear your pouch inside the underwear.
- Pouch covers add to your comfort and help absorb perspiration.

Will a Weight Gain or Loss Affect the Way the Pouch Fits?

- Yes. An excessive weight gain or loss (from 10 to 15 pounds) can change the fit of your pouching system or alter the wearing time of the pouching system. Be sure to contact your surgeon or enterostomal therapy nurse if weight gain or loss becomes a concern.

(Continued)

Table 93-6 Frequently Asked Questions for Ostomy Care—cont'd

Are There Any Special Traveling Recommendations?

- Always carry your ostomy supplies with you. Do not check them with your luggage in case it becomes lost, delayed, or damaged.
- Take twice the normal amount of ostomy equipment you usually need so that you are prepared for an emergency.
- Carry a list of retailers and United Ostomy Association (UOA) chapters in your travel case. They are a good resource if ostomy help is needed while traveling.
- Ask the Wound, Ostomy and Continence Nurses Society (WOCN) for a list of local enterostomal therapy nurses if you think you might need one when traveling.

What Do I Need to Know about Ordering Equipment?

- Allow enough time for delivery when ordering supplies.
- Remeasure your stoma before ordering precut pouches during the first 6 months.
- Always keep an extra 2-week supply of pouch equipment. There is no good substitution for the products if you should run out.
- Keep a list of your equipment along with the order numbers, manufacturers, and sources of supply. Give a duplicate of this list to a family member or friend in case their help is needed in an emergency.
- Check several retailers for the best equipment prices. Some suppliers will assist you with Medicare and insurance forms.
- Consider how long you wear your pouch when calculating the cost of your equipment.

Table 93-7 Selected Categories of Wound Care Dressings

TYPE	DESCRIPTION/USES
Transparent films	Elastomeric copolymers with an adhesive contact surface
	Maintain a moist wound environment
	Nonabsorptive; can be primary or secondary dressing
	Use on superficial wounds, wounds with necrosis or slough, and wounds with little or no exudate
Hydrogel	Water- or glycerin-based amorphous gels, impregnated gauze, or sheets
	Absorb minimal to moderate amounts of exudate; soothing; some require secondary dressing
	Use on partial- and full-thickness wounds, burns and tissue damaged by radiation, wounds with necrosis or slough, clean wounds
Hydrocolloid	Composed of gelatin, pectin, or carboxymethylcellulose in wafer or paste form
	Semiocclusive to occlusive
	Retain moisture
	Varying degrees of absorption
	Use on clean wounds, those with necrosis or slough, noninfected wounds, light to moderate exudate
Foam dressings	Semipermeable; provide varying degrees of absorption of exudate
	Most are nonadherent
	Can use with infected wounds
	Absorb drainage around tubes
	Use as primary dressing for absorption, secondary dressing for wounds with packing
Alginates	Material derived from brown seaweed
	Need secondary dressing
	Available in rope and sheet forms
	Forms a soft gel in wound
	Absorbs moderate to large amounts of exudate
	Use on partial- and full-thickness draining wounds, infected wounds
Exudate absorbers	Variety of products that absorb exudate, obliterate dead space, keep wound surface moist
	Most require secondary dressing
	Available in rope, powder, paste, or "pillow"
	Use on wounds with moderate to large amounts of exudate, infected exuding wounds, those with combination of exudate or necrosis
Gauze	Woven or nonwoven
	Primary or secondary dressing
	Nonadherent or adherent
	Wide range of uses
Combination dressing	Layered occlusive dressings that provide increased absorption and exudate management
Adjunctive therapy	Occlusive wound dressing with negative pressure to facilitate deposition of granulation tissue,
Negative-pressure wound closure	wound closure, and moist wound healing

Table 93-8 Recommended Basic Inventory List for Outpatient Setting

One-piece cut-to-fit flat drainable pouch with attached skin barrier
One-piece cut-to-fit flat urostomy pouch with attached skin barrier
Two-piece cut-to-fit pouching system
Skin barrier wafers
Skin barrier paste
Skin barrier powder
Stoma measuring guides
Wound measuring guides
Stationery binder clips
Nonadherent gauze
Sterile and nonsterile gauze
Scissors
Enterostomal therapy nurse resource contact numbers
Ostomy/wound product supplier catalogs
Manufacturer representative contact numbers

Table 93-9 Criterion Checklist for Colostomy Stimulation Procedure

1. Explain procedure and rationale to patient.
2. Wash hands.
3. Assemble equipment at bedside.
4. Apply nonsterile gloves.
5. Assemble irrigation set.
   a. Fill bag with normal saline (NS) (500 to 1000 mL).
   b. Attach indwelling catheter to tip of tubing; if enema bag is used, cut off tip of catheter to ensure snug fit to indwelling catheter.
   c. Open control valve to fill tubing with solution.
6. Position patient comfortably in supine or semi-Fowler's position.
7. Protect bed linen with pads.
8. Attach irrigation sleeve.
9. Position drainage receptacle next to patient so that sleeve end lays within receptacle.
10. Lubricate tip of catheter with water-soluble lubricant; gently insert catheter into the stoma while allowing the NS solution to flow through the catheter.
11. Instill 100–200 mL NS and observe for return around catheter; if no return, disconnect the catheter from the tubing and observe for return; if still no return, reassess patient; stop procedure if any increase in discomfort or distention is noted.
12. Using an in-and-out motion, slowly advance catheter while gradually instilling the remaining NS solution; it may be necessary to advance the catheter up to its bifurcation so long as no resistance or pain is encountered and some return is seen.
13. Measure the amount of solution and stool return; subtract the lesser amount from the greater amount to find the true output or retained volume.
14. Remove irrigation sleeve when immediate return has completed and stoma output has subsided.
15. Apply a new pouch according to the pouching procedure.
16. Remove gloves.
17. Discard waste in appropriate container.
18. Wash hands.
19. Document in progress notes response to stimulation and record true output in I & O (intake and output) sheet.

Table 93-10 Criterion Checklist for Colostomy Irrigation Procedure

1. Explain procedure to the patient.
2. Wash hands.
3. Assemble equipment at bedside; procedure can be done with patient in bed or sitting in bathroom.
4. Attach cone to irrigation bag tubing or place catheter through nipple sleeve.
5. Close tubing clamp and fill irrigation bag with 500–1000 mL tepid water.
6. Remove air from tubing by running water through the tip of cone/catheter and clamp immediately.
7. Hang irrigation bag on hook, above shoulder level.
8. Apply nonsterile gloves.
9. Place linen protector pads on bed.
10. Remove patient's pouching system, clean area, and apply irrigation sleeve.
11. Place end of irrigation sleeve in bedpan or in toilet if patient is in bathroom.
12. Through top open end of irrigation sleeve, insert cone/catheter into lumen of stoma.
13. Open clamp and allow water to flow slowly, evenly, and gently.
14. Push cone/nipple sleeve against stoma.
15. Regulate water flow with clamp.
16. If cramping occurs; slow flow of water and instruct patient to breathe slowly through mouth.
17. If cramps continue, stop flow of water but *do not* remove cone/catheter.
18. When entire volume of solution is instilled, slowly withdraw cone/catheter.
19. Initial return occurs in 15–20 minutes; secondary returns can take up to 1 hour; leave irrigation sleeve on until returns are complete.
20. Remove irrigation sleeve, wash and dry area, and reapply pouching system.
21. Remove gloves.
22. Discard waste in appropriate container.
23. Wash hands.
24. Document in progress notes.

Table 93-11 Criterion Checklist for Ileal Lavage Procedure

1. Explain procedure to the patient.
2. Wash hands.
3. Medicate if patient discomfort indicates.
4. Assemble equipment at bedside.
5. Position the patient comfortably.
6. Protect bed linen.
7. Apply nonsterile gloves and other protective garb as necessary.
8. Position drainage receptacle next to the patient; direct drainage spout of pouch into receptacle.
9. Lubricate tip of the catheter and connect to bulb syringe which is filled with saline (40–60 mL).
10. Insert the catheter into the stoma while gently injecting 40–60 mL saline; a maximum volume of 100 mL may be instilled at one time.
    a. If no resistance is met, slowly advance the catheter using an in-and-out motion.
    b. The catheter may be advanced its entire length, so long as no resistance is encountered.
11. Separate the catheter and syringe.
12. Remove the catheter intermittently.
13. Repeat steps 10 through 12 until there is relief or a negative response.
14. When lavage is completed, apply clean pouching system.
15. Remove gloves.
16. Discard waste in appropriate container.
17. Wash hands.
18. Document procedure in progress notes.

94

OUTCOMES ANALYSIS AND MEASUREMENT OF QUALITY OF LIFE

James M. Church, MBChB, M Med Sci, FRACS

Over the last 10 years, the practice of medicine increasingly has been subject to external forces and movements that threaten to change its very nature. The advent and progression of managed care along with the drive to contain Medicare costs have focused attention on the concepts of outcome measurement and management. When the supply of physicians exceeds the demand for their services, or when a variety of specialists can provide a similar service, consumers are going to use outcomes to determine where their money is best spent. If outside agencies use outcomes in contracting and paying for medical care, it is important that the providers of that care be familiar with the concepts involved. At a clinical level, outcomes assessment is essential to the evaluation of various treatments and a prerequisite to quality improvement. This chapter is intended to introduce the field of outcomes, defining the concepts involved in general terms and then applying them to the field of colorectal surgery.

■ DEFINITIONS

An *outcome* is the result of a process. Outcomes in colorectal surgery are the result of the doctor/patient interaction in which the doctor is a colorectal surgeon and the patient has a colorectal concern or complaint. *Outcomes measurement* involves quantifying the results of this interaction to allow comparison of surgeons, patients, specialties, diagnoses, and therapies. *Outcomes management* means changing the doctor/patient interaction so that the outcome is improved. Colorectal surgeons must have a vital interest in all three areas.

Three aspects of the doctor (or other health care professional)/patient interaction can be used to measure the quality of health care:

1. Structure: all human and physical resources used in delivery of health care (e.g., medical records, equipment, credentials)
2. Process: the procedures and activities involved in delivering health care (surgical procedures, clinical procedures, administration)
3. Outcome: the result of delivering health care (e.g., morbidity rates, mortality rates, recurrence rates, survival time, patient satisfaction, quality of life)

■ HISTORY

Interest in the outcome of health care is not new. During the Crimean War (1854) Florence Nightingale measured morbidity and mortality rates and related them to the quality of the nursing care given to wounded soldiers. She found that adequate care reduced the mortality rate by 32%. Early in the 20th century Dr. Emory Groves suggested that guidelines for postoperative follow-up could reduce adverse outcomes. At Massachusetts General Hospital in 1914 Dr. E. A. Codman recommended prophetically that the result of patient care should be used as an indicator of the quality of that care. Some 50 years later Donabedian was the first to refer to the three aspects of measuring quality in health care: structure, process, and outcome. He said that these three were complementary and equally important.

Further development of the concept of outcomes in health care is shown in the timeline given in Figure 94-1. Government became involved, first in the process of health care and then in its structure. The Healthcare Financing Administration's (HCFA) 1986 report on hospital mortality rates, based on Medicare data, first sparked interest in outcomes. As a result, the Joint Commission on Accreditation of Healthcare Organizations (JCAHO) produced its Agenda for Change in which it called for both clinical and organizational outcomes measurements. In the early 1990s managed care organizations (MCOs) began using outcomes measures as ways of defining quality of care. At the same time, specialist societies (including the American Society of Colon and Rectal Surgeons) became involved, producing Clinical Practice Guidelines and working on outcomes research on behalf of their members.

JCAHO continues to increase its focus on outcomes management during hospital accreditation. HCFA has established the Health Care Quality Improvement Initiative (HCQII), which uses the Medicare database to examine quality of care. This initiative will emphasize variation research, peer review, new quality improvement models, and practice guidelines with the ultimate aim of producing a uniform clinical dataset against which to compare the practice pattern of individual physicians. Today, in the new century, outcomes research, measurement, and management are an inherent part of the business of health care. Health care providers, including colorectal surgeons, are involved in this field, whether they realize it or not.

■ MEASURING OUTCOMES

Types of Data

There are many outcomes of the doctor/patient interaction, and many perspectives from which this interaction can be viewed. The following are some examples:

■ A disease-related approach, traditionally adopted by the physician, looks at accuracy of diagnosis, the complications, and the effectiveness of treatment.

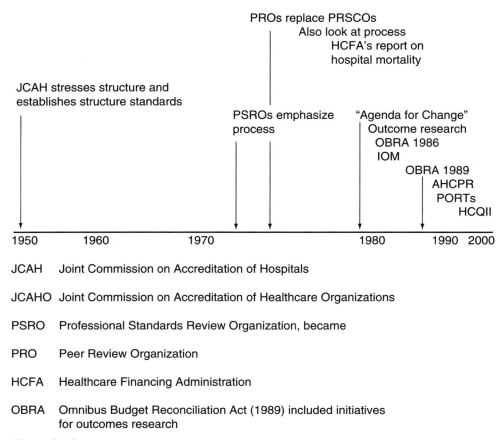

JCAH   Joint Commission on Accreditation of Hospitals

JCAHO   Joint Commission on Accreditation of Healthcare Organizations

PSRO   Professional Standards Review Organization, became

PRO   Peer Review Organization

HCFA   Healthcare Financing Administration

OBRA   Omnibus Budget Reconciliation Act (1989) included initiatives
        for outcomes research

Figure 94-1
A timeline for outcomes in health care.

- From the patient's view, the specifics of the clinic visit (ease of appointment making, parking, waiting for the doctor, professional courtesy) may be as important as the relief of pain and anxiety and the resolution of symptoms.
- The hospital manager looks at length of stay, unnecessary testing, cost-effectiveness of care, and the way in which medical outcomes affect the hospital's "bottom line."
- Specialist societies are interested in the degree to which their guidelines are followed, and the credentialing and recredentialing of their members.
- Payers consider value for money, and how patient satisfaction and good quality care can be achieved at minimal cost.

Some outcomes are easier to measure than others. Careful audit of morbidity and mortality rates associated with care has been part of routine clinical practice for years. Recently such data have been used by nonphysician groups as an indicator of quality of care. Hospitals record data on outcomes by patient and by physician. Which outcomes are measured will depend on the individual or organization doing the measuring, and the reason for the study. For example, measurement of local recurrence rate in rectal cancer may be done to show surgeons their performance relative to accepted standards and to that of their colleagues. A high recurrence rate may lead to referral of low rectal cancers elsewhere or provision of specialized instruction to improve technique. Measurement of length of stay and complication rates may be used by a health maintenance organization (HMO) to determine which physicians are added to their plan. Hospital administrators use cost per case data to identify physicians who may be extravagant with supplies.

Although these examples sound simple, measurement of outcomes is complex. Many factors may influence local recurrence rates after rectal cancer resection; many factors potentially affect length of stay, or cost per case. Case-mix index, hospital and physician referral patterns, associated morbidity rates, and the acute physiology and chronic health evaluation (APACHE) are examples of other variables that may need to be taken into account during outcomes measurement.

Methods

First, an outcome measurement should actually measure an outcome. Death from rectal cancer as an outcome of proctectomy must be distinguished from deaths from other diseases and then standardized according to the comorbidity of the patients. Outcome measurements must be reliable, valid, and appropriate. The data should be collected objectively, and with minimal errors. It must then be standardized, according to indices such as those already mentioned.

Purpose

The primary purpose of measuring outcomes is to improve them. Doctors want better results of care and greater patient satisfaction; patients want to be cured with the least amount of inconvenience; payers want these clinical outcomes achieved with the least cost. Measured outcomes are therefore compared to desired outcomes, be they national standards or guidelines, arbitrary goals, or established norms, and the results of this comparison are used to influence the original behavior that produced the outcome. Continuous quality improvement (CQI) programs use outcome measurement to pinpoint deficiencies in the structure and process of the health care interaction, and to correct them. This process is outcomes management.

■ OUTCOMES MANAGEMENT

The aim of outcomes management from a doctor's perspective is to improve the health of the patient and provide effective health care. From an administrator's view the aim is cost-efficient health care. The government is interested in minimal cost health care, and the private insurance companies are concerned with profitable health care. In a global sense it is hard to reconcile these agendas. Outcomes management, however, is a global concept, involving all aspects of the process and structure that underpins the doctor/patient interaction. Management can occur on many levels, but the levels are related. The efficiency of appointment scheduling may influence patient satisfaction and may affect cost to the patient, the health care provider, and the health care payer. Good chart documentation does not necessarily affect patient satisfaction but can change reimbursement and affect quality of care (Fig. 94-2).

■ QUALITY OF LIFE

Traditional outcome measures for colorectal surgeons include postoperative length of stay, intraoperative

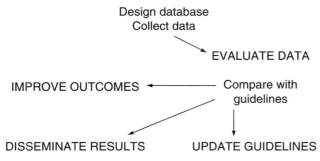

Figure 94-2
A model for outcomes management.

blood loss, postoperative complications, healing rates, mortality rates, disease-specific survival times, stool frequency, and fecal continence. In the 1980s the concept of "quality of life" as an index of outcome appeared. Since then, measurement of quality of life has become a science of its own.

Defining Quality of Life

Defining quality of life (QOL) is like trying to bottle early morning mist. It is nebulous and subjective. QOL involves more than just quality of health; it includes the ability to function in all areas of life and calls for an expression of contentment or happiness. In addition, QOL implies a comparison between the status at the time of measurement and a previous time when quality was "normal," better, or worse. Approaches to defining QOL can be summarized under three topics:

1. Happiness and satisfaction: QOL is expressed by the degree of satisfaction with those aspects of life that are important to the individual at the time of measurement. This value is subjective and dependent on the ability of the patient to express feelings.
2. Goal achievement: QOL depends on the degree to which the patient has achieved personal goals. It is related to satisfaction as this depends to some extent on achievement of goals.
3. Social utility and natural capacity: QOL reflects the degree to which a patient lives a "socially useful" life. This description focuses on mental and physical abilities and the extent to which they are impaired by a disease process or treatment.

Measuring Quality of Life

Measurement of QOL involves a more detailed assessment of factors that may contribute to each of these global concepts. Such factors can be grouped into four categories. For each category given, some examples are listed as follows:

1. Physical status: energy, strength, and ability to function physically.
2. Mental status: perception of health, self-image, depression, anxiety.
3. Social status: interpersonal relationships.
4. Symptoms: pain, nausea, shortness of breath.

There are two main approaches to measuring QOL, the utility approach and the psychometric approach.

Utility Approach

The concept of utility requires the patient to rate a preference for a particular outcome (e.g., death, continence, stool frequency) under various conditions. This preference is expressed on a scale from zero (e.g. death, complete incontinence) to one (e.g., perfect health, perfect continence). If quantity of life is multiplied by the utility value, quality-adjusted life-years are obtained.

Utility values can be determined by rating scales, standard gamble, or time trade-off techniques. Rating scales provide a linear scale representing patient preference between two distinct end points of health (e.g., perfect continence and complete incontinence). The standard gamble asks the patient to choose between two alternatives, with the probability of each being varied until the patient is indifferent to the choices. The time trade-off is similar in that the patient is asked to choose between two alternatives but is asked to sacrifice a variable amount of life to avoid an unpleasant health outcome. For example, would a patient choose to live 20 years with incontinence of solid stool or 15 years with perfect control?

The advantage of these utility methods is that they produce objective data on patient preferences in terms of years of life and alternate health outcomes. However, they are demanding in terms of time and work, and are complex.

Psychometric Approach

The psychometric approach to QOL uses questionnaires to assess patients' attitudes, feelings, or perceptions about a variety of items concerned with general aspects of patients' lives or specific aspects of a disease state. Most QOL scales contain multiple questions or statements with which the patient is asked to agree or disagree. Each item has an underlying measurement continuum, and questions have no "right" or "wrong" answer. Items are grouped according to the dimension of health they assess. Aggregation of answers produces a health profile, and the entire scale gives a health index.

Examples of generic QOL scales include the SF-36 Health Status Survey, the Sickness Impact Profile (SIP), and the Nottingham Health Profile. In colorectal surgery one of these scales is usually combined with a disease-specific instrument such as the Gastrointestinal Quality of Life Index (GIQLI), the, European Organization for Research and Treatment of Cancer (EORTC) Quality of Life Questionnaire, or the Inflammatory Bowel Disease Questionnaire (IBDQ). Recently, some disease-specific instruments for colorectal diseases have been constructed and validated. Examples include the Cleveland Clinic Quality of Life Score for patients undergoing ileal pouch–anal anastomosis, the IBDQ for assessment of the results of treatment of inflammatory bowel disease, and a Fecal Incontinence Quality of Life Scale for patients with fecal incontinence.

When constructing a psychometric QOL instrument, reliability and validity are of prime concern.

Reliability is the degree to which a scale gives the same results when used repeatedly. If the same instrument is given to the same sample under the same conditions on two different occasions, test-retest reliability can be evaluated (usually by using an intraclass correlation coefficient). If two different but parallel forms of the scale are used on the same group of patients, parallel form reliability is measured. An analysis of relationships between items within the scale shows internal consistency.

Validity is the degree to which the scale measures what it is meant to measure. Content validity is determined by review of the questions by a panel of experts. Construct validity looks at the performance of the scale in different groups of patients for whom different results would be expected. For example, if a scale designed to assess the impact of incontinence on QOL gave equal scores for a group of normal subjects and a group of incontinent patients, it would not be valid. Another way of measuring construct validity is to use multiple scales purported to measure the same construct, looking for at least a reasonable correlation.

Quality of life and outcomes measurements come together in current studies in colorectal surgery such as those cited in the suggested readings list.

Suggested Readings

Al-Assaf AF: Healthcare outcomes management and quality improvement. J R Soc Health 1996;116:245–252.

Brenneman FD, Wright JG, Kennedy ED, Mcleod RS: Outcomes research in surgery. World J Surg 1999;23:1220–1223.

Dedhiya S, Xianodong Kong S: Quality of life: An overview of the concept and measures. Pharm World Sci 1995;17:141–148.

Fazio VW, O'Riordain MG, Lavery IC, et al: Long-term functional outcome and quality of life after stapled restorative proctocolectomy. Ann Surg 1999;230:578–586.

Gough IR: Quality of life as an outcome variable in oncology and surgery. Aust NZ J Surg 1994;64:227–235.

Irvine EJ, Feagan B, Rochon J, et al: Quality of life: A valid and reliable measure of therapeutic efficacy in the treatment of IBD. Gastroenterology 1994;106:287–296.

McLeod RS: Quality-of-life measurement in the assessment of surgical outcome. Adv Surg 1999;33:293–309.

Rockwood TH, Church JM, Fleshman JW, et al: Fecal incontinence quality of life scale: Quality of life instrument for patients with fecal incontinence. Dis Colon Rectum 2000;43(1):9–16.

95

DOCUMENTATION AND USE OF THE CPT CODING SYSTEM FOR COLORECTAL SURGERY

Anthony J. Senagore, MD, MBA, MS, FACS
Tricia J. Bardon, BBA, ABA
Conor P. Delaney, MD, MCh, PhD,
FRSCI (Gen), FACS

The appropriate and optimal use of the Current Procedural Terminology (CPT) code system developed by the American Medical Association and adopted by most governmental and commercial health care payers requires a thorough understanding of all its components. The selection of a code begins with the performance of a medically necessary service by the surgeon and ends with the requisite documentation. Failure to understand the key components of the system and inappropriate use of these components can adversely affect reimbursement, practice management analysis, and legal risk. It obviously follows that accurate coding for all work performed will lead to appropriate and optimized reimbursement. Accurate coding also improves the revenue cycle because code submission will be correct, which results in rapid reimbursement and decreases payment denials. Analysis of code patterns and individual volumes can be an important practice management tool to assign resource consumption and identify practice variation. Code patterns can also provide a tool to compare reimbursement patterns by payer, assess the implications of specific patient volumes within various contractual relationships, and analyze the merits of maintaining a contractual relationship. Finally, a clear understanding of the components of a code and the documentation required in the medical record can remove all risk of Medicare fraud prosecution under a variety of federal statues.

■ CODE DEVELOPMENT FOR THE CPT SYSTEM

The system used to translate physician work into physician reimbursement is the Current Procedural Terminology code system. These codes are developed by the American Medical Association (AMA) in conjunction with representatives from virtually all medical specialties. The steps for code development are as follows. First, the CPT committee of the AMA accurately defines the components of a procedure or evaluation and management encounter, in conjunction with the recommending medical specialty. The second step involves presentation of the code and supporting documentation to the Relative Value Units Update Committee (RUC) of the AMA, whose responsibility is to define the work and practice expense involved in providing the service. The RUC's recommendation comes in the form of relative value units (RVUs) and is submitted to the Center for Medicare and Medicaid Services (CMS). It is the CMS's responsibility to accept, reject, or modify this recommendation, which defines the payment. CMS accepts over 95% of codes referred by the RUC, and the new code can be used once published in the CPT book. The code's final value as determined by CMS is published in the federal register. The relative values for physician work, practice expense, and malpractice, as well as the total values for facility and nonfacility site of service are in the federal register. An individual practice can use this information to perform impact analysis based upon the frequency with which that code is used.

■ EVALUATION AND MANAGEMENT ENCOUNTERS

This set of codes resides in the 99xxx range of the CPT manual and is used to describe the components of evaluation and management (E/M) encounters for new patients, consultations, and existing patients within your practice. Codes exist for all sites of service settings, such as your office, the hospital, and the extended care facility. The descriptors for levels of evaluation and management services recognize seven components used for describing the specific code level:

1. History
2. Examination
3. Medical decision making
4. Counseling
5. Coordination of care
6. Nature of presenting problem
7. Time

Codes also exist for describing counseling sessions and telephone management of complex long-term care patients; however, individual payers may not accept some of these codes, especially those for phone calls. This chapter will address only two sites of service typically used by surgeons: the physician's office and the hospital.

At the time of this writing, three potential processes or systems can be employed for determining which E/M code level should be used. These rules are referred to by the year the Health Care Financing Authority (HCFA; now CMS) published the final rule for that system: 1995, 1997, or the time-based system. The 1995 and 1997 rules are based upon a similar list of data elements used to describe specific organ systems; however, the counting of the elements used is slightly different. The criteria for time-based encounters are shown below; however, the time in and out of the room should be recorded in the medical record and include only face-to-face time with the patient.

Table 95-1 defines the values by code level when time is used as the parameter. The major deficiency of this system

Table 95-1 Time of Consultation and Level of Coding for Time-Based Billing Criteria

CODE	LEVEL 1	LEVEL 2	LEVEL 3	LEVEL 4	LEVEL 5
New patient	10	20	30	45	60
Established	5	10	15	25	30
Consult	15	30	40	45	60
Inpatient, initial	30	50	70		
Inpatient, subsequent	15	25	35		
Inpatient, consult	20	40	55		
Home visit, new	20	30	45	60	75
Home visit, estab.	15	25	40	60	

is that the amount of physician work is not measured or valued. For example, one could bill at the highest possible level for a patient with the common cold simply by spending the requisite 60 minutes. The impracticality of using these codes is obvious when time is of the essence, as in the typical day in the office. The one advantage of this system, however, is that certain encounters do primarily involve discussion or consultation with little or no physical examination. These encounters are most appropriately coded based upon the time used, although it is essential that the time in and out of the examination room be recorded on the chart when using this approach.

The 1995 and 1997 systems describe the elements of the three major components of an E/M visit: history, physical examination, and medical decision making. Each major component is further subdivided to allow assignment of a correct code level. The physical examination is scored a little differently for the two versions and accounts for the major differences between 1995 and 1997 rules.

It is important that the physician utilize the specific, approved nomenclature in the medical record. This information will survive an audit and is particularly true for the inclusion of the approved organ systems for a review of systems. The history data elements can be obtained by several means: (1) a patient completed form; (2) office personnel recorded information; or (3) review of the referring physician's history. In each case, the document obtained from a source other than the physician should be dated, signed, and maintained within the current medical record.

The patient history includes history of present illness (HPI), review of systems (ROS), past medical history (PH), family history (FH), and social history (SH). The present illness is used to describe location, quality, severity, duration, timing, context, modifying factors, and associated signs and symptoms. A brief HPI includes one

to three elements and an extended HPI includes more than three elements. The ROS includes the following organ systems: constitutional (weight loss, fatigue, etc.); eyes; ear, nose, throat, mouth; cardiovascular; respiratory; gastrointestinal; genitourinary; musculoskeletal; skin and breast; neurologic; psychiatric; endocrine; hematologic and lymph; and allergy and immune system. Reference to the ROS should include all positive findings and a reference to each negative finding by area or a general statement that all remaining ROS is negative. A problem-pertinent ROS includes 1 element, extended includes 2 to 9 elements, and a complete ROS reviews 10 or more elements. PH includes past surgical procedures, chronic medical illnesses, current medications, and allergies. FH and SH are self-explanatory. A pertinent PFSH includes one element, and complete PFSH includes two or three areas. The scoring system for the history component is shown in Table 95-2.

The physical examination also includes an extensive list of accepted elements for the general multisystem examination. The complete listing for single specialty examinations using the 1997 guidelines can be obtained directly from CMS or the AMA and will not be listed here. The examination elements are noted in the following list:

- *Constitutional.* General appearance; measurement of three vital signs (includes pain score)
- *Eyes.* Inspection of lids/conjunctivae; examination of pupils and iris; funduscopic evaluation
- *Ears, nose, mouth, throat.* External inspection of ears/nose; otoscopic; hearing assessment; inspection of nasal mucosa; inspection of lips, gums, and teeth; examination of oropharynx (tongue, tonsils, mucosa)
- *Neck.* Masses/symmetry; thyroid
- *Respiratory.* Assessment of respiratory effort; percussion of chest; auscultation

Table 95-2 Scoring System for History Component of CPT Billing

HISTORY	PROBLEM FOCUSED	EXPANDED	DETAILED	COMPREHENSIVE
HPI	Brief	Brief	Extended	Extended
ROS	None	Problem pertinent	Extended	Complete
PFSH	None	None	Pertinent	Complete

HPI, history of present illness; PFSH, past family and social history; ROS, review of systems.

- *Cardiovascular.* Palpation of heart; auscultation of heart; examination of carotids; examination of abdominal aorta; examination of femoral pulses and pedal pulses; assessment of extremities (edema, varicosities, deformities)
- *Chest (breast).* Inspection of breasts; palpation of breasts and axillae
- *Gastrointestinal.* Examination of abdomen (masses/tenderness), liver, and spleen; abdominal/groin hernias; examination of anus, perineum, and rectum
- *Lymphatic.* Palpation of two or more areas (neck, axilla, groin, other)
- *Genitourinary.* Males—examination of scrotal contents, penis, digital rectal examination of prostate; females—examination of external genitalia and vagina, urethra, bladder, cervix, uterus, adnexa
- *Musculoskeletal.* Examination of gait and station; inspection of digits and nails; examination of joints for range of motion, deformity, strength
- *Skin.* Inspection of skin; palpation of skin
- *Neurologic.* Test cranial nerves; examine deep tendon reflexes; examination of sensation
- *Psychiatric.* Orientation to time, person, place; recent/remote memory; mood and affect; description of patient's judgment and insight

All positive findings must be described; negative findings do not need to be individually documented necessarily, except as appropriate for the patient's care. For negative findings a notation indicating the system is negative is acceptable; the name of each system that is reviewed must be documented. An acceptable example follows:

Pulmonary: cough x 5 weeks, otherwise negative
Cardiac: negative
ROS: endocrine, neurologic, GI, GU all negative

Table 95-3 documents the major differences between the 1995 and 1997 documentation requirements and notes some problems with each. An ongoing process is in place to better define the rules and give guidance.

The 1995 guidelines for history only have two levels:

- *Problem focused.* 1 to 3 elements from 1 or more systems
- *Extended.* 4 or more elements from 1 or more systems

The scoring of the physical examination (1997 rules) components is shown below and follows the same template as used for the history component of the encounter.

- *Problem focused.* 1 to 5 elements from 1 or more systems
- *Expanded.* 6 to 11 elements from 1 or more systems
- *Detailed.* 12 to 17 bullets from 2 or more systems
- *Comprehensive.* 2 or more elements from 9 systems

The final component of the E/M encounter is decision making, which is the most important of the three major components because it drives medical necessity and therefore the overall maximum level that can be attained for any given encounter. This important point should be recalled at the start of any E/M visit. If the medical problem is simple, then regardless of the amount of data recorded, the level of the code will be 1 to 3. Conversely, evaluating a patient for a neoplasm or severe medical illness will likely be very complex; however, the encounter will only justify such a code based upon the data elements recorded. The precise distinction between individual levels of medical decision making are not as clearly quantified as the history and physical examination requirements. The important aspect of decision making is to accurately record potential diagnoses, diagnostic tests reviewed or ordered, medical procedures ordered or scheduled, and additional consultations ordered. All these aspects will provide documentation of the issues reviewed by the physician in ultimately determining a treatment course (Table 95-4).

The overall scoring of an E/M visit requires a review of the documentation of the three components of the encounter: history, physical examination, and medical decision making. A grid is provided in Table 95-5 as guidance for the selection of the appropriate code. Recall that

CODE COMPONENT	**1995 REQUIREMENTS**	**1997 REQUIREMENTS**
Hx—history of present illness	Specific requirements	Specific requirements
Hx—history of systems	Specific body area or organ system requirements	Specific body area or organ system requirements
Hx—past family social history	Brief information required	Brief information required
Physical examination	Specifically referenced general multisystem examination	General multisystem examination and 10 single system examinations
	Description of single system examinations inadequate	Four levels
		Very prescriptive
	Four levels	Confusing shading and bullets format
	Requirements not clear	Requirements often not relevant
Medical decision making	Four levels	Only three levels
	Laundry list of examples not reflective of clinical assessments and plans	Physician tailors documentation to assessment and plan of treatment
		Vignette examples

Table 95-3 Comparison of 1995 and 1997 Code Component Requirements

Table 95-4 Components for Determining Level of Complexity of Patient Presenting for an Office Visit

	DIAGNOSTIC/TREATMENT	DATA	RISK
Straightforward	Self-limited	Laboratory tests, x-rays	Nonprescription drugs/treatment
Low	2 minor acute/1 stable chronic illness	Nonstress tests; superficial biopsy	Physical therapy, minor surgery with no risk factors
Moderate	Uncomplicated acute illnesses, new condition, 2 chronic stable illnesses	Endoscopy, stress tests	Minor surgery with risk factors; major surgery no risk factors
Highly complex	Chronic illness with exacerbation; threat to life or bodily function	Endoscopy or testing with contrast medium	Major surgery with risk factors; changes in drug treatment with monitoring

for an existing patient code, only the lowest of the two highest components must achieve a given level; conversely, for a new or consultation patient code, the ultimate level is defined by the lowest of any of the three components.

■ PROCEDURE CODING

These code sets are used to describe all forms of medical procedures, both diagnostic and therapeutic, performed by physicians. It is essential to understand that the procedure performed must be accurately described by the terminology in the CPT manual. In the event that a given procedure is not represented by a code, then the unlisted code within that family should be used. New procedure codes are constantly brought forward by specialty societies to redefine or describe changes in medical practice and utilize the same process described earlier for code recognition and valuation. If a code is not represented in the CPT book, the physician can contact the specialty society's economic committee and ask them to put forth the code that is missing.

Code selection actually begins with an accurate operative report that describes all the components defined by a given procedural code(s). A complete report is essential to allow for accurate billing and ensures that all performed procedures are captured. In fact, claim submission should be based upon review of the medical record by the biller to avoid false claims, allow capture of all billable procedures, and as a quality review of the medical record. This approach also encourages dialogue between the physician and biller that can be a learning experience for both.

A variety of scenarios can alter payment for procedural codes that require the use of one or more code modifiers. The reader is referred to the actual CPT manual for a complete description of the potential modifiers. The codes are self-explanatory and should be clearly understood by all members of the practice.

Another component of the billing process that must be understood by the physician is the correct coding initiative (CCI) edits. These changes are published quarterly and describe code pairs that are mutually exclusive and therefore not paid when submitted together on a bill. This system need not be memorized. Instead, the physician should either purchase the software to perform these edits or ensure that the billing service employs this process. Using the proper software will avoid unnecessary payment denials. These edits are defined both at the national level and by local carriers. The only method to ensure an accurate use of the system is to update this software and to scrupulously review coding denials. The latter process allows for early recognition of new code edits and the rapid identification of erroneously applied denial rules.

■ SUMMARY

The purpose of this chapter is not to make the physician a trained CPT coder, but rather to increase the awareness of what is required in the medical record to define a given code. The advantages of correct documentation will allow the physician to be accurately and rapidly reimbursed for services rendered, avoid performing unnecessary work, and avoid legal entanglements related to inaccurate coding. If the physician works with the billing office, many of the errors in bill submission can be avoided and the physician will be able to obtain a much more accurate reflection of the sources of practice revenue. The individual physician is encouraged to develop a paper or computer template that allows the easy recognition of data elements and the

Table 95-5 Determination of Office CPT Code Based on History, Physical Examinations, and Decision Making Involved

CODE	HISTORY	PHYSICAL EXAMINATION	DECISION MAKING
992xx1	Problem focused	Problem focused	Straightforward
992xx2	Expanded	Expanded	Straightforward/low
992xx3	Detailed	Detailed	Low
992xx4	Comprehensive	Comprehensive	Moderate
992xx5	Comprehensive	Comprehensive	High

recording of those elements. A focus on a practice-friendly means of recording the data from each encounter will streamline the work efficiency and the overall revenue of the practice. The physician must always be aware of the office's billing abilities and problems that occur so that rejections are minimized and reimbursement is optimized.

Suggested Readings

CPT Assistant: American Medical Association, 515 N. State St., Chicago, IL 60610.

CPT 2002 Professional Edition: American Medical Association, 515 N. State St., Chicago, IL 60610.

Medicare Part B News (weekly publication): 11300 Rockville Pike, Suite 1100, Rockville, MD 20852-3030.

Specialty CPT books are available from various sources.

The preceding publications can be ordered or found on the following Web sites:

www.partbnews.com

www.ama-assn.org/ama/pub/category/3113.htm

Index

Note: Page numbers followed by f indicate figures; those followed by t indicate tables.